Textbook of Anaesthesia

EDITED BY

Alan R Aitkenhead BSc MD FRCA
Professor of Anaesthesia
University Department of Anaesthesia and Intensive Care
Queen's Medical Centre
Nottingham
UK

David J Rowbotham MD MRCP FRCA
Professor of Anaesthesia and Pain Management
University Department of Anaesthesia, Critical Care and Pain Management
Leicester Royal Infirmary
Leicester
UK

Graham Smith BSc (Hons) MD FRCA
Professor of Anaesthesia
University Department of Anaesthesia, Critical Care and Pain Management
Leicester Royal Infirmary
Leicester
UK

FOURTH EDITION

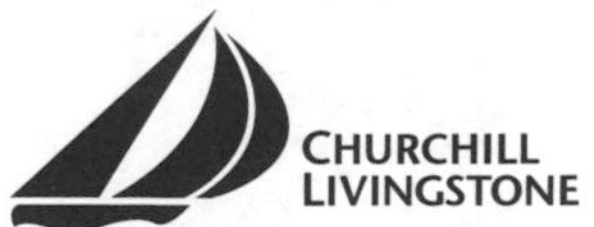

EDINBURGH LONDON NEW YORK OXFORD PHILADELPHIA ST LOUIS SYDNEY TORONTO 2001

Churchill Livingstone
An imprint of Elsevier Science Limited

First published 1985
Second edition 1990
Third edition 1996
Fourth edition 2001

Main edition
ISBN 0443063818
Reprinted 2002, 2003

International edition
ISBN 0443063915
Reprinted 2002, 2003

British Library Cataloguing in Publication Data
A catalogue record for this book is available from the British Library

Library of Congress Cataloging in Publication Data
A catalog record for this book is available from the Library of Congress

Note
Medical knowledge is constantly changing. As new information becomes available, changes in treatment, procedures, equipment and the use of drugs become necessary. The editors/authors/contributors and the publishers have, as far as it is possible, taken care to ensure that the information given in this text is accurate and up to date. However, readers are strongly advised to confirm that the information, especially with regard to drug usage, complies with the latest legislation and standards of practice.

The publisher's policy is to use **paper manufactured from sustainable forests**

Printed in Spain

Preface

This fourth edition of Textbook of Anaesthesia has been designed with the same objectives as those underlying former editions; the aim has been to provide a readable, comprehensive, and concise text to satisfy the needs of new recruits into anaesthesia during the first two years of training and also present this clinical discipline as an integrated development from basic sciences. We hoped that this approach in the first edition would also provide a satisfactory primer for trainees in those countries where examinations feature in the early stages of training. The response to the first edition clearly demonstrated that it did provide suitable reading for anaesthetists studying for the Part I FFARCS (later Part 1 FRCA) examination, the European Diploma of Anaesthesiology, and equivalent examinations in other parts of the world. The book also proved to be useful for a wider audience including medical practitioners giving occasional anaesthetics in rural areas or developing countries and non-medical staff involved full-time in anaesthesia such as operating department practitioners, anaesthetic assistants, and nurse anaesthetists.

In 1990, the Royal College of Anaesthetists changed the syllabus for its FRCA examination by reverting to a two-part examination. The Primary, intended to be taken twelve to eighteen months after commencing training, has a very broad syllabus encompassing both basic science and clinical practice of anaesthesia, whilst the Final FRCA examination is designed to examine knowledge and practice in clinical measurement and more specialised aspects of clinical anaesthesia.

In order to achieve our basic objective of producing within a single book a text suitable as both an introduction to the clinical practice of anaesthesia and also one which is appropriate reading for the Primary FRCA examination, we have made substantial changes to this fourth edition of Textbook, most noticeably by increasing the basic science content. The changes produced, in comparison with the third edition, are evident most ostensibly by a marked increase in size by incorporation of an additional 19 chapters. For editorial convenience we have divided the book into two main sections: Principles of Anaesthesia and Practice of Anaesthesia. This is not intended to separate or compartmentalise basic science and clinical practice; indeed both basic science and clinical practice are intertwined in most chapters.

In the section on Principles of Anaesthesia, we have incorporated most of the new chapters in order to cover areas which were not addressed in previous editions and which are now part of the syllabus for the Primary FRCA examination. There are new chapters on statistics, cellular physiology and pharmacology, three additional chapters on the cardiovascular system, three on the nervous system, three on the gastrointestinal tract, and others on immunology, the kidney, metabolism, and endocrinology. In addition, we have rearranged chapters throughout the book in an attempt to produce a more logical structure. In the second section on Practice of Anaesthesia, we have retained much of the content of previous editions but following the policy introduced in the third edition, we have changed approximately one third of the authors. We again emphasise that this is not a reflection of the quality of the contributions of the previous authors, to whom we are extremely grateful; our intentions are simply to ensure that fresh minds are applied to the subject matter and to avoid the risks which could be associated with asking authors merely to update their contributions. As in past editions, we are grateful to the authors of all our chapters for the quality of the revisions which they have made in this edition and we are also indebted to the many reviewers and readers of the book who have been sufficiently interested to provide helpful comments and draw our attention to mistakes and typographical errors.

We are grateful to all our contributors for allowing us to undertake widespread revision of manuscripts in an attempt to achieve uniformity of style. In addition we are indebted to the publishers who have arranged for redrawing of all figures and incorporation of a large number of new additional figures in a standardised format. Our gratitude must be recorded to Mrs Christine Gethins in Leicester and Ms Lynne Chapman in Nottingham for substantial secretarial assistance. Because of the additional work involved in this larger fourth edition and to provide some youth to the editorial team, we have also invited David Rowbotham to join the editors.

We hope that this fourth edition will continue to be as popular as the previous editions of Textbook, and that it will continue to serve as a useful introductory text for those beginning a career in anaesthesia. Our aim has been to try to encompass, as far as is possible within a readable text, the syllabus for the new Primary FRCA examination, and hopefully this aim will also have been achieved. Previous anaesthetic trainees have also found our book useful as a revision manual for the Final FRCA examination; although that is not the primary purpose of this text, nonetheless it may be helpful in this context. The incorporation of useful appendices and practical information on the conduct of anaesthesia within most specialist areas of anaesthesia should ensure that it remains useful both as a practical guide in the operating theatre and also a foundation of theoretical knowledge.

Alan R Aitkenhead, Nottingham
Graham Smith and David J Rowbotham, Leicester
2001

Preface

Contributors

Alan R Aitkenhead BSc MD FRCA
Professor of Anaesthesia, University Department of Anaesthesia and Intensive Care, Queen's Medical Centre, Nottingham, UK

John I Alexander FRCA
Consultant Anaesthetist, Department of Anaesthesia, Bristol Royal Infirmary, Bristol, UK

Robert Atcheson MD FRCA
Consultant Anaesthetist, Department of Anaesthesia, Royal Hallamshire Hospital, Sheffield, UK

Bryn R Baxendale FRCA
Consultant Anaesthetist, Department of Anaesthesia, Queen's Medical Centre, Nottingham, UK

Jennifer Benton FRCA
Associate Specialist in Anaesthesia, Department of Anaesthesia, Derriford Hospital, Plymouth, UK

Tim Bourne FRCA
Consultant Anaesthetist, Department of Anaesthesia, University Hospitals of Leicester NHS Trust, Leicester Royal Infirmary, Leicester, UK

Donal Buggy MSc MRCPI (Dublin) DME FFARCSI
Senior Lecturer, University Department of Anaesthesia, Critical Care & Pain Management, Leicester General Hospital, Leicester, UK

Aiden Byrne FRCA
Consultant Anaesthetist, Department of Anaesthesia, Morriston Hospital, Swansea, UK

D Paul Cartwright FRCA
Consultant Anaesthetist, Department of Anaesthesia, Derby City General Hospital, Derby, UK

Paul R Clarke MRCP FRCA
Consultant Anaesthetist, Academic Unit of Anaesthesia, St James's University Hospital, Leeds, UK

Beverley J Collett FRCA
Consultant Anaesthetist, Department of Anaesthesia, University Hospitals of Leicester NHS Trust, Leicester Royal Infirmary, Leicester, UK

John Curran PhD FRCA
Consultant Anaesthetist, Department of Anaesthesia, Nottingham City Hospital, Nottingham, UK

Eric de Melo FRCA
Consultant Anaesthetist, Department of Anaesthesia, University Hospitals of Leicester NHS Trust, Leicester Royal Infirmary, Leicester, UK

David R Derbyshire FRCA
Consultant Anaesthetist, Department of Anaesthesia, Warwick General Hospital, Warwick, UK

Christopher Dodds FRCA
Consultant Anaesthetist, Department of Anaesthesia, South Cleveland Hospital, Middlesbrough, UK

David J R Duthie MD FRCA
Consultant Anaesthetist, University Department of Anaesthesia, Critical Care and Pain Management, Glenfield General Hospital, Leicester, UK

Neil D Edwards FRCA
Consultant Anaesthetist, Department of Anaesthesia, Royal Hallamshire Hospital, Sheffield, UK

Christopher D Elton FRCA
Consultant Anaesthetist, Department of Anaesthesia, University Hospitals of Leicester NHS Trust, Leicester Royal Infirmary, Leicester. UK

David Fell FRCA
Consultant Anaesthetist, Department of Anaesthesia, University Hospitals of Leicester NHS Trust, Leicester Royal Infirmary, Leicester, UK

Helen F Galley PhD
Senior Lecturer, Academic Unit of Anaesthesia, University of Aberdeen, Aberdeen, UK

Keith J Girling FRCA
Consultant Anaesthetist, Department of Anaesthesia, Queen's Medical Centre, Nottingham, UK

Neville W Goodman FRCA
Consultant Anaesthetist, Department of Anaesthesia, Southmead Hospital, Bristol, UK

Ian S Grant FRCP (Edin-Glasg) FRCA
Consultant Anaesthetist and Medical Director, Intensive Therapy Unit, Western General Hospital, Edinburgh, UK

Andrew P Hall MRCP FRCA
Consultant Anaesthetist, Department of Anaesthesia, University Hospitals of Leicester NHS Trust, Leicester Royal Infirmary, Leicester, UK

Christopher D Hanning BSc MD FRCA
Consultant Anaesthetist, Department of Anaesthesia, University Hospitals of Leicester NHS Trust, Leicester General Hospital, Leicester, UK

Anne M Heffernan FFARCSI
Clinical Research Fellow, University Department of Anaesthesia, Critical Care and Pain Management, Leicester Royal Infirmary, Leicester, UK

Greg Hobbs DipRACOG FRCA
Consultant Anaesthetist, Department of Anaesthesia, Queen's Medical Centre, Nottingham, UK

Philip M Hopkins MD FRCA
Senior Lecturer, Academic Unit of Anaesthesia, St James's University Hospital, Leeds, UK

Jennifer M Hunter MD FRCA
Professor of Anaesthesia, University of Liverpool, Royal Liverpool University Hospital, Liverpool, UK

Gareth W Jones BSc MRCP FRCA
Consultant Anaesthetist, Department of Anaesthesia, University Hospitals of Leicester NHS Trust, Leicester Royal Infirmary, Leicester, UK

Michael J Jones BSc MRCP FRCA
Consultant Anaesthetist, Department of Anaesthesia, University Hospitals of Leicester NHS Trust, Glenfield General Hospital, Leicester, UK

Nisha Kumar MRCP FRCA
Consultant Anaesthetist, Department of Anaesthesia, University Hospitals of Leicester NHS Trust, Leicester Royal Infirmary, Leicester, UK

Jo M Lamb FRCA
Consultant Anaesthetist, Department of Anaesthesia, Queen's Medical Centre, Nottingham, UK

David G Lambert BSc (Hons) PhD
Senior Lecturer in Anaesthetic Pharmacology, University Department of Anaesthesia, Critical Care and Pain Management, Leicester Royal Infirmary, Leicester, UK

Jeremy A Langton MD FRCA
Consultant Anaesthetist, Department of Anaesthesia, Derriford Hospital, Plymouth, UK

Ravi P Mahajan MD FRCA
Senior Lecturer, University Department of Anaesthesia and Intensive Care, Nottingham City Hospital, Nottingham, UK

Anne E May FRCA
Consultant Anaesthetist, Department of Anaesthesia, University Hospitals of Leicester NHS Trust, Leicester Royal Infirmary, UK

Rosemary McDonald PhD FRCA
Formerly Consultant Obstetric Anaesthetist, St Jame's University Hospital, Leeds; Postgraduate Dean (Yorkshire), Department of Postgraduate Medical Education, Seacroft Hospital, Leeds, UK

Mary C Mushambi FRCA
Consultant Anaesthetist, Department of Anaesthesia, University Hospitals of Leicester NHS Trust, Leicester Royal Infirmary, Leicester, UK

Michael H Nathanson FRCA
Consultant Anaesthetist, Department of Anaesthesia, Queen's Medical Centre, Nottingham, UK

Martin Nicol FRCA
Consultant Anaesthetist, Department of Anaesthesia, Queen's Medical Centre, Nottingham, UK

Graham R Nimmo MD MRCP (UK) FFARCSI
Consultant Physician, Emergency Medicine and Intensive Care, Western General Hospital, Edinburgh, UK

Andrew J Ogilvy FRCA
Consultant Anaesthetist, Department of Anaesthesia, University Hospitals of Leicester NHS Trust, Leicester General Hospital, Leicester, UK

Susan R Pavord MRCP MRC Path
Consultant Haematologist, Department of Haematology, Leicester Royal Infirmary, Leicester, UK

Ian Power MD FRCA
Professor of Anaesthesia
University Department of Anaesthesia, Critical Care and Pain Management, Royal Infirmary, Edinburgh, UK

Charles S Reilly MD FRCA
Professor of Anaesthesia, Department of Surgical and Anaesthetic Sciences, Royal Hallamshire Hospital, Sheffield, UK

Bernard Riley FRCA
Consultant Anaesthetist, Department of Anaesthesia, Queen's Medical Centre, Nottingham, UK

David J Rowbotham MD MRCP FRCA
Professor of Anaesthesia and Pain Management, University Department of Anaesthesia, Critical Care & Pain Management, Leicester Royal Infirmary, Leicester, UK

Colin J Runcie FRCA FRCP (Glas)
Consultant Anaesthetist, Department of Anaesthesia, Western Infirmary, Glasgow, UK

Andrew R A Rushton FRCA
Consultant Anaesthetist, Department of Anaesthesia, Derriford Hospital, Plymouth, UK

Peter J Simpson MD FRCA
Consultant Anaesthetist, Department of Anaesthesia, Frenchay Hospital, Bristol; Senior Clinical Lecturer in Anaesthetics, University of Bristol, Bristol, UK

Graham Smith BSc (Hons) MD FRCA
Professor of Anaesthesia, University Department of Anaesthesia, Critical Care and Pain Management, Leicester Royal Infirmary, Leicester, UK

Justiaan C Swanevelder FRCA
Consultant Anaesthetist, Department of Anaesthesia, University Hospitals of Leicester NHS Trust, Glenfield General Hospital, Leicester, UK

Jonathan P Thompson FRCA
Senior Lecturer, University Department of Anaesthesia, Critical Care & Pain Management, Leicester Royal Infirmary, Leicester, UK

Douglas A B Turner FRCA
Consultant Anaesthetist, Department of Anaesthesia, University Hospitals of Leicester NHS Trust, Leicester Royal Infirmary, Leicester, UK

Peter G M Wallace FRCA
Consultant Anaesthetist, Division of Anaesthesia, Western Infirmary, Glasgow, UK

John Walls FRCP
Professor of Nephrology, Department of Nephrology, Leicester General Hospital, Leicester, UK

Jennifer Warner FRCA
Consultant Anaesthetist, Department of Anaesthesia, Nottingham City Hospital, Nottingham, UK

Nigel Webster PhD FRCA
Professor of Anaesthesia, Institute of Medical Sciences, University of Aberdeen, Aberdeen, UK

John A W Wildsmith MD FRCA
Professor of Anaesthesia, Department of Anaesthesia, Ninewells Hospital and Medical School, Dundee, UK

Sheila M Willatts MD FRCA FRCP
Clinical Reader in Anaesthesia, University of Bristol, Bristol, UK

J Keith Wood FRCP FRCPE FRCPath
Formerly Consultant Haematologist, Leicester Royal Infirmary, Leicester, UK

David A Zideman BSc FRCA
Consultant Anaesthetist and Honorary Senior Lecturer, Department of Anaesthesia, Hammersmith Hospital, London. UK

Contents

1 Clinical trials and statistics

'A clinical trial is a carefully and ethically designed experiment with the aim of answering some precisely framed question.' This definition by Sir Austin Bradford Hill, a pioneer of clinical trials, is worth remembering: careful, ethical, precisely framed. There are many types of research that provide information on which medical practice is based. The clinical trial is one of these types, but the one known to most practising anaesthetists. Statistics are important in the interpretation of clinical trials and pragmatically candidates for examinations in anaesthesia know they must 'learn some statistics'. But it is a knowledge of good study design, not of statistics, that is the key to good clinical research.

TERMINOLOGY

There is some confusion and overlap of terms. Scientific research may be observational or experimental. Although a clinical trial is, as Bradford Hill defines, an experiment, there are undercurrents to the word that make 'experiment' better avoided. A clinical trial is better described as a series of experiments: each patient is the subject of an experiment, providing a set of observations. If those observations are numerical, they are often termed *data*. The noun 'data' is in the plural ('the data are shown in the table...'), although many now accept that modern usage allows the singular ('the data is shown in the table...'). *Measurements* and *findings* are other words applied to the *outcomes* of a clinical trial.

The words *trial* and *study* may be synonymous – a 'clinical trial' or a 'clinical study' – and synonymous also with 'research project'. This meaning is implied in 'study design' and 'study protocol'. 'Study' is the better word here: 'trial' is applicable only to some types of experimental clinical research, whereas design and protocol are important in all scientific research. But a term is needed for each episode (i.e. each patient) in a clinical trial, and 'study' is often used in that sense ('the study period started at induction of anaesthesia and lasted until the patient left the recovery ward...').

STUDY DESIGN

The study design is the framework ensuring that, as far as possible, difficulties have been sorted out before the study starts. Formally, for any research involving humans or human material or patient records, a study design is needed for submission to an ethics or grant-awarding committee. Informally, there should be a design for any research, even if only a loose one, otherwise the research is likely to lack discipline.

Because this chapter is largely about clinical trials, it is helpful to use simple practical examples: a study of a new antiemetic in the treatment of postoperative nausea and vomiting; the effect of an intravenous induction agent on systolic arterial pressure; a comparison of the effect of two intravenous induction agents on arterial pressure; and a study of the effect of duration of surgery on patients' body temperature. These examples are used to illustrate principles and tests. Because the purpose of clinical trials is in some way to improve the management of patients, underlying most aspects of study design is the need to be as sure as possible that the improvement was indeed due to the investigators' intervention, and not to confounding factors. The purpose of good study design is the avoidance of bias.

BACKGROUND

Good study design starts long before the first patient is recruited, with a comprehensive survey of previous similar studies. Even in these days of electronic databases, the best starting place is a recent textbook or review. There are several reasons why investigators need to know what has been done before: to know what remains unknown; to frame their question precisely; to improve the chances of the study providing valid answers; and to prevent needless repetition. Even after their study has started, investigators must remain aware of new relevant work, but any alteration to study design at that stage may affect the validity of the findings.

SPECIFIC OBJECTIVES

After the initial survey, the specific objectives of the study should be clear: postoperative nausea after laparoscopic cholecystectomy in women; induction arterial pressure in patients already taking a β-blocking drug for hypertension; temperature changes during elective aortobifemoral reconstruction.

PATIENT SELECTION CRITERIA

For some studies, any patient presenting for the chosen operation is suitable, but that is unusual. Almost always, some unsuitable patients have to be excluded, if only on grounds of extremes of age. A study of postoperative nausea might exclude patients with a history of hiatus hernia; one of arterial pressure changes might exclude patients with a defined degree of hypertension; and one of temperature changes might exclude patients who have had amputations of the lower limb. Exclusions must be defined in the study design; some study designs contain long lists of both inclusion and exclusion criteria. Exclusions (patients predetermined as ineligible) differ from eligible patients refusing consent and differ again from withdrawals (eligible patients who failed to complete the study). All three categories of patients not included in the study must be admitted in the final report, and remembered when drawing conclusions from the findings. Generalization of the findings may be unsafe if only women aged less than 65 years are studied, if half the patients refuse consent, or if equipment failure forces withdrawal of patents.

TREATMENT SCHEDULES

The only difference between the groups in a clinical trial should be the study treatment. Everything else should be standardized: premedicant drugs, induction agents, neuromuscular blocking agents, infusion fluids, and use of techniques such as epidurals. Clearly, the degree of standardization depends on the trial: in almost all anaesthetic studies, the induction of anaesthesia is standardized; but the size and site of an intravenous cannula may not be important if it can have no influence on the outcome of the study.

Study treatment is best given so that neither clinician nor patient is aware of which treatment the patient is receiving: a *double-blind trial.* Sometimes the clinician knows but not the patient, which is termed a *single-blind trial.* If different anaesthetists are giving the anaesthetics and making the observations in a study, all those involved should remain unaware. If it is not possible to blind all those involved, care should be taken to avoid implicit or explicit clues being leaked to the supposedly blinded investigators. Many simple drug trials are easy to make blind, but blinding is less easy if the interventions are more complex. Sometimes investigators get clues even though technically the study is blind; it is easy to prepare and inject from masked syringes that may contain either thiopental or propofol, but patients complaining of pain during the injection may be presumed to be receiving propofol. Study design might include a questionnaire for the investigators, to determine to what extent blinding was successful.

A non-blinded study is not invalid; some studies are impossible to blind. But non-blinded studies tend to overestimate treatment effects – in other words, these studies are inevitably biased. Put simply, investigators find what they want to find; patients feel how they expect to feel. This is part of human nature.

Other terms to mention under this heading are *placebo*, *control* and *baseline*. In a comparison of a new treatment with the accepted standard treatment, the control group receives the standard treatment. If there is not yet an effective treatment for a condition – prophylaxis of postoperative nausea and vomiting is a good example – there is a place for a placebo group; the best study design would be for three groups: placebo, established drug and new drug. A placebo does not contain active drug but should otherwise be the same, e.g. in appearance and taste, as the test treatments. Placebos are a way of trying to negate the effect of simply doing something: the non-specific effect of medical treatment. Placebos are an obvious ethical issue (see below). Prophylaxis for postoperative nausea and vomiting is in general ineffective and not everyone prescribes it, so it can be argued that giving a placebo does not deprive patients of effective treatment. However, treatment of established nausea and vomiting is more effective and a placebo may be considered unethical.

The terms control and baseline are sometimes confused. A placebo group is a control group; in a two-group study of standard and new antiemetics, the standard group is the control group. In the study of the effect of anaesthetic induction on arterial pressure, readings taken before induction are not control readings but baseline readings with which post-induction readings are compared.

Patients *act as their own controls* if they receive both treatments in a trial. In practice, this is rarely feasible in a study of antiemetics, and uncommon in anaesthetic studies. In a *crossover* trial, patients receive first one and then the other drug, blinded and in random order. These trials may be complicated, including placebo periods and also periods of receiving one or other test drug. There may also be *wash-in periods* to establish drug effect and *wash-out periods* to remove that effect before the next drug is given. These trials are expensive, and unlikely without the backing of the pharmaceutical industry.

PATIENT EVALUATION

In a clinical trial, investigators measure variables (such as arterial pressure and temperature) and seek outcomes (such as postoperative nausea). The techniques and scales must be standardized as rigorously as the treatments, even for variables and outcomes that can be measured objectively, such as arterial pressure (but see measurement bias below). In a study of postoperative nausea, investigators need to decide, for example, whether to record nausea and vomiting separately, whether to record vomiting as yes/no or as number of vomits, whether to use a visual analogue score, and for how long and over what periods to record observations from each patient. The best way to decide how to evaluate patients is from reports of previous similar studies, because using similar methods makes comparison with those studies easier. But it is wise first to check that those methods are feasible in the investigators' own circumstances.

When there are few patients to study and research is difficult, such as in intensive care, the temptation is to record as much as possible from each patient. The danger is of ending up with a welter of figures and overcomplicated analyses, which obscure instead of clarifying. Investigators should refine and simplify their question to define a *primary outcome variable*, and not become distracted by collecting data.

TRIAL DESIGN

The examples of the antiemetic and induction arterial pressure studies are both *experimental* studies in which the investigators are looking for the effect of interventions; that of operative temperature is an *observational* study, although that term is reserved, more correctly, for epidemiological research in which the investigators study factors outside their control, such as the effects of smoking. All are *prospective* studies: the investigators define the conditions and the observations come after the question. In a *retrospective* study, observations are sought from pre-existing records, such as patients' notes; the investigators cannot define the conditions. In general, the greatest value of retrospective studies is in defining rather than in answering questions.

Studies may be *longitudinal*, in which patients are studied over time, or *cross-sectional*, of which a simple example is a snapshot postoperative survey of satisfaction. A *cohort* study is a long-term, longitudinal, prospective study, e.g. of a group of patients who all have the same disease. A cohort is a special type of sample (see below). A *case–control* study is a retrospective study in which patients with a disease are compared for pre-existing risk markers with people who do not have the disease. These definitions are sometimes used rather loosely, and studies may use more than one form of design.

RANDOMIZATION

Allocation to treatments by randomization is an important way of avoiding bias. *Randomized double-blind controlled trials* (RCTs) are probably the best way of determining which of two treatments, on average, gives the better outcome. It must be stressed, however, that just because a trial is randomized and double-blind does not, of itself, mean that the conclusions are justified or generalizable.

Randomization ensures that neither investigators nor patients know which treatment they receive until the time comes to give that treatment: there is no pre-selection. Randomization makes it less likely that, in an anaesthetic study, preoperative factors determine which treatment is given. Another important reason for randomization is that much of medical statistics is based on the assumption that the samples are random and that differences between them therefore behave similarly to the differences between truly random samples.

Randomization by flipping a coin is random but is open to the manipulation, sometimes subconscious, of saying that the coin 'wasn't flipped properly'. Random number tables or a computer's random number generator (all statistical computer programs include these) are better methods of true randomization: an odd number denotes treatment A, an even number treatment B. Clearly, the investigators must not see the next number in the table until the next patient is ready for treatment. This is usually managed by putting codes into sealed envelopes, taken sequentially by the investigators.

Simply using a coin or random numbers causes problems in small studies because of the likelihood of generating unequal groups, which cause statistical difficulties. The usual remedy is *block randomization*. In an intended study of 40 patients, which is probably an average-sized clinical study but in statistical terms is small, block randomization ensures two groups of 20 receive each treatment. If there are known important preoperative factors that affect outcome, e.g. smoking in a study of postoperative chest infections, randomization can be *stratified*, so that smokers and non-smokers are allocated by separate randomization.

Investigators should always describe their method of randomization, or, if they have not randomized treatments, they should explain why. Randomization is difficult when patients or investigators have clear views about which treatment they think is better.

PATIENT CONSENT

Patients must be given all the information necessary to make the decision as to whether to give freely their fully *informed consent* to enter the study. The information must be given in a non-coercive way, in words they understand. For all except the simplest of studies, patients are given a written information sheet. Discussion of possible risks of the study include far smaller risks than customarily discussed before non-research clinical procedures (although customs and attitudes change, and informed consent to treatment and to research are converging as informed consent to treatment demands more and more detail). Patients sign a consent sheet, which is kept with the study paperwork; ideally there should also be a copy filed in patients' notes.

Much of the work of ethics committees (see below) is concerned with the what and how of information provided to patients.

REQUIRED SIZE OF STUDY

The size of the study (i.e. the number of patients that need to be recruited) determines the power of the study (i.e. the likelihood of obtaining an answer). This is discussed in some detail below (see type II error), but is mentioned now because these *power calculations* are part of study design and are an important ethical issue. The notation for size of study group is n.

DESIGN DEVIATIONS

Sometimes investigators discover faults with the collection of information in a trial which imply that the patient can no longer be included. There are serious risks of introducing bias if patients are withdrawn from a study after randomization. Data from withdrawn patients must always be admitted, but it may not be possible to include those data in the general calculations. It is always best, before the trial begins, to think very carefully about how protocol violations may arise, and to have some plans for what to do in that eventuality. If it is important that a particular number of patients are recruited, one plan is to have some extra randomized envelopes available to replace patients who have dropped out. It infringes randomization and blinding simply to replace patients who drop out of one treatment group with additional patients having the same treatment. It is better to include enough patients in the original design, so that a few withdrawals do not matter.

Patients sometimes start in one group and, for clinical reasons, are transferred to a different treatment. A patient whose epidural is ineffective and who is prescribed intramuscular analgesia must, for the purposes of analysis, remain in the epidural group; this is known as analysis by *intention-to-treat*.

PLANS FOR STATISTICAL ANALYSIS

A medical statistician should be contacted early. The more complex the analysis – the more treatments being compared, the more groups of patients, the less well known the intended statistical test – the more important is good statistical advice. It is not a good idea to make casual inquiries of non-specialized statisticians. A statistician will advise about randomization and n, as well as plans for analysis, which must be drawn up before the data are generated.

The fewer measurements that are made, and the fewer comparisons that are made between them, the easier is the statistical analysis. Investigators must be especially wary of making *subgroup analyses* not set out in the original design. An example would be looking for different nausea scores between men and women, or in people above or below a certain weight, when all that was originally intended was to compare the two treatments. Subgroup analyses after the event ('post hoc') risk type I errors (see below).

ADMINISTRATION

Each investigator's job during the study must be defined: who gives the anaesthesia, who makes the measurements or observations, who undertakes the analysis. In a simple study, one investigator may do everything, but there are few clinical trials in which this is possible. There must be plans for monitoring the progress of the trial; forms must be filled in and stored properly, with efficient indexing so that any patient's records can be found quickly if needed. Any supporting institution – drug company, grant-giving body or government agency – can come at any time and demand to see the records. There are recommendations that records from a clinical study should be kept for 15 years.

In the United Kingdom (UK), the Data Protection Act must be complied with if personal information from any patient is stored in a computer file.

ETHICAL ISSUES

The protocol is submitted to a research ethics committee. In the UK, each hospital or group of hospitals has a local research ethics committee (LREC). A research project being done in five or more UK centres must be submitted first to a regional multicentre research ethics committee (MREC).

EXPERIMENTAL DATA AND SOME TYPES OF BIAS

EXPERIMENTAL DATA

Data are either *categorical* or *numerical*; categorical data are often referred to as *lower-order* data. Categorical data may be nominal or ordinal. The simplest type of ***nominal categorical data*** allocates observations to one of two possibilities, e.g. yes or no, male or female, general anaesthesia or local anaesthesia. Nominal data may be of more than two categories, e.g. the categorizing of diabetes as diet-controlled, tablet-controlled or insulin-controlled.

In ***ordinal categorical data***, the categories are ranked, e.g. when pain is assessed as none, mild, moderate or severe. These categories can be ranked by number, as 0, 1, 2 or 3. The common method of measuring pain in millimetres along a ***visual analogue scale*** (VAS) still produces ordinal categorical data. The essence of this type of data is that, whereas within one patient at one time, mild is less than moderate, or 1 is less than 2, there is no certainty that, even for that patient, mild today is the same as mild tomorrow, or that 1 is less than 2 by the same degree as 2 is less than 3; and there is no way of knowing whether one patient's mild is the same as another patient's. Without the need for statistical theory, this is the reason why it is illogical to deal with numbers measured on an ordinal scale arithmetically in the same way as higher-order data.

Numerical data are either discrete or continuous. An example of ***discrete numerical data*** is number of children: one child is less than two children by the same degree as two is less than three. Whereas no family can have 2.4 children, it is now logical to speak of an average-sized family as having 2.4 children: discrete numerical data can be dealt with arithmetically.

Examples of continuous numerical data are arterial pressure and serum sodium concentrations; an increase or decrease of 10 mmHg or 3 mmolL^{-1} is the same, whatever level the change occurs from. In practice, we treat most continuous data as discrete data in the sense that we usually measure to the nearest unit. Clearly, this depends on the precision of our instruments, the units and whether or not it makes clinical sense to measure to greater precision. Measuring arterial pressure in mmHg, it makes little sense to record with more precision than to the nearest 5 mmHg; measuring arterial gas tensions, it does make sense to measure to fractions of a kilopascal (kPa). Whatever precision is chosen, if the data are theoretically continuous, they can be dealt with arithmetically.

Continuous data may be treated as if they were categorical: patients can be categorized as normotensive or hypertensive. This is sometimes a reasonable approach for input variables (i.e. baseline characteristics) to a study, when it is useful to stratify randomization (see above) according to entry baseline arterial pressure. If applied to outcome variables, it causes statistical problems, one of which is the serious loss of information that occurs when all arterial pressures are lumped together above whatever arbitrary cut-off is chosen.

BIAS

Table 1.1 lists some types of bias, and some examples of how they arise. Bias has already been discussed (see under study design, above) but it is appropriate to discuss it further here.

It is a common problem that patients studied in clinical trials are unrepresentative of the population from which they are drawn (selection bias) and to which it is hoped to apply the conclusions of the trials. This problem has two causes, both of which are difficult to circumvent. First, most clinical trials are performed in large centres, but most patients are treated in more peripheral units. For many reasons, it is likely that neither the patients nor the treatments they receive are the same in these different settings. The best example of this effect is the two- to threefold difference in mortality among patients included in trials of treatments of myocardial infarction (commonly 7–10% mortality) and patients treated in the community (commonly 15–20%). Patients in trials are often the most favourable patients treated in the most favourable conditions. To a lesser extent, this probably happens in most trials. The second cause is the well-known phenomenon that even in the same institution, patients included in trials do better than patients who are not included.

A good example of intervention bias might occur in an unblinded comparison of epidural and intramuscular analgesia. Patients know epidural analgesia is more complicated, and might expect it to be better; anaesthetists are likely to spend more time optimizing epidural analgesia.

Follow-up bias, when patients are lost to the study for whatever reason, causes the same statistical difficulties as other withdrawals after randomization. There is the added difficulty that the patients cannot be analysed by intention-to-treat (see above), because the data are not available for analysis.

Examples of causes of measurement or information bias are investigators' transcribing readings incorrectly, inaccurate instruments or patients' mistaken recollections. Instruments and monitors used for research must always be calibrated before use, and researchers should know the limits of measurement of any apparatus they use. For some instruments, e.g. non-invasive arterial pressure monitors, it is adequate to read the technical parts of the manual, but it is sensible to use a recently serviced machine. Better, although probably not practical in most hospitals, is to use dedicated research machines. However, many pieces of equipment that we take for granted in clinical practice, e.g. blood gas analysers, must be calibrated specially if they are used for research. If a blood

Table 1.1 Types of bias in clinical trials

Type of bias	Stage of bias	Example of how bias can occur
Selection	Entering patients into the trial	Sample unrepresentative of population Controls not comparable with study group Exaggeration of a factor
Intervention	Applying treatments	Patients receiving more attention because of their treatment group, e.g. epidural trials
Follow-up	Assessing treatments	Subjects 'lost' to follow-up
Measurement or information	Collecting data Making measurements Making observations	Investigators' conscious or subconscious action Inaccurate or uncalibrated instruments Patients' mistaken recollection
Analysis	Collating data Statistical analysis	Withdrawals or design violations 'Massaging' data
Interpretation	Putting results into context	Prejudices of the investigator

sample is analysed by the hospital's laboratory, the technicians should be asked for the limits of accuracy; for any special analyses, e.g. those used in pharmacokinetic studies, the investigators may have to construct their own *standard curves* when measuring plasma concentrations of drugs.

When considering the accuracy of a measurement, there are two indices: *precision* (an indication of the variability when the concentration in a single sample is measured repeatedly) and *offset* (the difference between the measured value and the true value). Confusingly, offset is often termed bias. Precision and offset need to be measured over the full range of expected values. Precision can be assessed for any instrument (and is often given as the *coefficient of variation* – see below), but offset can be assessed only when there is some way of knowing the true value. The accuracy of non-invasive arterial pressure can be measured against invasive intra-arterial measurement, which is taken as the true arterial pressure.

It is at the analysis stage that investigators must be especially careful not to introduce bias. The unexpected and the peculiar must be reported together with the expected and routine, even though sometimes there are valid reasons for rejecting a measurement, e.g. accidental contamination of a sample.

As long as humans are involved in research, investigators will be biased when they interpret their findings. At this stage of a research project, the caution passes from the investigators to the readers.

STATISTICS

Even when doing research, clinicians need not know any calculations, because they are now performed by computer programs. Clinicians do need to know the principles underlying the calculations, or risk applying an incorrect statistical test.

There are two types of statistics: *descriptive statistics* describe data, and include the mean and standard deviation; *inferential statistics* allow conclusions to be drawn from observations, and include the standard error of the mean, confidence limits, correlation coefficients, and the special statistics of the Student's *t*-test and the chi-squared test (Student was the pseudonym of the statistician who described the *t*-distribution).

PROBABILITY

A correct understanding of probability is essential to understanding statistics.

A coin, when flipped, may land heads or tails. This is a random event. We can work out the expected probabilities for any sequence of heads or tails in a given number of flips. In an exactly analogous way, we make the assumption that when we draw samples of patients from the population for our clinical trials, and when we make measurements from those patients, the patients and measurements will behave with random variability. We may therefore compare our measurement from the real world of clinical trials with the expected behaviour of random numbers, derived from statistical theory that we need know nothing about.

Probability is denoted by P: a 50% probability, such as obtaining a head from flipping a coin, is written as $P = 0.5$. The convention for statistical significance is $P < 0.05$. If the likelihood is less than 1 in 20 that the findings of a clinical trial occurred by chance, then by convention we are prepared to accept that the finding did not occur by chance, but occurred because of whatever intervention we made in the clinical trial.

It is stressed here and later that $P < 0.05$ does not ensure that the findings did not occur by chance. In fact, one in 20 times that is precisely what will have happened (a type I error – see below). One in 20 is taken as the cut-off of statistical significance only as a convention, although it is regarded by many investigators – mistakenly – as the magic figure of respectability.

To help appreciate this, consider what happens if a coin is flipped five times: what is the chance of a run of five heads? There is a one in two chance for each flip, and probabilities are multiplied. The chance of two heads in a row is one in two times two (1/4 or $P = 0.25$), and thus of five heads is one in two × two × two × two × two (1/32 or $P = 0.031$). This probability is less than the magic figure. The logic of declaring the outcome of a clinical trial on a probability of $P < 0.05$ is thus the same as declaring that a coin is biased from observing just five flips. The correct logic is that the coin *might be* biased and the more times the coin is flipped the more certain one becomes, analogous to clinical trials in which the larger the number of patients studied the more certain one is about the treatment.

Increasingly, journals are asking for results to be presented as *confidence intervals* (see below). Probabilities are dimensionless and difficult to interpret clinically. Confidence intervals are expressed in the same units as the measurements and are thus readily understood by clinicians. Confidence intervals of 95% and a probability of 0.05 are equivalent, and the underlying mathematical calculations are the same (and in these days of computers there is no need to know them).

A SIMPLE OUTLINE

Table 1.2 appears here for reference while reading the remainder of the chapter. It shows how to handle the data from the four simple example studies. For each question, there are measurements, a representation of those measurements (by descriptive statistics) and an analysis (by inferential statistics). At the end of this process, the investigators know the probability of their findings having occurred by chance, and the 95% confidence intervals on those findings.

DESCRIPTIVE STATISTICS

When an experimental sample is small, e.g. fewer than six, all the data should be shown. Information is lost as soon as any summary statistics are used, but there are too many data in most clinical trials for it to be practical to show them all. Data are described by an *index of central tendency* – the *median* or the *mean*; and an *index of dispersion* – the *range*, the *interquartile range* or the *standard deviation*. Both these indices are needed; giving the index of central tendency of a measurement without any indication of its dispersion (i.e. of its variability) is misleading. It is not unusual for investigators to omit variability to make results look less messy, but science, especially clinical science, is often messy.

Although the discussion of types of data (above) went from lower-order to higher-order, it is more convenient to deal with mean and standard deviation first, because most people are already familiar with them. It is also useful to understand them before trying to explain why they are sometimes inappropriate.

(There is another index of central tendency: the *mode*. This is the most commonly occurring value. It is not useful statistically and is not discussed in detail.)

The mean

The mean is the average value: it is the sum of the values divided by the number of values. Thus for a sample of five observations (x_1 to x_5) – 24, 27, 28, 31 and 34 – the sum (notation: $\sum x$) is 144, and the mean (notation: $\bar{x}$) is 28.8. It is reasonable to present the mean and other statistics to one significant figure more than the data; here that is to one decimal place. Computer packages present data to as many significant figures as requested, but too many is spurious precision. (Note that presenting the mean of a sample of only five could be criticized as unnecessary statistics but is used here for ease of calculation.)

The standard deviation

The simplest index of dispersion is the full range (24 to 34 for our sample of five), but full range is easily distorted by outliers, which exaggerate the range of values likely to be seen. The most familiar index of dispersion is the standard deviation (SD). Clinicians need know only a few statistical calculations, but it is worth reading how to calculate the SD.

If we take our sample, calculate how each observation varies from the mean (–4.8, –1.8, –0.8, 2.2, 5.2), and sum these deviations, the sum is zero. (The sum of deviations from the mean is always bound to be zero: readers who cannot see intuitively that this is so are likely to have some difficulties with the mathematical aspects of anaesthesia and should seek help to improve their understanding.) The mathematical trick is then to square the deviations, which removes the minus values (23.04, 3.24, 0.64, 4.84, 27.04). The

Table 1.2 Four simple clinical questions: type of data, the measurements, representation and analysis (see text for details).

Question	Type of data	Measure	Representation and graph	Analyse
Two drugs for postoperative sickness	Categorical Nominal	Yes/no	Proportions	Chi-squared (χ^2) → P
Two drugs for postoperative sickness	Categorical Ordinal	Score 0–10	Medians Interquartile ranges Ranges Box-and-whisker plot	Mann–Whitney U → P
Induction of anaesthesia and arterial pressure	Numerical Continuous	Arterial pressures before and after	Means Standard deviations Dots and error (SD) bars	Student's t → P
Two anaesthetic agents and arterial pressure	Numerical Continuous	Arterial pressures at various times	Means Standard deviations Dots and error (SD) bars	ANOVA, Student's t → P
Duration of surgery and change of body temperature	Numerical Continuous	Times and temperatures	Scatter plot	Correlation (r) Regression (m) → P

sum of these squared deviations is 58.8, and the mean squared deviation is 58.8 divided by 5, which is 11.76. The mean squared deviation is a statistic known as the ***variance***, which is central to much statistical theory (it is the variance referred to in the ANOVA, see below), but is not much used practically in an obvious way.

The last step is to take the square root of the variance (3.43), and this is the standard deviation; it is the square root of the average squared deviation from the mean.

There is one refinement. Because small samples (small here implies less than 30) tend to underestimate the true SD, the summed squared deviation is divided not by the number in the sample (n), but by one less ($n - 1$), which gives 3.83.

So our sample has a mean of 28.8 with a standard deviation of 3.8 (the SD should have the same number of significant figures as the mean). This is usually printed as 28.8 ± 3.8, but it is better to put the SD in brackets: 28.8 (3.8). The implication of this description is that we would expect to find 95% of the observations within two standard deviations of the mean. Most anaesthetists are familiar with this idea, although it needs discussion of the normal distribution to understand it more fully (see below).

The ***coefficient of variation*** is the standard deviation divided into the mean. It is a useful comparator, e.g. for instruments used in chemical analyses, because scaling the standard deviation to the mean gives a relative idea of an instrument's precision.

The median

The median is the middlemost value: for our sample it is 28. As there cannot be a true middlemost value of an even-numbered sample, the median is taken as the average of the two values bracketing the middle of the sample. Note that if one peripheral value were different (say, 24, 27, 28, 31 and 44), the median would still be 28 but the mean would be 30.8 and the SD 7.8.

The interquartile range

This is the index of dispersion that goes with the median. It is not sensible to describe an interquartile range for a sample of only five (in fact, a mean and SD are scarcely more sensible, but this number was chosen only for convenience). The interquartile range is described most easily for a sample of 100. If the observations, e.g. 100 nausea scores, are ranked in order from 1 to 100, the quartiles are the 1st to 25th scores (which will be the lowest scores), 26th to 50th, 51st to 75th, and 76th to 100th (which will be the highest scores). The interquartile range is the 26th to 75th score. For $n \neq 100$, the quartiles are the equivalent proportions of the sample.

Which descriptive statistics are appropriate?

Taking a sample of 12 nausea scores – 0, 0, 0, 0, 1, 1, 1, 4, 4, 10, 10, 10 – the mean and SD can be calculated; they are 3.4 (4.2). These statistics can be calculated from any sample consisting of numerical values, but what meaning do these calculations have? They imply that 95% of the observations are within 2 SDs of the mean: but that implies that 95% of the nausea scores are expected within the range –5 to 11.8. Both these values are off the scale and are clinically meaningless, which is why mean and SD should not be used for these data. Certainly, the data are far from normally distributed, which is the technical reason for not using mean and SD; but these 12 nausea scores give the commonplace, clinically evident reason. On the other hand, the median is 1, and the interquartile range is 0–7; these numbers make clinical sense and can be sensibly compared with another sample.

THE NORMAL DISTRIBUTION

Further consideration of which descriptions to use requires some understanding of the normal distribution, which is the behaviour of many of the variables measured in anaesthesia research. That a variable follows the normal distribution does not imply that the variable is normal in the everyday sense; nor is a variable abnormal just because it does not follow the distribution. The distribution is sometimes known as the Gaussian distribution (after the mathematician, Gauss).

The familiar smooth bell-shaped curve of the normal distribution is an example of a ***frequency histogram***. These diagrams, in which the value of the variable is put on the x-axis and the number of observations with that value on the y-axis, are useful when first surveying research data. Systolic arterial pressure is normally distributed: the upper part of Figure 1.1 could be the frequency histogram of arterial pressure in a healthy, young population. The notation for the population mean is μ, and for the population SD is σ. Two-thirds of the observed arterial pressures are within 1 SD (σ is the mathematical symbol; SD is the conventional abbreviation) of the mean, 95% within 2 SDs, and 99% within 3 SDs (these numbers are accepted approximations). The conventional acceptance of $P < 0.05$, the 95% confidence intervals of the observations, is thus the range covered by two standard deviations each side of the mean: this does not imply that any measurement or patient outside this range is necessarily abnormal. Note that in the normal distribution, the mean and median (and the mode) are the same.

These proportions have to be remembered, and the question why they should be so is not easy to answer. The curve is described by a mathematical equation, from which the proportions are worked out, and from which can also be worked out how many observations are expected in whatever part of the curve is under consideration. Clinicians need not know the equation, except to know that this mathematical description of the normal distribution depends on the mean and the standard deviation: if these are known, then the distribution is completely described. Thus, the mean and standard deviation are the ***parameters*** of the normal distribution. This is where the terms parameter and parametric in statistics come from; they imply that the variable in question behaves according to a mathematically described distribution. It need not be the normal distribution. Variables can follow the Poisson distribution, for which the only parameter is the mean. An example is bed occupancy in intensive care units. Knowing the mean bed occupancy allows inferences to be made about how many beds will be occupied for how many days, and what the likelihood is of any number of beds being occupied on any one day. (For a near guarantee of an available bed in a six-bedded unit, mean occupancy should be no more than 2.7 patients. The Poisson distribution tells us that most units in the UK have too few beds!)

The values of t and χ^2 (see Table 1.2 and below) are also parametric, although familiarity with the shape of the distributions is not necessary. One other distribution clinicians may encounter is the ***binomial distribution***, which describes the frequency of occurrence of coin flips, dice rolls and hands of playing cards. The binomial distribution is non-parametric.

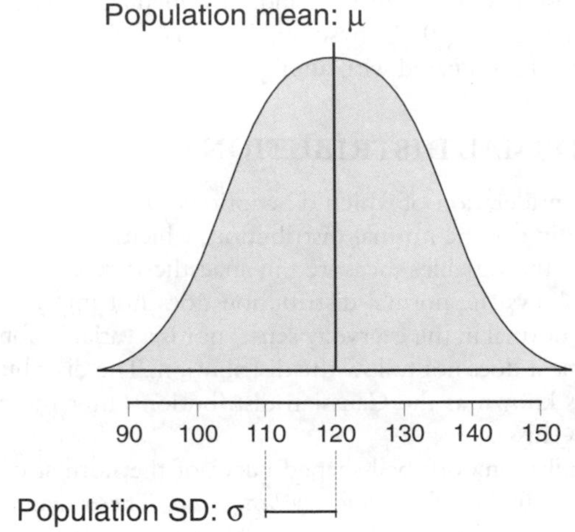

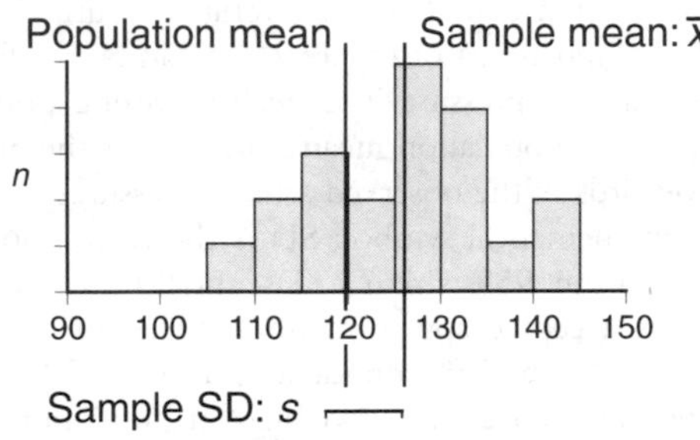

Fig. 1.1
The normal distribution. Frequency histograms of arterial pressure measurements from the population and from a sample. The known values are the sample mean ($\bar{x}$) and the sample standard deviation (s). The standard error of the mean (SEM) is calculated from s, and the confidence intervals (CI) from the SEM. This allows an estimate of the population mean from the sample mean or, if the population mean is known, indicates the likelihood that the sample came from the population. See text for more details.

As a further explanation of the word 'parameter', pharmacokinetic parameters determine the concentration of a drug in the body compartments. Another way of thinking of parameters is via the equation of a straight line: $y = mx + c$ (see regression, below). Here, y and x are the variables; m and c are the constants in the equation and may be thought of as the parameters that control the relationship between y and x. To avoid confusion, the distinction between variables (which are measured directly in clinical trials) and parameters (which are not) is important.

More on the representation of data

We know from previous research that arterial pressure is normally distributed. Sometimes investigators do not know what distribution a variable follows, and this is determined in a pilot study before the main study. There are formal tests for normality, but looking at the frequency histogram is often enough. Another check is that the mean and median are the same, and that the range of observations is approximately five standard deviations.

Parametric data, described by the mean and SD, are shown in diagrams by the familiar dot and error bars. (This is not an error in the sense of mistake; they would be better termed variability bars.)

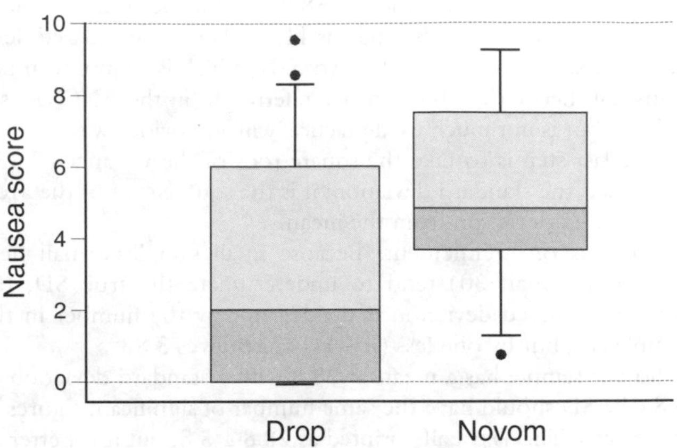

Fig 1.2
Box-and-whisker plots are shown for an imaginary clinical trial of the antiemetics droperidol and novom. The central horizontal line of the box is the median, the lower line the 25th centile and the upper line the 75th centile. The 'whiskers' usually represent the 10th–90th centile range. The dots beyond the whiskers are outliers, beyond the 10th–90th centiles. If outliers are not shown in this way, the whiskers should represent the full range.

The bars must always be defined, in case they are not one standard deviation but some other index. Data that are known not to be parametric are best shown by *box-and-whisker plots* (see Fig. 1.2). If there is any doubt, it is better to assume the data do not conform to a particular distribution, and to use a non-parametric description. This is also probably the best way to deal with small samples (e.g. less than 10) of parametric data.

Skewed distributions and transforming data

Some distributions, although smooth, are *skewed*: they have a tail. A good example is wake-up times after anaesthesia. Most patients wake up in a few minutes, but some take longer, and a few take much longer. The effect of this is that the longer times 'drag' the mean towards the tail (as in the simple calculation above), and the mean wake-up time is longer than the median (a *positive skew*). Such data can be analysed using non-parametrically based statistics, but parametrically based statistics are more *powerful* (see below). Skewed data can sometimes be *transformed*, by taking logarithms or by other mathematical manipulations, so that they assume the normal distribution. The decision to transform data should ideally be taken before the study is done.

INFERENTIAL STATISTICS

From sample to population

It is unusual that we know the population mean and standard deviation, and they are usually *inferred* from a sample. The inferential statistic is the *standard error of the mean* (SEM), which is used to estimate the mean of the population or, if the population mean is known, to decide whether or not the sample is likely to be drawn from that population. The SEM is one of the least understood and most misused statistics; it is not an index of dispersion, although it is often used as such because it is smaller than the SD and looks better on graphs. The SEM is also the key to understanding much of inferential statistics and the comparing of samples that underlies most clinical trials. If the explanation here is too abbreviated, readers are advised to look at Rowntree (1981).

Stating first an extended definition:

> The standard error of the mean is the standard deviation of all possible sample means of a given size, and from it can be calculated the confidence limits around the mean of the measured sample. These limits indicate, to the chosen probability, the likely mean of the population.

If the measured sample is the whole, large, population, then the sample mean *will be* the population mean. If the sample is half the population, the sample mean will still be extremely close to the population mean. However, the smaller the sample, the less likely it is that its mean will be exactly the population mean, and sometimes it will be substantially different. It should be intuitively obvious that the mean of a smaller sample – even if selected in a correctly random fashion – is more likely to misrepresent the mean of the population.

There is another way of expressing this. If many samples of the same size are taken (instead of the usual single sample of that size) the *means of those samples* are more similar to one another if the samples are large than if they are small. The means of these samples can themselves be treated as data, and a frequency histogram constructed: the sample means follow the normal distribution, and the larger the samples, the narrower is the distribution. In exactly the same way that the SD of the distribution of data is calculated, so may the SD of the sample means be calculated. The larger the value of n, the smaller the SD of the sample means. This SD of the sample means is the SEM (see definition, above). Thus, 95% of sample means (of a given n) will be within 2 SEMs of the population mean (and 99% within 3 SEMs), in exactly the same way that 95% of observations are within 2 SDs (and 99% within 3 SDs) of the population mean.

This logic is applied to a single trial sample, because statistical theory allows calculation of the SEM from the sample standard deviation (notation s): SEM = $s\sqrt{n}$. Then the 95% confidence intervals of the sample mean are 2 SEMs and there is 95% confidence that the population mean lies within that range.

(The *central limit theorem* of statistics states that the distribution of samples is normal whatever the distribution of the original data. This theorem is often used to justify applying parametrically based statistics to non-parametric data, but the clinical nonsense of parametric descriptions of these data is more important than statistical theory. The central limit theorem is beyond basic statistical knowledge.)

Probability and samples

An important implication of 95% of sample means lying within 2 SEMs of the population mean is that 5%, i.e. 1 in 20, do not. If 20 samples are drawn at random from a normally distributed population, on average one of them will be statistically significantly different from the population. This effect of pure chance is a type I error (see below). The size of the sample does not matter: at a probability of 0.05, on average one of 20 samples drawn at random from a normally distributed population will be statistically significantly different. However, the larger the sample, the smaller the absolute difference will be. It is thus less likely that a difference due to chance will be clinically important.

Comparing samples: the null hypothesis

Although the research question may be 'Is novom better than droperidol?' or 'Does propofol cause greater hypotension than thiopental at induction?', the statistical approach is via the *null hypothesis.* A hypothesis must be grounded (i.e. based on previous knowledge) and testable (otherwise it is not a hypothesis but a speculation), and the essence of the test is that the hypothesis is falsifiable. The philosophy of this (due to Popper) is that we can never know the truth, but progression in knowledge takes us further towards the truth. Thus, we start with the null hypothesis that novom and droperidol have the same effect. If we show a difference, then we reject the null hypothesis and accept that one of the drugs is a better antiemetic - *at our chosen level of probability* (but we can be wrong: see Type I error). If we fail to show a difference, we support the null hypothesis (but we can be wrong: see Type II error).

Comparing proportions: a new drug for postoperative sickness by 'yes/no'

If 17 patients of 40 given droperidol and 11 of 40 given novom vomit, the data are described as *proportions* (17/40 and 11/40) (data should not be described as percentages). These two proportions are then tested by the chi-squared test for the probability of these proportions having happened by chance. As with all statistical tests, it is not necessary to know the details of the test, the essential knowledge is knowing which test to apply. The principle of the chi-squared test is a comparison of the proportions that actually occurred in the study with the proportions that would have occurred if there had been no difference between the groups. (Here there are two groups, but the test can be applied to any number of groups.) The calculation gives chi-squared (notation: χ^2), and the value is looked up in tables (or provided by the computer program) to give the probability. The larger the number of tested groups, the larger χ^2 needs to be to reach the chosen P. The tables account for this; χ^2 is checked against the number of *degrees of freedom* in the data (degrees of freedom is a difficult statistical idea, and not necessary to a simple knowledge of statistics).

Comparing two samples of ordinal data: a new drug for postoperative sickness by nausea score

Comparisons of two samples of non-parametric data such as these (or of numerical data whose distribution is unknown or uncertain) is by a ranking test. When the two groups are of different patients, the data are *unpaired*, and the *Mann–Whitney U-test* is appropriate. Before computers, such tests were tedious. The calculations for the *t*-test (see below) are easy with pencil and paper by substituting in equations. There are no equations for ranking tests, and no alternative to the laborious listing and ranking of all the data.

The data are ranked from lowest to highest to determine the median and interquartile ranges (see above); the procedure is the same for the statistical test, but the rankings are summed and compared between the two groups (imagine doing that for two samples of 100 patients). This is best explained by example.

The first few nausea scores in a trial of droperidol (group D) and novom (group N) using a 100 mm visual analogue scale are:

Group D	0	5	12	13	15...
Group N	3	6	9	10	12...

These scores are ranked and the scores from novom are identified by underlining:

Rank order:	0	$\underline{3}$	5	$\underline{6}$	$\underline{9}$	$\underline{10}$	12	$\underline{12}$	13	15...
Ranking:	1	$\underline{2}$	3	$\underline{4}$	$\underline{5}$	$\underline{6}$	7.5	$\underline{7.5}$	9	10...

The rankings are then summed for each group. Shared scores rank equal, which is why the scores of 12 each rank 7.5:

Group sum of ranks:

Group D	=	1 + 3 + 7.5 + 9 + 10	=	30.5
Group N	=	$\underline{2} + \underline{4} + \underline{5} + \underline{6} + \underline{7.5}$	=	$\underline{24.5}$

If the null hypothesis is true, the rank sums are equal; the more unequal they are, the less support there is for the null hypothesis. *P* is read from a table of expected rank sums against *n*. The whole procedure is now done by computer, with no need to read from tables.

A paired test, the *Wilcoxon signed rank test*, is appropriate when a study is done within-patient, each patient being his or her own control. The pair differences are ranked and the rank sums calculated for the positive and negative differences from control. Again, the less equal these sums are, the more likely it is that the null hypothesis will be rejected. This is the paired equivalent of the Mann–Whitney. Some confusion arises because the Mann–Whitney test is also known as the *Wilcoxon two-sample test*.

Comparing two samples of numerical, normal, data: the effect of an induction agent on arterial pressure

When samples are very large, e.g. more than 150, they can be compared simply by referring to the normal distribution. It follows from the description above that two samples, the means of which are separated by more than 2 SEMs, are statistically significantly different at $P < 0.05$. The familiar Student's *t*-test extends this idea to small samples, when direct reference to the normal distribution becomes inaccurate (the reasons for this do not matter). Assumptions of the *t*-test are that the data are drawn from a normal population (although the samples themselves do not have to be rigidly normal) and that the variances (and hence the SEMs) of the two samples are not too different.

Analogous with the Mann–Whitney and the Wilcoxon tests, the *unpaired t-test* is for data from two different groups of patients and the *paired t-test* is for two groups of data from the same patients (e.g. before and after induction). The paired test is more powerful because the calculations are on the differences between the paired readings, which gives a smaller SEM and, as mentioned above, *t* is the ratio of the difference between the means and the SEM. For samples of about 30, *t* is about 2.05 at $P = 0.05$; for samples of 10, *t* is 2.26. Thus if *t* is larger than this value, we reject the null hypothesis at $P = 0.05$.

The basic question asked by the *t*-test is whether the samples could come from the same population, or whether they are better described as coming from two different populations.

The *t*-test can be one- or two-tailed. This commonly causes confusion. The safe option is always to do a two-tailed test. A one-tailed test is appropriate only when a comparison can only move in one direction (i.e. the two outcomes comparing groups A and B are A = B or A > B, but A < B is impossible). This is almost never true in clinical trials, and the commonest reason for using a one-tailed test is that $P < 0.05$ is more easily achieved.

Comparing more than two samples: a comparison of the effects of two induction agents on arterial pressure

A graph from this type of trial is likely to show means and standard deviations for each drug before induction and at intervals after induction. The obvious way to analyse these data is by repeated *t* testing, comparing arterial pressures with baseline arterial pressure and between the two groups at each time of measurement.

This *multiple testing* is incorrect because of the additive risk of a difference occurring by chance: 10 comparisons each at $P < 0.05$ gives an overall $P < 0.5$. One approach is first to do an ANOVA. This is the acronym for *analysis of variance*, which is a way of assessing the probability that there are measurements within the data that are statistically different from the rest. If ANOVA gives $P < 0.05$, then Student's *t* can be used to tease out the precise differences. The non-parametric equivalent of ANOVA is the *Kruskal–Wallis test*, which would be suitable for nausea scores measured at intervals postoperatively.

Multiple testing is a recurring problem and statistical advice should be sought. Another approach to the problem is to use a so-called *summary statistic*, so that for each patient the change in arterial pressure is represented by a single number such as the area enclosed by the graph of arterial pressure against time. (The most familiar way that anaesthetists might compare areas under curves, although this has nothing to do with multiple testing, is probably in the measurement of bioavailability, see page 27).

Relating variables to one another: correlation and regression – the relationship between duration of surgery and body temperature

Analysis aiming to link two variables should start with a *scatter plot* – a graph in which the *independent variable*, e.g. time, is plotted on the *x*-axis and the *dependent variable*, e.g. temperature, on the *y*-axis (see Fig. 1.3). If the relationship is linear, *least-squares statistics* are applied. The *correlation coefficient* (*r*), sometimes termed the Pearson correlation coefficient, describes the amount of scatter: it is the degree of agreement between the two variables. The *regression coefficient* (*m*) describes how *y* depends on *x*: it is the slope, or gradient, of *the line of best fit* (as in the equation for a straight line, see above). Whether correlation or regression is appropriate depends on whether it is sensible to predict *y* from *x*.

Thus, if weight is plotted against height for a sample of men, taller men are, on average, heavier, but the relationship does not allow sensible prediction of the weight of an individual man who is 1.83 m tall. Calculating *r* is sensible, but not *m*. On the other hand, if a subject breathes carbon dioxide mixtures, the resulting alveolar ventilation in that subject is predictable from the arterial tension, and *m* is a sensible measurement. As *m* is a constant in an equation, clearly it can have any value at all, can be positive or negative, and its units depend on *x* and *y* . However, *r* is a dimensionless measure of scatter. It is +1 for a perfect line of positive gradient, −1 for a perfect negative line, and zero if there is no correlation.

The statistics *r* and *m* are only best estimates of the true relationship between *x* and *y*, in the same way that $\bar{x}$ is an estimate of the true mean. Their probabilities and, better, confidence intervals must be given. Confidence intervals are shown graphically as an 'envelope' showing the 95% (or 99%) range around the line of best fit.

The relationship between two variables need not be linear. Least-squares statistics are used to fit any line, e.g. for the well

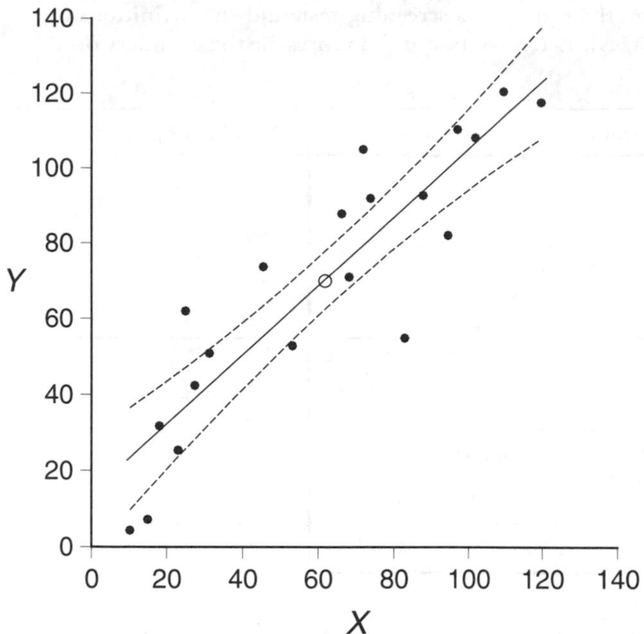

Fig 1.3
A scatter plot of two variables: *X* is the independent (or 'known') variable; *Y* is the dependent (or 'unknown') variable. Using least-square statistics, the correlation coefficient (r) is 0.90 and the line of best fit (shown by the solid line) is $Y = 0.90X + 14.6$. All three coefficients (of correlation, gradient and intercept) are only best estimates, and their confidence intervals should be reported. The 95% confidence 'envelope' is shown by the dotted lines: with the restraint that the line must pass through the means of *X* and *Y* (marked by the open circle), there is 95% confidence that the true relation between *Y* and *X* is defined by this envelope. Note that the lines should not extend horizontally beyond the measured values of *X*.

known exponential relation between drug concentration and time after injection (see Ch. 3). Or *y* may depend on several variables, so the data fit an equation of the form $y = m_1x_1 + m_2x_2 + m_3x_3 \ldots$ This is *multiple regression*. Sometimes the variables are nominal data. For example, if *y* is the likelihood of postoperative nausea, one of the terms may be for sex, which is represented in the equation as 0 or 1, and the coefficient applied to each term is often termed the 'weighting'. This is *logistic regression*. Regression using more than one term is not for amateurs in statistics.

Regression is inappropriate for ordinal data because the relationship between the variables cannot be described by equation. There are non-parametrically based estimates of *r*, e.g. Spearman's rank correlation.

Clinicians must beware of confusing *association* between variables, whether correlation or regression, with *causation*. For example, alcohol consumption and incidence of lung cancer are correlated, but alcohol does not cause lung cancer. The *confounding variable* is tobacco use. A common cause of false association is both variables changing with time.

Type I and type II errors

Type I error is best thought of as a *false positive*. A difference is found (or a gradient is described, etc.) when there is not one: the null hypothesis is rejected when it is in fact true. It is impossible to avoid type I error, but it is less likely if *P* is smaller or, as explained above, *n* is larger. Type I errors can occur despite the best study design. They come to light only if a study is repeated.

Type II error is a *false negative*. A difference is not found but there is one: the null hypothesis is not rejected when it should have been. The commonest cause of type II error is that *n* is too small. Type II error is linked with the *power* of a study, and power calculations are important in study design; the convention is that *n* should be large enough to give at least an 85–90% chance of finding a difference that exists. Underpowered studies risk rejecting treatments that are actually effective. Investigators need to know the variability of the data (which for normal data is the SD), to choose *P* and to decide what clinically important difference they are seeking. For simple, two-sample studies, *n* is then read from tables or nomograms. The sample will need to be larger if *P* is smaller, the SD is larger, or the sought difference is smaller. For a study to have 90% power at $P < 0.05$ when the sought difference is equal to the SD of the data, there should be two samples of 20. For more complicated studies, investigators should seek statistical advice.

Tests of prediction

As screening for diseases becomes more common, clinicians need to know the language of prediction. Examples from anaesthesia are the prediction of postoperative cardiac complications and of death on the intensive care unit; a test is done or a score is applied on a sample of patients and the result is correlated with the outcome. The test may predict the outcome (true positive or true negative) or may fail to predict (false positive or false negative). There is the risk of patients testing as false positives becoming the 'worried well', who may undergo unpleasant investigations to rule out the diagnosis. Patients testing as false negatives miss out on treatment and may sue their doctors when the diagnosis becomes apparent. False positives and false negatives are inevitable in screening, although too often they are taken as evidence of faults in the screening service.

Sensitivity is the proportion of true positives correctly identified by the test, and *specificity* is the proportion of true negatives correctly identified (see Table 1.3). Confusingly, specificity is also termed *selectivity*. (These are not synonymous terms for false-positive rate and false-negative rate, which are ambiguous and should be avoided.) *Positive predictive value* is the proportion of patients testing positive who are correctly diagnosed. There are no agreed 'acceptable' proportions for these indices, because they depend on the nature of the disease and the investigations or treatments made necessary by diagnosis. It is arguable that incurable diseases should not be screened for at all.

One important factor in screening is the *prevalence* of the disease in the population (cases per unit number), in other words how common the disease is (note that *incidence* is occurrence per unit number in a given time). The less common the disease, the more likely are false negatives. A test that is 95% specific (which is extremely high for any screening test) for a disease that occurs in only one person per 1000 will turn up 50 false positives if all 1000 people are screened.

Presenting the results of clinical trials

The results of most clinical trials are presented as percentage changes in outcome ('15% less vomiting with novom').

Table 1.3 Prediction and screening. A two-by-two table showing the results of a screening test, and the definitions of sensitivity and specificity (which are usually expressed as percentages). Letters a, b, c and d represent the numbers of patients in each box.

	Patient has disease	Patient does not have disease	Number of patients
Test says 'Yes, patient has disease'	True positive a SENSITIVITY: proportion with disease correctly forecast = a/(a + c)	False positive b	= a + b
Test says 'No, patient does not have disease'	False negative c	True negative d SPECIFICITY: proportion without disease correctly forecast = d/b + d	= c + d
	a + c	b + d	a + b + c + d = n

Increasingly, more clearly defined indices are presented, especially when results are pooled from single trials for *meta-analysis. Absolute risk reduction* is the actual percentage change in outcome; *relative risk reduction* is the percentage change in outcome related to the prevalence or incidence of the condition. Odds ratio is a comparison of outcomes with two treatments, or of treatment with control, but is not an easy number for clinicians to deal with. The clearest way of presenting numerical results from a clinical trial is by *numbers-needed-to-treat* (NNT). This describes the number of patients who have to be treated for one patient to have a favourable outcome. As with prediction, the acceptable NNT depends on the seriousness of the disease and the possible complications (and cost) of the treatment. All these indices should be presented with their confidence intervals.

INTERPRETATION OF CLINICAL TRIALS

It is unfortunately true that the standard of clinical trials (in the whole of medicine) is generally poor. A continuing problem is that many trials are too small, risking both type I and type II errors. Because investigators are understandably more enthusiastic when things go well, trials with positive results are more likely to be published than those with negative results, so-called *publication bias.* Other common problems are overcomplexity and data dredging (looking at different subgroups and with different statistical tests in an effort to find 'significant' results).

Statistical significance does not imply clinical significance. Whatever the statistical calculations produce, only clinicians are capable of interpreting whether a treatment is worth applying. Always remember that statistics, unlike mathematics, cannot prove or disprove anything. All they can do is to present probabilities, and the observer must then decide what action to take, based on these probabilities.

FURTHER READING

Altman D G 1991 Practical statistics for medical research. Chapman & Hall, London

Browner W S 1994 A simple recipe for doing it well. Anesthesiology 80: 923

Cruikshank S 1998 Mathematics and statistics in anaesthesia. Oxford Medical Publications, Oxford

Goodman NW 1998 Anaesthesia and evidence based medicine. Anaesthesia 53: 353

Greenhalgh T 1997 How to read a paper. BMJ Publishing Group, London

Rowntree D 1981 Statistics without tears. Penguin, London

2 Cellular physiology/ pharmacology relevant to anaesthesia

This chapter is divided into four main sections: a description of receptors (including second messengers); representation of drug–receptor interaction (receptor pharmacology); intracellular Ca^{2+} as a vital signalling molecule; and, finally, potential targets(s) for anaesthetic action are discussed.

RECEPTORS

Receptors recognize specific small signalling molecules to produce a biological effect. In the unbound state, a receptor is functionally silent. Excluding the intracellular receptor for inositol(1,4,5) triphosphate and the ryanodine receptor (discussed below) there are four main classes of receptor: G-protein coupled (GPCR), ligand-gated ion channels, tyrosine kinase coupled and intracellular steroid receptors. It has been estimated that 60% of the drugs routinely given to patients target the GPCR.

G-PROTEIN COUPLED

G-protein coupled receptors have been, and continue to be, the subject of intense research. Some examples are shown in Table 2.1. As the name suggests, the signal produced upon activation is transduced by a guanine nucleotide binding (or G) protein. The receptor spans the plasma membrane seven times with the N-terminus extracellular and the C-terminus intracellular (Fig. 2.1). Once activated, the receptor undergoes a conformational change such that the G-protein is able (in most circumstances) to interact with the third intracellular loop and the C-terminus.

G-proteins

These proteins form the link between receptor and effector to generate a second messenger. As the name suggests, G-proteins bind guanine nucleotides (guanosine triphosphate-GTP and guanosine diphosphate-GDP). The protein is composed of three subunits, α, β and γ, with the α subunit defining the G-protein (Fig. 2.1). For example, there are inhibitory G-proteins (G_i/G_o) and stimulatory G-proteins (G_s and G_q). In the past, G-protein activity was defined using two bacterial toxins: pertussis toxin, which inhibits the action of the G_i/G_o class of G-protein, and cholera toxin, which persistently activates the G_s class of G-proteins. However, the use of specific antibodies has made G-protein classification more precise. The α subunit is extremely important in the control of signalling via GPCRs; it is the site of GTP/GDP binding and is also an intrinsic GTPase. When an agonist binds to a GPCR, the G-protein can then interact with the C-terminus and the third intracellular loop of the (activated) receptor. In the inactive state, the G-protein has GDP bound to the α subunit. Following activation with agonist, GDP is exchanged for GTP and the G-protein is activated. Gα dissociates from Gβ/γ and activates an appropriate effector molecule. As the α subunit displays GTPase activity, there is a marked tendency to cleave GTP to GDP and hence inactivate the G-protein. In essence, the Gα subunit acts as an 'off' switch.

Table 2.1 Examples of G-protein coupled receptors (GPCRs) and their characteristics

Receptor	G-protein	Effector	Second messenger
α_1-Adrenoceptor	G_q	PLC	Increased $Ins(1,4,5)P_3/Ca^{2+}$
α_2-Adrenoceptor	$G_{i/o}$	Adenylyl cyclase	Decreased cAMP
		VSCC	Decreased Ca^{2+} influx
		K^+ channel	Increased K^+ efflux
β-Adrenoceptor	G_s	Adenylyl cyclase	Increased cAMP
μ, δ and κ opioid[a]	$G_{i/o}$	Adenylyl cyclase	Decreased cAMP
		VSCC	Decreased Ca^{2+} influx
		K^+ channel	Increased K^+ efflux
MgluR			
Class I	G_q	PLC	Increased $Ins(1,4,5)P_3/Ca^{2+}$
Class II/III	$G_{i/o}$	Adenylyl cyclase	Decreased cAMP
Bradykinin	G_q	PLC	Increased $Ins(1,4,5)P_3/Ca^{2+}$

[a]Similar effects can be observed for muscarinic m2/4 and cannabinoid.
MgluR, metabotrophic glutamate receptor; PLC, phospholipase C; VSCC, voltage-sensitive calcium channel.

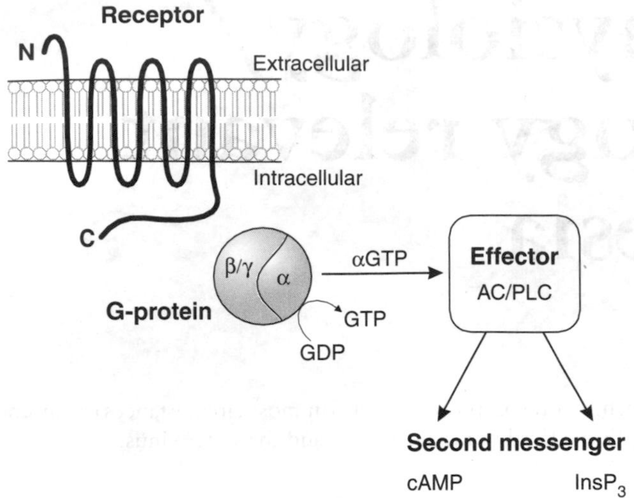

Fig. 2.1
Schematic representation of G-protein receptor–effector coupling. The seven transmembrane spanning G-protein coupled receptor (GPCR) is depicted coupling to an effector enzyme (e.g. adenylyl cyclase, phospholipase C) via a guanine nucleotide binding (G) protein. The G-protein comprises three subunits, α, β and γ. αGTP interacts with the effector enzyme to produce a second messenger. These second messengers modulate cellular activity (see text for details).

When αGTP is converted to αGDP, the α subunit can re-associate with the β/γ subunits and the G-protein is then free to interact with another receptor. One activated receptor may interact with multiple G-proteins.

Effectors

In this chapter, adenylyl cyclase, phospholipase C and ion channels (Ca^{2+} and K^+) are considered as examples of effector enzymes. Guanylyl cyclase, the target for nitric oxide, is not discussed in detail. Adenylyl cyclase is the enzyme responsible for the conversion of intracellular adenosine triphosphate (ATP) to cyclic adenosine monophosphate (cAMP). The enzyme is variably sensitive to G-protein α subunits, Ca^{2+} and G-protein β/γ subunits. Adenylyl cyclase is activated by the G_s class of G-proteins (e.g. by norepinephrine acting at β-adrenoceptors) to increase the formation of cAMP, or inhibited by the G_i class of G-proteins (e.g. by norepinephrine acting at α_2-adrenoceptors) to reduce cAMP formation (Fig. 2.2). Phospholipase C is the plasma membrane-bound enzyme responsible for the conversion of the membrane phosphoinositide, PIP_2 (phosphatidyl inositol 4,5 bisphosphate), to two second messengers, inositol(1,4,5)triphosphate [$Ins(1,4,5)P_3$] and diacylglycerol (DAG). In common with adenylyl cyclase, the enzyme is variably sensitive to Gα subunits of the G_q class (e.g. norepinephrine acting at α_1-adrenoceptors) of G-proteins, Ca^{2+} and G-protein β/γ subunits. Members of the G_i/G_o G-protein coupled class of receptors (e.g. opioid, α_2-adrenoceptor, cannabinoid) are capable of closing voltage-sensitive Ca^{2+} channels and activating K^+ channels (inward rectifiers – K_{ir}) to enhance an efflux of K^+, resulting in membrane hyperpolarization. This ion channel interaction is, as for the events described above, mediated by Gα subunits. One activated G-protein can potentially interact with multiple effector molecules.

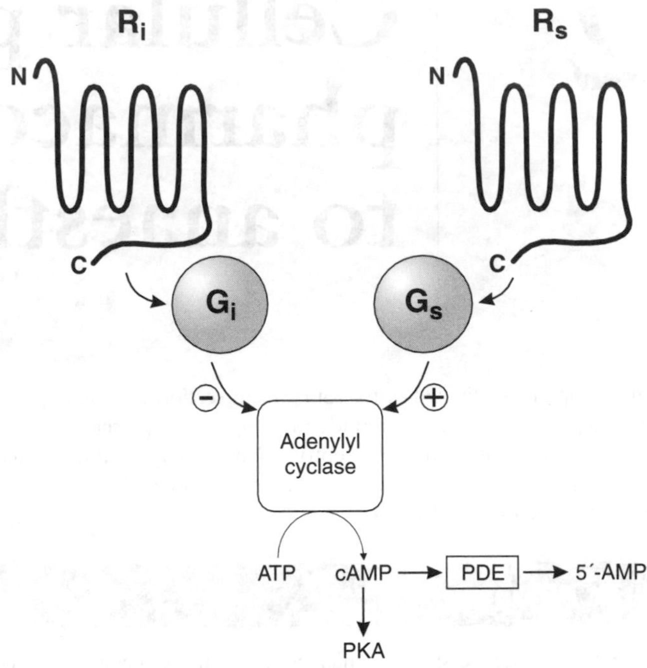

Fig. 2.2
Control of cyclic adenosine monophosphate (cAMP) formation. Stimulatory GPCRs (R_s) and inhibitory GPCRs (R_i) couple to adenylyl cyclase via stimulatory G-proteins (G_s) and inhibitory G-proteins (G_i), respectively. Activation of G_s activates adenylyl cyclase to increase the formation of cAMP. Activation of G_i inhibits adenylyl cyclase to inhibit the formation of cAMP. cAMP activates protein kinase A (PKA) and the cAMP signal is terminated by a phosphodiesterase (PDE).

Second messengers

Adenylyl cyclase and phospholipase C are responsible for the generation of cAMP and $Ins(1,4,5)P_3$/DAG, respectively. The action of cAMP is usually mediated by a cytosolic enzyme, protein kinase A, although this is not always the case. cAMP-sensitive target sites include elements of the contractile apparatus in muscle and metabolic enzymes. In addition, the I_h K^+ channel, which is involved in repolarization after action potential firing, is sensitive to cAMP. Prostaglandins increase and opioids decrease cAMP in addition to being pronociceptive and antinociceptive, respectively. It is thought that activation of I_h by increased cAMP in nociceptive neurones leads to more rapid repolarization, and hence an increased rate of firing may be involved in the pronociceptive actions of prostaglandins. Conversely, opioids reduce cAMP, thereby reducing I_h activity and delaying repolarization, and hence decreasing nociceptive transmission. However, with opioids, the antinociceptive action also involves closure of voltage-sensitive calcium channels (VSCCs) and activation of K_{ir}. Activated adenylyl cyclase is capable of producing many molecules of cAMP.

The discovery that $Ins(1,4,5)P_3$ releases Ca^{2+} from the endoplasmic reticulum provided the link between agonist-stimulated phosphoinositide turnover and agonist-stimulated increases in intracellular Ca^{2+}. $Ins(1,4,5)P_3$ binds to an intracellular receptor located on the endoplasmic reticulum membrane and occupation leads to a release of intracellular stored Ca^{2+} and a rise in cytosolic free Ca^{2+} (see below).

Table 2.2 Examples of ligand-gated ion channels

Receptor	Ligand	Ion and direction of flow
Nicotinic	Acetylcholine	Na^+ inward
$GABA_A$	GABA	Cl^- inward
Glycine	Glycine	Cl^- inward
NMDA	Glutamate	Ca^{2+} inward
AMPA	Glutamate	Na^+ inward
$5HT_3$	Serotonin	Ca^{2+} inward

The fact that one activated receptor can interact with many G-proteins, and in turn many effectors, to generate many molecules of second messenger allows this system to amplify receptor input.

The actions of cAMP are terminated by phosphodiesterase activity converting cAMP to the inactive 5′-AMP. cAMP-dependent phosphodiesterase is inhibited by methylxanthines such as caffeine. Termination of the Ins(1,4,5)P_3 signal is more complex but still involves metabolism. Ins(1,4,5)P_3 can be phosphorylated (3-kinase) to Ins(1,3,4,5)P_4, which may have some biological activity. Ins(1,3,4,5)P_4 and Ins(1,4,5)P_3 are both dephosphorylated by a 5-phosphatase to yield Ins(1,3,4)P_3 and Ins(1,4)P_2, respectively, both of which are inactive. Further dephosphorylation reactions yield inositol which is then re-incorporated into the membrane pool of phosphoinositides. Various stages in the dephosphorylation pathway are inhibited by Li^+, and it is believed that interruption of the phosphoinositide cycle underlies the antimanic action of this monovalent cation.

LIGAND-GATED ION CHANNELS

This class of receptor is found on the plasma membrane and is composed of four or five subunits in various combinations depending on the particular receptor. The protein doubles as both a receptor and an ion channel with distinct structural motifs encoding the ligand binding site, ion channel pore and modulatory site(s). When the receptor is activated by the appropriate agonist, a range of mono- and divalent ions flow along their concentration gradient either into or out of the cell (Table 2.2, Fig. 2.3A). This class of receptor is very important from the anaesthetic viewpoint in that the nicotinic acetylcholine receptor is the target for neuromuscular relaxants, the *N*-methyl-D-aspartate (NMDA) receptor is the target for ketamine, and the $GABA_A$ receptor is a major target for a range of inhalation and intravenous general anaesthetic agents (excluding ketamine).

TYROSINE KINASE COUPLED

In this class of receptor, the protein is a monomer that spans the plasma membrane only once. The extracellular domain binds the ligand and the intracellular domain possesses tyrosine kinase activity. Agonists for this receptor class include insulin and growth factors (Fig. 2.3B). When activated, the intracellular domain autophosphorylates, the receptor dimerizes and then activates a range of intracellular target proteins. These include enzymes/transporters involved in glucose metabolism (insulin) and phospholipase C.

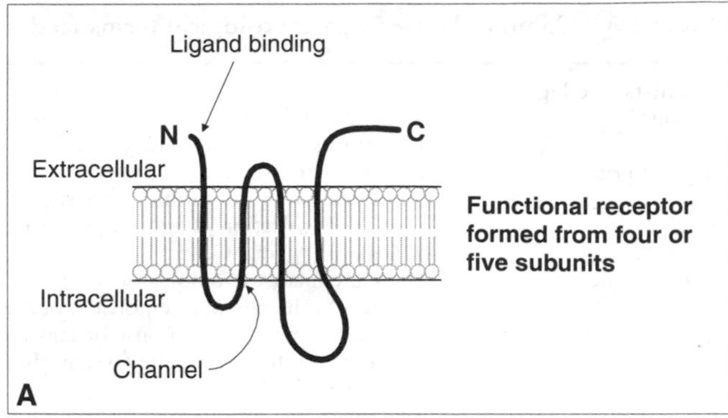

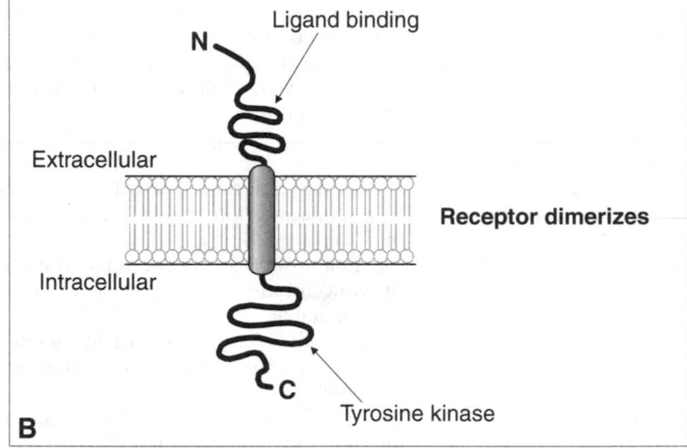

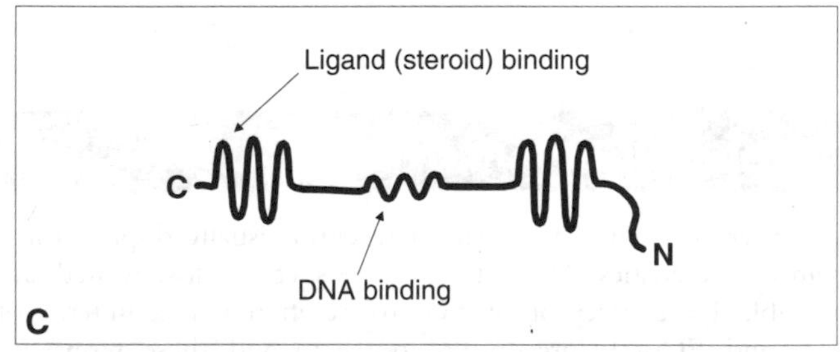

Fig. 2.3
Schematic representation of the structure of non-G-protein coupled receptors. **A.** A single subunit of a ligand-gated ion channel. A functional channel results from the combination of four or five of these subunits. **B.** A tyrosine kinase receptor. When activated, these receptors usually dimerize. **C.** A steroid receptor. Unlike in (A) and (B), the receptor is not located on the plasma membrane and resides in the cytoplasm. Upon activation, the receptor translocates to the nucleus and initiates gene transcription (see text for details).

INTRACELLULAR STEROID RECEPTORS

These monomeric receptors are not found on the plasma membrane. Examples of agonists for this class of receptor include sex hormones, thyroid hormones and adrenal hormones. The receptor possesses a ligand binding domain, a catalytic domain and a set of 'zinc fingers'. In the inactive (no ligand bound) state, the receptor is located in the cytosol of the cell. When the receptor is activated, it translocates to the nucleus and via the 'zinc fingers' binds to DNA and initiates gene transcription and new protein synthesis (Fig. 2.3C). Responses produced via activation of this receptor are slow compared with the other three receptor types.

Table 2.3 Commonly used pharmacological terms to describe drug–receptor interaction

Term	Description
Agonists (see Fig. A)	
Agonist	A ligand that binds to a receptor to produce a functional response. This results from an increase in the proportion of active receptors
Agonist potency	The ability to produce a response expressed in terms of concentration of the agonist. This should be defined further with: EC_{50}: concentration of agonist producing 50% maximal response pEC_{50}: $-\log_{10}$ of EC_{50}
Agonist efficacy	There are many definitions for this term. In its simplest form, it relates to the size of a response. For example, an agonist that produces a maximum response of 100% has higher efficacy than an agonist in the same tissue/system that produces a maximum response of 50%
Full agonist	An agonist that produces a 'maximum' response in a particular tissue/cellular system. Typically, full agonists produce this at low levels of receptor occupancy
Partial agonist	An agonist that produces a lower than maximum (than a full agonist) response. Even at full receptor occupancy, a full response cannot be elicited
Antagonists (see Fig. B)	
Antagonist	A drug that reduces the activity of another drug (usually an agonist)
Antagonist potency	IC_{50}: concentration of an antagonist that reduces a specified response by 50% pIC_{50}: $-\log_{10}$ of IC_{50}
Competitive antagonist	The inhibitory effect of the antagonist can be overcome by increasing the concentration of the agonist. The effect is competitive or surmountable
pA_2	$-\log_{10}$ of the concentration of an antagonist that makes it necessary to double the agonist concentration in order to elicit the original response
Non-competitive antagonist	The inhibitory effect of the antagonist cannot be overcome by increasing the concentration of the agonist

(A) Agonist concentration–response curve

Response (%) 100 0; Maximum response; Full agonist; Maximum response; Partial agonist; pEC_{50}; Log_{10} Concentration

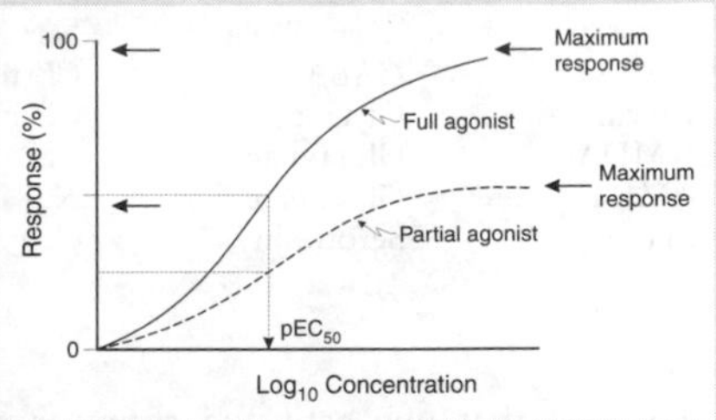

Full agonist has higher efficacy than partial agonist. In this example both have the same potency (pEC_{50}).

(B) Effect of antagonist on agonist concentration–response curve

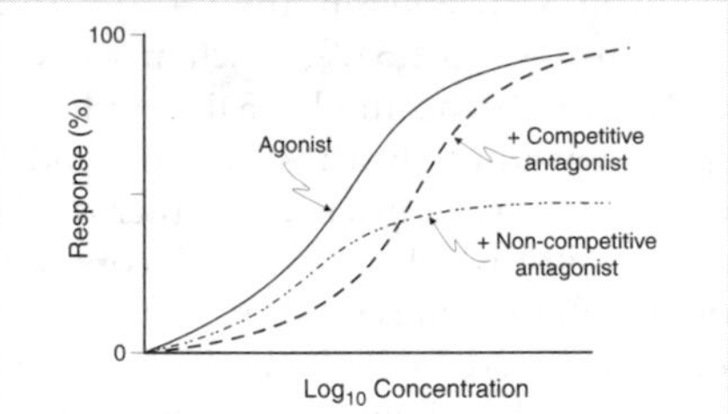

Response (%) 100 0; Agonist; + Competitive antagonist; + Non-competitive antagonist; Log_{10} Concentration

DRUG–RECEPTOR INTERACTION

The interaction of a drug with a receptor usually displays three main characteristics. This interaction is specific, dose-related and saturable. Drug–receptor interactions are often defined in terms of IC_{50} and EC_{50} (expression of potency) and these terms are obtained from a dose–response curve (see Table 2.3 for a description of some of the more commonly encountered basic pharmacological terms). A dose–response curve describes the administration of a dose of drug to a patient or animal. A concentration–response curve describes the incubation of an isolated tissue or a cell preparation with various concentrations of various drugs. Ignoring allosterism, drugs used in anaesthetic practice can be simply classified as agonists or antagonists.

Agonists

A drug that binds to a receptor to produce a functional response is an agonist, and the ability to produce a functional response is termed 'efficacy'. Efficacy depends on receptor numbers and type of coupling. An agonist that produces a maximum possible response is termed a full agonist. An agonist that produces a maximum response in the same tissue that is lower than that of a full agonist is termed a partial agonist. Antagonists have no efficacy. Agonists may have very different potencies but equal efficacies and vice versa. Potency and efficacy are not interchangeable, e.g. a high-potency drug may have lower efficacy than a low-potency drug (Table 2.3).

Relationship between receptor occupation and response and receptor reserve

In general, full agonists elicit maximal responses at low levels of receptor occupancy. Partial agonists cannot elicit a full response even when the entire receptor complement is occupied. If a full response is observed at low occupancy, this system is said to have a receptor reserve (this is commonly found for drugs that elicit smooth muscle contraction, relaxation or cardiac stimulation). These spare receptors are not hidden away; there are simply more than are needed.

Antagonists

There are two main classes of antagonist (see Table 2.3):

Competitive. For this class of antagonists, the effect is surmountable, i.e. increasing the agonist concentration will overcome the antagonist effect. This is the most common type of antagonism. Examples include propranolol antagonism of the effects of isoprenaline or atropine antagonism of methacholine in the heart.

Non-competitive. For this class, the effect cannot be overcome, i.e. increasing the agonist concentration does not overcome the antagonist effect. In tissues with a receptor reserve, low concentrations of non-competitive antagonists appear competitive (because the maximum response declines only when the receptor reserve is gone, i.e. when using a higher concentration). Non-competitive antagonism is sometimes termed irreversible. The concentration–response curves look similar but the explanation is different. Irreversible antagonists are usually experimental drugs that bind to and modify a receptor. In contrast, non-competitive block usually occurs at a site distal to the ligand binding site on the receptor. For example, ketamine inhibits NMDA receptor activity by occupying the ion channel pore – it does not alter binding.

Mixed agonist–antagonist

Where receptor subtypes exist, the potential for mixed agonist–antagonist behaviour exists, e.g. nalorphine: δ-agonist and μ-antagonist; pentazocine: μ-antagonist and δ/κ-partial agonist.

CONTROL OF INTRACELLULAR Ca^{2+}

(Fig. 2.4)

A plethora of physiological responses are dependent on Ca^{2+}, including muscle contraction, neurotransmission and cell division. Altered Ca^{2+} homeostasis is involved in the pathophysiology of malignant hyperthermia and underlies neuronal death resulting from ischaemic episodes.

GRADIENT MAINTENANCE

Intracellular Ca^{2+} concentration is maintained at approximately 100 nM in the presence of an enormous concentration gradient, with extracellular Ca^{2+} being around 1 mM. This concentration gradient is maintained by three main mechanisms, i.e. extrusion, sequestration and binding. Ca^{2+} is extruded across the plasma membrane utilizing the Ca^{2+}-ATPase enzyme (PMCA) which, as the name suggests, is an energy-requiring process. Ca^{2+} also leaves in exchange for Na^+ via the Na^+–Ca^{2+} co-transporter. At face value, this does not appear to be energy-requiring. However, for activity there needs to be a concentration gradient for Na^+ (in the inward direction) and this is set up via the Na^+/K^+-ATPase system. Therefore, Ca^{2+} entering the cell down its concentration gradient will be actively pumped out and/or exchanged for Na^+ (entering down its concentration gradient) (Fig. 2.4). In addition, Ca^{2+} may be

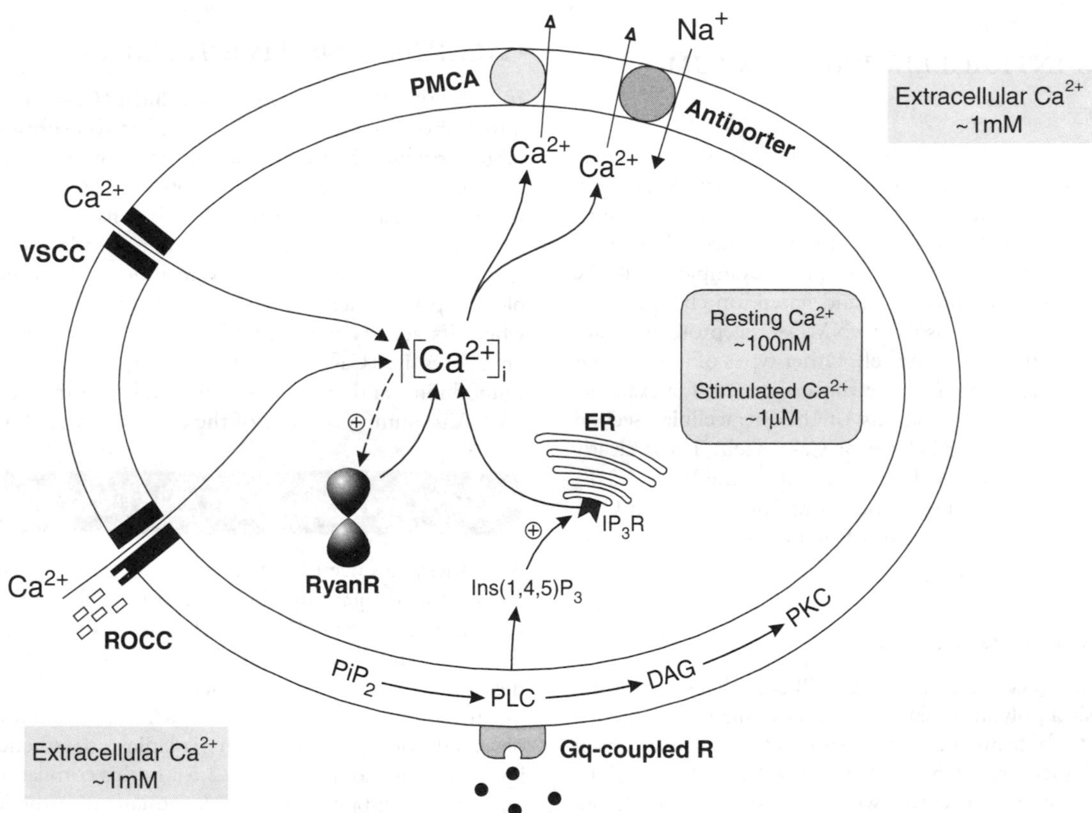

Fig. 2.4
Schematic representation of the regulation of intracellular Ca^{2+} concentrations ($[Ca^{2+}]_i$). Extracellular Ca^{2+} concentration is approximately 1 mM. As a result of plasma membrane Ca^{2+}-ATPase (PMCA) and antiporter activity coupled with sequestration into intracellular organelles, $[Ca^{2+}]_i$ is maintained at approximately 100 nM. Typically, agonist stimulation or depolarization increases $[Ca^{2+}]_i$ up to 1 μM. This increase can arise from extracellular sources via plasma membrane Ca^{2+} channels. These may be voltage-sensitive (VSCCs) or receptor-operated (ROCCs). Additionally, $[Ca^{2+}]_i$ may increase via release from intracellular stores. G_q-coupled GPCRs activate phospholipase C to produce Ins(1,4,5)P_3 and diacylglycerol (DAG). Ins(1,4,5)P_3 activates an Ins(1,4,5)P_3 receptor (IP_3R) on the endoplasmic reticulum (ER) to release stored Ca^{2+}. DAG activates protein kinase C (PKC). Ca^{2+} can also be released from ryanodine-sensitive stores via activation of the ryanodine receptor (RyanR) via increased Ca^{2+}. Ca^{2+} entering via the plasma membrane or released from intracellular stores is either pumped back across the membrane and/or resequestered into the intracellular stores (see text for details).

Table 2.4 Classification of voltage-sensitive Ca^{2+} channels including predominant location(s) and some examples of functions ascribed to their activity

	L	N	P/Q	R	T
Specific inhibitor	DHPs	ω-CgTx	ω-Aga-IVA[a]	None	None
HVA/LVA	HVA	HVA	HVA	NVA	LVA
Location	Heart	Neuronal	Neuronal	Neuronal	Heart
Function	Contraction	Release	Release	Release	Pacemaker
Anaesthetic interaction					
Volatile	Sensitive	Sensitive	Controversial	Unknown[b]	Sensitive
Intravenous	Sensitive	Sensitive	Controversial	Unknown	Controversial

[a]P-channels blocked by low concentrations of Agatoxin and Q-channels blocked by high concentrations.
[b]Unaware of any studies.
NT, neurotransmitter; DHPs, dihydropyridines; ω-CgTx, ω-conotoxin GVIA/VIIA; ω-Aga-IVA, ω-Agatoxin-IVA; LVA/HVA, low/high voltage-activated.

sequestered into intracellular organelles including mitochondria and the endo/sarcoplasmic reticulum. The former store is described as non-releasable, whereas the latter store(s) are releasable (see below). Ca^{2+} is also bound to intracellular proteins. Intracellular Ca^{2+} concentration may be elevated by opening membrane Ca^{2+} channels or releasing Ca^{2+} from intracellular (releasable) storage sites.

ELEVATING INTRACELLULAR CALCIUM

Calcium entry

Ca^{2+} can enter the cell across the plasma membrane via two classes of Ca^{2+} channels: voltage-sensitive and receptor-operated. Classification of the predominant voltage-sensitive Ca^{2+} channel classes is noted in Table 2.4. Ca^{2+} can also enter through a receptor-operated Ca^{2+} channel, of which a good example would be the glutamate NMDA receptor (a ligand-gated ion channel – see above). When glutamate binds to the NMDA receptor, the channel opens and Ca^{2+} flows into the cell. Other types of less obvious receptor-operated Ca^{2+} channels are those that are, for example, opened by increased concentrations of the intracellular second messenger Ins(1,4,5)P_3 (see below) or Ca^{2+} itself. These clearly require receptor activation for the production of the Ins(1,4,5)P_3 or Ca^{2+} signal (Fig. 2.4). These types of receptor-operated Ca^{2+} channels can be found in a variety of neurones and cells of the immune system.

Release of sequestered calcium

Activation of the G_q coupled class of GPCR stimulates the formation of the inositol polyphosphate second messenger Ins(1,4,5)P_3 which releases Ca^{2+} from the endoplasmic reticulum. Ca^{2+} itself also acts as a co-factor, further enhancing release. Ins(1,4,5)P_3 activates an intracellular receptor, which is distinct from steroid receptors, located on the endoplasmic reticulum membrane. This receptor is also an intrinsic Ca^{2+} channel and Ca^{2+} flows down its concentration from the endoplasmic reticulum lumen to the cytoplasm. The stores are also equipped with a Ca^{2+}-ATPase to enable them to refill. An additional intracellular Ca^{2+}-channel receptor is the ryanodine receptor, which responds to increased $[Ca^{2+}]_i$ to release its store contents (Fig. 2.4). There is currently much controversy as to whether a natural 'Ins(1,4,5)P_3-like' activator for this receptor is present. One candidate is cyclic ADP ribose. This channel also interacts with the classic dihydropyridine receptor (L-channel) and is involved in excitation–contraction coupling. Moreover, it is thought that a mutation in the ryanodine receptor is present in malignant hyperthermia-susceptible patients, increasing the sensitivity of the receptor to triggering agents like halothane.

CALCIUM-SENSITIVE TARGETS

In order that the increase in intracellular $[Ca^{2+}]_i$ can be translated into a physiological response, cells need to express Ca^{2+}-sensitive target proteins. These interactions may be direct, e.g. by a direct Ca^{2+} interaction such as with protein kinase C or phospholipase C. However, a large number of Ca^{2+}-sensitive targets require the activation of calmodulin. Calmodulin binds four molecules of Ca^{2+} and then goes on to activate a range of proteins. For example, the plasma membrane Ca^{2+}-ATPase is sensitive to calmodulin where its activity is increased. This is a feedback mechanism to limit rises in $[Ca^{2+}]_i$. In this model, Ca^{2+} rises and activates calmodulin, and the Ca^{2+}-calmodulin complex activates the PMCA to pump Ca^{2+} out of the cell and lower $[Ca^{2+}]_i$.

MECHANISM(S) OF ANAESTHESIA

Anaesthesia has been practised for over a century. Despite this, little is known regarding the target site(s) for anaesthetic agents. Over the years, many have searched for a single anaesthetic target site, with limited success. If there was a single anaesthetic target, then all anaesthetic agents would behave in essentially the same manner – this is clearly not the case. Early theories relied on the observed correlation between (volatile) anaesthetic potency and lipid (olive oil) solubility (Fig. 2.5). In this correlation, agents with high lipid solubility were more potent anaesthetic agents than those with lower lipid solubility. This led many authors to suggest that membrane lipids were the target for anaesthetic agents. However, lipids *per se* do not modify cellular activity. This led to the thought that it was the lipid surrounding integral membrane proteins that was important, with the anaesthetic modulating protein activity indirectly as a consequence of lipid interaction. In support of a specific protein target site for anaesthetic agents, there is the observation that some anaesthetics exist as stereoisomers and that one isomer is in general more potent than the other. This is

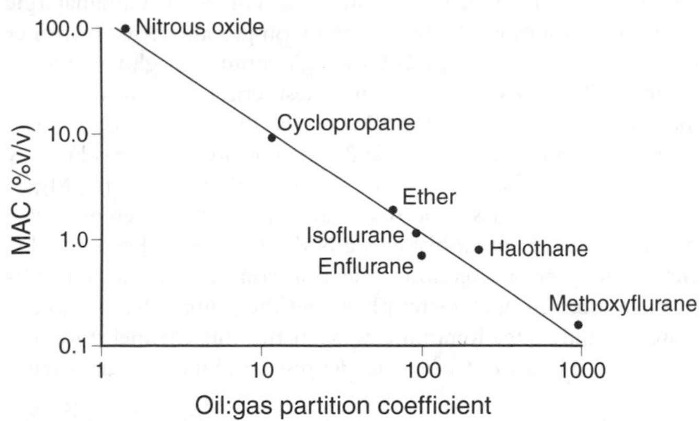

Fig. 2.5
Correlation between anaesthetic potency, expressed as minimum alveolar concentration (MAC), and lipid solubility, expressed as oil:gas partition coefficient.

the case for isoflurane [S(+) more potent than R(−)], barbiturates (in general S more potent than R) and ketamine [S(+) more potent than R(−)]. The literature reveals three potential (protein) target sites: $GABA_A$ receptors, VSCCs and excitatory amino acid transmission/receptors.

$GABA_A$ receptors

GABA receptors are classified into A and B subtypes (with a third type C suggested) (Table 2.5), and are activated by the major inhibitory transmitter in the brain, γ-aminobutyric acid (GABA). $GABA_A$ receptors are hetero-oligomeric protein ligand-gated ion channels and $GABA_B$ receptors are GPCRs. $GABA_A$ receptors comprise five subunits assembled in various combinations. $GABA_A$ receptor subunits used to assemble a functional channel arise from a number of families (α, β, δ and γ) and there are several genes encoding these subunits. This clearly allows much diversity in the make-up of individual $GABA_A$ receptors and can make comparative studies of $GABA_A$ receptor function difficult.

Table 2.5 Characteristics of GABA receptors[a]

	$GABA_A$[b]	$GABA_B$
Receptor type	LGIC	GPCR
Effector	Cl^- influx	K^+ efflux
Close VSCC		
Location	Postsynaptic	Presynaptic
Action	Inhibitory	Inhibitory
Agonist		
Endogenous	GABA	GABA
Pharmacological	Muscimol	Baclofen
Antagonist	Bicuculline	Phaclofen

[a]There is good evidence for $GABA_C$ receptors, which are similar to $GABA_A$.
[b]$GABA_A$ receptor action is potentiated by benzodiazepines.
LGIC, ligand-gated ion channel.

Indeed, it has been suggested that there may be in excess of 100 000 possible permutations in a functional channel, although in nature only a tiny number of these permutations exist. The $GABA_A$ receptor has been championed by many authorities as the major and unifying anaesthetic target site. With the exception of ketamine, all anaesthetic agents tested to date appear to interact with the $GABA_A$ receptor at clinically relevant concentrations. The effect produced is to potentiate $GABA_A$-mediated Cl^- influx, leading to hyperpolarization. This effect on Cl^- conductance requires the presence of GABA.

Voltage-sensitive calcium channels

Voltage-sensitive Ca^{2+} channels are involved in the control of neurotransmitter release. If we accept that anaesthetic agents inhibit neurotransmission without affecting axonal conduction, then blockade of VSCCs represents a logical target site for anaesthetic agents (Table 2.4).

Several in vivo studies have suggested that the L-channel may contribute to the mechanism of anaesthesia. However, with the exception of nimodipine, passage through the blood–brain barrier of L-channel blockers is poor, making clinical studies difficult. The

Table 2.6 Characteristics of glutamate receptors

	Ionotrophic			Metabotrophic
	NMDA	AMPA	Kainate	
Receptor type	LGIC	LGIC	LGIC	GPCR
Main effector	Ca^{2+}	Na^+	Na^+	PLC (+AC)
Location	Postsynaptic[a]	Postsynaptic[a]	Postsynaptic[a]	Presynaptic Postsynaptic
Agonist				
Endogenous	Glutamate	Glutamate	Glutamate	Glutamate
Pharmacological	NMDA	AMPA	?	Various[b]
Antagonist	D-AP5	CNQX	CNQX	Various[b]

PLC, phospholipase C (the activation of PLC leads to the formation of $Ins(1,4,5)P_3$ and release of stored intracellular Ca^{2+}); AC, adenylyl cyclase; AMPA, α-amino-3-hydroxy-5-methylisoxazole-4-propionic acid; NMDA, *N*-methyl-D-aspartate (the NMDA receptor channel is blocked by Mg^{2+}, dizoclipine (MK 801) and ketamine); D-AP5, 2-amino-5-phosphopentanoic acid; CNQX, 6-cyano-7-nitroquinoxaline-2,3-dione.
[a]May be some evidence for presynaptic action.
[b]Depends on subtype, eight (mGluR1-8) identified.

minimum alveolar concentration (MAC) for halothane in dogs is reduced by verapamil, and verapamil, flunarizine and nitrendipine augmented the general anaesthetic potencies of ethanol and pentobarbital. In addition, a range of intravenous anaesthetic agents have been shown to bind to L-channels, although no functional correlates were made in these studies. It is not possible to determine whether these actions at L-channels contribute to the anaesthetic state and it should be remembered that L-channels are not normally involved in neurotransmitter release. However, L-VSCCs are found in the heart and these anaesthetic actions at L-VSCCs may explain some of the cardiovascular side-effects of anaesthesia. In the absence of any antagonists for use in humans/whole animals, it is difficult to determine a role for N- and P-VSCCs (and others) in anaesthesia, although in electrophysiological studies, a range of anaesthetic agents are capable of inhibiting Ca^{2+} influx through N- and P-VSCCs, although the latter remain controversial. T-channel block is unlikely to be of any significance to anaesthesia. The major problem for the acceptance of VSCC block as a target for anaesthesia can be found by comparing the concentration–response curve for anaesthetic block of VSCCs with the dose–response curve for determination of MAC. In general, the latter curve lies to the left of the former, indicating that clinically relevant/achievable concentrations have little or no effect on VSCC activity. However, it should be borne in mind that the comparison is very artificial in that the dose of anaesthetic required to reduce movement to surgical stimulation in 50% of a population of individuals is compared with the electrophysiological measurement of single channel currents. In addition, as very small amounts of Ca^{2+} influx are capable of supporting neurotransmitter release, the question of how much inhibition of influx is functionally relevant remains unresolved.

Excitatory transmission

In contrast to a potentiation of GABA-ergic inhibition, it would also be advantageous to depress excitatory transmission. Indeed, glutamate (the major excitatory transmitter in the mammalian CNS) release from a variety of preparations is inhibited by a range of intravenous and volatile anaesthetic agents. This inhibition could be via an action on glutamate receptors on glutamatergic neurones, inhibition of VSCC activity on glutamatergic neurones or secondary to enhanced GABA-ergic input into glutamatergic-synapses. The most well known anaesthetic target in the glutamate receptor family is the NMDA receptor. This receptor is a ligand-gated ion channel (Table 2.6) and is under the modulatory control of a number of different agents, including glycine, Mg^{2+}, Zn^{2+} and polyamines. The dissociative anaesthetic ketamine is a non-competitive antagonist at the NMDA receptor. From the discussion in previous sections, the non-competitive block results from an interaction at a site other than the primary ligand (glutamate) binding site. Ketamine 'sits' in the ion channel pore and prevents the influx of Ca^{2+}, thus depressing glutamatergic (excitatory) transmission.

It is likely that anaesthesia results from an interaction of the three target groups described above and further research is needed to define the extent of interaction at each site for different classes of anaesthetic agents.

FURTHER READING

Barritt G J 1994 Communication within animal cells. Oxford Science Publications, Oxford

Calvey T N, Williams N E 1997 Principles and practice of pharmacology for anaesthetists, 3rd edn. Blackwell Scientific Publications, Oxford

Franks N P, Lieb W R 1994 Molecular and cellular mechanisms of anaesthesia. Nature 367: 607–614

Hudspith M J 1997 Glutamate: a role in normal brain function, anaesthesia, analgesia and CNS injury. British Journal of Anaesthesia 78: 731–747

International Union of Pharmacology (IUPHAR) 1998 The IUPHAR compendium of receptor characterization and classification. IUPHAR Media, London

Mehta A K, Ticku M K 1999 An update on $GABA_A$ receptors. Brain Research. Brain Research Reviews 29: 196–217

Rang H P, Dale M M, Ritter J M 1999 Pharmacology, 4th edn. Churchill Livingstone, London

Tanelian D L, Kosek P, Mody I, MacIver B 1993 The role of the $GABA_A$ receptor/chloride channel complex in anesthesia. Anesthesiology 78: 757–776

Various 1993 British Journal of Anaesthesia (Postgraduate issue) 71(1): 1–163

3 General principles of pharmacology and pharmacokinetics

HOW DO DRUGS ACT?

Drugs have an effect because of their physicochemical properties, activity at receptors, inhibition of enzyme systems or influence on nucleic acid synthesis.

PHYSICOCHEMICAL PROPERTIES

Sodium citrate neutralizes acid and is given frequently to reduce the likelihood of pneumonitis after inhalation of gastric contents. Chelating agents combine chemically with metal ions, reducing their toxicity and enhancing elimination, usually in the urine. Such drugs include desferoxamine (iron, aluminium), dicobalt edetate (cyanide toxicity), sodium calcium edetate (lead) and penicillamine (copper, lead). Stored blood is prevented from coagulating by sodium hydrogen citrate. This chelates calcium ions and may cause hypocalcaemia after massive blood transfusion.

ACTION ON RECEPTORS

A receptor is a complex structure on the cell membrane which can bind selectively with endogenous compounds or drugs, resulting in changes within the cell. Receptor function is reviewed in detail in Chapter 2.

A compound which binds to a receptor and changes intracellular function is termed an agonist. The classic dose–response relationship of an agonist is shown in Figure 3.1. As the concentration of the agonist increases, a maximum effect is reached as the receptors in the system become saturated (Fig. 3.1A). Conventionally, log-dose is plotted against effect, resulting in a sigmoid curve which is approximately linear between 20 and 80% of maximum effect (Fig. 3.1B). Three agonists are shown in Figure 3.2. Agonist A produces 100% effect at a lower concentration than agonist B. Therefore, compared with A, agonist B is less potent but has similar efficacy. Drug C is termed a partial agonist as the maximum effect is less than that of A or B. Buprenorphine is a partial agonist (at the μ-opioid receptor), as are some of the β-blockers with intrinsic activity, e.g. oxprenolol, pindolol, acebutalol.

Antagonists combine selectively with the receptor but produce no effect. They may interact with the receptor in a competitive (reversible) or non-competitive (irreversible) fashion. In the presence of a competitive antagonist, the dose–response curve of an agonist is shifted to the right but the maximum effect remains unaltered (Fig. 3.3A). Examples of this effect include the displacement

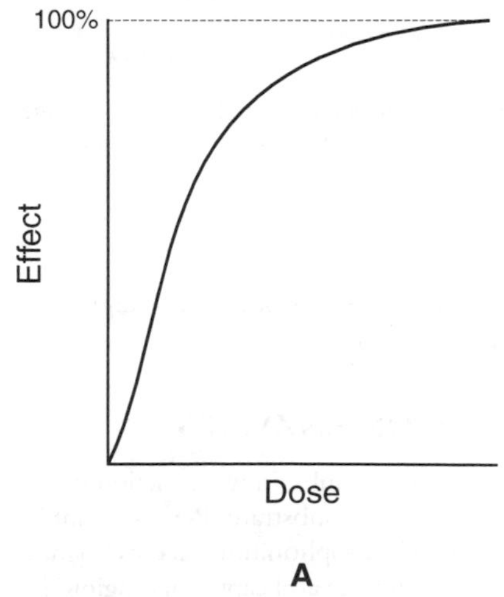

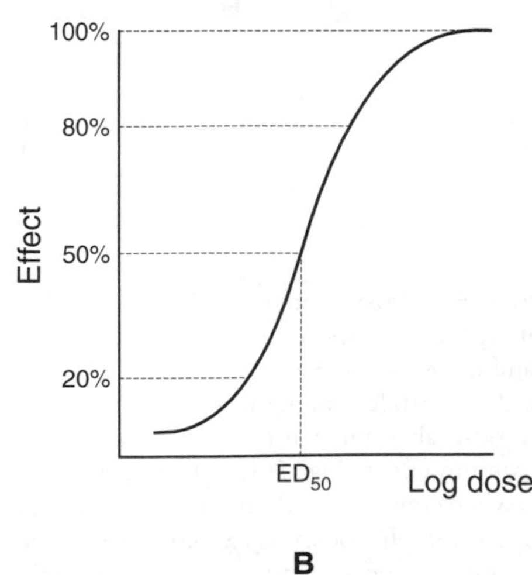

Fig. 3.1
(**A**) The effect of an agonist peaks when all the receptors are occupied. (**B**) A semilog plot produes a sigmoid curve which is linear between 20% and 80% effect. ED_{50} is the dose which produces 50% of maximum effect.

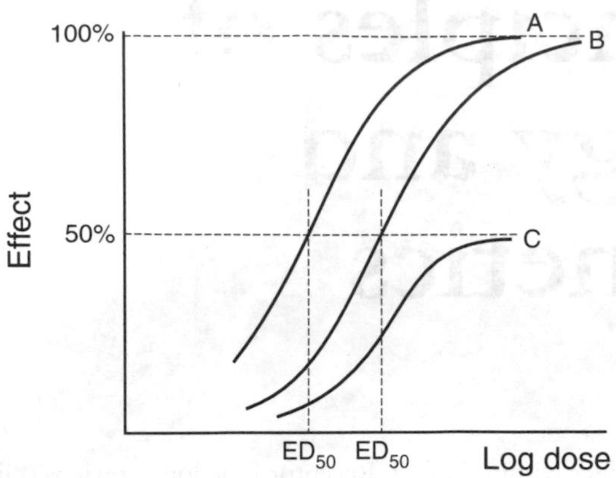

Fig. 3.2
Agonist B has a similar dose–response curve to A but is displaced to the right. A is more potent than B (smaller ED_{50}) but has the same efficacy. C is a partial agonist which is less potent than A and B and less efficacious (maximum effect 50% of A and B).

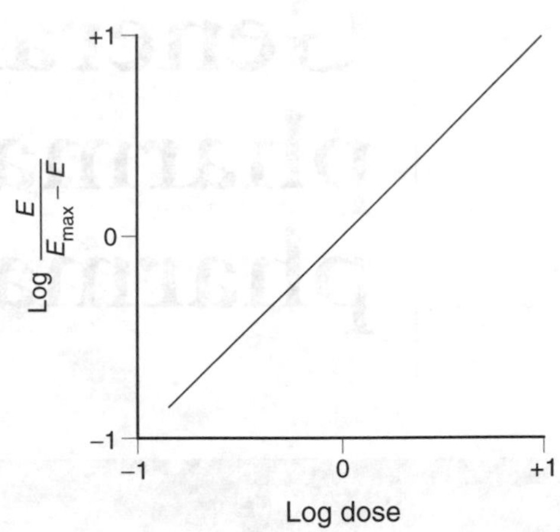

Fig. 3.4
A Hill plot. The Hill coefficient is the slope of the line (+1 for this drug). E_{max}, maximum effect; E, effect at different doses.

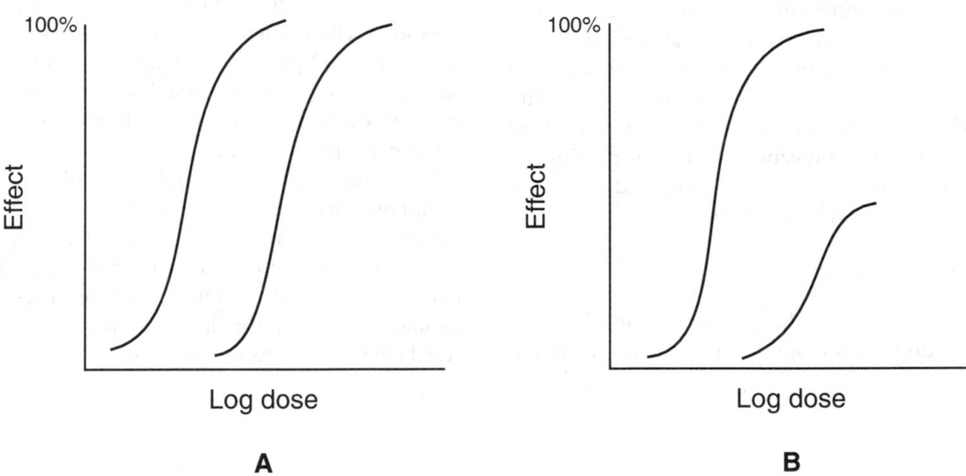

Fig. 3.3
(**A**) The dose–response curve of an agonist is displaced to the right in the presence of a reversible antagonist. There is no change in maximum effect but the ED_{50} is increased. (**B**) The dose–response curve is displaced to the right also in the presence of an irreversible antagonist but the maximum effect is reduced.

of morphine by naloxone, 5-hydroxytryptamine (5-HT) by 5-HT_3 antagonists in the gut wall and chemoreceptor trigger zone, and endogenous catecholamines by β-blockers.

A non-competitive (irreversible) antagonist shifts the dose–response curve to the right also but, with increasing concentrations, reduces the maximum effect (Fig. 3.3B). For example, the α_1-antagonist phenoxybenzamine, used in the preoperative preparation of patients with phaeochromocytoma, has a long duration of action because of the formation of stable chemical bonds between drug and receptor.

The relationship between drug dose and response is often described by a Hill plot (Fig. 3.4). A typical agonist such as that shown in Figure 3.1 produces a straight line with a slope (i.e. Hill coefficient) of +1.

ACTION ON ENZYMES

Drugs may act by inhibiting the action of an enzyme or competing for its endogenous substrate. Reversible inhibition is the mechanism of action of edrophonium (acetylcholinesterase), aminophylline (phosphodiesterase) and captopril (angiotensin-converting enzyme). Irreversible enzyme inhibition occurs when a stable chemical bond is formed between drug and enzyme, resulting in prolonged or permanent inactivity, e.g. omeprazole (gastric hydrogen-potassium

ATPase), aspirin (cyclooxygenase) and organophosphorus compounds (acetylcholinesterase).

Neostigmine inhibits acetylcholinesterase in a reversible manner, but the mechanism of action is more akin to that of an irreversible drug as the enzyme is carbamylated by the formation of covalent chemical bonds.

ACTION ON NUCLEIC ACID SYNTHESIS

Drugs may act via receptors on the cell nucleus influencing protein synthesis by stimulating the production of messenger RNA. Consequently, drugs acting in this manner, e.g. corticosteroids, have a slow speed of onset.

THE BLOOD–BRAIN BARRIER AND PLACENTA

Most drugs used in anaesthetic practice must cross the blood–brain barrier in order to reach their site of action. The brain is protected from most potentially toxic agents by tightly overlapping endothelial cells which surround the capillaries and interfere with passive diffusion. Enzyme systems are present in the endothelium which may also break down many potential toxins. Consequently, only relatively small, highly lipid-soluble molecules (e.g. intravenous and volatile anaesthetic agents, opioids, local anaesthetics) have access to the central nervous system (CNS). Compared with most opioids, morphine takes some time to reach its site of action because it has a relatively low lipid solubility. Highly ionized drugs (e.g. muscle relaxants, glycopyrronium) do not cross the blood–brain barrier.

The chemoreceptor trigger zone is situated in the area postrema near the base of the fourth ventricle (Ch. 21). It is not protected by the blood–brain barrier as the capillary endothelial cells are not bound tightly in this area and allow relatively free passage of large molecules. This is an important afferent limb of the vomiting reflex and stimulation of this area by toxins or drugs in the blood or cerebrospinal fluid often leads to vomiting. Many antiemetics act at this site.

The transfer of drugs across the placenta is of considerable importance in obstetric anaesthesia (Ch. 52). In general, all drugs which affect the CNS cross the placenta and affect the fetus. Highly ionized drugs (e.g. muscle relaxants) pass across less readily.

PLASMA PROTEIN BINDING

Many drugs are bound to proteins in the plasma. This is important as only the unbound portion of the drug is available for diffusion to its site of action. Changes in protein binding may have significant effects on the active unbound concentration of a drug and therefore its actions.

Albumin is the most important protein in this regard and is responsible mainly for the binding of acidic and neutral drugs. Globulins, especially α_1-glycoprotein, bind mainly basic drugs. If a drug is highly protein bound (> 80%), any change in plasma protein concentration or displacement of the drug by another with similar binding properties may have clinically significant effects. For example, most NSAIDs displace warfarin, phenytoin and lithium from plasma binding sites, leading to potential toxicity.

Plasma albumin is often decreased in the elderly, in neonates and in the presence of malnutrition, liver, renal or cardiac failure and malignancy. α_1-Glycoprotein is decreased during pregnancy and in the neonate but may be increased in the postoperative period and other conditions such as infection, trauma, burns and malignancy.

METABOLISM

Most drugs are lipid-soluble and many are metabolized in the liver into more ionized compounds which are inactive pharmacologically and excreted by the kidneys. However, metabolites may be active (Table 3.1). The liver is not the only site of metabolism. For example, succinylcholine and mivacurium are metabolized by plasma cholinesterase, esmolol by erythrocyte esterases, remifentanil by tissue esterases and, in part, dopamine by the kidney and prilocaine by the lungs.

A substance is termed a ***prodrug*** if it is inactive in the form in which it is administered, pharmacological effects being dependent on the formation of active metabolites. Examples of this are codeine (morphine), diamorphine (6-monoacetyl morphine, morphine) chloral hydrate (trichlorethanol) and methyldopa (methylnorepinephrine). Midazolam is ionized and dissolved in an acidic solution in the ampoule; after intravenous injection and exposure in the blood to pH 7.4, the molecule becomes lipid-soluble.

Drugs undergo two types of reactions during metabolism: phase I and phase II. Phase I reactions include reduction, oxidation and hydrolysis. Drug oxidation occurs in the smooth endoplasmic reticulum, primarily by the cytochrome P450 enzyme system. This system and other enzymes also perform reduction reactions. Hydrolysis is a common phase I reaction in the metabolism of ester and amide drugs.

Phase II reactions involve conjugation of a metabolite or the drug itself with an endogenous substrate. Conjugation with glucuronic acid is a major metabolic pathway, but others include acetylation, methylation and conjugation with sulphate or glycine.

ENZYME INDUCTION AND INHIBITION

Some drugs may enhance the activity of enzymes responsible for drug metabolism, particularly the cytochrome P450 enzymes and

Table 3.1 Examples of active metabolites

Drug	Metabolite	Action
Morphine	Morphine-6-glucuronide	Potent opioid agonist
Diamorphine	6-Monoacetyl morphine Morphine	Opioid agonist
Pethidine	Norpethidine	Epileptogenic
Codeine	Morphine	Opioid agonist
Diazepam	Desmethyldiazepam Temazepam Oxazepam	Sedative
Tramadol	O-desmethyltramadol	Opioid agonist

glucuronyl transferase. Such drugs include phenytoin, carbamazepine, phenylbutazone, barbiturates, ethanol, steroids and some inhalation anaesthetic agents (halothane, enflurane).Cigarette smoking also induces cytochrome P450 enzymes.

Drugs with mechanisms of action other than on enzymes may also interfere significantly with enzyme systems. For example, etomidate inhibits the synthesis of cortisol and aldosterone – an effect which probably explains the increased mortality in critically ill patients which occurred when it was used as a sedative in intensive care. Cimetidine is a potent enzyme inhibitor and may prolong the elimination of drugs such as diazepam, propranolol, oral anticoagulants, phenytoin and lidocaine.

DRUG EXCRETION

Ionized compounds, with a low molecular weight (MW), are excreted mainly by the kidneys. Most drugs diffuse passively into the proximal renal tubules by the process of glomerular filtration, but some are secreted actively, e.g. penicillins, aspirin, many diuretics, morphine, lidocaine and glucuronides. Ionization is a significant barrier to reabsorption at the distal tubule. Consequently, basic drugs are excreted more efficiently in acid urine and acidic compounds in alkaline urine.

Some drugs and metabolites, particularly those with larger molecules (MW > 400D), are excreted in the bile, e.g. glycopyrronium, vecuronium, alcuronium, pancuronium and the metabolites of morphine and buprenorphine.

PHARMACOKINETIC PRINCIPLES

Pharmacokinetics is the study of how the body handles a drug, in contrast to pharmacodynamics which describes the drug's action on the body. An understanding of the basic principles of pharmacokinetics is an important aid to the safe use of drugs in anaesthesia, pain management and intensive care medicine. Pharmacokinetics is an attempt to fit observed changes in plasma concentration of drugs into mathematical equations which may then be used to predict concentrations.

Derived values describing volume of distribution (V), clearance (Cl) and half-life ($t_{1/2}$) give an indication of the likely properties of a drug. However, even in healthy individuals of the same sex, weight and age, there is significant variability which makes precise prediction very difficult. Values quoted are usually the mean of several observations and it is of great value to note the standard deviation or range.

VOLUME OF DISTRIBUTION

Volume of distribution is a good example of the abstract nature of pharmacokinetics; it is not a real volume but merely a concept which helps us to understand what we observe. Nevertheless, it is a very useful concept which enables us to predict certain properties of a drug and also calculate other pharmacokinetic values.

Imagine that a patient receiving an intravenous dose of an anaesthetic induction agent is a bucket of water and that the drug is distributed evenly throughout the water immediately after injection. The volume of water represents the initial volume of distribution (V). It may be calculated easily:

$$C_0 = \frac{\text{dose}}{V} \tag{1}$$

where C_0 is the initial concentration. Therefore:

$$V = \frac{\text{dose}}{C_0} \tag{2}$$

A more accurate measurement of V is possible during constant rate infusion when the distribution of the drug in the tissues has time to equilibrate; this is termed volume of distribution at steady state (V_{ss}).

Drugs which remain in the plasma and do not pass easily to other tissues have a small V and therefore a large C_0. Relatively ionized drugs, e.g. muscle relaxants, or drugs highly bound to plasma proteins, e.g. non-steroidal anti-inflammatory drugs (NSAIDs), often have a small V. Drugs with a large V are often lipid-soluble and therefore penetrate and accumulate in tissues outside the plasma, e.g. intravenous induction agents. Some drugs accumulate outside the plasma such that values for V are greater than total body volume (a reminder of the abstract nature of pharmacokinetics). Large V values are often observed for drugs highly bound to proteins outside plasma (e.g. local anaesthetics, digoxin).

Several factors may affect initial V and therefore C_0 on bolus injection of a drug. Patients who are dehydrated or have lost blood have a significantly greater plasma C_0 after normal doses of intravenous induction agent, increasing the likelihood of severe side-effects, especially hypotension. Neonates have a proportionally greater volume of extracellular fluid compared with adults, and water-soluble drugs (e.g. muscle relaxants) tend to have a proportionally greater V. Factors affecting plasma protein binding (see above) may also affect V.

Finally, V can give some indication as to the half-life. A large V may be associated with a relatively slow decline in plasma concentration; this relationship is expressed below in a useful pharmacokinetic equation (eqn 4).

CLEARANCE

Clearance is defined as the volume of blood or plasma from which the drug is removed completely in unit time. Drugs may be eliminated from the blood by the liver, kidney or occasionally other routes (see above). The relative proportion of hepatic and renal clearance of a drug is important. Most drugs used in anaesthetic practice are cleared predominantly by the liver, but some rely on renal clearance. Excessive accumulation of a drug occurs in patients in renal failure if its renal clearance is significant. For example, morphine is metabolized primarily in the liver and this is not affected significantly in renal impairment. However, the active metabolite morphine-6-glucuronide is excreted predominantly by the kidney. This accumulates in renal insufficiency and is responsible for increased morphine sensitivity in these patients.

As with volume of distribution, clearance may suggest likely properties of a drug. For example, if clearance is greater than hepatic blood flow, factors other than hepatic metabolism must account for its total clearance. Values greater than cardiac output may indicate metabolism in the plasma (e.g. succinylcholine) or other tissues (remifentanil). Clearance is an important, but not the only, factor affecting $t_{1/2}$ and steady-state plasma concentrations achieved during constant rate infusions (see below).

ELIMINATION HALF-LIFE

The administration of a drug is influenced considerably by its plasma $t_{1/2}$, as this often reflects duration of action. It is important to remember that $t_{1/2}$ is influenced not only by clearance (Cl) but also by V:

$$t_{1/2} \propto \frac{V}{\mathrm{Cl}} \tag{3}$$

or

$$t_{1/2} = \text{constant} \times \frac{V}{\mathrm{Cl}}$$

The constant in this equation (elimination rate constant) is the natural logarithm of 2 (ln 2), i.e. 0.693. Therefore:

$$t_{1/2} = 0.693 \times \frac{V}{\mathrm{Cl}} \tag{4}$$

Half-life often reflects duration of action but not if the drug acts irreversibly (e.g. some NSAIDs, omeprazole, phenoxybenzamine) or if active metabolites are formed (e.g. morphine, diazepam).

So far, we have considered metabolic or elimination $t_{1/2}$ only. The initial decrease in plasma concentrations after administration of many drugs, especially if given intravenously, occurs primarily because of redistribution into tissues. Therefore, the simple relationship between elimination $t_{1/2}$ and duration of action does not apply in many situations (see below, 'two-compartment models').

CALCULATING $t_{1/2}$, V AND CLEARANCE

We shall calculate these values for a drug after intravenous bolus administration and regular blood sampling for plasma concentration measurements. In this example, we assume that the drug remains in the plasma and is removed only by metabolism, e.g. a one-compartment model. After achieving C_0, plasma concentration (C_p) declines in a simple exponential manner as shown in Figure 3.5A. If the natural log of the concentrations is plotted against time (semi-log plot) a straight line is produced (Fig. 3.5B). The gradient of this line is the elimination rate constant k, which may be related to $t_{1/2}$ in the following equation:

$$\mathrm{k} = \frac{\ln 2}{t_{1/2}} \tag{5}$$

We may calculate V using equation (2) and then clearance from equation (4). C_p may be predicted at any time from the following equation:

$$C_p = C_0 e^{-kt} \tag{6}$$

where t is the time after administration.

Clearance may be derived also by calculation of the area under the concentration-time curve extrapolated to infinity (AUC_∞) and substitution in the following equation:

$$\mathrm{Cl} = \frac{\text{dose}}{\mathrm{AUC}_\infty} \tag{7}$$

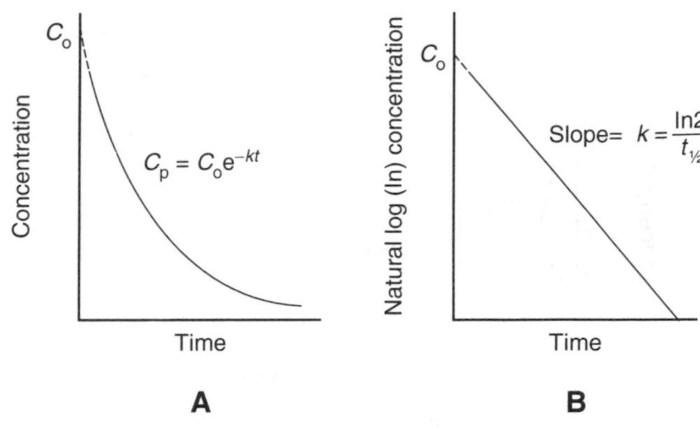

Fig. 3.5
A. Exponential decline in plasma drug concentration (C_p) in a one compartmental model. The equation predicts C_p at any time (t)
B. Semilog plot enables easy calculation of $t_{1/2}$(0.693). Extrapolation of this line enables C_0 and AUC_∞ to be derived easily.

TWO-COMPARTMENT MODELS

The body is not, of course, a single homogeneous compartment and plasma concentrations of drug are the result of elimination by metabolism and redistribution to and from tissues such as brain, heart, liver, muscles, fat, etc. Mathematics describing the real situation are extremely complex. However, plasma concentrations of many drugs behave approximately as if they were distributed in two or three compartments. Applying these mathematical models is a reasonable compromise.

Let us consider a two-compartment model; one compartment may be thought of as representing the plasma and the other, the remainder of the body. When an intravenous bolus is injected into this system, C_p decreases because of an exponential decay resulting from elimination and another exponential decay resulting from redistribution into the tissues. Therefore, when C_p is plotted against time, the curve may be described by a biexponential equation. If plotted on a semi-logarithmic plot (Fig. 3.6), two straight lines may be identified. Their gradients are the elimination rate constant dependent on elimination (α) and that dependent on redistribution (β).

Redistribution kinetics are not only of theoretical interest, because it is often the decline in C_p resulting from redistribution which is responsible for the cessation of an observed effect of a drug; intravenous induction agents and *initial* doses of intravenous fentanyl are good examples of this.

Calculating the separate pharmacokinetic values is easy; one curve is simply subtracted from the other. Consider Figure 3.6 where natural log concentration is plotted against time and two slopes are seen. The second and less steep slope represents decline in plasma concentration caused by elimination of the drug by metabolism. From this, the elimination half-life ($t_{1/2}{}^{\beta}$) may be calculated. In order to calculate the half-life of the redistribution phase ($t_{1/2}{}^{\alpha}$), the elimination slope is extrapolated back to time 0. If data on this imaginary part of the elimination slope are subtracted from those on the real line above it, another imaginary line may be constructed which represents that part of the decline in plasma concentration which is the result of redistribution. From

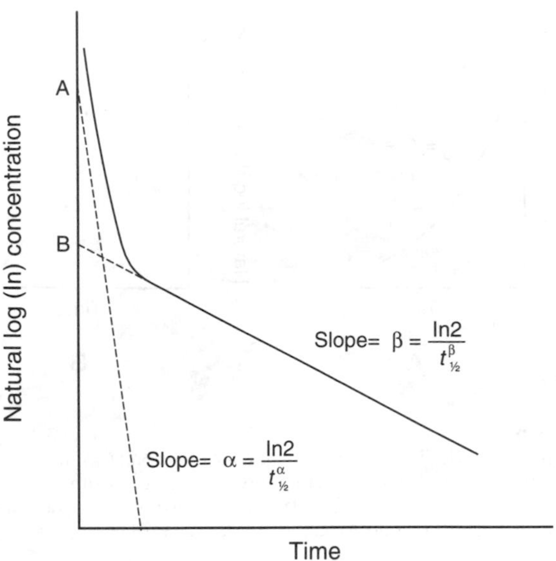

Fig. 3.6
Semilog plot of a two-compartment model. α, rate constant for exponential decay resulting from redistribution; β, rate constant for exponential decay resulting from elimination.

this line, the redistribution half-life ($t_{1/2}{}^{\alpha}$) may be calculated.

The equation for C_p at any time in a two-compartment model after bolus intravenous administration is therefore:

$$C_p = Ae^{-\alpha t} + Be^{-\beta t} \qquad (8)$$

where α and β are the redistribution and elimination rate constants, respectively, and A and B are values derived by back extrapolation of the redistribution and elimination slopes to the y-axis.

Some drugs, e.g. propofol, are best fitted to a triexponential, three-compartment model which reveals half-lives for two processes of redistribution ($t_{1/2}{}^{\pi}$ and $t_{1/2}{}^{\alpha}$) and one for elimination ($t_{1/2}{}^{\beta}$).

CONTEXT-SENSITIVE HALF-LIFE

This concept refers to plasma half-life (time for plasma concentration to decline by 50%) after an intravenous drug infusion and 'context' refers to the duration of infusion. The amount of drug accumulating in body tissues increases with duration of infusion for most drugs. Consequently, on stopping the infusion, time for the plasma concentration to decline by 50% depends on duration of infusion. The longer the infusion, the more drug accumulates and the longer the plasma half-life becomes, because there is more drug to enter the plasma on stopping the infusion.

Figure 3.7 shows the effect of duration of infusion on half-life for alfentanil, fentanyl and remifentanil. Alfentanil, and especially fentanyl, accumulates during infusion and this is reflected by an increase in context-sensitive half-lives. In other words, time to recovery from alfentanil- or fentanyl-based anaesthesia depends on duration of infusion. Remifentanil is metabolized by tissue esterases and does not accumulate. Therefore, time for plasma concentration of remifentanil to decline by 50% is independent of duration of infusion, i.e. recovery times after remifentanil-based anaesthesia are short and predictable, no matter how long the infusion has run.

METHODS OF DRUG ADMINISTRATION

ORAL

The oral route of drug administration is important in modern anaesthetic practice, e.g. premedication, postoperative analgesia. It is often necessary also to continue concurrent medication during the perioperative period, e.g. antihypertensives, anti-anginal medication. It is therefore important to appreciate the factors involved in the absorption of oral medication.

The formulation of tablets or capsules is very precise, as their consistent dissolution is necessary before absorption can take place. The rate of absorption, and therefore effect of the drug, may be influenced significantly by this factor. Most preparations dissolve in the acidic gastric juices and the intact drug is absorbed in the upper intestine. However, some drugs are broken down by acids (e.g. omeprazole, benzylpenicillin) or are irritant to the stomach (e.g. aspirin, phenylbutazone) and may be given as enteric-coated preparations. Drugs given in solution are often absorbed more rapidly but this may induce nausea or vomiting immediately after anaesthesia.

Gastric emptying

Most drugs are absorbed only when they have left the stomach and, if gastric emptying is delayed, absorption is affected. Furthermore, if oral medication is given continuously during periods of impaired emptying, it may accumulate in the stomach, only to be delivered to the small intestine *en masse* when gastric function returns, resulting in overdose. Many factors influence the rate of gastric emptying and these are described in Chapter 20.

Any factor increasing upper intestinal motility, e.g. prokinetic drugs such as metoclopramide, reduces the time available for absorption and may reduce the total amount of drug absorbed.

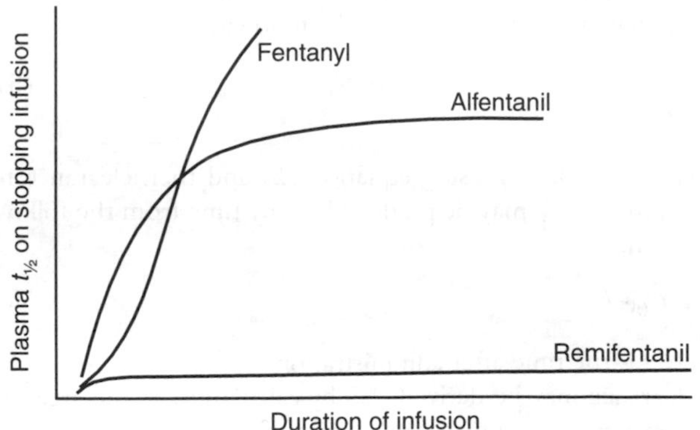

Fig. 3.7
Context-sensitive half-life. The time for plasma concentrations to decline by 50% increases with duration of infusion for alfentanil and fentanyl. This is not the case for remifentanil.

First-pass effect

Before entering the systemic circulation, the drug must pass through the portal circulation and, if metabolized extensively by the liver or even the gut wall, absorption may be reduced significantly, i.e. first-pass effect. For example, compared with intramuscular administration, significantly larger doses of oral morphine are required for the same effect. Other drugs susceptible to first-pass metabolism include most opioids (except methadone), dopamine, isoprenaline, propranolol and glyceryl trinitrate.

Bioavailability

This is the percentage of the oral dose of a drug which is absorbed into the systemic circulation. It is calculated by giving the same individual, on two separate occasions, the same dose of a drug orally and then intravenously. The resulting plasma drug concentrations are plotted against time and the area under the curve after oral administration is divided by the area under the intravenous curve.

LINGUAL AND BUCCAL

This is a useful method of administration if the drug is lipid-soluble and crosses the oral mucosa with relative ease. First-pass metabolism is avoided. Glyceryl trinitrate and buprenorphine are available as sublingual tablets and morphine as a buccal preparation.

INTRAMUSCULAR

This is still a popular route of administration in anaesthesia. It may avoid the problems associated with large initial plasma concentrations after rapid intravenous administration, is devoid of first-pass effects and may be administered relatively easily. However, absorption may be unpredictable, some preparations are particularly painful and irritant (e.g. diclofenac) and complications include damage to nervous and vascular tissue and inadvertent intravenous injection. An important disadvantage is the often intense dislike of injections, particularly by children.

Administration of postoperative analgesia by this route is still used frequently but the variation in absorption may be great. For example, peak plasma concentrations of morphine may occur at any time from 5 to 60 min after intramuscular administration, an important factor in the failure of this method to produce good reliable analgesia (see Ch. 42).

SUBCUTANEOUS

Absorption is very susceptible to changes in skin perfusion, and tissue irritation may be a significant problem. However, this method is used in several centres for providing postoperative pain relief, particularly in children, and has the advantage that difficult intravenous access is not required. A small cannula is placed subcutaneously during anaesthesia and can be replaced, if necessary, with relative ease. Even patient-controlled analgesia (PCA) (see below) has been used effectively by this route. Prophylactic heparin is, of course, administered subcutaneously.

INTRAVENOUS

Bolus

The majority of drugs used in anaesthetic practice are given intravenously as boluses and the pharmacokinetics are described in some detail above. The major disadvantage of this method is that dangerously high drug concentrations may occur readily, particularly with drugs of narrow therapeutic index and large interpatient pharmacodynamic and pharmacokinetic variations (i.e. most drugs used in anaesthetic practice). Therefore, it is an important general rule that all drugs administered intravenously should be given slowly. Manufacturers' recommendations in this regard are often surprising; for example, a 10 mg dose of metoclopramide should be given over 1–2 min.

Only two factors have a major influence on the plasma concentrations achieved during a bolus intravenous injection: speed of injection and cardiac output. Therefore, an elderly, sick or hypovolaemic patient undergoing intravenous induction of anaesthesia is likely to suffer significant side-effects if the drug is given at the same rate as would be given to a normal, healthy young adult.

Infusion

Drugs may be given by constant-rate infusion, a method used frequently for propofol, neuromuscular blocking agents, opioids and many drugs administered to patients in intensive care units. Plasma concentrations achieved during infusions may be described by a simple wash-in exponential curve (Fig. 3.8). The only factor influencing time to reach steady-state concentration is $t_{1/2}$. Maximum concentration is achieved after approximately 4–5 half-lives. Therefore, this method of administration is best suited to drugs with short half-lives such as remifentanil, glyceryl trinitrate, epinephrine and dopamine. However, in practice, it is often used for drugs such as morphine. Assuming a morphine $t_{1/2}$ of 4 h, it will be 24 h before steady-state concentration is reached. Therefore, vigilant observation is required with this method of delivery, especially if active metabolites are involved – in this example, morphine-6-glucuronide.

There is a simple equation describing the concentration achieved at steady state during a constant-rate infusion; this is based on the principle that, at steady state, the amount of drug cleared from the plasma is equal to that delivered:

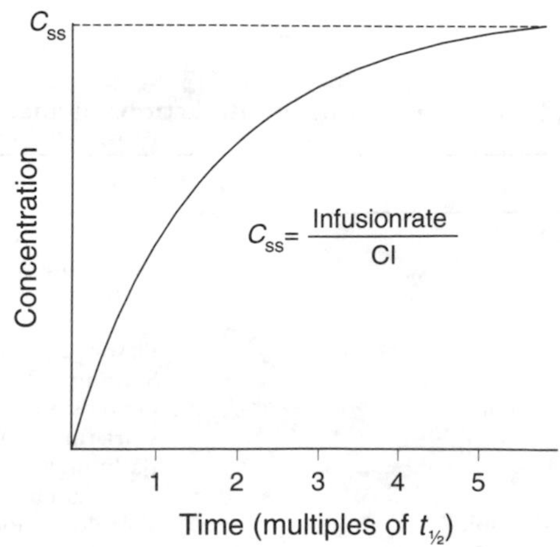

Fig. 3.8
Plasma concentrations during a constant-rate intravenous infusion against time expressed as multiples of $t_{1/2}$. C_{ss} = concentration at steady state, Cl = clearance.

$$\text{Rate of infusion} = \text{Cl} \times C_{ss} \quad (9)$$

where C_{ss} is the concentration at steady state.

Many pathological conditions reduce drug clearance and may therefore result in unexpectedly large plasma concentrations during infusions. Half-life does not influence C_{ss}, only how quickly it is achieved.

Patient-controlled analgesia

The use of PCA for the treatment of postoperative pain has become widespread and is described in detail in Chapter 42. The patient titrates opioid delivery to requirements by pressing a button on a PCA device which results in the delivery of a small bolus dose. A lockout time is set which does not allow another bolus to be delivered until the previous dose has had time to have an effect. There is an enormous interpatient variability in the pharmacodynamics and pharmacokinetics of opioids; PCA allows for this and produces superior analgesia.

RECTAL

This technique reduces the problems of first-pass metabolism and the need for injections. It is used in children (paracetamol, diclofenac) and adults (diclofenac) for postoperative analgesia. The rectal preparation of diclofenac is particularly useful, as the intramuscular route is painful.

TRANSDERMAL

Drugs with a high lipid solubility and potency may be given by this route. The pharmacological properties of glyceryl trinitrate render it ideal for this technique, i.e. potent, highly lipid-soluble, short half-life. Transdermal hyoscine is used for travel and other causes of sickness. Fentanyl transdermal delivery systems are effective in the treatment of pain, particularly in patients with cancer.

It may take some time before a steady-state plasma concentration is achieved and many devices incorporate large amounts of drug in the adhesive layer in order to provide a loading dose which reduces this period. At steady state, transdermal delivery has several similarities to intravenous infusions. However, on removing the adhesive patch, plasma concentrations may decline relatively slowly because of a depot of drug in the surrounding skin; this occurs with transdermal fentanyl systems.

INHALATION

The delivery of inhaled volatile anaesthetics is discussed below, but other drugs may be given by this route, especially bronchodilators and steroids. Atropine and epinephrine are absorbed if injected into the bronchial tree and this offers a route of administration in emergencies if no other method of delivery is possible. Opioids such as fentanyl and diamorphine have been given as nebulized solutions but this technique is not routine.

EPIDURAL

This is a common route of administration in anaesthetic practice. The epidural space is very vascular and significant amounts of drug may be absorbed systemically, even if any vessels are avoided by the needle or cannula. Opioids diffuse across the dura to act on spinal opioid receptors, but much of their action when given epidurally is the result of systemic absorption. Complications include subdural haematoma and infection and inadvertent dural puncture with consequent headache or spinal administration of the drug.

SPINAL (SUBARACHNOID)

When given spinally, drugs have free access to the neural tissue of the spinal cord and small doses have profound rapid effects; an advantage and also disadvantage of the method. Protein binding is not a significant factor as CSF protein concentration is relatively low.

DRUG INTERACTIONS

There are three basic types of drug interactions; examples are listed in Table 3.2.

Table 3.2 Examples of drug interactions in anaesthesia

Type	Drugs	Effect
Pharmaceutical	Thiopental: succinylcholine	Hydrolysis of succinylcholine
	Ampicillin: glucose, lactate	Reduced potency
	Blood: dextrans	Rouleaux formation Crossmatching difficulties
	Plastic: glyceryl trinitrate	Adsorption to plastic
	Sevoflurane: soda lime	Compound A
Pharmacokinetic	Opioids: most drugs	Delayed oral absorption
	Warfarin: NSAIDs	↑ Free warfarin
	Barbiturates: warfarin	↑ Warfarin metabolism
	Neostigmine: succinylcholine	↓ Succinylcholine metabolism
Pharmacodynamic	Volatiles: opioids	↓ MAC
	Volatiles: benzodiazepines	↓ MAC
	Volatiles: N_2O	↓ MAC
	Volatiles: muscle relaxants	↑ Relaxation
	Morphine: naloxone	Reversal (receptor antagonism)
	Muscle relaxants: neostigmine	↓ Relaxation

Pharmaceutical

In this type of interaction, drugs, often mixed in the same syringe or infusion bag, react chemically with adverse results. For example, mixing succinylcholine with thiopental (pH 10–11) hydrolyses the former, rendering it inactive. Before mixing drugs, data should be sought on their compatibility.

Pharmacokinetic

Absorption of a drug, particularly if given orally, may be affected by other drugs because of their action on gastric emptying (see above). Interference with protein binding (see above) is a common cause of drug interaction. We have discussed drug metabolism in some detail and there are many potential sites in this process where interactions can occur, e.g. competition for enzyme systems, enzyme inhibition or induction.

Pharmacodynamic

This is the most frequent type of interaction in anaesthetic practice. A typical anaesthetic is a series of pharmacodynamic interactions. It may be adverse, e.g. increased respiratory depression with opioids and volatile agents, or advantageous, e.g. reversal of muscle relaxation with neostigmine. An understanding of the many subtle pharmacodynamic interactions in modern anaesthesia accounts for the difference in the quality of anaesthesia and recovery associated with the experienced compared with the novice anaesthetist.

VOLATILE ANAESTHETIC AGENTS

MECHANISM OF ACTION

The exact mechanism of action of volatile anaesthetic agents is at present unknown. Potency is, in general, related to lipid solubility (Meyer–Overton relationship, see Fig. 2.5 and Table 3.3) and this has given rise to the concept of volatile agents dissolving in the lipid cell membrane in a non-specific manner, disrupting membrane function and thereby influencing the function of proteins, e.g. ion channels. However, it is now appreciated that volatile agents may bind selectively to receptor sites, e.g. $GABA_A$ receptor.

POTENCY

Potency is defined classically in terms of minimum alveolar concentration (MAC). MAC is the alveolar concentration of a volatile agent that produces no movement in 50% of spontaneously breathing patients after skin incision. MAC is inversely related to lipid solubility (Table 3.3).

Table 3.3 MAC in oxygen and lipid solubility (expressed as oil/gas solubility coefficient)

Agent	MAC (%) in O_2	Oil/gas solubility
N_2O	104	1.4
Desflurane	6.6	29
Sevoflurane	1.8	80
Enflurane	1.63	98
Isoflurane	1.17	97
Halothane	0.75	224

Table 3.4 Solubility of volatile agents in blood (expressed as blood/gas solubility coefficients)

Agent	Blood/gas solubility coefficient
Desflurane	0.45
N_2O	0.47
Sevoflurane	0.65
Isoflurane	1.4
Enflurane	1.8
Halothane	2.4

ONSET OF ACTION

When considering onset of action of volatile agents, there is a fundamental difference compared with intravenous agents. Effects of non-volatile drugs are related to plasma or tissue concentrations; this is not so with volatile agents. Of importance in this case is the partial pressure of the agent, not the concentration. If a volatile agent is highly soluble in blood, partial pressure increases slowly as large amounts dissolve in the blood. Consequently, onset of anaesthesia is slow with agents soluble in blood and rapid with agents which are relatively insoluble. The same applies to recovery from anaesthesia. Table 3.4 lists the most commonly used volatile agents (in order of speed of onset) and their relative blood/gas solubilities.

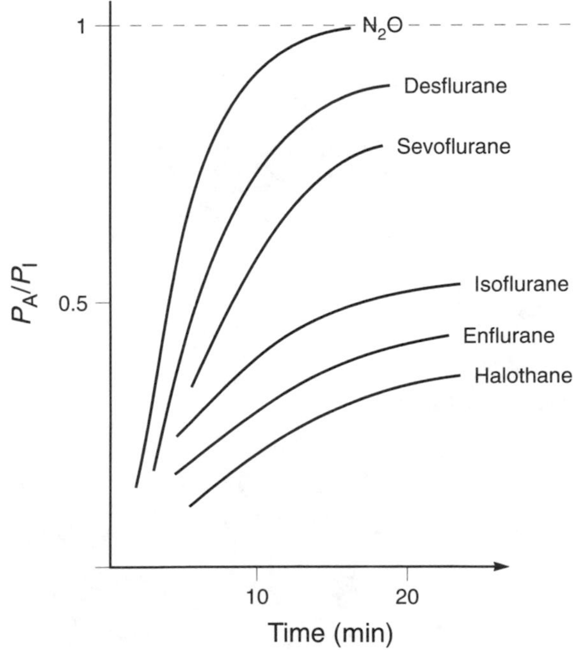

Fig. 3.9
The rate at which P_A reaches P_I is related to speed of induction of anaesthesia. Agents insoluble in blood equilibrate more rapidly.

Alveolar partial pressure (P_A) is assumed to be equivalent to cerebral artery partial pressure and therefore depth of anaesthesia. At a fixed inspired partial pressure (P_I), the rate at which P_A approaches P_I is related to speed of onset of effect (Fig. 3.9). This is rapid with agents of low blood solubility, e.g. N_2O, and relatively slow with more soluble agents, e.g. halothane.

Clearly, solubility of the agent in blood is a major determinant of the speed of onset of anaesthesia, but other factors can have significant effects. The rate of delivery of the agent to the alveoli is important; therefore increasing P_I by adjusting the vaporizer (a factor limited by irritant effects on the airway in spontaneously breathing patients), reducing apparatus dead space and increasing alveolar ventilation increase speed of induction of anaesthesia. If cardiac output is reduced, relatively less agent is removed from the alveolus and P_A increases towards P_I more rapidly. Consequently, induction of anaesthesia is more rapid in patients with reduced cardiac output. Both rate of delivery and cardiac output have particularly significant effects with agents that are relatively soluble in blood but less so with insoluble agents, e.g. N_2O.

Ventilation/perfusion mismatch may reduce the speed of induction, an effect more significant in agents of low solubility. For example, if one lung is collapsed, i.e. perfused but not ventilated, increasing ventilation or inspired concentration of agents such as halothane helps to compensate. However, this is not the case for N_2O.

FURTHER READING

Calvey T N, Williams N E 1997 Principles and practice of pharmacology for anaesthetists, 3rd edn. Blackwell Scientific Publications, Oxford

4 Anatomy of the cardiovascular system

A sound knowledge of anatomy is important to the anaesthetist. This chapter describes the anatomy of the heart and the great vessels. In addition, the vascular anatomy of the upper and lower limbs and the neck in relation to venepuncture is described.

THE HEART

The heart is the muscular pump of the systemic and pulmonary circulations. Irregularly conical in shape, it lies obliquely across the lower mediastinum behind the sternum, suspended by the great vessels.

BORDERS AND SURFACES

The borders and surfaces of the heart may be understood easily if the 'schematic' heart (two atria over two ventricles) is placed on its left side and turned clockwise (Fig. 4.1). It can then be seen that the right atrium forms the right border of the heart; the lower part of the atrium, the right ventricle and the apex of the left ventricle form the lower border; and the left atrium and ventricle form the left border.

The anterior surface, from right to left, consists of the right atrium and ventricle, the atrioventricular groove, the anterior interventricular groove and the left ventricle. Of the ventricular surfaces, two-thirds consists of the right ventricle and one-third the left ventricle (Fig. 4.2). This proportion is reversed on the diaphragmatic surface, i.e. one-third consists of the right ventricle, and two-thirds of the left ventricle separated by the posterior interventricular groove. The left atrium, with the pulmonary veins, and a small portion of the right atrium form the base or the inferior surface of the heart (Fig. 4.3).

SURFACE MARKINGS

The heart lies obliquely across the mediastinum behind the sternum (Fig. 4.4). The right border extends from the third costal cartilage to the sixth costal cartilage, 1.25 cm from the right sternal edge. The inferior border runs from the right sixth intercostal cartilage to the left fifth intercostal space, approximately 9 cm from the midline. It is at this point that the apex beat of the heart may be felt. The left border runs from the apex to the second intercostal space, 1.25 cm from the left sternal edge.

CHAMBERS

Right atrium

This is a thin-walled narrow chamber, which is derived embryologically from two sources: the embryonic right atrium and the horn of the sinus venosus. In the adult, these two components are separated by the crista terminalis. The smooth portion

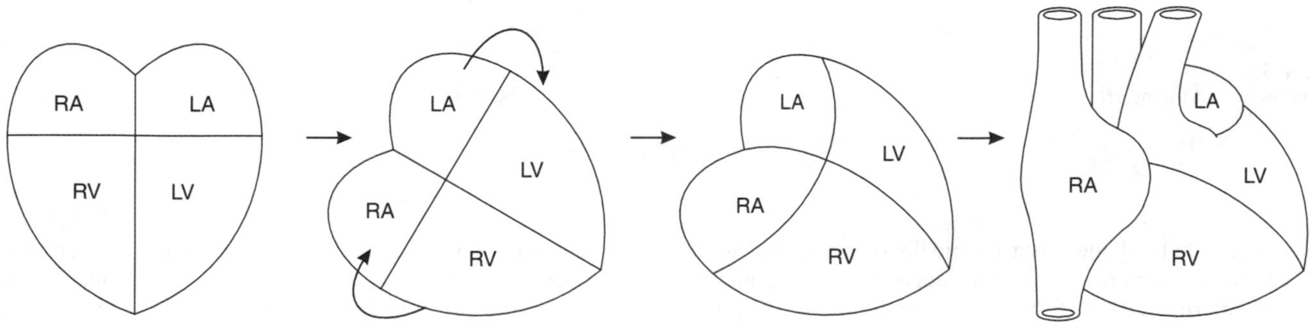

Fig. 4.1
Borders and surfaces of the heart. (After Moffat 1993, with permission).

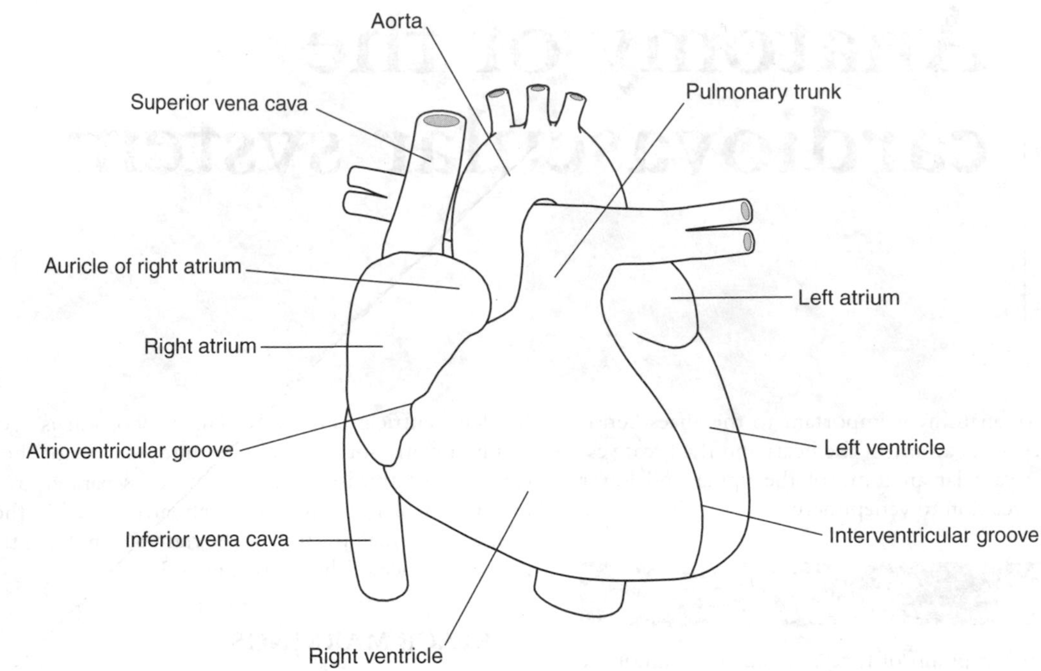

Fig. 4.2
Anterior surface of the heart.

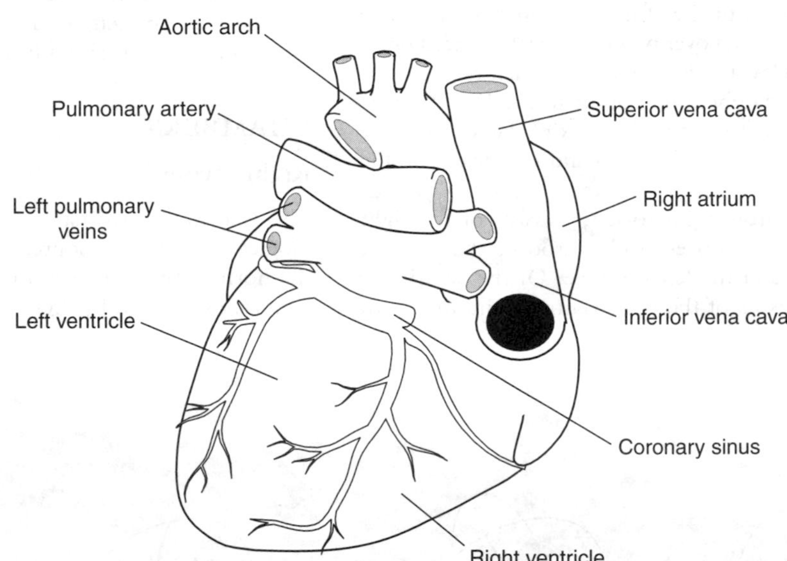

Fig. 4.3
Posterior view of the heart.

of the atrium behind the crista terminalis is the sinus venosus and receives the superior vena cava superiorly and the inferior vena cava inferiorly. The left horn of the sinus venosus develops into the coronary sinus, the opening of which is near the inferior vena cava. The rough-walled portion of the atrium in front of the crista terminalis is derived from the true embryonic right atrium, as is the auricular appendage. The caval orifices do not contain functioning valves, although rudimentary valves mark the opening of the inferior vena cava and the coronary sinus. A shallow depression on the interatrial septum, the *fossa ovalis*, marks the site of the *foramen ovale*, which allows the flow of oxygenated blood from the right atrium to the left atrium in the fetal circulation. A small percentage of adults continue to possess a patent foramen ovale.

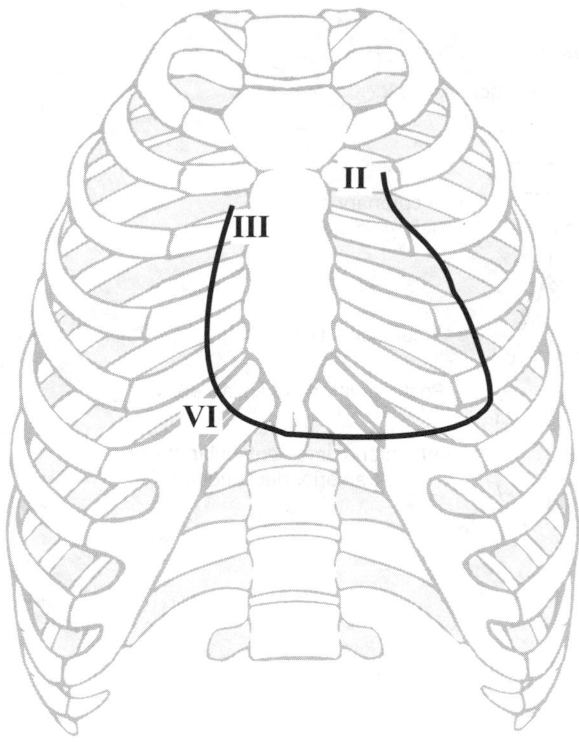

Fig. 4.4
Surface markings of the heart.

Right ventricle

This is a thick-walled elongated chamber, which makes up most of the anterior and one-third of the diaphragmatic surface of the heart. The atrioventricular orifice separates the right atrium from the right ventricle and lies postero-inferiorly near the base of the ventricle. Oval in shape and surrounded by a fibrous ring, it contains the tricuspid valve, so termed because it has three cusps or leaflets. These are triangular in shape and consist of a thin layer of fibrous tissue sandwiched between two layers of endocardium. The leaflets are connected not only at their bases to the fibrous ring surrounding the orifice but also to each other, thereby forming a continuous annular membrane. The cusps or leaflets vary in size and are named according to the position they occupy within the orifice (anterior, inferior and medial). The central part of the leaflet is thick, becoming thin and translucent at the lateral margins.

The anterior surface of the valve is smooth. On its ventricular surface, delicate tendinous chords, the chordae tendineae, connect the free margins of the leaflets to the ventricle. The points of attachment are the papillary muscles, muscular projections from the inner surface of the ventricle, itself containing irregular muscular ridges, the trabeculae carnae. The papillary muscles are situated on the anterior and posterior walls of the cavity. The chordae tendineae and papillary muscles anchor the tricuspid valve such that the valve is prevented from ballooning back into the atrium during right ventricular systole.

The pulmonary valve guards the pulmonary orifice and consists of three semilunar leaflets (right anterior, left anterior and posterior). A muscular ridge, the infundibuloventricular crest, lying between the atrioventricular and the pulmonary valves separates the inflow and outflow tracts of the ventricle. The outflow tract of the ventricle, the infundibulum, is smooth-walled and directed upwards and to the right towards the pulmonary trunk.

Left atrium

This is a rectangular chamber that lies behind the right atrium and forms most of the base of the heart. Smaller than the right atrium and with a thicker wall, it receives the superior and inferior pulmonary veins from the lungs. These enter on the posterior surface, two on either side, so that there are four openings into the atrium.

Left ventricle

This is a longer, more conical shaped chamber than the right atrium. It lies behind the right ventricle and forms a small part of the anterior surface of the heart, much of the inferior portion and also the apex. It is thicker walled but otherwise similar to the right ventricle. Most of its walls are covered with thick muscular ridges, trabeculae carnae, except for a smooth area just below the aortic orifice, the vestibule. The bicuspid mitral valve guards the atrioventricular orifice. The anterior and posterior leaflets of the valve are attached to the papillary muscles via the chordae tendineae. The aortic orifice is a fibrous ring lying behind and to the right of the pulmonary orifice. It contains the aortic valve, which has three semilunar cusps (anterior, right posterior and left posterior). The ventricles are separated by the interventricular septum. The right ventricle, into which the septum bulges, lies anterior and the left ventricle posterior. The septum is muscular except for a small area just distal to the atrioventricular valves, where it is membranous.

CONDUCTING SYSTEM

The conducting system of the heart consists of specialized cardiac muscle cells found in the sinoatrial node, atrioventricular node and the bundle of His. The sinoatrial node (the physiological pacemaker of the heart), located at the top of the right atrium at the upper end of the crista terminalis and to the right of the superior vena caval opening, initiates the impulse for cardiac contraction. From there the impulse spreads through the atrium to reach the atrioventricular node, in the lower part of the interatrial septum, immediately above the opening of the coronary sinus. The impulse is then conducted to the ventricles by the atrioventricular bundle (of His). This bundle divides at the junction of the membranous and muscular parts of the interventricular septum into its right and left branches, which pass down either side of the septum subendocardially. The left bundle branch further divides into anterior and posterior fascicles. The branches ramify and Purkinje fibres spread from the ends of the branches to the papillary muscles and the ventricular walls (Fig. 5.6).

BLOOD SUPPLY

Arterial supply to the heart is via the left and right coronary arteries, so termed because they form a circle (corona) around the atrioven-

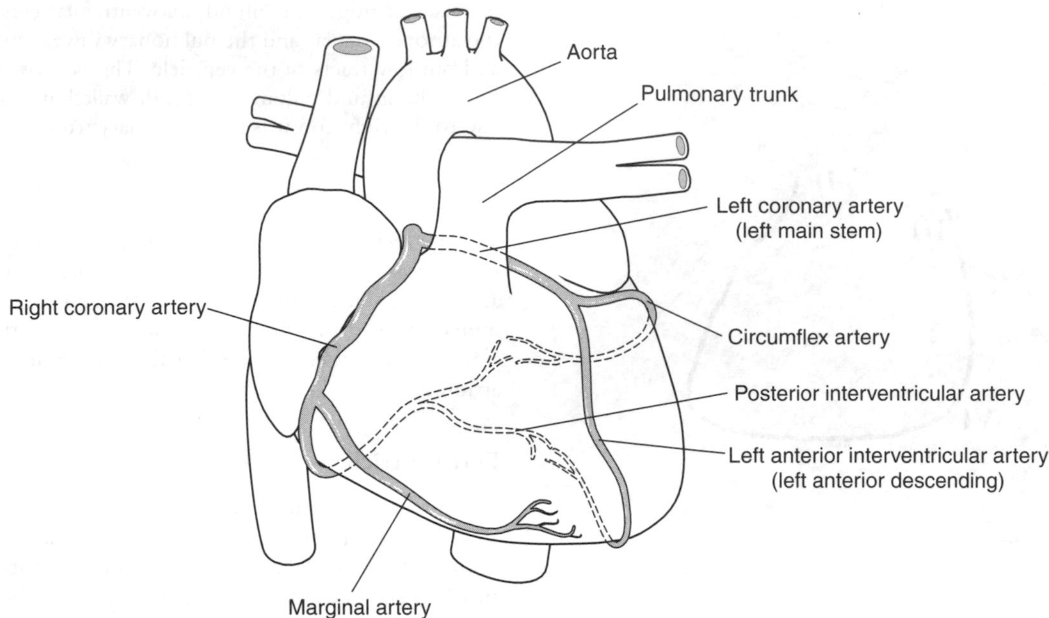

Fig. 4.5
Arterial supply of the heart.

tricular groove (cf. coronet). While these arteries and their branches do anastomose with each other, the anastomoses are not sufficiently large to maintain a collateral circulation if a major branch is occluded. They are therefore functional, if not anatomical, end arteries. Thus the sudden occlusion of a major artery may result in sudden death, but more slowly developing occlusion of smaller branches may allow time for a collateral circulation to develop.

Arterial (Fig. 4.5)

The right coronary artery arises from the anterior aortic sinus or right sinus of Valsalva, just above the anterior cusp of the aortic valve. It passes forwards between the right atrium and pulmonary trunk and descends along the right atrioventricular groove to the inferior border of the heart where it turns round to the posterior surface and anastomoses with the left coronary artery at the posterior interventricular groove. It gives a marginal branch at the lower border of the heart, which runs to the left towards the apex, and in 80% of cases it terminates as the posterior interventricular branch, which supplies the interventricular septum. In view of the fact that the interventricular septum contains the bundle of His and its branches, the interventricular arteries are of particular importance (especially the inferior one). The right coronary artery supplies the sinoatrial node in 60% of individuals and, in 85%, the atrioventricular node and the posterior and inferior parts of the left ventricle. Conduction abnormalities are commonly associated with occlusion of the right coronary artery.

The left coronary artery arises from the posterior aortic sinus or left sinus of Valsalva. It passes forward behind the pulmonary trunk and then divides in the space between the aorta and pulmonary artery into the left anterior interventricular artery (anterior descending artery) and the circumflex branch. The anterior interventricular artery passes along the anterior interventricular groove towards the apex, turns round the lower border and anastomoses with the posterior interventricular artery. The major branches of the left anterior interventricular artery are the diagonal branches, which supply the free walls of the left ventricle, and the septal branches, which supply the interventricular septum. The diagonal and septal branches are important landmarks in the description of lesions in the left anterior descending artery.

The circumflex artery passes laterally around the left border of the heart to reach the posterior interventricular groove. It supplies the sinoatrial node in 40% of individuals and the lateral wall of the ventricle via the marginal arteries.

Generally, therefore, the left coronary artery supplies the left ventricle and the right coronary artery the right ventricle; both supply the interventricular septum and the atria are supplied in a variable manner. Variations on this anatomical pattern do occur. In less than 20% of individuals, the circumflex artery gives rise to the posterior descending artery and the left coronary artery supplies the whole of the interventricular septum and the atrioventricular node. Thus the left coronary artery is the most important supply for the left ventricle unless the posterior descending artery arises from the right coronary artery.

Venous drainage (Fig. 4.6)

The veins of the heart follow the pattern of the arteries although they have different names. Approximately two-thirds of the myocardial venous drainage is via the coronary sinus and anterior cardiac veins into the right atrium. The remaining blood drains by means of small veins (venae cordae minimae) that open directly into the cavities of the heart. The coronary sinus, a continuation of the great cardiac vein, is formed at the left border of the heart and passes to the right in the posterior interventricular groove. It enters the right atrium near the orifice of the inferior vena cava.

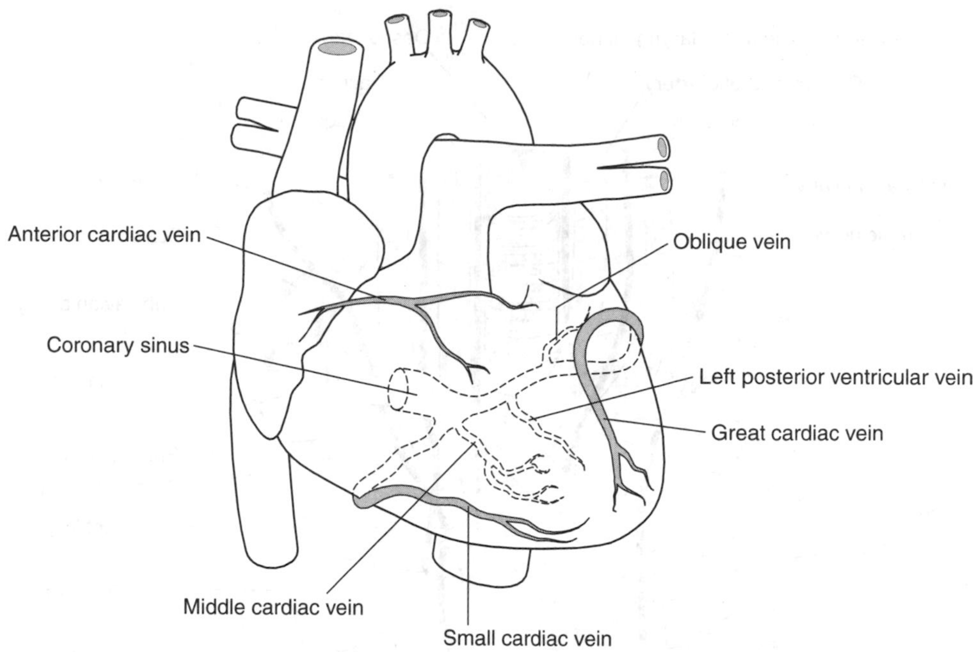

Fig. 4.6
Venous drainage of the heart.

The coronary sinus receives the following:

- Great cardiac vein – drains both ventricles; it ascends in the anterior interventricular groove, turns around the left border of the heart and becomes the coronary sinus
- Middle cardiac vein – lies in the posterior interventricular groove
- Small cardiac vein – this is a continuation of the right marginal vein, which runs along the lower border of the heart
- Oblique vein – this descends obliquely on the back of the left atrium and opens near the left extremity of the coronary sinus; it is a remnant of the left superior vena cava.

The anterior cardiac vein crosses in the anterior cardiac groove. It drains most of the anterior surface of the heart and opens directly into the right atrium.

The coronary venous blood draining (via the thebesian, anterior sinusoidal and the anterior luminal veins) directly into the left ventricle constitutes a fixed shunt and contributes to the dilution of oxygenated blood.

NERVE SUPPLY

The heart is innervated by the autonomic nervous system. The parasympathetic innervation is derived from the vagus nerve and is distributed to the nodal tissue and atrial musculature. The sympathetic innervation is derived from the upper thoracic (T1–T4, cardioaccelerator fibres) segmental roots of the spinal cord. These nerves form the superficial and deep cardiac plexuses. Fibres from here are distributed with the coronary arteries to supply heart muscle, coronary arteries and the conducting system of the heart. Ischaemic pain sensation transmitted by the afferent sympathetic nerves is manifested as referred pain in the somatic distribution of the T1–T4 segmental sensory roots, e.g. radiation of substernal chest pain to the neck and the arms.

THE AORTA

The aorta is the main arterial trunk of the systemic circulation and consists of an ascending part, an arch, a descending part and an abdominal part. The ascending aorta leaves the left ventricle above the aortic valve and passes to the right around the pulmonary trunk up to the level of the sternal angle. Above each of the semilunar folds of the aortic valve is a dilatation, an aortic sinus from which the coronary arteries arise. The aortic arch is formed as the aorta curves back and slightly to the left over the root of the left lung and then descends to reach the left side of the fourth thoracic vertebra. This gives rise to the characteristic knuckle seen in radiographs of the chest. The brachiocephalic, left common carotid and subclavian arteries arise from the aortic arch. The principal relations of the arch of the aorta are shown in Figure 4.7.

The descending aorta begins at the lower border of T4 and descends to the left of the midline, moving medially to pierce the diaphragm in the midline at the level of T12. The bodies of the vertebrae T4–T8 are therefore slightly flattened on their left side.

The branches of the descending aorta are the posterior intercostal arteries (3rd to 11th), two or three bronchial arteries, four or five oesophageal arteries, mediastinal and diaphragmatic arteries. Where the aorta lies left of the midline, right posterior intercostal arteries have to cross the bodies of the vertebrae behind the oesophagus to reach the right intercostal spaces. The posterior intercostals also give off spinal branches to supply the spinal cord. These anterior radicular arteries are variable in both size and number, and while they anastomose along the longitudinal axis of the

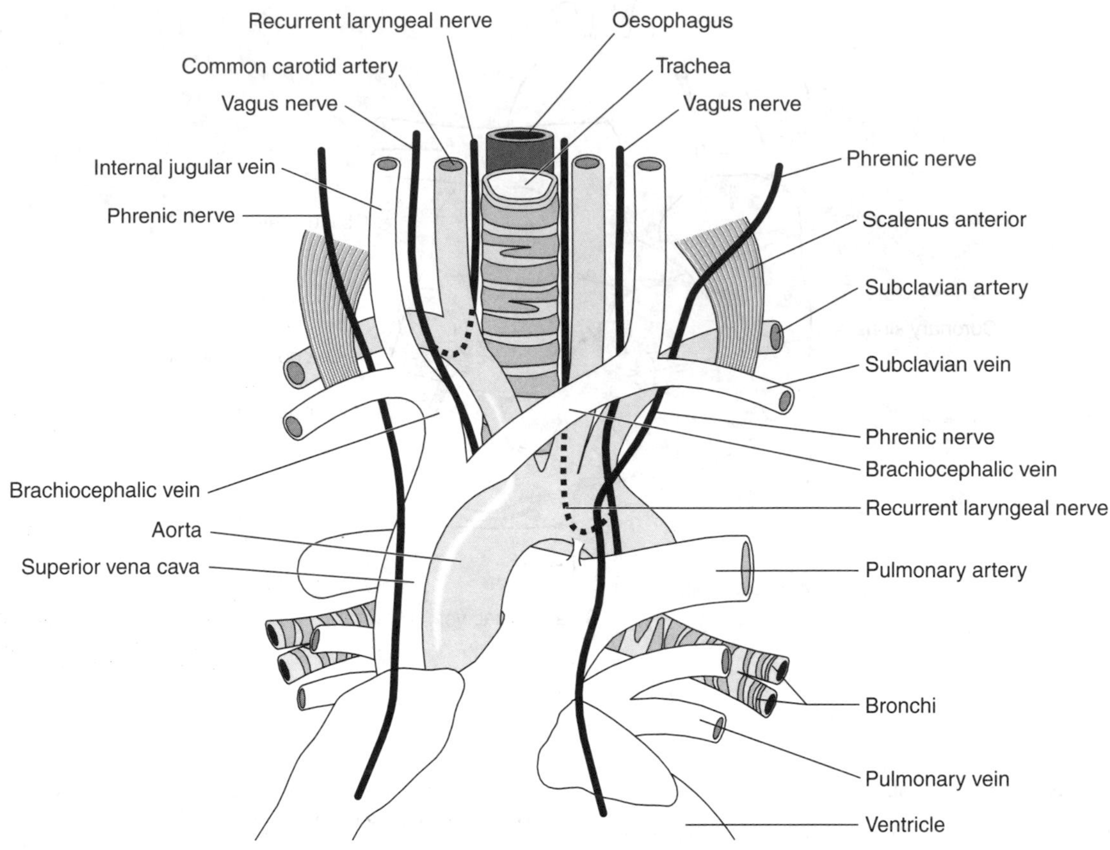

Fig. 4.7
Principal relations of the arch of the aorta.

spinal cord, this may be inadequate. Often, however, one of the anterior radicular arteries is of considerable size and is termed the artery of Adamkiewicz. Its position is variable and it arises usually in the lower thoracic or lumbar region, on the left side. On reaching the spinal cord, this artery sends a branch to the anterior and posterior spinal arteries and may be responsible for the blood supply to two-thirds of the spinal cord. Occlusion of this vessel during thoracic aortic cross-clamping or aortic dissection may compromise blood supply to the cord.

The relations of the descending aorta anteriorly are the root of the left lung, the left atrium, the oesophagus and the diaphragm. Posteriorly it lies on the vertebral column and the hemiazygous veins. On the right side, it is in contact with the oesophagus above and the right lung and pleura below, while on the left it is in contact with the left pleura and lung. The thoracic duct and the azygous vein lie to its right.

THE PULMONARY TRUNK

Beginning at the pulmonary orifice of the right ventricle to the left and slightly in front of the ascending aorta, this runs upwards and backwards to divide in the concavity of the aortic arch into the right and left pulmonary arteries. It is covered anteriorly by the left lung; the right and left coronary arteries surround its base. A short fibrous band, the ligamentum arteriosum, connects the left pulmonary artery to the lower surface of the aortic arch. This is the remains of the ductus arteriosus which short-circuits blood

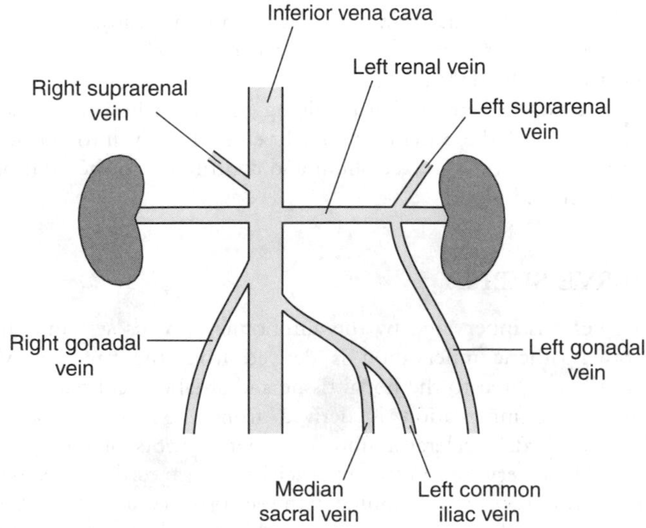

Fig. 4.8
Schematic diagram of the inferior vena cava and its branches.

into the aorta to prevent it going through the lungs in the fetal circulation. This usually closes within hours of birth, although failure to do so gives rise to a patent ductus arteriosus, one of the commonest congenital abnormalities.

In the lung, the pulmonary arteries accompany the bronchi and bronchioles.

THE LARGE VEINS

The pulmonary veins open into the left atrium, usually two (upper and lower) from each lung. At the hilum of the lung, they lie below and in front of the pulmonary artery. On the right, the upper passes behind the superior vena cava, and the lower behind the right atrium.

The union of the corresponding internal jugular and subclavian veins, behind the sternoclavicular joints, forms the brachiocephalic veins (Fig. 4.7). The left brachiocephalic vein crosses the midline just above the arch of the aorta. As the arch is entirely behind the manubrium sterni, the left brachiocephalic vein lies only just below the suprasternal notch and is above it in children. There is the potential, therefore, for major haemorrhage during procedures such as tracheostomy in children.

The right brachiocephalic vein passes vertically downwards behind the right border of the manubrium, anterolateral to the brachiocephalic artery. The phrenic nerve runs down along its lateral surface between it and the pleura. The brachiocephalic veins unite to form the superior vena cava, at the middle of the right border of the manubrium. The brachiocephalic veins receive a number of tributaries, including the left superior intercostal vein, which crosses the aortic arch to enter the left brachiocephalic vein, the inferior thyroid veins, which come down from the neck in front of the trachea, the vertebral veins and the internal thoracic veins. The vertebral veins drain the neck muscles at the back and the vertebral column, and the internal thoracic veins drain the anterior chest wall and the diaphragm.

The superior vena cava is formed by the union of the brachiocephalic veins at the middle of the right border of the manubrium. It lies to the right of the ascending aorta just before opening into the right atrium at the level of the third costal cartilage. The transverse sinus of the pericardium separates it from the aorta and pulmonary trunk. Anteriorly are the right lung and pleura, and posteriorly is the right lung root. The right phrenic nerve and right lung lie laterally and the ascending aorta and brachiocephalic vein medially.

The inferior vena cava begins at the body of the fifth lumbar vertebra and ascends on the posterior abdominal wall to the right of the aorta to pierce the central tendon of the diaphragm at the level of T8. After a short intrathoracic course, it opens into the right atrium. It receives the renal veins, the hepatic vein and the right suprarenal vein. From the posterior abdominal wall, it also receives the inferior phrenic and lumbar veins (Fig. 4.8).

UPPER LIMB VEINS

The superficial veins form varying patterns, but the common arrangements are shown in Figures 4.9 and 4.10.

The arrangement of the arteries is less varied than that of the veins. However, developmental anomalies do occur and it is wise to inspect and palpate for arterial pulsation before undertaking venepuncture. An 'ulnar' artery may leave the brachial artery in the arm and, passing superficial to the common attachment of the

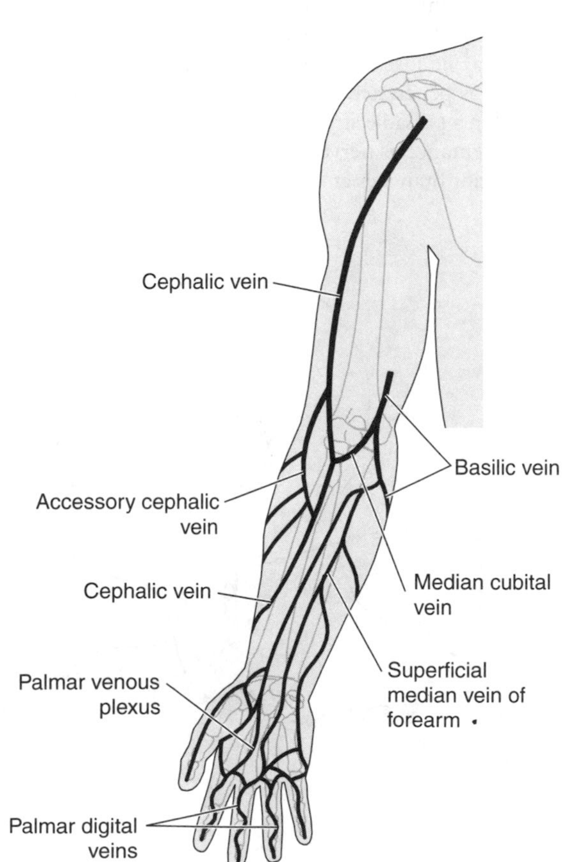

Fig. 4.9
Superficial veins of the right upper limb.

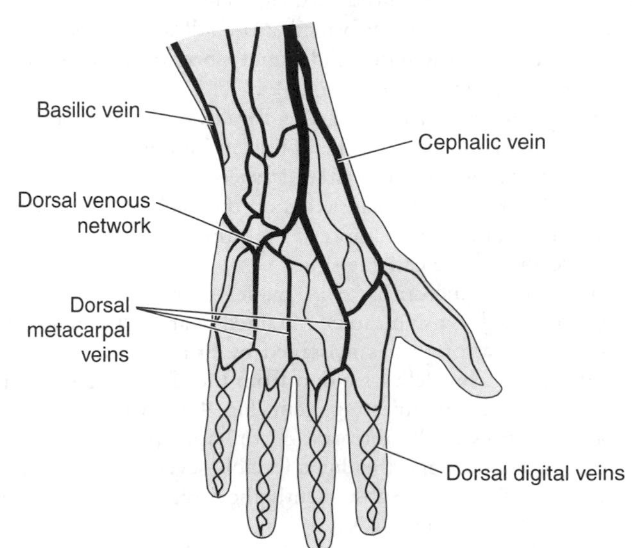

Fig. 4.10
Dorsal metacarpal veins of the right hand.

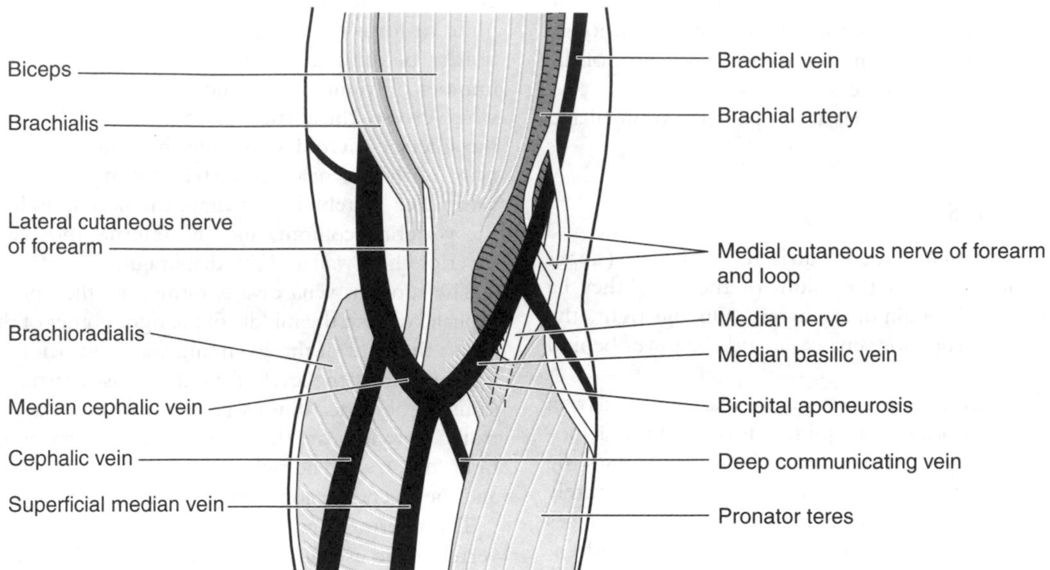

Fig. 4.11
Veins at the right elbow.

superficial flexor muscles of the forearm, lie immediately deep to the median cubital vein – without the intervention of the bicipital aponeurosis. Similarly, a 'radial' artery may arise proximally and be situated superficially in the forearm. Metacarpal veins, lying superficially on the back of the hand, drain blood from the digits and hand (Fig. 4.10). These veins join together to form the dorsal venous arch. From the lateral and medial ends of the dorsal venous arch, the blood is carried centripetally by the cephalic and basilic veins, respectively. These veins also receive tributaries from the skin and superficial tissues of the forearm, thus draining, respectively, the pre- and postaxial borders of the upper limb. The basilic vein, having received the brachial veins, continues as the axillary vein. The cephalic vein, after passing through the deltopectoral groove, drains into the axillary vein.

Venepuncture may be performed at the following sites:

On the back of the hand and lateral aspect of the wrist in one of the dorsal metacarpal veins (Fig. 4.11).

On the anterior aspect of the forearm in the cephalic or median veins (Fig. 4.10), or one of their tributaries. Usually there are useful veins also on the posterior aspect.

It is preferable to cannulate veins on the back of the hand and on the forearm rather than those at the elbow because the cannula may be secured more easily in situ.

When a venepuncture is to be made at or below the elbow, greater venous distension can be obtained in an obstructed vein if the front of the forearm is massaged by firm pressure from the wrist upwards. This delivers blood from the superficial veins and from the deep (communicating) vein (Fig. 4.11) which drains the deeper structures of the forearm. A conscious patient should be asked to flex and extend the digits forcibly several times and then to clench the fist firmly. Subsequently the forearm should be massaged from the wrist upwards.

At the elbow in either the cephalic or median cubital vein (Fig. 4.11). Usually the median cubital vein is the larger and more mobile of the two, but, if used inexpertly, there may be complications. If the needle is inserted too deeply, it may pass through the bicipital aponeurosis and penetrate the brachial artery. The pulsation of this artery can be felt immediately medial to the tendon of the biceps. Medial to the brachial artery lies the median nerve. An anomalous ulnar artery may lie just deep to the median cubital vein and be at risk if the vein is penetrated too deeply (Fig. 4.11). Withdrawal of arterial blood in a pulsatile stream indicates that this has happened.

The medial cutaneous nerve of the forearm divides into its anterior and posterior branches at the elbow (Fig. 4.11) and sometimes

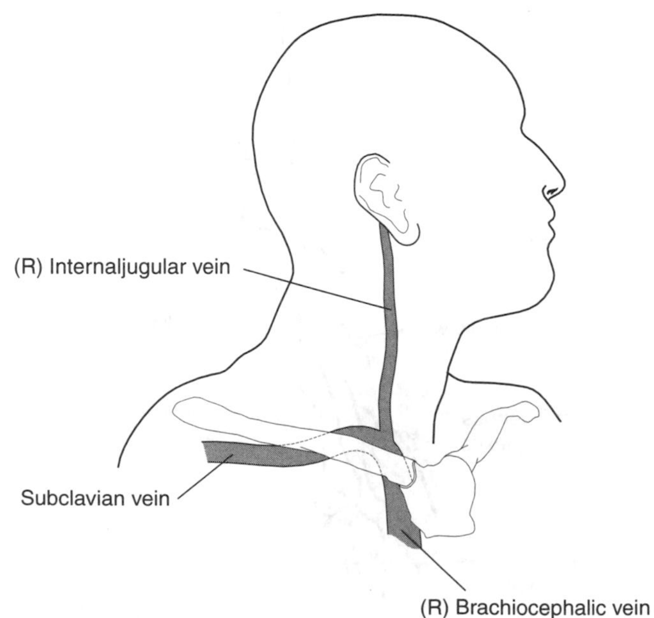

Fig. 4.12
Right subclavian and jugular veins.

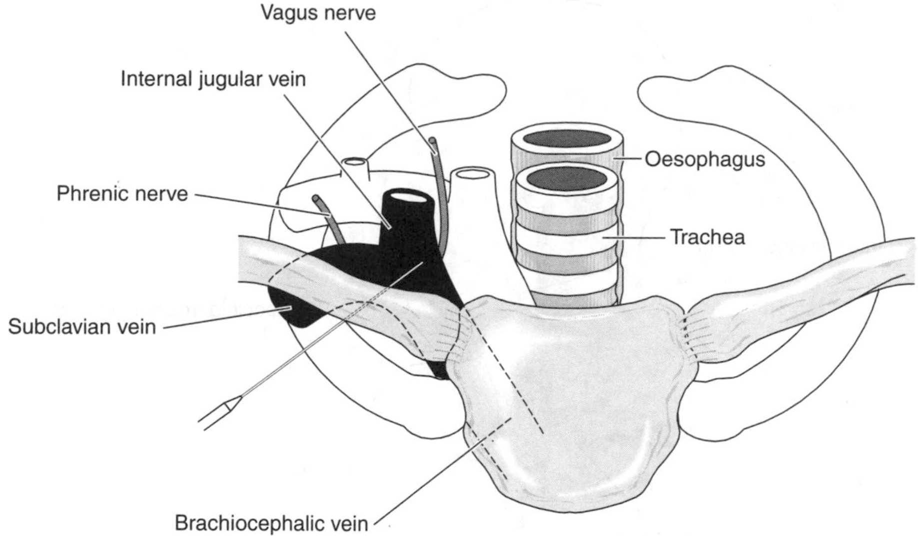

Fig. 4.13
Right subclavian vein.

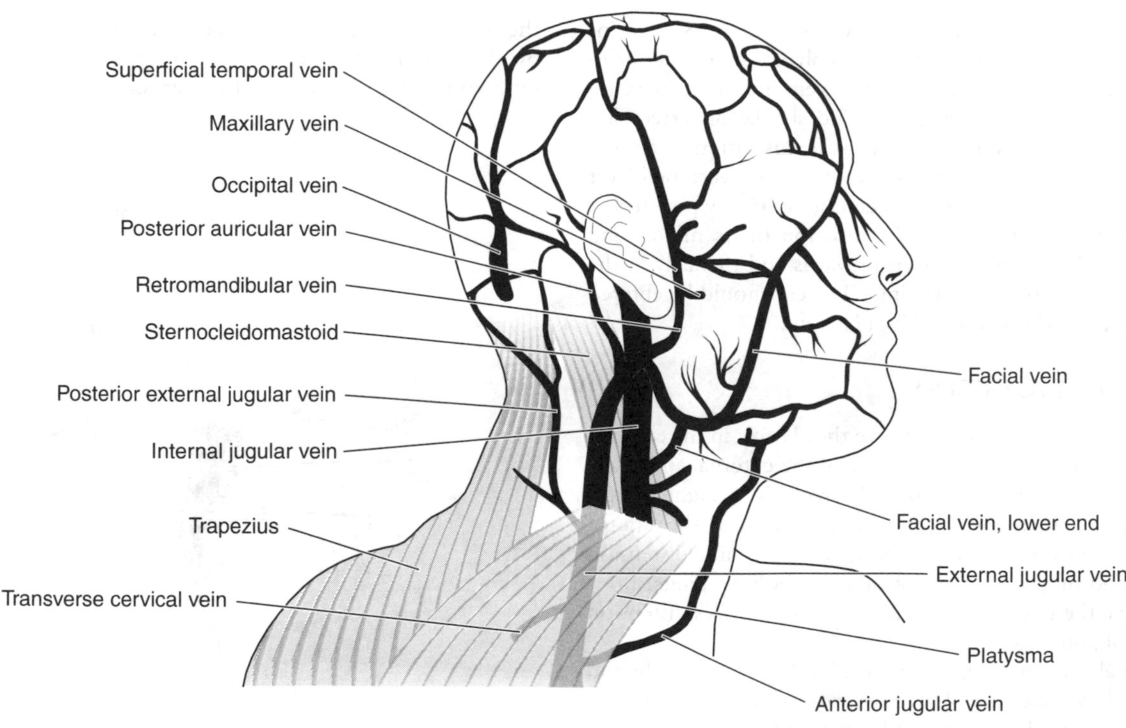

Fig. 4.14
Veins of the right side of the head and neck.

these form a loop around the median cubital vein. Thus perivenous piercing with the needle, extravasation of fluid, or the occurrence of a haematoma at this site may damage nerve fibres and in the conscious patient cause acute pain along the inner border of the forearm.

Below the clavicle in the subclavian vein (Fig. 4.12). Use of the right subclavian rather than the left provides easier access to the superior vena cava and right atrium. The subclavian vein – the continuation of the axillary – runs from a point just below and medial to the midclavicular point. From here it arches upwards,

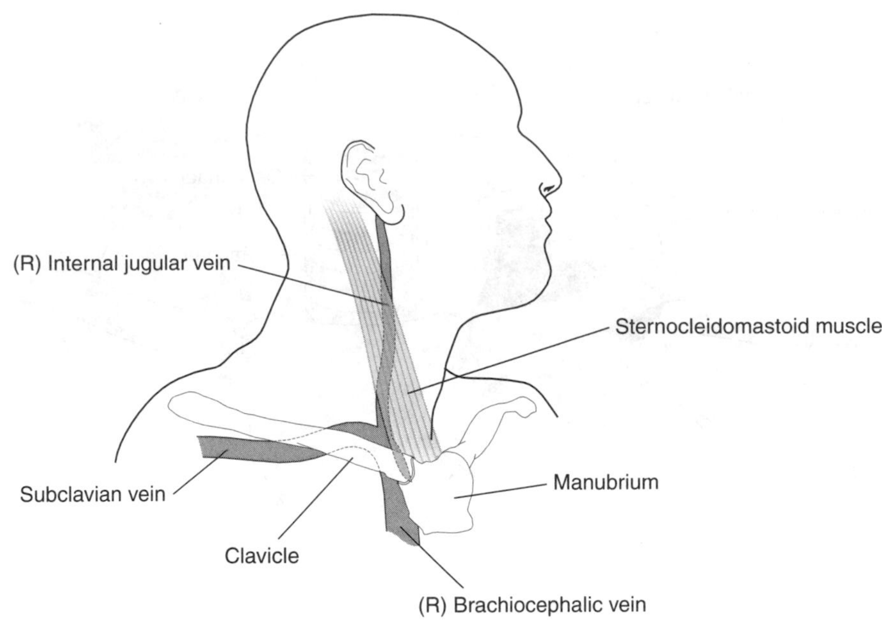

Fig. 4.15
Right internal jugular vein.

and then, passing downwards and forwards (Fig. 4.13), it joins the internal jugular to form the brachiocephalic vein posterior to the sternoclavicular joint. The subclavian vein lies in a groove on the superior surface of the first rib. The subclavian artery lies above and behind the vein with the scalenus anterior tendon intervening. The phrenic nerve lies deep to the prevertebral layer of the cervical fascia covering the scalenus anterior. By puncturing the skin below the clavicle – at the junction of its middle and medial thirds – the needle is passed upwards and medially in the direction of the sternoclavicular joint. The vein should be entered at its confluence with the internal jugular vein.

NECK AND HEAD VEINS

Venepuncture may be performed above the clavicle in the external and internal jugular veins. For puncture of the external and internal jugular veins, the patient should be lying in a slight Trendelenburg position with the head turned away from the side of puncture. This position provides easy access to and distension of the veins and minimizes the risk of air embolism. Finger pressure just above the middle of the clavicle also produces distension of the external jugular vein.

The external jugular vein, receiving blood from the scalp and face, is formed by the union of the posterior auricular vein and the posterior division of the retromandibular vein (Fig. 4.14). It runs vertically downwards from just behind the angle of the mandible to pass posterior to the clavicle lateral to the sternocleidomastoid tendon, where it terminates in the subclavian vein. In its course, it lies deep to the skin and the platysma muscle, and superficial to the investing layer of the deep cervical fascia and sternocleidomastoid muscle. Puncture of the vein should be made one finger's breadth above the clavicle.

The internal jugular vein (Fig. 4.14) is the continuation of the sigmoid sinus. It runs from its superior bulb (dilation) just below the base of the skull to terminate posterior to the sternoclavicular joint, where its inferior bulb is joined by the subclavian vein to form the brachiocephalic vein. The internal jugular lies deep to the sternocleidomastoid muscle on

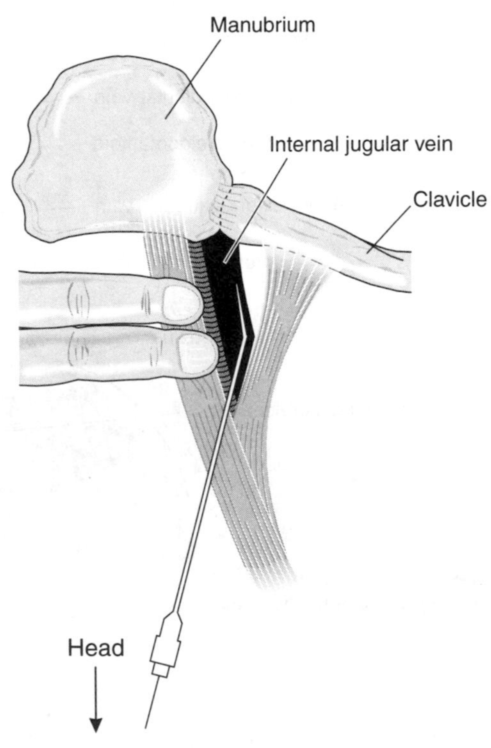

Fig. 4.16
Approach to the right jugular vein. Catheter inserted through cannula.

the lateral side of the internal and common carotid arteries (Fig. 4.15).

It is safest to puncture the internal jugular vein using a 'high approach'. A common technique is to approach the vein at the apex of the triangle formed by the sternal and clavicular heads of sternocleidomastoid muscle (Fig. 4.16). This is usually found at the level of the cricoid cartilage where it may be crossed by the external jugular vein. At this point a needle is directed downwards at an angle of 30° to the skin in the direction of the ipsilateral nipple. If the internal jugular vein is not encountered, the needle is redirected medially. Complications include entry of the common carotid artery, branches of the costocervical trunk, the thoracic duct (on the left side) and damage to the sympathetic trunk. The 'high approach' reduces the chance of injury to the pleura and lung.

On the right side, central venous cannulation is easy as the right internal jugular vein, brachiocephalic vein, superior vena cava and right atrium lie almost in a straight line.

LOWER LIMB VEINS

There are several different patterns of the superficial saphenous system. Various direct and indirect communications exist between the long (great) and short (small) saphenous veins (Fig. 4.17). Throughout their courses, these veins both receive tributaries from the skin and subcutaneous tissues and also give off perforating branches which join the deep veins. The perforating veins normally convey blood from the superficial to the deep system. All the veins of the lower limb have bicuspid valves which are arranged so that blood is directed towards the heart. The flow of blood may be reversed when varicosity of the veins is present.

Dorsal metatarsal veins, which receive blood from the toes, run together to form a dorsal venous arch which lies across the foot over the heads of the metatarsal bones. This dorsal network of veins also receives blood from the sole and sides of the foot. The medial end of the dorsal venous arch is continued as the long saphenous vein, the lateral end continues as the short saphenous. These veins respectively mark the pre- and postaxial borders of the lower limb.

The long saphenous vein lies, with the saphenous nerve, immediately anterior to the medial malleolus at the ankle (Fig. 4.17). As the vein ascends (still accompanied by the saphenous nerve) along the medial side of the leg, it passes obliquely across the lower part of the tibia to become posteromedial at the medial condyles of the tibia and femur. From here, often accompanied by branches of the medial femoral cutaneous nerve, the vein passes upwards and obliquely forwards to pass through the saphenous opening of the deep fascia which lies two finger breadths below and lateral to the pubic tubercle to enter the femoral vein, which lies medial to the femoral artery. When puncturing the long saphenous vein, any perivenous probing with the needle or spread of injection fluid, or the occurrence of a haematoma, may damage the accompanying nerve and cause acute pain in the conscious patient.

Venepuncture may be performed:

- On the dorsum of the foot in the dorsal venous arch or one of its tributaries (Fig. 4.17). This provides the best site in the lower limb for i.v. infusions in the operating theatre.
- On the anteromedial aspect of the leg using either the long saphenous vein or one of its tributaries (Fig. 4.17). The saphenous vein has a thick wall and therefore a sharp needle is required. The lowest part of the vein, in its own fascial sheath, lies in direct contact with the periosteum over the tibia and care should be taken to avoid injuring these structures.

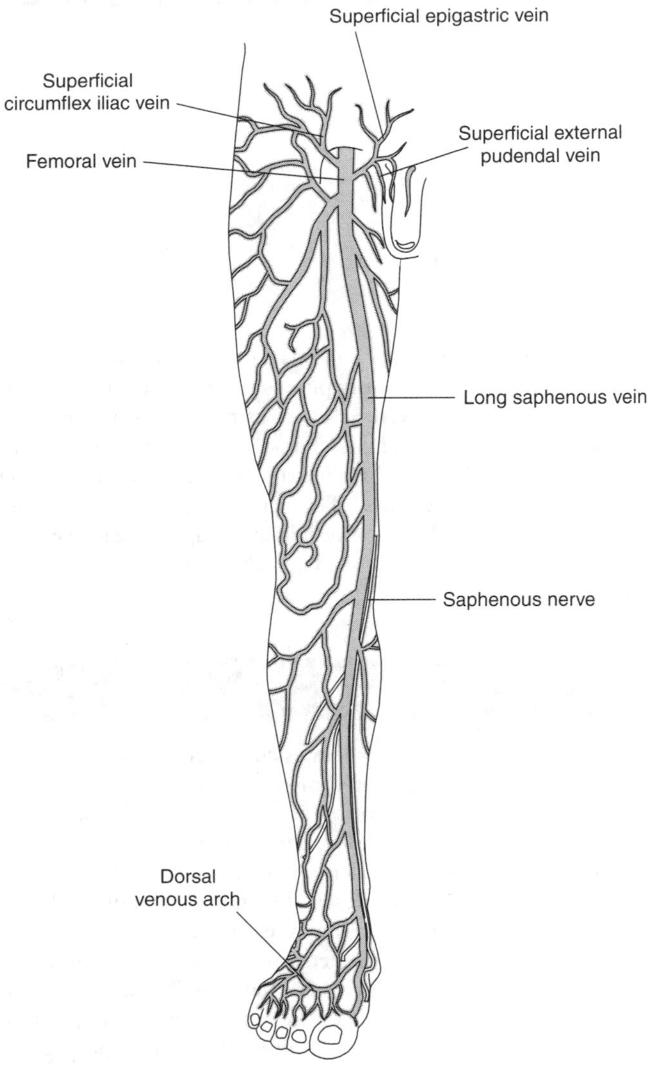

Fig. 4.17
Superficial veins of the right lower limb.

FURTHER READING

Ellis H, Feldman S 1996 Anatomy for Anaesthetists, 7th edn. Blackwell Scientific Publications, Oxford

Moffat DB 1993 Lecture notes in anatomy, 2nd edn. Blackwell Scientific Publications, Oxford

Lumley JSP, Craven JL, Aitken JT 1995 Essential anatomy, 5th edn. Churchill Livingstone, New York

Hwang NC, Sinclair M 1997 Cardiac anaesthesia: a practical handbook, 1st edn. Oxford University Press, New York

5 The heart

The heart consists of four chambers. The two atria serve as reservoirs for blood and as accessory pumps to augment ventricular filling. The right and left ventricles act as pumps propelling blood around the pulmonary and systemic circulations. To function effectively, the full heart chambers must be excited rhythmically and in the proper sequence. The ventricular muscle cells must contract synchronously, with the cells at the apex of each ventricle contracting first to squeeze blood into the pulmonary and the systemic circulations.

THE CARDIAC CELL

The cardiac muscle cell incorporates characteristics of both skeletal and smooth muscle. Striated myofibrils occupy about half the cell volume, the basic unit of the myofibril being the sarcomere. Each sarcomere consists of an orderly array of two proteins, actin and myosin, similar but not identical to skeletal muscle. However, unlike the fibres of striated muscle, the individual muscle fibres in the heart are contained within discrete cell membranes. These cell membranes contain extensive networks of folds which interdigitate and form mechanical links between muscle fibres via special connections termed intercalated discs. In addition, gap junctions between laterally adjacent muscle fibres allow rapid propagation of action potentials between cells.

MYOCARDIAL CONTRACTION

Myocardial contraction is caused by the interaction of actin and myosin, which are seen as thin and thick filaments when viewed under the electron microscope. Individual actin fibres combine to form long-chain double helix structures or thin filaments. These surround thick filaments made from myosin from which protrude cross-bridges with globular heads. Regularly spaced along the thin filament is a complex of two more proteins, tropomyosin and troponin. These proteins regulate the interaction between actin and myosin. Troponin consists of three polypeptides: troponin T (TnT), troponin I (TnI) and troponin C (TnC). TnT binds to tropomyosin, TnI binds to actin to inhibit the reaction of actin with myosin, and TnC binds calcium.

When the myocardial myofibrils are relaxed, tropomyosin lies in a position on the actin helix, and this prevents interaction between the actin and the myosin heads. To initiate myofibril contraction, action potentials at the outer cell membrane are transmitted into the cytoplasm of the cardiac cell by a system of transverse tubules (t-tubules).

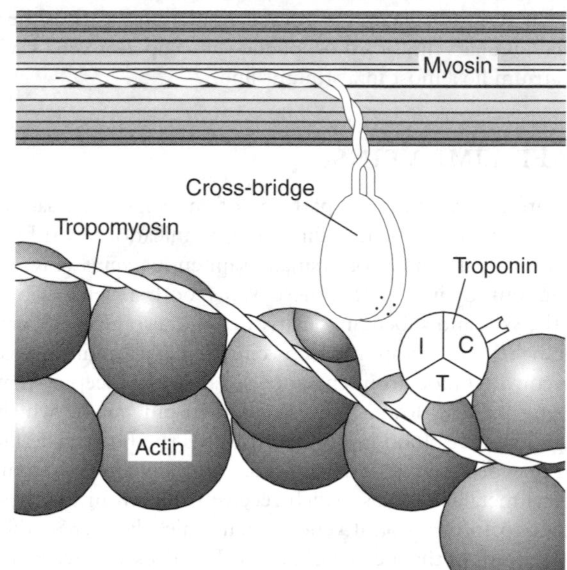

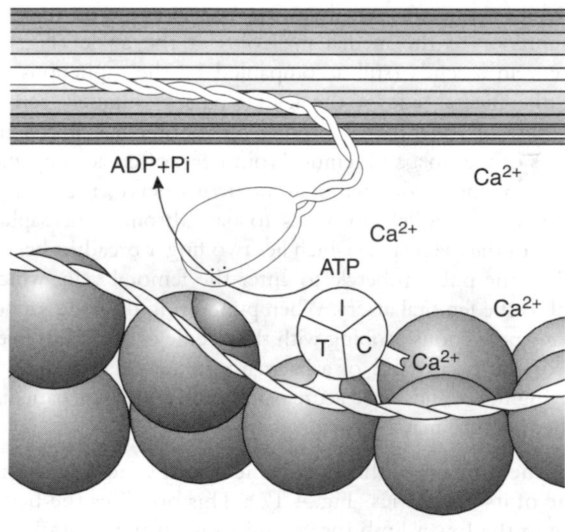

Fig. 5.1
Initiation of muscle contraction. The binding of calcium displaces tropomyosin from actin to troponin, allowing the myosin cross-bridge to bind to actin. (Reproduced with permission from Katz 1975.)

The initial entry of calcium ions into the cell stimulates the release of more calcium ions from the sarcoplasmic reticulum. Intracellular calcium ion concentration then increases from less than 10^{-7} to more than 10^{-5} mmol L^{-1}. These free calcium ions bind to TnC, resulting in a conformational change in troponin such that TnI becomes detached from actin. Tropomyosin then rotates away from its position on the actin helix, allowing a complex cycle of interactions between the actin and myosin and myocardial contraction (Fig. 5.1). The interaction between actin and myosin requires ATP, which is hydrolysed to ADP by a magnesium-dependent ATPase.

Termination of the contraction occurs as calcium is returned to the sarcoplasmic reticulum by an active transport mechanism utilizing a calcium/magnesium ATPase pump, again allowing inhibition of the actin–myosin interaction by using tropomyosin. The ATP required for the whole process is produced by oxidative phosphorylation within the high concentrations of mitochondria present in cardiac cells.

ELECTRICAL PROPERTIES OF CARDIAC MUSCLE CELLS

Action potentials in cardiac muscle cells last much longer than in other electrically excitable cells. The cardiac action potential consists of five phases, which always seem numbered somewhat out of order, i.e. phase 4 (resting), phase 0 (rapid depolarization), phase 1 (partial repolarization), phase 2 (plateau period) and phase 3 (repolarization). Cardiac action potentials vary between non-pacemaker and pacemaker cells and also between cells in different areas of the heart (Fig. 5.2). These differences between cells lie in their permeability to various ions, resulting in differences in cell resting membrane potential and rate of depolarization, which alter the rate of propagation of the action potential through different parts of the heart.

Non-pacemaker cell potentials

Phase 4: resting potential. The resting membrane potential (RMP) of an ordinary ventricular muscle cell is about –90 mV. Essentially, it is the concentration gradient of potassium ions across the membrane which determines the cell resting membrane potential. This may be explained in terms of four interdependent processes.

1. At rest, the cardiac cell membrane has a low permeability to sodium and calcium and a much higher permeability to potassium (about 100 times greater). Consequently, there is little movement of sodium or calcium across the cell membrane at rest, whereas potassium ions are able to cross the cell membrane down their concentration gradient.
2. An active transport sodium/potassium ATPase pump in cardiac cells extrudes sodium ions from the cell in exchange for potassium ions at a ratio of 3:2. As a result, the concentration of potassium ions inside the cell is far greater than that outside.
3. Potassium ions therefore have a tendency to leak out of the cell down this concentration gradient, leaving an accumulation of non-diffusible, negatively charged ions within the cell (proteins, phosphates etc.).
4. As the negative charge increases within the cell, potassium ions are subject to an increasing electrochemical force preventing them from leaving the cell. A balance is finally reached where the tendency for potassium to pass down its concentration gradient is balanced by the resultant electrochemical gradient. Increased permeability of the resting cell membrane to potassium results in a larger (more negative) RMP. Reduced cell membrane permeability to potassium decreases RMP.

Phase 0 (rapid depolarization). The opening of 'fast' sodium channels and 'slow' L-type voltage-dependent calcium channels brings about rapid depolarization. Sodium ions diffuse into the cell causing rapid depolarization. The membrane potential rapidly changes from –90 to +20 mV. The rate of change of potential is dependent on the resting potential. The more negative the resting potential, the more steeply phase 0 increases and the greater the velocity of propagation of the action potential.

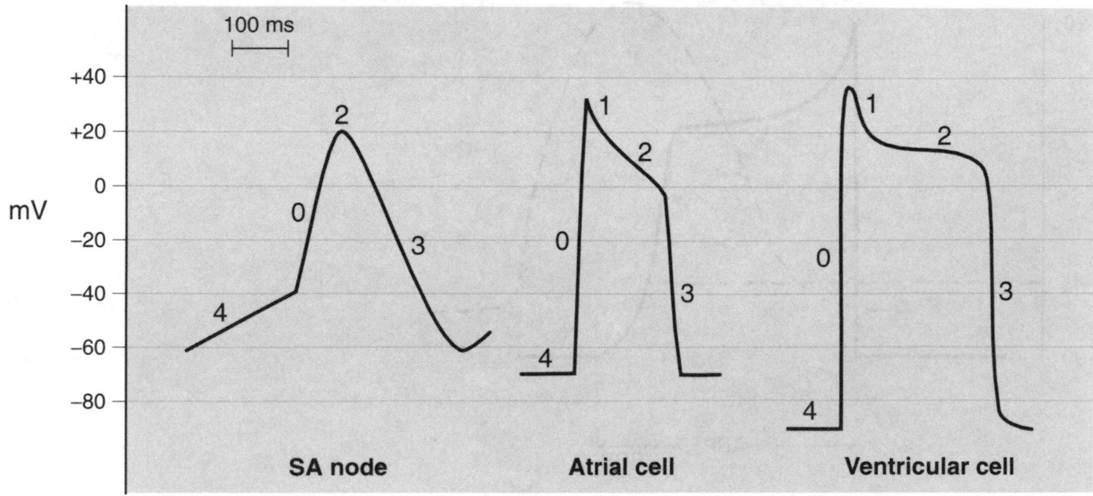

Fig. 5.2
Typical action potentials in different cardiac cells.

Phase 1 (partial repolarization). At the end of phase 0, the fast sodium channels close rapidly, although the permeability of the cell membrane to sodium still remains several times higher than its resting level. As a consequence, the positive potential decreases.

Phase 2 (plateau). Following the initial decline in potential, the membrane potential plateaus at around 0 mV. During phase 2, sodium ion permeability decreases, but the 'slow' calcium channels, which initially open at about –40 mV during phase 0, remain open. Calcium ions therefore continue to enter the cell, keeping the cell polarized. Towards the end of phase 2, calcium ion permeability decreases and this leads to the onset of phase 3.

Phase 3 (rapid repolarization). This is characterized by a rapid fall in potential because of increasing permeability of the membrane to potassium ions. As the cell membrane potential decreases, increasing numbers of potassium channels open. Potassium ions tend to leave the cell, allowing the membrane potential to return to its resting level. The resulting repolarization causes further closure of calcium and sodium channels.

During the action potential, myocardial cells gain sodium and calcium ions and lose potassium ions. The intracellular levels of these ions are restored during phases 3 and 4 of the action potential. Calcium ion concentrations are restored by an active sodium/calcium pump in the cell membrane, which exchanges one ion of intracellular calcium for three ions of extracellular sodium (further increasing intracellular sodium). In addition, a calcium/magnesium ATPase returns calcium ions into the sarcoplasmic reticulum. The sodium/potassium pump, extruding sodium in exchange for potassium, restores sodium and potassium ion concentrations.

Pacemaker cell potentials

Whilst all cardiac cells are capable of producing spontaneous action potentials, these are produced more rapidly in the sinoatrial (SA) node cells, resulting in its function as the pacemaker of the heart. The membrane potentials of cells in the SA node differ significantly from other cardiac cells, having a much larger number of calcium slow channels and a less negative resting membrane potential (–60 mV).

During phase 4, pacemaker cells exhibit spontaneous depolarization. This may occur as a result of two mechanisms:

- There is a progressive reduction in potassium ion permeability, resulting in less potassium leak from the cells and a less negative interior.
- There is a gradual increase in calcium ion permeability, with an increased flow of calcium ions into the cell.

When the membrane potential reaches a critical threshold potential of about –40 mV, many more calcium channels open, resulting in phase 0 depolarization. Thus, in contrast to other cardiac cells, the depolarization phase of the action potential in the SA node cells results mainly from the increase in calcium ion permeability and fast sodium channel involvement is negligible. Partial repolarization and the plateau period are far less pronounced in SA node cells. Phase 3 depolarization is similar to that in non-pacemaker cells, although the absolute refractory period in pacemaker cells is longer.

The action potential of cells in the atrioventricular (AV) node is also dependent upon slow calcium channels rather than on fast sodium channels. This acts to slow conduction through the AV node, allowing sufficient delay between atrial and ventricular contraction.

Refractory period (Fig. 5.3)

While the resting membrane potential remains more positive than about –45 mV, the cardiac muscle cell is insensitive to further

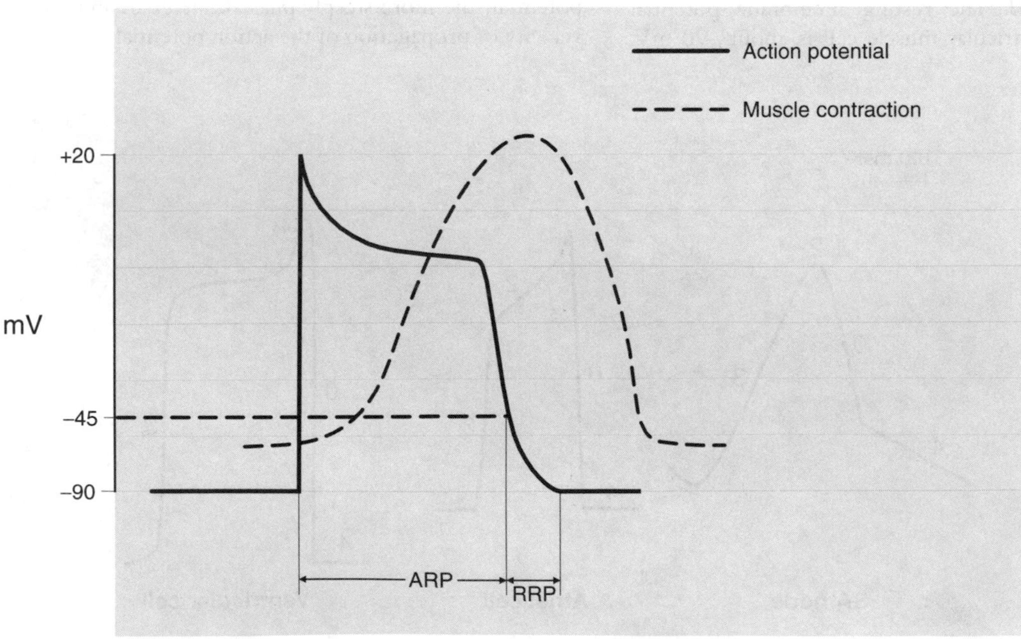

Fig. 5.3
Refractory periods in a ventricular cell. ARP, absolute refractory period; RRP, relative refractory period.

stimulation (absolute refractory period), and for a short period following this, the cell shows reduced sensitivity to additional stimulation (relative refractory period). Contraction of the muscle cell begins soon after the onset of the action potential and peaks towards the end of the plateau phase. Contraction, therefore, occurs entirely within the refractory period and consequently heart muscle cannot be tetanized.

Non-pacemaker action potentials vary between different cardiac cells. Atrial cells have a shorter and less well maintained plateau than do ventricular cells. Purkinje cells have a very rapid phase 0 and the longest plateau.

REGULATION OF HEART RATE

This occurs through the pacemaker cells within the SA node. Electrophysiological alteration of heart rate can occur in one of three ways (Fig. 5.4):

- altering the rate of phase 4 depolarization
- altering the threshold potential
- altering the resting membrane potential.

Many factors influence SA node activity; in particular the SA node has an extensive autonomic innervation. Vagal stimulation results in slowing of the heart rate. Acetylcholine released from vagal nerve endings has two effects:

- It increases the permeability of the cell membrane to potassium, increasing the leak of positively charged potassium ions from the cell and thereby increasing the negative cell resting potential.
- It reduces the cell membrane permeability to calcium ions, reducing the slope of phase 4 depolarization.

Sympathetic nerve stimulation and circulating catecholamines increase the heart rate by increasing the rate of phase 4 depolarization (by increasing calcium ion permeability) and by lowering the threshold potential.

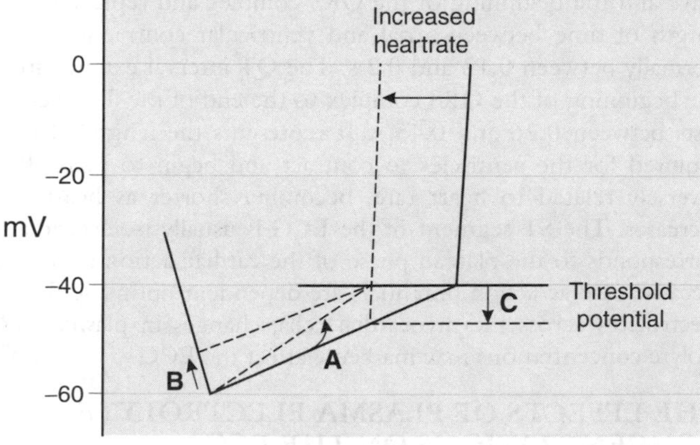

Fig. 5.4
Mechanisms for altering heart rate in a pacemaker cell. A, slope of phase 4; B, resting membrane potential; C, threshold potential.

CARDIAC PERFORMANCE

Cardiac performance may be considered in terms of factors that affect the contraction of isolated heart muscle, and how these factors can be related to the intact heart within the circulating system.

ISOLATED HEART MUSCLE

The three major factors affecting the force, velocity and extent of isolated heart muscle contraction are preload, contractility and afterload.

Preload

When the preload or resting cardiac muscle length is increased, the force of contraction is increased (Starling's law). Increasing the preload increases the maximum force a muscle develops, but does not alter the velocity of force development at a given load.

Contractility

Increasing the inotropic state of cardiac muscle (contractility) produces an increase in the maximum force a muscle develops *and* an increase in the velocity of force development with no change in resting muscle length.

Afterload

When the load against which cardiac muscle is contracting is increased, both the maximum force and the velocity of force development are decreased.

THE INTACT HEART

Within the intact heart, it is much harder to measure preload, afterload or force of contraction directly, so alternative measures are required. Preload is probably best reflected by end-diastolic volume, but ease of measurement has meant that end-diastolic pressures have been used much more widely. Afterload is usually reflected by vascular resistance. For cardiac contractility, many different, variables have been used, including stroke volume (SV), speed of contraction, maximum rate of rise of ventricular pressure, peak ventricular pressure, ejection fraction (SV/end-diastolic volume) and stroke work (SV × [mean arterial pressure (MAP) – mean venous pressure (MVP)]).

Ventricular function curves

By plotting indices of cardiac contractility against indices for preload, a curve is derived which may give an indication of ventricular function, and which may be useful clinically in assessing the response to treatment (Fig. 5.5). A shift of the curve upwards and to the left indicates improved contractility or reduced vascular resistance (afterload). A shift downwards and to the right indicates myocardial depression or increased vascular resistance.

When such curves are plotted using filling pressures rather than volumes, great care is needed in interpretation, because end-diastolic pressure does not relate directly to fibre length and end-diastolic volume. In addition, alterations may occur in ventricular

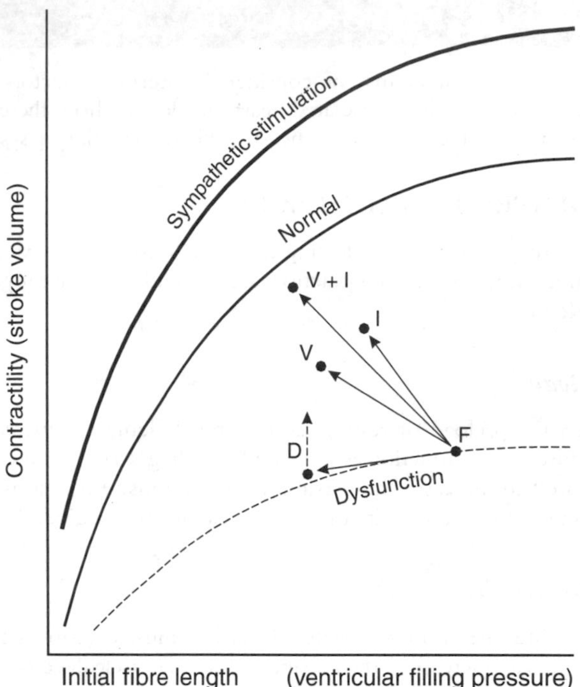

Fig. 5.5
Starling's law of the heart and changes in myocardial contractility. Letters and arrows signify effects of different treatments in cardiac failure. I, inotropic drugs; V, vasodilator drugs; V + I, combined use; D, diuretics; the broken line indicates that ventricular function may improve later.

compliance, changing the relationship between end-diastolic pressure and volume such that a similar end-diastolic pressure represents a significantly different end-diastolic volume.

THE CONDUCTION PATHWAY

Specialized tissues initiate and conduct rhythmic depolarization, causing the myocardial cells to contract in an ordered way (Fig. 5.6). The SA node lies in the wall of the right atrium medial to the superior vena cava (SVC). Spontaneously generated action potentials from pacemaker cells in the SA node sweep through the atrium via anterior, middle and posterior internodal tracks to the AV node. Impulses also pass from cell to cell within the atrium via gap junctions. Impulses spread throughout the atria at a rate of 0.5–1 ms^{-1}.

The AV node lies in the right atrium just above and medial to the tricuspid valve and gives rise to the AV bundle (bundle of His). Conduction in the AV node is slow and the impulse is delayed 0.1–0.2 s, before passing rapidly (1–4 ms^{-1}) down the AV bundle. The AV bundle passes through a fibrous opening into the interventricular septum and divides into the right and left bundle branches, which pass to the apices of the right and left ventricles. The right bundle supplies the right ventricle. The left bundle further divides within the interventricular septum into anterior superior and posterior inferior divisions (fascicles), to supply the left ventricle. At their terminal ends, these bundles continue to divide to form the Purkinje fibres, which consist of broad cells with sparse myofibrils but extensive intercalated discs. These cells do not contract forcefully, but the action potentials travel along them much more rapidly than other cardiac cells and allow rapid conduction of impulses to all parts of the ventricle.

The wave of depolarization initiates cardiac muscle contraction. The right atrium contracts just before the left atrium. The delay in the AV node allows time for the atria to empty into the ventricles, before they in turn contract, with the left preceding the right by 10–30 ms. Within the ventricles, excitation of muscle fibres spreads from endocardium to epicardium. The interventricular septum is activated first, followed by the apical regions and finally the bases. The interventricular septum and papillary muscles are therefore the first parts of the ventricles to contract. Septal contraction anchors the heart and papillary muscle tightening prevents prolapse of the tricuspid and mitral valves during ejection. Apical contraction occurring just before basal contraction ensures maximal efficiency in ventricular ejection.

THE ELECTROCARDIOGRAPH (ECG)

The electrical currents generated by cardiac muscle during depolarization and repolarization may be measured at the skin surface. The ECG reflects the summated electrical activity of cardiac action potentials. It may indicate rate and rhythm, abnormal conduction pathways, myocardial damage and hypertrophy or atrophy of areas of the heart. It does not reflect the adequacy of mechanical contraction. Normal complexes may be observed in the absence of mechanical activity. The normal ECG consists of a P wave, QRS complex and T wave (Fig. 5.7).

The P wave is the electrical current produced by atrial depolarization. It lasts between 0.07 and 0.14 s, and signals the onset of atrial contraction. The QRS complex results from ventricular depolarization and signals the onset of ventricular contraction. Normally the complex is narrow, lasting between 0.06 and 0.1 s. Widening of the QRS occurs if the conduction pathway is abnormal. The height of the QRS complex is increased with ventricular hypertrophy and may also be increased when conduction is altered, e.g. by ischaemia or electrolyte imbalances. The T wave represents repolarization of the ventricles and precedes ventricular relaxation. Following the T wave, there is sometimes a small after-potential (U wave).

The PR interval is the time between the beginning of the P wave and the beginning of the QRS complex and represents the length of time between atrial and ventricular contraction. It is normally between 0.12 and 0.2 s. The QT interval extends from the beginning of the QRS complex to the end of the T wave and lasts between 0.26 and 0.45 s. It represents the length of time required for the ventricles to contract and begin to relax. It is inversely related to heart rate, becoming shorter as heart rate increases. The ST segment of the ECG is usually isoelectric and corresponds to the plateau phase of the cardiac action potential. Because cardiac action potentials are dependent upon the flux of electrolytes across the myocardial cells, changes in plasma electrolyte concentrations may markedly affect the ECG.

THE EFFECTS OF PLASMA ELECTROLYTE CONCENTRATIONS ON THE ECG

Calcium

Calcium affects depolarization (phase 4 and phase 0) in the SA and AV nodes, and the plateau (phase 2) period in other myocardial

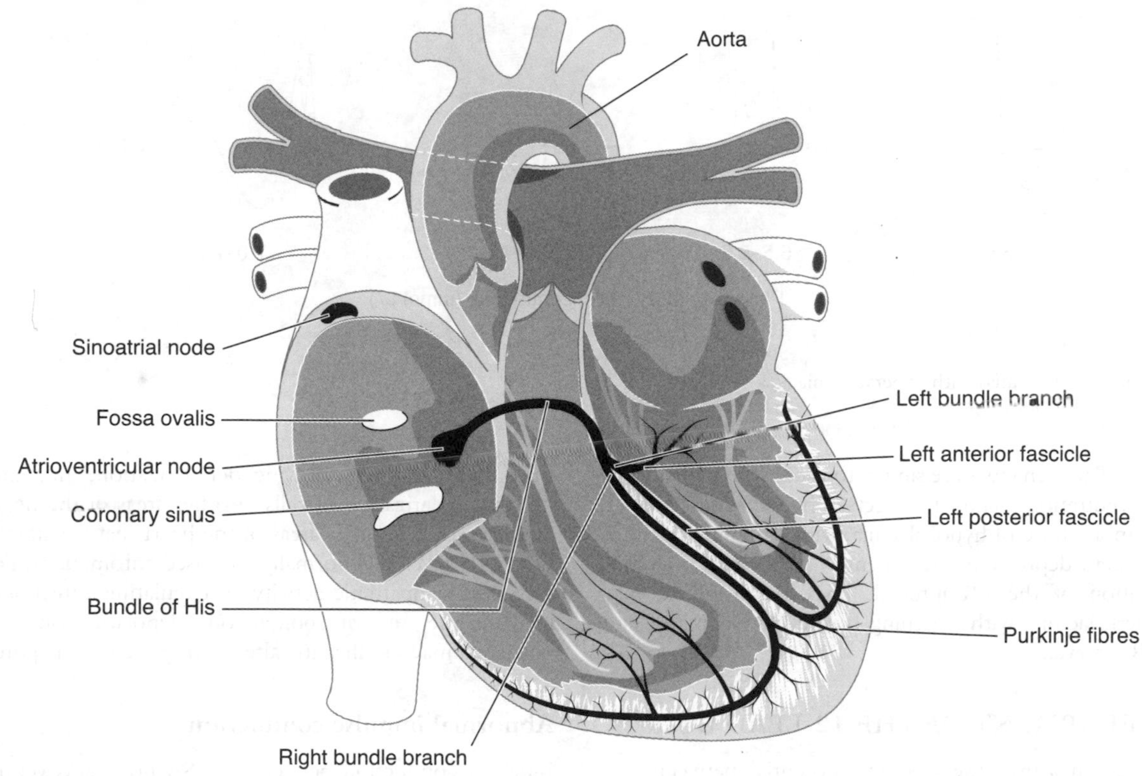

Fig. 5.6
The cardiac conducting system.

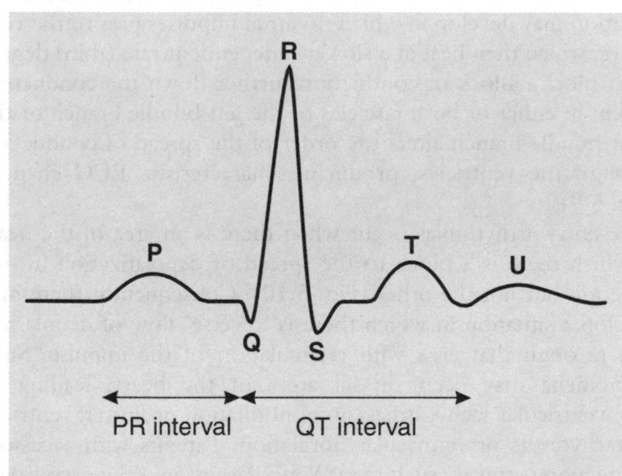

Fig. 5.7
The ECG.

cells. The main effects of abnormal plasma calcium ion concentrations on the ECG are the result of changes in the plateau phase of the action potential, which affects the QT interval.

Hypercalcaemia increases the rate at which calcium passes into the cell when calcium channels are open. This results in a reduction in the duration of the plateau and shortening of the QT interval. Conversely, hypocalcaemia prolongs the QT interval.

Potassium

The effects of changes in plasma potassium ion concentrations on the ECG are the result mainly of alterations in the cell resting potential. In hyperkalaemia, increasing plasma concentrations of potassium reduce the tendency for potassium to leave the cell down its concentration gradient. As a result, more positive ions remain inside the cell and there is a reduction in the myocardial cell resting membrane potential. This decreases the rate of phase 0 depolarization, slowing impulse conduction. In addition, during phase 3 repolarization, when the cell membrane potential is positive, and potassium channels are open, potassium ions tend to leave the cell more quickly. This accelerates repolarization, leading to tall peaked narrow T waves. Further increases in plasma potassium levels lead to increasingly prolonged impulse conduction. There is broadening and flattening of the P wave, a decrease in R wave height, widening of QRS complexes, and ST segment changes. Intraventricular block may then develop, and ultimately asystole or ventricular fibrillation (Fig. 5.8).

Hypokalaemia increases the cell resting membrane potential, increasing the rate of depolarization but reducing the rate of repolarization. This leads to flattening and widening of the T wave and increased U wave height. Increased cardiac irritability increases the risk of cardiac arrhythmias.

Magnesium

Magnesium is essential for intracellular cardiac cell function, and minor ECG changes may be associated with altered plasma

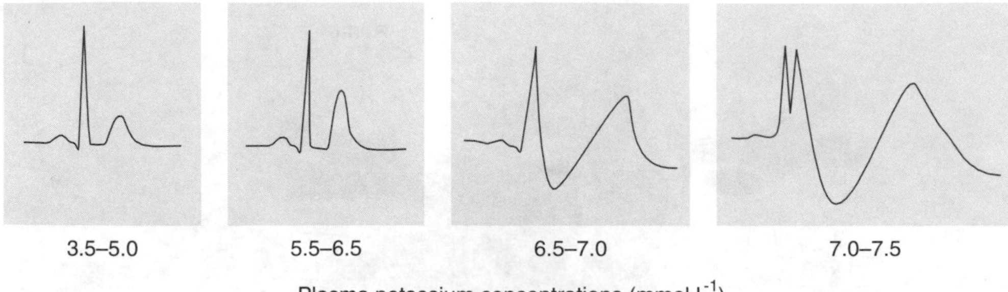

Fig. 5.8
Typical ECG changes associated with hyperkalaemia.

concentrations. These changes are similar to those seen with altered potassium concentrations. Thus the effects of hypomagnesaemia on the ECG resemble those of hypokalaemia, with flattening of the T waves, ST-segment depression, prominent U waves and, occasionally, prolongation of the PR interval. Hypermagnesaemia may resemble hyperkalaemia, with widening of the QRS complex and prolonged PR interval.

THE DEVELOPMENT OF THE 12-LEAD ECG

Each ECG lead measures the electrical potential between two electrodes, one negative and one positive. Current flowing towards the positive electrode results in an upward deflection of the ECG, and current flowing away from the positive electrode results in a downward deflection.

Eindhoven originally described the detection of current between electrodes placed on the right arm, left arm and left leg. This resulted in three bipolar limb leads, I, II and III, which formed an equilateral triangle around the heart (lead I: right arm negative, left arm positive; lead II: right arm negative, left leg positive; lead III: left arm negative, left leg positive). Unipolar leads were then added which measured the potential between an exploring positive electrode and a central terminal located at the centre of the heart, which was formed by combining the right arm, left arm and left leg leads. It was subsequently found that for the limb leads, the amplitude of the recorded potential was augmented if the connection to the limb for which the potential was being recorded was omitted from the combined electrode, and these leads were termed augmented limb leads (aVR, aVL and aVF). The addition of these three augmented leads and six unipolar precordial leads (V_1 to V_6) gave rise to the modern 12-lead ECG.

MECHANISMS OF CARDIAC ARRHYTHMIAS

Arrhythmias may be caused by either abnormal impulse initiation or abnormal impulse conduction. Either problem may lead to brady- or tachyarrhythmias.

Abnormal impulse initiation

Many cells have the potential for automatic depolarization. Normally, impulses generated in the sinus node and spreading through the heart cause depolarization of these cells before they depolarize spontaneously. Disease of the SA node or excessive vagal stimulation, by slowing depolarization, may allow spontaneous depolarization of cells in other areas of the heart to occur. Similarly, cells in other areas of the heart may be altered in such a way as to develop abnormally increased automaticity. For example, increased sympathetic activity or circulating catecholamines may increase the rate of spontaneous depolarization in cells, and ischaemia may significantly alter resting membrane potential.

Abnormal impulse conduction

Block of conduction between the SA node and ventricular cells may be partial or complete. Slowing of conduction near the AV node or in the AV bundle results in prolongation of the PR interval on the ECG (first degree heart block). If the block worsens, this can progress to a situation where some atrial beats are not followed by ventricular beats (second degree heart block). Finally a situation may develop in which no atrial impulses pass to the ventricles, which then beat at a slower independent rate (third degree heart block). Block of conduction further down the conducting system in either or both fascicles of the left bundle branch or the right bundle branch alters the order of the spread of conduction through the ventricles, producing characteristic ECG changes (Fig. 5.9).

Re-entry arrhythmias occur when there is an area of the heart in which there is a block to the spread of depolarization in one direction but not the other (Fig. 5.10). Consequently, there may develop a situation in which there is 'reverse' flow of depolarization through that area with recirculation of the impulse. Such phenomena may occur in all areas of the heart, leading to supraventricular tachycardias, atrial fibrillation or flutter, ventricular tachycardia or ventricular fibrillation. Patients with accessory conduction pathways such as in Wolff–Parkinson–White syndrome are particularly at risk of developing arrhythmias by this route.

CORONARY BLOOD SUPPLY

Myocardial cells receive an abundant blood supply, contain numerous mitochondria in which energy is produced, and have an increased myoglobin content which acts as an oxygen store. The great majority of the energy used by cardiac cells is provided by aerobic metabolism in the form of ATP. At rest, less than 1% of energy is produced anaerobically, although this proportion can

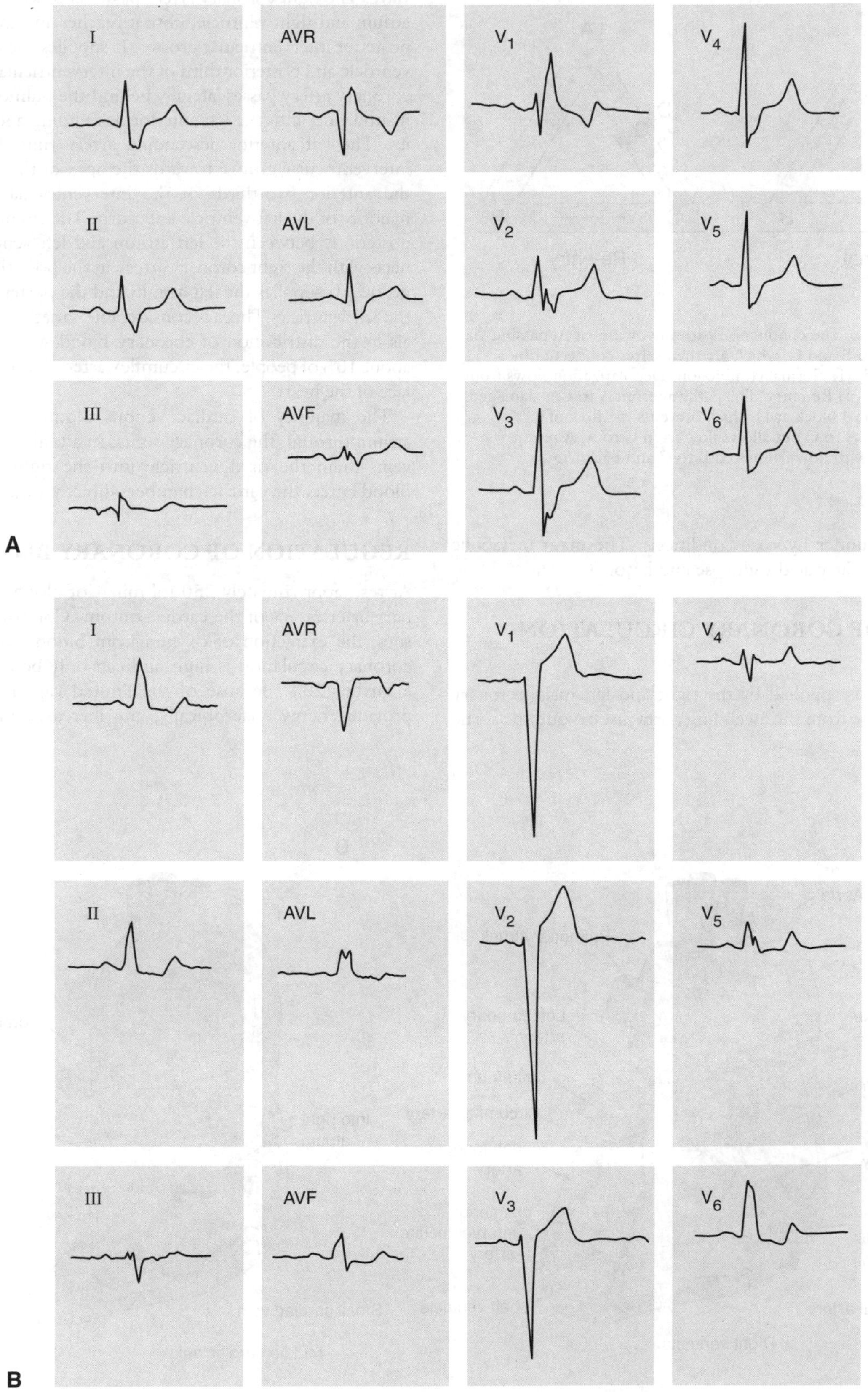

Fig. 5.9
Typical 12-lead ECG seen in bundle branch block. **A.** Right bundle branch block. **B.** Left bundle branch block.

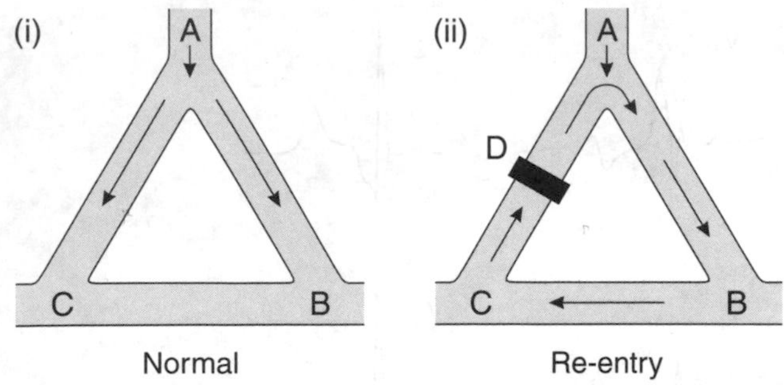

Fig. 5.10
Re-entry arrhythmias. The conduction pathway divides at A, passing via separate pathways to B and C, which are themselves connected by a conduction pathway. (i) Normal conduction. Depolarization flows from A to both B and C. (ii) Re-entry. The pathway from A to C is damaged. There is unidirectional block at D which prevents the flow of depolarization from A to C but allows flow from C to A. A re-entry circuit is produced with flow from A to B to C and back to A.

increase to 10% under hypoxic conditions. The main metabolic substrates are free fatty acids, glucose and ketones.

ANATOMY OF CORONARY CIRCULATION (Fig. 5.11)

The myocardium is supplied by the right and left main coronary arteries, which arise from the ascending aorta just beyond the aortic valve. The right coronary artery passes anteriorly between the right atrium and right ventricle, until it reaches and then runs down the posterior interventricular groove. It supplies the right atrium, right ventricle and posterior third of the interventricular septum. The left coronary artery passes laterally behind the pulmonary artery where it subdivides into the left anterior descending and circumflex arteries. The left anterior descending artery runs down the anterior interventricular groove towards the apex of the heart and supplies the anterior two-thirds of the interventricular septum and the majority of the left ventricle anteriorly. The circumflex artery passes posteriorly between the left atrium and left ventricle until it connects with the right coronary artery in the posterior interventricular groove. It supplies the left atrium and the posterolateral portion of the left ventricle. There is considerable variation between individuals in the distribution of coronary blood supply. For example, in about 10% of people, the circumflex artery supplies the inferior surface of the heart.

The majority of cardiac venous blood returns to the right atrium through the coronary sinus. In addition, anterior coronary veins drain the right ventricle into the right atrium and some blood enters the cardiac chambers directly via the thebesian veins.

REGULATION OF CORONARY BLOOD FLOW

At rest, approximately 250 ml min^{-1} of blood perfuses the coronary arteries, 5% of the cardiac output. Compared with other tissues, the extraction of oxygen from blood passing through the coronary circulation is high and can only be increased by about a further 20%. Because of the limited capacity of the heart to provide energy anaerobically, any increased myocardial oxygen

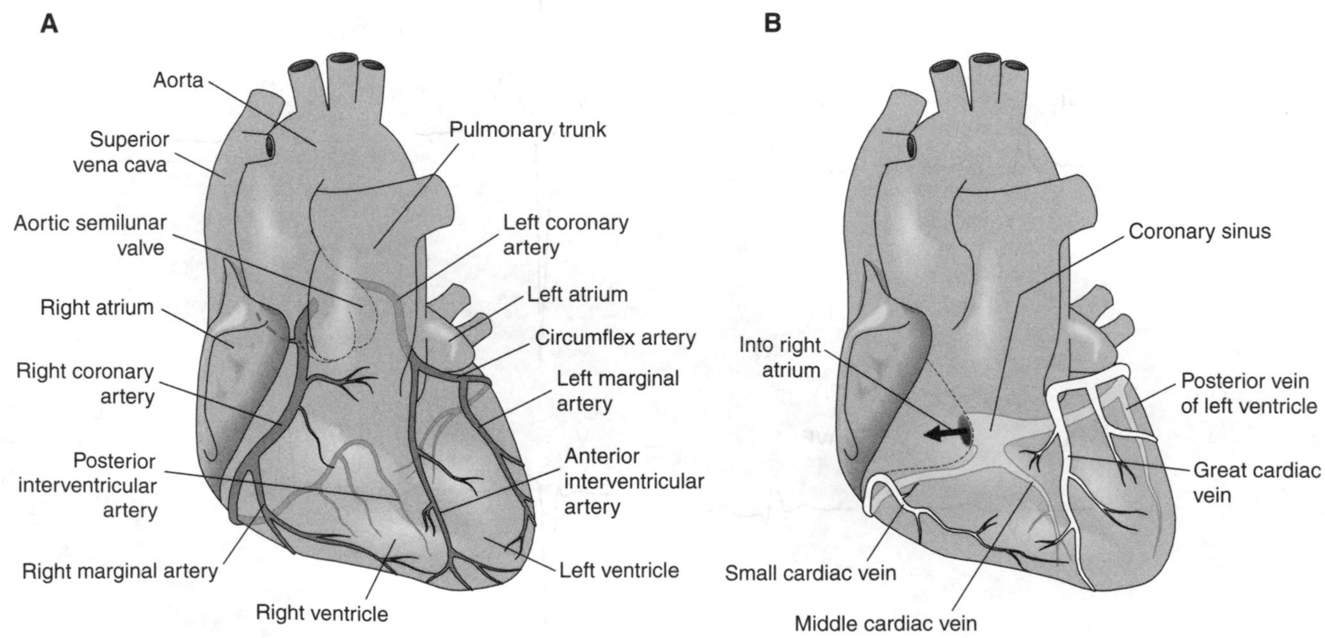

Fig. 5.11
The coronary circulation. **A.** Arterial supply. **B.** Venous drainage. (Reproduced with permission from Seeley et al 1999.)

demand must be met by improving the oxygen supply by altering coronary blood flow.

At rest, the coronary vasculature is relatively constricted. Increased metabolic demands are therefore met by appropriate coronary vasodilatation, which increases coronary blood flow up to fivefold. There are two mechanisms involved in the regulation of coronary blood flow, localized metabolic control and neurohumoral control.

Metabolic control of coronary blood flow

Inadequate blood supply to areas of the heart results in hypoxia and the accumulation of myocardial metabolites (such as carbon dioxide, phosphate, adenosine, prostaglandins, hydrogen ions and potassium ions). Some of these metabolites have a major effect on the coronary vasculature, dilating small arterioles and precapillary sphincters to increase local coronary flow. Local metabolism thus has a major role in regulating coronary blood flow.

Neurohumoral control of coronary blood flow

The coronary vessels are innervated by both sympathetic and parasympathetic fibres, but the role of the autonomic nervous system in controlling coronary blood flow is probably minor compared with local effects.

DISTRIBUTION OF CORONARY BLOOD FLOW

Differences in intraventricular pressures created during cardiac systole result in significant differences in the pattern of perfusion between right and left ventricles. During left ventricular systole, myocardial contraction results in the production of a large intraventricular pressure. This pressure is transmitted across the ventricular wall, progressively increasing from epicardium to endocardium to subendocardium. The pressure in the subendocardial layer of the myocardium exceeds systolic arterial pressure. Consequently, there is no subendocardial blood flow during systole, and flow occurs in the arteries supplying the subendocardium of the left ventricle only during diastole. Lower pressures in the outer muscle layers of the left ventricle result in some systolic blood flow. In the right ventricle, the lower intraventricular pressures result in flow to all areas of the heart throughout the cardiac cycle.

MYOCARDIAL ISCHAEMIA

Myocardial ischaemia occurs when oxygen demand outstrips supply. Heart rate, myocardial contractility and ventricular wall tension determine myocardial oxygen demand. Myocardial oxygen supply is determined mainly by coronary blood flow.

As a result of differences in blood flow distribution, the subendocardium of the left ventricle is the area most vulnerable to ischaemia. As blood flow to this area occurs only during diastole, its oxygen supply effectively depends upon:

- the difference between aortic diastolic pressure and left ventricular end-diastolic pressure (the perfusion pressure)
- the duration of diastole (time available for flow).

Obviously, coronary artery vasodilatation usually compensates for reduced flow. However, when it reaches its limit, myocardial ischaemia occurs.

The risk of myocardial ischaemia is increased in conditions of increased myocardial oxygen demand and/or reduced coronary blood flow. Some situations therefore increase the risk of patients developing myocardial ischaemia. The obvious patients at risk are those with coronary artery disease, where obstruction to flow reduces myocardial perfusion. However, other conditions also put patients at risk of ischaemia. The hypertensive patient is at risk because of the increased work of the heart pumping against a higher afterload. The patient with chronic heart failure is at risk because increased left ventricular end-diastolic pressure (LVEDP) reduces perfusion pressure. Patients with aortic stenosis are at risk because of the decreased perfusion pressure that exists in the post-stenotic dilatation, where the origins of the coronary arteries (coronary ostia) lie. In such conditions, increased myocardial demand (tachycardia, profound hypertension, use of inotropic agents) or further reductions in supply (hypotension, reduced diastolic time in tachycardia) add further to the risk of myocardial ischaemia. In addition, anaemia and hypoxaemia, by reducing the oxygen content of blood, may also precipitate myocardial ischaemia in at-risk individuals.

ECG changes in myocardial ischaemia

As discussed previously, the heart has very limited capacity for anaerobic metabolism and there is no capacity for developing oxygen debt. With cessation of coronary arterial supply, the oxygen stores in myoglobin are rapidly exhausted and contraction stops. Hydrogen ions, adenosine and other compounds accumulate, and there is accelerated opening of potassium channels, resulting in more rapid repolarization of the damaged muscle cells. The sodium/potassium pump then begins to fail, and as their resting membrane potential decreases, ischaemic myocardial cells show a slower rate of increase of the action potential and a poorly sustained plateau. Consequently, during systole, ischaemic cells have a less positive potential than normal cells and there is flow of current from normal to ischaemic cells. This may be seen as ST-segment changes in an ECG electrode overlying the ischaemic area. During diastole, ischaemic cells have a less negative potential than normal cells and current flows from ischaemic to normal cells, resulting in reciprocal QT segment changes on the overlying ECG, exaggerating the ST changes already seen. Generally, subendocardial ischaemia produces ST-segment depression and subepicardial ischaemia ST elevation. Mild ischaemia may result in T-wave changes only, if it is just the repolarization phase of the action potential that is affected, with the resting membrane potential of affected cells remaining normal.

THE CARDIAC CYCLE

The orderly contraction and relaxation of cardiac muscle cells results in cyclical changes in pressures and volumes within the heart chambers (the cardiac cycle) (Fig. 5.12). Obviously, atrial contraction follows atrial depolarization and ventricular contraction follows ventricular depolarization. Thus atrial systole starts just after the P wave of the ECG; ventricular systole starts at the end of the R wave and ends just after the T wave. In describing the events of the cardiac cycle, it is easiest to divide the cycle into three stages: ventricular filling, ventricular systole, and isovolumic ventricular relaxation.

Ventricular filling

During ventricular diastole, the ventricular muscle relaxes and ventricular pressure decreases below atrial pressure. The AV valves open and blood which has accumulated in the atria enters the ventricles, which begin to fill. Most ventricular filling occurs during the first third of ventricular diastole. As the pressures in the atria and ventricles equalize, the flow into the ventricles is reduced so that there is little ventricular filling during the second third of ventricular diastole. This rapid initial filling of the ventricle is important because, as a consequence, the heart rate may increase without significantly reducing filling.

Atrial systole begins during the final third of ventricular diastole. Atrial contraction therefore completes ventricular filling. At normal heart rates, atrial contraction does not contribute much to ventricular filling. However, as the heart rate increases, atrial contraction adopts an increasingly important role. Consequently, when atrial contraction is ineffectual, such as in atrial fibrillation, the heart is able to function satisfactorily at lower ventricular rates, but may become compromised at higher ventricular rates.

Ventricular systole

Ventricular contraction leads to a rapid increase in ventricular pressure. When ventricular pressure exceeds atrial pressure, the AV valves close, leading to the first heart sound. The pressure within the ventricle continues to increase, but at this stage there is little muscle shortening. This period is termed isovolumetric contraction.

When the pressure in the ventricle exceeds that in either the pulmonary artery or the aorta depending upon the ventricle, the semilunar valves open and blood flows into the corresponding artery. This period is termed ventricular ejection. Ejection is initially rapid and then slows. Towards the end of ventricular systole, intraventricular pressure starts to decrease.

Isovolumic ventricular relaxation

At the end of ventricular systole, the ventricles suddenly relax. The already declining ventricular pressure now decreases rapidly. When the pressure in the ventricle is lower than that in the pulmonary artery or aorta, the semilunar valves close, leading to the second heart sound. The ventricular pressure continues to decrease as the ventricular muscle relaxes. However, at this stage there is no flow of blood into or out of the ventricle until the ventricular pressure decreases below atrial pressure. At this point, the AV valves open again and ventricular filling commences.

Although one tends to think of the two ventricles as contracting and relaxing together, there are slight differences in the timing of their contractions and in the opening and closing of the cardiac valves. The left ventricle begins to contract just before the right. Left ventricular pressure therefore increases slightly before right ventricular pressure, and the mitral valve closes before the tricuspid valve. However, because pulmonary artery pressure is much lower than aortic pressure, the pulmonary valve opens first and right ventricular ejection begins before the left. Similarly, the higher aortic pressures result in the aortic valve closing before the pulmonary valve at the end of ventricular systole. At the end of isovolumic relaxation, the lower right ventricular pressures lead to the tricuspid valve opening before the mitral valve.

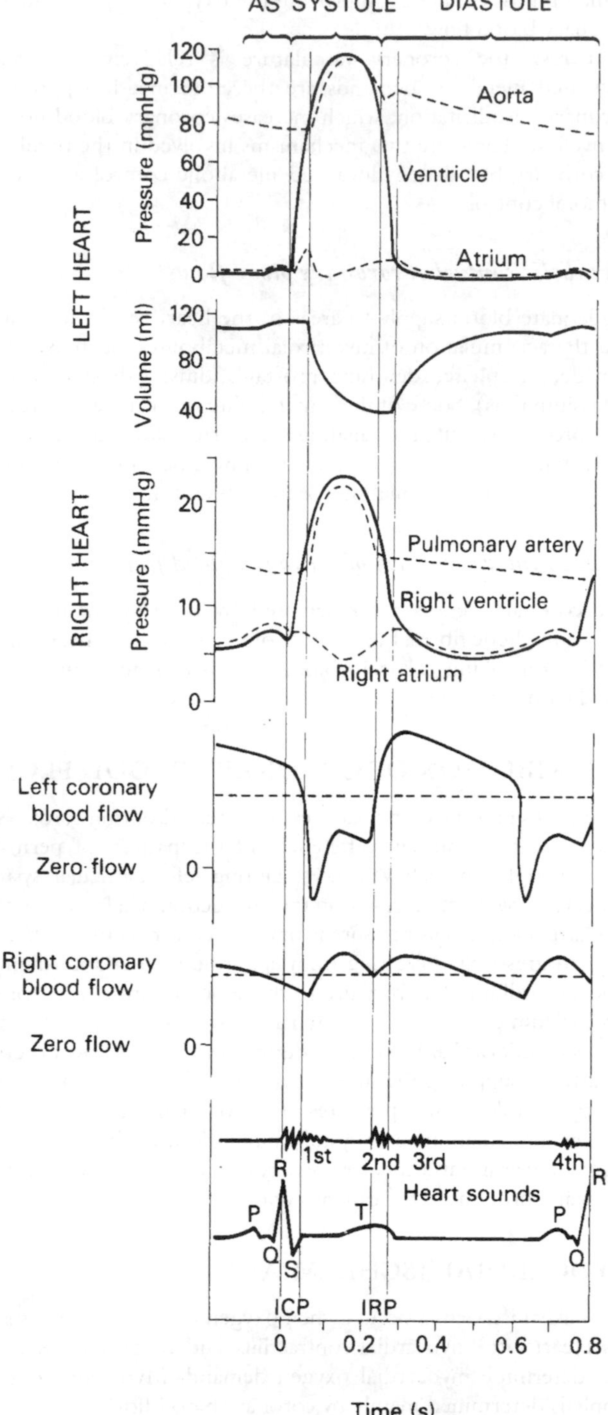

Fig. 5.12
The cardiac cycle.

ATRIAL PRESSURE CHANGES DURING THE CARDIAC CYCLE

Pressures within the right and left atrial chambers show several fluctuations during the cardiac cycle, producing characteristic waveforms, which may be seen during central venous and pulmonary artery monitoring. The waveform is described in terms of a-, c- and v-waves, and x- and y-descents.

The a-wave occurs just after the P wave on the ECG and is caused by atrial contraction at the end of ventricular filling. Ventricular systole then follows, and as the ventricles contract, the AV valves are pulled downwards, lowering atrial pressures and resulting in the x-descent. When ventricular pressure exceeds atrial pressure, the AV valves snap closed, bulging into the atria and resulting in a temporary increase in atrial pressure seen as the c-wave. The v-wave represents increasing atrial pressure during atrial diastole as refilling of the atria occurs. The y-descent then follows, representing the decrease in atrial pressure which occurs at the end of isovolumic ventricular relaxation, when the AV valves open to allow ventricular filling to begin.

AORTIC PRESSURE CHANGES DURING THE CARDIAC CYCLE

As the left ventricle contracts and then relaxes, blood enters the aorta and flows around the body. However, the pressure waveform in the aorta differs significantly from that in the left ventricle, because of the aortic valve and the elastic properties of the aorta itself.

During left ventricular contraction, the walls of the aorta stretch as blood is forced out of the left ventricle, with a resulting pressure wave that is similar to left ventricular pressure. However, as left ventricular pressure decreases towards the end of ventricular systole and the beginning of ventricular relaxation, the elastic recoil of the aorta forces blood back towards the heart. Consequently, the aortic valve closes. This leads to a temporary increase in the falling aortic pressure, seen as the dicrotic notch in the pressure waveform. The aortic pressure then continues to decrease throughout ventricular diastole. However, the elastic recoil of the aorta and other large arteries maintains a much higher pressure in the arterial tree during diastole than is seen in the ventricles. This allows continuing forward flow of blood into the peripheral vessels and capillaries towards the low-pressure venous system.

FURTHER READING

Katz A M 1975 Congestive heart failure: role of altered myocardial cellular control. New England Journal of Medicine 293: 1184–1191

Seeley R R, Stephens T D, Tate P 1999 Essentials of anatomy and physiology, 3rd edn. McGraw Hill, London

6 Peripheral circulation and control of cardiac output and arterial pressure

The function of the cardiovascular system is to provide blood flow through the capillaries of the organs of the body at a pressure that allows adequate tissue perfusion in order to deliver oxygen and nutrients and to remove products of metabolism. It also acts as a conduit for the cells of the immune system and hormones.

STRUCTURE OF THE PERIPHERAL CIRCULATION

The peripheral circulation comprises arteries, arterioles, capillaries, veins and venules. Each of these components has an important role in maintaining the function of the cardiovascular system and possesses a structure consistent with its role. The structure of the typical vessel (Fig. 6.1) consists of an endothelial layer of cells separated from a layer of smooth muscle by the internal elastic lamina; the outer border of the smooth muscle is separated from the thick adventitia by the external elastic lamina.

VASCULAR ENDOTHELIUM

Endothelium was, until recently, thought to be a metabolically inert permeability membrane lining blood vessels. It is now known that it is a metabolically dynamic tissue with diverse functions.

The patency of blood vessels and prevention of thrombogenesis are maintained by the production of thrombomodulin, tissue plasminogen activator, heparin, prostacyclin and nitric oxide.

The endothelium is central to the manifestation of the acute inflammatory response by facilitating the adherence of activated neutrophils and their subsequent migration from the circulation to the tissues. This is due to the expression of cellular adhesion molecules [vascular cellular adhesion molecules (VCAMs) and intercellular adhesion molecules (ICAMs)] on the endothelial cell surface.

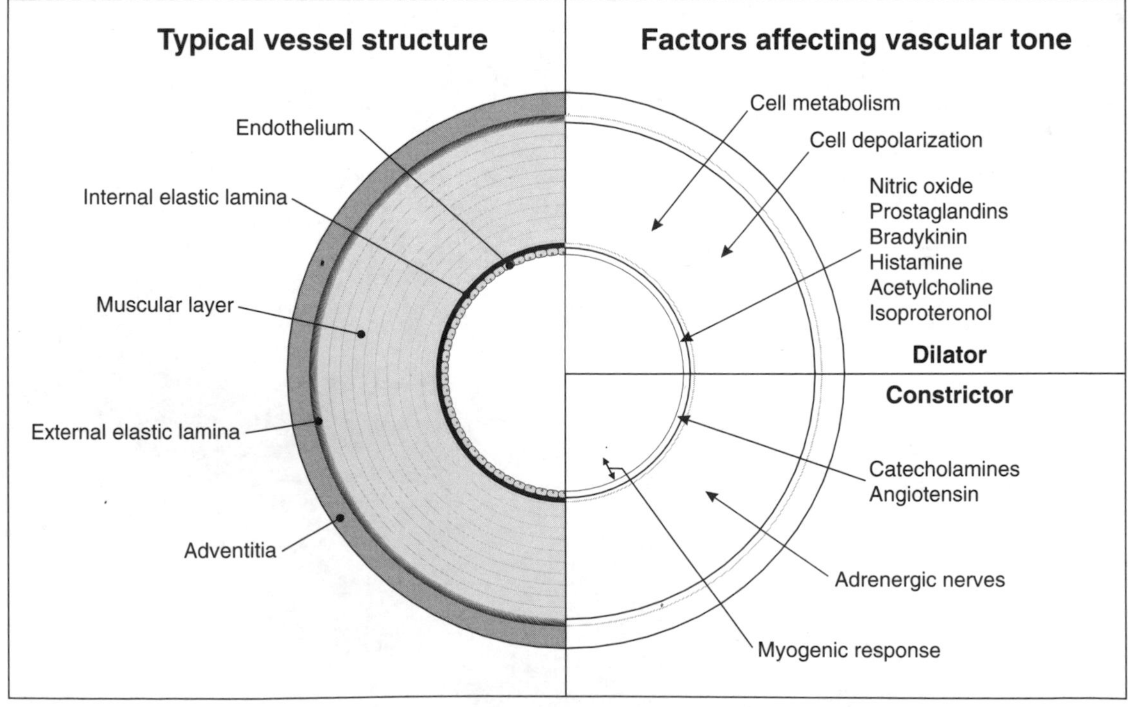

Fig. 6.1
Cross-section of a blood vessel.

The endothelium also produces substances that diffuse into the smooth muscle layers to alter vascular tone. Nitric oxide, formerly termed endothelium-derived relaxing factor (EDRF), is produced from L-arginine by the enzyme nitric oxide synthase in the endothelial cell. The nitric oxide synthase enzyme has several isoforms. It is present in the endothelium in both its constitutive (calcium and calmodulin-dependent enzyme) form, which is probably responsible for basal release of nitric oxide, and an inducible form (independent of calcium and calmodulin) responsible for increased nitric oxide release in the presence of lipopolysaccharide and cytokines. The production of nitric oxide results in smooth muscle relaxation and vasodilatation. The endothelium also produces endothelins that act either as potent vasoconstrictors or as vasodilators. Three distinct endothelin molecules have been described (ET-1, ET-2 and ET-3) and two receptor subtypes (A and B) have been cloned. Only the ETB receptor is found on the vascular endothelium.

SMOOTH MUSCLE AND ELASTIC TISSUE

Although present to some extent in venules and veins, these tissues are much more predominant in arteries and arterioles. Elastic tissue predominates in the major arteries, and smooth muscle in the peripheral arteries.

Elastic tissue in the artery wall allows the kinetic energy of pulse generation by the heart to be converted to potential energy. This effectively damps the systolic pressure wave generated by the ventricle. This reduces both the peak pressure that would be generated and the diastolic pressure decrease that would occur in a non-elastic vessel.

Smooth muscle controls the calibre of the vessels. The calibre is dependent on the inherent tone of the muscle, the activity of the autonomic nervous system, circulating hormones and the local concentration of metabolites. Smooth muscle generally exhibits spontaneous contraction in the absence of other stimuli and this is the likely source of inherent tone. Mechanical stretching of the muscle by pulsatile internal pressure may also initiate contractions. In general, tissues with the least sympathetic innervation have the greatest inherent tone. For example, vessels in skeletal muscle, brain and myocardium have a high tone, whereas those in skin have a low inherent tone.

Autonomic nervous system innervation of blood vessels

Sympathetic adrenergic (Fig. 6.2)

The adrenergic sympathetic innervation of blood vessels forms the predominant pathway through which the systemic circulation is controlled. The vasomotor area in the medulla sends descending fibres to the preganglionic cells in the thoracolumbar segment of the spinal cord. The preganglionic fibres synapse in the ganglia of the sympathetic chain, and postganglionic fibres travel to vascular smooth muscle. Norepinephrine is the transmitter that acts on the α_1-receptors in the vascular smooth muscle.

The activity of the vasomotor centre is influenced by afferent impulses from many sensory areas, including baroreceptors, chemoreceptors and skin, and from higher centres in the cortex and hypothalamus. The preganglionic cells in the spinal cord may also be influenced directly by higher centres and by reflex activity

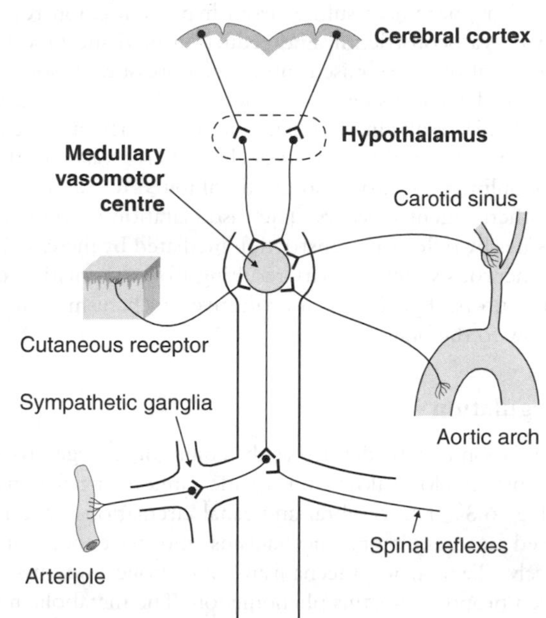

Fig. 6.2
The vasomotor centre and its connections.

at spinal level. The vasomotor centre is active continuously, resulting in a resting tone in vascular smooth muscle. Increased sympathetic activity does not affect all tissues equally. Tissues with the highest intrinsic vascular tone respond less well than those with a lower tone. Vascular smooth muscle in skeletal muscle, heart and liver also possesses β_2-adrenergic receptors that have a vasodilator effect. Thus, with increased adrenergic sympathetic activity, there is a redistribution of blood from skin, muscle and gut to brain, heart and kidney.

Sympathetic cholinergic

Activation of sympathetic cholinergic fibres results in vasodilatation in skeletal muscle. These fibres are represented centrally in the cerebral cortex and are involved in the anticipatory response to exercise (the 'fight or flight' reaction). Stimulation of the appropriate area of the brain initiates redistribution of blood flow from the skin and viscera to skeletal muscle.

Dopaminergic receptors

Dopamine is a precursor of norepinephrine and has been shown to have a vasodilator effect on splanchnic and renal vessels mediated through specific D_1 receptors. This response may be useful pharmacologically, but the physiological role of such receptors is unclear.

Metabolic control

Several metabolites, including CO_2, K^+ and H^+, influence the calibre of blood vessels. Adenosine, bradykinin and prostaglandins are among the endogenous chemicals known to cause vasodilatation. It is likely that different tissues respond more readily to some compounds than to others.

Induced hypocapnia resulting from hyperventilation results in generalized vasoconstriction and reduction in tissue blood flow. In some situations, e.g. raised intracranial pressure, vasoconstriction may be deleterious because it increases the risk of ischaemia.

Hypoxaemia results in vasodilatation in all parts of the circulation except the pulmonary vessels, where vasoconstriction (hypoxic pulmonary vasoconstriction, inhibited to varying extents by anaesthetic agents) occurs. The vasodilatation is countered in most tissues by reflex vasoconstriction mediated by increased sympathetic nervous system activity resulting from stimulation of the chemoreceptors. This acts as a protective mechanism to increase blood flow to the brain.

Autoregulation

Autoregulation may be defined as the ability of an organ to maintain a constant blood flow over a wide range of perfusion pressures (Fig. 6.3). The cerebral and renal circulations have highly developed autoregulatory mechanisms and have been studied extensively. Two major mechanisms, metabolic and myogenic, have been proposed for this phenomenon. The metabolic mechanism depends on the accumulation and washout of vasodilator metabolites. During periods of decreased perfusion pressure, a temporary reduction occurs in tissue blood flow, resulting in accumulation of vasodilator metabolites, e.g. H^+, CO_2 and lactic acid; this results in local vasodilatation and blood flow returns to a normal level. The myogenic mechanism of autoregulation depends on the intrinsic tone of the vascular smooth muscle. During periods of increased perfusion pressure, vascular smooth muscle is stretched; the muscle tone increases, causing a degree of vasoconstriction, and flow is maintained at a constant level.

Many factors affect cerebral autoregulation. For example, the autoregulatory curve is shifted to the right in the presence of persistent hypertension; minor or severe head injury results in impairment of cerebral autoregulation; and some anaesthetic agents (e.g. desflurane) significantly reduce cerebral autoregulatory capacity while others (e.g. sevoflurane) have almost no effect.

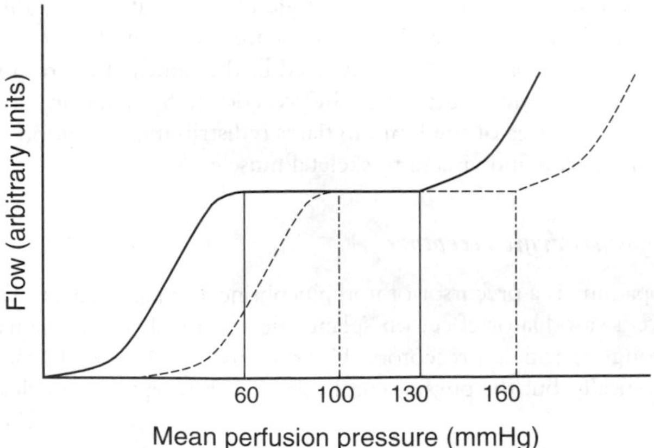

Fig. 6.3
Cerebral autoregulation, showing the normal limits for autoregulation and the effect of long-standing hypertension on the curve position (dashed line). Linear axis indicating in bold line the normal maintenance of flow between perfusion pressures of 60–130mmHg. The dashed line represents the hypertensive patient in whom flow is maintained constant at a higher range of perfusion pressures e.g. 100–160mmHg.

CAPILLARIES

These are composed of a single layer of endothelial cells which permits free exchange of nutrients and metabolites between tissues and blood. Capillaries are organized in capillary beds and arise from metarterioles rather than arterioles themselves (Fig. 6.4). Precapillary sphincters (thickenings of the smooth muscle in the metarteriole wall) control the flow of blood passing through the capillaries. The metarterioles and precapillary sphincters are in intimate contact with the tissues that they serve, and their diameters are altered significantly by local products of metabolism.

The density of capillaries in any tissue is related to the maximum oxygen consumption of the tissue. Although the surface area available for gas exchange in each capillary is small, the vast number of capillaries (equal to approximately 300 m^2 in the systemic circulation at rest) ensures that there is a very significant area available for exchange purposes.

The exact nature of the junctions between endothelial cells differs among tissues and determines the function of the endothelium in different organs. For example, in the brain, the endothelial cells are held closely together by tight junctions. This limits transendothelial exchange to substances that are able to pass through these tight junctions (the so-called blood–brain barrier). However, in renal glomerular capillaries, the endothelium is fenestrated. This allows molecules up to the size of albumin to be filtered. In the spleen, the endothelium is distracted further and has large gaps between the endothelial cells, allowing significantly larger substances, including cells, to pass through.

The forces responsible for the exchange of fluids across the capillary are given by Starling's equation:

$$J_v = K_f(P_i - P_o) - r(COP_i - COP_o)$$

where J_v is the transcapillary fluid filtration rate, K_f is the ultrafiltration coefficient, P_i is the hydrostatic pressure inside the capillary, P_o

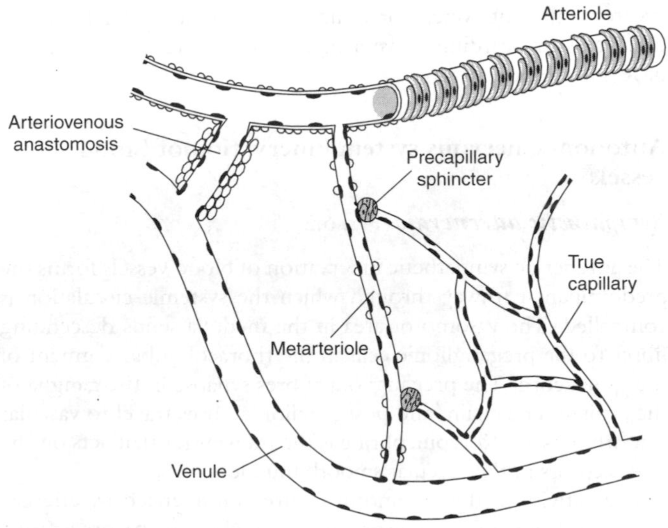

Fig. 6.4
Diagrammatic representation of the microcirculation.

is the hydrostatic pressure outside the capillary, r is the reflection coefficient, COP_i is the colloid osmotic pressure inside the capillary, and COP_o is the colloid osmotic pressure outside the capillary.

At the arterial end of the capillary, the high hydrostatic pressure in the capillary compared with that outside tends to move fluid out of the capillary. The capillary pressure is technically difficult to determine accurately but it is of the order of 25–30 mmHg inside the capillary compared with an interstitial pressure of approximately −2 to −5 mmHg. The ultrafiltration coefficient (K_f) of the capillary is determined by the exchange surface area and the nature of the capillary endothelial junctions as described above. The value of K_f in the brain endothelium is therefore lower than that of the renal or splenic endothelium.

The colloid osmotic pressure (COP) at the arterial end of the capillary favours movement of fluid from the interstitium to the capillary. The colloid osmotic pressure in the capillary is approximately 28 mmHg compared with an interstitial value of approximately 6 mmHg. Taking these forces into account, the net filtration force across the capillary into the interstitial fluid at the arterial end is approximately 10–15 mmHg (Fig. 6.5). At the venous end of the capillary this situation changes; the capillary hydrostatic pressure is now of the order of 10 mmHg, whereas the interstitial and colloid osmotic pressures are unchanged. Thus at this end of the capillary, the net filtration force across the capillary into the vessel is of the order of 5–8 mmHg.

The reflection coefficient is a value that indicates the permeability of the endothelium in a specific capillary bed to the molecules that contribute to the colloid osmotic pressure. This value varies from nearly zero to almost 1.0. It is a comparison of the ability of the capillary membrane to exclude molecules of a specific size and charge density from passage across the membrane relative to the movement of water across the membrane.

The COP is generated almost exclusively by dissolved proteins. In the healthy subject, the serum albumin concentration makes a very significant contribution to the COP. Factors affecting the intravascular COP include hepatic function (determining the rate of albumin production), the rate of filtration of albumin into the interstitium (determined by the reflection coefficient) and the rate of loss of albumin by excretion and metabolism. Previously, maintenance of intravascular COP was one reason for transfusion of albumin in the critically ill patient in whom the serum albumin concentration had decreased. However, in this clinical situation, it is acute-phase proteins rather than albumin that maintain the intracapillary COP.

Interstitial COP varies in different tissues, with a value close to zero in the brain and approximating to the intravascular COP in the liver.

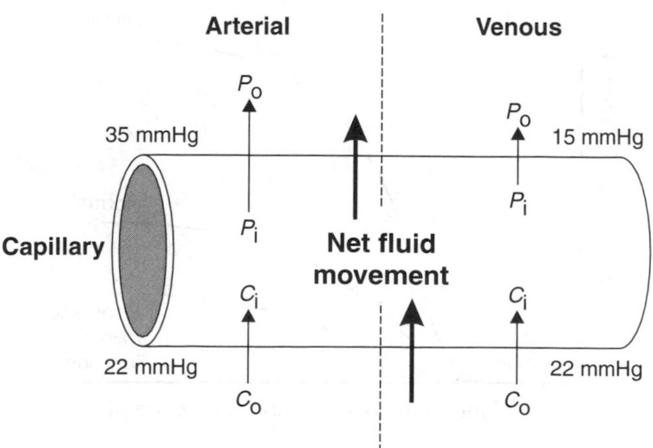

Fig. 6.5
Diagrammatic representation of the forces across a capillary membrane.

CAPACITANCE AND RESISTANCE VESSELS

The highly muscular layers in the peripheral arterial system enable the arterioles (defined as vessels with an internal diameter of less than 0.5 mm) to act as resistance vessels. The relationships between pressure, flow and resistance detailed below in the control of arterial pressure also hold true at the tissue level. The resistance generated in the peripheral arterioles, in the face of an adequate cardiac output, controls capillary (and therefore tissue) perfusion pressure. These vessels therefore control the local tissue blood flow, the total peripheral resistance and the movement of fluid across capillary membranes (by Starling forces described above) by varying the pressure at the arterial end of the capillary.

The lack of any significant muscle layer and the greater distensibility of the veins imply that they can be regarded as capacitance vessels in an analogous manner to an electrical capacitor. At rest, approximately 75% of the circulating blood volume is in the venous part of the circulation. A vein has a compliance 24 times greater than that of a corresponding artery because of a larger volume and distensibility.

The smooth muscle of the vein wall is innervated richly with sympathetic vasoconstrictor fibres. Venoconstriction and dilatation adjust the capacity of the circulation to maintain and balance the blood volume. For example, during initial hypovolaemia, venoconstriction occurs, so that the venous return is maintained by mobilizing blood from the venous reservoir, tending to maintain cardiac output. If volume loss continues in the presence of maximal venoconstriction, there are sudden and dramatic reductions in cardiac output and arterial pressure when venous return can no longer be maintained. This is the physiological basis by which compensated hypovolaemia is converted to uncompensated shock.

During changes in posture, alterations in venous capacitance provide the mechanism for maintaining and limiting changes in cardiac output. Impairment of venoconstriction by disease or drugs, e.g. antihypertensive agents, leads to a reduction in cardiac output, and hypotension on standing (postural hypotension).

SUMMARY

The peripheral circulation comprises different types of vessels, each with a structure dictated by its physiological role. Endothelium is metabolically active, maintains vessel patency and produces substances that alter vascular tone locally. Smooth muscle layers control vessel diameter and therefore, to a large extent, the flow through them. Capillaries are highly specialized vessels which, in addition to performing endothelial functions, allow transfer of nutrients and waste products to and from the interstitial tissues. The amount of fluid passing across a capillary may be calculated by determining the balance of the hydrostatic pressure forcing fluid out of the capillary and the COP drawing fluid in. Allowances have to be made for the surface area of exchange, the nature of the capillary junctions and the molecular size and charge density.

CONTROL OF CARDIAC OUTPUT

Cardiac output is the volume of blood pumped from the heart into the aorta each minute. The venous return is the volume of blood returning to the right atrium from the great veins each minute. The value for each of these two values (cardiac output and venous return) should be equal except for the few heartbeats that follow a change in cardiac output.

The cardiac output ($\dot{Q}$) is the product of the stroke volume (SV) and the heart rate (HR) and may be summarized as:

$$\dot{Q} = SV \times HR$$

A heart rate of 70 beat min^{-1} and a stroke volume of 70 ml would therefore equate to a cardiac output of approximately 5 L min^{-1}. Cardiac output is known to vary with body size, and therefore in order to compare values obtained from different patients, the cardiac output per square metre of body surface area may be calculated. This is termed cardiac index. The normal value in adults is approximately 3.0 L min^{-1} m^{-2}. Body surface area is calculated from standard charts relating height and weight.

Cardiac index changes with age, reaching a peak resting value of approximately 4 L min^{-1} m^{-2} at 10 years of age and declining to about 2.5 L min^{-1} m^{-2} at 80 years of age.

FACTORS CONTROLLING CARDIAC OUTPUT

These can be classified as either cardiac or peripheral factors.

Cardiac factors are those that may affect heart rate or stroke volume. Increased sympathetic stimulation of the heart causes both an increased heart rate and an increase in the force of contraction of the ventricles, resulting in an increase in cardiac output. Failure of the myocardium to contract normally (e.g. after a myocardial infarction, during administration of cardiodepressant drugs such as general anaesthetic agents or in the presence of cardiotoxic cytokines) results in a decrease in stroke volume, reducing cardiac output unless there is a compensatory increase in heart rate. Although depressed cardiac function during pathological processes may significantly decrease the cardiac output, the heart is not the major determinant of cardiac output in normal physiology. In the normal situation, peripheral factors, including tissue metabolism, circulatory volume and venous return, play a major role in the regulation of cardiac output.

The metabolic rate of any tissue determines the flow of blood through it. Therefore, increased metabolic requirements of the tissues result in an increased cardiac output. Strenuous exercise may result in a cardiac output that is seven times greater than normal. Cardiac output parallels oxygen consumption during exercise as shown in Figure 6.6. Reduced peripheral resistance, e.g. opening an arteriovenous fistula, results in an increase in cardiac output; after 24 h, the cardiac output will have increased by the same amount as the flow through the fistula.

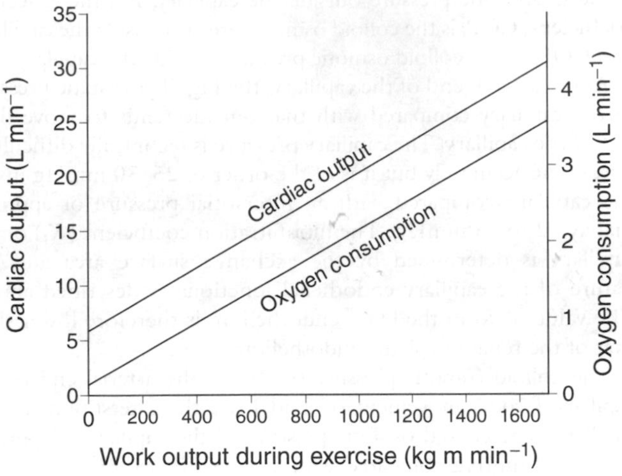

Fig. 6.6
Relationship between exercise, cardiac output and oxygen consumption.

Cardiac output and right atrial pressure

Cardiac output is controlled by a combination of both cardiac and peripheral factors. Cardiac output increases with increasing right atrial pressure until it reaches a plateau (Fig 6.7). Previous suggestions that cardiac output decreases with further increases in right atrial pressure are almost certainly investigative methodological errors rather than real changes. The position of the curve changes with varying levels of sympathetic stimulation. Maximal sympathetic stimulation results in the plateau increasing to approximately 170% of its resting value. This is as a result of changes in both rate and contractility.

Parasympathetic stimulation has a minimal effect on contractility and therefore stroke volume does not change significantly. Decreases in cardiac output on parasympathetic stimulation are a result mainly of a reduction in heart rate, and the position of the curve shown in Figure 6.7 changes only slightly.

The position of the curve is also influenced by factors which reduce myocardial contractility, e.g. myocardial ischaemia, myocarditis, general and regional anaesthesia, and sepsis.

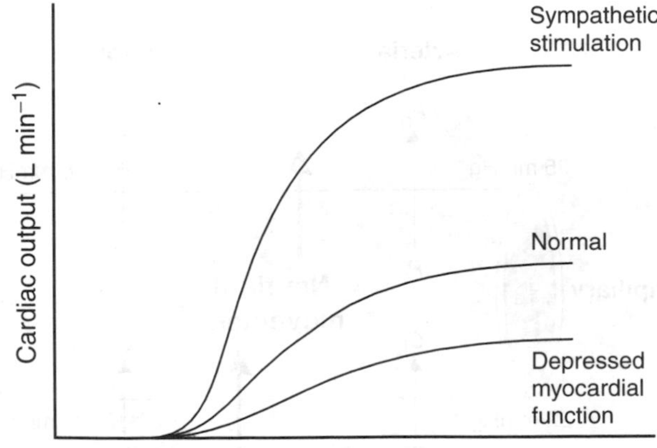

Fig. 6.7
Relationship between cardiac output and right atrial pressure for the normal heart, during sympathetic stimulation and for the heart with depressed myocardial function.

It is important to recognize that although the curves in Figure 6.7 are represented by right atrial pressure as a measure of initial fibre length, it is the transmural pressure that determines the effective filling pressure of the heart. The transmural pressure is the difference between the right atrial pressure and the intrapleural pressure. Thus, changing from spontaneous to positive pressure ventilation results in the cardiac output curve being shifted to the right. That is, in the presence of a positive intrathoracic pressure, a higher right atrial pressure is required to obtain the same cardiac output.

Venous return and cardiac output

It is obvious that if there is no venous return of blood to the right atrium, there can be no cardiac output. Except in conditions of dynamic change of cardiac output, the cardiac output and venous return must be equal. For blood to pass into the right atrium, there must be a venous driving pressure that is greater than the right atrial pressure. This venous driving pressure has been termed the mean circulatory filling pressure and makes an important contribution to the control of cardiac output.

A useful analogy to explain the concept of the mean circulatory filling pressure is to consider the venous system as an elastic band (Fig. 6.8). When totally empty, the band is flaccid. A certain volume is required to distend it to its resting circular position; however, at this point there is no tension in the elastic band. Further distension results in the band being stretched beyond its resting position. The band tension increases as intraluminal band volume increases. This gives rise to the concept of the stressed and non-stressed volume. The volume in the venous system that distends the vessels to their resting positions is the unstressed volume. Any further increase in volume results in stretching of the vessel such that the wall tension and intraluminal pressure increase; this additional volume is the stressed volume. It is only the stressed volume that is responsible for the venous pressure gradient returning blood to the right atrium.

If this hypothesis were true, the majority of the circulating volume would not contribute to the mean circulatory filling pressure. Experiments in animals and humans have indicated that the stressed volume is approximately one-third of the normal circulating volume. The remaining two-thirds of the circulating volume contributes only to the non-stressed volume and therefore makes no contribution to the venous pressure gradient.

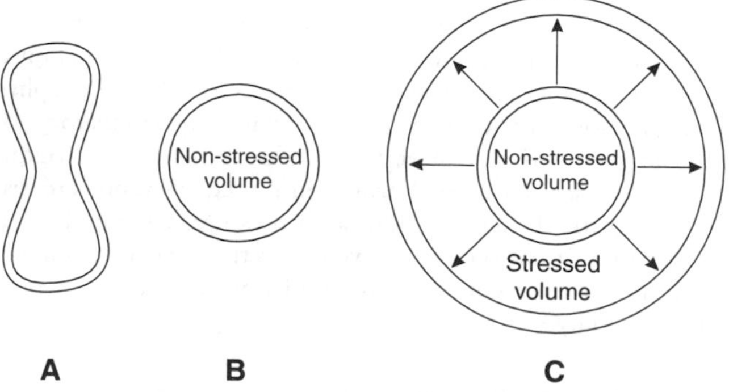

Fig. 6.8
Diagrammatic representation of the stressed and non-stressed volume as shown by the elastic band. **A.** The band is flaccid. **B.** The contained volume has been increased such that the band is circular but with no wall stress. **C.** The intraluminal volume has been increased and wall stress now increases with volume; stressed and non-stressed volumes are indicated.

In addition to the physical properties of the blood vessels, mechanical factors aid venous return. The venous system contains valves to encourage unidirectional flow of blood. This becomes particularly important during exercise when muscle contraction forces blood through the venous system. The venous valves then ensure that the blood is moved in a unidirectional manner to return blood to the right atrium. Respiration also assists venous return, particularly while standing. Negative intrathoracic pressure together with positive intra-abdominal pressure during inspiration result in a pressure difference that tends to drive blood back to the heart.

Venous return and right atrial pressure

If the mean circulatory pressure is equal to the right atrial pressure, no blood returns to the right atrium. As shown in Figure 6.9, as right atrial pressure decreases, venous return increases until it reaches a plateau. The plateau is due to the effect of transmural pressure. As right atrial pressure decreases to values below intrapleural pressure, the great veins entering the right heart collapse. This effectively limits the venous return possible at each level of systemic venous pressure.

Because venous return and cardiac output must be equal, Figures 6.7 and 6.9 may be drawn together on the same axis, as shown in Figure 6.10. The point at which the two lines cross

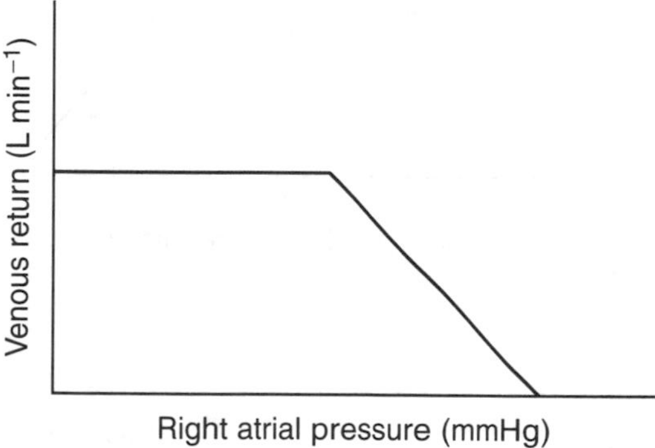

Fig. 6.9
Relationship between venous return and right atrial pressure.

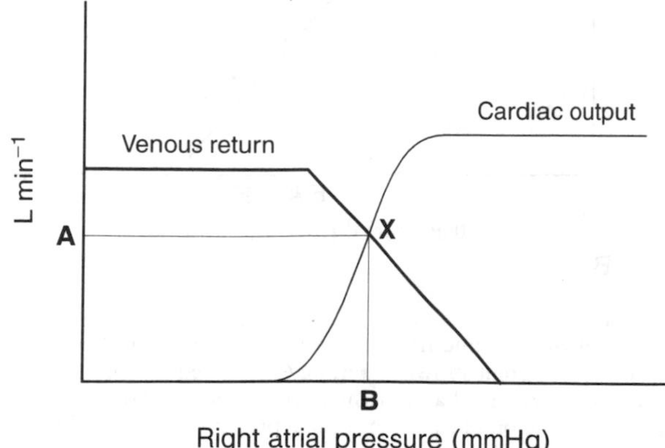

Fig. 6.10
Combined representation of venous return and cardiac output with respect to right atrial pressure. The intersection of the lines (X) represents the cardiac output A at the right atrial pressure B.

must represent the cardiac output generated at a specific value of right atrial pressure. Factors affecting either the venous return or the cardiac output change the positions of the lines and therefore the point of intersection. This graphical relationship becomes helpful in the understanding of changes in these cardiovascular variables. The effects of altering circulating filling pressure by increasing circulating volume are shown in Figure 6.11A. Changes in cardiac contractility are shown in Figure 6.11B. It may be seen from Figure 6.12 that if a patient has depressed myocardial function with a normal circulating filling pressure, the administration of additional fluid does not result in an increased cardiac output. However, following the use of inotropic drugs to increase myocardial contractility, administration of additional fluid may then result in an increase in cardiac output.

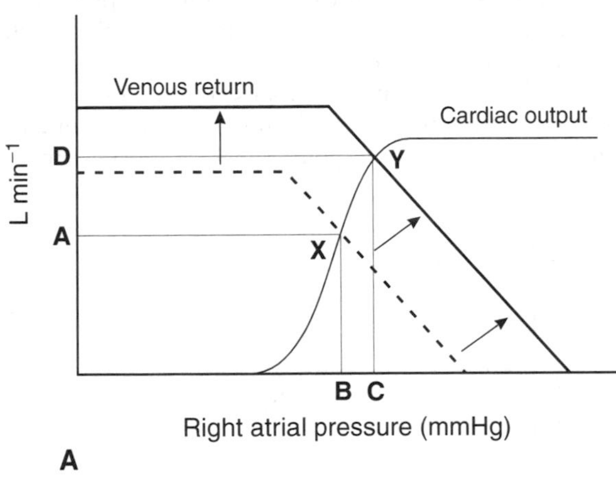

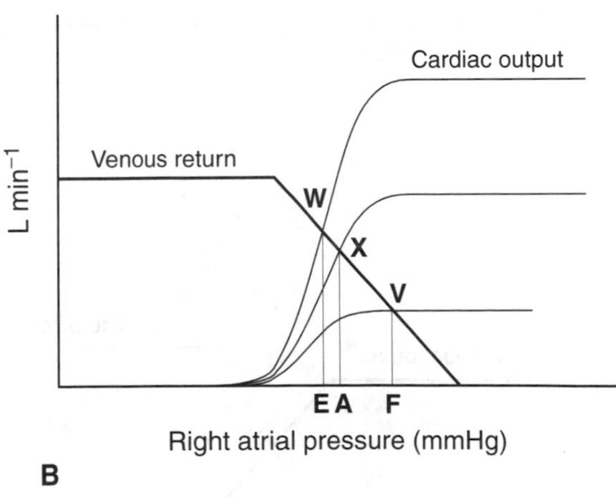

Fig. 6.11
A. The circulating volume has been increased by administration of fluid from the starting point shown in Figure 6.10. The position of the venous return curve has changed and the intersection of the two curves is now at Y; the new cardiac output and right atrial pressure are shown by points D and C, respectively. **B.** The cardiac output is changed from normal (X) to an augmented level (W) and a depressed level (V), resulting in new points of intersection and reduced (E) or increased (F) values of right atrial pressure.

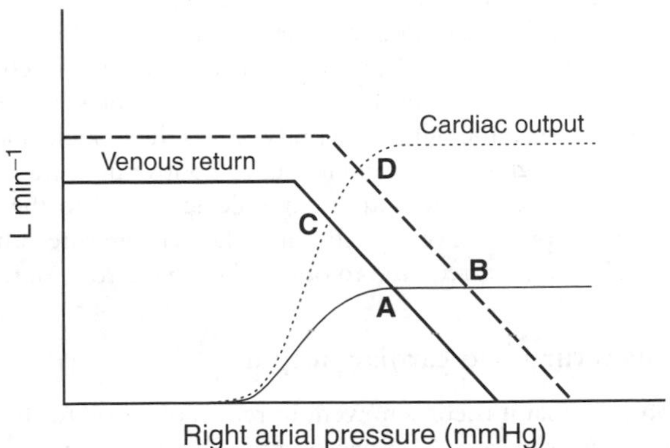

Fig. 6.12
Graphical representation of a subject with diminished cardiac output due to depressed myocardial function. Intersection of venous return and cardiac output curves occurs at A. Administration of intravenous fluids would move the intersection to B with no change in the cardiac output. Administration of inotropic agents initially would move the intersection point from A to C, with an increased cardiac output and decrease in right atrial pressure. At this point, the use of intravenous fluids would now move the intersection to D, with a further increase in cardiac output and the right atrial pressure returning approximately to the starting position.

Peripheral resistance and cardiac output

The relationships between arterial pressure, peripheral resistance and cardiac output are considered in detail later in this chapter. Cardiac output is related inversely to peripheral resistance. Therefore, in situations of low peripheral resistance (e.g. systemic sepsis), if mean arterial pressure remains constant, cardiac output increases.

Increasing the peripheral resistance by administration of a vasopressor drug, e.g. norepinephrine, results in a decrease in cardiac output. In situations of poor myocardial contractility and normal or increased peripheral resistance, administration of a vasopressor drug may cause significant decreases in cardiac output and mean arterial pressure.

SUMMARY

Cardiac output is the volume of blood pumped from the heart into the aorta each minute. It is controlled by a combination of both cardiac and non-cardiac (peripheral) factors. In normal physiology, the non-cardiac factors (tissue metabolism, circulatory volume and venous return) have more influence on cardiac output than do the cardiac factors. Cardiac output equals venous return. Both vary with changes in right atrial pressure. Graphical representations of cardiac output and venous return may be combined to indicate the effects of changing circulating volume and myocardial contractility.

CONTROL OF ARTERIAL PRESSURE

Systemic arterial pressure is normally controlled closely in order to maintain the driving pressure needed for tissue perfusion. Normal values vary depending on both age and gender (Table 6.1), in

Table 6.1 Changes in arterial pressure, cardiac output and systemic vascular resistance with age

Age (years)	Arterial pressure (mmHg)		Blood flow		Peripheral vascular resistance[b]	
	Systolic/diastolic	Mean	Cardiac index[a] ($L\ min^{-1}\ m^{-2}$)	Cardiac output ($L\ min^{-1}$)	($mmHg\ L^{-1}\ min^{-1}$)	($dyn\ s\ cm^{-5}$)
10	100/65	75	4.0	4.8	15	1150
20	110/70	85	3.7	6.7	12	950
30	115/75	90	3.4	6.1	14	1100
40	120/80	92	3.2	5.8	15	1200
50	125/82	95	3.0	5.4	17	1300
60	130/85	98	2.8	5.0	19	1500
70	135/88	102	2.6	4.7	21	1650
80	140/90	105	2.5	4.5	22	1800

[a]Assuming a body surface area of 1.2 m^2 at age 10 and 1.8 m^2 thereafter.
[b]Assuming a CVP of 5 mmHg.

addition to physiological changes including sleep. However, measurement of a 'normal' or even elevated arterial pressure is no guarantee of adequate tissue perfusion.

Mean arterial pressure (MAP) is the average pressure throughout each cardiac cycle (Fig. 6.13) and is generally regarded as being more important than systolic pressure as an indicator of tissue perfusion. A reasonable approximation may be calculated from the formula:

$$\text{MAP} = \text{diastolic arterial pressure} + (1/3) \times \text{pulse pressure}$$

The values recorded for systemic arterial pressure may also be influenced by both the technique of measurement (e.g. the use of Korotkoff sounds IV or V using a sphygmomanometer) and the site of measurement (e.g. femoral vs. radial/dorsalis pedis arteries). The passage of the arterial pressure waveform through the peripheral vessels tends to result in a higher systolic pressure reading, although the curve becomes narrower (see Fig. 6.13B) and consequently the MAP remains constant.

The interrelationships between pressure, flow and resistance are fundamental to the understanding of the control of arterial pressure. Flow through a tube is determined entirely by the pressure difference between the two ends of the tube and the resistance to flow through the tube (Fig. 6.14). This relationship may be expressed using Ohm's law, a central relationship in cardiovascular physiology:

$$\text{Flow} = \frac{\text{Pressure difference along the tube}}{\text{Resistance to flow through the tube}}$$

The resistance to blood flowing through a blood vessel is dependent on four factors: calibre and length of the vessel, viscosity of blood and the nature of the flow (turbulent or laminar).

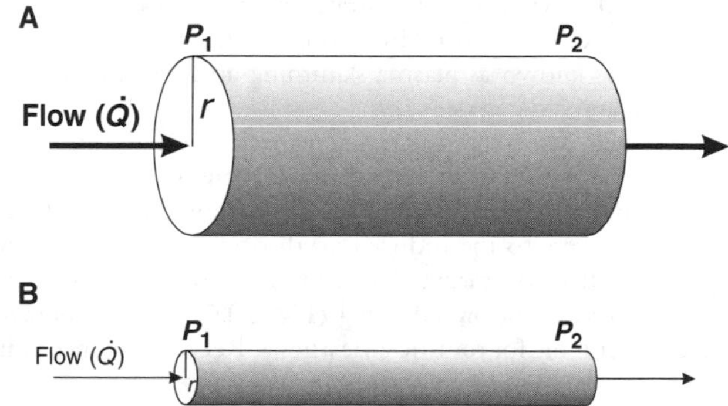

Fig. 6.14
Diagrammatic representation of flow ($\dot{Q}$) through a tube. The flow is dependent on the pressure applied along the tube ($P_1 - P_2$) and the resistance of the tube. Resistance is determined by a number of factors (see text), the most important of which is the radius (r). In (**B**), the pressure difference is the same, the radius is markedly reduced and the flow is decreased.

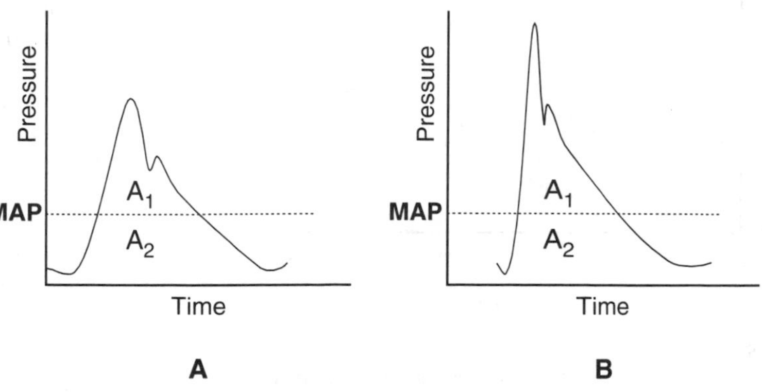

Fig. 6.13
Graphical representation of aortic (**A**) and peripheral (**B**) arterial pressure waveforms. The point at which area A_1 is equal to area A_2 gives the mean arterial pressure (MAP). In (B), the pressure waveform is narrower and has a higher peak pressure, but the MAP remains unchanged.

In the absence of irregularities in the vessel wall (resulting from atheroma), flow in blood vessels is laminar. The relationship between the driving pressure and flow under these conditions may be expressed by the Hagen–Poiseuille formula:

$$\dot{Q} = \Delta P \pi r^4 / 8 \eta l$$

where ($\dot{Q}$) is the flow rate, r is the radius of the vessel, l is its length, ΔP is the driving pressure and η is the blood viscosity. This relationship holds true only for steady flow of Newtonian fluids, i.e. those with viscosity independent of flow rate. These conditions do not apply to the cardiovascular system, where flow is pulsatile and blood viscosity is determined by flow rate. It is therefore an oversimplification but it does illustrate the critical role of the vessel radius in determining the flow rate.

Viscosity

Blood is a mixture of solutes (e.g. electrolytes and proteins) and particles (e.g. cells and chylomicrons). At low flow rates, the cells tend to aggregate, thus increasing viscosity. In addition, cells tend to concentrate in the centre of the blood vessel, where the velocity is greatest. The haematocrit is therefore lowest at the periphery of the lumen, where the velocity is lowest. Thus blood tends to act much more as a Newtonian fluid in vivo than in vitro. The tendency of erythrocytes to concentrate in the centre of a vessel results in a lower haematocrit in blood that enters side branches. This process is known as plasma skimming and has implications for flow rate and oxygen delivery.

Anaemia reduces oxygen-carrying capacity and results in an increase in cardiac output to maintain oxygen delivery. The increased flow rate through blood vessels is facilitated by reduced viscosity secondary to the reduced erythrocyte count. Clinically, there is little effect on cardiac index until the haemoglobin concentration decreases below 10 g dl^{-1} (Fig. 6.15), the traditionally accepted lower limit for routine anaesthesia. Recent evidence indicates that maintaining the haemoglobin concentration between 7 and 9 g dl^{-1}, even in critically ill patients, is not associated with adverse outcomes.

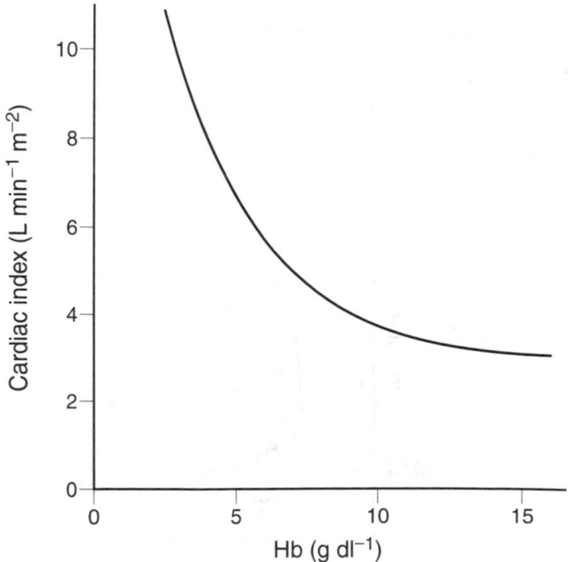

Fig. 6.15
Relationship between haemoglobin concentration and cardiac index in chronic anaemia.

FACTORS AFFECTING ARTERIAL PRESSURE

The relationships between flow, pressure and resistance through a tube described above can be rearranged as follows:

$$\text{Arterial pressure} = (\text{flow} \times \text{resistance}) + \text{venous pressure}$$

If it is accepted that the venous pressure is usually low, this value has impact on the overall value for arterial pressure, and therefore for the systemic circulation:

$$\text{MAP} = \text{CO} \times \text{SVR}$$

where MAP is given in mmHg and cardiac output (CO) in L min^{-1}. Systemic vascular resistance (SVR) is traditionally expressed in dyne s cm^{-5}, necessitating the inclusion of a correction factor of 80:

$$\text{SVR} = 80 \times \text{MAP}/\text{CO}$$

Thus for a patient with MAP = 100 mmHg and CO = 5 L min^{-1}, SVR = 1600 dyne s cm^{-5}. As indicated above, cardiac output is usually expressed as cardiac index to allow comparison between individuals. Similarly, SVR can be expressed as systemic vascular resistance index (SVRI):

$$\text{SVRI} = 80 \times \text{MAP}/\text{CI}$$

The normal SVRI is in the range 2000 ± 500 dyne s cm^{-5} m^{-2}.

REGULATION OF ARTERIAL PRESSURE

The cardiovascular system controls mean arterial pressure within a very small range despite a wide range of stimuli that would otherwise result in very significant arterial pressure swings. In order to achieve this control, several mechanisms exist, some acting rapidly for short-term control and others more slowly for longer-term regulation.

Neural control mechanisms

These include the arterial baro- and chemoreceptor mechanisms. Arterial baroreceptors are located in the carotid sinus and the wall of the aortic arch. They are not strictly pressure sensors but rather are stretch receptors. An increase in arterial pressure results in stretching of the major arteries and an increase in the frequency of impulses generated by the baroreceptors. These impulses are transmitted via the vagus nerve to the medulla of the brain stem. The carotid sinus receptors transmit impulses only at a mean arterial pressure above 60 mmHg, and reach a maximal response at 180 mmHg. The aortic arch receptors respond between 90 and 210 mmHg. The baroreceptors are exceptionally sensitive to small changes in pressure and respond much more dramatically to a dynamic change in pressure than to a static pressure.

When the brain stem is stimulated by the baroreceptors, the output from the vagal centre is increased, resulting in slowing of the heart rate and a decrease in the force of cardiac contraction. In addition, the vasoconstrictor centre is inhibited, resulting in peripheral vasodilatation. The combination of reduced heart rate and reduced cardiac contractility results in reduced cardiac output. The combination of reduced peripheral resistance and decreased cardiac output reduces mean arterial pressure. However, if the original stimulus to pressure change persists for 1–2 days, the baroreceptors 'reset' at that level. Thus, the baroreceptor system is not a mechanism that controls long-term changes in arterial pressure, but it is vital in the control of arterial pressure during the normal activities of daily living.

Assessment of baroreceptor responses

The loss of baroreceptor reflex control of arterial pressure affects normal activities of daily living, resulting, for example, in postural hypotension. During anaesthesia, the loss of these reflexes (e.g. in patients with an autonomic neuropathy secondary to diabetes mellitus) results in impairment of the normal cardiovascular responses to events such as positive pressure ventilation of the lungs.

The integrity of the baroreceptor response may be assessed simply either by the arterial pressure response to a change in posture or by the Valsalva manoeuvre. The Valsalva manoeuvre (Fig. 6.16), a forced expiration against the closed glottis, results in increased intrathoracic pressure, increased central venous pressure and decreased venous return to the heart. The baroreceptors sense the decrease in cardiac output and arterial pressure. In the normal individual, the result is peripheral vasoconstriction and a reflex increase in heart rate to maintain the arterial pressure. On release of the raised intrathoracic pressure, venous return to the heart increases. There is transient hypertension and bradycardia until the peripheral vasoconstriction is reversed. The heart rate response is easier to detect and may be measured at the bedside.

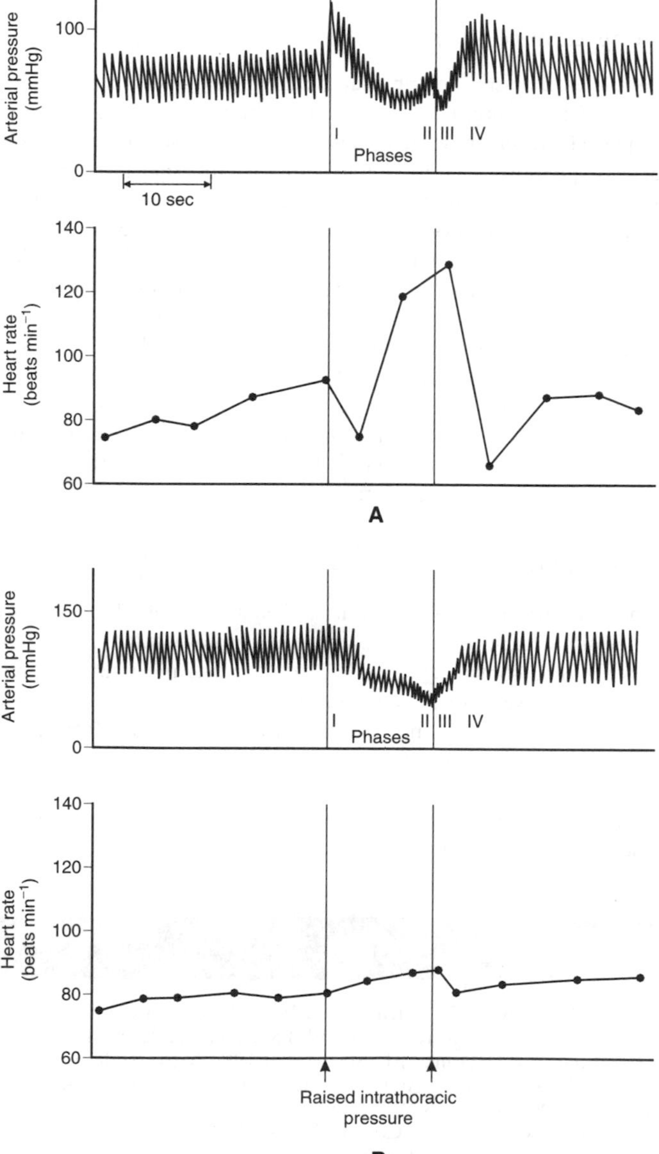

Fig. 6.16
Valsalva manoeuvre. **A**. Normal response. **B**. Patient with impaired cardiovascular control. (See text for details.)

Chemoreceptors are located within the carotid and aortic bodies. These cells have an extremely high blood supply and respond to changes in oxygen and carbon dioxide tensions and pH. During periods of hypotension, they become relatively ischaemic and hence detect changes in the local concentration of these substances.

Stretch receptors are also found in the atria and have both renal and hypothalamic effects. The renal effects include afferent arteriolar dilatation and a consequent increase in glomerular filtration. This is coupled with a reduction in the secretion of antidiuretic hormone from the posterior pituitary secondary to hypothalamic stimulation. This decreased secretion results in less of the increased glomerular filtrate being reabsorbed, promoting a diuresis. This in turn reduces the atrial volume and thus reduces cardiac output and MAP.

Humoral control mechanisms

In addition to the rapid-onset neural control mechanisms, several hormones are involved in the early control of changes in arterial pressure. These include catecholamines, renin, angiotensin, vasopressin, atrial natriuretic peptide and nitric oxide.

Catecholamines

Stimulation of the sympathetic nervous system results not only in direct effects on blood vessels but also in an indirect effect via catecholamines released from the adrenal medulla. The cells of the adrenal medulla are analogous to postganglionic neurones and stimulation results in the release primarily of epinephrine (80%), but also of norepinephrine.

The circulating catecholamines have the same peripheral effect as direct stimulation of the sympathetic nervous system, i.e. peripheral vasoconstriction and cardiac inotropy. However, the duration of effect is significantly longer for the circulating catecholamines (up to 3 min) than for direct stimulation of the autonomic nervous system. Circulating catecholamines are also able to reach parts of the circulation such as the metarterioles that have no direct sympathetic innervation.

Renin–angiotensin system

Renal artery pressure is sensed by the juxtaglomerular cells located in the afferent renal arteriole. These cells also synthesize renin which they release into the circulation if renal artery pressure decreases, if sodium delivery to the distal tubule decreases, or on sympathetic nervous system stimulation. Renin cleaves angiotensinogen, formed in the liver, to angiotensin I which is hydrolysed by angiotensin-converting enzyme (found predominantly in the lungs) to the metabolically active angiotensin II. This compound is a potent vasoconstrictor. In addition, angiotensin II stimulates the adrenal cortex directly to synthesize and secrete aldosterone.

Thus the renin–angiotensin system elevates arterial pressure both by increasing the systemic vascular resistance and by causing salt and water retention to increase cardiac output. This control system is vitally important in the hypovolaemic or sodium-depleted individual, and in patients with a low cardiac output. However, it is not as rapid in response as the neural or catecholamine systems. It takes approximately 20 min to become fully active, but it has a longer duration of effect when stimulated.

Vasopressin (antidiuretic hormone, ADH)

This peptide is synthesized in the supraoptic and paraventricular nuclei of the brain stem. It is then transported through the pituitary stalk to the posterior pituitary gland from where it is released. Release of vasopressin is triggered by several stimuli. These include an increase in plasma osmolality, a decrease in plasma volume or increased plasma concentration of angiotensin II. Vasopressin acts as a direct vasoconstrictor (hence its use in the management of bleeding oesophageal varices), increasing the systemic vascular resistance and tending to elevate the arterial pressure. The vasoconstrictor effect is relatively rapid in onset but is supplemented by an indirect and longer-term control via its effect on the kidneys. Vasopressin binds to specific receptors, causing the collecting ducts of the kidneys to reabsorb more free water and thereby to reduce urine output. Again, the result is to increase circulating blood volume, cardiac output and arterial pressure.

Atrial natriuretic peptide

This peptide is synthesized and stored in the atrial myocytes. Release is triggered by atrial distension or by circulating epinephrine, ADH or morphine. It acts directly on vascular smooth muscle, causing vasodilatation and therefore reductions in systemic vascular resistance and arterial pressure. In addition, it inhibits the release of renin, aldosterone and ADH.

Nitric oxide

In 1987, nitric oxide was identified as the substance previously termed endothelium-derived relaxing factor. It is now known that this substance has a wide range of physiological effects, including control of vessel tone. Nitric oxide is produced from the substrate L-arginine, an abundant amino acid, in the endothelial cells. The enzyme nitric oxide synthase is required to bring about the production of nitric oxide. Nitric oxide synthase has two isoforms. The constitutive form is calcium/calmodulin-dependent and is present in normally functioning tissues; the inducible form is not calcium/calmodulin-dependent and is found in pathological states such as septic shock. The nitric oxide produced in endothelial cells diffuses into smooth muscle cells where it stimulates the enzyme guanylate cyclase, causing cyclic guanosine monophosphate (cGMP) to be formed from guanosine triphosphate (GTP). This reaction activates a phosphorylation cascade, resulting in smooth muscle relaxation and vasodilatation with reductions in systemic vascular resistance and arterial pressure.

This pathway may be inhibited in several ways. First, a substrate analogue may be provided in the place of L-arginine. Two such compounds have been described: nitro-L-arginine methyl ester (L-NAME) and L-N-monomethyl-arginine (L-NMMA). These substances may be infused intravenously and counteract the nitric oxide. However, they have a significantly longer half-life than other currently used vasopressors and they have resulted in myocardial ischaemia owing to increased peripheral resistance and myocardial work. Second, a guanylate cyclase inhibitor may be administered, e.g. methylene blue. This also results in inhibition of the nitric oxide pathway, and results in similar side-effects.

Nitric oxide regulation of vascular tone tends to be in response to local metabolic changes, the presence of bradykinin or acetylcholine, or to local shearing stress in the vessel wall. Nitric oxide has a systemic effect only when the stimulating mechanism is very widespread, such as in systemic sepsis. The local response tends to be very rapid and very short-lived; nitric oxide combines with haemoglobin to form methaemoglobin and this gives it a systemic half-life of less than 5 s.

Long-term control

All the mechanisms described above are rapid responses to changes in arterial pressure, tending to return the pressure to the normal range. However, these mechanisms adapt to sustained changes in arterial pressure and do not produce useful long-term control, which is almost entirely under the influence of renal mechanisms.

The renal control of circulating volume affects each of the factors controlling arterial pressure, except heart rate. At its simplest level, renal output of salt and water is dependent on perfusion pressure. An increase in renal perfusion pressure results in increased salt and water output by the kidney; this results in a decrease in blood volume, and decreases in cardiac output and arterial pressure. A decrease in renal perfusion pressure has the opposite effects. In addition, changes in arterial pressure affect the renin–angiotensin system, which has direct effects on the kidneys to cause salt and water retention.

SUMMARY

The product of cardiac output and systemic vascular resistance determines mean arterial pressure. The cardiovascular system possesses several control systems that maintain the mean arterial pressure within a very small range. Short-term control systems function via neural mechanisms initiated via baro- and chemoreceptor pathways and humoral control systems, including the renin–angiotensin, vasopressin, atrial natriuretic peptide and nitric oxide pathways. Long-term control of mean arterial pressure is almost exclusively under the influence of renal mechanisms.

FURTHER READING

Guyton A C, Jones C E, Coleman T G 1973 Circulatory physiology: cardiac output and its regulation. W B Saunders, Philadelphia

Lowenstein C J, Dinerman J L, Snyder S H 1994 Nitric oxide: a physiologic messenger. Annals of Internal Medicine 120: 227–237

Magder S, De Varennes B 1998 Clinical death and the measurement of stressed vascular volume. Critical Care Medicine 26: 1061–1064

Priebe H-J, Skarvan K 2000 Cardiovascular physiology, 2nd edn. BMJ Books, London

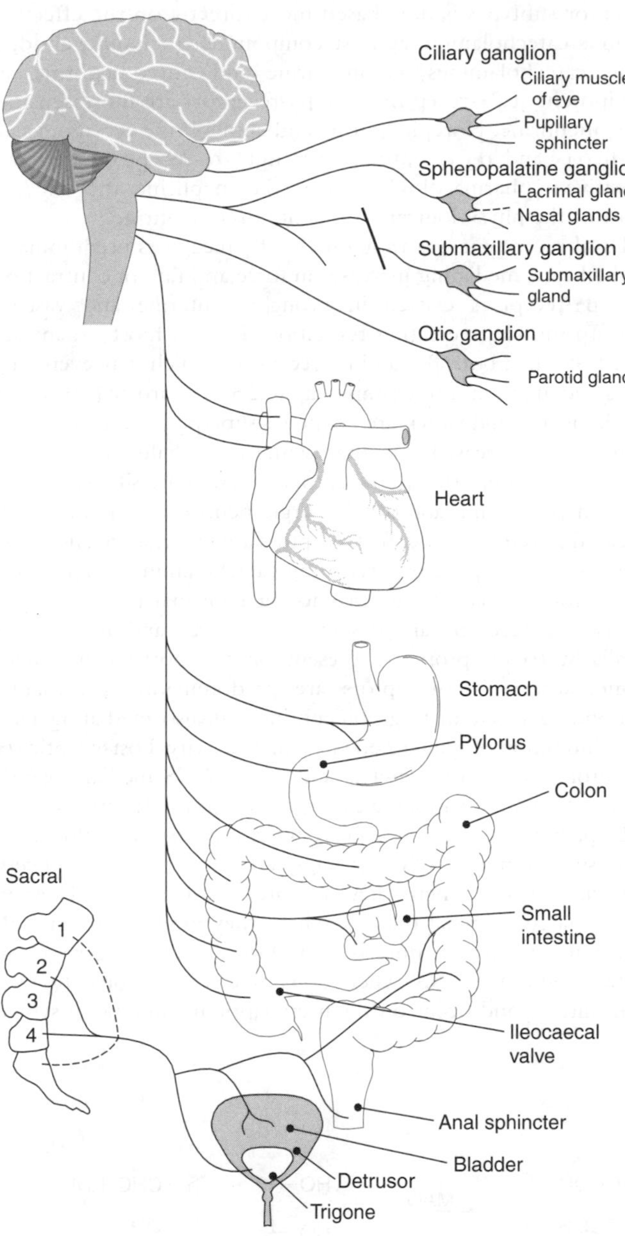

Fig. 7.2
The parasympathetic nervous system.

HO, HO, NH_2, Catechol Nucleus, Amine Side chain

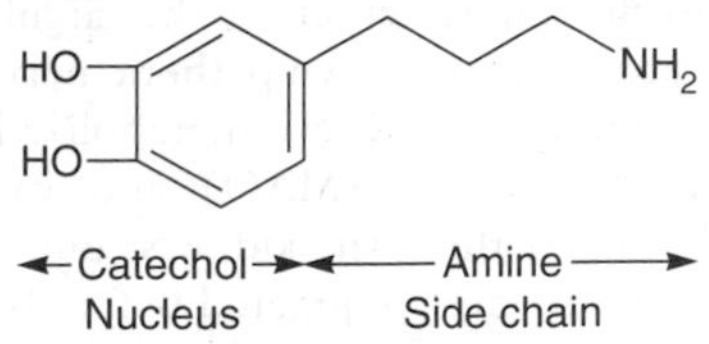

Fig. 7.3
Standard molecular structure of catecholamines, composed of a catechol ring with –OH substitution in the 3 and 4 positions relative to the amine side chain.

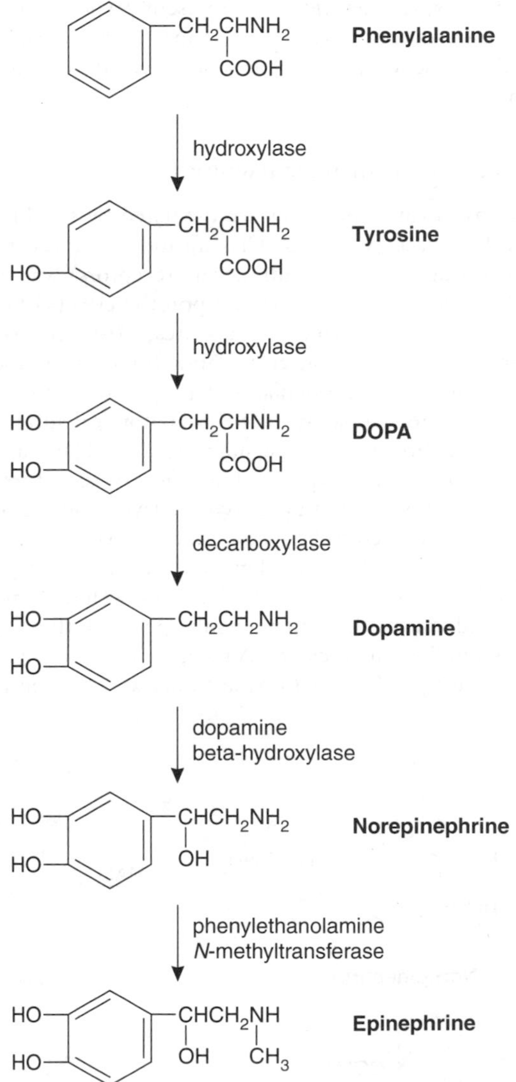

Fig. 7.4
Synthesis of endogenous catecholamines from the essential amino acid phenylalanine.

acid phenylalanine. Their structure is based on a catechol ring (i.e. a benzene ring with -OH groups in the 3 and 4 positions), and an ethylamine side chain (Figs 7.3 and 7.4). The -OH groups in positions 3 and 4 on the benzene ring designate the compound a *catechol*, and substitutions in the side chain produce the different compounds. Dopamine may act as a precursor for both epinephrine and norepinephrine when administered exogenously (see below).

The action of norepinephrine released from sympathetic nerve endings is terminated in one of three ways:

- re-uptake into the nerve terminal
- diffusion into the circulation
- enzymatic destruction.

Most norepinephrine released from sympathetic nerves is taken back into the presynaptic nerve ending for storage and subsequent reuse. Re-uptake is by active transport back into the nerve terminal cytoplasm and then into cytoplasmic vesicles. This mechanism of presynaptic re-uptake, termed *uptake*$_1$, is dependent on adenosine triphosphate (ATP) and Mg^{2+}, is enhanced by Li^+ and may be blocked by cocaine and tricyclic antidepressants.

Endogenous catecholamines entering the circulation, by diffusion from their site of action at sympathetic nerve endings or by release from the adrenal gland, are metabolized rapidly by the enzymes monamine oxidase (MAO) and catechol-o-methyl transferase (COMT) in the liver, kidneys, gut and many other tissues. The metabolites are conjugated before being excreted in the urine as 3-methoxy-4-hydroxymandelic acid, metanephrine (from epinephrine) and normetanephrine (from norepinephrine) (Fig. 7.5). Norepinephrine taken up into the nerve terminal may also be deaminated by cytoplasmic MAO.

Another mechanism for the postsynaptic cellular re-uptake of catecholamines, termed *uptake$_2$*, is present predominantly at the membrane of smooth muscle cells. It may be responsible for the termination of action of catecholamines released from the adrenal medulla.

Adrenergic receptor pharmacology

The actions of catecholamines are mediated by specific postsynaptic cell surface receptors. Classification of these receptors into two groups (α- and β-adrenergic receptors) was first suggested by Ahlquist in 1948, based upon the effects of epinephrine at peripheral sympathetic sites, α-receptors being responsible for vasoconstriction and β-receptors mediating effects on the heart, bronchial and intestinal smooth muscle. However, it is now apparent that this anatomical subdivision of the receptor subtypes is an oversimplification. There are several subtypes of α- and β-receptors in addition to receptors specific for dopamine (DA_1 and DA_2 subtypes). Two subtypes of α- and β-receptors have been well characterized to date on functional, anatomical and pharmacological grounds (α_1 and α_2, β_1 and β_2). A third subtype of β-receptor, β_3, has been well documented in humans, and at least three further subtypes of both α_1- and α_2-receptors and five subtypes of DA receptor have been identified, although their precise functions are unclear. Differentiation of receptor subtypes is now based more directly on the effects of various catecholamine agonist compounds (including endogenous catecholamines). Epinephrine and norepinephrine are equipotent at β_1-receptors, but β_2-receptors are more sensitive to epinephrine. Norepinephrine and epinephrine are agonists at both α_1- and α_2-receptors. Although α_1-receptors are more sensitive in pharmacological terms to epinephrine, they mediate most of the physiological actions of norepinephrine.

Until recently it was thought that β_1-receptors predominated in the heart, mediating increases in force and rate of contraction, and β_2-receptors existed in bronchial, uterine and vascular smooth muscle, mediating relaxation. In fact, most organs and tissues contain both β_1- and β_2-receptors, which may even serve the same function. For example, up to 25% of cardiac β-receptors in the normal individual are of the β_2 subtype , and this proportion may be increased in patients with cardiac failure (see below). It is now apparent that β_1-receptors in tissues are situated on the postsynaptic membrane of adrenergic neurones and respond to released norepinephrine. β_2-Receptors are presynaptic and, when stimulated principally by circulating catecholamines, they modulate autonomic activity by promoting neuronal norepinephrine release. β_3-Receptors are present on adipocytes and other tissues. Similarly, α_1-receptors are present on the postsynaptic membrane, whereas α_2-receptors are predominantly presynaptic, responding to circulating epinephrine but also mediating feedback inhibition of sympathetic neuronal activity. Postsynaptic α_2-receptors present on platelets and in the CNS mediate platelet aggregation and membrane hyperpolarization, respectively.

Dopamine receptors (DA_1) are present postsynaptically in vascular smooth muscle of the renal, splanchnic, coronary and cerebral circulations, where they mediate vasodilatation. They are also situated on renal tubules, where they inhibit sodium reabsorption, causing natriuresis and diuresis. DA_2-receptors are widespread in the CNS (where dopamine is an important neurotransmitter), and occur on the presynaptic membrane of sympa-

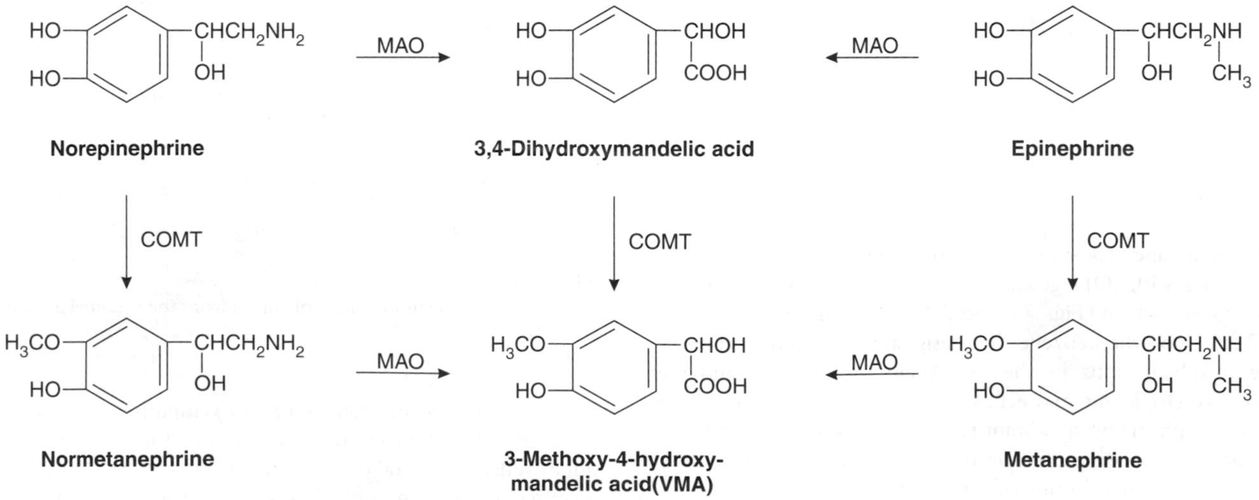

Norepinephrine —MAO→ 3,4-Dihydroxymandelic acid ←MAO— Epinephrine

COMT ↓ (each)

Normetanephrine —MAO→ 3-Methoxy-4-hydroxy-mandelic acid(VMA) ←MAO— Metanephrine

Fig. 7.5
The metabolites (metabolized by MAO and COMT) of endogenous catecholamines are excreted in the urine as 3-methoxy-4-hydroxymandelic acid, metanephrine (from epinephrine) and normetanephrine (from norepinephrine). MAO = monoamine oxidase; COMT = catechol-o-methyl transferase.

thetic nerves and in the adrenal gland. Stimulation of presynaptic DA_2-receptors inhibits dopamine release by negative feedback.

Postganglionic sympathetic fibres supplying sweat glands and arterioles in some areas of skin and skeletal muscle are cholinergic. Vascular smooth muscle also contains non-innervated cholinergic receptors which mediate vasodilatation in response to circulating agonists. Cholinergic effects on vascular smooth muscle are usually minimal but may be involved in the mechanism of vasovagal attacks.

These subdivisions are summarized in Table 7.1.

Table 7.1 Effects of the sympathetic and parasympathetic nervous systems on peripheral effector organs, and receptor subtypes mediating these functions (where known). All postganglionic parasympathetic fibres are muscarinic (M), but in many sites the subtype has not been identified.

	Sympathetic		Parasympathetic	
Organ	Receptor subtype	Effect	Receptor subtype	Effect
Heart	β_1 also β_2, ? also α and DA_1 α_1	↑ Heart rate ↑ Force of contraction ↑ Conduction velocity ↑ Automaticity (β_2) ↑ Excitability ↑ Force of contraction	M_2	↓ Heart rate ↓ Force of contraction Slight ↓ conduction velocity
Arteries	β_1 β_2 α_1, α_2 DA_1, β_2	Coronary vasodilatation Vasodilatation (skeletal muscle) Vasoconstriction (coronary, pulmonary, renal and splanchnic circulations, skin and skeletal muscle) Splanchnic and renal vasodilatation	M[a]	Vasodilatation in skin, skeletal muscle, pulmonary and coronary circulations
Veins	α_1, also α_2 β_2	Vasoconstriction Vasodilatation		
Lung	β_2 α_1	Bronchodilatation Inhibition of secretions Bronchoconstriction	M_3	Bronchoconstriction Stimulation of secretions
GI tract	α_1,α_2, β_2 α_1,α_2	Decreased motility Contraction of sphincters Inhibition of secretions	M	Increased motility Relaxation of sphincters Stimulation of secretions
Pancreas	β_2 α_1, α_2	Increased insulin release Decreased insulin release		
Kidney	β	Renin secretion		
Liver	β_2, α β_2, ?α	Glycogenolysis Gluconeogenesis	M	Glycogen synthesis
Bladder	β_2 α	Detrusor relaxation Sphincter contraction	M	Detrusor contraction Sphincter relaxation
Uterus	α_1 β_2	Myometrial contraction Myometrial relaxation		
Adipocytes	β_3	Lipolysis		
Eye	α_1	Mydriasis (radial muscle contraction) Ciliary muscle relaxation for far vision	M	Miosis Ciliary muscle contraction for near vision
Platelets	α_2	Promote platelet aggregation		
Sweat glands	M[b]	Sweating		

[a]Muscarinic receptors are present on vascular smooth muscle, but they are independent of parasympathetic innervation and have little or no physiological role in the control of vasomotor tone.
[b]Sympathetic cholinergic fibres supply sweat glands and arterioles in some sites.

Presynaptic receptors

Autonomic nerve terminals (whether adrenergic, dopaminergic or cholinergic) possess receptors on the presynaptic membrane in addition to the α_2-, β_2- and DA_2-receptors outlined above, which modulate neuronal transmission. These respond to a variety of endogenous substances which may facilitate or inhibit activity of the nerve (Fig. 7.6). The function of presynaptic β_2-receptors may include maintaining basal levels of norepinephrine release when sympathetic activity is low, and augmenting neuronal norepinephrine transmission in response to high circulating catecholamine concentrations. Several compounds may be stored in vesicles within the presynaptic sympathetic nerve terminal. These include enkephalins, substance P, vasoactive intestinal peptide, somatostatin, nitric oxide, dopamine and neuropeptide Y. The function of these substances is not defined, but they may modulate the synthesis or release of particular neurotransmitters. Alternatively, they may be released alone or in conjunction with the neurotransmitter to act directly on the postsynaptic receptor.

Structure of adrenergic receptors

Both α- and β-adrenergic receptors are proteins with a similar basic structure, comprising seven hydrophobic transmembrane domains and an intracellular chain. Differences in amino acid sequences of the intracellular chain differentiate α- and β-receptors. Both are linked to guanine nucleotide binding proteins (G-proteins) in the cell membrane which mediate the generation of second messengers which activate intracellular events. These second messenger systems include enzymes (adenylate cyclase, phospholipases) and ion channels (for calcium and potassium) (see Ch. 2).

Second and third messenger systems

In addition to functional differences, α- and β-receptors differ in the intracellular mechanisms by which they act. Stimulation of β_1- and β_2-receptors activates G_s-proteins, which activate adenylate cyclase and cause the generation of intracellular cyclic adenosine monophosphate (cAMP) (Fig. 7.7). cAMP activates intracellular enzyme pathways (the third messengers) to produce the associated alteration in cell function (e.g. increased force of cardiac muscle contraction, liver glycogenolysis, bronchial smooth muscle relaxation). In cardiac myocytes, the intracellular pathway involves the activation of protein kinases to phosphorylate intracellular proteins and increase intracellular Ca^{2+} concentrations. Intracellular cAMP concentration is modulated by the enzyme phosphodiesterase, which breaks down cAMP to inactive 5′AMP. The balance between production and degradation of cAMP is an important regulatory system for cell function. α_2-Receptors interact with G_i-proteins to ***inhibit*** adenylate cyclase and Ca^{2+} channels, but activate K^+ channels, phospholipase C and phospholipase A_2. Cholinergic M_2-receptors and somatostatin affect G_i-proteins in the same way.

In contrast, α_1-receptor stimulation does not affect cAMP levels within the cell directly, but causes coupling with another G-protein, G_q, to activate membrane-bound phospholipase C. This in turn hydrolyses phosphatidylinositol biphosphate (PIP_2) to inositol triphosphate (IP_3), which produces changes in intracellular Ca^{2+} concentration and binding. These lead, for example, to smooth muscle contraction.

Functions of the sympathetic nervous system

There is constant activity of both the sympathetic and parasympathetic nervous systems even at rest, mediated by the control centres in the medulla (see below). This is termed sympathetic or parasympathetic tone and allows alterations in autonomic activity to produce rapid two-way regulation of physiological effect. For example, a decrease in sympathetic tone produces decreased vasoconstriction, i.e. vasodilatation. Coordinated activation of the sympathetic nervous system produces the ‘fight or flight’ response to threatening or noxious stimuli, which results in an increased cardiac output and

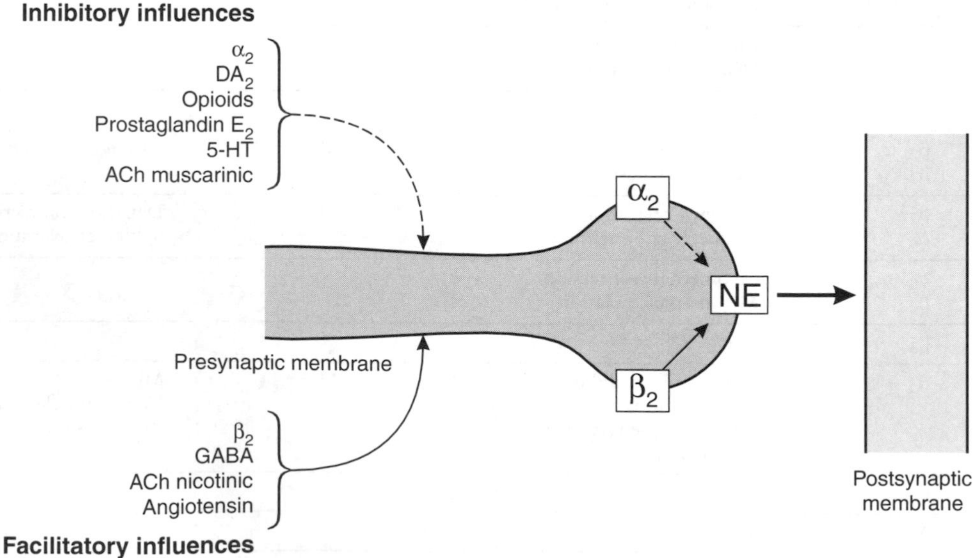

Fig. 7.6
Influences on sympathetic nervous transmission.

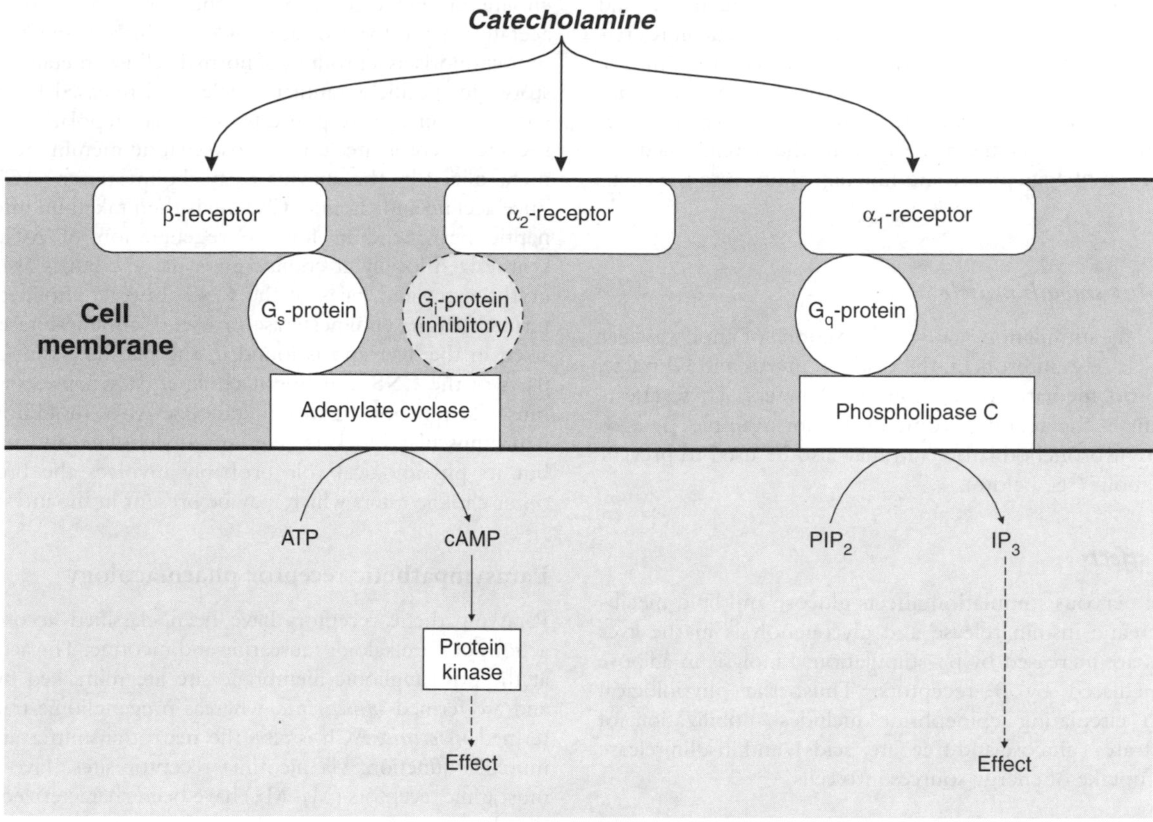

Fig. 7.7
Intracellular mechanisms of action of adrenergic receptors. Activation of β-receptors stimulates adenylate cyclase to catalyse the conversion of adenosine triphosphate (ATP) to cyclic adenosine monophosphate (cAMP) via a membrane-bound G_s-protein. Activation of α_2-receptors inhibits adenylate cyclase via an inhibitory (G_i) protein. α_2 Receptor stimulation also activates K^+ channels, inhibits Ca^{2+} channels, and activates phospholipases A_2 and C. α_1-Adrenergic stimulation interacts with a G_q-protein to activate phospholipase C, to promote the production of inositol triphosphate (IP_3).

blood flow to skeletal muscle, and increased energy production to fuel increased metabolic activity. Most of the effects of sympathetic stimulation are mediated by sympathetic nerves, but some are mediated by non-innervated receptors in response to circulating epinephrine. The effect of sympathetic stimulation on a particular organ depends on the balance of adrenergic receptors present (Table 7.1).

Cardiovascular effects

Sympathetic stimulation produces increases in heart rate and contractility, mediated predominantly by β_1-receptors, although β_2-, α- and possibly DA-receptors are also involved. The diameter of blood vessels (and thus the resistance to blood flow) depends on the state of contraction of vascular smooth muscle; normal sympathetic tone is α-mediated. Sympathetic activity at α-receptors therefore controls the peripheral resistance to blood flow (by effects on the arterial side of the circulation) and the circulating volume (venous constriction increases blood flow returning to the heart). The redistribution of blood between skeletal muscle and other tissues is determined by activation of β-receptors and is mediated physiologically by circulating epinephrine; β-stimulation produces vasodilatation in skeletal muscle, the brain and the coronary circulation. Dopaminergic (DA_1) and β_2-receptors in the splanchnic and renal circulations also mediate regional vasodilatation. The overall effect of catecholamines on cardiac output and arterial pressure depends on the interaction between effects on cardiac rate, contractility and peripheral vascular resistance. This may be used therapeutically by using drugs with specific effects at α-, β- and dopaminergic receptors or at a combination of receptors. For example, drugs which increase peripheral resistance in addition to cardiac contractility are most effective in increasing arterial pressure, although cardiac output may actually decrease and intense vasoconstriction may cause ischaemia elsewhere.

Overall, cardiovascular homeostasis is coordinated in the medulla and lower third of the brain stem. The ventrolateral medulla is traditionally referred to as the vasomotor centre because it is the primary site regulating sympathetic outflow, with rostral portions containing excitatory neurones and the caudal portions initiating sympatho-inhibitory neurones. It is now known that cardiovascular function is controlled by several regions or groups of cells with specific interconnections, responsible for different aspects of cardiovascular activity, although these cells act in a coordinated manner. Afferent signals from baroreceptors, pulmonary stretch receptors, cardiac and respiratory mechanoreceptors and visceral receptors synapse in the nucleus tractus solitarius in the posterolateral portions of the medulla. Efferent preganglionic fibres originate in the upper five or six thoracic spinal segments and terminate in the corresponding ganglia of the sympathetic trunk and cervical ganglia. Postganglionic fibres reach the heart via the superior, middle and inferior cardiac branches of the cervical portion of the sympathetic trunk, and through varying numbers of thoracic cardiac nerves. The fibres terminate in the sinoatrial and atrioventricular nodes, on cardiac muscle fibres and in coronary vessels; they cause increased heart rate, contractility and coronary vasodilatation. Sympathetic nerve impulses are usually transmitted at the same time to the adrenal medulla, causing secretion of epinephrine and norepinephrine into the circulation.

Non-vascular smooth muscle

In general, β_2-stimulation causes relaxation of non-vascular smooth muscle (e.g. in bronchi, the bladder, uterus and GI tract), and α-receptors mediate contraction of sphincters. These effects are important in the action of some drugs; for example, β_2-agonists are potent bronchodilators and may also be used to prevent premature labour (see below).

Metabolic effects

Sympathetic nervous stimulation affects glucose and lipid metabolism. Pancreatic insulin release and glycogenolysis in the liver and muscles are increased by β_2-stimulation. Lipolysis in adipose tissue is mediated by β_3-receptors. Thus, the physiological response to circulating epinephrine includes mobilization of energy substrates (glucose and free fatty acids), and insulin release to promote uptake of energy sources into cells.

THE PARASYMPATHETIC NERVOUS SYSTEM

Parasympathetic neurones arise from cell bodies of the motor nuclei of the cranial nerves III, VII, IX and X in the brain stem, and from the sacral segments of the spinal cord (the 'craniosacral outflow') (Fig. 7.2). The preganglionic fibres run almost to the organ innervated and synapse in ganglia within the organ, giving rise to postganglionic fibres, which supply the relevant tissues. The ganglion cells may be well organized (e.g. in the myenteric plexus of the intestine) or diffuse (e.g. in the bladder or blood vessels).

Parasympathetic neurotransmitters

The chemical neurotransmitter at both pre- and postganglionic synapses is ACh, although transmission at postganglionic synapses may be modulated by other substances, including GABA, serotonin and opioid peptides. ACh is synthesized in the cytoplasm of cholinergic nerve terminals by the combination of choline and acetate (in the form of acetyl-CoA, which is synthesized in the mitochondria as a product of normal cellular metabolism). ACh is stored in specific agranular vesicles and released from the presynaptic terminal in response to neuronal depolarization to act at specific receptor sites on the postsynaptic membrane. It is rapidly metabolized by the enzyme acetylcholinesterase (AChE) to produce acetate and choline. Choline is then taken up into the presynaptic nerve ending for the regeneration of ACh. AChE is synthesized locally at cholinergic synapses, but is also present in erythrocytes and parts of the CNS. Butyryl cholinesterase (also termed plasma cholinesterase or pseudocholinesterase) is synthesized in the liver and is found in the plasma, skin, GI tract and parts of the CNS, but not at cholinergic synapses or the neuromuscular junction. It may metabolize ACh, in addition to some neuromuscular blockers (e.g. succinylcholine and mivacurium), but its physiological role probably involves the breakdown of other choline esters which may be present in the intestine.

Parasympathetic receptor pharmacology

Parasympathetic receptors have been classified according to the actions of the alkaloids muscarine and nicotine. The actions of ACh at the postganglionic membrane site are mimicked by muscarine and are termed *muscarinic*, whereas preganglionic transmission is termed *nicotinic*. ACh is also the neurotransmitter at the neuromuscular junction, via nicotinic receptor sites. Five subtypes of muscarinic receptors (M_1–M_5) have been characterized by molecular cloning techniques, and specific antagonists developed for M_1–M_3 receptors. All five receptor subtypes exist in the CNS, but there are differences in their peripheral distribution and function (Table 7.2). M_1-receptors are found in the stomach where they mediate acid secretion, whereas M_2-receptors predominate in the myocardium, where they modulate heart rate and impulse conduction. Prejunctional M_2-receptors may also be involved in the regulation of synaptic norepinephrine and ACh release. M_3-receptors are present in classic postsynaptic sites in glandular tissue (of the GI and respiratory tract) and probably in bronchial smooth muscle. M_4-receptors have been isolated in cardiac and lung tissue in animal models and may have inhibitory effects, but the distribution and functions of M_5-receptors are not yet defined.

In common with adrenergic receptors, muscarinic receptors are coupled to membrane-bound G-proteins and thus comprise seven transmembrane domains, of which the third intracellular domain interacts with the G-protein. The subtypes differ in the second

Table 7.2 Properties of muscarinic (M_1-M_5) receptors (adapted with permission from Lambert & Appadu 1995)

	M_1	M_2	M_3	M_4	M_5
Second messenger	IP_3	cAMP	IP_3	cAMP	IP_3
Location	CNS Stomach	Heart CNS	CNS Glands	CNS Heart	CNS
Important clinical effects	Gastric acid production	Bradycardia	Secretion	?	
Clinically selective agent	Pirenzepine	None	None	None	None

IP_3 stimulates inositol triphosphate production.
cAMP inhibits adenylate cyclase to decrease cAMP formation.

messenger system with which they interact. M_1-, M_3- and M_5-receptors couple to phospholipase C via a G_q-protein to generate IP_3. M_2- and M_4-receptors uncouple adenylate cyclase via interaction with a G_i-protein and decrease the formation of cAMP, activate K^+ channels and inhibit Ca^{2+} channels. Apart from pirenzepine (a specific M_1-antagonist which is used to decrease gastric acid secretion in patients with peptic ulcer disease), currently available drugs acting on cholinergic transmission are thought to act non-specifically at muscarinic receptor subtypes. However, antimuscarinic drugs, e.g. atropine and hyoscine, differ in their clinical spectra (see below), suggesting that they may have differing effects at different muscarinic receptor subtypes and that more specific drugs might be useful clinically.

Functions of the parasympathetic nervous system

The parasympathetic nervous system controls vegetative functions, i.e. the digestion and absorption of nutrients, excretion of waste products, and the conservation and restoration of energy. As the majority of all parasympathetic nerves are contained in branches of the vagus nerve, which innervates the viscera of the thorax and abdomen, increased parasympathetic activity is characterized by signs of vagal overactivity. Parasympathetic fibres also pass to the eye via the oculomotor (IIIrd cranial) nerve, and to the lacrimal, nasal and salivary glands via the facial (VIIth) and glossopharyngeal (IXth) nerves. Fibres originating in the sacral portion of the spinal cord pass to the distal GI tract, bladder and reproductive organs (Fig. 7.2).

Cardiovascular system

The parasympathetic nervous system plays only a minor role in cardiovascular regulation overall, but is involved in the regulation of heart rate via the vagus nerve. Cell bodies of preganglionic neurones are mainly in the brain stem (the nucleus ambiguus and dorsal motor nucleus of the vagus). Fibres enter cardiac branches of the vagus and synapse with the postganglionic neurones in the cardiac plexuses and scattered cell clusters in the walls of the atria. Postganglionic fibres supply the sinoatrial (SA) and atrioventricular (AV) nodes to decrease heart rate; fibres supplying atrial and ventricular muscle decrease contractility, and those supplying coronary arteries cause vasoconstriction. Cardiac effects are blocked by muscarinic antagonists (e.g. atropine) but are not physiologically significant, being obscured by sympathetic activity and by baroreceptor and other reflexes. Muscarinic receptors mediating vasodilatation are present on vascular smooth muscle but are independent of parasympathetic nerves. They have minimal effects on the physiological control of vascular tone, but may be involved in the mechanism of vasovagal attacks.

Gastrointestinal system

The parasympathetic nervous system controls the secretomotor activity of the GI tract. Stimulation produces increased tone, amplitude of contractions and peristaltic activity via postganglionic fibres in the myenteric nerve plexus. Relaxation of gastric and intestinal sphincters, biliary contraction, and salivary, gastric, exocrine pancreatic and intestinal secretions are also stimulated. Parasympathetic stimulation increases ureteric peristalsis, contracts bladder detrusor muscle and relaxes bladder sphincters, thus encouraging micturition.

Bronchial tree

Bronchoconstriction is produced in addition to increased mucus secretion. These effects may be a problem in asthmatic and allergic subjects in whom cholinergic drugs should be used with caution. Induction of bronchospasm by reflex cholinergic (vagal) effects in some asthmatics has led to the use of anticholinergics as bronchodilators (see Ch. 13).

Eye

Miosis and spasm of the ciliary muscle occur so that the eye is accommodated for near vision. Intraocular pressure decreases as a result of increased reabsorption of intraocular fluids.

DRUGS ACTING ON THE SYMPATHETIC NERVOUS SYSTEM

SYMPATHOMIMETIC DRUGS

Drugs which partially or completely mimic the effects of sympathetic nerve stimulation or adrenal medullary discharge are termed sympathomimetic. They may act:

- directly on the adrenergic receptor, e.g. the catecholamines, phenylephrine, methoxamine
- indirectly, causing release of norepinephrine from the adrenergic nerve ending, e.g. amphetamine
- by both mechanisms, e.g. dopamine, ephedrine, metaraminol.

The major clinical effects of most sympathomimetic drugs are produced via α-, β- or DA-receptors. The drugs may be classified according to their structure (catecholamine/non-catecholamine), their origin (endogenous/synthetic) and their mechanism of action (via adrenergic receptors or a via a non-adrenergic mechanism) (Table 7.3).

Drugs that affect myocardial contractility are termed inotropes, although this term is usually applied to those drugs which increase

Table 7.3 Classification of sympathomimetic drugs

Catecholamines		Non-catecholamines	
Endogenous	Synthetic	Acting via adrenergic receptors	Acting via non-adrenergic mechanisms
Epinephrine	Isoproterenol	Ephedrine	Phosphodiesterase inhibitors
Norepinephrine	Dobutamine	Phenylephrine	Digoxin
Dopamine	Dopexamine	Methoxamine	Glucagon
		Metaraminol	Calcium salts

cardiac contractility (strictly 'positive inotropes'). Myocardial contractility may be increased by the following (Fig. 7.8):

- increasing intracellular cAMP by activation of the adenylate cyclase system (e.g. catecholamines and other drugs acting via the adrenergic receptor)
- decreasing breakdown of cAMP (e.g. phosphodiesterase inhibitors)
- increasing intracellular calcium availability or increasing the response of contractile proteins to calcium (e.g. digoxin, calcium salts, glucagon).

Inotropes may also be classified into positive inotropic drugs which also produce systemic vasoconstriction ('inoconstrictors'), and those which also produce systemic vasodilatation ('inodilators'). Inoconstrictors include norepinephrine, epinephrine and ephedrine. Inodilators are dobutamine, dopexamine, isoproterenol and phosphodiesterase inhibitors. Dopamine is an inodilator at low dose, and an inoconstrictor at higher doses.

Catecholamines

The catecholamines are based on a catechol ring (i.e. a benzene ring with -OH groups in the 3 and 4 positions) and an ethylamine side chain (Figs 7.3 and 7.4). Substitutions in the side chain produce the different compounds. The endogenous catecholamines are epinephrine, norepinephrine and dopamine; synthetic catecholamines include dobutamine, dopexamine and isoproterenol Several other drugs with a non-catecholamine structure produce sympathomimetic effects via adrenergic receptors. These include ephedrine, methoxamine and phenylephrine. All the exogenous (and endogenous) catecholamines are inactivated in the gut by MAO and are usually only administered parenterally. They all have very short half-lives in vivo, and so when given by intravenous infusion, their effects may be controlled by altering the infusion rate.

Endogenous catecholamines

Epinephrine accounts for 80–90% of the catecholamine content of the adrenal medulla and is also an important neurotransmitter in the CNS. It is a powerful agonist at both α- and β-adrenergic receptors, being more potent than norepinephrine at α-receptors, and more potent than isoproterenol at β-receptors. It is the treatment of choice in acute allergic (anaphylactic) reactions and is used in the management of cardiac arrest and shock, and occasionally as a bronchodilator. Except in emergency situations, i.v. injection is avoided because of the risk of inducing cardiac arrhythmias. Subcutaneous administration produces local vasoconstriction and so smoothes out its own effect by slowing absorption.

The effects of epinephrine on arterial pressure and cardiac output are dependent on dose (usual range 0.01–0.2 $\mu g\ kg^{-1}\ min^{-1}$). Although both α- and β-receptors are stimulated, β_2 vasodilator effects are most sensitive. Heart rate and contractility, cardiac output and systolic pressure are increased by β_1 effects. In low dosage, vasodilatation in skeletal muscle and splanchnic arterioles (β_2) is prominent; systemic vascular resistance and diastolic pressure may decrease, pulse pressure widens, but mean arterial pressure remains stable. At higher doses, α-mediated vasoconstriction occurs in the precapillary resistance vessels of skin, mucosa and

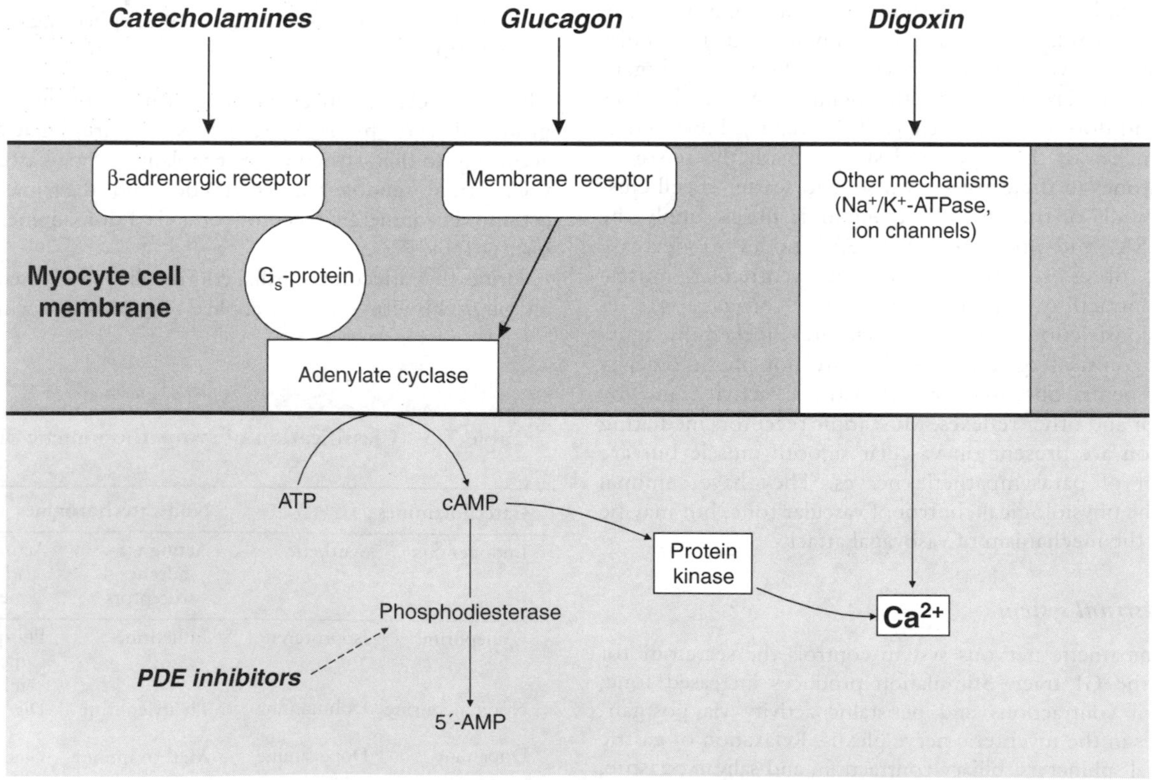

Fig. 7.8
Intracellular action of positive inotropic drugs.

kidney. Systolic pressure increases further, and cardiac output may decrease. Epinephrine causes marked decreases in renal blood flow, but coronary blood flow is increased. In contrast to other sympathomimetics, epinephrine has significant metabolic effects. Hepatic glycogenolysis and lipolysis in adipose tissue increase (β_1 effects), and insulin secretion is inhibited (α_1 effect) so that hyperglycaemia occurs.

In the treatment of acute anaphylactic reactions, epinephrine 0.5–1 mg i.m. (0.5–1.0 ml of 1:1000 solution) or 100 μg increments i.v. to a dose of 1 mg (1–10 ml of a 1:10 000 solution) are used. Epinephrine is important in the management of cardiac arrest, (in doses of 1 mg i.v., repeated every 3 min), mostly because of its α effects: widespread systemic vasoconstriction occurs, increasing aortic diastolic pressure and coronary and cerebral perfusion. Pure α-agonists are less effective than epinephrine in the management of cardiac arrest, and the β_2 effects of epinephrine may contribute to improved cerebral perfusion. In emergency situations, it may also be administered via the tracheal route, in doses of 2–3 mg diluted to a volume of 10 ml. It is effective by aerosol inhalation in bronchial asthma but has been superseded by the newer β_2-agonists (see below). Unlike indirect-acting sympathomimetics that cause norepinephrine release, tachyphylaxis should not occur with epinephrine. Epinephrine is also used as a topical vasoconstrictor to aid haemostasis and is incorporated into local anaesthetic solutions to decrease systemic absorption and prolong the duration of local anaesthesia.

Norepinephrine acts as a potent arteriolar and venous vasoconstrictor, which acts almost exclusively at α-receptors, although it is less potent here than epinephrine. Infusions of norepinephrine increase systolic and diastolic systemic and pulmonary arterial pressures and central venous pressure. Heart rate decreases because of baroreflex activity. Despite some stimulatory effects on cardiac contraction, the widespread intense vasoconstriction leads either to no change or to a decrease in cardiac output at the cost of increased myocardial oxygen demand. The usual dose range is 0.01–0.1 μg kg^{-1} min^{-1}; at higher doses renal blood flow and glomerular filtration rate are reduced. In clinical practice its use is limited by cardiac arrhythmias, adverse effects on renal function and intense vasoconstriction (leading to peripheral ischaemia), but it may be useful in the management of septic shock when systemic vascular resistance is very low.

Dopamine is the natural precursor of epinephrine and norepinephrine. It stimulates both α- and β-adrenergic receptors in addition to specific dopamine (DA_1) receptors in renal and mesenteric arteries. Dopamine has a direct positive inotropic action on the myocardium via β-receptors and also by release of norepinephrine from adrenergic nerve terminals. However, the overall effect of dopamine is related to dosage. In low dosage (< 3 μg kg^{-1} min^{-1}), renal and mesenteric vascular resistance is reduced by an action on DA_1-receptors, resulting in increases in splanchnic and renal blood flows, glomerular filtration rate and sodium excretion. Thus low-dose infusions have been used in an attempt to prevent acute renal failure in intensive care patients or those undergoing high-risk surgery. However, despite its theoretical attractions, there is no firm evidence that dopamine is either effective or superior to any other inotrope for this indication. At slightly higher doses (5–10 μg kg^{-1} min^{-1}), the increasing direct β-mediated inotropic action becomes apparent, with little or no peripheral vasoconstrictor effects. This combination of increased cardiac output and renal vasodilatation is useful in the management of cardiogenic, traumatic, septic and hypovolaemic shock, where excessive use of direct sympathomimetics associated with a major increase in physiological sympathetic activity may lead to severe compromise of renal blood flow and peripheral circulation. At these doses, direct cardiac chronotropic action is usually minimal, and tachyarrhythmias are less common than with other sympathomimetics. Systolic pressure is increased, with little effect on diastolic arterial pressure. Total peripheral resistance is usually unchanged. However, at higher doses (> 15 μg kg^{-1} min^{-1}), α-receptor activity predominates, with direct vasoconstriction and increased cardiac stimulation (similar to norepinephrine). Renal and splanchnic blood flow decreases, and arrhythmias may occur. Dopamine receptors are widely present in the CNS, particularly in the basal ganglia, pituitary and chemoreceptor trigger zone (CTZ) on the floor of the fourth ventricle. They mediate pituitary prolactin secretion and nausea and vomiting at the CTZ. Decreased CNS dopamine concentrations are a feature of Parkinson's disease. Dopamine antagonists (e.g. phenothiazines, butyrophenones) have been used widely as antipsychotics and antiemetics, although extrapyramidal side-effects may limit their use. Recently, dopamine infusions have been associated with decreased prolactin secretion, and the use of 'prophylactic' dopamine infusions in an attempt to preserve renal function in critically ill patients is declining.

Synthetic catecholamines

Isoproterenol is a β_1- and β_2-agonist, with virtually no activity at α-receptors. It acts via cardiac β_1-receptors, and β_2-receptors in the smooth muscle of bronchi, vasculature of skeletal muscle and the gut. After intravenous infusion, heart rate increases and peripheral resistance is reduced. Cardiac output is increased by a combination of increased venous return, heart rate and contractility. Systolic pressure may increase, but diastolic pressure decreases and coronary perfusion may be impaired. Myocardial oxygen consumption is increased and arrhythmias are common. Other β_2-mediated effects include relaxation of bronchial smooth muscle and stabilization of mast cells. It has been widely used in the treatment of severe asthma, although newer specific β_2-agonists with fewer cardiac effects are now preferred. Isoproterenol is usually administered by intravenous infusion or aerosol. Its most important current indication is in the treatment of bradyarrhythmias or atrioventricular heart block associated with low cardiac output (e.g. following acute myocardial infarction), because it increases heart rate and conduction by a direct action on the subsidiary pacemaker. This indication is usually an interim measure before insertion of a temporary pacing wire.

Dobutamine resembles isoproterenol and dopamine chemically, but is primarily a β_1-agonist, with moderate β_2- and mild α_1-agonist activity, and no action at DA-receptors. The dose range is 2.5–25 μg kg^{-1} min^{-1}. Its primary effect is an increase in cardiac output via increased contractility (β_1 effect) augmented by a reduction in afterload. Heart rate also increases (β_2 effect). Systolic arterial pressure may increase, but peripheral resistance is reduced or unchanged. There is no direct effect on venous tone or renal blood flow, but preload may decrease and urine output and sodium excretion increase as a consequence of the increased cardiac output. Dobutamine increases SA node automaticity and conduction velocity in the atria, ventricles and AV node, but to a lesser extent than isoproterenol. Dobutamine infusion produces a progressive increase in cardiac output which is greater than with comparable doses of dopamine, although arterial pressure may initially remain unchanged. At higher doses, tachycardia and arrhythmias may occur, but dobutamine has less effect on myocardial oxygen consumption compared with other catecholamines. It is used alone or in combination with vasodilator drugs in the treatment of cardiac failure when peripheral resistance is high. Conversely, it is useful in the management of some low cardiac output states in combination with dopamine or norepinephrine.

Dopexamine is a synthetic dopamine analogue which is an agonist at β_2- and DA_1-receptors. It is also a weak DA_2-agonist and it inhibits the neuronal re-uptake of norepinephrine (uptake$_1$), but has no direct effects at β_1- or α-receptors. Its principal effect is β_2-agonism, producing vasodilatation in skeletal muscle; it is less potent at DA_1-receptors, but a more potent β_2-agonist than dopamine. It produces mild increases in cardiac contractility (effect on β_2-receptors and norepinephrine uptake), renal and mesenteric vasodilatation (β_2 and DA_1 effects), and natriuresis (DA_1 effect). Coronary and cerebral blood flows are also increased. At doses of 0.5–6.0 $\mu g\ kg^{-1}\ min^{-1}$, heart rate and cardiac output increase, and systemic vascular resistance decreases. Arterial pressure may decrease if intravascular volume is not maintained. Dopexamine has theoretical advantages in maintaining splanchnic blood flow in patients with systemic sepsis, cardiac failure or those who are undergoing major surgery, but definitive data are lacking. It also has anti-inflammatory effects (in common with other β-agonists) that are independent of its effects on gut mucosal perfusion. It is metabolized by hepatic methylation and conjugation and is eliminated mostly via the kidneys.

Fenoldopam. This is a dopamine (DA_1) agonist that causes peripheral vasodilatation and increases renal blood flow and sodium and water excretion. It has been used in the treatment of hypertensive emergencies. Unlike some other vasodilators (e.g. sodium nitroprusside) it does not cause rebound hypertension after stopping the infusion.

Ibopamine is a non-selective DA_1- and DA_2-agonist with similar pharmacological effects to dopamine. Ibopamine is a prodrug, which is converted to epinine (*n*-methyldopamine) after oral administration, and produces a diuresis and natriuresis in patients with cardiac failure.

Non-catecholamine sympathomimetics

Synthetic sympathomimetic drugs may mimic the effect of epinephrine at adrenergic receptors (direct-acting) or may produce effects by causing release of endogenous norepinephrine from postganglionic sympathetic nerve terminals (indirect-acting). Some drugs have direct and indirect sympathomimetic effects (e.g. ephedrine, metaraminol). Direct-acting compounds may affect α- or β-receptors selectively, whereas indirect-acting compounds have predominantly α- and β_1-agonist effects (as norepinephrine is only a weak β_2-agonist). Indirect-acting compounds are taken up into the nerve terminal via the norepinephrine re-uptake pathway, and so their effect is reduced by drugs which block norepinephrine re-uptake (e.g. tricyclic antidepressants). Conversely, the effect of direct-acting drugs is enhanced. In patients treated with drugs that decrease sympathetic nervous system activity (e.g. clonidine, reserpine), the cardiovascular response to indirect-acting drugs is diminished; however, upregulation of adrenergic receptors occurs and an increased response to direct-acting sympathomimetics is seen. Drugs with selective α-adrenergic receptor effects (e.g. phenylephrine, methoxamine) are potent vasoconstrictors.

Ephedrine

Ephedrine is strictly a naturally occurring sympathomimetic amine (it is the active constituent of some Chinese herbal medicines), but it is now produced synthetically. It acts directly and indirectly as an agonist at α-, β_1- and β_2-receptors. The indirect actions are increased endogenous norepinephrine release and inhibition of MAO. Its cardiovascular effects are similar to those of epinephrine, but the duration of action is up to 10 times longer. It causes increases in heart rate, contractility, cardiac output and arterial pressure (systolic > diastolic). It may predispose to arrhythmias. Systemic vascular resistance is usually unchanged, as α-mediated vasoconstriction in some vascular beds is balanced by β-mediated vasodilatation in others – e.g. blood flow is increased in coronary and skeletal muscle, but renal and splanchnic blood flows decrease. It relaxes bronchial and other smooth muscle, and is occasionally used as a bronchodilator. It is active orally as it is not metabolized by MAO in the gut, and is useful by intramuscular injection as muscle blood flow is preserved. Ephedrine undergoes hepatic deamination and conjugation but significant amounts are excreted unchanged in the urine. This accounts for its long duration of action and elimination half-life (3–6 h). Tachyphylaxis (a decreased response to repeated doses of the drug) occurs because of persistent occupation of adrenergic receptors and depletion of norepinephrine stores.

Ephedrine is useful to prevent or treat hypotension resulting from sympathetic blockade during regional anaesthesia or from the effects of general anaesthesia. It is particularly indicated during regional anaesthesia in obstetric patients, as uterine blood flow is maintained (whereas pure vasoconstrictors may restore systemic blood pressure at the expense of uterine blood flow). The usual intravenous dose is 3–12 mg, or 15–30 mg i.m. Oral or topical ephedrine is also useful as a nasal decongestant.

Phenylephrine

Phenylephrine is a potent synthetic direct-acting α_1-agonist, which has minimal agonist effects at α_2- and β-receptors. It has similar effects to those of norepinephrine, causing widespread vasoconstriction, increased arterial pressure, bradycardia (as a result of baroreflex activation) and a decrease in cardiac output. Venoconstriction predominates, and diastolic pressure increases more than systolic pressure, so that coronary blood flow may increase. It may be administered as slow intravenous boluses of 20–50 μg, repeated after 5 min, or as an infusion (10 mg in 500 ml 5% dextrose) at a rate of 20–50 $\mu g\ min^{-1}$ titrated to effect. It is also used topically as a nasal decongestant and mydriatic. Absorption of phenylephrine from mucous membranes may occasionally produce systemic side-effects.

Methoxamine

Methoxamine is a direct-acting α_1-agonist which also has a weak β-antagonist action. It produces vasoconstriction, increases in systolic and diastolic arterial pressures, and decreases in cardiac output and heart rate. Venoconstriction is minimal, and the bradycardia results from baroreflex activation and the mild β-blocking effect. It is a useful vasopressor for the treatment of hypotension during regional or general anaesthesia in intravenous doses of 2–5 mg. Its onset of action is 2 min, with effects lasting for 20 min or more.

Metaraminol

Metaraminol is a direct and indirect-acting α- and β-agonist, which acts partly by being taken up into sympathetic nerve terminals and acting as a false transmitter for norepinephrine. Its α effects predominate, and vasoconstriction is more evident than with ephedrine; reflex bradycardia may occur. Both systolic and diastolic arterial pressures increase. The recommended dose is 1–5 mg i.v., which acts within 3 min and lasts for 25 min.

Phosphodiesterase inhibitors

Phosphodiesterase inhibitors increase intracellular cAMP concentrations by inhibition of the enzyme responsible for cAMP breakdown (Fig. 7.8). Increased intracellular cAMP concentrations promote the activation of protein kinases, which lead to an increase in intracellular Ca^{2+}. In cardiac muscle cells, this causes a positive inotropic effect and also facilitates diastolic relaxation and cardiac filling (termed 'positive lusitropy'). In vascular smooth muscle, increased cAMP decreases intracellular Ca^{2+} and causes marked vasodilatation. Several subtypes of phosphodiesterase (PDE) isoenzyme exist in different tissues. Theophylline is a non-specific PDE inhibitor, but the newer drugs (e.g. amrinone, enoximone and milrinone) are selective for the PDE type III isoenzyme which occurs in the myocardium, vascular smooth muscle and platelets. PDE III inhibitors are positive inotropes and potent arterial, coronary and venodilators. They decrease preload, afterload, pulmonary vascular resistance and pulmonary capillary wedge pressure (PCWP), and increase cardiac index. Heart rate may increase or remain unchanged. In contrast to sympathomimetics, they improve myocardial function *without* increasing oxygen demand or causing tachyphylaxis. Their effects are augmented by the co-administration of β_1-agonists (i.e. increases in cAMP production are synergistic with decreased cAMP breakdown). They have particular advantages in patients with chronic cardiac failure, in whom downregulation of myocardial β-adrenergic receptors occurs, so that there is a decreased inotropic response to β-sympathomimetic drugs. A similar phenomenon occurs with advanced age, prolonged (>72 h) catecholamine therapy and possibly with surgical stress.

They are indicated for acute refractory cardiac failure, e.g. cardiogenic shock, or pre- or post-cardiac surgery. However, long-term treatment with oral PDE III inhibitors is associated with increased mortality in patients with congestive cardiac failure. All PDE III inhibitors may cause hypotension, and tachyarrhythmias may occur. Other adverse effects include nausea, vomiting and fever. Amrinone may cause thrombocytopenia and is available only as a parenteral preparation. The half-life of all PDE III inhibitors is prolonged several-fold in patients with cardiac or renal failure and they are commonly administered as an i.v. loading dose over 5 min with or without a subsequent i.v. infusion.

Amrinone and *milrinone* are derived from bipyridines, whereas *enoximone* is an imidazole derivative. Enoximone undergoes substantial first pass metabolism, and is rapidly metabolized to a sulfoxide compound, which is excreted via the kidneys. The elimination $t_{1/2}$ of enoximone is 1–2 h in healthy individuals but up to 20 h in patients with cardiac failure. The sulfoxide metabolite is active and is less protein bound than the parent drug; its elimination may also be prolonged in cardiac or renal failure. The loading dose of enoximone is 0.5 mg kg^{-1} followed by an infusion of 5 μg kg^{-1} min^{-1}.

Glucagon

Glucagon is a polypeptide secreted by the α cells of the pancreatic islets; its physiological actions include stimulation of hepatic gluconeogenesis in response to hypoglycaemia, amino acids and as part of the stress response. These effects are mediated by increasing adenylate cyclase activity and intracellular cAMP, by a mechanism independent of the β-adrenergic receptor (Fig. 7.8). It increases cAMP in myocardial cells and so increases cardiac contractility. Glucagon causes nausea and vomiting, hyperglycaemia and hyperkalaemia and is not used as an inotrope except in the management of β-blocker poisoning (see below).

Calcium

Calcium ions are involved in excitation, excitation–contraction coupling, and contraction in cardiac, skeletal and smooth muscle cells. Increased extracellular calcium increases intracellular calcium concentrations and consequently the force of contraction of cardiac myocytes and vascular smooth muscle cells in vitro. Massive blood loss and replacement with large volumes of calcium-free fluids or citrated blood (which chelates calcium) may cause a decrease in serum calcium concentration, especially in the critically ill. Therefore calcium salts (e.g. calcium chloride, calcium gluconate) have been used as an inotrope, particularly during and after cardiopulmonary bypass. Intravenous calcium 5 mg kg^{-1} may increase mean arterial pressure, but the effects on cardiac output and systemic vascular resistance are variable and there is little evidence for the efficacy of calcium salts. Moreover, high calcium concentrations may cause cardiac arrhythmias and vasoconstriction, may be cytotoxic and may worsen the cellular effects of ischaemia. Calcium salts may be indicated for the treatment of hypocalcaemia (ionized Ca^{2+} < 0.8 mmol L^{-1}), hyperkalaemia and calcium channel blocker toxicity.

Selective β_2-agonists

Specific β_2-receptor agonists relax bronchial, uterine and vascular smooth muscle whilst having much less effect on the heart than isoproterenol. They include salbutamol, terbutaline, fenoterol, rimiterol and salmeterol. These drugs are partial agonists, (their maximal effect at β_2-receptors is less than that of isoproterenol) and are only partially selective for β_2-receptors. They are used widely in the treatment of bronchospasm (see Ch. 10). Although less cardiotoxic than isoproterenol, in high doses, β_2-mediated tremor, tachyarrhythmias, hyperglycaemia, hypokalaemia and hypomagnesaemia may occur. β_2-Agonists are resistant to metabolism by COMT and therefore have a prolonged duration of action (mostly 3–5 h). Salmeterol is highly lipophilic and has a strong affinity for the β_2-adrenergic receptor; it is longer acting than the other β_2-agonists, permitting twice-daily dosage. β_2-Agonists may be administered by several routes (inhaled, oral, i.v., intramuscular or subcutaneous). However, absorption may be unpredictable and they have a high hepatic extraction ratio, so the inhaled (by metered dose inhaler or nebulizer) and intravenous routes are used most commonly. When inhaled, only 10–20% of the administered dose reaches the lower airways; this proportion is reduced further when administered to a patient with a tracheal tube. Nevertheless, systemic absorption does occur, although adverse effects are less common during long-term therapy.

Salbutamol

Salbutamol is the β_2-agonist used most commonly for the prevention and treatment of bronchospasm. When administered by metered dose inhaler (1–2 puffs, each delivering 100 μg), it acts within a few minutes, with a peak action at 30–60 min and a duration of 3–5 h. In severe cases, it may be given by nebulizer (2.5 mg given as 2.5 ml of a 0.1% solution), repeated if required. The intravenous dose is either 250 μg by slow i.v. injection or as an infusion at 5μg min^{-1}, titrated to response, the usual range being 3–20 μg min^{-1}. Larger doses may be required in the presence of a tracheal tube. It is metabolized in the liver and excreted in the urine both as metabolites and as unchanged drug; the proportions are dependent on the route of administration.

Ritodrine

Ritodrine is commonly used as a tocolytic to stop uterine contractions in premature labour. Its action is predominantly via β_2-receptors, but ritodrine infusions often cause tachycardia, which is mediated partly by β_1-agonism. It is administered as an infusion starting at 50 μg min^{-1}, increasing to a maximum of 350 μg min^{-1} (the usual dose range being 150–350 μg min^{-1}), and is continued until labour has stopped for 12 h before continuing oral ritodrine therapy. Adverse effects are common, and include tachycardia, increased cardiac output and vasodilatation. Renin secretion is stimulated, causing sodium and water retention; fatal pulmonary oedema has been reported. Hypokalaemia and hyperglycaemia may also occur, with the potential for reactive fetal hypoglycaemia. Careful monitoring of ECG, fluid balance, blood glucose and electrolytes is necessary in patients receiving a ritodrine infusion, and diabetic parturients may require an intravenous insulin regimen. Ritodrine is contraindicated in patients with pre-eclampsia, antepartum haemorrhage requiring immediate delivery, or maternal cardiac disease.

Selective β_1-agonists

Drugs with selective β_1 effects have been developed from the group of β-adrenergic receptor antagonists with intrinsic sympathomimetic (partial agonist) activity (see below). Enhancing the intrinsic activity of the β-blocking drugs produces compounds which in low doses have stimulant activity at the β-adrenergic receptor, whilst at high doses they act as pure β-antagonists, blocking the effects of circulating catecholamines. The degree to which the properties of agonist or antagonist are expressed depends on the compound itself and also the degree of sympathetic nervous system activation in the patient. In theory, drugs in this category would be potentially useful as positive inotropic agents in cardiac failure. Thus, at low doses, they would produce mild stimulation to contractility without the excessive chronotropic effects seen with the full agonists such as isoproterenol. At high doses, they should act more as β-blocking drugs. The most studied drug in this class is xamoterol, which is a β_1-selective partial agonist with approximately 45% of the intrinsic activity of isoproterenol in animal models and in humans. Initially, xamoterol was found to be of some benefit in patients with mild to moderate heart failure, but in patients with more severe heart failure, in whom sympathetic drive is high, xamoterol acted more as a full antagonist and has now been withdrawn. These drugs have been superseded in the management of heart failure by the third-generation β-blockers (see below).

SYMPATHOLYTIC DRUGS

Drugs which antagonize the effects of the sympathetic nervous system are termed sympatholytic. They may act at central adrenergic neurones, at peripheral autonomic ganglia or neurones, or at postsynaptic α- or β-receptors. Most are hypotensive drugs, although they now have several other indications.

Centrally acting sympatholytic drugs

Centrally acting sympatholytic drugs (e.g. α-methyldopa, clonidine) were among the first drugs shown to be effective in the treatment of hypertension. Their use for this purpose has declined because of the increasing availability of alternative agents with few adverse effects.

α_2-Adrenergic receptor agonists

Clonidine and α-methyldopa act by stimulation of brain stem α_2-receptors (in the nucleus tractus solitarius and nucleus reticularis lateralis region of the rostroventrolateral medulla) to decrease sympathetic tone. It is now known that their hypotensive action is mediated partly by an agonist effect at central imidazoline (I_1) receptors.

The α_2-adrenergic receptor is coupled via a G-protein to several effector mechanisms, including inhibition of adenylate cyclase and effects at K^+ and Ca^{2+} channels. At least three subtypes of α_2-receptor have been identified. Central α_2 stimulation causes decreases in arterial pressure, peripheral resistance, venous return, myocardial contractility, cardiac output and heart rate by inhibition of sympathetic outflow. Plasma and CNS catecholamine concentrations are decreased, but baroreceptor reflexes are preserved, and the pressor response to ephedrine or phenylephrine may be exaggerated. Stimulation of peripheral α_2-receptors on vascular smooth muscle causes direct arteriolar vasoconstriction, although the central effects of these drugs predominate overall. However, severe rebound hypertension may occur on stopping chronic oral therapy.

Centrally acting α_2-agonists produce analgesia by activation of descending spinal and supraspinal inhibitory pathways; they also potentiate the effect of opioids. α_2-Receptors in the dorsal horn of the spinal cord modulate upward transmission of nociceptive signals by modifying local release of the nociceptive neurotransmitters substance P and CGRP. The analgesic effects are greatest when administered by the epidural or spinal route, although a transdermal preparation of clonidine is available. Other effects include dry mouth, sedation and anxiolysis, mediated by stimulation of α_2-receptors in the locus coeruleus and a decrease in CNS catecholamine concentrations.

Clonidine is a partial agonist at central and peripheral α_2-receptors, and has agonist effects at central imidazoline (I_1) receptors. I_1 receptors are also present in several peripheral tissues including the kidney. Clonidine has some effects at α_1-receptors ($\alpha_2:\alpha_1 > 200:1$); dexmedetomidine and azepexole are more α_2-selective alternatives. Transient hypertension and bradycardia may occur after i.v. injection, caused by direct stimulation of peripheral vascular α_2-receptors; an α_1-agonist effect may also contribute. Clonidine has synergistic analgesic effects with centrally administered opioids and potentiates the MAC of inhalation anaesthetic agents by up to 50%. The augmentation of opioid effects may be partly a pharmacokinetic effect, as the elimination half-life of opioids is increased. Clonidine is well absorbed orally, with peak plasma concentrations after 60–90 min. It is highly lipid-soluble and approximately 50% is metabolized in the liver to inactive metabolites; the rest is excreted unchanged via the kidneys, with an elimination half-life of 9–12 h. Clonidine 5 $\mu g\ kg^{-1}$ as premedication attenuates reflex sympathetic responses and may improve cardiovascular stability during anaesthesia. It is also used in the treatment of opioid withdrawal and perioperative shivering. Epidural clonidine 1–2 $\mu g\ kg^{-1}$ increases the duration and potency of analgesia provided by epidural opioid or local anaesthetic drugs. α_2-Agonists also have some antiarrhythmic effects, decreasing both the incidence of catecholamine-related arrhythmias and the toxicity of bupivacaine and cocaine.

Methyldopa crosses the blood–brain barrier easily and is converted to α-methyl norepinephrine, the active molecule, which is a full agonist at α_2-receptors with α_2:α_1 selectivity of 10:1. Its adverse effects include peripheral oedema, hepatotoxicity, depression and a positive direct Coombs' test; some patients develop haemolytic anaemia. It may have a place in the management of pregnancy-associated hypertension, but is otherwise rarely used.

Moxonidine

Moxonidine is a moderately selective imidazoline I_1-receptor agonist ($I_1 > \alpha_2$) which reduces central sympathetic drive by stimulation of medullary I_1-receptors. Systemic vascular resistance is reduced, but heart rate, stroke volume and pulmonary artery pressures are not affected. Cardiac output remains unchanged or increases slightly. Plasma epinephrine, norepinephrine and renin concentrations decrease. Moxonidine has minimal α_2-related adverse affects (e.g. sedation, dry mouth, rebound hypertension) and no effects on lipid and carbohydrate metabolism and it may even improve insulin sensitivity by direct cellular effects. It increases urine flow rate and sodium excretion, lowers intraocular pressure and has possible antiarrhythmic actions. It may be beneficial in patients with congestive heart failure, although the evidence is conflicting. It may potentiate bradycardia and is contraindicated in SA, second- or third-degree AV block. Bioavailability is almost 90%, maximum plasma concentrations occur after approximately 1 h, and it is excreted via the kidneys. Half-life is 2.5 h, but, in common with other antihypertensive drugs, its pharmacological effect lasts longer than this, suggesting possible retention in the CNS.

Peripherally acting sympatholytic drugs

Ganglion blocking drugs

Nicotinic receptor antagonists (e.g. hexamethonium, pentolinium, trimetaphan) competitively inhibit the effects of ACh at autonomic ganglia and block both parasympathetic and sympathetic transmission. Sympathetic blockade produces venodilatation, decreased myocardial contractility and hypotension, but the effects are variable, depending on pre-existing sympathetic tone. Tachyphylaxis develops rapidly, but trimetaphan is still used occasionally as part of a hypotensive anaesthetic technique.

Adrenergic neurone blocking drugs

Guanethidine decreases peripheral sympathetic nervous system activity by competitively binding to norepinephrine binding sites in storage vesicles in the cytoplasm of postganglionic sympathetic nerve terminals. Further uptake of norepinephrine into the vesicles is inhibited and it is metabolized in the cytoplasm by monoamine oxidase, so that the nerve terminals become depleted of norepinephrine. Guanethidine has local anaesthetic properties, and does not cross the blood–brain barrier. It is used to produce intravenous regional sympathetic blockade in the treatment of chronic limb pain associated with excessive autonomic activity (reflex sympathetic dystrophy or complex regional pain syndromes). Bretylium has a similar mode of action; it is used in the treatment of resistant ventricular arrhythmias (see below).

α-Adrenergic receptor antagonists

α-Adrenergic antagonists (α-blockers) selectively inhibit the action of catecholamines at α-adrenergic receptors. They are used mainly as vasodilators for the second-line treatment of hypertension or as urinary tract smooth muscle relaxants in patients with benign prostatic hyperplasia. They also have an important role in the preoperative management of phaeochromocytoma (see Ch. 55).

α-Blockers diminish vaso- and venoconstrictor tone causing venous pooling and a decrease in peripheral vascular resistance. In common with other vasodilators, they may have indirect positive inotropic actions as a result of reduction in afterload and preload; cardiac output may increase. They may be classified according to their relative selectivity for α_1- and α_2-receptors. Non-selective α-blockers commonly induce postural hypotension and reflex tachycardia, partly because α_2-blockade blocks the feedback inhibition of norepinephrine on its own release at presynaptic α_2-receptors, and neuronal norepinephrine concentrations increase. The action of norepinephrine at cardiac β-receptors then limits the hypotensive effects of non-selective α-blockers. In addition, the proportions of pre- and postsynaptic α_2-receptors in the arterial and venous smooth muscle may be different, so that α_1-selective drugs have a more balanced effect on venous and arterial circulations. The co-administration of a β-blocker may attenuate reflex tachycardia and produces a synergistic effect on arterial pressure.

α_1-Selective antagonists

Selective α_1-blockers include prazosin, doxazosin, indoramin, phenoxybenzamine and urapidil. *Doxazosin* has succeeded prazosin as the most commonly used agent in this class as it has a more prolonged duration of action. Reflex tachycardia and postural hypotension are less common than with direct-acting vasodilators (e.g. hydralazine) and the non-selective α-blockers, but may still occur on initiating therapy. Nasal congestion, sedation and inhibition of ejaculation may occur. *Phenoxybenzamine* binds covalently (i.e. irreversibly and non-competitively) to the receptor so that its effects last up to several days, and may be cumulative on repeated dosing. It is used for the preoperative preparation of patients with phaeochromocytoma (see Ch. 55).

Labetalol (see below) is a competitive α_1-, β_1- and β_2-antagonist, which is more active at β than at α-receptors. However, at low doses (e.g. 5–10 mg i.v.), it produces a controlled decrease in arterial pressure without tachycardia. At higher doses, the β effect becomes more prominent, with negative inotropic and chronotropic effects. Carvedilol is also an antagonist at α_1- and β-receptors (see above).

Urapidil is a peripheral postsynaptic α_1-selective antagonist, which is also an agonist at central serotonin 5-HT_1A receptors in the rostral ventrolateral medulla. It reduces blood pressure by arterio- and venodilatation, with little effect on heart rate or cardiac output. This is because $5HT_1A$ receptor stimulation suppresses central autonomic activity and attenuates the reflex tachycardia triggered by vasodilatation. It has less adverse effects than other α_1-blockers. Intravenous urapidil as a bolus of 0.5–2 mg kg^{-1} may be useful in patients with pre-eclampsia, hypertensive crises or perioperative hypertension.

α_2-Selective antagonists

Drugs of this type, e.g. yohimbine, are not used because of the unacceptable incidence of adverse effects.

Non-selective α-antagonists

Non-selective α-blockers, e.g. phentolamine or tolazoline, block α_1- and α_2-receptors equally and produce more postural hypotension, reflex tachycardia and adverse gastrointestinal effects (e.g. abdominal cramps, diarrhoea) than α_1-selective drugs. However, i.v. phentolamine 2–5 mg produces a rapid decrease in arterial pressure lasting 10–15 min and is used for the treatment of hypertensive crises, e.g. during surgery for removal of phaeochromocytoma.

β-Adrenergic receptor antagonists

β-Adrenergic receptor antagonists (β-blockers) are structurally similar to the β-agonists, e.g. isoproterenol. Variations in the molecular structure (primarily of the catechol ring) have produced compounds that do not activate adenylate cyclase and the second messenger system despite binding avidly to the β-adrenergic receptor. Most are stereoisomers and the L-form is generally more potent (as an agonist or antagonist) than the D-form. β-Blockers are competitive antagonists with high receptor affinity, although their effects are attenuated by high concentrations of endogenous or exogenous agonists. They may be classified according to:

- their relative affinity for β_1- or β_2-receptors
- agonist/antagonist activity
- membrane-stabilizing effect
- ancillary effects (e.g. action at other receptors).

β_1- or β_2-adrenergic receptor affinity

The relative potency of β-blockers is less important than their relative effects on the different β-receptor subtypes. Compounds are available which block preferentially either β_1- or β_2-receptors, although in clinical practice the β_1-selective drugs are more important. The first generation of β-blockers (e.g. propranolol, timolol) were non-selective; second-generation drugs (e.g. atenolol, metoprolol, bisoprolol) are selective for β_1-receptors but have no ancillary effects. The third generation of β-blockers are β_1-selective, but also have effects on other receptors (e.g. labetalol and carvedilol are antagonists at α_1-adrenergic receptors, and bucindolol produces vasodilatation by a cGMP-dependent mechanism). β_1-Selective (or 'cardioselective') drugs have theoretical advantages, as some of the adverse effects of β-blockers are related to β_2-antagonism, but it is important to remember that the selectivity of both drugs and tissues is only relative. All β_1-selective drugs antagonize β_2-receptors at higher doses, and 25% of cardiac β-receptors are of the β_2 subtype. However β_1-selective drugs appear to have *less* adverse effects on blood glucose control in diabetics, less effect on serum lipids, and less effect on bronchial tone in patients with chronic obstructive pulmonary disease.

Partial agonist activity

Some β-blockers are partial agonists. Dichloroisoproteronol, the first drug shown to be capable of blocking β-receptors, has a very similar structure to isoproterenol. It has some stimulant or β-agonist activity, (approximately 50% of that of isoproterenol), i.e. it exhibits partial agonist activity (formerly termed as having 'intrinsic sympathomimetic activity' [ISA]). This stimulant effect is apparent at low levels of sympathetic activity, but at high levels of sympathetic discharge, blockade of endogenously released catecholamines is the major clinical effect. Partial agonists may be advantageous in patients with a low resting heart rate, and have theoretical advantages in patients with peripheral vascular disease or hyperlipidaemia. However, only β-blockers *without* partial agonist activity have been shown to be beneficial after myocardial infarction.

Membrane-stabilizing effect

Some β-blockers have a quinidine-like action, inhibiting sodium transport in nerve and cardiac conducting tissue ('membrane-stabilizing effect'). This may be demonstrated in vivo as a stabilizing effect on the cardiac action potential, reducing the slope of phase 4 noticeably, and thus decreasing excitability and automaticity of the myocardium (see below). However, the membrane-stabilizing activity probably has little clinical significance, as it occurs only at plasma concentrations above the therapeutic range, and the antiarrhythmic effect of β-blockade occurs via inhibition of the effects of catecholamines.

Ancillary effects

Some of the newer β-blocking drugs have other effects, e.g. action at α_1-receptors, vasodilatation, free radical scavenging and other actions. The relevance of these properties is discussed below.

Pharmacological properties of β-blockers

The pharmacological properties of β-blockers are summarized in Table 7.4. All β-blockers are weak bases and most are well absorbed to produce peak plasma concentrations 1–3 h after oral administration. The more lipid-soluble drugs are almost completely absorbed, but are metabolized to a greater extent and tend to have a marked first-pass effect through the liver. This reduces the bioavailability of the lipophilic drugs, but is offset by the fact that the 4-hydroxylated metabolites so formed are also active. The first-pass metabolism also tends to become saturated, so that proportionately higher plasma

Table 7.4 Pharmacological properties of beta blockers

Drug	β_1 selectivity	Partial agonist activity	Membrane-stabilizing effect	Lipid solubility	Absorption (%)	Bioavailability (%)	Protein binding (%)	Terminal half-life (h)	Significant active metabolites?	Elimination
Acebutolol	±	+	+	Medium	90	50	20	8–10	Yes	Hepatic, renal
Atenolol	+	–	–	Low	50	40	5	6–8	No	Renal
Bisoprolol	++	–	–	Low	>90	90		10–12	No	Hepatic, renal
Carvedilol	–	–	?	High	>90	25	98	6–10	Yes	Hepatic
Celiprolol	+	+	?	Low	30	30				
Esmolol	+	–	–	High			55	0.15	No	Plasma hydrolysis
Labetalol	–	±	+	High	70	30	50	4	No	Hepatic
Metoprolol	+	–	±	High	90	50	10–20	4	No	Hepatic
Nadolol	–	–	–	Low	30	30	20	20–24	No	Renal
Oxprenolol	–	+	+	High	80	50	80	2	No	Hepatic
Pindolol	–	++	±	Medium	90	90	50	4	No	Hepatic
Propranolol	–	–	++	High	90	30	90	5	Yes	Hepatic
Sotalol	–	+	+	Low	80	60	0	8–15	No	Renal
Timolol	–	+	±	High	90	50	10	4	No	Hepatic, renal

concentrations of the parent drug are achieved at higher oral doses. The first-pass effect is also a source of wide interindividual variation in plasma concentrations achieved from the same dose of primarily metabolized drugs; it is less with renally excreted drugs. β-Blockers have a flat dose–response curve, so that large changes in plasma concentration may give rise to only a small change in degree of β-blockade. However, differences in individual plasma concentration–response relationships may occur, possibly as a result of variations in sympathetic tone or the formation of active metabolites. All β-blockers are distributed widely throughout the body and significant concentrations occur in the CNS, particularly for the more lipid-soluble drugs (e.g. propranolol).

The less lipid-soluble drugs (e.g. atenolol, nadolol) are less well absorbed, are metabolized to a lesser extent and are excreted via the kidneys. They tend to have longer half-lives. Atenolol, nadolol and sotalol are excreted largely unchanged in the urine and so are little affected by impairment of liver function. Although propranolol depends less on the kidney for elimination than do other β-blockers, active metabolites which are excreted via the kidneys may accumulate when β-blockers are used in patients with renal failure. Plasma concentrations of *unchanged* propranolol are also increased in uraemia. Propranolol decreases the clearance of amide local anaesthetics (by decreasing hepatic blood flow and inhibiting metabolism) and the pulmonary first-pass uptake of fentanyl.

Clinical indications for β-blockade (Tables 7.5 and 7.6)

Hypertension. β-Blockers are regarded as first-line therapy for the treatment of hypertension, either alone or in combination with other drugs (see below). They are of proven benefit in reducing the incidence of stroke and the morbidity and mortality from coronary heart disease in hypertensive patients. The antihypertensive effect results from a combination of factors:

- *Reductions in heart rate, cardiac output and myocardial contractility.*
- *A reduction in central sympathetic nervous activity.* The significance of this is uncertain, as different drugs vary widely in their lipophilicity and consequent CNS penetration, but have similar effects on arterial pressure control.
- *An effect on plasma renin concentration.* β-Blockers decrease resting and orthostatic release of renin to a variable extent. The non-selective drugs propranolol and timolol cause the greatest reduction, while partial agonists (oxprenolol, pindolol) or β_1-selective drugs are less effective. However, no correlation has been found between renin-lowering effect and antihypertensive activity or dosage of β-blocker used.
- *An effect on peripheral resistance.* β-Blockade does not reduce peripheral resistance directly and may even cause an increase by allowing unopposed α stimulation. As the vasodilating effect of catecholamines on skeletal muscle is β_2-mediated, unopposed α stimulation would be expected to be lower with cardioselective drugs or partial agonists. However, cardioselectivity decreases with dosage and, as hypertensive patients often require a large dose of β-blocker, little real advantage is

Table 7.5 Clinical indications for β-blockade

Hypertension
Ischaemic heart disease
Secondary prevention of myocardial infarction
Obstructive cardiomyopathy
Congestive cardiac failure
Arrhythmias
Miscellaneous

Table 7.6 Specific perioperative indications for β-blockers

Prevention or treatment of intraoperative hypertension, tachycardia and supraventricular tachyarrhythmias associated with excessive sympathetic activity
Treatment of postoperative hypertension
Controlled hypotension
Prophylaxis or treatment of perioperative myocardial ischaemia
Pre- and perioperative management of phaeochromocytoma
Pre- and perioperative management of thyrotoxic patients

offered. Drugs with partial agonist activity may not increase peripheral resistance as much as those without.

Arterial pressure reduction begins within an hour of administration of a β-blocker, but several days may elapse before the plateau is reached, and the full hypotensive effect of oral β-blockers takes about 2 weeks, suggesting the involvement of several mechanisms including readjustment of central and peripheral cardiovascular reflexes. During chronic administration, the hypotensive effects of β-blockers last longer than the pharmacological half-life, so that single daily dosage is adequate therapeutically. However, upregulation of receptors may occur, leading to adverse effects (e.g. tachycardia, hypertension, myocardial ischaemia) on abrupt withdrawal of β-blockers. This may be important in the perioperative period. They are all equally effective as hypotensive drugs; patients unresponsive to one β-blocker are generally unresponsive to all. β-Blockers are particularly indicated for patients with hypertension and angina or coincident arrhythmias.

Ischaemic heart disease. β-Blockers improve symptoms in patients with ischaemic heart disease, and decrease the frequency and severity of silent myocardial ischaemia, which otherwise occurs in 60–100% of patients with angina. The incidence of perioperative myocardial ischaemia (PMI) in high-risk patients is reduced by perioperative β-blocker administration. PMI is associated with perioperative and long-term cardiac morbidity, and recent data suggest that perioperative β-blockade may improve long-term outcome. β-Blockers reduce heart rate and cardiac contractility, with consequent decreases in wall tension and myocardial oxygen demand. A slower heart rate also permits longer diastolic filling time and hence potentially greater coronary perfusion. The perfusion of ischaemic regions may be improved by redistribution of myocardial blood flow. However, other mechanisms may be involved in this perioperative cardioprotective effect.

β-Blockade also reduces exercise-induced increases in arterial pressure, velocity of cardiac contraction and oxygen consumption at any workload. Drugs with partial agonist activity have less effect on the resting heart rate; this is of benefit particularly in patients with an existing low heart rate, as it reduces the risk of AV conduction disturbance. Partial agonists may theoretically increase the metabolic demand of the myocardium and may be less effective in patients with angina at rest or at very low levels of exercise. In contrast to effects on blood pressure, there is a more direct relationship between plasma concentration and anti-anginal effect. To achieve effective plasma concentrations over a sustained period as a single daily dosage, either the long-half-life drugs (e.g. atenolol, nadolol) or slow-release preparations (e.g. oxprenolol-SR, propranolol-LA, metoprolol-SR) are required.

Secondary prevention of myocardial infarction (see Ch. 35). Early i.v. administration after acute myocardial infarction can decrease infarct size, the incidence of ventricular and supraventricular arrhythmias and mortality in both lower and higher risk groups (e.g. elderly patients or those with left ventricular dysfunction). Mortality is reduced by 20–40%, and the risk of re-infarction is reduced if oral therapy is continued for 2–3 years.

Obstructive cardiomyopathy. β-Blockers improve exercise tolerance and alleviate symptoms in hypertrophic obstructive cardiomyopathy by decreasing heart rate, myocardial work, contractility and thus outflow tract obstruction. However, the incidence of sudden death in this condition is not affected. The incidence of cyanotic episodes caused by pulmonary outflow obstruction in patients with Fallot's tetralogy is reduced by a similar mechanism.

Congestive cardiac failure (see below). It is now established that morbidity and mortality in patients with chronic congestive cardiac failure are reduced by β-blockade with second- or third-generation drugs.

Arrhythmias (see below). β-Blockers are effective in the treatment of arrhythmias caused by sympathetic nervous overactivity, or after myocardial infarction. The mechanisms are related to β-blockade itself rather than any membrane-stabilizing effect, i.e. antagonism of catecholamine effects on the cardiac action potential and muscle contractility. The result is a slowing of rate of discharge from the sinus and any ectopic pacemaker, and slowing of conduction and increased refractoriness of the AV node. β-Blockers also retard conduction in anomalous pathways of the heart. They may be used i.v. to terminate an attack of supraventricular tachycardia, or decrease the ventricular rate in atrial fibrillation and flutter; conversion to sinus rhythm may also be achieved. If given within 30 min of i.v. verapamil, there is a danger of severe bradycardia or asystole. Most β-blockers have similar antiarrhythmic effects in adequate dosage, but esmolol has the advantage of a short half-life (see below) so that adverse effects are limited. They are sometimes useful as second-line alternatives for the treatment of ventricular tachycardia. Sotalol has both class 2 and class 3 antiarrhythmic activity, and is licensed for use only for its antiarrhythmic action, in particular for the treatment of supraventricular and ventricular tachycardias. However, sotalol may cause torsades de pointes and other life-threatening arrhythmias, particularly in the presence of hypokalaemia.

Miscellaneous. β-Blockers are occasionally prescribed for migraine prophylaxis, essential tremor or anxiety states. They decrease intraocular pressure, probably by reducing the production of aqueous humour, and are widely used in the treatment of glaucoma. Topical preparations (e.g. timolol, betaxolol, carteolol) are used in an attempt to decrease adverse effects, but significant systemic absorption may still take place; bradycardia, hypotension and bronchospasm may occur, particularly during anaesthesia.

Adverse reactions to β-blockers

All available β-blockers have similar adverse effects, although their magnitude depends on β_1-selectivity and the presence or absence of partial agonist activity. They may be classified into the following:

Reactions resulting from β-blockade

Cardiovascular effects. β-Blockers may precipitate heart failure in patients with compromised cardiac function, and accentuate AV block. Their negative inotropic and chronotropic effects may be additive with other drugs affecting cardiac conduction or drugs used during anaesthesia. They prevent the compensatory tachycardia which accompanies hypovolaemia, and therefore severe hypotension may occur if intravascular replacement is delayed. Bradycardia caused by excessive β-blockade may be treated by atropine, β-agonists (e.g. dobutamine or isoproterenol), glucagon or calcium chloride. Glucagon (1–10 mg i.v.) increases intracellular cAMP concentrations by a mechanism independent of β-receptors and may be the treatment of choice for β-blocker poisoning. Occasionally cardiac pacing may be required.

Induction of bronchospasm in patients with asthma or chronic bronchitis who rely on sympathetically (β_2) mediated bronchodilatation. Theoretically, β_1-selective drugs are less likely to aggravate bronchospasm in asthmatics, but as their selectivity is only relative, they should not be considered completely safe.

Raynaud's phenomenon and peripheral vascular disease are relative contraindications to the use of β-blockers, as symptoms of cold extremities may be exacerbated

Diabetes mellitus. Cardiovascular (tachycardia-β_1) and metabolic (hepatic glycogenolysis-β_2) responses to insulin-induced hypoglycaemia are impaired. These effects may be more marked with non-selective drugs.

Increased muscle fatigue, possibly resulting from blockade of β_2-mediated vasodilatation in muscles during exercise.

A withdrawal phenomenon may occur after abrupt cessation of long-term therapy for angina, causing rebound tachycardia, worsening angina or precipitation of myocardial infarction.

Impotence occurs commonly during chronic β-blocker therapy.

Idiosyncratic reactions

Central nervous system effects occur with some β-blockers, including nightmares, hallucinations, insomnia and depression. These effects are more common with the lipophilic drugs (e.g. propranolol, acebutolol, oxprenolol and metoprolol). Gastrointestinal reactions include nausea, vomiting and diarrhoea.

Oculomucocutaneous syndrome affects the eye, mucous and serous membranes and was recognized in association with practolol therapy. There is no firm evidence that any other β–lockers may provoke a similar reaction and practolol is no longer available.

Newer β-blockers

Recently, third-generation β-blockers which also have vasodilating effects have been introduced (e.g. labetalol, bucindolol and carvedilol). All are non-selective ($\beta_1 > \beta_2$) antagonists and carvedilol has been used in the management of cardiac failure (see below). Labetalol and carvedilol are also α_1-antagonists; bucindolol produces direct vasodilatation by a cGMP-dependent mechanism.

Labetalol is a competitive α_1-, β_1- and β_2-antagonist, which is a partial agonist at β_2-receptors. It is four to seven times more potent at β- than at α-receptors and is useful for the prevention and treatment of perioperative hypertension, or to produce controlled hypotension (see Ch. 56). It is also available as an oral preparation for the treatment of chronic hypertension or the preoperative management of phaeochromocytoma (see Ch. 55). Intravenous labetalol in small increments (e.g. 5–10 mg) produces a controlled decrease in arterial pressure over 5–10 min with no change in cardiac output or reflex tachycardia, suggesting that at this dose the vasodilating action predominates. At higher doses, the β-effect becomes more prominent, with negative inotropic and chronotropic effects.

Carvedilol is also an antagonist at α- and β-receptors (with relative $\beta:\alpha_1$ selectivity of 10:1), but it has other effects, including significant antioxidant activity and possibly calcium channel blockade in higher doses; these may account for some of its beneficial activity in patients with cardiac failure. Carvedilol is a stereoisomer which undergoes extensive first-pass metabolism with the production of active metabolites.

Bucindolol is a β-blocker which also produces vasodilatation by a cGMP-dependent mechanism. Systemic and cardiac concentrations of norepinephrine are decreased and it produces little inverse agonism.

Nebivolol is a lipophilic β_1-selective blocker, administered as a racemic mixture of equal proportions of D- and L-enantiomers, which has no membrane-stabilizing activity but which appears to have nitric oxide-mediated vasodilatory effects. It is used for the treatment of hypertension.

Celiprolol is a β_1-selective blocker which is a weak β_2-agonist. It therefore has advantages in patients with reactive airways disease (COPD or asthma) or peripheral vascular disease. β_1-Selective antagonists have theoretical advantages in these patients, but selectivity is not complete and adverse effects may occur at high doses. Celiprolol is excreted unchanged.

Esmolol is a rapid-onset, short-acting β_1-selective blocker with no membrane-stabilizing or partial agonist activity which is only available for i.v. use. It has an onset time of 1–2 min and is rapidly metabolized by red cell esterases (distinct from plasma cholinesterases); its elimination half-life is 9 min. The rapid onset and offset of effect are an advantage in the perioperative period, as any effects such as dose-dependent bradycardia or hypotension are short-lived. It is effective in preventing or controlling intraoperative tachycardia and hypertension, and is also useful for the treatment of supraventricular tachyarrhythmias, e.g. atrial fibrillation or flutter. It may be given as a slow i.v. bolus of 0.5–2.0 mg kg^{-1} or an infusion of 25–500 μg kg^{-1} min^{-1}; its effects terminate within 10–20 min of stopping the infusion.

DRUGS ACTING ON THE PARASYMPATHETIC NERVOUS SYSTEM

The major drugs in use which act on the parasympathetic nervous system are muscarinic antagonists (e.g. atropine, hyoscine and propantheline), and parasympathetic agonists (e.g. the anticholinesterases neostigmine and pyridostigmine). The pharmacology of neuromuscular blocking drugs, which act at nicotinic receptors, is described in Chapter 19. Ganglion-blocking drugs, which modify preganglionic (nicotinic) autonomic transmission, are now rarely used clinically and this chapter focuses primarily on drugs acting at postganglionic muscarinic receptors.

Parasympathetic antagonists

Parasympathetic antagonists act by blocking muscarinic ACh receptors. They are either tertiary or quaternary amine compounds, which differ in their ability to cross biological membranes. Tertiary amines, e.g. atropine and hyoscine, are more lipid-soluble and cross the blood–brain barrier. Therefore, they may affect central ACh receptors and produce sedative or stimulatory effects. Similar antimuscarinic drugs, e.g. benzatropine and procyclidine, are useful anti-Parkinsonian agents because of their predominant central action; procyclidine is useful for the reversal of acute dystonic reactions to dopaminergic drugs (e.g. phenothiazines, droperidol). Many other parasympathetic antagonists developed as gastrointestinal or urinary antispasmodics are quaternary amines; they are poorly absorbed after oral administration but produce minimal central effects.

Atropine

The muscarinic-blocking action of atropine affects a wide range of parasympathetic autonomic nervous functions, depending upon dosage. Salivary secretion, micturition, heart rate and visual accommodation are impaired sequentially. CNS effects (sedation or excitation, hallucinations and hyperthermia) may occur at high doses. Atropine is administered intravenously in doses of 0.6–3.0 mg to counteract bradycardia in the presence of hypotension and to prevent bradycardia associated with vagal stimulation or the use of anticholinesterase drugs. Adverse cardiac effects of atropine include an increase in cardiac work and ventricular arrhythmias. Occasionally, atropine may produce a transient bradycardia, before tachycardia supervenes. The initial bradycardia is thought to be caused by increased ACh release mediated by M_2-receptor antagonism. In therapeutic dosage, effects mediated by M_3-receptors (tachycardia, bronchodilatation, dry mouth, mydriasis) predominate.

Hyoscine

Hyoscine has less effect on heart rate than atropine but crosses into the brain more readily and may cause confusion, sedation and ataxia, particularly in the elderly. This may result in the 'central anticholinergic syndrome' described in Chapter 34. It has greater antisialagogue and mydriatic effects than atropine and is also useful as an antiemetic, particularly for the prophylaxis of motion sickness. Hyoscine is available as a transdermal patch for this purpose.

Glycopyrronium bromide (glycopyrrolate)

This is a quaternary amine which has similar anticholinergic actions to those of atropine. It is used as an alternative to atropine during the reversal of neuromuscular blockade or for its antisecretory actions. Some other quaternary amines, e.g. propantheline and dicycloverine, have a mainly peripheral parasympathetic antagonist action and are used as gastrointestinal and urinary antispasmodics.

Ipratropium bromide is used as an inhaled anticholinergic bronchodilator.

Antimuscarinic drugs in premedication

Subcutaneous or oral atropine and hyoscine have been used as premedicant drugs, usually in combination with an opioid or sedative, to decrease salivary and respiratory secretions, and counteract vagally mediated reflexes (see Ch. 18). Their use has declined with the decreased use of ether, and the side-effects of dry mouth and blurred vision may be unpleasant. However, if an antisialagogue is particularly indicated, glycopyrrolate is effective in a dose of 0.2 mg i.m., with minimal central or cardiovascular effects.

Parasympathetic agonists

Synthetic parasympathetic agonists (e.g. carbachol, bethanechol) produce predominantly muscarinic effects and have been used historically as gastrointestinal tract and bladder smooth muscle stimulants. *Bethanechol* is not hydrolysed by AChE and its action lasts several hours. *Pilocarpine* is a naturally occurring agonist which is used as a topical miotic in the treatment of glaucoma. Bradycardia, flushing, sweating and excessive salivation are predictable adverse effects, which may occur after topical or systemic administration.

Anticholinesterase drugs

These drugs (e.g. *neostigmine*, *pyridostigmine*) antagonize acetylcholinesterase, thereby decreasing the breakdown of released ACh; they exert both nicotinic and muscarinic effects. The action on the ANS tends to appear at low doses, as nicotinic effects are dose-related. They are used in anaesthesia to reverse the neuromuscular blockade of non-depolarizing muscle relaxants (see Ch. 19). Their other uses include the diagnosis and symptomatic management of myasthenia gravis, where pyridostigmine is a useful, relatively long-acting agent. Anticholinesterases are used occasionally for their muscarinic effects to increase gastrointestinal and bladder smooth muscle tone; topical anticholinesterases are also used in ophthalmology as miotic agents.

Physostigmine differs from neostigmine and pyridostigmine in being a tertiary amine, which is therefore well absorbed from the gastrointestinal tract and may cause CNS effects, producing CNS excitation. It has been used to treat poisoning with anticholinergic agents, ketamine, diazepam or tricyclic antidepressants, which have anticholinergic effects. However, physostigmine may induce convulsions and may exacerbate any cardiac bradyarrhythmias associated with tricyclic antidepressant toxicity.

VASODILATORS

Drugs which dilate arteries or veins are used alone or in conjunction with inotropic agents in the management of acute left ventricular failure (Table 7.7). Some are also used in the treatment of hypertension, angina and ischaemic heart disease, including acute myocardial infarction. Vasodilators are useful in the treatment of acute hypertensive episodes and as part of a controlled hypotensive anaesthetic technique to reduce haemorrhage during surgery (see Ch. 56).

Vasodilators may reduce afterload or preload, or both. Acute and chronic cardiac failure are both associated with a reflex increase in sympathetic tone and an increase in systemic vascular resistance. By lowering this resistance (afterload), the work and oxygen requirements of the heart are reduced. Vasodilators which act on the venous side of the circulation (e.g. nitrates) increase venous capacitance, reduce venous return to the heart and so decrease the left ventricular filling pressure (preload). This in turn decreases the degree of stretch of myocardial fibres and reduces myocardial oxygen consumption for the same degree of cardiac work performed.

Vasodilators may be classified into those acting directly on arterial smooth muscle (nitroprusside, nitrates, hydralazine, diazoxide, minoxidil, calcium channel blockers) and neurohumoral antagonists (α-blockers and ACE inhibitors). They may also be classified according to which side of the heart they act on preferentially. Hydralazine, calcium channel blockers and minoxidil act mainly on afterload. Nitrates principally affect preload. Nitroprusside, α-blockers and ACE inhibitors have a balanced effect on arteries and veins.

Table 7.7 Indications for vasodilators
Acute and chronic left ventricular failure
Prophylaxis and treatment of unstable and stable angina
Treatment of acute myocardial ischaemia and infarction
Chronic hypertension
Acute hypertensive episodes
Elective controlled hypotensive anaesthesia

Nitrates

The organic nitrates (*glyceryl trinitrate* and *isosorbide mononitrate and dinitrate*) cause systemic and coronary vasodilatation. They act primarily on systemic veins, causing venodilatation, sequestration of blood in venous capacitance beds, and a reduction in preload. At higher doses (> 2 mg h^{-1}), arteriolar dilatation occurs and afterload is reduced; tachycardia, hypotension and headaches may occur. Systolic pressure decreases more than diastolic pressure so that coronary perfusion pressure tends to be preserved. In left ventricular failure, venodilatation is beneficial, reducing pulmonary congestion; cardiac dynamics may be improved so that stroke volume and cardiac output increase. Nitrates are used widely for the prevention and treatment of angina and myocardial infarction as they cause vasodilatation in stenotic coronary arteries and redistribution of myocardial blood flow. Effects on systemic vessels also cause a reduction in myocardial wall tension and oxygen consumption, and consequently they may be beneficial after myocardial infarction. Glyceryl trinitrate (GTN) is a powerful myometrial relaxant. Nitrates also inhibit platelet aggregation in vitro.

Nitrates are converted to the active compounds nitric oxide (NO) and nitrosothiols by a denitration mechanism involving reduced sulphydryl groups. NO and nitrosothiols activate guanylate cyclase in the cytoplasm of vascular smooth muscle cells to increase intracellular cGMP. This leads to phosphorylation of a protein kinase and a decrease in intracellular calcium ions, causing relaxation of vascular smooth muscle and vasodilatation. During continuous therapy, tolerance to nitrates develops rapidly (within 24 h), caused by depletion of reduced sulphydryl groups or activation of neurohormonal counter-mechanisms, and a nitrate-free period of 8–12 h is required. Nitrates may be administered by oral, buccal, transdermal and intravenous routes; the last three may be useful in the perioperative period. Intravenous nitrates may be used during coronary artery bypass surgery for the treatment of perioperative hypertension or myocardial ischaemia and as part of a hypotensive anaesthetic technique. However, attempts to demonstrate a beneficial effect of prophylactic GTN on perioperative myocardial ischaemia in cardiac or non-cardiac surgery have proved inconclusive. Nitrates are absorbed by rubber and plastics (especially PVC infusion bags), so are best administered by syringe pump.

Sodium nitroprusside

Sodium nitroprusside (SNP) is reduced to NO on exposure to reducing agents, and in tissues including vascular smooth muscle cell membranes, by a non-enzymatic process. It therefore has a similar ultimate mechanism of action to that of nitrates (via increased cGMP). SNP produces similar effects on capacitance and resistance vessels so that preload and afterload are equally reduced, and it is useful in the management of acute left ventricular failure. Systolic and diastolic pressures are decreased equally in a dose-dependent manner. In larger doses (e.g. when used for hypotensive anaesthesia), heart rate increases.

Release of NO from nitroprusside is accompanied by release of cyanide ions, which are detoxified by the liver and kidney to thiocyanate (requiring thiosulphate, vitamin B_{12}, and the enzyme rhodanase), which is excreted slowly in the urine. It has an immediate, short-lived effect (lasting only for a few minutes) so it must be given by intravenous infusion. Arterial pressure can then be manipulated simply by adjustment of the infusion rate. SNP is photodegraded to cyanide ions; infusion solutions should be protected from light and not used if they have turned dark brown or blue. There is an additive effect with other vasodilators. In practice, nitroprusside is well tolerated and most symptoms are associated with too rapid a decrease in arterial pressure.

If the total dose of SNP exceeds 1.5 mg kg^{-1} or the infusion rate exceeds 1.5 μg kg^{-1} min^{-1}, cyanide and thiocyanate may accumulate, with the risk of metabolic acidosis; plasma bicarbonate concentrations should be monitored. The risks of cyanide toxicity are increased in the presence of impaired renal or hepatic function, but symptoms may be delayed until after the SNP infusion has been discontinued. Plasma cyanide or thiocyanate concentrations may also be monitored if the drug is used for more than 2 days. Thiocyanate is potentially neurotoxic and may cause hypothyroidism. In cases of suspected cyanide toxicity, sodium thiosulphate (which promotes conversion to thiocyanate), dicobalt edetate (which chelates cyanide ions) and hydroxocobalamin (which combines with cyanide to form cyanocobalamin) may be given. The use of sodium nitroprusside in hypotensive anaesthesia is considered in Chapter 56.

Potassium channel activators

Hydralazine, minoxidil and diazoxide are direct-acting arteriolar vasodilators which have largely been superseded by newer agents. Minoxidil and diazoxide activate ATP-sensitive potassium channels in vascular smooth muscle cells, causing potassium efflux and membrane hyperpolarization. This leads to closure of calcium channels, reduced intracellular calcium availability and consequently smooth muscle relaxation and arterial vasodilatation. Hydralazine may act via a similar mechanism. All these drugs reduce afterload, with little or no effect on preload. Their effects are limited by reflex tachycardia and a tendency to cause sodium and water retention (by activation of the renin–angiotensin system and a direct renal mechanism). Consequently, they are usually administered during long-term therapy with a β-blocker and a diuretic.

Hydralazine is the most widely used of these drugs. Its half-life is short (approximately 2.5 h), but its antihypertensive effect is relatively prolonged. It may be given as a slow i.v. bolus of 5–10 mg, with appropriate monitoring, for the treatment of hypertensive emergencies.

Minoxidil is only available orally. It has a long duration of action (12–24 h), unrelated to its plasma half-life, and it causes hypertrichosis; T-wave abnormalities on ECG are observed in 60% of patients.

Diazoxide has a similar structure to thiazide diuretics. It causes sodium retention, increases plasma glucose concentrations and may be used orally for the treatment of intractable hypoglycaemia. In hypertensive emergencies, diazoxide 1–3 mg kg^{-1} i.v. may be given rapidly (over 30 s) for effects lasting 4–24 h. However, it is difficult to control the action or duration of action of repeated doses, and it is rarely used.

Nicorandil

Nicorandil is a recently introduced vasodilator used for the treatment of angina. It activates potassium channels in vascular smooth muscle, but also causes nitric oxide release and increases intracellular cGMP in vascular endothelium, causing venous dilatation. It therefore reduces preload as well as afterload. Nicorandil causes coronary vasodilatation with no effect on heart rate or contractility, and improves coronary blood flow in patients with coronary artery disease. In experimental models it protects against ischaemia and reduces infarct size. It is well absorbed orally with a duration of action of 12 h, although the plasma half-life is approximately 1 h. It is metabolized in the liver, excreted via the kidneys, and does not cause tolerance. Nicorandil may be useful for the treatment of angina e.g. in nitrate-tolerant patients or those unresponsive to β-blockers. There is potential for an additive hypotensive effect with other vasodilators, which may be important in patients presenting for anaesthesia and surgery, although few data are available.

CALCIUM CHANNEL BLOCKERS

MECHANISM OF ACTION

The normal function of cardiac myocytes and conducting tissues, skeletal muscle, vascular and other smooth muscle, and neurones depends on the availability of intracellular calcium ions. Under physiological conditions, calcium entry into the cell induces further calcium release from the sarcoplasmic reticulum, which facilitates conduction of the cardiac action potential and excitation–contraction coupling by interaction with calmodulin (in smooth muscle) or troponin (within cardiac muscle). Calcium enters the cell via several ion channels situated on the plasma membrane, the most important being voltage-gated calcium channels, which are activated by nerve impulses or membrane depolarization. Other types of calcium channel are receptor-operated and stretch-activated channels. Calcium channel blockers (calcium antagonists) are a diverse group of compounds (see Table 7.8) which decrease calcium entry into cardiac and vascular smooth muscle cells through the L-subtype (long-lasting inward calcium current) of voltage-gated calcium channels. The L-type channel consists of several subunits. Calcium channel blockers bind in several ways to the α_1 subunit of L-type channels to impede calcium entry. Phenylalkylamines (e.g. verapamil) bind to the intracellular portion of the channel and physically occlude it, whereas dihydropyridines modify the extracellular allosteric structure of the channel. Benzothiazepines (e.g. diltiazem) act on the α_1 subunit, although the mechanism has not been fully elucidated and may have further actions on sodium–potassium exchange and calcium–calmodulin binding.

Cardiac cells in the SA and AV nodes are dependent on the slow inward calcium current for depolarization. Calcium channel blockers which act here decrease calcium entry during phase 0 of the action potential of SA node and AV node cells, decreasing heart rate and AV node conduction. Calcium entry during phase 2 of the action potential of ventricular myocytes may be decreased (see Fig. 7.10, p. 92) and excitation–contraction coupling inhibited, causing decreased myocardial contractility. There is experimental evidence to suggest that some calcium antagonists have favourable effects on endothelial function.

CLINICAL EFFECTS

Calcium channel blockers differ in their selectivity for cardiac muscle cells, conducting tissue and vascular smooth muscle, but to some degree they all decrease myocardial contractility and produce coronary and systemic vasodilatation with a consequent decrease in arterial pressure. Therefore, they have been used widely for the treatment of hypertension, angina and vasospastic disorders, but have been superseded in some areas by newer drugs. Verapamil and diltiazem also decrease SA node activity, AV node conduction and heart rate, and they are useful in the treatment of paroxysmal supraventricular tachyarrhythmias. Calcium channel blockers may also inhibit platelet aggregation, protect against bronchospasm, and improve lower oesophageal sphincter function. The non-dihydropyridines are contraindicated in the presence of second- or third-degree heart block and should not be combined with β-blockers as they may cause bradycardia or heart block. With the exception of amlodipine and felodipine, calcium channel blockers should not be used in patients with cardiac failure.

CLASSIFICATION

Calcium channel blockers are a diverse group of compounds which have been classified in several ways, according to their structure, mechanism of action and specificity for slow calcium channels. In this chapter, they are described in accordance with a

Table 7.8 Classification of calcium channel blockers

Group	Prototype/ first-generation drugs	Second and third generation drugs	Effects on:				
			SA node	AV node conduction	Myocardial contractility	Peripheral arteries	Coronary arteries
Benzothiazepine	Diltiazem		+/−	+	+	+	++
Phenylalkylamine	Verapamil		++	++	+	+	+
Dihydropyridine	Nifedipine		−	−	+	++	++
		Nicardipine	−	−	+/−	++	+++
		Nimodipine	−	−	+/−	++	+/−
		Felodipine	−	−	−	+++	+
		Isradipine	−	−	−	+++	+
		Amlodipine[a]	−	−	−	+++	++
		Lacidipine[a]	−	−	−	++++	+/−
Phenylalkylamine/ benzimidazoyl	Mibefradil		−	−	−	+	++

[a]Third-generation calcium antagonists.

recent classification which broadly groups the drugs according to their basic structure (thus distinguishing drugs with different affinities at different sites, e.g. cardiac conducting tissue or arterial vasculature) and then divides them into first-, second- or third-generation compounds according to pharmacokinetic differences. This classification therefore accounts for chemical structure, tissue selectivity and pharmacokinetic properties (Table 7.8).

The first-generation calcium channel blockers, verapamil, diltiazem and particularly nifedipine, have a rapid onset of action which may reduce arterial pressure acutely and produce reflex sympathetic activation. They have marked negative dromotropic and inotropic effects (especially verapamil and diltiazem), and they should not be used in patients with left ventricular (LV) dysfunction or after myocardial infarction. Their intrinsic duration of action is short, requiring multiple daily dosing, but slow-release formulations have been developed (see below). All are well absorbed from the GI tract, but undergo a significant first-pass effect leading to low bioavailability. All are highly protein-bound, most are metabolized extensively by hepatic demethylation and dealkylation, and some produce active metabolites. Plasma concentrations are increased in the elderly, by hepatic impairment, decreased hepatic blood flow or drugs affecting hepatic function, and there is wide individual pharmacokinetic variability.

Some of these problems were addressed by the development of second- and third-generation drugs which have an improved pharmacokinetic profile with slower onset and longer duration of action (leading to less sympathetic activation) and greater selectivity for vascular smooth muscle (see Tables 7.8 and 7.9).

First-generation calcium channel blockers

Nifedipine

Nifedipine is a dihydropyridine derivative which is a systemic and coronary arterial vasodilator. It is effective in countering coronary artery spasm, thought to be an important component of all forms of angina, and it may bring symptomatic relief in patients with peripheral vasospastic (e.g. Raynaud's) disease. Its anti-anginal effect is additive with that of β-adrenergic blocking drugs and nitrates. Adverse effects related to the vasodilating action of nifedipine include flushing, headaches, ankle oedema, dizziness, tiredness and palpitations. Nifedipine is absorbed rapidly, particularly when the stomach is empty, with an onset of action of 20 min. This may produce reflex tachycardia and increased myocardial contractility, although nifedipine is cardiopressant in vitro. It is well absorbed (> 90%), but undergoes significant hepatic first-pass metabolism. It is metabolized in the liver to inactive metabolites and is excreted mainly via the kidneys with an elimination half-life of 3–5 h. Kinetics are not affected significantly by renal impairment.

Verapamil

Verapamil is a phenylalkylamine which has more pronounced effects on the SA and AV nodes than other calcium antagonists, and is used mainly as an antiarrhythmic (see below). However, it has vasodilator, anti-anginal and negative inotropic properties and has been used for the treatment of angina and hypertension. It is also indicated for hypertrophic obstructive cardiomyopathy.

Verapamil is well absorbed but its bioavailability is low. It is metabolized in the liver and excreted via the kidneys; the elimination half-life is 5 h. Both verapamil and diltiazem inhibit the hepatic metabolism of several drugs; plasma concentrations of digoxin, carbamazepine and theophyllines are increased by verapamil. Verapamil has a marked negative inotropic action and may cause bradycardia, hypotension, AV block or cardiac failure when combined with β-blockers or other cardiodepressant drugs (including disopyramide and the volatile anaesthetic agents). It may also potentiate the effects of neuromuscular blocking drugs. Most calcium channel blockers possess one or more chiral centres, and the different enantiomeric forms have different pharmacokinetic and pharmacodynamic properties. For example, L-verapamil undergoes higher first-pass metabolism than the D-form, so that after intravenous administration, plasma concentrations of L-verapamil are relatively higher, producing more pronounced negative inotropic and chronotropic effects.

Diltiazem

Diltiazem is a benzothiazepine which has less effect on conducting tissue but a greater effect on coronary arteries than verapamil, and is used mainly in the treatment of hypertension and angina. It is well absorbed with low bioavailability, is metabolized in the liver producing active metabolites, and excreted via the kidneys. Its half-life is approximately 5 h.

Second- and third-generation calcium antagonists

The second-generation calcium antagonists are mostly dihydropyridine derivatives which have a slower onset and longer duration of action and greater selectivity for vascular smooth muscle than the first-generation drugs. They are either sustained-release formulations (e.g. diltiazem SR, nifedipine SR) or new compounds. The slow onset results in less sympathetic activation and reflex tachycardia. The new compounds (e.g. felodipine, nisoldipine, nicardipine) have less effect on AV conduction and less negative inotropic and chronotropic effects. All second- and

Table 7.9 Pharmacokinetic properties of some commonly used calcium channel blockers

Drug	Nifedipine	Verapamil	Diltiazem	Nicardipine	Felodipine	Amlodipine	Lacidipine
Bioavailability (%)	50	20	25–50	30	15	65–80	10
Elimination half-life (h)	3–5	5–8	2–6	3–8	25	35–50	13–19
Route of elimination	Renal, hepatic	Renal, hepatic,	Hepatic	Renal, hepatic	Renal, hepatic	Renal	Hepatic, renal
Time to peak plasma concentration (h)	1–2	4–8	3–4	1	12–24	6–12	1–3

third-generation calcium antagonists have little effect on lipid or glucose metabolism and may be used in patients with renal dysfunction. Some have special features.

Nimodipine is selective for cerebral vasculature and is used to prevent vasospasm after subarachnoid haemorrhage. *Nicardipine* causes less reduction in myocardial contractility than other calcium antagonists. *Felodipine* acts predominantly on peripheral vascular smooth muscle and has negligible effects on myocardial contractility, although it does produce coronary vasodilatation. It also has a mild diuretic and natriuretic effect. It is indicated for the treatment of hypertension, but has been used in patients with impaired LV function. Felodipine is formulated in a hydrophilic gel which limits the release of drug and prolongs its absorption. Hence bioavailability is low and plasma concentrations are stable after 12–24 h.

The third generation of calcium antagonists (lacidipine, amlodipine) are new dihydropyridines which bind to specific high-affinity sites in the calcium channel complex. They have a particularly slow onset and long duration of action, and so reflex sympathetic stimulation is not evident. However, adverse effects related to vasodilatation (headache, flushing, ankle oedema) do occur. Both are extensively metabolized in the liver to inactive metabolites which are excreted via the kidneys and liver. *Lacidipine* is highly lipophilic, so that it is sequestered in the lipid bilayer of vascular smooth muscle cells. It has low bioavailability and reaches peak plasma concentrations in 1–3 h, but its elimination half-life is 13–19 h. *Amlodipine* is well absorbed, with peak concentrations after 6–12 h, and has a half-life of 35–50 h.

Some calcium antagonists, in particular lacidipine, may delay the development of atherosclerosis via effects on modulators of vascular smooth muscle and platelet function. Lacidipine may augment the action of endothelium-derived relaxing factors, e.g. nitric oxide, which has vasodilator, antiplatelet and antiproliferative effects, and antagonize the effects of endothelin-1, a potent vasoconstrictor which also stimulates endothelial proliferation.

Mibefradil is a tetralol derivative which selectively blocks T-type calcium channels and was recently introduced for the treatment of hypertension and angina. It causes coronary artery vasodilatation without suppressing myocardial contractility, and heart rate is decreased. Although generally well tolerated, mibefradil was associated with multiple drug interactions and has now been withdrawn from clinical use.

INDICATIONS FOR CALCIUM CHANNEL BLOCKERS

The indications for calcium channel blockers have evolved over the last decade. Currently accepted indications are detailed below:

Hypertension

Calcium antagonists are now considered as first-line antihypertensive drugs only in certain circumstances:

- isolated systolic hypertension in the elderly (long-acting dihydropyridines)
- hypertension with angina (long-acting dihydropyridines)
- cyclosporin-induced hypertension
- hypertension with coexisting atrial fibrillation or supraventricular tachycardia (non-dihydropyridines)
- acute hypertension – sublingual nifedipine has been used for the rapid treatment of acute hypertension but, following reports of serious adverse effects resulting from precipitous decreases in arterial pressure, it is no longer recommended. Verapamil 5–10 mg or diltiazem 0.3 mg kg^{-1} i.v. are effective.

Angina

Calcium channel blockers, particularly the non-dihydropyridines, are effective in angina as they decrease myocardial oxygen consumption by decreasing afterload, heart rate and contractility. They also decrease coronary artery spasm and improve blood flow to ischaemic myocardium. Amlodipine and felodipine, combined with a diuretic or ACE inhibitor, may be beneficial in patients with angina and impaired LV function, but the other calcium channel blockers should not be used. In addition, there has been increasing concern over the association of short-acting dihydropyridines with cardiac and cerebral ischaemic events, and with an apparent increase in mortality after MI when used in higher doses.

Subarachnoid haemorrhage

Nimodipine, used by the i.v. or nasogastric routes, is selective for cerebral arteries and improves outcome after SAH by the prevention of vasospasm.

Arrhythmias

Verapamil 5–10 mg i.v. (or diltiazem 0.15 mg kg^{-1} i.v.) are class 4 antiarrhythmic drugs used for the treatment of paroxysmal supraventricular tachycardias (see p. 94).

Hypertrophic obstructive cardiomyopathy

Verapamil improves exercise tolerance and decreases symptoms but has no effect on the incidence of sudden death.

Miscellaneous

Some non-dihydropyridines, when combined with ACE inhibitors, may decrease proteinuria in diabetic nephropathy. Nifedipine may be useful in the management of peripheral vasospastic disease (e.g. Raynaud's).

ANAESTHESIA AND CALCIUM CHANNEL BLOCKERS

Both intravenous and volatile anaesthetic agents block conduction through L-type calcium channels in neuronal and cardiac tissues, and may therefore interact with calcium antagonists through pharmacokinetic and pharmacodynamic mechanisms. Verapamil (and to a lesser extent diltiazem) has additive effects with halothane on cardiac conduction and contractility, with the potential for bradycardia and myocardial depression. Calcium channel blockers potentiate the hypotensive effects of volatile anaesthetics, particularly enflurane. Verapamil has been shown to decrease the MAC of halothane, and, in an animal model, nifedipine enhances the analgesic effects of morphine by stimulation of spinal 5-HT_3 receptors.

Plasma concentrations of verapamil are increased during anaesthesia with volatile agents, possibly because of decreased hepatic blood flow.

Calcium antagonists potentiate the effects of depolarizing and non-depolarizing neuromuscular blockers in experimental conditions, although the clinical relevance of this is uncertain.

DRUGS ACTING VIA THE RENIN–ANGIOTENSIN-ALDOSTERONE SYSTEM

The renin–angiotensin–aldosterone system (RAS) is intimately involved with cardiovascular and body fluid homeostasis. Angiotensin II (A-II), produced from inactive precursors, is the major regulator of the renin–angiotensin system. It is a potent vasoconstrictor, which has several renal and extrarenal effects. A-II has an important role in the maintenance of circulating volume in response to several stressors, whilst direct renal effects are mostly responsible for long-term regulation of body fluid volume and blood pressure.

Renin is a proteolytic enzyme produced by the juxtaglomerular cells in the kidney. Renin cleaves four amino acids from angiotensinogen, an α_2-globulin produced by the liver, to form the decapeptide angiotensin I (A-I). Angiotensin I is further cleaved of two amino acids by a non-specific carboxypeptidase, angiotensin-converting enzyme (ACE), to form the octapeptide A-II. A-II is then metabolized by several peptidases to several breakdown products including angiotensin III (A-III), which has some activity at angiotensin (AT) receptors, although this is minimal compared with that of A-II. The production of A-I and A-II takes place in the walls of small blood vessels in the lungs, kidneys and other organs, and in the plasma. The rate-limiting step for this cascade is the plasma concentration of renin (see Fig. 7.9).

There are at least two subtypes of angiotensin receptors: type 1 (AT_1) and type 2 (AT_2). AT_1 receptors are found principally in vascular smooth muscle, adrenal cortex, kidney, liver and some areas of the brain, and mediate all the known physiological functions of A-II. The function of the AT_2 receptor is unclear; AT_2 receptors are also present in the kidney, and predominate in the adrenal medulla, uterus, ovary and other parts of the brain. AT_1 receptors show a greater affinity for angiotensin II. AT_2 receptors show similar affinity for A-II and A-III and may play a role in cell growth and differentiation.

AT_1 receptors are typical G-protein-coupled receptors which, when stimulated, activate phospholipase C, with the production of DAG and IP_3. IP_3 causes the release of intracellular Ca^{2+}, which activates enzymes to cause the phosphorylation of intracellular proteins. A-II also increases Ca^{2+} entry through membrane channels. The intracellular mechanism of action of AT_2 receptors is not defined.

ACTIONS OF ANGIOTENSIN-II

Angiotensin-II has several effects (Fig. 7.9). It is a potent vasoconstrictor (direct action on vascular smooth muscle of arterioles and veins) and it promotes sodium reabsorption both by direct action at the proximal tubules and by stimulating aldosterone secretion from the zona glomerulosa of the adrenal cortex. Aldosterone causes further sodium reabsorption by exchange for potassium and, to a lesser extent, hydrogen ions, at the distal tubule. A-II produces preglomerular vasoconstriction and vasoconstriction of the efferent arterioles, and so maintains glomerular filtration rate in response to a decrease in renal blood flow. It also affects the local regulation of blood flow in other vascular beds, e.g. the splanchnic circulation. In addition, A-II stimulates the sympathetic nervous system via direct and indirect methods to increase norepinephrine and epinephrine release; it may also inhibit the cardiac vagus. A-II stimulates erythropoiesis and has direct trophic effects on vascular smooth muscle and cardiac muscle, promoting cellular proliferation, migration and hypertrophy. There is some evidence for relative downregulation of AT_1 receptors and upregulation of AT_2 receptors in cardiac failure, with AT_2 receptors being responsible for some cardioprotective effects.

RAS activity tends to be low in the resting state, but is activated by several stimuli, e.g. depletion of circulating volume, haemorrhage or sodium depletion. These cause renin secretion and increased production of A-II, leading to vasoconstriction, increased cardiac output, arterial pressure and sodium retention. Renin production, the rate-limiting step in the production of A-II, is stimulated by the following mechanisms:

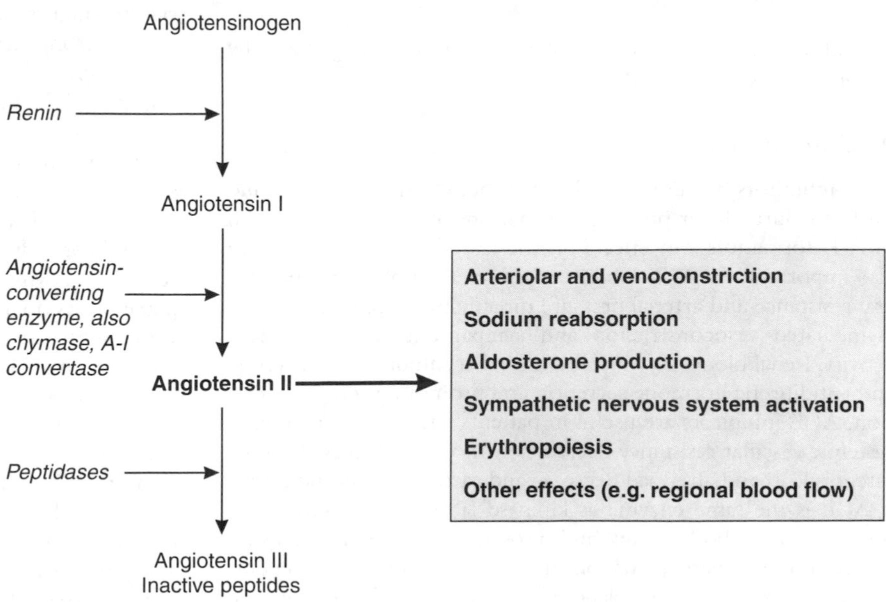

Fig. 7.9
The renin–angiotensin system showing the biochemical cascade for the production of angiotensin II and its actions at AT_1 receptors.

- sympathetic activity (mediated by β_1-receptors responding to circulating catecholamines and direct renal nerve stimulation)
- decreased renal perfusion pressure (via renal baroreceptors)
- decreased right atrial pressure (mediated by vagal afferents to the kidney)
- decreased tubular sodium concentration in the macula densa.

Renin secretion is inhibited by:

- negative feedback by A-II
- negative feedback by aldosterone
- vasopressin
- atrial natriuretic factor.

The RAS may be involved in the pathogenesis of hypertension, but the relationship is complex; RAS activity may be high (e.g. in renal artery stenosis), low (as in primary aldosteronism) or variable (essential hypertension).

DRUGS ACTING ON THE RENIN–ANGIOTENSIN SYSTEM

The activity of the RAS may be inhibited at three key points, by various mechanisms:

- *Suppression of renin release or inhibition of renin activity.* Renin secretion may be inhibited by sympatholytic drugs (e.g. β-blockers or central α-antagonists). This mechanism is partly responsible for the hypotensive effects of β-blockers. Renin inhibitors competitively inhibit the reaction between renin and its substrate, angiotensinogen, preventing the production of A-II. Because renin release still occurs, the consequent reduction of plasma A-II concentrations leads to a secondary increase in renin secretion, limiting the effect of such drugs.
- *Inhibition of ACE.* The primary mechanism of action of ACE inhibitors is to block the conversion of A-I to A-II, although effects on kinin and prostaglandin metabolism also contribute.
- *Blockade of A-II receptors.* AT_1-receptor antagonists competitively block A-II receptors.

In addition, the effects of aldosterone may be antagonized by spironolactone (see Ch. 26).

ACE inhibitors

ACE inhibitors are used for the treatment of hypertension and cardiac failure. Their principal mechanism of action is inhibition of A-II formation, but effects on the kallikrein–kinin system are also important. All ACE inhibitors reduce arteriolar tone, peripheral resistance and arterial pressure directly by decreasing both A-II-mediated vasoconstriction and sympathetic nervous system activity. Renal blood flow increases, further inhibiting aldosterone and antidiuretic hormone secretion and promoting sodium excretion. ACE inhibitors are useful in patients with cardiac failure, as systemic vascular resistance decreases without an increase in heart rate; preload and afterload decrease and cardiac output increases.

ACE is the same enzyme as kininase II and is involved in the metabolism of both kinins and prostaglandins. ACE inhibitors therefore block the degradation of kinins, substance P and endorphins, and increase prostaglandin concentrations. Bradykinin and other kinins are highly potent peptides which cause arterial and venous dilatation by stimulating the production of arachidonic acid metabolites, NO and endothelial-derived hyperpolarization factor, via specific bradykinin B_2 receptors in vascular endothelium. Bradykinin also enhances the uptake of circulating glucose into skeletal muscle and has a protective effect on cardiac myocytes by a mechanism involving prostacyclin stimulation. Kinins counteract the vasoconstriction induced by A-II, and therefore ACE inhibitors, which potentiate the actions of endogenous kinins by about 50-fold, promote kinin-induced vasodilatation. Kinins have no major effect on arterial pressure regulation in normotensive individuals or those with low-renin hypertension, but they account for up to 30% of the effects of ACE inhibitors in renovascular hypertension. The adverse effects of dry cough and angioneurotic oedema sometimes associated with ACE inhibitors may be kinin-dependent. ACE is widely distributed in tissues and plasma; ACE inhibitors may differ in their affinity for ACE at different sites. Other tissue enzymes (A-I convertase and chymase) may also produce A-II, from A-I or directly from angiotensinogen, so that inhibition of the renin–angiotensin system by ACE inhibitors is incomplete.

Clinical applications of ACE inhibition

ACE inhibitors are established in the treatment of hypertension; they decrease morbidity and mortality in congestive cardiac failure, and improve left ventricular dysfunction after myocardial infarction. They delay the progression of diabetic nephropathy and have a protective effect in non-diabetic chronic renal failure, although they are associated with proteinuria in approximately 1% of patients. ACE inhibitors improve vascular endothelial function by their effects on A-II and bradykinin; the clinical importance of this in patients with vascular disease is unknown.

ACE inhibitors have a common mechanism of action, differing in the chemical structure of their active moieties, in potency, bioavailability, plasma half-life, route of elimination, distribution and affinity for tissue-bound ACE (Table 7.10). However, the efficacy of most ACE inhibitors is similar. Most of the newer compounds are prodrugs, converted to an active metabolite by the liver, and have a prolonged duration of action. Most are excreted via the kidneys, and dosage should be reduced in the elderly and those with impaired renal or cardiac function. Enalapril is available as the active drug, enalaprilat, and may be administered intravenously (1.25 mg over 5 min) for the treatment of hypertensive emergencies.

ACE inhibitors are generally tolerated well, with no rebound hypertension after stopping therapy and few metabolic effects. Symptomatic first-dose hypotension may occur, particularly in hypovolaemic or sodium-depleted patients with high plasma renin concentrations. Symptomatic hypotension was more common with the higher doses originally used. ACE inhibitors have a synergistic effect with diuretics (which increase the activity of the renin–angiotensin system), but are less effective in patients taking NSAIDs.

The adverse effects of ACE inhibitors may be classified into those that are class-specific (related to inhibition of ACE) and those that relate to specific drugs. Class-specific effects include hypotension, renal insufficiency, hyperkalaemia, cough (10%) and angioneurotic oedema (0.1–0.2%). ACE inhibitors may cause renal impairment, particularly if renal perfusion is decreased (e.g. because of renal artery stenosis, congestive cardiac failure or hypovolaemia) or there is pre-existing renal disease. Renal impairment is also more likely in

Table 7.10 Pharmacology of ACE inhibitors

	Captopril	Lisinopril	Enalapril	Perindopril	Quinapril	Trandolapril	Ramipril	Fosinopril
Zinc ligand	Sulphhydryl	Carboxyl	Carboxyl	Carboxyl	Carboxyl	Carboxyl	Carboxyl	Phosphinyl
Prodrug	No	No	Yes	Yes	Yes	Yes	Yes	Yes
Bioavailability (%)	75	25	60	65	40	70	50	35
t_{max} (h)[a]	0.8	6–8	3–4	3–4	2	4–6	2–3	3–6
$t_{1/2}$ (h)[a]	2	12	11	25[b]	20–25[b]	16–24[b]	4–50[b]	12
Metabolism[a]	Oxidation (50%)	Minimal	Minimal	Prodrug	Prodrug	Prodrug	Prodrug	Prodrug
Elimination	Renal	Renal	Renal	Renal	Renal	Renal, hepatic	Renal	Renal, hepatic

[a]The prodrugs are metabolized in the gut mucosa and liver to active compounds. Pharmacokinetic data refer to the active compounds.
[b]These drugs have polyphasic pharmacokinetics, with a dose-dependent prolonged terminal elimination phase from plasma of over 24 h.

the elderly or those receiving NSAIDs, and renal function should be checked before starting ACE inhibitor therapy, and monitored subsequently. Hyperkalaemia (plasma K^+ concentration usually increases by 0.1–0.2 mmol L^{-1} because of decreased aldosterone concentrations) may be more marked in those with impaired renal function or in patients taking potassium supplements or potassium-sparing diuretics. The mechanism of cough is not known but is mediated by C fibres and may be related to bradykinin or substance P production. It is reversible on stopping the ACE inhibitor. Other adverse effects include upper respiratory congestion, rhinorrhoea, gastrointestinal disturbances, and increased insulin sensitivity and hyperglycaemia in diabetic patients.

Some adverse effects – skin rashes (1%), taste disturbances, proteinuria (1%) and neutropenia (0.05%) – are related to the presence of a sulphydryl group (e.g. captopril). ACE inhibitors may cause fetal abnormalities and are contraindicated in pregnancy.

Although anaesthesia *per se* has no direct effect on the RAS or ACE inhibitors, the RAS is activated by several stimuli which may occur during the perioperative period. These include blood or fluid losses and the stress response to surgical stimulation. Activation of the RAS contributes to the maintenance of arterial pressure after haemorrhage, or during anaesthesia. The incidence of hypotension during anaesthesia is increased in patients receiving long-term antihypertensive treatment with ACE inhibitors, and it has been argued that they should be stopped before surgery if significant blood loss or fluid shifts are likely. ACE inhibitors improve ventricular function in patients with cardiac failure or after myocardial infarction, but it is not known whether acute cessation before surgery is harmful. Conversely, they may have beneficial effects on regional blood flow and have been associated with improved renal function in patients undergoing aortic surgery. There is no consensus on the optimum perioperative management of patients receiving ACE inhibitors.

A-II receptor antagonists

Angiotensin II receptor antagonists selectively block the type 1 A-II receptor (AT_1 receptor). They inhibit the RAS independently from the source of A-II and block any effects of A-II resulting from compensatory stimulation of renin, such as reflex activation of the sympathetic nervous system. Hence, they do not cause tachycardia or an increase in cardiac contractility and are used in the treatment of hypertension. However, they are ineffective in primary hyperaldosteronism. Their antihypertensive effect is similar to that of ACE inhibitors and they may be useful in the management of cardiac failure, as they reduce afterload and increase cardiac output. AT_1 antagonists have no effect on bradykinin metabolism or prostaglandin synthesis, so they do not produce the cough or rash associated with ACE inhibitors. They are generally well tolerated and produce few adverse effects, although angio-oedema has been reported. However, plasma concentrations of renin, A-I and A-II increase, and aldosterone concentrations decrease during long-term therapy; hyperkalaemia may occur if potassium-sparing diuretics are also administered.

The prototype AT_1 antagonist was saralasin, a peptide analogue of A-II, which is rapidly inactivated in the gut and therefore used only for experimental or diagnostic purposes. All clinically available AT_1-receptor antagonists are non-peptide imidazole compounds. The active compounds bind specifically and non-competitively to the AT_1 receptor without agonist activity. They are highly protein-bound, with a prolonged duration of action exceeding their plasma half-life, and a maximum antihypertensive effect 2–4 weeks after starting therapy. Their antihypertensive effect is enhanced when combined with a thiazide diuretic; combination formulations are available. In common with ACE inhibitors, they are contraindicated in pregnancy and are likely to have an adverse effect in patients with renal artery stenosis or those taking NSAIDs. The pharmacological properties of some AT_1-receptor antagonists are shown in Table 7.11.

There are few data describing the effects of AT_1-receptor antagonists in the perioperative period, but caution would be appropriate when large fluid or blood losses are expected.

ANTIARRHYTHMIC DRUGS

Cardiac arrhythmias are defined as irregular or abnormal heart rhythms, including bradycardias or tachycardias outside the physiological range. Patients may present for surgery with a pre-existing arrhythmia; alternatively, arrhythmias may be precipitated or

Table 7.11 Pharmacology of AT_1 antagonists

Drug	Losartan	Candesartan	Irbesartan	Valsartan
Prodrug	No[a]	Yes	No	No
Bioavailability (%)	33	14–40	60–80	23
t_{max} (h)	1[a]	3–4	1.5–2	2–4
$t_{1/2}$ (h)	2[a]	9	11–15	9
Metabolism	Hepatic	Minimal	Hepatic	Minimal
Elimination	Renal, hepatic	Renal, hepatic	Renal, hepatic	Bile, urine

[a]Undergoes significant first-pass metabolism, producing an active metabolite EXP 3174, which is more potent than the parent compound. Peak concentrations and elimination half life of EXP 3174 are 3–4 and 6–9 h, respectively.

accentuated during anaesthesia by several surgical, pharmacological or physiological factors (Table 7.12). Although several drugs (including anaesthetic drugs) have effects on heart rate and rhythm, the term antiarrhythmic is applied to drugs which primarily affect ionic currents within myocardial conducting tissue. Antiarrhythmic drugs are classified according to their effects on the action potential (see below), and knowledge of the normal electrophysiological events of the cardiac cycle is required to understand their effects.

THE CARDIAC ACTION POTENTIAL

The cardiac action potential (Fig. 7.10) is generated by movement of charged ions across the cell membrane and comprises five phases. At rest, the cells are polarized and the resting membrane potential is negative (–50 to –60 mV in sinus node pacemaker cells and –80 to –90 mV in Purkinje, atrial and ventricular muscle fibres). The action potential is triggered by a low intracellular leak of sodium ions (and calcium ions at the AV node) until a threshold point is reached, when sudden rapid influx of sodium ions causes an increase in positive charge within the cell and generates an impulse (phase 0, depolarization). The action potential starts to reverse (phase 1), but is sustained because of slower inward movement of calcium ions (phase 2). Efflux of potassium ions brings about repolarization (phase 3) and the gradual termination of the action potential. Thereafter, re-equilibration of sodium and potassium takes place and the resting membrane potential is restored (phase 4). The action potential spreads between adjacent cells and is transmitted through the specialized conducting system from the AV node to the bundle of His and ventricular muscle fibres via the Purkinje fibres. The SA node pacemaker cells have the fastest spontaneous discharge rate and usually initiate the coordinated action potential. However, action potentials may also be generated by the AV node and other cells in the conducting system.

Table 7.12 Precipitants of arrhythmias during anaesthesia

Myocardial ischaemia
Hypoxia
Hypercapnia
Halogenated hydrocarbons (volatile anaesthetic agents, e.g. trichloroethylene, cyclopropane, halothane)
Catecholamines (endogenous or exogenous)
Electrolyte abnormalities (hypo- or hyperkalemia, hypocalcaemia, hypomagnesaemia)
Hypotension
Autonomic effects (e.g. reflex vagal stimulation, brain tumours or trauma)
Acid–base abnormalities
Mechanical stimuli (e.g. during CVP or PAFC line insertion)
Drugs (toxicity or adverse reactions)
Medical conditions (e.g. pneumonia, alcohol abuse)

MECHANISMS OF ARRHYTHMIAS

Arrhythmias are caused by abnormalities of impulse generation or conduction, or both, by a number of mechanisms:

- *Altered automaticity.* Increased pacemaker activity in the SA node (e.g. caused by increased sympathetic tone) may cause

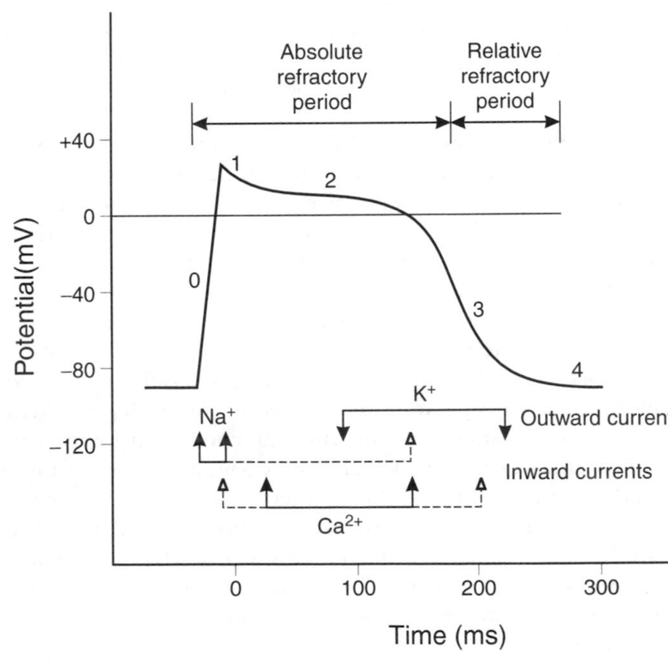

Fig. 7.10
Diagrammatic representation of a cardiac action potential denoting its phases, the main ion fluxes and the refractory periods. The plateau phase (2) is characteristic of ventricular myocardium. Phase 0 corresponds to the rapid depolarization; phase 3 to repolarization; and phase 4 to the diastolic plateau.

sinus tachycardia, or atrial or ventricular tachyarrhythmias. Decreased SA node automaticity (e.g. as a result of enhanced vagal activity) may allow the emergence of latent pacemaker activity in distal conducting tissues, e.g. AV node or the bundle of His–Purkinje system, causing sinus bradycardia, AV nodal or idioventricular escape rhythms. These rhythms are common during halothane anaesthesia.

- *Unidirectional conduction block.* Interruption of the normal conduction pathways caused by anatomical defects, alterations in refractory period or excitability may cause heart block and favours arrhythmias caused by abnormal re-entry or automaticity.
- *Ectopic foci.* Ectopic foci may give rise to arrhythmias in a variety of circumstances. In the presence of bradycardia or SA node block, pathological damage in cardiac muscle cells or conducting tissues may augment the generation of arrhythmias from ectopic foci, via:
  —increased automaticity
  —re-entry phenomena
  —pathological after-depolarizations.

These mechanisms are thought to be responsible for the production of many ventricular and supraventricular tachyarrhythmias, including the Wolff–Parkinson–White (WPW) syndrome. Increased automaticity in atrial, ventricular or conducting tissues as a result of ischaemia or electrolyte disturbances (e.g. hypokalaemia) may cause depolarization before the SA node and permit the generation of an arrhythmia. Re-entrant arrhythmias arise from retrograde conduction along a branch of tissue in which anterograde conduction has been blocked by disease. If there is a discrepancy in the refractory periods of the two branches, retrograde conduction may occur in cells that have already discharged and repolarized, triggering a further action potential which is both premature and ectopic. These premature action potentials become self-sustaining (circus movements), leading to atrial or ventricular tachycardia or fibrillation. Pathological after-depolarizations are spontaneous impulses arising just after the normal action potential, but are dependent on the prior impulses for their generation. They occur mostly in ischaemic myocardium (e.g. after myocardial infarction) and are more likely in the presence of hypoxaemia, increased catecholamine concentrations, digoxin toxicity or electrolyte abnormalities.

ARRHYTHMIAS AND ANAESTHESIA

Arrhythmias are common in patients during anaesthesia and in intensive care, especially in those with ischaemic heart disease, preoperative arrhythmias, valvular heart or pericardial disease or cardiomyopathies. They may be precipitated by several factors. Some arrhythmias are immediately life-threatening, but all arrhythmias warrant attention because they usually imply the presence of other disturbances, and the effects of specific therapy (e.g. drugs, electrical cardioversion or cardiac pacing) are enhanced by prior corrective measures. Specific antiarrhythmic treatment is usually reserved for arrhythmias that affect cardiac output or may progress to dangerous tachyarrhythmias.

In addition to volatile agents, several drugs used during anaesthesia may facilitate arrhythmias by direct toxicity (e.g. local anaesthetics), autonomic effects (e.g. succinylcholine, pancuronium), by enhancing the effects of catecholamines (e.g. nitrous oxide, thiopental, cocaine), or as a result of histamine release. These are discussed in the appropriate chapters. Opioids potentiate central vagal activity, decrease sympathetic tone and have direct negative chronotropic effects on the SA node. They may therefore cause bradycardia but conversely decrease the incidence of ventricular arrhythmias.

MECHANISMS OF ACTION OF ANTIARRHYTHMIC DRUGS

An arrhythmia may be controlled either by slowing the primary mechanism or, in the case of supraventricular arrhythmias, by reducing the proportion of impulses transmitted through the AV node to the ventricular conducting system. The cardiac action potential may be pharmacologically manipulated in three ways:

- The *automaticity* (tendency to spontaneous discharge) of cells may be reduced. This result can be achieved by reducing the rate of leakage of sodium (reducing the slope of phase 4), by increasing the electronegativity of the resulting membrane potential or by decreasing the electronegativity of the threshold potential.
- The *speed of conduction* of the action potential may be suppressed as reflected by a lowering of the height and slope of the phase 0 discharge. A reduction in the electronegativity of the membrane potential at the onset of phase 0 reduces both the amplitude and the slope of the phase 0 depolarization. This situation occurs if the cell discharges before it has been completely repolarized.
- The *rate of repolarization* may be reduced, which prolongs the refractory period of the discharging cell.

All antiarrhythmic drugs may themselves induce arrhythmias. Many (particularly class 1 antiarrhythmics) have a narrow therapeutic index and some have been associated with no benefit or even an increase in mortality in large-scale studies. In addition, non-pharmacological techniques (e.g. DC cardioversion, implantable pacemakers or cardioverter defibrillators, and radiofrequency ablation) have become more widespread. Consequently, the use of antiarrhythmic drugs for chronic therapy has declined in recent years. However, owing to the frequency of arrhythmias during anaesthesia, knowledge of the available drugs and their interactions is important for the anaesthetist.

Antiarrhythmic agents may be classified empirically on the basis of their effectiveness in supraventricular tachycardias (e.g. digoxin, β-blockers and verapamil) or in ventricular arrhythmias (lidocaine, mexiletine, tocainide, phenytoin and bretylium). Many agents (disopyramide, amiodarone, quinidine and procainamide) are effective in both supraventricular and ventricular arrhythmias. The Vaughan Williams classification (Table 7.13) is based on electrophysiological mechanisms. Although this classification has limitations (some drugs belong to more than one class, some arrhythmias may be caused by several mechanisms, some drugs, e.g. digoxin, adenosine, do not fit into the classification) it remains in common use, and is therefore described below.

Class 1 drugs inhibit the fast sodium influx during depolarization; they inhibit arrhythmias caused by abnormal automaticity or re-entry. All class 1 antiarrhythmics decrease the maximum rate of rise of phase 0, and decrease conduction velocity, excitability and automaticity to varying degrees. In addition to these local anaes-

Table 7.13 Vaughan Williams classification of anti-arrhythmic drugs

Class	Examples	Mechanism	Effects	Indication
1a	Quinidine Disopyramide	Na^+ channel blockade (moderate) ↓ Conduction velocity Prolonged duration of action potential	Moderate ↓ V_{MAX} ↑ Action potential duration ↑ Refractory period QRS widened	Prevention of SVT, VT, atrial tachycardia WPW
1b	Lidocaine Bretylium	Na^+ channel blockade (mild) ↓ Conduction velocity Shortened repolarization	Mild ↓ V_{MAX} ↓ Action potential duration ↓ Refractory period QRS unchanged	Prevention of VT/VF during ischaemia
1c	Flecainide Propafenone	Na^+ channel blockade (marked) ↓ Conduction velocity No change in repolarization	Marked ↓ V_{MAX} Minimal change in action potential duration and refractory period QRS widened	Conversion/prevention of SVT/VT/VF
2	β-Blockers	β-Adrenergic receptor blockade	Decreased automaticity (SA and AV nodes)	Prevention of sympathetic-induced tachyarrhythmias, rate control in AF, 2° prevention after MI, prevention of AV node re-entrant tachycardia
3	Amiodarone Bretylium Sotalol	Inhibition of inward K^+ current	Markedly prolonged repolarization ↑ Action potential duration ↑ Refractory period QRS unchanged	Prevention of SVT/VT/VF
4	Diltiazem	Calcium channel blockade	↓ Depolarization and V_{MAX} of slow response cells in SA and AV nodes ↓ Action potential duration ↓ Refractory period of AV node	Rate control in AF Prevention of AV node re-entrant tachycardia

thetic properties, some have membrane-stabilizing effects. Class 1a drugs antagonize primarily the fast influx of sodium ions and so reduce conduction velocity through the AV node and His–Purkinje system, whilst prolonging the duration of the action potential and the refractory period. They also have antimuscarinic and sympathomimetic effects, to varying degrees. Class 1b drugs have much less effect on conduction velocity in usual therapeutic doses and they shorten the refractory period. Agents in class 1c affect conduction profoundly without altering the refractory period.

β-Blockers (class 2) depress automaticity in the SA and AV nodes, and attenuate the effects of catecholamines on automaticity and conduction velocity in the sinus and AV nodes. Class 3 drugs prolong the action potential and so lengthen the refractory period. Verapamil (class 4) also prolongs the action potential, in addition to depressing automaticity (especially in the AV node) (see Tables 7.14 and 7.15).

Class 1 antiarrhythmics

Class 1a

These drugs are used for the treatment and prevention of ventricular and supraventricular arrhythmias. Their use in the prevention of atrial fibrillation has declined because of pro-arrhythmic effects and increased mortality in several large studies, in particular in patients with ischaemic heart disease or poor LV function. However, torsade de pointes (a form of polymorphic ventricular tachycardia) may be induced even in patients without structural heart disease.

Quinidine is an isomer of quinine formerly used in the treatment of atrial and supraventricular tachycardias. It has antimuscarinic and α-blocking properties, the latter causing vasodilatation and decreased myocardial contractility; severe hypotension may occur after i.v. administration. It may cause conduction defects or accelerate AV node conduction, accelerating ventricular rate and leading to ventricular arrhythmias. Visual and auditory disturbances with vertigo and gastrointestinal symptoms are signs of toxicity. Idiosyncratic reactions (rashes, thrombocytopenia and agranulocytosis) may also occur. Quinidine enhances digoxin toxicity by increasing plasma concentrations. It has an additive effect with other cardiodepressant drugs (e.g. disopyramide, β-blockers and calcium channel blockers) and potentiates the effects of non-depolarizing neuromuscular blockers.

Table 7.14 Drug treatments for specific arrhythmias

Atrial fibrillation	Paroxysmal atrial fibrillation	Atrial flutter	Paroxysmal SVT	WPW	Ventricular arrhythmias
Digoxin β-Blockers Verapamil Amiodarone Flecainide	Disopyramide Amiodarone Quinidine	Digoxin Amiodarone	Adenosine Verapamil β-Blockers	Disopyramide Amiodarone Flecainide β-Blockers	Lidocaine Amiodarone Mexiletine Disopyramide Magnesium

Table 7.15 Classification of anti-arrhythmics by site of action

SA node	Atria	AV node	Ventricles	Accessory pathways
Class 2 Class 4 Digoxin Adenosine	Class 1a and 1c Class 2 Class 3	Class 1c Class 2 Class 4 Digoxin (Adenosine)	Class 1 Class 3	Class 1a Class 3

Disopyramide is useful in supraventricular tachycardias and as a second-line agent to lidocaine in ventricular arrhythmias. It has less action on the His–Purkinje system than quinidine, but greater antimuscarinic and negative inotropic effects, especially if combined with β-blockers, quinidine, procainamide or verapamil. Its half-life (8 h) is prolonged in renal impairment and after myocardial infarction. Side-effects result mainly from the anticholinergic effect of the parent drug and a major metabolite, which can produce urinary retention and blurred vision.

Procainamide has similar effects to those of quinidine and may cause hypotension after i.v. administration. It may be used i.v. to terminate ventricular arrhythmias, or as an oral antiarrhythmic, although it has a short half-life (3 h), and requires frequent administration or the use of a sustained-release oral preparation. In common with quinidine, it is metabolized by the liver to active and inactive metabolites, but is restricted usually to short-term use because of the high risk of drug-induced systemic lupus erythematosus.

Ajmalin is a quinidine-like drug derived from the alkaloid rauwolfia which is available in European countries. It inhibits intraventricular conduction and prolongs AV conduction time, and is used for the treatment of WPW syndrome.

Class 1b

Class 1b drugs are useful for the prevention and treatment of premature ventricular contractions, ventricular tachycardia and ventricular fibrillation, particularly associated with ischaemia.

Lidocaine is the first choice drug for ventricular arrhythmias resistant to DC cardioversion. It decreases normal and abnormal automaticity and decreases action potential and refractory period duration. The threshold for ventricular fibrillation is raised, but it has minimal haemodynamic effects. The antiarrhythmic properties of lidocaine are enhanced by hypoxaemia, acidosis and hyperkalaemia, so that it is particularly effective in ischaemic cells, e.g. after acute myocardial infarction, during cardiac surgery, or in arrhythmias associated with digitalis toxicity. The usual loading dose is 50–100 mg, followed by a continuous infusion, titrated to response. Lidocaine redistributes rapidly after i.v. injection and it may be necessary to repeat the loading dose after 5–10 min. Close adjustment of the infusion rate is required to avoid CNS toxicity (confusion, dysarthria, tremor, numbness, dizziness and convulsions). Cardiotoxic effects (bradycardia, hypotension, asystole) occur at higher doses and are potentiated by hypoxaemia, acidosis and hypercapnia. It has a short half-life (less than 2 h), is 70% bound to plasma proteins and is metabolized in the liver. Clearance is decreased if hepatic blood flow is decreased (e.g. in the elderly, those with congestive cardiac failure, after myocardial infarction), and also by β- blockers, cimetidine and liver disease. In these circumstances, the dose should be reduced by 50%. It is less effective in the presence of hypokalaemia.

Mexiletine is a longer-acting, orally effective lidocaine analogue, which is well absorbed orally, with peak plasma concentrations after 2 h and an elimination half-life of 10–15 h. It undergoes hepatic metabolism and is excreted via the kidneys. Hypotension, bradycardia and heart block may occur after i.v. administration. Most frequent adverse effects involve the CNS and include tremors, nystagmus, confusion, speech disturbances, tinnitus, paraesthesiae and convulsions. Gastrointestinal effects are also common during oral treatment.

Tocainide is another lidocaine analogue that may be given orally or parenterally. It is used only in patients with poor LV function in whom other drugs have been unsuccessful or are contraindicated, because it frequently causes blood dyscrasias; other adverse effects resemble those of mexiletine. Arrhythmias unresponsive to lidocaine are unlikely to respond to tocainide.

Phenytoin has effects similar to those of lidocaine, but uniquely accelerates intraventricular conduction and may suppress re-entrant arrhythmias. It was formerly used for the treatment of digoxin-induced ventricular arrhythmias, but has been superseded.

Class 1c

Class 1c drugs are used for the prevention and treatment of supraventricular and ventricular tachyarrhythmias and junctional tachycardias with or without an accessory pathway. They are pro-arrhythmogenic, particularly in patients with myocardial ischaemia, poor LV function or after myocardial infarction, and although effective in chronic atrial fibrillation, they are reserved for life-threatening arrhythmias.

Flecainide is a procainamide derivative which has little effect on repolarization, the refractory period or action potential duration, but unlike other drugs in this class, it decreases automaticity and produces dose-dependent widening of the QRS complex. Its half-life is 14 h, but this may be prolonged up to 30 h in renal or congestive cardiac failure. In acute atrial fibrillation, intravenous flecainide usually restores sinus rhythm and is useful prophylaxis against further episodes of atrial fibrillation. However, it increases the risk of ventricular arrhythmias after myocardial infarction, especially in patients with structural cardiac disease. Long-term therapy may worsen cardiac failure and is associated with adverse gastrointestinal and CNS effects. It interacts with several drugs, e.g. plasma concentrations of both digoxin and propranolol are increased.

Propafenone has a complex pharmacology including weak antimuscarinic, β-adrenergic receptor and calcium channel blocking effects. It should be used with caution in patients with reactive airways disease. Interaction with digoxin may increase plasma digoxin concentrations.

Class 2 antiarrhythmic drugs

β-Blockers are used mainly for the treatment of sinus and supraventricular tachycardias, especially those provoked by endogenous or exogenous catecholamines, emotion or exercise. They decrease mortality after myocardial infarction and in chronic heart failure. Their antiarrhythmic effects are an intrinsic property of β-blockade, i.e. reduced automaticity in ectopic pacemakers, and prolonged AV node conduction and refractory period, although some β-blockers have class 1 activity in high doses ('membrane-stabilizing activity'). Their negative inotropic effects are a disadvantage in patients with acute left ventricular dysfunction.

Class 3 antiarrhythmic drugs

Class 3 antiarrhythmics prolong the action potential in conducting tissues and myocardial muscle. In particular, they prolong repolarization by K^+ channel blockade, decreasing outward K^+ conduction in the bundle of His, atrial and ventricular muscle, and accessory pathways. They are used for the treatment of supraventricular and ventricular tachyarrhythmias, including those associated with accessory conduction pathways. Some drugs have other actions (e.g. sotalol also produces β-blockade, and disopyramide has class 1 effects). All class 3 drugs in high doses or in the presence of electrolyte disturbance may prolong the QT interval and precipitate torsade de pointes.

Sotalol is a non-selective β-blocker with class 3 antiarrhythmic effects. Action potential duration and refractory period are lengthened, and it is effective in the treatment of supraventricular and ventricular tachyarrhythmias. In particular, atrial flutter and fibrillation may be converted to sinus rhythm. It also suppresses ventricular tachyarrhythmias and ventricular ectopic beats. In common with other β-blockers it has negative inotropic effects, but it does not usually precipitate cardiac failure. However, sotalol may cause torsades de pointes and other life-threatening arrhythmias, and it is recommended only for its anti-arrhythmic (rather than its β blocking) effects. It is water-soluble and is excreted via the kidneys. The usual intravenous dose is 20–120 mg administered over 10 min.

Amiodarone is primarily a class 3 drug; it acts by inhibition of inward K^+ current. It also blocks sodium and calcium channels, and has competitive inhibitory actions at α- and β-adrenoceptors, and may therefore be considered to have class 1, 2 and 4 antiarrhythmic activity. It prolongs action potential duration, repolarization and refractory periods in the atria and ventricles. In addition, AV node conduction is markedly slowed and refractory period increased. Ventricular conduction velocity is slowed. Amiodarone is very effective against a wide variety of supraventricular and ventricular arrhythmias, including WPW syndrome, and is preferred to other drugs in the presence of impaired left ventricular function. Intravenous amiodarone should be diluted and administered slowly (5 mg kg^{-1} over at least 5–10 min) to avoid bradycardia, hypotension (particularly if LV function is poor) and thrombophlebitis. It prolongs PR and QT intervals; AV block may also occur. It is contraindicated in the presence of bradycardia or AV block, and should not be combined with diltiazem, verapamil or drugs which prolong the QT interval (e.g. phenothiazines, sotalol or class 1a antiarrhythmics). Bradycardia unresponsive to atropine, and hypotension have been reported during general anaesthesia in patients receiving amiodarone therapy. Oral amiodarone is absorbed slowly, is highly protein-bound, widely distributed in the tissues, and one of the hepatic metabolites is active. Its half-life is extremely prolonged (up to 50 days) but shows significant interpatient variation; oral doses are reduced after initial loading. Long-term therapy produces reversible corneal microdeposits, cutaneous photosensitivity and pigmentation, pulmonary fibrosis and hepatotoxicity. Amiodarone is an iodinated compound, which binds within the thyroid gland, interfering with conversion of T_4 to T_3 and the action of T_3 itself. Continued treatment may cause clinical hyperthyroidism or, less commonly, hypothyroidism, and the interpretation of thyroid function tests may be confounded during amiodarone therapy. Amiodarone may decrease the clearance of digoxin and potentiate the effects of heparin and warfarin.

Bretylium is a quaternary ammonium compound which prevents norepinephrine uptake into sympathetic nerve endings. It prolongs action potential duration and refractory period with no effect on automaticity, and is used as second line to lidocaine for resistant life-threatening ventricular tachycardias or fibrillation. It may also facilitate electrical defibrillation to sinus rhythm and is useful for the treatment of ventricular arrhythmias associated with local anaesthetic toxicity. Catecholamine concentrations increase initially, causing increases in heart rate and arterial pressure, but after 20–30 min, heart rate, systemic vascular resistance and arterial pressure decrease. The initial dose is 5 mg kg^{-1} as a rapid i.v. bolus; the effect is apparent within 5–15 min. Bretylium is excreted unchanged in the urine. Bradycardia or asystole occasionally occurs and ventricular arrhythmias may be worsened, particularly those caused by cardiac glycosides.

Class 4 antiarrhythmic drugs

Class 4 drugs (calcium channel blockers) prevent voltage-dependent calcium influx during depolarization, particularly in the SA and AV nodes. Verapamil is more selective for cardiac cells than other calcium channel blockers, but it is also a coronary and peripheral vasodilator, and decreases myocardial contractility. It depresses AV conduction and is effective in cases of supraventricular or re-entrant tachycardia. Similarly, it controls the ventricular rate in atrial fibrillation. However, it is contraindicated in WPW syndrome, as conduction through the accessory pathway may be encouraged, leading to ventricular fibrillation. Intravenous administration may reduce arterial pressure (by vasodilatation), and caution is necessary in low-output states and in patients treated with negative inotropic drugs, e.g. β-blockers, disopyramide, quinidine or procainamide. Verapamil and diltiazem are both effective by the i.v. and oral routes.

Other antiarrhythmics

Adenosine is an endogenous purine nucleoside which mediates a variety of natural cellular functions via membrane-bound receptors. Several adenosine receptor subtypes (A_1–A_4) have been identified. Myocardial A_1 receptors activate potassium channels and decrease cAMP by activating inhibitory G_I-proteins; A_2 receptors mediate coronary vasodilatation by stimulating endothelial-derived relaxing factor and increasing intracellular cAMP. Increased potassium conductance induces membrane hyperpolarization in the SA and AV nodes, reducing automaticity, and blocking AV node conduction. Adenosine also has an anti-adrenergic effect in calcium-dependent ventricular tissue. It effectively converts paroxysmal supraventricular tachyarrhythmias (including those associated with WPW syndrome) to sinus rhythm, and is used in the diagnosis of broad complex tachycardias when the origin (ventricular or supraventricular) is uncertain. It is ineffective in the conversion of atrial flutter or fibrillation. In patients unable to exercise, adenosine is used as a coronary vasodilator in combination with myocardial perfusion scanning to diagnose coronary artery disease. The duration of action of adenosine is very short (half-life < 10 s), as it is metabolized to AMP or inosine by erythrocytes and vascular endothelial cells. Adenosine is given as a rapid i.v. bolus of 3 mg, which may be repeated in increasing doses after 1–2 min. Adverse effects are short-lived but include dyspnoea, flushing, bronchospasm, bradycardia and, occasionally, ventricular standstill or malignant tachyarrhythmias.

Magnesium sulphate. Intravenous magnesium sulphate (8 mmol over 10–15 min followed by a continuous i.v. infusion) is the treatment of choice for *torsade de pointes*, a type of ventricular tachycardia occasionally induced by class 1a or class 3 antiarrhythmic drugs which prolong the QT interval. It may be useful as a second-line treatment for supraventricular and ventricular arrhythmias, particularly those associated with digoxin toxicity or hypokalaemia, or as an anticonvulsant in patients with pre-eclampsia. Its role in the prevention of arrhythmias after myocardial infarction has not been confirmed.

Cardiac glycosides

Digoxin and digitoxin are cardiac glycosides whose structure consists of a cyclopentanophenanthrene nucleus, an aglycone ring (responsible for the pharmacological activity) and a carbohydrate chain made up of sugar molecules (which solubulize the drug). They are all derived from plant sources, principally ***digitalis purpura*** and ***digitalis lanata***. Digitalis compounds have been used for over 200 years for the treatment of cardiac failure but have now been largely superseded and are principally indicated for the control of ventricular rate in supraventricular arrhythmias, particularly atrial fibrillation. Cardiac glycosides have several actions, including direct effects on the myocardium and both direct and indirect actions on the ANS. They increase myocardial contractility and decrease conduction in the AV node and bundle of His. Action potential and refractory period duration in atrial cells are reduced, and the rate of phase 4 depolarization in the SA node is decreased. The refractory periods of the AV node and bundle of His are increased, but in the ventricles, refractory period is decreased and spontaneous depolarization rate increases. This latter effect (increased ventricular excitability) is more marked in the presence of hypokalaemia and may lead to the appearance of ectopic pacemaker foci. The principal direct cardiac action is inhibition of membrane Na^+/K^+-ATPase activity. Intracellular Na^+ concentration and Na^+/Ca^{2+} exchange increase, leading to increased availability of intracellular Ca^{2+} and increased myocardial contractility. Increased local catecholamine concentrations as a result of decreased neuronal reuptake and increased central sympathetic drive may also contribute to this positive inotropic action.

The actions of cardiac glycosides at the SA node (decreased automaticity), atria (reduced refractory period) and AV node (decreased conduction and increased refractory period) are mediated directly, but direct and indirect effects on the vagus are also involved. Central vagal tone, cardiac sensitivity to vagal stimulation and local myocardial concentrations of acetylcholine are all increased by digitalis. Thus these effects may be antagonized to some extent by atropine.

Cardiac glycosides are well absorbed orally along the principles of first-order kinetics, and are distributed throughout the body. They have a large apparent volume of distribution and long half-lives, and so a loading ('digitalizing') dose based approximately on lean body weight is usually required. Most are eliminated unchanged via the kidney by filtration and tubular secretion, and doses should be reduced in renal impairment or elderly patients. Their therapeutic index is low. Plasma concentrations are a poor guide to toxicity, as the drugs are concentrated in cardiac and other tissues. However, toxicity is more likely at plasma concentrations greater than 2.5 ng ml^{-1}. Even at therapeutic plasma concentrations, digitalis affects the ECG causing repolarization abnormalities, which may be wrongly interpreted as ischaemia. The classic 'digoxin effect' on ECG is of 'reverse tick' (downsloping) ST-segment depression with inversion of T waves. These changes are usually widespread, are not confined to the territory of one coronary artery, and do not indicate digitalis toxicity.

Digitalis toxicity usually causes cardiac, CNS, visual and gastrointestinal disturbances, including almost any arrhythmia, although ventricular arrhythmias (particularly extrasystoles, bigeminy and trigeminy) and various degrees of heart block are commonest. Supraventricular arrhythmias also occur, often with some degree of conduction block. Cardiac glycosides should be avoided in the presence of second-degree heart block, ventricular tachycardia or aberrant conduction pathways (e.g. WPW syndrome), as arrhythmias may be precipitated, and used with caution after myocardial infarction. Sensitivity to glycosides is increased by hypokalaemia, hypomagnesaemia, hypercalcaemia, renal impairment, chronic pulmonary or heart disease, myxoedema and hypoxaemia. There is decreased sensitivity in thyrotoxicosis. Quinidine, amiodarone, verapamil, nicardipine and erythromycin tend to increase plasma digoxin concentrations. β-Blockers and verapamil have combined effects on the AV node. Digoxin should be administered cautiously in situations where AV conduction is already suppressed.

Other symptoms of digoxin toxicity are rather unpredictable and in chronic toxicity include fatigue, weakness of arms or legs, agitation, nightmares, various visual disturbances, anorexia and nausea or abdominal pain. Treatment of serious arrhythmias involves careful administration of potassium chloride under ECG control (especially in the presence of heart block or renal impairment). Lidocaine and phenytoin are useful for ventricular arrhythmias, β-blockade for supraventricular arrhythmias, and bradyarrhythmias may be treated with atropine. Digoxin should be stopped for at least 48 h before elective DC cardioversion, as ventricular fibrillation may be precipitated. If cardioversion is required, the initial dose should be low (e.g. 10–25 J) and increased if necessary.

Digoxin is the commonest cardiac glycoside. It has a half-life of approximately 36 h (which is sensitive to changes in renal function), and in the absence of a loading dose, effective plasma concentrations occur after approximately 5–7 days. Although the effect of an i.v. injection begins within 30–60 min, distribution into cardiac tissue takes place slowly over the first 6 h after oral or i.v. administration. The maximum response occurs 4–6 h after i.v. administration and digoxin measurements in blood samples taken before this 6-h period cannot be interpreted correctly. Intramuscular injections are painful and absorption is unreliable. Rapid digitalization may be achieved with a dose of 250–500 μg i.v. over 10–20 min, followed by further doses after 4–8 h to a maximum of 1 mg. The usual oral starting dose is 125–250 μg day^{-1} for 1 week, reducing to a maintenance dose according to heart rate, plasma concentrations and renal function

Digitoxin is metabolized by the liver, and is less dependent upon renal function for its elimination. It has a very long half-life (4–6 days) so that maintenance doses may be required only on alternate days, but this is also a disadvantage as toxic effects are very persistent.

Ouabain is a cardiac glycoside derived from *strophanthus*, which has a more rapid onset than digoxin when given intravenously

DRUGS USED FOR THE TREATMENT OF HYPERTENSION

A wide variety of drugs are used to treat hypertension, including α- and β-blockers, diuretics, calcium channel blockers, ACE inhibitors, AT_1-receptor antagonists, and vasodilators (Table 7.16). Non-pharmacological strategies include weight reduction, a decrease in alcohol intake and the institution of a low-sodium (with or without high potassium) diet with regular exercise. If these measures fail, drug therapy is indicated. Recent guidelines from the UK and the USA have emphasized the need for antihypertensive treatment in patients with a sustained systolic pressure ≥ 160 mmHg or sustained diastolic pressure ≥ 100 mmHg. Drug treatment may also be indicated in cases where sustained systolic and diastolic pressures are ≥ 140 and ≥ 90 mmHg, respectively, in the presence of diabetes, end-organ damage or cardiovascular disease.

Individual antihypertensive drugs have similar efficacy when used in isolation, but therapy with a single drug may only be adequate in 50–60% of patients. Combining lower doses of two drugs produces additive or synergistic effects (e.g. ACE inhibitors or β-blockers with diuretics or calcium channel antagonists) on arterial pressure, with fewer adverse effects than monotherapy. Alternatively, the adverse effects of one drug may be neutralized by administration of a drug with opposing physiological effects (e.g. sympathetic activation caused by direct-acting vasodilators is attenuated by β-blockade). The choice of antihypertensive drug also depends on coexisting disease (e.g.

Table 7.16 'Compelling' and 'possible' indications and contraindications for the major classes of antihypertensive drugs (Adapted with permission from Ramsay LE *et al* 1999.)

	Indication		Contraindications	
Class of drug	**Compelling**	**Possible**	**Possible**	**Compelling**
α-Blockers	Prostatism	Dyslipidaemia	Postural hypotension	Urinary incontinence
ACE inhibitors	Heart failure Left ventricular dysfunction Type I diabetic neuropathy	Chronic renal disease[a] Type II diabetic nephropathy	Renal impairment[a] Peripheral vascular disease[b]	Pregnancy Renovascular disease
AT_1-receptor antagonists	Cough induced by ACE inhibitor[c]	Heart failure Intolerance of other antihypertensive drugs	Peripheral vascular disease[b]	Pregnancy Renovascular disease
β-Blockers	Myocardial infarction Angina	Heart failure[d]	Heart failure[d] Dyslipidaemia Peripheral vascular disease	Asthma or chronic obstructive pulmonary disease Heart block
Dihydropyridine Calcium channel blockers	Isolated systolic hypertension in elderly patients	Angina Elderly patients	—	—
Rate-limiting calcium channel blockers	Angina	Myocardial infarction	Combination with β-blockade	Heart block Heart failure
Thiazide diuretics	Elderly patients	–	Dyslipidaemia	Gout

[a]Angiotensin-converting enzyme (ACE) inhibitors may be beneficial in chronic renal failure but should be used with caution. Close supervision and specialist advice are needed when there is established and significant renal impairment.
[b]Caution with ACE inhibitors and angiotensin II receptor antagonists in peripheral vascular disease because of association with renovascular disease.
[c]If ACE inhibitor indicated
[d]β-Blockers may worsen heart failure, but in specialist hands may also be used to treat heart failure (see text).

ACE inhibitors may be preferred in patients with cardiac failure, or diabetes mellitus with proteinuria, but avoided in those with renal artery stenosis). Conversely, the action of diuretics and ACE inhibitors may be attenuated by NSAIDs. The newer agents are often longer-acting, with a more favourable therapeutic profile, but patients may still be receiving long-term therapy with older drugs.

In the absence of other considerations (e.g advanced age, coexisting medical disease, adverse effects or the effects of other medication), the first choice drugs are usually diuretics, as they are the longest proven and cheapest available class of drugs. They are used in lower doses than previously with a consequent reduction in adverse effects, and if not used as initial therapy they are usually considered as second-line drugs, as they augment the effects of β-blockers and ACE inhibitors. β-Blockers are an alternative initial choice. They are well established and have been shown to decrease mortality in hypertensive patients, but are contraindicated in those with asthma, bradycardia or grade II AV block. β-Blockers or long-acting calcium channel blockers are advantageous in patients with hypertension and angina, and β-blockers or ACE inhibitors are preferable after myocardial infarction. ACE inhibitors are particularly indicated in those with LV dysfunction, or diabetes mellitus with proteinuria. AT_1-receptor antagonists are useful for those intolerant of ACE inhibitors, e.g. because of cough or angio-oedema. Their mechanism of action is probably similar to that of ACE inhibitors, although the incidence of adverse effects may be lower.

Fluctuations in heart rate and arterial pressure during anaesthesia and surgery are exaggerated in hypertensive patients. Antihypertensive medication attenuates these responses and should be continued throughout the perioperative period, although ACE inhibitors may be associated with perioperative hypotension. In addition, β-blockers may afford some protection against myocardial ischaemia.

Drugs which attenuate sympathetic nervous system activity may cause exaggerated decreases in systemic arterial pressure in response to decreased venous return, e.g. caused by haemorrhage, positive pressure ventilation or adoption of a head-up position. Long-term sympathetic blockade may cause upregulation of α-adrenergic receptors and an exaggerated response to exogenous catecholamines and direct-acting sympathomimetics. Conversely, drugs which cause depletion of norepinephrine from nerve endings or which act on vascular smooth muscle may decrease the sensitivity to indirect-acting sympathomimetic drugs (e.g. ephedrine).

DRUGS USED FOR THE TREATMENT OF CONGESTIVE CARDIAC FAILURE

Congestive cardiac failure may be caused by impaired systolic function (when ejection fraction is low), impaired diastolic function (occurring mainly in the elderly; ejection fraction is normal, and there may be hypertension), or by a mixture of the two. The decrease in cardiac output causes sympathetic nervous stimulation and increased plasma and cardiac norepinephrine concentrations, increasing cardiac output, systemic vascular resistance and afterload.

Table 7.17 Drugs used for the treatment of cardiac failure

Diuretics
ACE inhibitors
Third-generation β-blockers
AT_1 antagonists
Spironolactone
Digoxin, amiodarone (if arrhythmias present)
Nitrates, inotropes (acute setting)

Plasma renin concentrations increase, particularly when diuretics are used. However, myocardial oxygen consumption is increased, and the increased peripheral resistance mediated by prolonged activation of the sympathetic nervous and renin–angiotensin systems leads to progression of the disease and a propensity to arrhythmias. Downregulation of myocardial β_1-adrenergic receptors occurs, and they become less responsive to circulating catecholamines.

Diuretics and ACE inhibitors are first line therapy in patients with LV failure associated with either systolic or diastolic dysfunction (see Table 7.17). When used in combination, they decrease morbidity, disease progression and mortality, particularly after acute myocardial infarction. AT_1 antagonists are an alternative when ACE inhibitors are not tolerated. The addition of spironolactone to a diuretic/ACE inhibitor combination can decrease mortality in refractory cardiac failure. In the presence of arrhythmias and systolic cardiac failure, digoxin, β-blockers or amiodarone may be used.

Recently, some second- and third-generation β-blockers, (e.g. bisoprolol, metoprolol and carvedilol) have been shown to be effective in the treatment of cardiac failure. All are non-selective ($\beta_1 >> \beta_2$) antagonists; carvedilol is also an α_1-antagonist. Their beneficial action may be from slowing of heart rate, reducing arrhythmias, or upregulation of β-receptor density or function, which leads to increases in myocardial contractility and ejection fraction. Angiotensin II concentrations also decrease (because of β_1 inhibition). When used in patients with cardiac failure, they must be introduced cautiously as symptoms may initially worsen, and ventricular function improves only after 1 month of therapy.

Amlodipine may be useful in non-ischaemic cardiomyopathy, but other calcium channel blockers are relatively contraindicated. Parenteral inotropes are useful in the acute setting (see above), but oral inotropes such as phosphodiesterase inhibitors (e.g. amrinone, milrinone) or dopamine agonists (fenodopam) have shown no benefit and some may be associated with increased mortality (e.g. milrinone).

FURTHER READING

ABPI Compendium 1999–2000 Datapharm Publications, London

Brown N, Vaughan D E 1998 Angiotensin converting enzyme inhibitors. Circulation 97(14): 1411–1120

Calvey T N, Williams N E 1997 Principles and practice of pharmacology for anaesthetists, 3rd edn. Blackwell Science, Oxford

Colson P, Ryckwaert F, Coriat P 1999 Renin angiotensin system antagonists and anesthesia. Anesthesia and Analgesia 89: 1143–1155

Coodley E 1999 Newer drug therapies for congestive cardiac failure. Archives of Internal Medicine 159: 1177–1183

Coriat P (ed) 1997 Clinical cardiovascular medicine in anaesthesia. BMJ Publishing Group, London

Lambert D G, Appadu B L 1995 Muscarinic receptor subtypes: do they have a place in clinical anaesthesia? British Journal of Anaesthesia 74: 497–499

Luscher T F, Cosentino F 1998 The classification of calcium antagonists and their selection in the treatment of hypertension. Drugs 55(4): 509–517

Maze M, Tranquilli W 1991 Alpha-2 adrenoceptor antagonists: defining the role in clinical anesthesia. Anesthesiology 74: 581–605

Ramsay L E et al 1999 British Hypertension Society guidelines for hypertension management 1999. British Medical Journal 319: 630–635

Skarvan K (ed) 1994 Vasoactive drugs. Baillière clinical anaesthesiology vol 8, no. 1. Baillière Tindall, London

Stoelting R K 1998 Pharmacology and physiology in anesthetic practice, 3rd edn. Lippincott Williams & Wilkins, Philadelphia

Van Gelder I C, Brugemann J, Crijns H J G M 1998 Current treatment recommendations in antiarrhythmic therapy. Drugs 55: 331–346

Velasquez M T 1996 Angiotensin II receptor blockers: a new class of antihypertensive drugs. Archives of Family Medicine 5: 351–356

8 Anatomy of the respiratory tract

The respiratory tract begins at the anterior nares (nostrils) and the lips and ends in the alveoli of the lungs. It is divided into an upper and lower airway at the level of the vocal cords. A detailed knowledge of the anatomy of the respiratory tract is of vital importance to an anaesthetist. It is an essential prerequisite for understanding respiratory physiology and the pharmacokinetics of volatile and gaseous anaesthetic agents. Instrumentation of the airway is part of anaesthetic daily routine, requiring great familiarity with the structures involved. Many clinical problems that confront the anaesthetist arise from compromised airway patency.

THE UPPER AIRWAY

THE NOSE AND NASAL CAVITY

The nasal airway extends from the anterior nares (nostrils) to the posterior nares (or choanae) before the nasopharynx. The nose itself contains the two nasal vestibules, each approximately 2 cm long and 1 cm wide, and leads to a nasal cavity. The skeleton of the nose is mainly cartilaginous, although the nasal bones contribute to the 'bridge' superiorly. It is lined by skin rich in sebaceous and sweat glands and bearing coarse hairs.

The nasal cavity is a narrow passage that extends back almost horizontally from the vestibule and is lined mainly by a ciliated columnar epithelium. Its arched ceiling extends superiorly to the olfactory area with olfactory epithelium overlying the cribriform plate. This ceiling is supported by the nasal, frontal, ethmoid (containing the cribriform plate) and sphenoid bones. The medial wall (nasal septum) separating the two nasal cavities is formed mainly by the plate of the ethmoid bone and by the vomer. The floor of the nose is formed by the palatine process of the maxilla and the palatine bone, which make up the hard palate, and by the soft palate posteriorly. The lateral wall of the nasal cavity (Fig. 8.1) is supported by the maxillary and ethmoid bones.
Its surface area is increased by three horizontally running bony folds: the superior, middle and inferior conchae (turbinates). The inferior concha runs 1 cm above the floor of the nasal cavity and is the largest; the nasolacrimal duct empties into its meatus beneath. The middle meatus receives the openings of the frontal, anterior

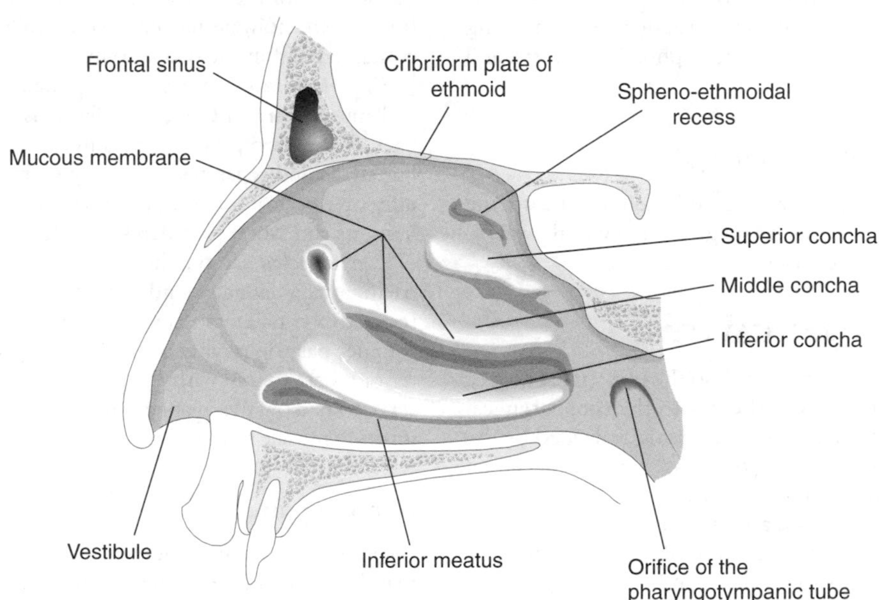

Fig. 8.1
Sagittal section of the nose and nasal cavity.

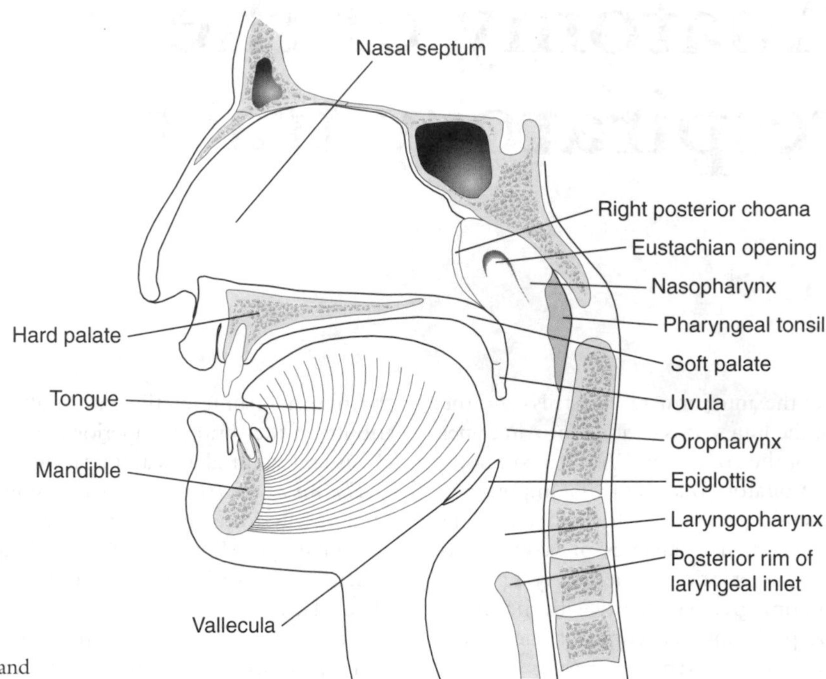

Fig. 8.2
Sagittal section of the mouth and pharynx.

ethmoidal, middle ethmoidal and maxillary sinuses. The posterior ethmoidal sinus opens into the superior meatus, while the sphenoid sinus joins the spheno-ethmoid recess situated above the superior concha.

These paranasal sinuses develop as diverticulae from the wall of the nasal cavity. They are also lined by mucus-secreting respiratory epithelium.

Nerve supply

The olfactory mucosa is supplied by the olfactory (Ist cranial) nerve. The trigeminal (Vth cranial) nerve supplies the remaining majority of the nasal cavity through its ophthalmic (first) and maxillary (second) divisions.

Blood supply and lymphatic drainage

The ophthalmic, maxillary and facial arteries contribute to the blood supply to the nose. Venous drainage is largely to the pterygoid venous plexus and to the facial vein.

THE MOUTH AND ORAL CAVITY

The mouth, while part of the airway, is also the uppermost part of the digestive tract. It extends from the lips to the oropharyngeal isthmus at the level of the palatoglossal folds and is divided by the teeth into an outer vestibule and the oral cavity proper. A sagittal section of the mouth is shown in Figure 8.2.

The oral cavity is lined by squamous epithelium containing mucus-secreting glands. It is bounded anterolaterally by the teeth and gums and superiorly by the hard and soft palates. The palatoglossal fold (anterior pillar of the tonsil) runs between the soft palate and the tongue and marks the oropharyngeal isthmus. It joins the tongue at the junction of its anterior two-thirds and posterior third.

The tongue sits on the floor of the mouth and resembles an inverted shoe in shape with its toe directed anteriorly. This muscular organ almost fills the closed mouth. It contains intrinsic muscle and several extrinsic muscles connecting it to associated structures: genioglossus, to the mandible; hyoglossus, to the hyoid bone; styloglossus, to the styloid process of the skull base; and palatoglossus, to the soft palate. The undersurface of the tongue is attached by a fold of mucous membrane, the frenulum, to the floor of the mouth in the midline anteriorly. The posterior third of the tongue has embryologically different origins and is contained within the oropharynx.

The soft palate consists of an aponeurotic sheet into which several muscles are inserted laterally. It is attached anteriorly to the back of the hard palate, and its free posterior edge bears the midline uvula and separates nasopharynx from oropharynx. While the inferior aspect of the soft palate is covered with a squamous epithelium, its superior aspect bears a ciliated columnar epithelium.

Five muscles act on the soft palate: tensor palati and levator palati attach laterally and act to tense and elevate the palate, respectively; palatoglossus passes in the palatoglossal fold to the tongue; palatopharyngeus lies in the palatopharyngeal fold (posterior pillar) to join with the pharyngeal constrictor muscle – both serve to narrow the oropharyngeal opening; musculus uvulae is an intrinsic muscle that acts to draw up the uvula.

Nerve supply

Common sensation is supplied by branches of the maxillary and mandibular divisions of the trigeminal nerve. The lingual nerve, a branch of the mandibular division, conducts afferent fibres from taste buds in the anterior two-thirds of the tongue and floor of the mouth. These fibres then pass along the chorda tympani to join the facial (VIIth cranial) nerve.

Parasympathetic secretomotor fibres to the submandibular and sublingual salivary glands pass in the opposite direction along the chorda tympani to join the lingual nerve [the secretomotor input to the parotid gland originates from the glossopharyngeal (IXth cranial) nerve].

All the muscles of the tongue are supplied by the hypoglossal (XIIth cranial) nerve with the exception of palatoglossus, which is supplied through the pharyngeal plexus by the vagus (Xth cranial) nerve. The pharyngeal plexus also supplies the other muscles of the soft palate with the exception of tensor palati. This striated muscle is supplied by a branch of the mandibular division of the trigeminal nerve.

Blood supply and lymphatic drainage

Arterial supply arises from the lingual, facial and maxillary branches of the external carotid artery and blood drains to corresponding veins. The soft palate drains to the pharyngeal venous plexus. Lymphatic drainage passes eventually to the deep cervical lymph chain. The anterior tongue and floor of mouth drain initially to submental and submandibular nodes.

THE PHARYNX

The pharynx is a fibromuscular tube at the 'crossroads' between mouth, nose, larynx and oesophagus. It extends from the skull base to the level of the sixth cervical vertebra, where it is in continuity with the oesophagus. The pharynx lies immediately anterior to the cervical spine and prevertebral fascia. A sagittal section through the pharynx is shown in Figure 8.2. Figure 8.3 shows a coronal section.

The pharynx is divided into three parts: the nasopharynx, the oropharynx and the laryngopharynx.

The nasopharynx sits behind the posterior nares (choanae) and is in continuity with the oropharynx at the level of the soft palate. In common with the nasal cavity, it is lined by a ciliated columnar epithelium. A Eustachian tube opens onto each lateral wall, and the posterior wall bears the pharyngeal tonsils (adenoids).

The oropharynx is in continuity below, with the laryngopharynx at the level of the tip of the epiglottis. Anteriorly it meets the oral cavity at the oropharyngeal isthmus formed by the palatoglossal folds. It is lined by a stratified squamous mucosa. The lateral wall contains the palatine tonsil in its fossa between the palatoglossal and palatopharyngeal folds. Beneath the oropharyngeal isthmus, the posterior third of the tongue sits anterior to the epiglottis. It is connected to the front of the epiglottis by a medial and two lateral glosso-epiglottic folds; the two pockets thus formed between the medial and each lateral fold are termed the valecullae. It is here at laryngoscopy (in adults) that the tip of the laryngoscope is placed before lifting the epiglottis.

The laryngopharynx is lined by stratified squamous epithelium. Anteriorly, in the midline, are the laryngeal opening and mucosa covering arytenoid and cricoid cartilages. The laryngopharynx extends anterolaterally around the larynx towards the laminae of the thyroid cartilage. The two longitudinal channels thus created are termed the pyriform fossae and are a common site for impaction of foreign bodies. Each fossa is bounded anterolaterally by mucosa overlying thyroid cartilage, and medially by the aryepiglottic folds and cricoid cartilage.

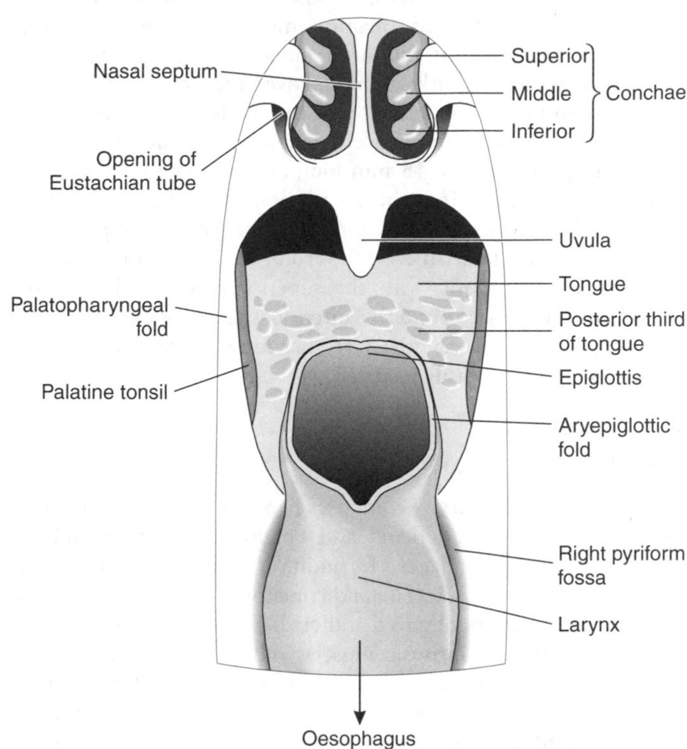

Fig. 8.3
Coronal section of the pharynx showing the view of the posterior choanae, the oropharyngeal isthmus, the larynx and laryngeal inlet from behind.

Beneath the mucosa of the pharynx is a fibromuscular sheath, the fibrous layer being relatively dense superiorly where muscle is absent. These muscles are intimately involved in the act of swallowing. The *superior*, *middle* and *inferior constrictor muscles* encircle the pharynx and overlie each other like a stack of paper cups. *Stylopharyngeus*, *salpingopharyngeus* and *palatopharyngeus* insert into the fibromuscular tube thus formed.

Nerve supply

The pharyngeal plexus supplies sensory, motor and autonomic nerves. Sensory fibres pass principally in the glossopharyngeal nerve which also carries taste sensation from the posterior third of the tongue. Motor supply arises mainly from the vagus nerve.

Blood supply and lymphatic drainage

Arterial supply comes from the ascending pharyngeal, superior thyroid, lingual, facial and maxillary arteries, all branches of the external carotid artery. Venous drainage is largely to the pharyngeal venous plexus and thus to the internal jugular vein. Lymphatic flow passes to retropharyngeal lymph nodes and to the deep cervical lymph node chain.

THE LARYNX

The larynx separates the pharynx and trachea. It sits at the junction of the specialized airway and common airway and digestive tract and has evolved beyond a pure sphincter function. It has a skeleton made of cartilages, ligaments and membranes. The larynx is lined by stratified squamous mucous membrane that is in continuity with that of the laryngopharynx. This membrane is thinner and more tightly adherent over the vocal cords where there are no mucous glands. Below the cords, the mucous membrane has a ciliated columnar epithelium. In the adult male, the larynx is approximately 45 mm long and has an anteroposterior diameter of 35 mm. It is smaller in the adult female; 35 mm by 25 mm. The larynx lies anterior to the proximal oesophagus in front of the third to sixth cervical vertebrae. Each carotid sheath is situated laterally along with the superior poles of the thyroid gland. Anteriorly are found the anterior strap muscles of the neck, the deep cervical fascia, the platysma muscle and skin through which the larynx is easily palpated.

Cartilages

The skeleton of the larynx comprises five major cartilaginous components: the thyroid, cricoid and epiglottic cartilages and the paired arytenoid cartilages. In addition, there are two smaller paired bodies: the corniculate and cuneiform cartilages. The cartilages articulate at cricothyroid and cricoarytenoid joints which are acted upon by the intrinsic muscles of the larynx (see below). These cartilages and their relative positions are depicted in Figure 8.4 together with their associated ligaments as viewed externally.

The thyroid cartilage is the largest and forms the main body of the larynx. It is composed of two laminae which are joined anteriorly at the thyroid prominence, visible in the anterior neck (the 'Adam's apple'). Posteriorly, each lamina extends superiorly and inferiorly to form the superior and inferior horns or cornua. Each inferior horn articulates with the posterolateral aspects of the cricoid cartilage.

The cricoid cartilage is found at the lower end of the larynx above the trachea. It is the only laryngeal structure that forms a complete circle. The shape of a signet ring with a posterior lamina and a narrow anterolateral arch, each posterolateral surface has an articular facet forming a joint with the inferior horn of the thyroid cartilage. The posterior lamina articulates superiorly with each arytenoid cartilage.

The epiglottic cartilage is leaf-shaped; it attaches inferiorly to the posterior aspect of the thyroid cartilage and anteriorly to the posterior aspect of the hyoid bone by the hyoepiglottic ligament. It projects superiorly behind the hyoid bone and the base of the tongue, and gives anterior support to the aryepiglottic folds that encircle the laryngeal inlet.

The arytenoid cartilages are the shape of a three-sided pyramid, the bases articulating with the posterior lamina of the cricoid inferiorly. Each has a medial, anterolateral and posterior surface. The projection anteriorly forms the vocal process and is the posterior attachment of the vocal cords. The lateral muscular process gives attachment to the posterior and lateral cricoarytenoid muscles.

The corniculate cartilage is little more than a small nodule at the apex of each arytenoid cartilage.

The cuneiform cartilage is a tiny strip of cartilage found within the margin of each aryepiglottic fold.

Ligaments and membranes

Extrinsic ligaments connect the larynx to other structures. The *thyrohyoid* and *hyoepiglottic ligaments* connect with the hyoid bone above, and the *cricotracheal ligament* joins with the trachea below. Two paired intrinsic membranes connect the cartilaginous components within the larynx (Fig. 8.5).

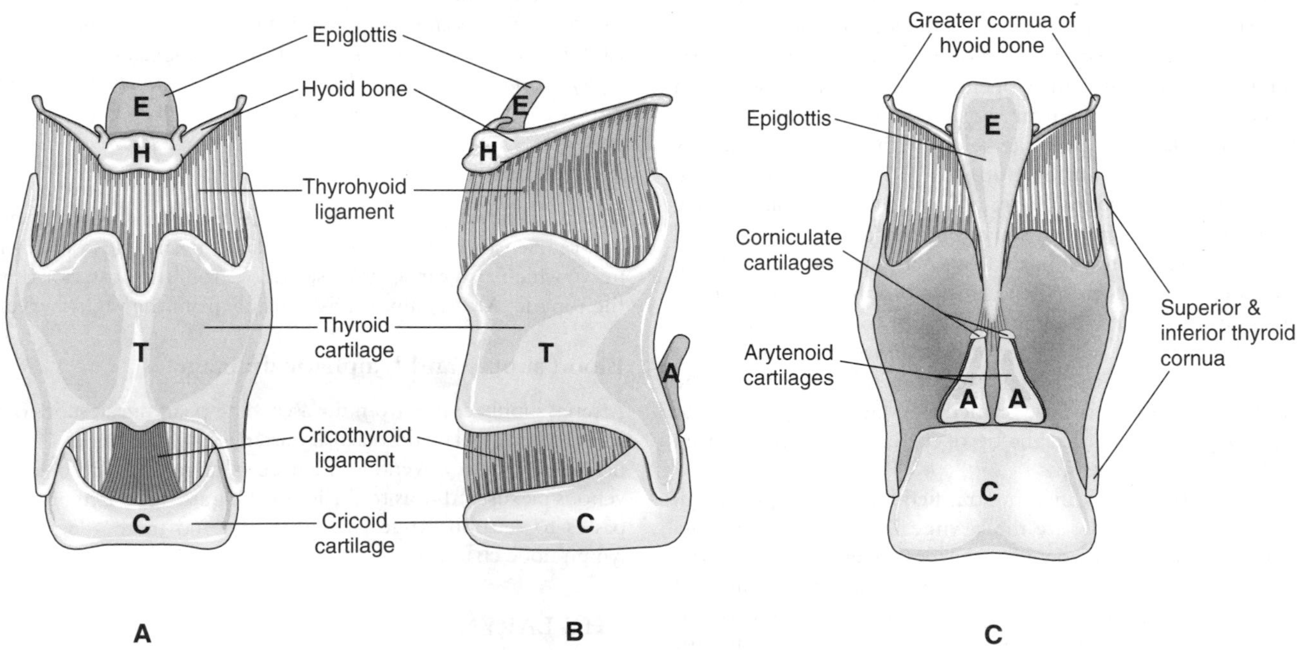

Fig. 8.4
The cartilages and ligaments of the larynx seen from its external surface; the hyoid bone is also shown. **A**. View from the front. **B**. View from the left. **C**. View from the back.

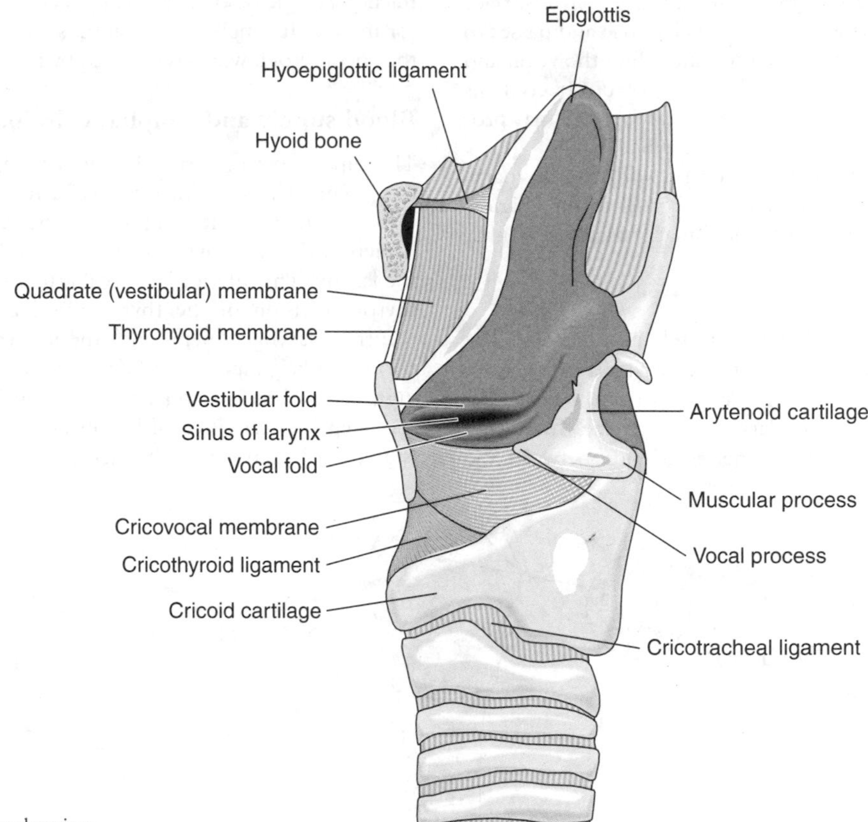

Fig. 8.5
Sagittal section of the larynx showing cartilages and ligaments.

The vestibular (quadrate) membrane joins the thyroid, epiglottic and arytenoid cartilages. At the laryngeal opening, its free upper border is contained within the aryepiglottic fold and incorporates the corniculate and cuneiform cartilages. The lower border runs between the thyroid and arytenoid cartilages and forms the framework for the vestibular fold (false vocal cord). The fissure between right and left vestibular folds is termed the rima vestibuli.

The cricothyroid (cricovocal) membrane joins the cricoid and arytenoid cartilages to the thyroid cartilage. Superiorly, it connects the thyroid prominence to the vocal process of the arytenoid cartilage, the free edge forming the 'skeleton' of the vocal cord (true vocal cord). The fissure between the cords forms the rima glottidis (the space between the rima vestibuli and the rima glottidis is termed the laryngeal sinus). Inferiorly, the cricothyroid membrane connects cricoid and thyroid cartilages and is readily palpated. This is an important site of access for securing an emergency surgical airway (cricothyroidotomy) when oro/nasotracheal intubation is not possible.

Muscles

Extrinsic muscles connect the larynx to neighbouring structures and include the *thyrohyoid* and *sternothyroid muscles* (which elevate and depress the larynx, respectively, and are supplied by the hypoglossal nerve) and the *inferior constrictor muscle* of the pharynx (no action on the larynx, see above). Other muscles act on the larynx through their attachments to associated structures. These include the indirect elevators – the mylohyoid, stylohyoid and geniohyoid muscles – and the indirect depressors – the sternohyoid and omohyoid muscles.

The intrinsic muscles of the larynx subserve a sphincter function and/or act on the vocal cords to facilitate cough and phonation.

The cricothyroid muscle is the only intrinsic muscle to lie outside the cartilaginous laryngeal skeleton. It originates from the anterior aspect of the cricoid arch and is inserted into the lower border of the thyroid lamina and its inferior cornua. It acts to increase vocal cord tension by tipping the lamina of the cricoid, and therefore the arytenoids, posteriorly.

The posterior cricoarytenoid muscle originates from the posterior aspect of the lamina of the cricoid and inserts into the muscular process of the arytenoid. It acts to externally rotate the arytenoid upon the cricoid and is the sole abductor of the vocal cords.

The lateral cricoarytenoid muscle arises from the superior aspect of the cricoid ring anterolaterally and passes to the lateral surface of the arytenoid. It acts to adduct the cords through internal rotation of the arytenoid cartilage.

The interarytenoid muscle is the other adductor of the vocal cords. The only unpaired muscle, it passes between the two arytenoid cartilages. Fibres from this muscle continue to become the aryepiglottic muscle.

The aryepiglottic muscle is contained within the aryepiglottic fold and has some sphincter function at the laryngeal inlet.

The thyroarytenoid muscle originates from the posterior surface of the thyroid cartilage at the junction of its laminae and passes to the anterolateral surface of the arytenoid, including the vocal and muscular processes. It acts to relax the vocal cords. It contains within it some fibres that insert within the vocal fold and may provide fine adjustment to cord tension (*vocalis muscle*).

The thyroepiglottic muscle shares its origin with the thyroarytenoid muscle and is attached to the lateral border of the epiglottis where it contributes to sphincter function at the laryngeal inlet.

Nerve supply

The vagus nerve supplies the larynx through its branches. The mucous membrane is supplied by the internal laryngeal nerve above the vocal cords and by the recurrent laryngeal nerve below. The internal laryngeal nerve enters the larynx through the thyrohyoid membrane. The recurrent laryngeal nerve ascends between the trachea and the oesophagus and passes deep to the inferior constrictor muscle. It supplies all the intrinsic muscles of the larynx except the cricothyroid, which is supplied by the external laryngeal nerve.

Blood supply and lymphatic drainage

The superior and inferior thyroid arteries contribute branches to the larynx. The superior laryngeal artery is a branch of the superior thyroid artery; it accompanies the internal laryngeal nerve as it pierces the thyrohyoid membrane and supplies the interior of the larynx. The inferior laryngeal artery is a branch of the inferior thyroid division of the thyrocervical trunk. It passes with the recurrent laryngeal nerve into the larynx. Venous drainage is via corresponding superior and inferior thyroid veins into the internal jugular and brachiocephalic veins. The lymphatic drainage is to the deep cervical chain of lymph nodes. The vocal cords form a 'watershed' from where channels pass up or down.

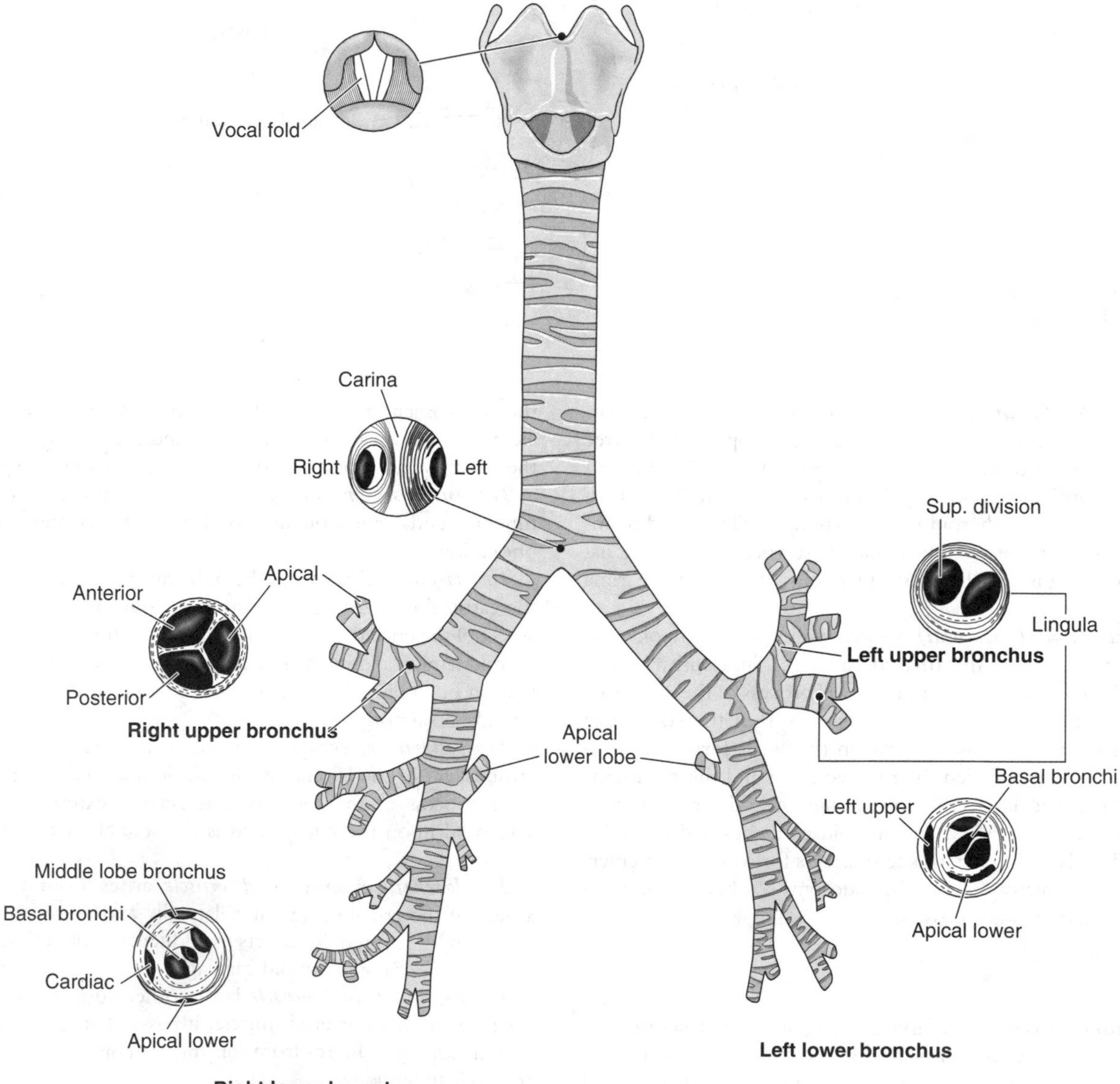

Fig. 8.6
The proximal bronchial tree and its appearance at bronchoscopy.

THE LOWER AIRWAY

The lower airway consists of the trachea, bronchi and bronchial tree, ending in the alveolar air spaces. In all but the smaller terminal branches, it is lined by mucous membrane with a ciliated columnar epithelium. Goblet cells produce mucus that traps debris, which is then swept proximally by the action of cilia to the laryngopharynx from where it is swallowed subconsciously.

THE TRACHEA AND BRONCHI

The trachea is a midline structure approximately 10–12 cm long, although this may increase by 3–5 cm in deep inspiration. The adult trachea has an internal diameter of about 2.5 cm. It is suspended from the cricoid ring above by the cricotracheal ligament, which fuses with the fibrous membrane investing the trachea (at the level of the sixth cervical vertebra). Inferiorly, the trachea bifurcates at the carina into right and left main bronchi. This bifurcation occurs at the level of the fourth/fifth thoracic vertebrae, which is also the level of the sternal angle (angle of Louis). The tracheal lumen is supported by a skeletal structure of 16–20 C-shaped rings. The ends of each ring are situated posteriorly and joined by the smooth trachealis muscle, which gives the posterior aspect of the trachea a flattened profile. Contraction of trachealis reduces the lumen and affords protection from overdistension due to raised intraluminal pressure, e.g. during coughing.

The trachea lies anterior to the oesophagus with the left recurrent laryngeal nerve ascending in the groove between them. In the chest, it is crossed anteriorly by the brachiocephalic artery and the left brachiocephalic vein. To the left lie the common carotid and subclavian arteries above and the aortic arch below. To the right are the mediastinal pleura, the right vagus nerve and the azygous vein. The right main bronchus is about 3 cm long. It is both wider and more vertically situated than the left, and thus foreign bodies and accidental endobronchial intubation are more likely in the right bronchus. The right upper lobe bronchus usually arises from the right main bronchus just before the hilum of the lung. However, in a significant number of individuals, the right upper lobe bronchus arises more proximally and may even branch from the trachea. The design of endobronchial and some tracheal tubes take this anatomical variability into consideration. The left main bronchus is about 5 cm long.

Blood supply and lymphatic drainage

The trachea is supplied from the inferior thyroid artery and from the bronchial arteries below. The bronchial arteries are branches of the descending aorta. Tracheal veins drain into the inferior thyroid venous plexus or directly into the brachiocephalic vein. Right bronchial veins drain to the azygous vein, and left bronchial veins to the left superior hemiazygous vein. Lymphatic drainage is to the deep cervical lymph nodes, the pre- and paratracheal nodes and the tracheobronchial lymph nodes.

Nerve supply

The autonomic nerve supply to the trachea and bronchi travels in the vagus nerve via its recurrent laryngeal branch and from the sympathetic chain (alongside the arterial supply). The sympathetic nerves originate in the second to fifth thoracic segments of the spinal cord and synapse in the upper four thoracic ganglia.

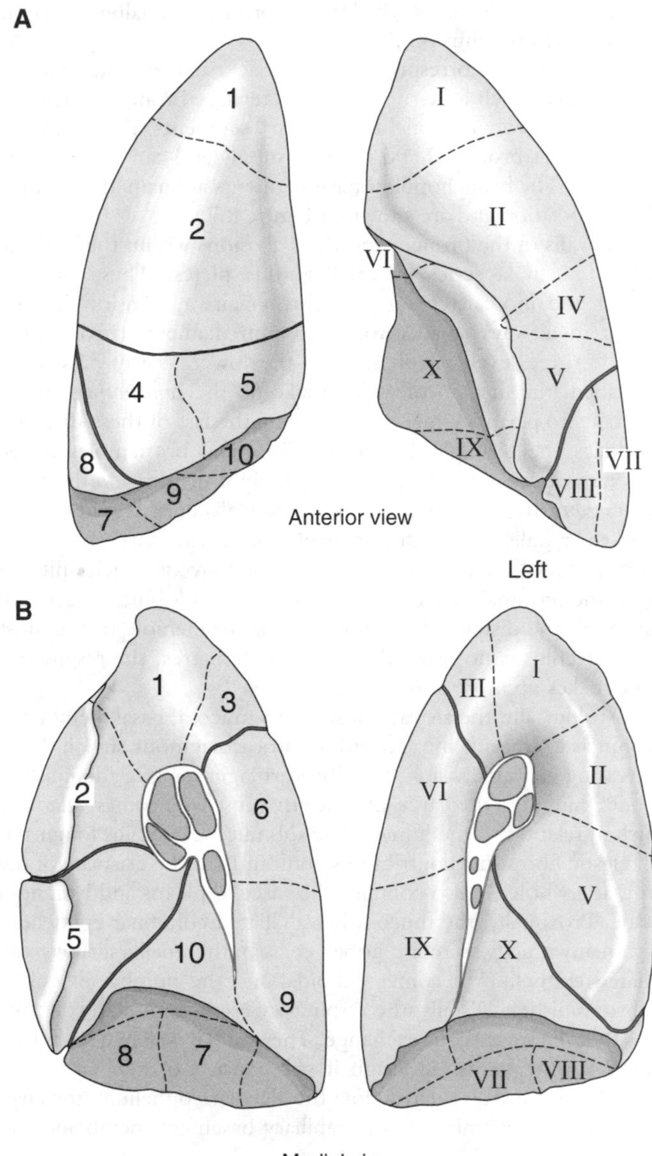

Fig. 8.7
The bronchopulmonary segments viewed from the front (**A**) and medial side (**B**). *Right upper lobe:* 1, apical; 2, anterior; 3, posterior. *Right middle lobe:* 4, lateral; 5, medial (cardiac). *Right lower lobe:* 6, apical; 7, lateral; 8, anterior; 9, posterior; 10, medial. *Left upper lobe:* I, apical; II, anterior; III, posterior; IV, superior lingular; V, inferior lingular. *Left lower lobe:* VI, apical; VII, lateral; VIII, anterior; IX, posterior; X, medial (cardiac).

THE LUNGS AND BRONCHIAL TREE

The right and left main (primary) bronchi divide further on entering each lung. Figure 8.6 illustrates the structure of the proximal bronchial tree and its appearance at bronchoscopy. The right main bronchus divides into secondary bronchi for right upper, middle and lower lobes of the right lung; the left main bronchus similarly divides into left upper and lower lobe bronchi. The left upper lobe bronchus rapidly gives off the lingular bronchus, analogous to the middle lobe bronchus on the right.

These divisions correspond to the lobar structure evident at the lung surface. Each lobe then supports tertiary bronchial divisions into units known as bronchopulmonary segments. Each segment has a distinct bronchial and vascular supply and can be separated surgically. The bronchopulmonary segments are named according to their position and are shown in Figure 8.7.

The walls of the bronchi and their divisions within the lung are supported by a series of cartilaginous plates. These become smaller and more irregular with further airway division and are absent in airways smaller than 0.6 mm diameter (bronchioli). Twenty-three levels of division of the lower airway have been described, the first 16 of which make up the *conducting airway* and take no part in actual gas exchange; the last of these divisions produces the terminal *bronchioles.* Terminal bronchioles divide into *respiratory bronchioles*, the first of eight divisions in the *respiratory zone.* Respiratory bronchioles have alveoli that bud directly from their walls, although principally they divide further through alveolar ducts, alveolar sacs and finally into alveoli. Each unit distal to the terminal bronchiole is described as a lobule (or acinus). Although the distance from the terminal bronchiole to the most distal alveolus is no more than a few millimetres, the respiratory zone makes up most of the lung volume.

Histologically, the airway consists of a mucosa, basal membrane, submucosa, smooth muscle and a fibrocartilaginous sheath. With increasing airway division, the fibrocartilaginous layer diminishes. While thinning, the layer of smooth muscle becomes relatively thick in relation to the lumen. The submucosa contains longitudinal elastic fibres that contribute significantly to the elasticity of the lung as a whole. It also contains the vascular plexus and lymphoid tissue. Proximally, the mucosa has a ciliated columnar epithelium with many mucus-secreting goblet cells. In the smaller airways, the ciliated epithelium becomes cuboidal and the number of goblet cells diminishes. Distally, the respiratory epithelium markedly flattens to facilitate gaseous exchange. The alveolar wall may be as thin as 0.2 μm in places, although it still consists of four layers discernible on electron microscopy: the alveolar epithelium, the alveolar basement membrane, the capillary basement membrane and the capillary wall. The alveolar wall also contains large vacuolated cells, the type II pneumocytes. These cells secrete the lipoprotein surfactant, which stabilizes the alveolar structure through reduction in fluid surface tension.

Blood supply and lymphatic drainage

The bronchial arteries arise from the descending thoracic aorta and supply the large airways and parenchyma within the lung. Corresponding bronchial veins drain to the azygous or accessory hemiazygous veins, although some of this blood returns to the heart via the pulmonary veins. Deoxygenated blood is delivered to each lung in the pulmonary artery; its branches accompany those of the bronchial tree. Terminal branches end in the capillary network surrounding the alveoli, and corresponding veins drain to the upper and lower pulmonary veins. Lymphatic drainage is via a superficial subpleural lymph plexus and a deep lymph plexus that follows the bronchial tree. Both systems drain to the hilar lymph nodes, which in turn drain to the tracheobronchial lymph nodes and then the mediastinal lymph trunks.

Nerve supply

The pulmonary plexus receives efferent nerve supply from the sympathetic chain (T2–4, bronchodilator) and from the vagus nerve (bronchoconstrictor and secretomotor). Sensory afferent fibres responsive to stretch pass mainly to the vagus nerve.

FURTHER READING

Abrahams P H, Hutchings R T, Marks S C 1998 McMinn's colour atlas of human anatomy, 4th edn. Mosby, London

Ellis H, Feldman SA 1996 Anatomy for anaesthetists, 7th edn. Blackwell, Oxford

West J B, 1999 Respiratory physiology–the essentials, 6th edn. Lippincott Williams & Wilkins, Philadelphia

Williams P L 1995 Gray's anatomy, 38th edn. Churchill Livingstone, Edinburgh

9 Respiratory physiology

The principal purpose of the respiratory system is the exchange of oxygen and carbon dioxide between the blood and the respired gas. It has secondary roles in the control of acid–base balance, the metabolism of hormones and the removal of compounds and particulate matter, taking advantage of its position as the only organ which receives the entire cardiac output.

Breathing is the most obvious attribute of the respiratory system and the sequence of events in a normal breath in the upright posture will be outlined as a basis for further consideration.

A BREATH

Initiation of a breath starts in the inspiratory neurones of the respiratory centre in the floor of the fourth ventricle. As expiration ends, increasing neuronal traffic develops in the descending motor neurones of the lateral and ventral columns which synapse with the anterior horn cells of the nerves supplying the respiratory muscles. As the muscles start to contract, muscle spindles sense the load and adjust anterior horn cell activity to achieve the required force.

The diaphragm is the main muscle of respiration, and contraction of its inverted J-shaped muscle fibres causes it to descend with a consequent decrease in intrapleural pressure. Simultaneously, the dilator muscles of the upper airway (alae nasi, tensor palatini, palatoglossus, myoglossus, posterior cricoarytenoid) constrict, opening the airway and resisting the developing subatmospheric collapsing force. The strap muscles and the intercostal muscles also contract, stabilizing the upper chest, preventing it from being indrawn and aiding the expansion of the lower rib cage by the 'bucket handle' movement of the ribs.

The increasing subatmospheric intrapleural pressure expands the lung and dilates the intrathoracic airways. Air is drawn through the nose, where it is warmed and humidified, through the pharynx, larynx, trachea and bronchi until it reaches the terminal bronchioles. The increase in total cross-sectional area of the airways is so great at this point that little further mass movement of gas occurs and transfer of gas to and from the alveoli is by diffusion. The distance is less than 5 mm and takes less than 1 s to reach equilibrium.

The inspired air is not distributed evenly around the lung but is directed preferentially to those areas which are best perfused, the dependent areas of the lung. Final matching of blood flow and gas exchange is achieved by the mechanism of hypoxic pulmonary vasoconstriction (HPV).

Oxygen diffuses from the terminal bronchioles, through the respiratory bronchioles and alveolar sacs into the alveoli. It then diffuses across the alveolar epithelium, basement membranes, capillary endothelium, plasma and red cell membrane before combining with haemoglobin. Carbon dioxide diffuses in the reverse direction.

As inspiration proceeds, increasing afferent neuronal traffic from stretch receptors in the lungs, rib cage and muscles, coupled with increasing feedback from the inspiratory neurones themselves, ultimately inhibits the inspiratory neurones so that inspiration ceases.

Expiration then generally proceeds passively with the stored elastic energy in the lung and chest wall providing the force to overcome the resistance to air flow through the bronchial tree and upper airway. As lung volume decreases to the functional residual capacity (FRC), activity in the expiratory neurones decreases and that in the inspiratory neurones increases, heralding the start of the next breath.

CONTROL OF RESPIRATION

Respiration is regulated by the respiratory neurones (often known as the respiratory centre) to maintain homoeostasis. Arterial carbon dioxide tension (P_aCO_2) is regulated at about 5.3 kPa (40 mmHg) and thus under normal circumstances the main determinant of the minute ventilation ($\dot{V}_E$) is the production of carbon dioxide ($\dot{V}CO_2$), which in turn is determined by the metabolic activity of the body and the energy substrate. Ventilation is greater on a carbohydrate-based diet [respiratory quotient (RQ) = 1.0] than on a fat-based diet (RQ = 0.7) as the energy produced per unit of CO_2 evolved is greater with the latter.

Respiration is modified by many other factors, particularly from higher centres in the brain, including the cortex. The pattern of respiration is modulated by speech and ingestion of food and drink. The anticipation of exercise as well as the activity itself increases respiration. The respiratory centre also balances the depth of respiration (tidal volume, V_t) against the rate, so that the least energy is spent on breathing ($\dot{V}O_{2\ resp}$). Increases in the elastic work of breathing (e.g. pulmonary oedema or fibrosis) tend to increase the respiratory rate, whereas increases in the resistive work (e.g. asthma) tend to increase V_t.

Respiration is also influenced by P_aCO_2, arterial pH and P_aO_2; P_aCO_2 acts on central chemoreceptors, P_aO_2 acts on peripheral chemoreceptors, and pH acts on both central and peripheral chemoreceptors.

CENTRAL CONTROL

The central chemoreceptors lie in the floor of the fourth ventricle and either are the neurones responsible for generation of the respiratory rhythm or are closely related to them. The cells are responsive to changes in the interstitial fluid pH and their sensitivity to changes in P_aCO_2 is in part due to the lesser buffering capacity of cerebrospinal fluid (CSF) compared with blood. The response is very rapid and injection of blood with an increased P_aCO_2 into the carotid artery of an experimental animal during inspiration results in an augmentation of that breath. The change in $\dot{V}_E$ with P_aCO_2 is approximately linear up to a P_aCO_2 of about 12 kPa (90 mmHg) and averages about 15 L min^{-1} kPa^{-1} (Fig. 9.1).

PERIPHERAL CHEMORECEPTORS

The peripheral chemoreceptors are located in the carotid and aortic bodies. They are best regarded as sensors of oxygen delivery as they respond to a decrease in both P_aO_2 and blood flow rate. The carotid bodies effectively monitor the oxygen supply to the brain, the organ most easily damaged by hypoxaemia. The mechanism is probably similar to the central chemoreceptors in that the sensor cells respond to changes in pH. The ventilatory response to hypoxaemia is shown in Figure 9.2 and, if the P_aCO_2 is kept constant, changes exponentially with P_aO_2. The response is linear when oxygenation is expressed as oxyhaemoglobin saturation (S_aO_2). The response is much greater if P_aCO_2 increases at the same time as it generally does in 'real life'.

RESPIRATORY REFLEXES

COUGH

A cough is one means of removing unwanted material from the respiratory tract. It complements the mucociliary escalator which clears small particulate matter and mucus. A cough may be induced voluntarily but is normally spontaneous from stimulation of receptors in the airways. It comprises a maximal inspiration followed by a forced expiration against a closed glottis, when intrathoracic pressures may reach 80 cmH$_2$O. The larynx then opens, allowing expiration to occur at maximum velocity. The increased intrathoracic pressure causes dynamic compression of the bronchi, thus further increasing the velocity of expired air within them, often approaching the speed of sound and creating shear forces which detach the mucus from the mucosa. A wave of dynamic compression sweeps from the smaller to the larger bronchi as the cough progresses.

An effective cough thus requires three elements: an adequate inspired volume, adequate expiratory power and a functioning glottis. Absence of any of these elements leads to impaired coughing and retention of secretions.

LARYNGOSPASM

Laryngospasm is, phylogenetically, a very primitive reflex and is intended to protect the lungs from inhalation of noxious substances. It is induced by stimulation of both chemical and touch

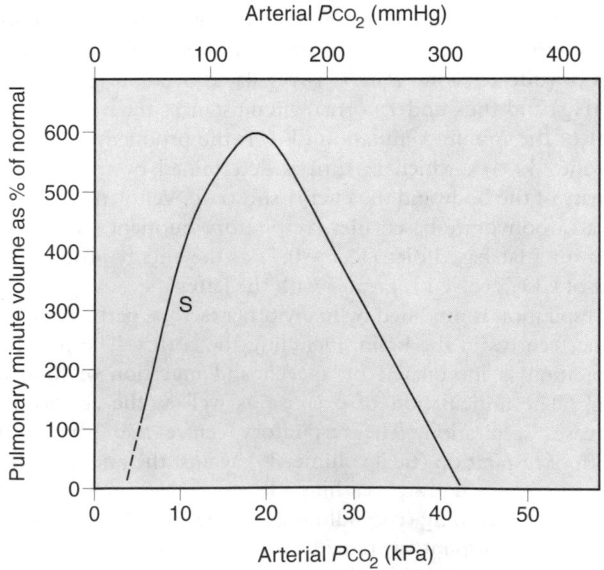

Fig. 9.1
The probable complete ventilatory response to carbon dioxide. Only the straight portion of the ascending limb has been determined in humans and the slope, s, is used to quantify the response.

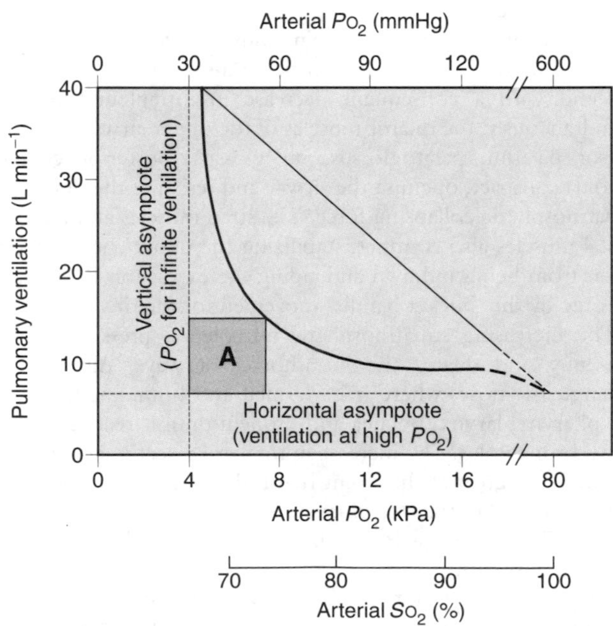

Fig. 9.2
The ventilatory response to hypoxaemia, expressed as P_aO_2 (heavy line) and as S_aO_2 (light line). It is a rectangular hyperbola described by the area A.

receptors above and below the glottis. The reflex is less vigorous in the elderly and is attenuated by sedative drugs of all types, including anaesthetic agents, benzodiazepines and opioids.

AROUSAL

The ability to arouse from sedation or sleep in response to apnoea, airway obstruction or the need to cough is an important respiratory response. It is obtunded during normal sleep and by sedative and analgesic drugs such as morphine and may be a major contributory factor in postoperative respiratory complications.

SLEEP

The onset of sleep leads to a reduction in $\dot{V}_E$ accompanied by a small increase in P_aCO_2 and a decrease in P_aO_2. The ventilatory response to hypercapnia and hypoxaemia is reduced, particularly in REM sleep. Brief periods of apnoea, both central and obstructive, are common during normal sleep in normal individuals. The diminution of upper airway muscle tone, particularly in the muscles of the tongue, commonly leads to partial airway obstruction, manifested by snoring which may progress to complete airway obstruction with arousal. Obstructive sleep apnoea (OSA) may complicate the postoperative period. The hypotonia of skeletal muscles which accompanies REM sleep may affect the distribution of air within the lungs leading to impaired V/Q matching and hypoxaemia. Any patient with disease of the airways, lungs or chest wall (e.g. OSA, asthma, COAD, pulmonary oedema and kyphoscoliosis) may be expected to be most hypoxaemic during REM sleep and this should be taken into account when assessing the condition.

MECHANICS OF RESPIRATION

The respiratory system may be regarded as a collapsible elastic sac (the lungs) surrounded by a semirigid cage (the thorax) with a piston at one end (the diaphragm) supplied through a branching set of semirigid tubes (the airway and bronchial tree). The volume of the system at rest, the FRC, is a balance between the tendency of the lungs to collapse, the thorax to expand and the position of the diaphragm.

LUNG VOLUMES

The total volume of the respiratory system (total lung capacity, TLC) when fully expanded by voluntary effort is about 5.0/6.5 L in the average adult and is related more to height than weight. It can be divided into the parts that participate in gas exchange (alveolar volume) and those that do not (dead space). The total lung volume may also be divided into that which can be measured at the lips (vital capacity, VC) and that which remains in the lungs after a maximal expiration (residual volume, RV) (Fig. 9.3). These volumes change little with body position, unlike the volume left in the lungs after a normal expiration (FRC). The FRC is influenced by body position, being greatest in the upright position and least when lying head downwards, the changes being mostly due to movement of the diaphragm. The closing capacity (CC) is that volume of the lung at which small airways in the dependent parts of the lung begin to collapse during expiration. Normally CC is less than FRC but greater than RV. This can be demonstrated by voluntary expiration to RV, which is inevitably followed by a sigh to re-expand the collapsed lung. CC increases with age and FRC is decreased by a number of factors (Table 9.1), and if CC is greater than FRC, dependent parts

Table 9.1 Factors influencing the functional residual capacity (FRC)

Factors decreasing FRC
Increasing age
Posture – supine and head-down
Anaesthesia – intraoperative
Abdominal and thoracic surgery – postoperative
Pulmonary fibrosis
Pulmonary oedema
Obesity
Abdominal swelling – pregnancy, tumour, ascites
Thoracic cage distortion
Reduced muscle tone
Factors increasing FRC
Increased intrathoracic pressure – PEEP, CPAP
Emphysema
Asthma

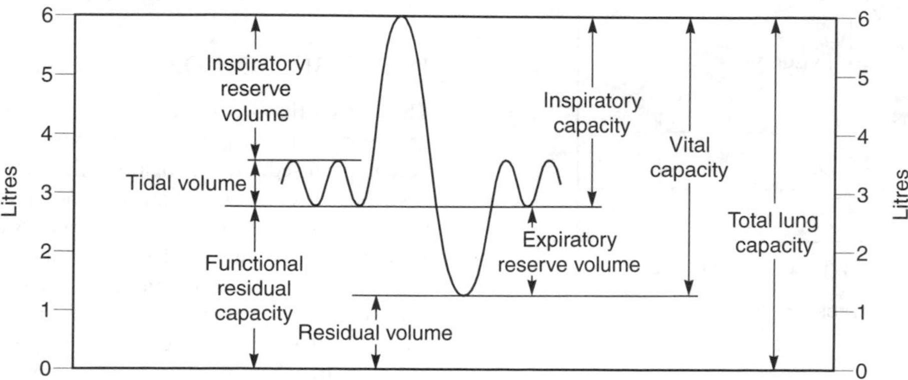

Fig. 9.3
The static lung volumes in a normal 70 kg adult male.

of the lung collapse during normal tidal breathing, resulting in hypoxaemia.

The volumes described above are obtained by slow breathing so that airway resistance is not important. For clinical evaluation of patients, dynamic lung volumes, such as the forced vital capacity (FVC) and the forced expiratory volume in the first second (FEV_1), are more useful. The limiting factor in a forced expiration is the dynamic compression of the intrathoracic airways by the raised intrathoracic pressure.

COMPLIANCE AND SURFACTANT

Expansion of both the lungs and the chest wall requires a distending force, expressed as volume change per unit of distending pressure (compliance) (ml cmH_2O^{-1}), the value of each is approximately 200 ml cmH_2O^{-1}. The compliance of the whole respiratory system (100 ml cmH_2O^{-1}) is clearly less than the individual components and is derived by adding the reciprocals (1/200 + 1/200). The compliance curve of the lung is shown in Figure 9.4. The compliance is approximately linear over most of the range but is lower when the lung is small and nearly fully inflated. The former is due to the added force needed to expand collapsed areas of the lung and overcome surface tension effects, and the latter is due to the elastic fibres in the lung reaching their limit

The lung exhibits hysteresis, i.e. the compliance differs during inflation and deflation. This is due to the effect of alveolar surfactant and is absent if the lung is inflated with a fluid. If the alveoli are regarded as a series of interconnected bubbles, then surface tension would ensure that the smaller bubbles emptied into the larger. However, the presence of a surface active material, dipalmitoyl lecithin, secreted by the type II alveolar cells, ensures that this does not occur. As the alveolus decreases in size, the concentration of surfactant in the surface layer of fluid increases, thus effectively reducing the surface tension. Collapsed lung and small airways have no air–liquid interface and thus additional force is required to open those areas.

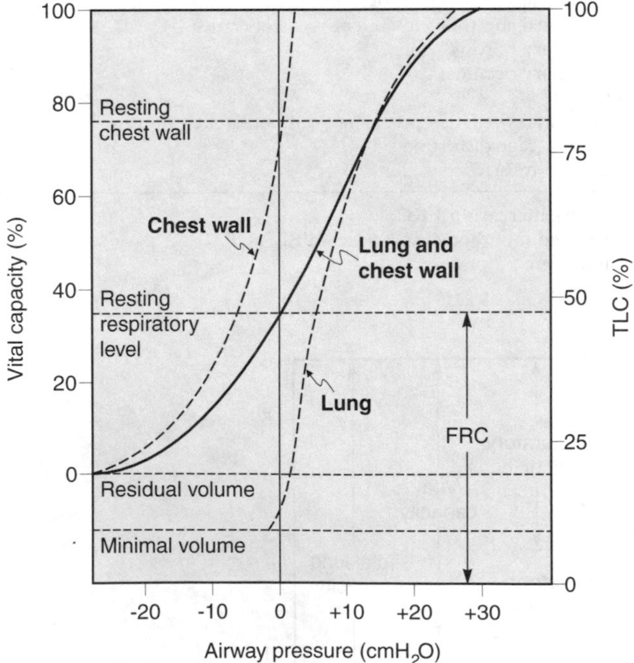

Fig. 9.4
The compliance curves of the lungs, chest wall and total respiratory system. The last is obtained by adding the individual curves. The FRC is determined by balance between the forces exerted by the lung and chest wall.

RESISTANCE

The flow of air into and out of the lungs is opposed by the frictional resistance of the airways and to a lesser extent by the inertia of the gas. The type of flow is important, with laminar flow offering less resistance than transitional or turbulent flow. Laminar flow occurs at low flow rates and in the smaller bronchi. In the larger airways and at branches in the bronchial tree, transitional and turbulent flow may occur.

Laminar flow rate ($\dot{V}$) is related to driving pressure (δP) by Poiseuille's equation:

$$\dot{V} = \frac{\delta P \pi r^4}{8 \eta L}$$

where r is the radius of the tube, L its length and η the viscosity of the gas. Note that the radius of the tube is critical, a halving of the tube diameter reducing the flow by a factor of 16 for the same δP, an important factor in paediatric practice.

Airway resistance is related to lung volume, decreasing as the lung expands. It is also related to bronchomotor tone and the thickness of the mucosal layer.

MATCHING OF VENTILATION AND PERFUSION

As noted earlier, the purpose of the lungs is to exchange gases by bringing the inspired gas into contact with pulmonary capillary blood. Under normal circumstances, the distributions of ventilation and blood flow are nearly perfectly matched, not least as the calibre of the supplying vessel and bronchus are proportional to the volume of that portion of lung. Fine-tuning of ventilation–perfusion matching, e.g. in response to changes in posture, is described below.

DISTRIBUTION OF PERFUSION

The distribution of blood flow within the lungs is influenced by gravity, with the dependent portions of the lung being relatively better perfused. In a helpful theoretical analysis, West has described three distinct zones in the erect posture (Fig. 9.5). In the upper zone, alveolar pressure exceeds both pulmonary arterial and venous pressures and there is no flow. This zone does not occur under normal conditions but may occur in the presence of hypovolaemia and with increased alveolar pressure. In the middle zone, alveolar pressure is exceeded by pulmonary arterial pressure but is greater than pulmonary venous pressure. In the lower zone, both pulmonary arterial and venous pressures exceed alveolar pressure. In the middle and lower zones, flow increases in the more dependent areas.

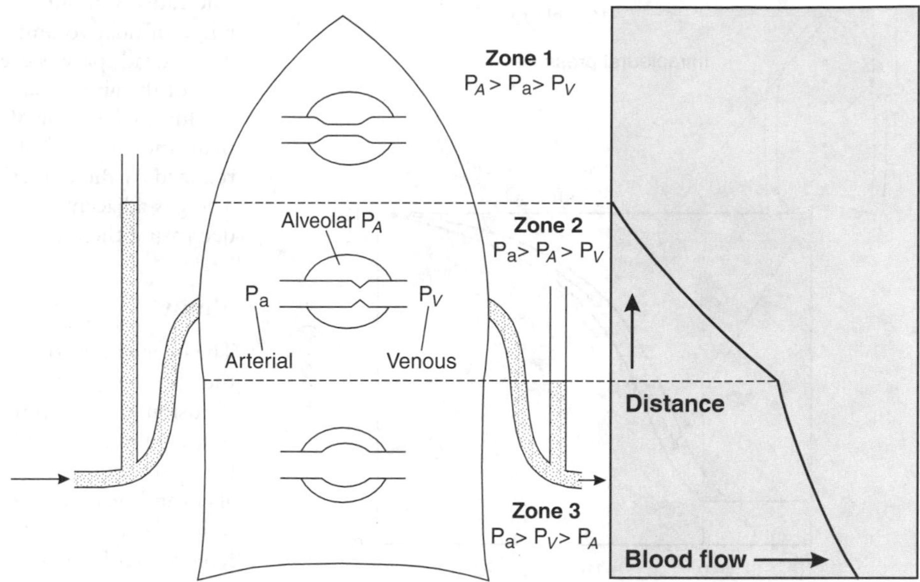

Fig. 9.5
Pressure flow relationships in different parts of the lung in the erect posture. The three zones are described in the text. (Adapted from West et al 1990.)

Within the substance of the lung, the pulmonary arteries divide and subdivide following the lobar pattern of the bronchi. The pulmonary capillaries form such a dense network around the alveoli that a red cell would 'see' an open space with supporting pillars rather than a network of tunnels. The nuclei of the endothelial cells and supportive collagen fibres are arranged so that they are on the opposite side to the alveoli and gas diffusion occurs through the thinned service wall which comprises just the flattened epithelial and endothelial cells and their fused basement membranes (Fig. 9.6).

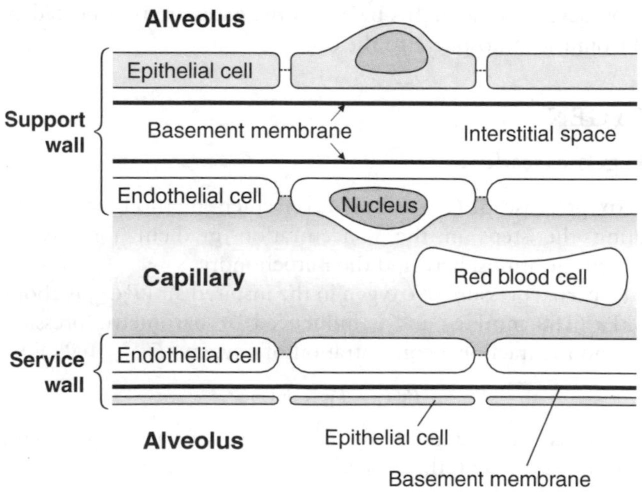

Fig. 9.6
Cross-section of the alveolar wall.

A red cell traverses two or three alveoli in its passage through the lung.

Diffusion of CO_2 and oxygen is very rapid, and under normal circumstances saturation of the haemoglobin with oxygen is complete before the red cell is halfway through its journey and is thus independent of cardiac output.

DISTRIBUTION OF VENTILATION

Several factors ensure that the inspired gas is directed towards the dependent parts of the lungs. The major factor is the compliance of the different parts of the lung. A pressure gradient exists from the top to the bottom of the pleural space due to the weight of the lung, such that it is less negative at the base compared with the apex. The different parts of the lung are thus on different parts of the compliance curve (Fig. 9.7). When inspiration occurs, the *change* in pleural pressure, typically about 5 cmH_2O for an average V_t, is the same for all parts of the lung but results in a greater increase in volume in the dependent parts of the lung than in the non-dependent parts.

HYPOXIC PULMONARY VASOCONSTRICTION

The mechanisms outlined above are very effective at matching blood flow and gas exchange but the local fine-tuning is achieved by a reflex vasoconstriction in the supplying pulmonary artery in response to alveolar hypoxia. This mechanism is of minor importance in the normal lung but is very important in the presence of disease such as pneumonia or during one-lung anaesthesia for thoracic surgery.

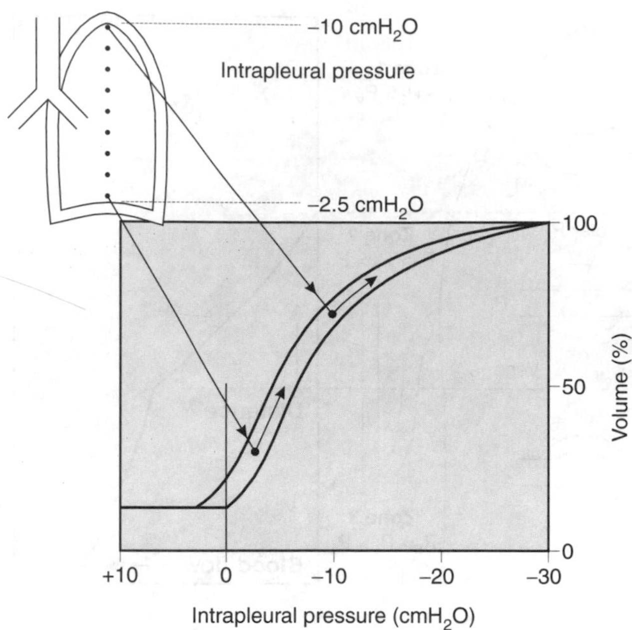

Fig. 9.7
Regional differences in the pressure–volume curve of the lung. The same change in pressure causes a greater change in volume at the base of the lung compared with the apex. (Adapted from West 1990.)

DEAD SPACE, V/Q MATCHING AND SHUNT

In ideally ventilated and perfused lung, the ratio between alveolar ventilation and perfusion (V/Q) is 1.0. If ventilation exceeds perfusion, the ratio is >1, and if perfusion is absent, the ratio is ∞. Conversely, if perfusion exceeds ventilation, the V/Q ratio is < 1, and if ventilation is absent, it is zero. The former condition comprises part of the dead space and the latter comprises part of the intrapulmonary shunt.

Dead space

The dead space of the respiratory system is that part which does not participate in gas exchange. It comprises the anatomical dead space, the upper airway and tracheobronchial tree down to the respiratory bronchioles and the physiological dead space (those parts of the lung whose V/Q ratio is > 1). The anatomical dead space is about 150 ml in the average adult and may be reduced by a tracheal tube. The more useful measure is the ratio of dead space (V_d) to tidal volume (V_t).

The volume of CO_2 expired in a single breath is the product of V_t and the mixed expired concentration ($F_{\bar{E}}CO_2$). This comprises gas from the alveoli (V_A) with a CO_2 concentration the same as that of arterial blood and the dead space gas which contains no CO_2. Gas concentrations can be converted into partial pressure if the barometric pressure is known. V_A is equal to $V_t - V_d$ and thus:

$$V_t \times P_{\bar{E}}CO_2 = (V_t - V_d) \times P_aCO_2$$

This can be rearranged to give Bohr's equation:

$$\frac{V_d}{V_t} = \frac{P_aCO_2 - P_{\bar{E}}CO_2}{P_aCO_2}$$

The ratio is about 0.3 under normal circumstances over a wide range of tidal volume from 50 ml to 1.5 L. At greater tidal volumes, dead space is greater than the anatomical because of dilatation of the airways and increased ventilation of the upper parts of the lung where the V/Q ratio is > 1. When tidal volume is less than the anatomical dead space, the apparent dead space is reduced by the tendency of the gas flow in the airway to be axial. The gas adjacent to the wall of the airway moves very little, thus decreasing the effective diameter of the airway.

Shunt

The oxygen tension in the arterial blood (P_aO_2) is less than that in the alveolus (P_AO_2). This difference ($P_AO_2 - P_aO_2$) is due to the diffusion gradient across the alveolar capillary membrane, dilution of the pulmonary capillary blood by blood which has bypassed the lungs (bronchial circulation, thebesian veins and cardiac anomalies) and that which has come from areas of the lung with a V/Q ratio of < 1. For convenience, the different causes of an A–a difference can be aggregated and the lung regarded as perfect but with a proportion of the cardiac output ($\dot{Q}_S$) bypassing or shunting past the lungs ($\dot{Q}_T$). The ratio $\dot{Q}_S/\dot{Q}_T$ (virtual shunt fraction) is derived in a similar way to the Bohr equation:

$$\frac{\dot{Q}_S}{\dot{Q}_T} = \frac{C_{c'}O_2 - C_aO_2}{C_{c'}O_2 - C_{\bar{v}}O_2}$$

where $C_{c'}O_2$, C_aO_2 and $C_{\bar{v}}O_2$ are the oxygen contents (ml 100 ml^{-1} blood) of end pulmonary capillary, arterial and mixed venous blood, respectively. The concept of virtual shunt, which is normally less than 4% of cardiac output, is useful in critically ill patients.

If the lungs are normal, decreases in mixed venous oxygenation, e.g. due to a decrease in cardiac output, have little effect on arterial oxygenation. However, in the presence of a shunt, such decreases can result in significant hypoxaemia.

GAS EXCHANGE AND CARRIAGE

Oxygen is utilized and CO_2 is produced in the mitochondria. This section describes the means by which the gases are transported to and from the atmosphere to the cells.

OXYGEN

Oxygen cascade

The oxygen cascade (Fig. 9.8) is a convenient method for demonstrating the steps in the concentration gradient for oxygen between the atmosphere and the mitochondria.

The partial pressure of oxygen in the inspired air (P_IO_2) is about 21 kPa (160 mmHg) and is influenced by barometric pressure (P_B) and the fractional concentration of oxygen (F_IO_2) (0.21):

$$P_IO_2 = P_B \times F_IO_2$$

The inspired gas is 'diluted ' by the presence of water vapour and, as it is fully saturated, the reduction is determined by:

$$P_IO_{2(sat)} = (P_B - P_{H_2O}) \times F_IO_2$$

where P_{H_2O} is the saturated vapour pressure of water at 37°C (normally 6.3 kPa, 47 mmHg).

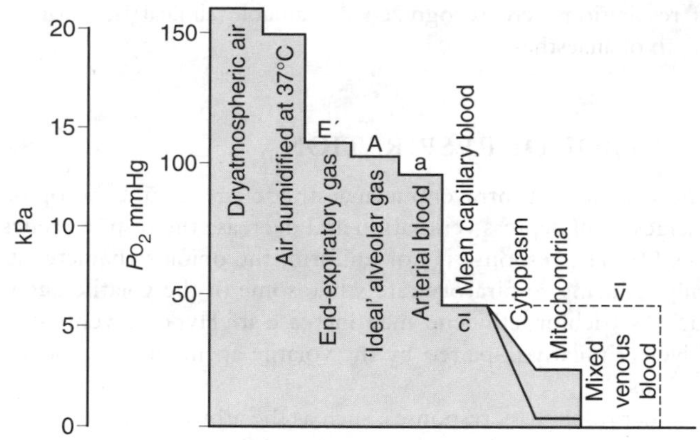

Fig. 9.8
The oxygen cascade.

The inspired gas is further 'diluted ' by the addition of carbon dioxide and the removal of oxygen in the alveolus. With a normal diet, slightly less CO_2 is produced than oxygen is consumed (RQ < 1.0) and the alveolar oxygen tension (P_AO_2) is given by the alveolar air equation:

$$P_AO_2 = P_IO_2 - \frac{P_ACO_2}{RQ}$$

As noted above, the difference between the P_ACO_2 and the P_aCO_2 is very small and the latter term may be substituted into the equation. This is an important equation; for example, it enables the effect of changing the minute ventilation (hyper- and hypoventilation) on P_aO_2 to be determined.

The relationship between alveolar ventilation ($\dot{V}_A$) and P_aCO_2 is shown in Figure 9.9 and is exponential. Thus a doubling of $\dot{V}_A$ results in a halving of P_aCO_2, and a halving of $\dot{V}_A$ results in a doubling of P_aCO_2. If this change is entered into the alveolar air equation then the relationship between $\dot{V}_A$ and P_aO_2 shown in Figure 9.9 becomes apparent. Two curves are shown, the lower for an F_IO_2 of 0.21 and the upper for an F_IO_2 of 0.3. It can be seen that hypoxaemia develops rapidly as $\dot{V}_A$ decreases but is readily corrected by a small increase in F_IO_2, while hyperventilation results in little increase in P_aO_2.

Oxygen then diffuses from the alveolus to the red cell where it binds with haemoglobin.

Haemoglobin

Each 100 ml of blood contains about 20 ml of oxygen, almost all of which is carried on the haemoglobin. Oxygen is poorly soluble in blood [0.023 ml 100 ml^{-1} blood kPa^{-1} (0.003 ml 100 ml^{-1} blood mmHg^{-1})]. The oxygen content of blood (C_{O_2}) is thus:

$$C_{O_2}\ (\text{ml } 100\text{ ml}^{-1}\text{ blood}) = 0.023 \times P_{O_2}\ (\text{kPa}) + 1.34 \times \text{Hb (g dl}^{-1}) \times S_{O_2}\ (\%)/100$$

where S_{O_2} is the oxyhaemoglobin saturation.

Each molecule of Hb can carry four molecules of oxygen, the relationship between P_{O_2} and S_{O_2} being the familiar sigmoid shape of the oxyhaemoglobin dissociation curve (Fig. 9.10). The normal P_aO_2 is about 13 kPa (100 mmHg) and S_aO_2 is 97%, while the mixed venous values ($P_{\bar{v}}O_2$ and $S_{\bar{v}}O_2$) are 6 kPa (45 mmHg) and 75%, respectively. Note that increasing the P_aO_2 above normal has little effect on arterial oxygen content because of the poor solubility of oxygen, and thus the venous point changes little even if 100% oxygen is respired. $P_{\bar{v}}O_2$ is determined by the balance between oxygen supply and demand. Thus an increased demand (e.g. shivering) or decreased supply

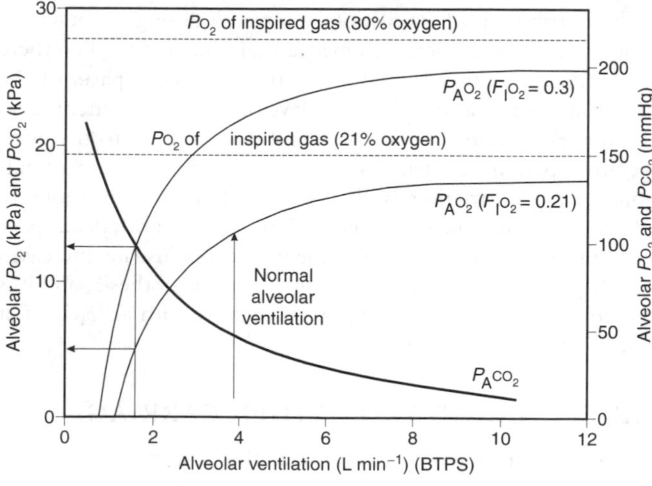

Fig. 9.9
The effect of changing alveolar ventilation on P_ACO_2 (heavy line) and on P_AO_2 (light lines). The effect of increasing the F_IO_2 from 0.21 to 0.3 on P_AO_2 is also shown.

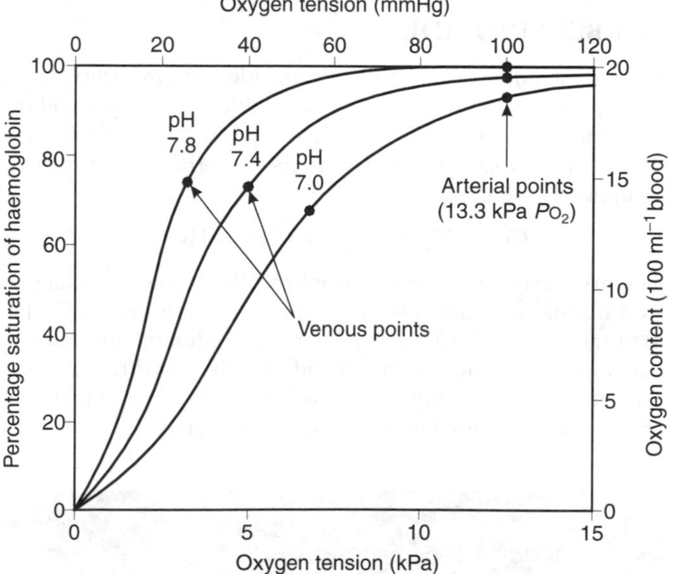

Fig. 9.10
The oxyhaemoglobin dissociation curves for normal adult haemoglobin at normal pH and with acidosis and alkalosis.

(e.g. cardiogenic shock) reduces $P_{\bar{v}}O_2$, while a decreased utilization (e.g. cyanide poisoning) or excessive supply (e.g. sepsis) increases it.

The position of the curve is best described by the P_{50}, the PO_2 at which the Hb is 50% saturated (normally 3.6 kPa, 27 mmHg). Several factors can influence the curve. Increases in temperature, PCO_2, hydrogen ion concentration (decrease in pH) and concentration of 2,3-diphosphoglycerate all shift the curve to the right, while decreases in these factors shift the curve to the left. Displacement of the curve to the right (acidosis) slightly decreases the affinity for oxygen in the lungs but increases the availability of oxygen in the tissues. Conversely, displacement to the left (alkalosis) slightly increases uptake in the lungs but renders the tissues relatively hypoxic in order to achieve the same oxygen extraction. A small shift of the curve with pH and PCO_2 occurs under normal physiological conditions in the lungs and tissues to facilitate oxygen transport and is known as the Bohr effect.

The final part of the diffusion pathway for oxygen is from the haemoglobin to the mitochondria where the PO_2 is only 0.5–3 kPa (4–23 mmHg).

The oxygen stores of the body are limited to about 1500 ml, of which about 750 ml is combined with Hb, 500 ml in the lungs and 250 ml combined with myoglobin. A glance at the oxyhaemoglobin dissociation curve shows that only about half the oxygen attached to Hb is available and almost none of that attached to myoglobin, and thus the available stores in the event of apnoea are less than 1000 ml. This would permit a period of apnoea of about 4 min at the normal $\dot{V}O_2$ of 250 ml min^{-1} before serious arterial hypoxaemia occurred.

Preoxygenation with 100% oxygen, if complete, increases the stores to about 4500 ml and thus increases the potential duration of apnoea at least fourfold. If cardiac arrest occurs, the stores in the lungs are unavailable and, as the brain has no oxygen stores, unconsciousness occurs within about 10 s.

CARBON DIOXIDE

Carbon dioxide passes in a reverse cascade from mitochondria to atmosphere. It is much more water-soluble than oxygen and diffuses more readily. CO_2 is mostly carried in the blood as bicarbonate ion (HCO_3^-) but is also attached to proteins as carbamino compounds and in solution:

$$CO_2 + H_2O \rightleftharpoons H_2CO_3 \rightleftharpoons H^+ + HCO_3^-$$

The first part of the reaction is inherently slow and is catalysed by carbonic anhydrase which is found in the red cells. The hydrogen ion is buffered by protein, predominantly reduced haemoglobin (Haldane effect) and the HCO_3^- diffuses out of the red cell in exchange for chloride (Hamburger shift). The reverse occurs in the lungs as CO_2 is eliminated.

EFFECTS OF ANAESTHESIA ON RESPIRATION

The depressant effect of anaesthetic drugs on respiration has been known since the earliest days when the depth, character and rate of respiration were recognized as valuable clinical signs of the depth of anaesthesia.

CONTROL OF RESPIRATION

The volatile and intravenous anaesthetic agents and the opioid analgesics all depress ventilation and decrease the responsiveness to CO_2. The response is not uniform, the opioids characteristically reducing respiratory rate while some of the volatile agents such as trichloroethylene may increase it. Hypoxic ventilatory drive is similarly impaired by the volatile agents in low concentrations.

Other respiratory responses, such as the arousal response to airway obstruction and cough, are reduced during anaesthesia. The pattern of respiration during anaesthesia tends to be regular without the intermittent sighs seen during wakefulness.

MECHANICS OF RESPIRATION

The induction of anaesthesia results in a reduction in the FRC of about 0.5 L, probably due to cranial displacement of the diaphragm. This effect is greatest after neuromuscular blockade. The thoracic contribution to inspiration also diminishes and expiratory abdominal muscle activity increases, giving the characteristic pattern often seen during anaesthesia with spontaneous respiration.

MATCHING OF VENTILATION AND PERFUSION

Induction of anaesthesia does not affect the distribution of perfusion, except that the increased intrathoracic pressure of mechanical ventilation may reduce cardiac output and increase or create the zone in the lung where alveolar pressure exceeds pulmonary arterial pressure, thus increasing dead space.

The distribution of ventilation is impaired during spontaneous respiration and worsened with mechanical ventilation, when there is a reduction in the ventilation to the dependent parts of the lung. Plate-like areas of atelectasis develop in the dependent areas within a few minutes of induction and may persist into the postoperative period, contributing to hypoxaemia. Hypoxic pulmonary vasoconstriction is abolished by low concentrations of volatile agents and the overall effect is to increase both dead space and shunt in the anaesthetized patient. P_aCO_2 is usually increased and P_aO_2 is usually decreased during general anaesthesia, and it is thus conventional to administer a gas mixture with an F_IO_2 of at least 0.3 during anaesthesia.

GAS EXCHANGE AND OXYGEN CARRIAGE

Gas exchange is impaired during anaesthesia, as outlined above, and oxygen carriage may be impaired by the reduced cardiac output. However, the reduced metabolic rate tends to compensate for the reduced oxygen delivery. By reducing the P_aCO_2, hyperventilation reduces oxygen delivery by shifting the oxyhaemoglobin dissociation curve to the left (see above). The associated vasoconstriction further impairs tissue oxygenation.

Increased oxygen consumption

Shivering commonly occurs in the postoperative period, causing a marked increase in oxygen consumption (see Ch. 14). Cardiac output cannot always increase to meet the demand and mixed venous oxygen tension decreases. This increases the impact of intrapulmonary shunting due to atelectasis and V/Q mismatching and worsens arterial oxygenation, setting up a 'vicious circle '.

Second gas effect

Under normal circumstances, only oxygen is taken up from the lungs and there is no net uptake of nitrogen. When a second gas that is absorbed rapidly, such as nitrous oxide, is introduced into the lungs, the uptake of that gas has the effect of 'concentrating ' the gases remaining in the alveoli. The effect on oxygen is of no clinical importance, but the increase in concentration of volatile anaesthetic agents speeds the induction of anaesthesia.

The reverse occurs when the administration of nitrous oxide is stopped. The elimination of the gas 'dilutes' the alveolar gases and may result in significant hypoxaemia unless the $F_{I}O_2$ is increased. This effect lasts for about 5 min after discontinuation of the nitrous oxide.

NON-RESPIRATORY FUNCTIONS

ACID–BASE BALANCE

Maintenance of a normal arterial pH is important for cellular function and the respiratory system provides a means for rapid adjustment by controlling the elimination of an important acid, carbonic acid.

Rearrangement of the equation for the buffering of CO_2 given above gives the familiar Henderson–Hasselbalch equation. It can be seen that alterations to the P_aCO_2 affect the pH:

$$pH = pK + \log \frac{[HCO_3^-]}{s \times P_aCO_2}$$

A decrease in plasma pH stimulates the respiratory centre via the central chemoreceptors, increasing alveolar ventilation and reducing P_aCO_2. This is well shown in diabetic ketoacidosis where the patient is usually found to be hyperventilating, demonstrating respiratory compensation for a metabolic acidosis.

The reverse occurs during a metabolic alkalosis when P_aCO_2 increases. Metabolic compensation also occurs for chronic changes in the respiratory component of acid–base balance. With a chronic reduction in P_aCO_2, e.g. following an ascent to high altitude when the reduced P_aO_2 has stimulated respiration, there is increased renal loss of bicarbonate ion, thus restoring the pH towards normal. Conversely, when P_aCO_2 is chronically increased with respiratory failure, the kidney retains bicarbonate to maintain the balance.

METABOLIC

The lungs have many of the enzyme systems found in the liver, but as their metabolic mass is considerably lower, their contribution to overall drug metabolism is small. Nevertheless, they have considerable synthetic and metabolic functions.

Synthesis

Surfactant is synthesized by the type II alveolar cells and is necessary for the stability of the alveoli (see above). Coagulation factors, including heparin and various components of the pulmonary defence mechanisms, are also produced and are discussed below.

Metabolism

The best-known metabolic function of the lung is the conversion of angiotensin I, which is inactive, to the active angiotensin II. Several other hormones are inactivated by passage through the lung, including norepinephrine, serotonin, bradykinin, prostaglandins and leukotrienes.

The cytochrome P450 general oxidative system is active in the lung and several largely basic drugs are metabolized to some extent. However, the contribution is generally small in comparison with the liver.

FILTRATION

Any particulate matter, including thrombi, released into the venous system passes to the lungs. The theoretical pore size of the lung as a filter is about 70 μm, although in practice, much larger particles can traverse the lungs, presumably through arterio-venous connections.

The lung possesses active proteolytic systems for dissolving fibrin clots and the endothelium contains plasmin activator which converts plasminogen to plasmin. It is also rich in heparin and thromboplastin and presumably plays a role in the regulation of coagulation.

PULMONARY DEFENCE MECHANISMS

Inhaled air contains particles of dust and airborne bacteria and viruses. The respiratory system contains several defence mechanisms to protect the lower airways and alveoli. The primary defence is the nose with its lining of mucus-producing ciliated epithelium. The turbinates ensure turbulence, thus avoiding streaming of the inhaled air. The nasal mucosa becomes engorged and secretes extra mucus in response to inhaled irritants, as every hay fever sufferer knows. The tracheobronchial tree is also lined with ciliated epithelium and equipped with mucus glands. The cilia sweep the mucus coat with the entrapped particles towards the pharynx where it is swallowed with the saliva. Coughing also contributes.

Pulmonary macrophages are found throughout the airways and alveoli. They phagocytose inhaled particles and microorganisms, producing several proteases to kill the bacteria. The lung contains α_1-antitrypsin to inactivate the proteases and prevent damage to itself. The macrophages also release highly reactive oxygen compounds, including the superoxide radical. Superoxide dismutase is produced in the lung to prevent damage from these compounds. IgA is secreted in pulmonary mucus and contributes to the killing of microorganisms.

FURTHER READING

Hlastala M P, Berger A J 1996 Physiology of respiration. Oxford University Press, New York

Lumb AB 2000 Nunn's applied respiratory physiology, 5th edn. Butterworth-Heinemann, Oxford

West J B 1999 Respiratory physiology – the essentials, 6th edn. Williams & Wilkins, Baltimore

West J B 1990 Ventilation, blood flow and gas exchange, 5th edn. Blackwell Scientific Publications, Oxford

10 Drugs acting on the respiratory system

Many drugs used in anaesthetic practice have effects on the respiratory system. For example, opioids depress the respiratory centre, inhalation agents and anticholinergics dilate bronchi, and anticholinesterases cause bronchial constriction. These are the secondary effects of these drugs. This chapter describes the pharmacology of drugs used primarily for their effects on the respiratory system. These may be classified in the following manner:

- drugs acting on the respiratory centre
- drugs acting on airway calibre
- drugs acting on pulmonary vascular resistance
- drugs acting on mucociliary function
- surfactant replacement therapy.

DRUGS ACTING ON THE RESPIRATORY CENTRE

These drugs may either be true stimulants of ventilation or reverse respiratory depression caused by opioids or benzodiazepines.

RESPIRATORY STIMULANTS

Several classes of drug stimulate ventilation and may be used when ventilatory drive is inadequate. These agents increase respiratory drive through a variety of mechanisms. For example, strychnine blocks central inhibitory pathways, acetazolamide increases hydrogen ion concentration in the extracellular fluid around the respiratory centre, and nikethamide and doxapram stimulate the respiratory centre directly. Only doxapram is now used clinically.

In general, respiratory stimulants should not be used if respiratory failure is caused by muscle exhaustion. The suggested clinical indications for the use of respiratory stimulants include the following:

- overdose with sedatives
- post-anaesthetic respiratory depression
- idiopathic hypoventilation
- opioid overdose
- acute exacerbation of chronic obstructive pulmonary disease (COPD).

It must be stressed that artificial ventilation is the best option for respiratory management in most of these circumstances and that respiratory stimulants should be used only as a short-term measure or when facilities for artificial ventilation are not immediately available. Respiratory stimulants are rarely indicated in the late stages of COPD because respiratory drive in these patients is already maximal.

Doxapram

At low doses (0.5 mg kg^{-1}), doxapram stimulates carotid chemoreceptors. At high doses, it also stimulates medullary respiratory centres. However, the effect of a single dose is transient and a continuous intravenous infusion may be required for sustained action.

Uses

In addition to the indications listed above, it has been suggested that doxapram may be used in the following situations:

- prevention of postoperative atelectasis and thus maintenance of better oxygenation
- prevention of postoperative chest complications
- facilitation of blind nasal intubation
- treatment of apnoea in premature babies.

When it is used to reverse opioid-induced respiratory depression, doxapram has the advantage in comparison with opioid antagonists in that it does not reverse the analgesic effect.

Dosage and administration

Doxapram is given intravenously as a slow bolus of 0.5 mg kg^{-1}. The effect lasts for 5–10 min. For sustained action, a continuous i.v. infusion of 1–2 mg min^{-1} may be used.

Adverse effects

In common with other analeptics (such as nikethamide), doxapram has central excitatory effects, although it affects the respiratory centre preferentially. The main adverse effects are listed in Table 10.1. In extreme cases, convulsions may occur; hypoxaemia and hypercapnia are predisposing factors.

Doxapram is metabolized by the liver and should be used with caution if liver function is impaired.

OPIOID ANTAGONISTS

Naloxone

Naloxone is not a respiratory stimulant *per se*. It is an oxymorphone derivative and is an opioid antagonist without significant intrinsic agonist activity. It reverses opioid-induced respiratory depression, analgesia and sedation; however, careful titration allows reversal of respiratory depression without reversing analgesia.

Uses

The main indication for naloxone is reversal of opioid-induced respiratory depression. It does not reverse the depressant effects of other drugs or depression of ventilation caused by neurological disease.

Although artificial ventilation is usually a safer option for treatment of opioid-induced respiratory depression, administration of naloxone is indicated particularly under the following circumstances:

- neonatal respiratory depression caused by administration of an opioid to the mother during labour
- as a diagnostic test if the cause of sedation and respiratory depression is not clear.

Dosage and administration

Naloxone may be given either intravenously or intramuscularly. In adults, a bolus dose of up to 0.4 mg can be given initially. The action is apparent in 2–5 min and lasts for about 30–40 min. This duration of action is shorter than that of most opioid agonists. Consequently, repeated doses are often required, and the patient's condition must be monitored closely so that recurrence of respiratory depression is detected promptly. Alternatively, a continuous i.v. infusion may be used in adults at a rate of 0.4–2 mg h^{-1}. The rate of infusion should be adjusted according to the response.

Adverse effects

Adverse effects are rare but include arrhythmia, hypertension and pulmonary oedema. The main undesirable effect is reversal of the analgesic effect of the agonist.

BENZODIAZEPINE ANTAGONISTS

Flumazenil

In common with naloxone, flumazenil is not a direct respiratory stimulant. It is an imidazobenzodiazepine, which is a competitive binder to the benzodiazepine receptors. Its administration reverses all the central effects of benzodiazepines, including sedation and depression of ventilation.

Uses

- To reverse sedation and respiratory depression induced by benzodiazepines such as diazepam and midazolam
- As a diagnostic tool in patients with sedation and/or respiratory depression of unknown origin.

Dosage and administration

Flumazenil is usually administered intravenously. An initial dose of 0.2 mg is appropriate in adults. Additional doses of 0.1 mg can be given every 15 min. The maximum recommended dose is 1.0 mg, although massive doses of up to 100 mg have been administered safely. The effect of each dose is short-lived (15–45 min) and unpredictable. The half-life is shorter than those of the benzodiazepine agonists, and sedation and depression of ventilation may recur, particularly if a large dose of agonist has been given; the patient must be monitored closely. For a longer duration of action, a continuous infusion of flumazenil at a rate of 0.1–1.0 mg h^{-1} may be used.

Table 10.1 Adverse effects of doxapram

Restlessness
Sweating
Anxiety
Agitation
Confusion
Headache
Hallucinations
Tachycardia
Hypertension
Convulsions

Adverse effects

Flumazenil has no direct effect on the central nervous system. It is a relatively safe drug even in doses higher than recommended. However, the dose should be reduced in the presence of liver disease, because flumazenil is almost completely metabolized by the liver. Its use in patients with epilepsy is not recommended because it may precipitate convulsions by rapidly reversing the central effects of benzodiazepines.

DRUGS ACTING ON CALIBRE OF THE AIRWAYS

The normal tone of airway smooth muscles is the result of a balance between the opposing effects of sympathetic (mainly β_2) and parasympathetic influences (Fig. 10.1). At the cellular level, β_2-adrenergic drugs bind to the cell membrane receptor to activate adenylate cyclase. This catalyses the conversion of adenosine triphosphate (ATP) to cyclic adenosine monophosphate (cAMP) within the cell. Through different enzyme systems (kinases), cAMP relaxes bronchial smooth muscle. Cyclic AMP is inactivated by the enzyme phosphodiesterase to produce 5′AMP. Thus drugs which increase the concentration of cAMP relax the bronchi (β_2-antagonists, phosphodiesterase inhibitors). Conversely, drugs which reduce the level of cAMP (β_2-antagonists) may cause bronchoconstriction.

Cholinergic drugs act on muscarinic receptors to activate guanylate cyclase, which converts guanosine triphosphate (GTP) into cyclic guanosine monophosphate (cGMP). Cyclic GMP, through kinases, causes bronchial constriction. Thus cholinergic drugs increase cGMP and cause bronchoconstriction, while anticholinergic drugs reduce the production of cGMP and cause bronchial dilatation. The bronchial smooth muscle tone at any given time is determined by the balance between the concentrations of cAMP and cGMP (Fig. 10.1).

Histamine and other mediators also play an important role in promoting bronchial constriction (H_1 receptors), especially during ana-

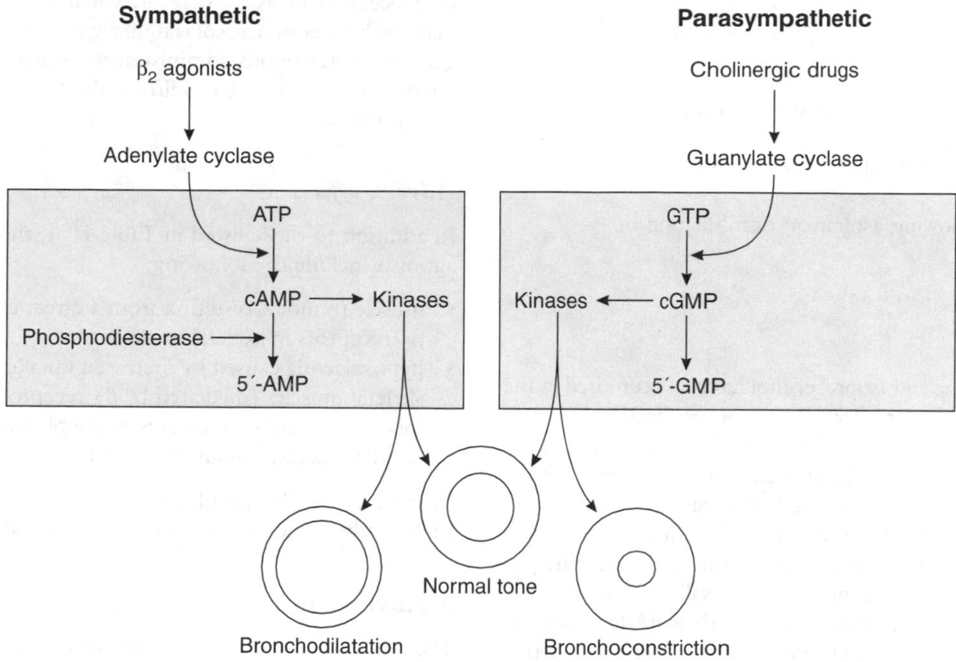

Fig. 10.1
Regulation of bronchomotor tone and mechanism of action of drugs. The relative quantities of cAMP and cGMP determine the state of bronchial tone; cAMP relaxes bronchial muscles and cGMP constricts them.

phylaxis, drug reactions, allergy, asthma and respiratory infections. Membrane stabilizers (sodium cromoglycate) and anti-inflammatory agents (steroids) may reduce or prevent bronchoconstriction in these conditions. Table 10.2 summarizes the factors that influence airway calibre.

BRONCHODILATORS

Bronchoconstriction leads to the following:

- increased difficulty in breathing
- inadequate ventilation
- V/Q mismatch
- hypoxaemia
- impaired ability to cough.

The goal of bronchodilator therapy is to reverse these effects. Depending upon the condition of the patient, bronchodilators may be used either in isolation or as a part of respiratory support with other measures such as oxygen therapy, humidification of inspired gases, antibiotics, physiotherapy and mechanical ventilation. Three types of bronchodilator are in clinical use:

- β-adrenergic agonists
- methylxanthines
- anticholinergics.

Membrane stabilizers such as sodium cromoglycate may prevent bronchoconstriction, but do not have a direct bronchodilator action. Therefore, these drugs are ineffective when bronchoconstriction has already occurred.

β-Adrenergic agonists

Epinephrine has been used in the treatment of asthma since the beginning of the 20th century. In addition to increasing the intracellular concentration of cAMP, β-agonists have other complementary effects on the airways, the most notable being inhibition of mast cell mediator release. Table 10.3 summarizes the effects of β-agonists on the airways. These effects are mediated via subtype β_2-receptors, which are spread throughout the larger and smaller airways; β_2-selective agents are now used commonly as bronchodilators.

Table 10.2 Factors influencing airway calibre
Bronchodilatation
Sympathetic stimulation – increased intracellular cAMP
β_2-Agonists
Methylxanthines
Anticholinergics
Bronchoconstriction
Parasympathetic stimulation – increased intracellular cGMP
Cholinergic drugs
β_2-Antagonists
Inflammatory mediators
Allergy and anaphylaxis
Prevention of bronchoconstriction
Membrane stabilizers – sodium cromoglycate
Steroids

Uses

- asthma
- COPD
- hyperreactive airways in patients undergoing mechanical ventilation
- bronchospasm caused by allergic reactions and anaphylaxis
- bronchospasm following aspiration or inhalation of toxins.

Choice of drug

Epinephrine, ephedrine and isoproterenol have all been used in the past for their bronchodilator effect. Their use has declined because of cardiovascular side-effects mediated by β_1-receptors; selective β_2-agonists are now preferred. However, epinephrine remains the drug of choice in anaphylaxis when a combination of β_1-, β_2- and α-agonist action is desirable. Some patients with acute asthma respond best to subcutaneous epinephrine, but in the large majority of patients, β_2 selective agonists such as salbutamol or terbutaline are the first drugs of choice because they are less likely to produce unwanted β_1 actions. However, it should be noted that the selectivity of β_2-agonists is only relative and that in high doses or in the presence of predisposing factors (hypoxaemia, hypercapnia), β_2-agonists may also produce β_1 effects (Table 10.4).

Dosage and administration

Inhalation is the method of choice because systemic side-effects are minimized. An inhaled drug may also be more effective because it reaches the surface cells (mast cells and epithelial cells) which are relatively inaccessible to a drug administered systemically. Salbutamol may be administered from a pressurized aerosol (100 µg per puff; dose 1–2 puffs). The effect lasts for 4–6 h. The drug may also be nebulized to be delivered with oxygen-enriched air using a face mask, or with inspiratory gases in patients undergoing mechanical ventilation. For this purpose, a dose of 2.5–5 mg (1 mg ml^{-1}) every 4–6 h is used. Side-effects are more likely when these drugs are used in nebulized form rather than a pressurized aerosol because aerosols deliver a smaller dose and a smaller proportion is absorbed systemically.

Oral administration has no advantage over inhalation and is associated with more side-effects. Intravenous administration is used occasionally as a last resort when bronchospasm is so severe that a nebulizer or aerosol is unlikely to deliver the drug to the target cells. Intravenous administration is associated with more frequent side-effects and should be used only when the patient is monitored intensively.

Table 10.3 Effects of β-agonists on the airways

Specific
Increase in intracellular cAMP and bronchodilatation
Non-specific but complementary
Inhibition of mast cell mediator release
Inhibition of plasma exudation and microvascular leakage
Prevention of airway oedema
Increased mucus secretion
Increased mucociliary clearance
Prevention of tissue damage mediated by oxygen free radicals
Decreased acetylcholine release in cholinergic nerves by an action on prejunctional β_2-receptors

Adverse effects

In addition to those listed in Table 10.4, the adverse effects of β-agonists include the following:

- muscle tremor – resulting from a direct effect on β_2-receptors in skeletal muscle
- hypokalaemia caused by increased uptake of potassium ions by skeletal muscles (mediated by β_2-receptors)
- metabolic effects – increases in the plasma concentrations of free fatty acids, insulin, glucose, pyruvate and lactate.

In high doses, β_1-stimulants may cause dangerous arrhythmias, particularly in the presence of hypoxaemia and hypercapnia.

Methylxanthines

The bronchodilator effect of strong coffee was described in the 19th century. Methylxanthines, which are related to caffeine, have been used widely to control asthma since 1930. Theophylline is the most commonly used parent compound. Aminophylline is a water-soluble salt that contains over 75% theophylline and is used as the injectable form of theophylline. Methylxanthines have widespread effects involving various organ systems. With regard to their bronchodilator effects, the following mechanisms have been proposed:

- phosphodiesterase inhibition – this leads to an increased level of intracellular cAMP (Fig. 10.1)
- adenosine receptor antagonism – adenosine, especially in asthmatic subjects, causes mast cell histamine release which is prevented by theophylline
- endogenous catecholamine release
- prostaglandin inhibition
- interference with calcium mobilization
- potentiation of β_2-agonists.

All these mechanisms have therapeutic effects on the airways and respiratory muscles, which are summarized in Table 10.5.

The net effect is reduced airways resistance, reduced work of breathing and increased efficiency of the respiratory muscles. Other effects of methylxanthines contribute to their side-effects.

Central nervous system effects. Stimulation of the CNS may lead to nausea, restlessness, agitation, insomnia, tremor and seizures. Some CNS effects (e.g. tremor) may occur even with therapeutic plasma concentrations of the drug.

Table 10.4 Adverse β_1 effects of β-agonists

Anxiety
Nausea and vomiting
Tachycardia and other tachyarrhythmias
Hypertension
Headache
Dizziness

Cardiovascular effects. Methylxanthines have positive chronotropic and inotropic effects on the heart. They are potent vasodilators and may have a beneficial effect in left ventricular failure. Tachyarrhythmias occur with therapeutic doses.

Renal effects. Methylxanthines cause increased urine output which may be related to an effect on tubular function or may be an indirect effect of the increased cardiac output.

Miscellaneous effects. Methylxanthines are known to increase gastric acid secretion and promote gastro-oesophageal reflux.

Uses

Methylxanthines are the second line of bronchodilators if β_2-agonists alone are not effective or are only partly effective. They are particularly useful in COPD. Recently, they have been shown to improve exercise tolerance in intensive care patients who are on a weaning programme.

Dosage and administration

Aminophylline is a strong alkaline solution and should *never* be given intramuscularly or subcutaneously. Oral sustained release tablets are available; the dosage is 225–450 mg (6–12 mg kg^{-1} in children) twice daily. For i.v. administration, the loading dose of aminophylline is 5 mg kg^{-1} (slow injection over 20 min) followed by an infusion of 0.5 mg kg^{-1} h^{-1}. If the patient is already taking theophylline, then half the loading dose should be given and the plasma concentration should be checked frequently.

There is a close relationship between the degree of bronchial dilatation and the plasma concentration of theophylline. A concentration of less then 10 mg L^{-1} is associated with a mild effect and a concentration of more than 25 mg L^{-1} is associated with frequent side-effects. Consequently, the therapeutic window is narrow and the plasma concentration should be maintained within the range 10–20 mg L^{-1}. Approximately 40% of the drug is protein-bound. Theophylline is metabolized mainly in the liver by cytochrome P450 and P448 microenzymes; 10% is excreted unchanged in urine. Factors which affect the activity of hepatic enzymes and thus the clearance of the drug are summarized in Table 10.6. The infusion rate of aminophylline should be adjusted accordingly (e.g. 1.6 times for smokers, 0.6 times for patients receiving cimetidine). Frequent estimation of plasma concentration is required to prevent undertreatment or toxicity.

Adverse effects

Adverse effects of methylxanthines are frequent (Table 10.7). They are more likely to occur in patients who are already receiving other β-agonist bronchodilators or sympathomimetic drugs. Extreme care should be exercised in the presence of hypoxaemia, hypercapnia, dehydration, hypokalaemia or cardiac arrhythmias. Patients receiving intravenous theophylline must be monitored closely. Death caused by gross hypokalaemia and cardiac arrhythmias has been reported.

If toxic symptoms develop, administration of the drug should be discontinued. Symptomatic treatment should be provided. The serum potassium concentration should be measured, and corrected if necessary. In some cases, haemodialysis may be required to hasten elimination of the drug.

Table 10.5 Respiratory effects of methylxanthines
Specific
Bronchodilatation by phosphodiesterase inhibition
Non-specific but complementary
Increased mucociliary clearance
Decreased mediator release
Decreased microvascular leakage
Decreased airway oedema
Increased contraction of fatigued respiratory muscles

Table 10.6 Factors affecting the plasma concentration of methylxanthines for a given dose
Factors which lower the plasma concentration
Children
Smoking
Enzyme induction – rifampicin, ethanol
Increased protein diet
Reduced carbohydrate diet
Factors which reduce clearance and thus increase plasma concentration
Old age
Congestive heart failure
Liver disease – cirrhosis
Pneumonia
Viral infection or vaccination
Increased carbohydrate diet
Enzyme inhibition – cimetidine, erythromycin

Table 10.7 Common adverse effects of methylxanthines
Nausea and vomiting
Gastrointestinal upset
Gastro-oesophageal reflux
Headache and restlessness
Diuresis
Arrhythmias
Seizures
Hypokalaemia

Anticholinergic drugs

The use of anticholinergic agents for their bronchodilator properties dates back two centuries when datura plants were smoked for the relief of asthma. Atropine was used later but the side-effects, particularly dry secretions, made it unpopular. Less soluble ammonia compounds such as ipratropium were then introduced. Ipratropium is active topically and there is little systemic absorption from the respiratory or gastrointestinal tract. It has been suggested that the cholinergic mechanism (increased intracellular cGMP) may be responsible for hyperreactive airways. Thus ipratropium is effective in both prevention and treatment of reflex bronchoconstriction. Mast cell stabilization has also been proposed as a complementary mechanism of action. The maximum effect occurs 30–60 min after inhalation. The effect may persist for up to 8 h.

Uses

Ipratropium is a second-line bronchodilator which has an additive effect when used with β-agonists. Its safety profile is well proven may it is used in both acute asthma and COPD. It is particularly effective in older patients with COPD.

Dosage and administration

Ipratropium is used as an aerosol, which delivers 20 μg per puff. The dose is 1–2 puffs three to four times daily. It may also be delivered in a nebulized form; 2–3 ml of a solution containing 250 $\mu g\ ml^{-1}$ is used.

Adverse effects

These are uncommon, but include dry secretions, a bitter taste and exacerbation of glaucoma (caused by direct effects of the nebulized drug on the eye).

MEMBRANE STABILIZERS

Disodium cromoglycate

This is a derivative of khellin, an Egyptian herbal remedy which was found to protect bronchi against allergens. It has no intrinsic bronchodilator effect.

The main mechanism of action of disodium cromoglycate is the stabilization of the mast cell membrane, which in turn inhibits the release of mediators by allergens. It closes the calcium channels and thus prevents the entry of calcium ions, which trigger mast cell degranulation. Long-term treatment with this drug reduces hyperreactivity of the bronchial tree. Other possible mechanisms include an interaction with sensory nerves and effects on other inflammatory cells including macrophages and eosinophils.

Uses

Disodium cromoglycate reduces or prevents bronchospasm in children and adults who suffer from mild asthma, especially if it is exacerbated by fog or exercise. It is also useful in allergic rhinitis and conjunctivitis. To be effective, it needs to be administered frequently (up to four times a day) even if the patient is symptom-free.

Dosage and administration

Disodium cromogylcate is not soluble and is not absorbed after oral administration. It is administered as an inhaled metered dose (50 μg per puff).

Adverse effects

These are rare, but include cough, wheeze (pre-treatment with a β_2-agonist prevents it), pharyngeal discomfort and a transient rash and urticaria in patients with pulmonary eosinophilia.

ANTI-INFLAMMATORY AGENTS

Steroids

Steroids remain the most effective anti-inflammatory agents for lung disease. A variety of mechanisms may be involved in achieving the anti-inflammatory effects (Table 10.8). There is growing evidence that hyperreactive airways are the result of an inflammatory process. Steroids reduce hyperreactivity of airways but have no direct bronchodilator effect. The anti-asthma property of an inhaled steroid is proportional to its anti-inflammatory potency. In addition to their anti-inflammatory actions, steroids sensitize β_2-adrenoceptors to the effects of agonists, increase the receptor population and prevent tachyphylaxis.

Uses

The main indications are

- asthma
- COPD
- sarcoidosis
- interstitial lung disease
- pulmonary eosinophilia.

Steroids are a second-line treatment in acute asthma. There is a delayed onset of action, with a peak effect about 6–12 h after intravenous administration. Steroids are of particular use in acute severe asthma (but not for an immediate effect) and in acute exacerbations of COPD. They are also effective in reducing the frequency and severity of acute episodes in chronic asthma. Intravenous hydrocortisone reduces the duration of hospital

Table 10.8 Sites of action and mechanisms of anti-inflammatory effects of steroids

Intracellular steroid receptors. Steroid-receptor complex alters the transcription of genes leading to altered protein synthesis
Lipocortin. Increase in production of lipocortin which inhibits the release of arachidonic acid metabolites and platelet-activating factor from lung and macrophages
Eosinophils. Decrease in the number of eosinophils and inhibition of degranulation
'T' lymphocytes. Reduction in the number of 'T' lymphocytes and the production of cytokines
Macrophages. Reduced secretion of leukotrienes and prostaglandin
Endothelial cells. Reduction of the leak around endothelial cells
Airway smooth muscle β_2-adrenoceptors. Increased sensitivity of β_2-adrenoceptors and therefore augmentation of the effect of agonists together with increase in receptor density and prevention of tachyphylaxis
Mucous glands. Reduced mucus secretions

admission in patients with asthma. Some patients with COPD also benefit from the long-term use of inhaled steroids.

Dosage and administration

Prednisolone may be administered orally in a dose of 30–40 mg daily, reducing later to 10–15 mg daily. Prednisolone is absorbed rapidly after oral administration. Ninety per cent of the drug is protein-bound and it is metabolized by the liver. Enzyme induction by ethanol or rifampicin reduces the half-life of prednisolone.

Hydrocortisone is the drug of choice for intravenous administration. The dose is 3–4 mg kg^{-1} 6-hourly.

Administration by inhalation is preferred for chronic use because it is associated with delivery of a lower dose and with a reduced incidence of systemic side-effects. Beclomethasone is used in a dose of 400–500 µg daily. Inhaled steroids may be absorbed systemically either by surface absorption or by swallowed pharyngeal deposits.

Adverse effects

Steroids are well known for their widespread side-effects, which involve almost every system. Systemic effects are less likely with inhaled steroids, but the local effects may be troublesome. The high incidence of adverse effects is the main factor which limits the long-term use of steroids in clinical practice. If it is necessary to use steroids, the dose should be adjusted to achieve the optimal balance between clinical benefit and adverse effects. The adverse effects of steroids are summarized in Table 10.9.

Table 10.9 Common adverse effects of steroids
Local (inhaled steroids)
Hoarseness
Oral pharyngeal candidiasis
Throat irritation and cough
Systemic
Adrenergic suppression
Fluid retention
Hypertension
Peptic ulceration
Diabetes mellitus
Increased appetite
Weight gain
Bruising and skin thinning
Increased bone metabolism, osteoporosis
Cataracts
Stunted growth in children
Psychosis

DRUGS ACTING ON PULMONARY VESSELS

A rational approach to manipulating pulmonary vascular tone relies on the understanding of the complex physiological and pathophysiological control of pulmonary resistance vessels. The underlying mechanisms are not fully understood, but there are several broad principles which have been recognized recently:

- Lungs and pulmonary vessels produce and metabolize many vasoactive substances.
- The adrenergic nerves innervate pulmonary vessels; α-stimulation causes vasoconstriction and β-stimulation causes vasodilatation.
- Arachidonic acid metabolites may cause vasoconstriction (thromboxane) or vasodilatation (prostaglandins PGI_2 and PGD_2).
- Oxygen has a strong influence on the pulmonary blood vessels; hypoxia constricts the vessels and oxygen inhalation dilates them.
- Acetylcholine, ATP and bradykinin cause vasodilatation via a specific receptor to produce endothelium-derived relaxing factor (EDRF) and/or endothelium-derived nitric oxide (EDNO), which diffuses into muscle cells to increase the concentration of cyclic GMP, resulting in vasodilatation.

The therapeutic value of drugs acting on pulmonary vessels is mainly as a means of reducing pulmonary vascular resistance. Occasionally, increased pulmonary vascular resistance may be desirable in order to obtain temporary relief in some congenital heart diseases with a large left-to-right shunt. A decrease in pulmonary vascular resistance causes a reduction in right heart afterload. Usually, oxygen inhalation is sufficient to obtain a moderate decrease in pulmonary vascular resistance, but drugs may be needed if more profound vasodilatation is required. It is important to remember that these measures are only helpful if there is a reversible element to the increased pulmonary vascular resistance.

Drugs affecting the pulmonary vascular resistance are summarized in Table 10.10. They may be used either for initial diagnostic or therapeutic evaluation, or for long-term management of pulmonary hypertension, in a variety of clinical conditions:

- primary pulmonary hypertension
- congenital heart disease
- mitral valve disease
- COPD and cor pulmonale
- acute respiratory distress syndrome (ARDS)
- acute respiratory failure
- acute pulmonary oedema.

Pulmonary vasodilators may be administered either by systemic vascular infusion or by inhalation (oxygen, nitric oxide). In patients with acute respiratory failure and/or ARDS, systemic pulmonary vasodilators may worsen the clinical situation, whilst inhaled pulmonary vasodilators may improve it.

INITIAL DIAGNOSTIC AND THERAPEUTIC EVALUATION

Initial evaluation aims to ascertain simply and safely whether significant and reversible pulmonary vasoconstriction is present. Accurate evaluation of pulmonary vascular reactivity requires direct measurement of pulmonary arterial pressure and pulmonary blood flow. Non-invasive approaches using Doppler techniques are not yet sufficiently accurate to obviate an invasive approach. However, an improvement in oxygenation is an indirect measure of the success of therapy. To evaluate vascular reactivity, the agents with the least side-effects and shortest duration of action should be used.

Table 10.10 Factors affecting pulmonary vascular resistance

Factors increasing pulmonary vascular resistance
Hypoxia
Acidosis
α-Adrenergic agonists
β-Adrenergic antagonists
Protamine
Histamine
Serotonin
Angiotensin II
Thromboxane
Factors decreasing pulmonary vascular resistance
Oxygen
Alkalosis
α-Adrenergic antagonists
β-Adrenergic agonists
Prostaglandins PGI_2 and PGD_2
Calcium channel blockers
ACE inhibitors
Acetylcholine
Aminophylline
Nitrates and nitrites
Nitric oxide
Sodium nitroprusside
Hydralazine
Diazoxide

Inhalation of 100% oxygen for at least 10 min is sufficient to demonstrate a change in most cases. Tolazoline hydrochloride (an α-antagonist and a directly acting vasodilator) in a dose of 0.5–1.0 mg kg^{-1} given over 30 s into the right atrium or pulmonary artery is probably the most commonly used agent for evaluating the pulmonary vascular response in individuals with congenital heart disease. It has the disadvantage of significant systemic effects (hypotension, tachycardia) which limit the dose that can be given. Other agents that have been used and are being evaluated include acetylcholine, prostaglandin PGI_2, nitroprusside and ATP-magnesium chloride infusion.

LONG-TERM MANAGEMENT WITH VASODILATORS

Oxygen

In acute forms of specific hypoxic pulmonary vasoconstriction such as high altitude pulmonary hypertension, increasing the inspired oxygen concentration immediately can be life-saving; descent to lower altitude is curative. In chronic forms of lung disease, particularly COPD, oxygen assists management by reducing pulmonary vascular resistance to varying degrees and therefore reducing the severity of cor pulmonale. In these patients, administration of oxygen should be as continuous as is feasible and should continue during sleep. In general, the beneficial effects are only modest and in most instances oxygen is supplemented by at least one other vasodilator.

Adrenergic agonists and antagonists

Tolazoline, phentolamine and prazosin have been used for their α-adrenergic blocking effect. Trials of long-term therapy have been inconclusive. β-Adrenergic stimulation by isoprenaline and terbutaline has also been used. These agents are not uniformly effective and are associated with significant side-effects including angina, tachycardia, arrhythmias and tremors. Children with congenital heart disease and pulmonary vascular disease often have hyperreactive pulmonary vessels and may develop a pulmonary hypertensive crisis postoperatively, especially during tracheal suction and weaning from the ventilator. These episodes may be managed with adequate sedation, intrathecal lidocaine before tracheal suction and systemic α-adrenergic blockade.

Calcium channel blockers

All three of the currently available agents (verapamil, diltiazem and nifedipine) prevent hypoxia-induced pulmonary vasoconstriction. Clinical trials of long-term oral treatment with diltiazem or nifedipine have shown some improvement in survival of a subset of patients with primary pulmonary hypertension.

Arachidonic acid metabolites

PGI_2 is a pulmonary vasodilator. Continuous infusion of PGI_2 has been used in pulmonary hypertension, but systemic hypotension may be a problem. Non-steroidal anti-inflammatory drugs such as indomethacin or aspirin inhibit production of PGI_2; these agents may accentuate hypoxic pulmonary vasoconstriction.

Directly acting agents

Hydralazine and tolazoline are direct pulmonary vasodilators (tolazoline has an α-blocking effect as well). Only tolazoline has been used with success (see above). Inhaled nitric oxide has gained immense popularity recently. Its pharmacology and clinical role are discussed below.

Miscellaneous agents

Theophylline, used mainly as a bronchodilator, also has a direct dilator effect on the pulmonary vasculature. Angiotensin II increases pulmonary vascular resistance, and captopril, an angiotensin II inhibitor, reduces pulmonary vascular resistance. Long-term treatment with captopril has proved beneficial in some studies.

Nitric oxide

Nitric oxide is produced endogenously by vascular epithelium. The production is modulated by shear stress in the vessel wall; this ensures a constant basal production. In 1991, it was first used therapeutically in patients who had pulmonary hypertension and respiratory failure.

Organic nitrates and nitrites relax smooth muscle in both arteries and veins. They release nitric oxide, which results in cyclic GMP-mediated smooth muscle relaxation. Studies have indicated that systemic administration of these agents results in significant relief of pulmonary hypertension. Intravenous glyceryl trinitrate is effective when relief is required immediately. On a long-term basis, sublingual isosorbide, in combination with another vasodilator, provides effective treatment. Intravenous sodium nitrite also appears to be an effective pulmonary vasodilator.

In some respiratory conditions, such as ARDS, a combination of hypoxaemia, hypercapnia and acidosis promotes excessive pulmonary vasoconstriction, particularly in hypoventilated areas of the lung. Other factors that may aggravate this disproportionate vasoconstriction include platelet aggregation, white cell aggregation and cytokine release. Pulmonary vasoconstriction in ARDS may be regarded either as an increased afterload on the right ventricle or as a locally protective mechanism which reduces ventilation–perfusion mismatch (i.e. hypoventilated areas receive less blood supply; Fig. 10.2). Intravenous systemic vasodilators act on pulmonary vasculature as a whole and induce vasodilatation simultaneously in well ventilated and poorly ventilated alveolar units. Thus the proportion of total pulmonary blood flow which perfuses the hypoventilated areas increases. This leads to an increase in shunt fraction and deterioration in the oxygenation of arterial blood.

In contrast, an inhaled vasodilator (nitric oxide) is delivered preferentially to the well ventilated areas and thus causes vasodilatation primarily in those areas. Consequently, the proportion of total pulmonary blood flow that perfuses the hypoventilated areas decreases. This leads to a decrease in shunt fraction and an improvement in oxygenation of arterial blood (Fig. 10.2). The other main site of action of inhaled nitric oxide is the bronchial tree; there, it causes bronchodilatation. These advantages of inhaled nitric oxide over intravenous vasodilators have led to the surge in its popularity in recent years. Administration of other vasodilators such as PGI_2 and tolazoline by inhalation is currently under investigation.

Table 10.11 The main clinical indications for administration of inhaled nitric oxide

Acute respiratory distress syndrome
Neonatal hypoxic respiratory failure
Lung transplant
Increased right heart afterload and impaired right ventricular function after cardiac surgery
Mitral valve disease
Right ventricular infarction
Heart transplant

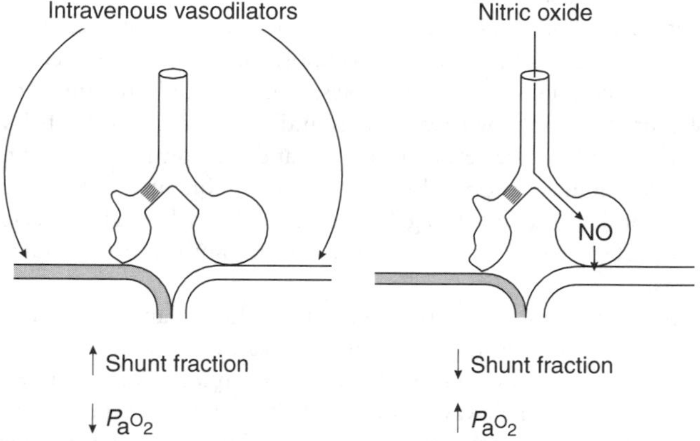

Fig. 10.2
Pulmonary vasodilators, on systemic administration, dilate the vessels supplying hypoventilated areas in addition to adequately ventilated areas; this may result in an increase in shunt fraction and deterioration in oxygenation of arterial blood. Inhaled vasodilators, such as nitric oxide, are delivered preferentially to the well ventilated areas; this results in a decrease in shunt fraction and an improvement in oxygenation of arterial blood.

Uses

In a dose of 40–80 ppm, nitric oxide has been used as a pulmonary vasodilator in a wide variety of conditions. The main indications for inhaled nitric oxide are shown in Table 10.11. In all these situations, inhaled nitric oxide has been shown to reduce pulmonary vascular resistance, reduce right ventricular wall stress, increase coronary artery blood flow, reduce the need for inotropic support, increase right ventricular output and increase systemic cardiac output.

In addition, bronchodilatation and reduction in shunt fraction result in an improvement in oxygenation in patients with ARDS. In neonates, nitric oxide also helps to keep the ductus arteriosus closed and has been shown to reduce the need for extracorporeal membrane oxygenation (ECMO).

Another advantage of inhaled nitric oxide is that it does not produce significant systemic effects. This is because inhaled nitric oxide first diffuses through the alveoli to reach vascular smooth muscle and then through the endothelial cells to reach the bloodstream, where it is inactivated rapidly by haemoglobin.

Dosage and administration

Nitric oxide is stored in concentrations of 1000 ppm in nitrogen (in oxygen it is converted into higher oxides). For clinical use, it is diluted in an air–oxygen mixture to produce concentrations of 20–100 ppm. It is delivered through a mechanical ventilator. In the pulmonary bloodstream, it is inactivated rapidly as it combines with haemoglobin to form mainly nitrosyl-haemoglobin (NOHb) but also some methaemoglobin and nitrates. Nitric oxide has an effective half-life of 0.5–1.0 s. NOHb is converted into nitrites and nitrates which are excreted by the kidney.

The toxicity of nitric oxide is related to the total amount delivered and to its concentration. Consequently, the design of the delivery system is crucial for the safety of patients. Several delivery systems are now available. Monitoring the levels of nitric oxide and higher oxides (NO_2) is essential with all systems.

Adverse effects

Because of its single unpaired electron, nitric oxide is also a free radical and is potentially harmful. Both endogenous and exogenous nitric oxide react readily with oxygen, water, superoxide, nucleotides, metalloproteins, amines and lipids. Biochemical end-products of these reactions can lead to an array of toxic effects. The following have been demonstrated in experimental and/or clinical settings:

- lipid peroxidation
- impaired mitochondrial function
- mutagenesis
- prolonged bleeding time
- impaired surfactant function.

It is difficult to wean some patients from nitric oxide. This difficulty is related mainly to rebound pulmonary hypertension on withdrawal of nitric oxide. Underlying mechanisms include lack of endogenous nitric oxide and the exaggerated constrictive response of pulmonary vessels to hypoxia. In some patients, sudden withdrawal of nitric oxide may precipitate life-threatening pulmonary hypertension and deterioration in gas exchange.

DRUGS ACTING ON MUCOCILIARY FUNCTION

The effectiveness of the mucociliary system depends upon the integrity of the mucus 'blanket' and ciliary motility. The 'blanket' is a high-viscosity mucopolysaccharide gel floating over a low-viscosity serous layer. In health, secretions from goblet cells and bronchial glands maintain the composition of airway secretions. The goblet cells secrete mucopolysaccharides and are stimulated by irritant factors; their response is under local control. Bronchial gland secretions are serous in nature and are controlled by vagal stimulation in addition to local factors. Consequently, both stimulation and blockade of vagal tone affect bronchial gland secretions. The secretions are reduced by administration of opioid drugs.

Cilia are important in propelling the outer 'blanket' of mucus (with entrapped dust, soot or microorganisms) over the serous layer. They act in unison to set the flow of mucus from peripheral airways to central airways from which the mucus is expectorated. Several factors affect ciliary movement and thus mucociliary function. These are summarized in Table 10.12. It is also important to realize that impaired mucociliary function has an indirect effect on the viability of surfactant. Drugs used to improve mucokinetics may be classified as hydrating agents or mucolytics.

HYDRATING AGENTS

Aerosolized water and good systemic hydration help mucociliary clearance. Aerosolized saline may provoke bronchospasm. Hypertonic saline is administered if irritation is desired to provoke ciliary clearance. Hypotonic saline is used for hydration.

Table 10.12 Factors affecting mucociliary function

Factors that depress mucociliary function
Extremes of temperature
Acidic environment
Smoking
Dehydration
Alcohol
Atropine
Anaesthetics
Dry gases
Opioids
Factors that optimize mucociliary function
Temperature (airway) range 29–34°C
Hydration
Humidification
Sympathomimetics
Methylxanthines

Humidification

In health, the upper airways warm and humidify the inspired gases. In disease or when the upper airway is bypassed (mouth breathing, tracheal intubation), inspiration of dry, cold gases results in increased viscosity of mucus, depressed ciliary function, impaired surfactant function, airway obstruction by tenacious secretions, tracheal inflammation and mucosal ulceration. For these reasons, the inspired gases delivered via a tracheal tube should be saturated with water vapour at body temperature.

Methods of humidification

A variety of methods may be used to achieve humidification of the inspired gases. These include condensers (heat and moisture exchangers), cold water bubble humidifiers, hot water bath humidifiers, and aerosol generators. The details of each method are beyond the scope of this chapter. Condensers are less efficient than heated humidifiers but are useful for short-term humidification. Cold water bubble humidifiers are inefficient and unnecessary; they also have an increased risk of microbial infection. Heated water bath humidifiers are commonly used in intensive care units; the disadvantages are condensation of water, risk of infection and thermostat malfunction. Aerosol generators are effective and may be used with a face mask or mechanical ventilator; the disadvantages include infection and overhydration.

MUCOLYTICS

Cysteine derivatives such as *n*-acetylcysteine may cause mucolysis. *n*-Acetylcysteine may be given systemically or by inhalation. However, because of its unpleasant odour, irritation of the upper airway and bronchospasm, its use seems to be associated with more problems than benefits. The results of trials in patients with COPD have been disappointing.

SURFACTANT REPLACEMENT THERAPY

Natural surfactant is produced by type II cells in the alveolar epithelium. It is a lipoprotein of complex structure. It lines the alveoli and reduces the surface tension at the air–alveolar interface to prevent the alveoli from collapsing during expiration. An inadequate quantity or quality of endogenous surfactant causes reduced compliance and atelectasis of the lungs, increased pressure gradient between capillaries and pulmonary interstitial space (leading to interstitial oedema), increased work of breathing, increased shunt fraction and hypoxaemia.

In order to reduce surface tension during expiration, natural surfactant forms a mobile and flexible surface film that expands and collapses with the change in alveolar surface area that occurs throughout the respiratory cycle. In order to do so, it must be capable of adsorbing rapidly to the surface of the air–liquid interface, re-spreading rapidly at the onset of inspiration and forming a stable film that is capable of lowering surface tension to a very low value. No single synthetic substance exhibits all of these properties of functional surfactant; this is one of the difficulties in replacing natural surfactant with an artificial compound. The most surface-active phospholipid (85% of surfactant) in natural surfactant is dipalmitoylphosphatidyl choline. However, when administer-

alone, this phospholipid is ineffective because it does not spread and absorb effectively under physiological conditions. It is necessary to co-administer various other protein components to achieve adequate spread and adsorption.

In infants with respiratory distress syndrome (RDS) the production of natural surfactant is inadequate. In ARDS there is either inadequate production or poor quality of natural surfactant caused by endogenous (capillary leak, endothelial damage, sepsis) or exogenous (smoke inhalation, drowning, aspiration of gastric contents) factors. Administration of artificial surfactant has established its role in RDS in neonates, but in ARDS there is no convincing evidence that it offers benefit.

To date, the following substances have been investigated for their potential to replace exogenous surfactant:

- natural surfactants isolated from human amniotic fluid aspirated during Caesarean section for term pregnancy
- natural preparations from minced calf or porcine lungs
- semi-synthetic mixtures of minced calf lung extract with surfactant phospholipid
- synthetic surfactant preparations containing a mixture of dipalmitoylphosphatidyl choline and dispersing and emulsifying agents.

Human surfactant from healthy subjects would be the ideal replacement, but practical difficulties in obtaining sufficient quantities and the risk of transmission of infections (cytomegalovirus, herpes, HIV) restrict its use. Bovine extracts have been used with some success in RDS of neonates, but the potential remains for infection and immunological reactions to the foreign protein content. Synthetic surfactants are protein-free and there is no threat of transmission of infection.

Exosurf

This is a sterile, protein-free, synthetic preparation which is presented as lyophilized powder stored in a vacuum. It contains 80% dipalmitoylphosphatidyl choline mixed with hexadecanol and tyloxapol. The blend of these three components achieves the biophysical properties necessary for pulmonary surfactant to prevent alveolar collapse during expiration. Dipalmitoyphosphatidyl choline decreases the surface tension and the other two compounds facilitate its rapid spread and adsorption to the air–fluid interface during the respiratory cycle.

Uses

In RDS in infants who weigh more than 700 g, the use of Exosurf has shown promise:

- 66% reduction in mortality from RDS
- 44% reduction in 1-year mortality from any other cause
- improvement in survival without bronchopulmonary dysplasia
- reduction in incidences of pneumothorax and pulmonary interstitial oedema
- reduction in the number of days of mechanical ventilation
- reduction in the incidence of patent ductus arteriosus
- no change in the incidence of infection or sepsis.

In ARDS, no definite advantage has been shown to date.

Adverse effects

In neonates, the use of Exosurf is associated with an increased incidence of apnoea. Other adverse effects include episodes of transient oxygen desaturation (followed by improvement) and mucus plugging.

FURTHER READING

Berge K H, Warner D O 2000 Drugs that affect the respiratory system. In: Hemmings H, Hopkins P (eds) Foundations of anaesthesia. Mosby, London

Laurence D R, Bennett P N, Brown M J 1997 Clinical pharmacology. Churchill Livingstone, London

Murphy A W, Platts-Mills T A E 1998 Drugs used in asthma and obstructive lung disease. In: Brody T M, Larner J, Minneman K P (eds) Human pharmacology molecular to clinical. Mosby, Philadelphia

11 Anatomy of the nervous system

This chapter describes the structure and blood supply of the brain and spinal cord, the major pathways in the central nervous system and the anatomy of the cranial nerves. Relevant information on the anatomy of peripheral nerves and major nerve plexuses is found in Chapter 43.

THE BRAIN

The brain comprises the brain stem, the cerebellum, the midbrain, and the paired cerebral hemispheres.

BRAIN STEM

The brain stem is formed from the medulla and the pons, with the medulla connected to the spinal cord below and with the cerebellum posteriorly. The medulla contains the ascending and descending nerve tracts, the lower cranial nerve nuclei and the respiratory and vasomotor (or vital) centres. It has two swellings on its anterior surface, termed the pyramids. These contain the fibres of the descending corticospinal tracts, which are therefore sometimes referred to as the pyramidal tracts. The majority of the descending fibres cross (or decussate) to the opposite side of the brain stem at the level of the lower medulla. The ascending sensory fibres from the posterior columns of the spinal cord also decussate in the medulla. The pons connects the medulla to the midbrain and is also connected to the cerebellum. Running through the brain stem is the reticular system which is associated with consciousness. The brain stem constitutes a great highway of information between the brain and the spinal cord and contains many important structures, including the vital centres. A lesion or compression of the brain stem secondary to raised intracranial pressure produces abnormal function of the vital centres that is rapidly fatal (coning).

CEREBELLUM

The cerebellum occupies the posterior fossa of the cranium below the tentorium cerebelli. The cerebellum consists of two cerebellar hemispheres joined together by the vermis and is connected to the midbrain and the brain stem. The cerebellum coordinates balance, posture and muscular tone. Cerebellar lesions cause signs on the same side of the body.

MIDBRAIN

The midbrain connects the pons and cerebellum to the hypothalamus, the thalamus and the cerebral hemispheres.

CEREBRUM

The cerebrum consists of the diencephalon and the two cerebral hemispheres.

Diencephalon

The diencephalon is the central part of the forebrain and consists of the thalamus and the hypothalamus. The thalamus contains the nuclei of the main sensory pathways. The hypothalamus coordinates the autonomic nervous system and the endocrine systems of the body. Below the hypothalamus is the pituitary gland. Pituitary tumours may produce the signs of a space-occupying lesion or restrict the visual fields by compressing the optic chiasma or give rise to an endocrine disturbance.

Cerebral hemispheres

The cerebral hemispheres comprise the cerebral cortex, the basal ganglia and the lateral ventricles. The two hemispheres are separated by a deep cleft into which the falx cerebri projects. The surface of the cortex is thrown into folds or gyri which are separated from each other by clefts or sulci. The central sulcus separates the main motor gyrus anteriorly from the main sensory gyrus posteriorly. Each hemisphere is divided into four areas or lobes. These are demarcated both anatomically and functionally. They are the frontal, parietal, temporal and occipital lobes. The medial part of the cortex also contains the limbic system which is associated with emotion and behaviour. The function of the four lobes is incompletely understood. However, the frontal lobe contains the motor cortex and areas concerned with intellect and behaviour. The parietal lobe contains the sensory cortex, the temporal lobe is concerned with auditory sensation and the integration of other stimuli, and the occipital lobe contains the visual cortex. Lesions of the cerebral hemispheres give rise to sensory and motor deficits on the opposite side of the body. The two hemispheres are linked through the fibres of the corpus callosum. The exact function of the basal ganglia is not known, but they are involved in controlling motor function. Between the basal ganglia and the thalamus lies the internal capsule containing the descending motor tracts from the cerebral cortex.

THE SPINAL CORD

The spinal cord is 45 cm long and passes from the foramen magnum, where it is continuous with the medulla, to a tapered end termed the conus medullaris at the level of the first or second lumbar vertebrae. The cord is roughly cylindrical in shape but expands at the cervical and lumbar levels corresponding with the origins of the brachial and the lumbosacral plexuses, respectively. At each spinal level, paired anterior (motor) and posterior (sensory) spinal roots emerge on each side of the cord. Each posterior root has a ganglion containing the cell bodies of the sensory nerves. The roots join at each intervertebral foramen to form a mixed spinal nerve. The roots lengthen progressively towards the lower end of the cord. The cervical roots (of which there are eight) arise from the cord opposite the corresponding intervertebral foramina. However, as the cord finishes at the upper lumbar level, the roots of the lower thoracic, the lumbar and especially the sacral levels must become progressively longer to pass down from where they exit the cord to their corresponding foramina. The collection of nerve roots below the end of the cord passing through cerebrospinal fluid (CSF) in the dural sac into the sacrum is termed the cauda equina.

The cord comprises a central canal containing CSF, surrounded by grey matter with anterior and posterior horns, which is itself surrounded by white matter containing the ascending and descending tracts in anterior, posterior and lateral columns (Fig. 11.1). The anterior horns of grey matter contain the motor nerve cells. Some peripheral sensory nerves synapse in the posterior horns. From the first thoracic to the second lumbar level, there is an additional lateral horn which contains the cell bodies of the first-order neurones of the sympathetic nervous system.

CEREBROSPINAL FLUID

Cerebrospinal fluid fills the cerebral ventricles and the subarachnoid space around the brain and the spinal cord. The CSF acts as a buffer separating the brain and spinal cord from the hard bony projections inside the skull and the vertebral canal. It is produced by the choroid plexus in the lateral, third and fourth ventricles by a combination of filtration and secretion (Fig. 11.2). The total volume of CSF is 150–200 ml. It flows from the lateral ventricles into the third ventricle through the interventricular foramina of Monro. The third ventricle is a narrow cleft between the two thalami. CSF passes from the third to the fourth ventricle along the cerebral aqueduct of the midbrain and leaves the fourth ventricle through the median foramen of Magendie and the two lateral foramina of Luschka to enter the subarachnoid space. The fourth ventricle also communicates with the central canal of the spinal cord. CSF passes back into the venous blood through arachnoid villi. These are diverticuli of the arachnoid mater through the dura mater into the dural venous sinuses. The normal CSF pressure, measured with the patient lying in the lateral position, is 7–15 cm H_2O. The CSF pressure fluctuates as a result of respiration and arterial pressure. Changes are also seen as a result of changes in venous pressure, e.g. an increase in pressure in the intrathoracic veins after coughing. Blockages which obstruct the normal flow of CSF through the ventricular system or prevent its reabsorption lead to a build-up in CSF pressure, dilatation of the ventricles and hydrocephalus.

MENINGES

Three meninges or membranes surround the brain and the spinal cord. These are the dura mater, the arachnoid mater and the pia mater.

BRAIN

Around the brain, the dura mater is a thick, strong, double membrane which separates into its two layers in parts to form the cerebral

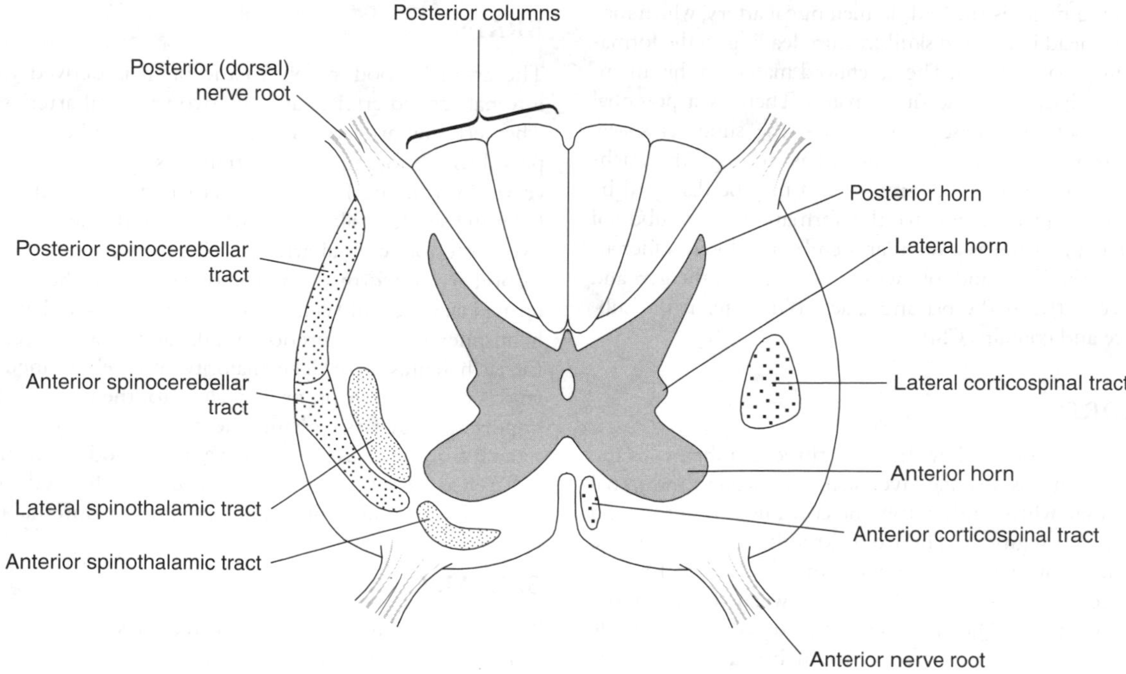

Fig. 11.1
Transverse section of the spinal cord at the mid-thoracic level.

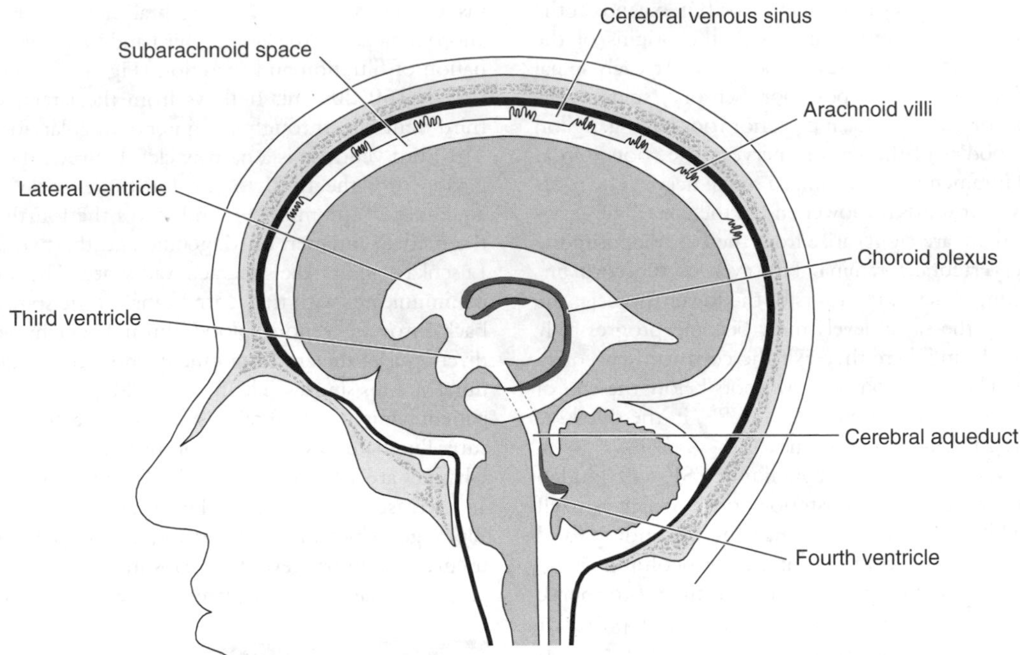

Fig. 11.2
The ventricular system and subarachnoid space.

venous sinuses. The outer or endosteal layer is strongly adherent to the skull bones and is the equivalent of the periosteum. The inner layer is continuous with the dura which surrounds the spinal cord. This inner layer has projections which help support the brain, including the falx cerebri which separates the two cerebral hemispheres and the tentorium cerebelli which separates the posterior fossa and its contents from the rest of the cranium. The major artery supplying the dura mater is the middle meningeal artery, which may be damaged in a head injury and skull fracture leading to the formation of an epidural haematoma. The arachnoid mater is a thin membrane normally adjacent to the dura mater. There is a potential space, however, between these two layers – the subdural space. Cortical veins from the surface of the brain pass through the arachnoid mater to reach dural venous sinuses and may be damaged by relatively minor trauma leading to the formation of a subdural haematoma. The pia mater is a vascular membrane closely adherent to the surface of the brain and follows the contours of the gyri and sulci. The space between the pia and arachnoid mater is the subarachnoid space and contains CSF.

SPINAL CORD

The spinal cord is surrounded by the same three membranes as the brain. The dura mater is a single-layer structure around the spinal cord. It forms a sac which ends below the cord, usually at the level of the second sacral segment. The dura extends along each nerve root and is continuous with the epineurium of each spinal nerve. There is an extensive subarachnoid space between the arachnoid mater and the pia mater. The pia mater is thickened on either side of the spinal cord and extends laterally to anchor the cord to the arachnoid and dura mater. The pia mater continues below the conus medullaris to the coccyx as the filum terminale. The space between the dura and the bony part of the spinal canal (the epidural space) is filled with fat, lymphatics, arteries and an extensive venous plexus.

VASCULAR SUPPLY

BRAIN

The arterial blood supply to the brain is derived from the two internal carotid arteries and the two vertebral arteries (Fig. 11.3). The vertebral arteries are branches of the subclavian arteries and pass through foramina in the transverse processes of the upper six cervical vertebrae. They join together anterior to the brain stem to form the single basilar artery which then divides again to form the two posterior cerebral arteries. These vessels and the two internal carotid arteries form an anastomotic system at the base of the brain termed the circle of Willis. The main arteries supplying the cerebral hemispheres are the anterior, middle and posterior cerebral arteries for each hemisphere. The majority of cerebral aneurysms are of vessels that are part of, or very close to, the circle of Willis. Other important vessels supplying the brain stem and the cerebellum branch from the basilar artery. Venous blood drains into the cerebral venous sinuses, the walls of which are formed from the dura mater. These sinuses join and empty into the internal jugular veins.

SPINAL CORD

The blood supply to the spinal cord comes from the single anterior spinal artery formed at the foramen magnum from a branch from each of the vertebral arteries, and from the paired posterior spinal arteries derived from the posterior inferior cerebellar arteries. The

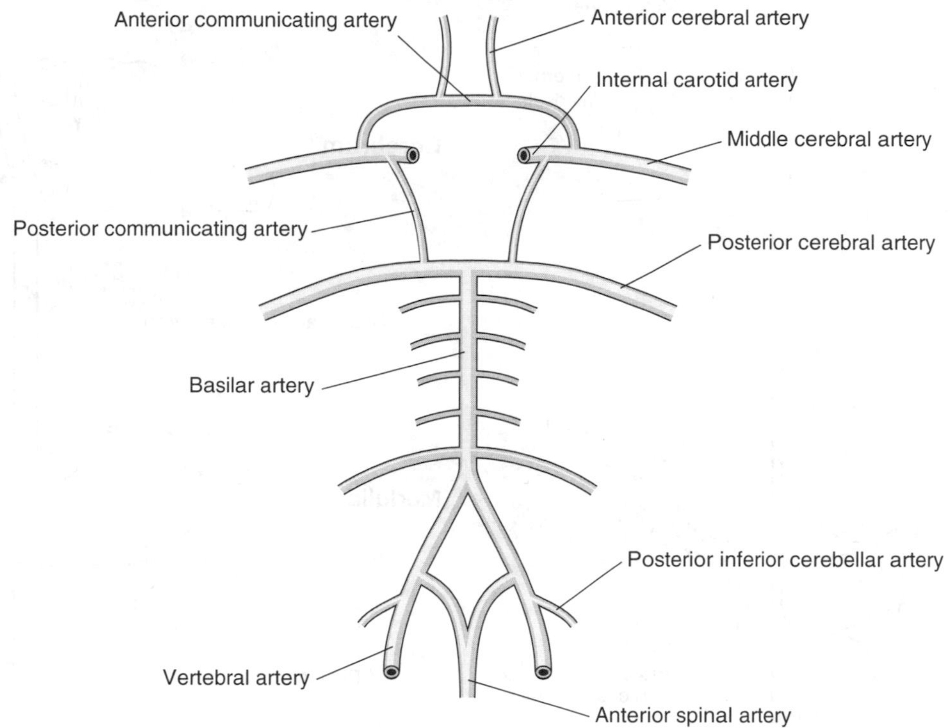

Fig. 11.3
The major arteries of the brain and the circle of Willis.

anterior artery supplies the anterior two-thirds of the cord. There are additional supplies from segmental arteries and also a direct supply from the aorta usually at the level of the 11th thoracic intervertebral space. This artery is termed the artery of Adamkiewicz and may be a major source of blood to the lower half of the spinal cord in some patients. The blood supply to the spinal cord is fragile and infarction of the cord may result from even minor disruption of the normal arterial supply.

ASCENDING AND DESCENDING NERVE TRACTS

MOTOR PATHWAYS

Efferent motor impulses pass along the descending or pyramidal tracts (Fig. 11.4). The first-order cells or upper motor neurones originate mostly from the motor (precentral) gyrus of the cerebral cortex. From here, fibres pass to the cranial nerve nuclei via the corticonuclear tracts and to the anterior horn cells in the spinal cord via the corticospinal tracts. The fibres pass between the basal ganglia and the thalamus in the internal capsule, which is supplied by the medial and lateral striate branches of the middle cerebral artery. These are frequently the site of the lesion producing a 'stroke'. Fibres passing to the spinal cord decussate mostly in the medulla and pass through the cord in the lateral corticospinal tract. Some fibres remain uncrossed in the anterior corticospinal tracts and cross to the opposite side at the level where they synapse in the anterior horn. Nerve fibres in the corticospinal tracts may synapse directly with the lower motor neurones, or synapse first with a short intermediate neurone in the anterior horn. The cell bodies of the lower motor neurones are in the anterior horn of the spinal cord and the fibres leave the cord in the anterior nerve root. Other descending tracts include the extrapyramidal tracts concerned with motor tone, coordination and posture. A lesion of the cord results in paralysis below the lesion on the same side of the body.

SENSORY PATHWAYS

The two main ascending sensory tracts are the spinothalamic tracts and the posterior columns (Fig 11.5). Usually these tracts contain three orders of neurones. The cell bodies of the first-order neurones are in the dorsal root ganglia with the peripheral part of the nerve ending either at a specialized receptor or a bare nerve ending. Many of the first-order neurones branch and contribute to reflex arcs within the spinal cord.

Spinothalamic tracts

There are two spinothalamic tracts – the anterior and the lateral – which mainly serve light touch, pain and temperature sensation. Fibres serving pain and temperature synapse in the substantia gelatinosa in the posterior horn of the cord. From here they cross the cord and ascend in the lateral spinothalamic tract. Light touch fibres follow the same path but ascend in the anterior spinothalamic tract. The second-order neurones synapse in the thalamus and the third-order neurones pass to the sensory (postcentral) gyrus of the cortex. Pain sensation from the head is carried in fibres in

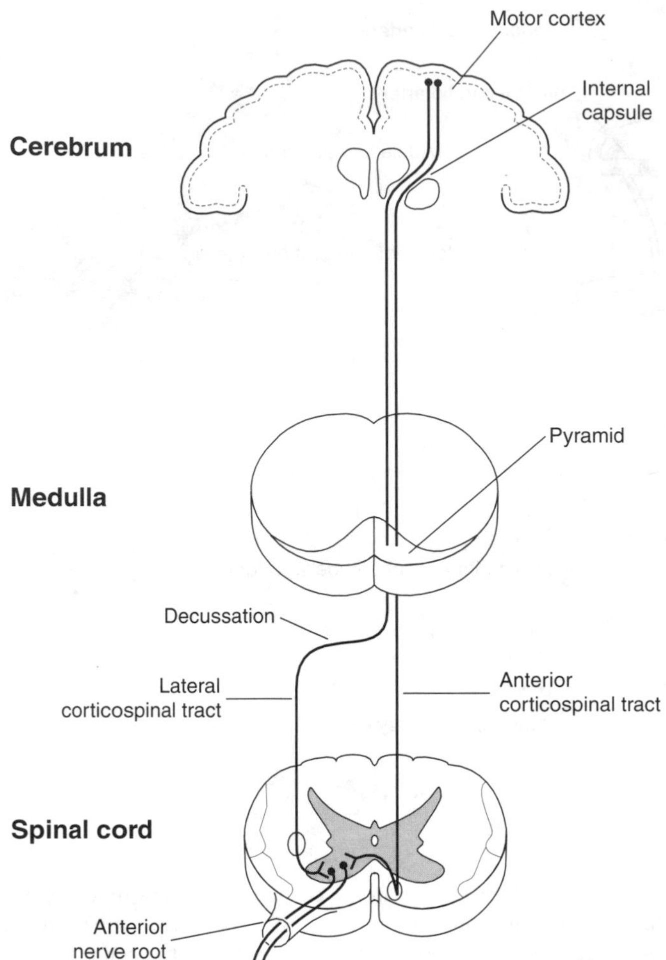

Fig. 11.4
The major descending motor pathways.

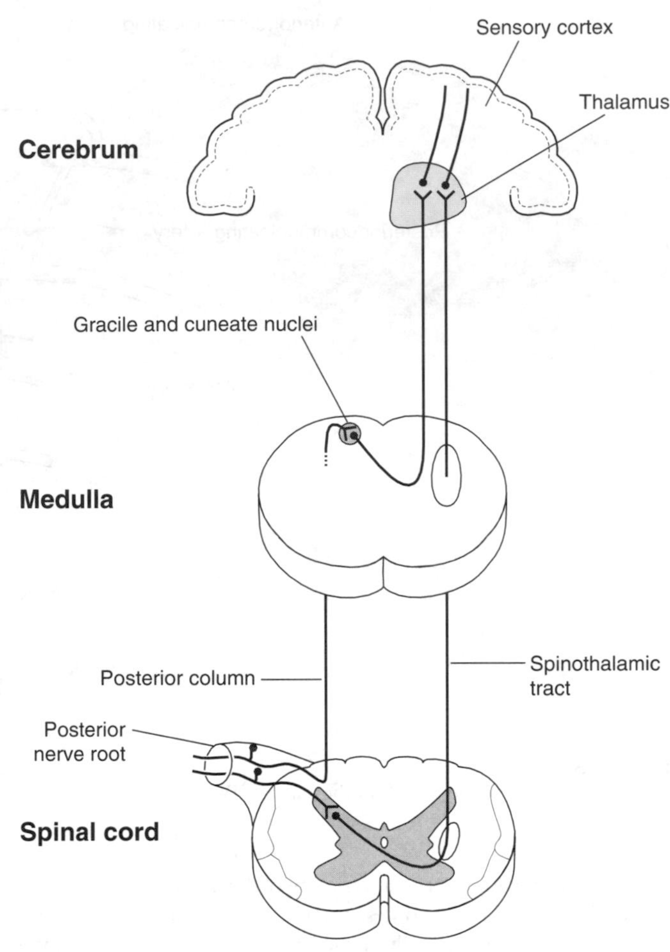

Fig. 11.5
The major ascending sensory pathways.

the Vth, VIIth and IXth cranial nerves (see below). Some areas of the brain are closely associated with modification of the sensation of pain – these are the periventricular area of the diencephalon, the periaqueductal grey matter of the midbrain and some nuclei in the brain stem. Fibres from these areas descend in the cord and modify function in the posterior horns.

Posterior columns

The posterior columns contain fibres which carry vibration sensation, fine touch and proprioception. They are uncrossed and pass through the cord without synapsing to end in the gracile and cuneate nuclei in the medulla. Second-order neurones decussate and pass to the thalamus where they synapse again and the tracts then pass to the sensory cortex. Other ascending tracts include the spinocerebellar tracts which carry sensation from the muscle, tendon and joint receptors to the cerebellum. Damage to the spinal cord results in loss of sensation of vibration and proprioception on the same side as the lesion and loss of pain and temperature sensation on the opposite side of the body.

AUTONOMIC NERVOUS SYSTEM

The autonomic nervous system is divided on anatomical and physiological grounds into the functionally opposing sympathetic and parasympathetic nervous systems. The central areas responsible for coordinating the autonomic nervous system are mostly in the hypothalamus and its surrounding structures, and in the frontal lobes.

Sympathetic nervous system (Fig. 7.1)

The sympathetic nervous system cells arise from the lateral horn of the thoracic and first two lumbar segments of the spinal cord. The first-order neurones supplying the gut synapse in the coeliac ganglia and the superior and inferior mesenteric plexuses. The supply to the rest of the body synapses in the ganglia of the sympathetic chain lying alongside the vertebral column, and the second-order neurones pass with spinal nerves or with the carotid vessels if they are supplying the head. There is also a sympathetic supply of first-order neurones to the adrenal medulla.

Parasympathetic nervous system (Fig. 7.2)

The neurones of the parasympathetic nervous system exit the central nervous system with the IIIrd, VIIth, IXth and Xth cranial nerves and from the second to fourth sacral segments of the spinal cord. The neurones usually synapse in ganglia or plexuses near or in the organ concerned. The autonomic nervous system also has an afferent component for both the sympathetic and parasympathetic systems which generally follows the same pathways as the efferent system.

CRANIAL NERVES

There are 12 paired cranial nerves, arising mostly from the base of the brain. Cranial nerves I, II and VIII are entirely sensory, nerves III, IV, VI, XI and XII are entirely motor and the rest are mixed. The nuclei of the cranial nerves are within the midbrain and the brain stem. The cortical supply to the motor nuclei comes via the corticonuclear tracts. Sensory nerve fibres have their cell bodies either in ganglia along the course of the nerve or in the sensory organ supplied. The central processes of these fibres end in the nuclei of the cranial nerves with second-order fibres passing to the thalamus and other structures.

Nerve I

The olfactory nerve is a specialized nerve carrying afferent fibres for smell sensation from the nasal mucosa to the olfactory lobes in the frontal lobe.

Nerve II

The optic nerve and the retina are derived from the developing forebrain and the nerve is not therefore a true nerve. The meninges and the subarachnoid space extend along the nerve and fuse with the structures of the sclera. The optic nerve has an intraorbital course, where inadvertent injection of local anaesthetic into the CSF may occur during attempted retrobulbar block. The two optic nerves join in the optic chiasma close to the pituitary gland. Fibres from the medial (nasal) half of the retina cross in the optic chiasma to enter the opposite optic pathway and join fibres from the ipsilateral lateral retina. Most fibres in the optic nerve pass to the occipital cortex via the thalamus, but some pass to the midbrain.

Nerves III, IV and VI

These are the oculomotor, trochlear and abducent nerves, respectively. They control the extrinsic eye muscles. The trochlear nerve controls the superior oblique muscle, the abducent nerve controls the lateral rectus muscle, and the oculomotor nerve controls the rest. The oculomotor nerve also carries fibres which control the intrinsic muscle of the eye and a supply to the levator palpebrae superioris muscle. Raised intracranial pressure causes compression of the oculomotor nerve leading to pupillary dilatation on the affected side. The abducent nerve has a long intracranial course and may be damaged in injuries to the skull base.

Nerve V

The Vth or trigeminal nerve is the largest cranial nerve and has important sensory and motor functions. It carries sensation from the face, orbit, nose and mouth. The face is supplied by ophthalmic, maxillary and mandibular divisions of the nerve. It also supplies motor fibres to the muscles of mastication in the mandibular branch.

Nerve VII

The VIIth or facial nerve is also a mixed sensory and motor nerve. The motor supply is to the muscles of facial expression and the stapedius muscle in the ear. The facial nerve has secretomotor fibres for the lacrimal, submandibular and sublingual glands, and transmits taste sensation from the anterior two-thirds of the tongue. That part of the facial nerve nucleus which controls the upper facial muscles receives innervation from both cerebral cortices. Hence, with a unilateral supranuclear palsy of the facial nerve, the muscles of facial expression of the upper part of the face are not affected, but a lesion at the level of the nucleus or below results in the upper part of the face on the affected side being paralysed.

Nerve VIII

The VIIIth or auditory nerve supplies the ear. In addition to cochlear fibres for hearing, there are vestibular fibres concerned with balance.

Nerve IX

The IXth or glossopharyngeal nerve contains sensory fibres for the pharynx and the posterior one-third of the tongue, secretomotor fibres for the parotid gland, innervation for the carotid body and carotid sinus, and motor fibres to the stylopharyngeus muscle.

Nerve X

The Xth cranial nerve is the vagus nerve. It carries motor, sensory and secretomotor fibres. Its motor supply is to the pharynx and larynx, heart and lungs, and the gut as far as the splenic flexure of the colon. The sensory supply is to the epiglottis, airway, heart and gut, and the secretomotor supply is to the bronchi and the gut.

Nerve XI

The XIth cranial or accessory nerve has two components – a cranial component which innervates the muscles of the pharynx and larynx via the vagus nerve, and a spinal component derived from the upper part of the cervical spinal cord which provides motor innervation to the sternomastoid and trapezius muscles.

Nerve XII

The hypoglossal or XIIth cranial nerve is entirely motor and supplies the muscles of the tongue.

FURTHER READING

Ellis H, Feldman S 1996 Anatomy for anaesthetists, 7th edn. Blackwell Scientific Publications, Oxford

Snell R S 1997 Clinical neuroanatomy for medical students, 4th edn. Lippincott-Raven, Philadelphia

12 Physiology of the nervous system

STRUCTURE AND FUNCTION

The function of the human nervous system is the acquisition of information from the external environment and its computation to produce an integrated response. The central nervous system (CNS) comprises the brain and spinal cord. The peripheral nervous system is composed of 43 pairs of nerves which contain afferent sensory fibres conducting impulses to the CNS from the periphery, and efferent motor fibres conducting in the reverse direction. There are 10^9–10^{12} neurones in the CNS, each surrounded by neuroglial cells. These cells are of two types:

- oligodendrocytes, which form myelin
- microglia, which phagocytose degenerating neurones.

The physiology of the nervous system is related intimately to membrane physiology and cell excitation. Excitability results from specialization of excitable cell membranes. The intracellular environment is controlled by cell membranes which exhibit selective permeability by virtue of channels or pores in the membrane. Excitable membranes undergo rapid reversible changes in permeability to some charged molecules or ions. At a pressure receptor, the membrane ionic permeability alters in response to mechanical deformation, and flow of ions occurs across the membrane.

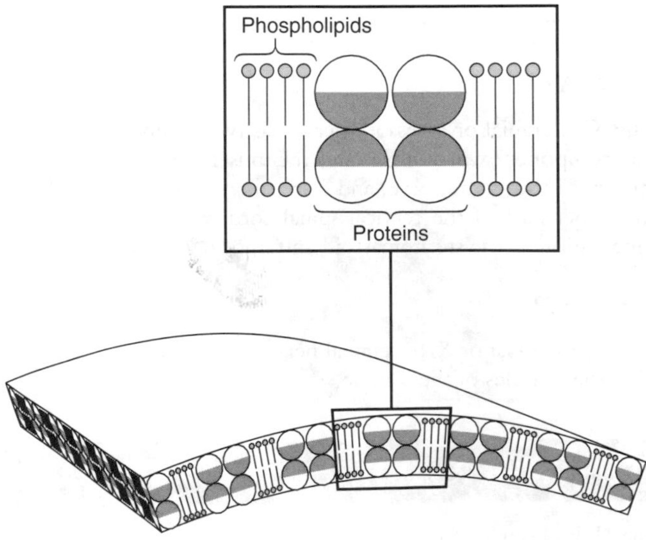

Fig. 12.1
Section of the cell membrane.

A cell membrane is composed of lipids and protein (Fig. 12.1). Phospholipid forms the major part of the cell membrane, which may be considered as a bilayer arranged such that a polar head is located on the outside of the cell membrane and one or two hydrocarbon chains, which are hydrophobic, constitute the inner part of the bilayer. Cell membrane proteins are composed of chains of amino acids with different side chains, either hydrophilic or hydrophobic, which by folding can 'hide' their hydrophobic amino acids on the interior.

A lipid bilayer is very impermeable to small ions; consequently, cell membrane permeability resides in the membrane proteins. The proteins confer specific ionic permeability on the membrane, whilst only a small part of the membrane appears to be directly involved in ion flow.

Membrane function

Ion movement across a cell membrane may occur against the electrochemical gradient and is therefore active. Membrane proteins which achieve active transport are termed ion pumps. All cell membranes contain a sodium pump (Fig. 12.2). Ionic permeability is of two types:

- constant resting ionic permeability to ions including potassium (K^+) and chloride (Cl^-), which is not affected by physiological stimuli
- non-constant permeability, which changes rapidly because of the action of a stimulus on an appropriate membrane protein.

Permeability is 'gated' by the stimulus. This is a characteristic of excitable membranes.

Several possibilities exist for the actual transport of an ion across the cell membrane. A protein may act as a carrier and ferry the ion across, or it may span the bilayer and produce a pore (Fig. 12.3). The latter mechanism produces much more rapid transport.

Electrochemical gradient

This is a measure of the force driving a specific ion into or out of the cell. It comprises an electrical component, which is the potential difference between the inside and outside of the cell (–60 mV). The chemical gradient is a simple concentration gradient. In certain conditions, these two components may oppose and cancel each other out, at which point the ion is in electrochemical equilibrium across

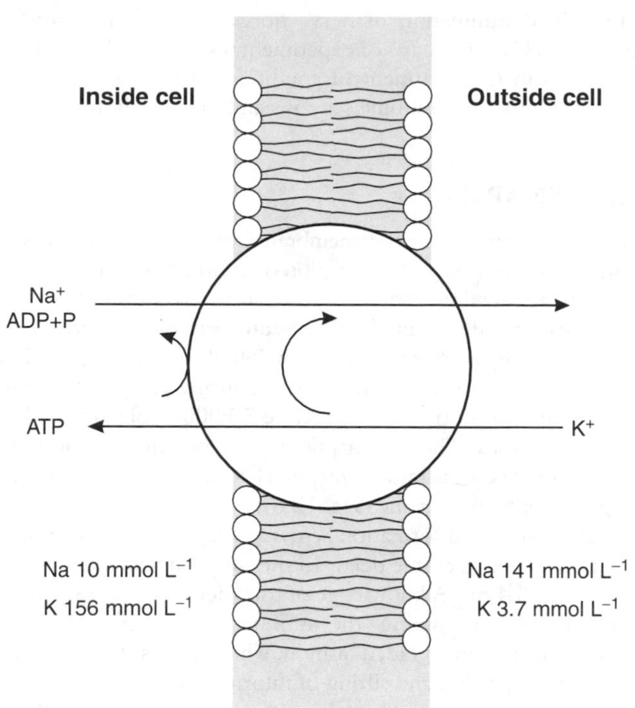

Fig. 12.2
The sodium pump. Na, sodium; K, potassium; ADP, adenosine diphosphate; ATP, adenosine triphosphate; P, phosphate.

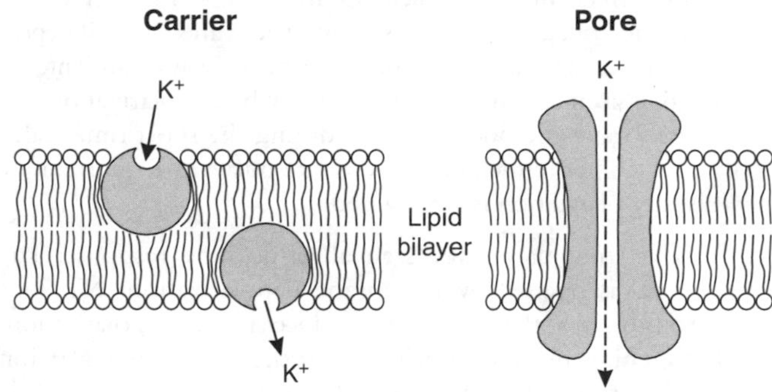

Fig. 12.3
Mechanisms of ion transport by proteins.

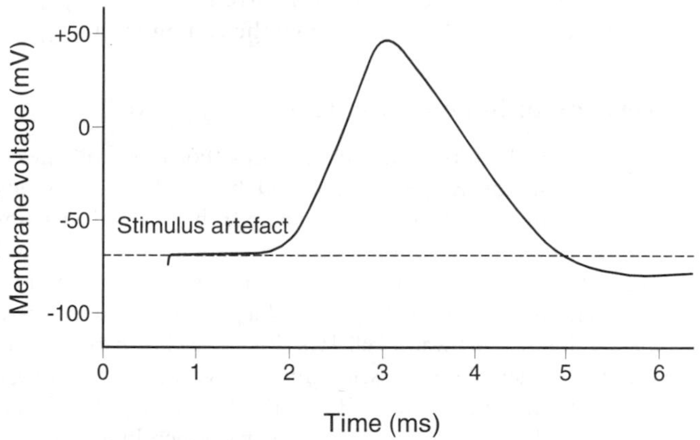

Fig. 12.4
The action potential.

the membrane and the Nernst equation applies. This is dependent upon the unequal distribution of ions across membranes. If permeability to sodium (Na^+) and Cl^- is assumed to be zero at the resting potential of biological membranes, then:

$$V = \frac{RT}{F} \log_e \frac{K_o^+}{K_i^+}$$

where V is the potential difference, R is the gas constant, F is Faraday's constant, T is temperature, K_o^+ is the concentration of K^+ in extracellular fluid (ECF), and K_i^+ is the concentration of K^+ in intracellular fluid (ICF).

Nerve impulse and conduction

Characteristic changes in membrane potential on passage of a nerve impulse constitute an action potential. Electrical stimulation of a nerve axon produces first a stimulus artefact and then an action potential (Fig. 12.4).

ACTION POTENTIAL

This is an all-or-none phenomenon. The least stimulus strength required to produce an action potential is termed the threshold stimulus. The transient reversal of the membrane potential propagates along an axon at constant velocity in a non-decremental manner. The refractory period is the period during which a second stimulating current does not elicit a second action potential. The absolute refractory period occurs immediately after the initial stimulus and lasts for approximately the same duration as the action potential itself. At this time, it is not possible to initiate a new impulse. Thereafter, the relative refractory period requires an increased threshold to initiate an impulse.

In the giant squid axon, the resting membrane potential (– 60 mV) is close to the Nernst potential for K^+ and results from selective permeability to K^+ in the axon membrane.

A change in resting potential is produced by changes in external and internal K^+ concentration. The resting potential is the result of two factors:

- ionic gradients produced by the sodium pump
- selective permeability of the resting axon to K^+ with respect to Na^+.

As an action potential passes, the axon membrane becomes active and the membrane voltage is reversed from negative to positive. This corresponds to depolarization with an overshoot up to +40 mV. The action potential results from an increase in membrane conductance to Na^+, resulting in an increase in membrane potential towards the Nernst potential for Na^+. Thus, if the external Na^+ concentration decreases, the action potential becomes smaller in amplitude and eventually is reduced to zero. Selective block of Na^+ ion current may be produced experimentally with tetrodotoxin, and that of K^+ with tetraethylammonium. Such studies show that the following events occur:

1. The sodium channel is opened rapidly by depolarization of membrane voltage and closes slowly (inactivates) even if depolarization is maintained. The open phase is always transient.
2. The potassium channel is opened slowly by depolarization of the membrane and does not close during the short time-scale of the action potential, i.e. there is late outward K^+ current whilst depolarization is maintained.

A threshold stimulus produces an all-or-nothing response. The Na^+ channel is opened by membrane depolarization; Na^+ ions pass through into the axon to produce more depolarization, thereby opening more channels and further increasing Na^+ ion influx and outward flux of K^+, which resists depolarization. Na^+ channels do not open until the membrane voltage has changed by 20 mV from the resting potential. Inactivated Na^+ channels take a few milliseconds to become functional again and therefore are not opened again by immediate depolarization. These are the underlying events of the refractory period. The increase in K^+ conductance always tends to increase K^+ ion current, which resists any change of membrane voltage away from the resting level.

Propagation of impulse (Fig. 12.5)

Large axons have high conduction velocities. For fibres of a given diameter, conduction is greatly increased by myelination. Axons from 1 to 25 μm in diameter are myelinated; those less than 1 μm are unmyelinated. Nerve fibres have a structure akin to a shielded electrical cable, in other words a central conducting core with insulation and an external conducting area which is ECF. In vertebrate myelinated fibres, a Schwann cell lays down myelin in concentric layers. Between neighbouring segments of myelin, there is a very narrow gap termed the node of Ranvier, which is less than 1 μm wide; here no obstacle exists between the axon membrane and the ECF. This accounts for conduction occurring in a saltatory manner. The myelin sheaths act as high-resistance barriers to current flow and excitation occurs only at the nodes of Ranvier. Thus, the impulse is propagated from node to node.

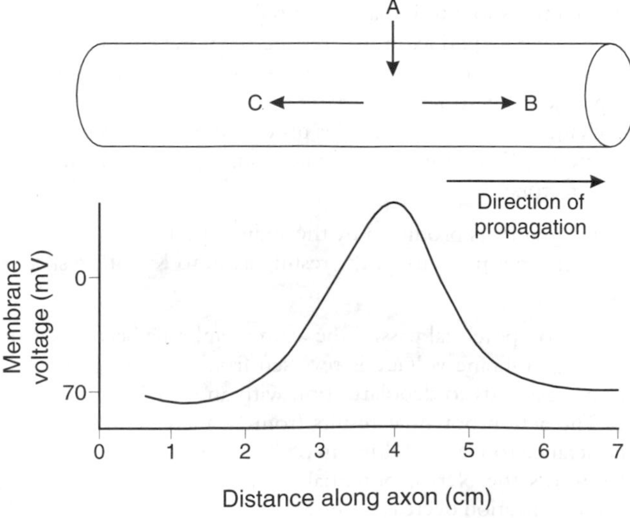

Fig. 12.5
Local circuit theory of impulse propagation. A, influx of Na^+ ions at active membrane; B, C, current flow. B propagates the impulse; C finds the membrane refractory.

Repetitive stimulation of nerve fibres induces an increase in their size. This is the basis of experimental spinal cord stimulation techniques in the treatment of conditions such as chronic pain, and in patients with multiple sclerosis and bladder dysfunction.

THE SYNAPSE

A synapse occurs where the membranes of two excitable cells are closely apposed to allow transmission of information. The transmitter is usually chemical, is released in a controlled amount by the cell and diffuses rapidly to bind to a receptor site on the second cell, where it produces rapid changes in ion flux. Presynaptic fibres divide into numerous fine branches, producing presynaptic knobs. A single anterior horn cell may receive 30 000 knobs from a large number of axons. The presynaptic membrane releases transmitter from synaptic vesicles into a synaptic cleft, 20–25 nm in width, to the postsynaptic membrane (Fig. 12.6).

Transmission of information across a synapse is usually undirectional and involves a time delay. In the spinal motor neurone, this amounts to 0.4 ms. A knowledge of total delay in a reflex pathway is useful in determining the number of synapses involved. Synapses operate in a graded fashion, which allows the neurone to carry out integration and sifting of information.

Enzymes break down the transmitter after release, usually but not always reducing its duration of action at the postsynaptic membrane.

Control of transmitter release

The arrival of an action potential produces depolarization of the terminal membrane, which opens voltage-sensitive calcium ion (Ca^{2+}) channels, resulting in flux of Ca^{2+} into presynaptic areas. This in turn stimulates transient exocytosis of the transmitter into the synaptic gap, where it diffuses rapidly to specific protein-binding sites (receptors) on the postsynaptic membrane. Ionic currents through these sites then alter the membrane potential of the post-

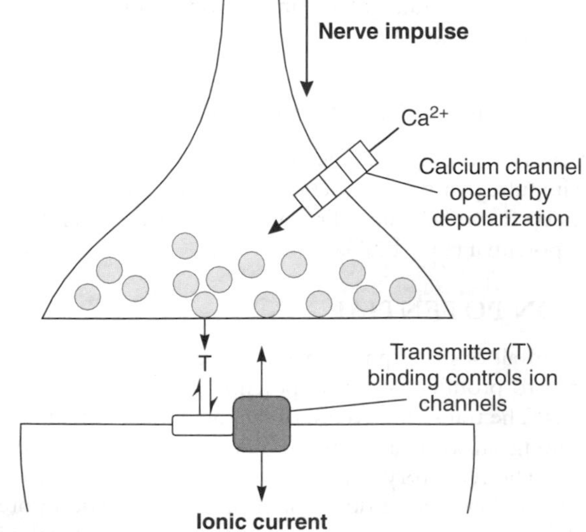

Fig. 12.6
Chemical synapse transmission.

synaptic cell in a direction determined by the ion selectivity of the channels concerned. Depolarization causes excitation, and hyperpolarization results in inhibition.

The postsynaptic membrane channels are gated by specific chemical stimuli. In the absence of nerve stimulation, miniature end-plate potentials (MEPPs) occur; these are produced by arrival of single transmitter vesicles. A propagative end-plate potential requires 100 transmitter vesicles. At the neuromuscular junction, one impulse produces 100 vesicles, each containing 50 000 molecules of acetylcholine (ACh). Of the 5 million transmitter molecules released, only 100 000 are required to open a postsynaptic channel, but this is sufficient to cause 10 billion Na^+ ions to enter muscle in 1 ms. Both excitatory and inhibitory postsynaptic potentials may be recorded intracellularly. Presynaptic inhibition may also occur from inhibitory terminals situated on excitatory presynaptic nerve endings; stimulation of these terminals reduces the amount of neurotransmitter released.

It is well known that antibiotics may interfere with neuromuscular conduction, often by decreasing end-plate transmitter. High concentrations of magnesium (Mg^{2+}) and some antibiotics decrease evoked release of ACh. Postjunctional effects include receptor or end-plate ion channel blockade. There is considerable variability between antibiotics in their neuromuscular blocking mechanisms. Aminoglycosides, polymyxin and tetracyclines produce neuromuscular block by a combination of pre- and postjunctional effects.

Information is processed by nerve networks by two basic mechanisms:

- *Spatial summation*. This occurs when stimulation of two afferent nerves together produces a response which neither can elicit alone. Both synapses may be excitatory for that particular nerve.
- *Temporal summation*. Stimulation of the same nerve twice in rapid succession produces a response where a single stimulus elicits none.

There are also electrical synapses (e.g. in the retina) and synapses at which transmitter release is controlled by graded depolarizations.

Neurotransmitters

Neurotransmitters are of three main types (amino acids, monoamines and peptides) which are present in widely differing concentrations. Synaptic transmission is more complex than simple transfer of excitation or inhibition from the presynaptic neurone to the postsynaptic cell. There is a great range of synaptic connections, and the possibility of chemical coding exists. Axoaxonal synapses may regulate the amount of transmitter released from presynaptic terminals; other inputs may trigger very long-lasting postsynaptic events (lasting for minutes) and therefore control the excitability of a target cell, rather than directly controlling its firing.

Fast chemical signalling in the CNS

Amino acids are fast neurotransmitters in the CNS. L-Glutamate (Glu) and L-aspartate (Asp) act at excitatory synapses and γ-aminobutyric acid (GABA) and glycine (Gly) act at inhibitory synapses.

Fast excitatory transmitters

Glutamate is the most important excitatory transmitter in the CNS. It acts on at least three types of receptor, two of which are coupled to ion channels (ionotropic receptors) and one which is coupled to second messenger-producing systems (metabotropic receptors). The ionotropic receptors are named after specific agonists γ-amino-3-hydroxy-5-methyl-4-isoxazole propionate (AMPA) and *N*-methyl-D-aspartate (NMDA; Table 12.1). The AMPA receptor is linked to an ion channel that is permeable to both Na^+ and K^+ ions, whereas the NMDA receptor, in addition to permitting flow of Na^+ and K^+, is also permeable to calcium ions. This receptor is usually blocked at the resting membrane potential with magnesium, which is removed from the channel by depolarization due to activation of AMPA receptors or other excitatory receptors. The channel can also be blocked by dissociative anaesthetics such as ketamine. The metabotropic receptors are coupled to different intracellular second-messenger systems and may lead to changes in intracellular calcium and activation of protein kinase C via hydrolysis of phosphatidylinositol 4,5 biphosphate (the PI system) or to activation of adenylate cyclase to alter cyclic adenosine monophosphate (cAMP) concentration.

L-Glutamate is widely distributed in the CNS and has been implicated with other excitatory transmitters in sensory processing, motor control and higher cortical functions, including mem-

Table 12.1 Excitatory amino acid receptors

	Ionotropic		Metabotropic
Other agonists	AMPA Glutamate Kainate	NMDA Glutamate Aspartate	ACPD Glutamate Quisqualate Ibotenate
Antagonists	Nitroquinoxalines	APV MK 801 Dissociative anaesthetics such as ketamine Magnesium	Phenylglycines

AMPA, γ-amino-3-hydroxy-5-methyl-4-isoxazole propionate; NMDA, *N*-methyl-D-aspartate; ACPD, (1*S*,3*R*)-1-aminocyclopentane-1,3-dicarboxylic acid; APV, 2-amino-5-phosphonopentanoic acid.

ory and learning. In neurological or pathological conditions such as stroke, anoxia or epilepsy, these transmitters are believed to have key roles, and drugs that antagonize their effects have great therapeutic potential. An example of this is the neuroprotective effect of lubeluzole. This drug limits neurotoxicity after acute stroke by inhibiting the glutamate-activated nitric oxide synthase pathway. The effect of this is to limit the damage to cells in the ischaemic penumbra.

Inhibitory amino acids

GABA is the main inhibitory neurotransmitter in the CNS, and acts at almost one-third of all synapses. There are two main GABA receptors: $GABA_A$ and $GABA_B$. $GABA_A$ receptors are associated with chloride channels and the receptor contains modulatory sites to which benzodiazepines and barbiturates can bind to enhance the actions of GABA (Fig. 12.7). The $GABA_B$ receptor is linked to a potassium channel. In status epilepticus, the pathophysiological process involves stimulation of excitatory transmission and reduction in inhibitory transmission. Glycine predominates as the inhibitory transmitter in the spinal cord.

Diffuse regulatory systems: monoamines

These are associated with diffuse neural pathways, mainly in the brain stem. Much of the monoamine release may be at non-synaptic sites.

Neuropeptides

Virtually all peptide hormones of the endocrine and neuroendocrine systems also exist in distinct systems of the CNS. Active peptides released from endocrine and neural tissue are called regulatory peptides. They are capable of producing an effect by acting as hormones, local regulators or neurotransmitters, or a combination of all of these. Vasoactive intestinal peptide (VIP), which acts as a neurotransmitter, is one example. Enteric nerves containing peptides belong to a non-adrenergic, non-cholinergic subdivision of the autonomic nervous system. The spinal cord contains a very large number of regulatory peptides, including substance P, VIP, enkephalin and neuropeptide Y. The latter is involved in reducing the threshold for epilepsy.

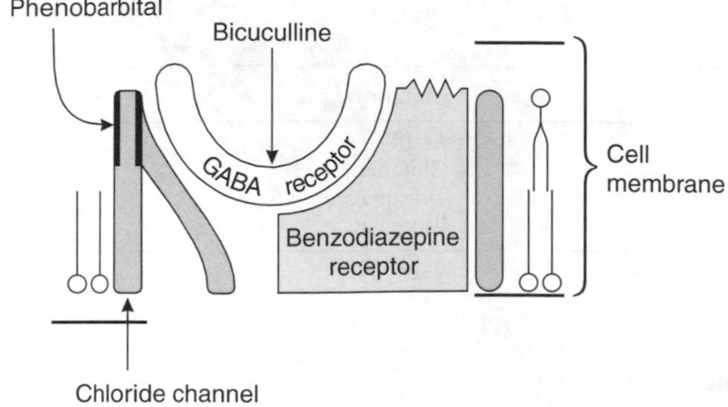

Fig. 12.7
γ-Aminobutyric acid (GABA) receptor, benzodiazepine receptor and chloride channel.

MEMBRANE RECEPTOR FUNCTION IN ANAESTHESIA

Most hormones and drugs produce effects by binding to cell recognition sites termed receptors. A receptor is an integral membrane protein which is recognized selectively by a precise hormone or neurotransmitter termed a ligand (Fig. 12.8). A ligand is an agonist if it activates a receptor to transduce a response, or an antagonist when the substance interacts with a receptor causing it to remain inactive and, by occupying the receptor, diminishes or aborts the effect of an agonist. The interaction between ligand and receptor is specific, reversible, saturable and is usually a high-affinity binding process. Binding is followed by alterations in metabolic events within the cell, e.g. ion flux, which produce the characteristic physiological effect.

A range of receptor types have been successfully cloned and sequenced in recent years. Positron emission tomography allows quantitative imaging of muscarinic, cholinergic, opioid and benzodiazepine receptors. Radioactive tracer molecules can be incorporated into substrates such as glucose or into a drug, and become bound to receptors so that serial images can be obtained from different areas of the brain. Such techniques allow measurement of regional oxygen metabolism, assist the differential diagnosis of coma and are useful in cases of epilepsy if surgery is being considered.

Adrenergic receptors

Molecular biology methods and radioligand binding have identified new adrenergic receptor subtypes all of which are linked to guanine nucleotide-binding proteins (G-proteins). Three types each of α_1-, α_2- and β-adrenergic receptors have now been identified but not their precise function because of lack of specific agonists and antagonists. There are also multiple types of G-protein, each of which can be used for signalling by more than one receptor, resulting in changes in intracellular concentrations of second messengers which modulate cellular events (see Ch. 2).

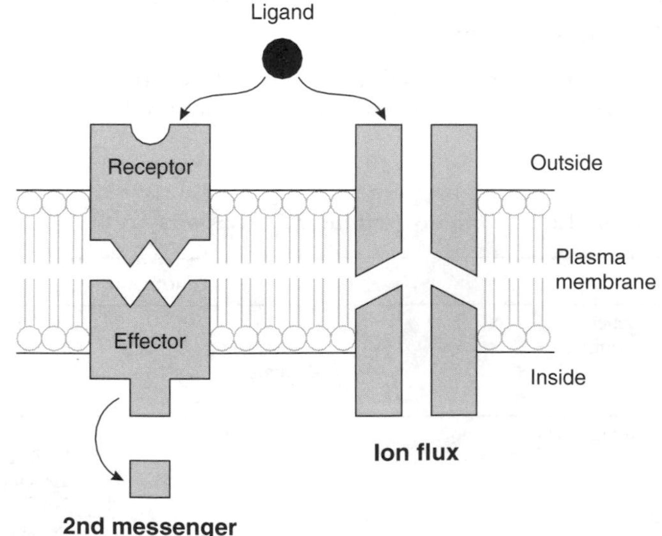

Fig. 12.8
Receptor–effector mechanisms: release of second messenger or promotion of ion flux.

Agonists at β-adrenoreceptors in order of potency include isoproterenol (isoprenaline), epinephrine, norepinephrine and dopamine. β_1-Receptors are found in the heart and are equally sensitive to epinephrine and norepinephrine; β_2-receptors are found in smooth muscle and are more sensitive to epinephrine than to norepinephrine. The effects are mediated by intracellular cAMP, the second messenger, which activates protein kinases (Fig 1.1). Thus the β-adrenergic agonist–receptor complex couples to adenylate cyclase (the effector molecule), which is then activated and catalyses synthesis of cAMP; this is subsequently hydrolysed by phosphodiesterase.

α-Adrenoceptors mediate control of smooth muscle in the vasculature of the uterus and gastrointestinal tract. The order of potency of agonists is: epinephrine, norepinephrine, isoproterenol. There are two classes of α-receptor (Fig. 12.9); α_1-receptors are postsynaptic and mediate constriction of smooth muscle. These are blocked selectively by prazosin and phenoxybenzamine. α_2-Receptors are presynaptic and mediate feedback inhibition of further neurotransmitter release by norepinephrine. These receptors are blocked selectively by yohimbine. α_2-Receptors are also found on platelets, where they mediate aggregation. Methoxamine and phenylephrine are selective α_1-agonists. There are at least two subtypes of presynaptic α_2-adrenoreceptors involved in norepinephrine release. Clonidine and dexmedetomidine, α_2-agonists, inhibit central sympathetic activity, producing sedation and a reduced requirement for anaesthetic agents (see Ch. 7).

Within the CNS, epinephrine is found in small groups of cells in the pons and medulla which project to the hypothalamus and brain stem and to the nucleus tractus solitarius, which may be important in central arterial pressure control. Norepinephrine is found in all areas of the brain and spinal cord, with a high density in the hypothalamus. Experimentally, norepinephrine in low doses enhances the response to excitatory amino acids, but in high doses it inhibits these responses. Adrenergic receptors in central and peripheral neurones are coupled to G-proteins linked to adenylate cyclase. Activation of β-adrenoreceptors increases cAMP production via G_s (stimulatory) protein and activation of α-receptors decreases cAMP via G_i (inhibitory) protein. Dexmedetomidine is a selective α_2-adrenoreceptor agonist with similar sedative effects to clonidine, and exerts its effects by inhibiting conductance through a G_I-protein-modulated potassium channel.

The regulation of adrenergic receptors by receptor-specific agonists and antagonists is important clinically. Treatment of normal subjects with β-adrenergic antagonists may increase the number of β-receptors on peripheral blood leucocytes, suggesting that the number of receptors expressed on the cell surface is probably regulated by the ambient catecholamine concentration. Persistent exposure to agonist may result in loss of receptors (downregulation). In patients with cardiac failure and dilated cardiomyopathy, cardiac β-desensitization occurs partly as a result of downregulation of β_1-receptors and partly as a result of uncoupling of β_2-receptors

Dopamine receptors

Dopamine receptors occur in basal ganglia, the substantia nigra, corpus striatum and the limbic system. In the basal ganglia, dopamine is antagonistic to ACh. Absence of dopamine is an important aetiological factor in Parkinsonism. In the hypothalamus, dopamine is concerned with release of prolactin. Dopamine suppresses prolactin secretion and dopamine antagonists (e.g. metoclopramide) increase hyperprolactinaemia.

A dopaminergic system connects the limbic cortex, basal ganglia and hypothalamus and is concerned with behaviour. This system is involved in the pathogenesis of schizophrenia (phenothiazines block dopamine receptors). Dopaminergic fibres are found in the chemoreceptor trigger zone; stimulation produces nausea and vomiting. Dopaminergic and sympathomimetic receptors have been identified in the coronary, renal, cerebral and mesenteric vessels. Dopamine receptors also occur on the presynaptic membrane of postganglionic sympathetic nerves and sympathetic ganglia where their physiological role is unclear.

Acetylcholine

Acetylecholine is found in motor neurones of the spinal cord and cranial nerve motor nuclei, where it acts as a fast chemical trans-

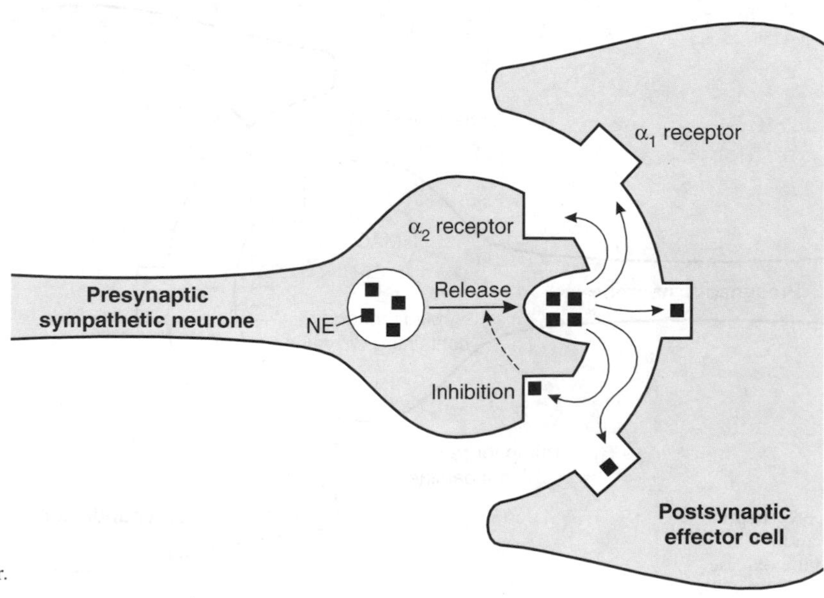

Fig. 12.9
Types of α-adrenergic receptor. NE, norepinephrine.

mitter for neuromuscular transmission. In intrinsic pathways in the CNS, it probably acts as a modulator in basal ganglia, the hippocampus and the diffuse ascending pathways to the cortex, and may represent what was known as the ascending reticular activating system. ACh probably plays an important part in cortical arousal and electroencephalographic (EEG) changes of rapid eye movement (REM) sleep. The effects of ACh are terminated by hydrolysis by cholinesterase. Its peripheral effects may be classified into two types:

- muscarinic effects at postganglionic parasympathetic fibres
- nicotinic effects at sympathetic and parasympathetic ganglia and the neuromuscular junction.

Muscarinic cholinergic receptors in the intestine stimulate electrolyte transport by acting directly on the enterocyte, whereas nicotinic agonists act indirectly to augment absorption by stimulating release of intermediary neurotransmitters.

Denervation of skeletal muscle enhances its sensitivity to ACh by development of a diffuse distribution of ACh receptors over postjunctional surfaces. Administration of succinylcholine in these circumstances results in severe hyperkalaemia.

Histamine receptors

H_1-Receptors are responsible for contraction of smooth muscle (e.g. in the gut and bronchi). H_2-Receptors stimulate acid secretion by the stomach and increase heart rate. These H_2 effects are not prevented by H_1-antihistamines, but by H_2-receptor blockers such as cimetidine and ranitidine. The vascular effects of histamine are mediated by both types of receptor. In some instances, H_1 and H_2 have opposing actions, e.g. H_1 produces pulmonary vasodilatation. Both H_1- and H_2-receptors occur in the brain.

5-Hydroxytryptamine (5-HT, serotonin)

This has been isolated from the brain stem, many forebrain sites and the dorsal horns of the spinal cord. It may represent one of the descending control pathways which modulate sensitivity of the spinal cord to pain input from the periphery, and therefore plays a key role in mediating analgesic actions of morphine and related opioid analgesics. In the forebrain, this system may be responsible for control of sleep and waking, central temperature regulation and control of aggressive behaviour.

Benzodiazepines

Although not endogenous substances, these drugs act at specific synapses in the CNS (including the spinal cord) at which GABA is the transmitter. Benzodiazepines selectively facilitate GABA action at synapses. Aminophylline may reverse diazepam sedation by its adenosine-blocking effect at GABA receptors. Adenosine is as potent a CNS-depressant mediator as GABA, and may have an amplifying effect on the GABA-receptor complex. Flumazenil is a benzodiazepine antagonist. Benzodiazepines exert their effects via a GABA–benzodiazepine receptor–chloride channel complex (Fig. 12.7), which is enclosed in the lipid bilayer of cell membranes and which may also mediate anxiety.

Neurotransmitters in disease

Anxiety probably involves many neurotransmitters including GABA, 5-HT, norepinephrine and dopamine. There are strong indications that central monoamine metabolism is disturbed in endogenous depression, and that the disturbance is causal. Tricyclic antidepressants inhibit the presynaptic uptake of 5-HT and norepinephrine (Fig. 12.10). All antidepressants facilitate synaptic activity of amines; however, tricyclic antidepressants also block cholinergic receptors. The anticholinesterase physostigmine can relieve manic symptoms.

In patients with affective disorders, cholinergic receptor density is increased. In schizophrenia, catecholamine activity may worsen symptoms. Neuroleptic drugs administered in small doses dramatically reverse amphetamine-induced psychoses; amphetamine induces schizophrenic exacerbations. This provides further support for the

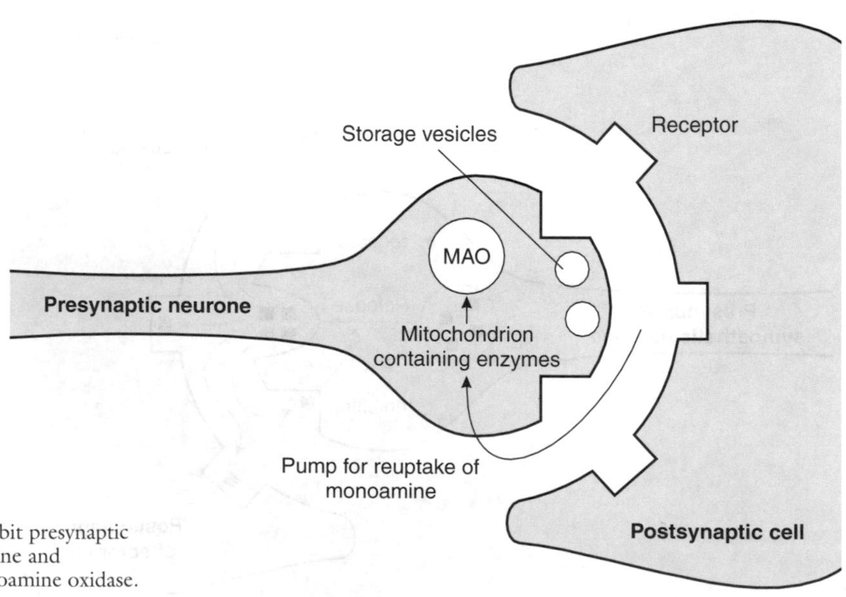

Fig. 12.10
Tricyclic antidepressants inhibit presynaptic uptake of 5-hydroxytryptamine and norepinephrine. MAO, monoamine oxidase.

concept of a dopaminergic abnormality in schizophrenia. Some symptoms of schizophrenia are reduced by naloxone, suggesting that opioid peptides (e.g. enkephalins) are involved, although naloxone also blocks GABA receptors. The brain of patients who have died with Alzheimer's disease contains reduced concentrations of choline acetyltransferase, norepinephrine, GABA and somatostatin, although the most severe abnormality is a cholinergic deficit.

Epilepsy

A binding site for phenytoin, which interacts with the GABA/chloride inophore benzodiazepine complex and an endogenous compound which binds to this site have been isolated from the brain. It is thought that one or more components of the GABA inhibitory system may be concerned with maintenance of a normal state. It may be that in epilepsy there is a lower threshold for seizure, but inhibitory systems within the brain terminate the seizure. Drugs which increase GABA in the CNS are useful in the control of epilepsy.

Hepatic encephalopathy

This may result from increased concentrations of false neurotransmitters, such as octopamine and 5-HT, which replace the normal dopamine and norepinephrine. GABA is produced in the gut by bacterial action on protein and may lead to coma by passing through the blood–brain barrier in liver failure. The number of binding sites for GABA, glycine and benzodiazepines on postsynaptic neurones is increased in acute liver failure; present data suggest that this mechanism is the most important contributor to hepatic encephalopathy. The benzodiazepine antagonists reverse hepatic encephalopathy temporarily. The hypersensitivity to benzodiazepines in patients with hepatic encephalopathy may be explained by an increase in the free drug concentration.

Asthma

In this condition, there is reduced β-adrenergic, and increased cholinergic and α-adrenergic, responsiveness.

Generally, treatment of disease states with agonists produces alterations in receptor density and desensitization, probably mediated via cAMP. In the case of β-adrenergic receptors, this is effected by phosphorylation. Abrupt discontinuation of a β-blocking drug such as propranolol may produce hypersensitivity to catecholamines and may precipitate angina or myocardial infarction.

Many intracellular events require release of a neurotransmitter, the action of which depends subsequently on activation of calmodulin by calcium binding. There are huge numbers of circuits, transmitters and coupled reactions within the CNS. Several must act simultaneously to produce coordinated CNS responses.

THE SENSORY SYSTEM

Detection of mechanical stimuli

Peripheral receptors exist in excitable tissues. Skin receptors appreciate touch, cold, warmth and pain, and deeper receptors appreciate pressure and proprioception. There are large numbers of different receptors and end-organs, and although end-organs are specialized for one form of sensation, the type of sensation does not depend on the type of stimulus arousing it. Information is transmitted to the CNS by varying the frequency and patterns of action potentials. There is often extensive branching of axons and a single fibre may be said to have a peripheral receptive field.

Adaptation

A sustained, mechanical stimulus produces only a transient response, i.e. there is processing of information at receptor level, so that the brain is not constantly informed of an unchanging stimulus.

Mechanical transduction

This consists of transfer of a mechanical stimulus through accessory structures to the nerve terminal itself. A graded electrical response is then produced equivalent to the generator or receptor potential, with initiation of an action potential.

A generator potential is produced by a mechanical stimulus and is a transient depolarization of the nerve terminal membrane, independent of the ion channels. The potential appears to be created by the nerve terminal itself and the important stimulus is distortion of the terminal.

Modalities of cutaneous sensation

There are four main modes of cutaneous sensation: touch, cold, warmth and pain. Pain registered by stimulation of the skin has a pricking, itching quality and is well-localized. The pain threshold may be increased by one-third by distracting the subject's attention and reduced by half in sunburned skin. The first sensation of pain arises abruptly and is carried by moderately large fibres, conducting impulses at 10 m s^{-1}. The second sensation is slower and of a burning nature, probably being carried by unmyelinated fibres. Pain nerve endings are distributed in a punctate fashion independent of the end-organs concerned with touch and temperature. Sensations from viscera and vessels travel in autonomic nerves and are often projected to a definite position on the surface of the body with the corresponding dermatome (referred pain; Fig. 12.11).

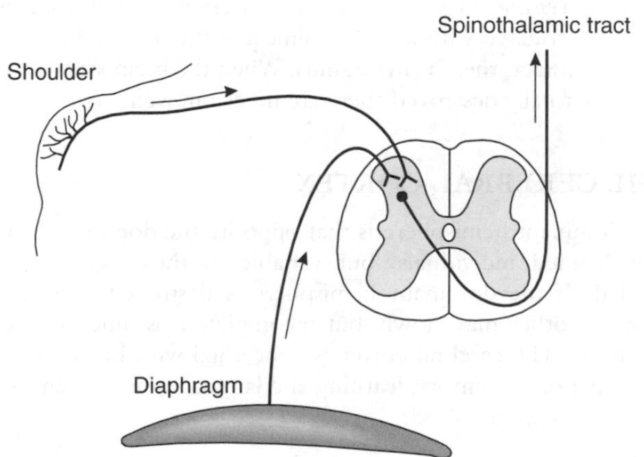

Fig. 12.11
Referred pain; irritation of the diaphragm is felt in the shoulder tip. Nerves from these areas synapse with common neurones in the spinal cord.

SPINAL CORD PATHWAYS

These may be divided into afferent (sensory), motor, cerebellar and autonomic pathways and are discussed in Chapter 11.

BRAIN STEM AND MIDBRAIN FUNCTION

The functions of the brain stem are crucial to the concept of brain stem death. An understanding of these functions requires some knowledge of anatomy.

The reticular formation

This constitutes the central core of the brain stem, projecting widely to the limbic system and cortex with many ascending connections. Stimulation activates the cortex, initiating an arousal reaction, i.e. this area is responsible for generating the capacity for consciousness. Attention and circadian rhythms are also dependent upon the correct functioning of the reticular formation.

Brain stem function tests

- Activity of nerves II–XII may be tested individually to permit localization of a lesion.
- All motor information from the cortex to the spinal cord and all sensory information in the opposite direction is transmitted through the brain stem. Although spinal reflexes may be active when the brain stem is destroyed, there should be no abnormal posture, either decorticate (flexed forearms and extended legs) or decerebrate (extended hyperpronated forearms and extended legs), nor trismus.
- *Control of ventilation.* In the absence of brain stem activity there is apnoea. Loss of vasomotor control also occurs.
- *Brain stem reflexes*
  - *Oculocephalic.* In the absence of brain stem function, when the head is rotated to one side and held there for 3–4 s and then rotated through 180° in the opposite direction, the head and eyes move together. In a patient with damaged cerebral hemispheres and an intact brain stem, there is deviation of the eyes to the opposite side as the head is rotated, followed by realignment of the eyes with the head.
  - *Vestibulo-ocular.* If the clear external auditory canal is irrigated with ice-cold saline and the brain stem is intact, there is nystagmus. When the brain stem is totally destroyed there are no eye movements.

THE CEREBRAL CORTEX

The dominant hemisphere is that opposite the dominant hand in right-handed individuals, but variable in those who are left-handed. If the dominant hemisphere is destroyed early in life, then the other may slowly but incompletely assume intellectual functions. The cerebral cortex is concerned with higher intellectual functions (memory, learning and language); in humans, three major areas are involved:

- frontal, in front of the motor cortex
- temporal, between the superior temporal gyrus and limbic cortex
- parieto-occipital, between the sensory and visual cortex.

These areas have complex connections from the thalamus, to each other and to the deeper cortex.

Coning

Brain swelling may cause part of a cerebral hemisphere, usually the temporal lobe, to become impacted under the falx cerebri or tentorial hiatus. Any expanding supratentorial lesion, e.g. middle meningeal haemorrhage, forces the medial aspect of the temporal lobe into the tentorial hiatus. Compression of the cerebral peduncle and oculomotor nerve causes ipsilateral pupillary dilatation with contralateral hemiparesis. Later, brain stem compression produces apnoea.

An expanding posterior fossa lesion may push the cerebellum into the tentorial hiatus. Medullary coning from high intracranial pressure forces the medulla and cerebellar tonsil down into the foramen magnum, and is rapidly fatal because of compression of the respiratory and vasomotor centres.

CEREBROSPINAL FLUID

Cerebrospinal fluid (CSF) is formed by secretory cells of the choroid plexus which project into the lateral, third and fourth ventricles (Fig. 12.12). CSF then flows via the third ventricle through the aqueduct and fourth ventricle to escape by two lateral foramina of Luschka and the median foramen of Magendie into the subarachnoid space around the brain and spinal cord.

The total volume of CSF is approximately 140 ml in the adult; approximately 50% is intracranial, and the remainder occupies the spinal canal. CSF is produced at a rate of 0.3–0.5 ml min^{-1}.

Production must match absorption to prevent an increase in pressure. Obstruction to the flow of CSF increases pressure, with dilatation of the ventricles upstream from the obstruction.

Resorption is mainly into the venous system via arachnoid villi, which are areas where the arachnoid invaginates into large venous sinuses. If the CSF pressure is less than venous pressure, the vac-

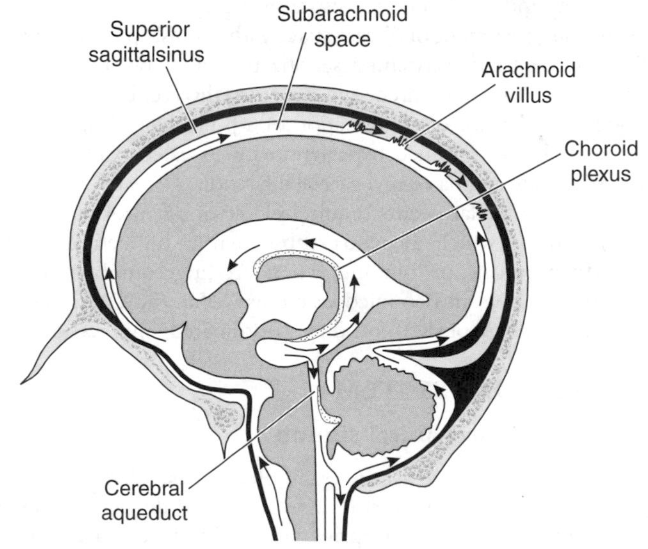

Fig. 12.12
The circulation of cerebrospinal fluid.

uoles collapse. Some CSF is probably absorbed around spinal nerves into spinal veins and through the ependymal lining of the ventricles. CSF acts as a cushion between the skull and the brain. It may accommodate some change in brain volume by displacement into the lumbar region. In conditions producing cerebral atrophy, there is an increase in CSF volume.

CSF is a clear, colourless liquid of specific gravity 1005, with fewer than 5 lymphocytes mm^{-3} and pH 7.33 (Table 12.2). It is produced from plasma, probably by a combination of secretion and ultrafiltration. The high concentration of chloride arises because carbon dioxide passes into glial cells where, by the action of carbonic anhydrase, it is hydrated to carbonic acid. Resulting bicarbonate ions are exchanged for chloride which passes into the CSF against a concentration gradient. CSF is slightly hypertonic; Na^+ and Mg^{2+} ions are actively transported into CSF. Lipophilic substances pass readily from blood to brain, but dissociated hydrophilic substances pass only very slowly.

The blood–brain barrier (Fig. 12.13) is composed of a lipid membrane of capillary walls, the endothelial cells of which are joined by tight junctions around the entire periphery of each cell. Solutes at higher concentration in the ECF of the brain diffuse into CSF and are carried into blood at the arachnoid villi. Some substances are transported actively by cells of the choroid plexus from CSF into blood.

CSF proteins are derived by filtration of plasma, from brain interstitial fluid and brain cells, and from cells of the CSF compartment itself. They may reflect abnormalities of the filtration mechanism, of barrier function, brain metabolism or activities of the CSF. Electrophoresis is used for investigat conditions such as multiple sclerosis, Guillain and neurosyphilis.

Table 12.2 Composition of plasma and cerebrospinal fluid

	Plasma (mmol L^{-1})	CSF (mmol L^{-1})
Urea	2.5–6.5	2.0–7.0
Glucose (fasting)	3.0–5.0	2.5–4.5
Sodium	136–148	144–152
Potassium	3.8–5.0	2.0–3.0
Calcium	2.2–2.6	1.1–1.3
Chloride	95–105	123–128
Bicarbonate	24–32	24–32
Protein	60–80 g L^{-1}	200–400 mg L^{-1}

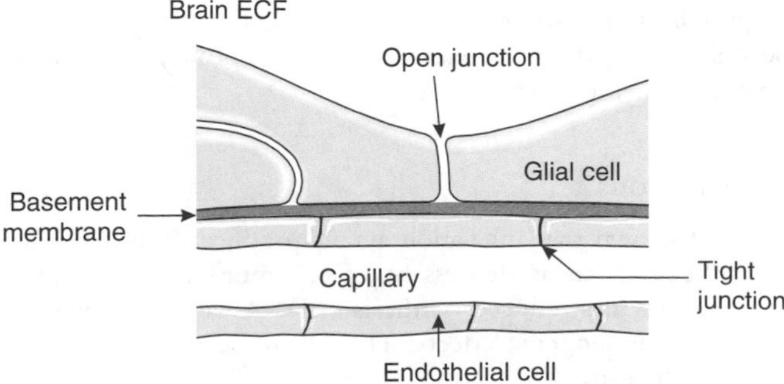

Fig. 12.13
Blood–brain barrier. ECF, extracellular fluid.

PAIN

Pain is a combination of severe discomfort, fear, autonomic ch reflex activity and suffering, and is discussed in Chapter 17.

MECHANISMS OF GENERAL ANAESTHESIA

The underlying mechanisms of general anaesthesia (a reversible loss of awareness and pain sensation) still await complete elucidation despite great progress in recent years. There is now a consensus that anaesthetics act on synaptic transmission rather than on axonal conduction and on proteins rather than lipids. At very high concentrations, general anaesthetics may act non-specifically at a wide variety of neuronal sites, but at clinical concentrations the primary effect is at a small number of targets. At these concentrations, the main effects are on ligand-gated targets rather than voltage-gated ion channels.

Previous concepts

The well-known correlation between anaesthetic potency and lipid solubility suggested that anaesthetics had a hydrophobic mechanism of action. Originally developed in 1901 by H. H. Meyer and E. Overton as the lipid solubility theory, this suggested a correlation between anaesthetic potency (minimum alveolar concentration, MAC) and oil/gas partition coefficient (Fig. 12.14). The

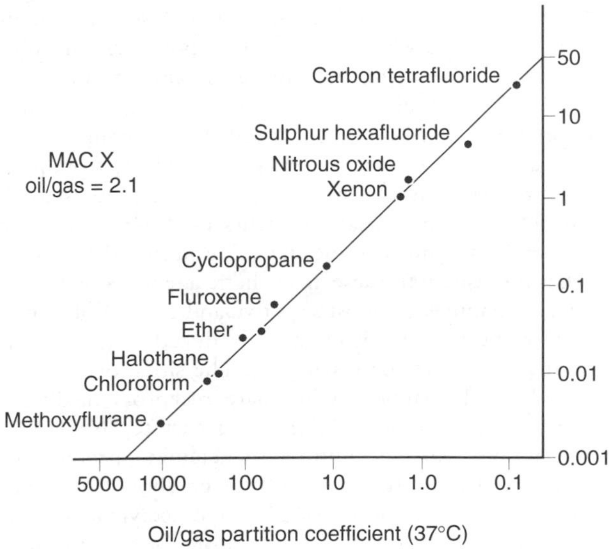

Fig. 12.14
Correlation of anaesthetic potency (minimum alveolar concentration, MAC) with oil/gas partition coefficient. Standard deviations are omitted.

ith decreasing temperature, stant relationship. v of anaesthetic action ıaesthetic partial pres- the gas hydrates ggested that anaes- as to reduce the anding the lipid mem- s. However, some potent athrates under the relevant condi- , e.g. fluorocarbons, do not fit this cor- is no mechanism for the additivity of otencies. Therefore the lipid region of the cell ne or the hydrophobic region of protein molecules was ought most likely to be the site of a common anaesthetic mechanism.

Pressure reversal and the critical volume hypothesis

If mice are placed in a pressure chamber and anaesthetized with halothane, the addition of helium to the chamber to increase the pressure to 50 atm allows the mice to wake up, although the partial pressures of halothane and oxygen are unaltered. In addition, high pressure reverses anaesthetic-induced depression of the evoked cortical response. The critical volume hypothesis proposed that there was a critical hydrophobic molecular site which is expanded by an anaesthetic and contracted by pressure. The percentage reduction in anaesthetic potency is linearly related to the total increase in pressure and the slope is the same for all agents. However, at very high pressures, this relationship no longer pertains and, in addition, not all agents behave in the same way at high pressure.

Anaesthetic action on cell membranes

Anaesthetics may block conduction by preventing channels from opening, altering the Na^+ flux, or by favouring the inactive state. Any agent which chronically depolarizes a membrane favours the inactive state, preventing channels from opening. However, K^+ channels may be blocked completely and an action potential may still be produced. Small changes in these voltage-gated Na^+ or K^+ channels seem unlikely, from present evidence, to play a significant part in the anaesthetic state. The inhibitory effects of inhalation agents on Ca^{2+} have recently been reviewed and most studies have found that these channels are rather insensitive to these anaesthetic agents. Some voltage-gated Ca^{2+} channels are most sensitive and their inhibition may account for the presynaptic effects of reduced neurotransmitter release that occurs at some synapses. The situation is different for ligand-gated channels. Glutamate receptors mediate fast excitatory transmission. *N*-Methyl-D aspartate (NMDA) is a selective agonist which is inhibited by ketamine, producing dissociative anaesthesia. It has recently been shown that volatile agents are potent inhibitors of nicotinic acetylcholine receptors. In addition to inhibiting excitatory neurotransmission, general anaesthetics could also potentiate inhibitory transmission and most anaesthetics are effective at potentiating responses to GABA.

Depression of the postsynaptic response

It is highly likely that this occurs in the anaesthetized patient. There is some evidence that anaesthetics may be selective for a specific type of synapse. Ketamine decreases synaptic transmission selectively at terminals of excitatory neurones. It preferentially depresses responses in the NMDA subtype of glutamate receptor. In contrast, methohexital enhances synaptic inhibition mediated by GABA. Such specific effects on particular synaptic processes do not support a common mechanism of anaesthesia. However, inhibition of postsynaptic currents by clinical concentrations of inhalation anaesthetics are consistent with prolonging receptor binding of GABA released presynaptically. Propofol also enhances the action of GABA so that in general almost all agents (except ketamine) potentiate postsynaptic currents induced by low concentrations of GABA, and the weight of evidence suggests that the GABA receptor channel complex is the major target for most general anaesthetics. Glycine may be equally important in the spinal cord and lower brain stem.

Multisite expansion hypothesis

The question of how general anaesthetics act at the molecular level is taxing. The effects of clinical concentrations of anaesthetic agents on lipid bilayers are far too small to account for the disruption of structure or dynamic function of the nerve membranes. This led to development of the multisite expansion hypothesis. Much of this is controversial, but the hypothesis may be summarized as follows:

- General anaesthesia may be produced by the expansion of more than one molecular site; the sites may have different physical properties.
- The physical properties of the molecular sites may be influenced by the presence of anaesthetics or pressure.
- The molecular sites have a finite size and limited degree of occupancy.
- Pressure need not necessarily act at the same site as the anaesthetic.
- Molecular sites for anaesthesia are not perturbed by a decrease in temperature in a manner analogous to an increase in pressure.

Lipids in membranes move and rotate within the bilayer and influence the activity of proteins which control ionic and neurotransmitter fluxes. Perhaps the presence of a general anaesthetic in the membrane increases the movement of lipid and is associated with an increase in its volume. This might effect conformational changes in the protein. Other studies suggest that anaesthetic agents increase the thickness of the lipid bilayer so that the protein pore cannot expand the membrane adequately.

Miscellaneous

It is well known that inhalation agents produce dose-dependent toxic effects, such as depression of cell multiplication, mitotic abnormalities and reduced synthesis of DNA with perhaps mutagenic and carcinogenic effects. These may be related to anaesthetic mechanisms.

Other areas of study have included the effect of anaesthetic agents on the microtubules which give rigidity to cytoplasm. These are rings of protein molecules bound longitudinally. Cold and hydrostatic pressure both reversibly depolymerize these microtubular proteins and produce narcosis. There remains the possibility that general anaesthetics reversibly depolymerize microtubular proteins by binding to non-polar sites on globular proteins.

Proton pump leak theory

Anaesthetic agents increase leakiness in presynaptic vesicles; this reduces pH gradients, and in turn affects the release and uptake of neurotransmitter. This concept is dependent primarily on intracellular pH. Cooling and high pressure reduce proton pump activity and neurotransmitter concentration. Anaesthetic effects of high concentrations of carbon dioxide (30%) in animals are not related to lipid solubility but to a direct action on intracellular pH. Complete anaesthesia occurs at a CSF pH of 6.7. Changes of ECF calcium concentration affect cell surface potential in a similar manner to addition of anaesthetic agents such as chloroform. Thus, it is possible that modulation of surface potential by variation in ECF composition is important for the function of excitable cells.

Sensorimotor modulation systems

Anaesthetic action on sensorimotor modulation systems switches off excitation and turns on inhibition such that messages between the periphery and brain are blocked mainly at thalamic level, with loss of motor control. Loss of consciousness occurs by a mechanism similar to an exaggerated sleep state. The number of synapses in such pathways is irrelevant, but the degree of supraspinal modulation of postsynaptic membrane excitation is important.

Somatosensory evoked responses in animals show four effects of anaesthetics. The older anaesthetics act by impeding transmission of information to the cerebral cortex at the level of thalamic relay nuclei, and impede the onward transmission of information to the cerebral cortex. The second group, represented by propofol and etomidate, act by blocking the access of information to the cortex. The third (the benzodiazepines) and fourth groups (the α_2-agonists) disrupt the transmission of sensory information at thalamic and cortical level, which distorts the coherence of cellular responses at these two sites.

Protein change

Nuclear magnetic resonance studies of volatile anaesthetic agents on haemoglobin provide evidence that anaesthetic agents interact with hydrophobic pockets within proteins at sites which appear to behave as bulk solvents. Conformational changes are then transmitted and detected in non-hydrophobic areas of the protein. Conformational changes specific to an individual anaesthetic have been observed in the same protein. Most drugs whose mode of action is known act by binding directly to proteins and it may be that anaesthetics act in the same way. The most direct evidence that general anaesthetic agents act by direct binding to proteins comes from observations of stereoselectivity shown by isoflurane. Anaesthetic binding sites have not yet been demonstrated on membrane proteins.

NEUROPHYSIOLOGICAL INVESTIGATIONS

Background activity of the brain may be recorded from the intact skull by scalp electrodes which may be unipolar or bipolar, the latter measuring the potential difference fluctuations between two electrodes. The EEG (Fig. 12.15) is a continuous recording of the immediate electrical responses from the underlying brain and represents excitatory and inhibitory postsynaptic potentials in the larger dendrites of neurones of the superficial cortex.

In the resting adult, with the eyes closed, the most prominent component is α rhythm (8–13 Hz, 50 μV amplitude), recorded best in the parieto-occipital region; β activity is 18–30 Hz, of lower voltage, and is mainly found over the frontal region; θ activity occurs in children at 4–7 Hz and is composed of large regular waves; δ activity is very slow (less than 4 Hz). If the eyes are open, fast, irregular low-voltage activity occurs with no dominant frequency. This is termed α block or desynchronization, and occurs with any form of sensory stimulation.

Deep sleep induces large, irregular δ waves interspersed with α-like activity. REM or paradoxical sleep occurs with rapid low-voltage irregular EEG activity, resembling arousal. Wakening during this period is associated with reports of dreaming. REM periods occur approximately every 50 min and occupy a total of 20% of the young adult's normal sleep time. They are associated with a marked reduction in skeletal muscle tone. Repeated awakening during REM sleep produces anxiety and irritability with an increased percentage of REM sleep in subsequent undisturbed nights.

Characteristic changes in the EEG occur in anaesthesia and other forms of coma. Increasing depth of anaesthesia with more potent agents produces slowing of the basic frequency of activity with a progressive increase in amplitude. Periods of isoelectricity appear, interspersed with bursts of activity. This is known as burst

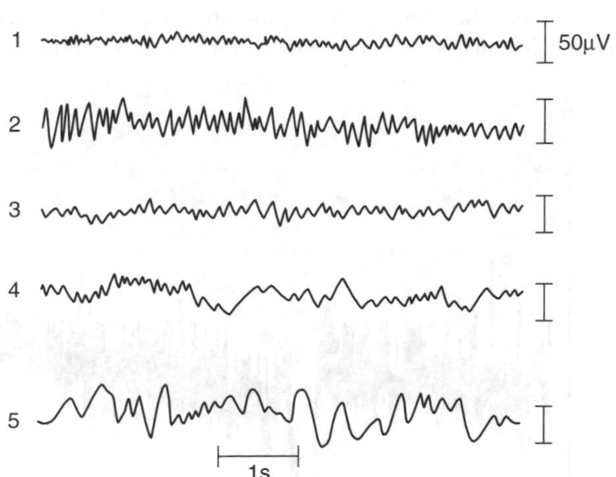

Fig. 12.15
Electroencephalogram. 1, excited; 2, relaxed; 3, drowsy; 4, asleep; 5, deep sleep.

suppression. With progressive depth of anaesthesia, there is increasing distance between bursts, resulting finally in an isoelectric line.

Characteristic changes with spike formation in the EEG occur during epilepsy. Hypoxaemia produces an acute increase in the amplitude of the EEG initially and then a marked reduction in amplitude, with the appearance of slow waves as hypoxaemia worsens.

There are problems with using the EEG to monitor the brain continuously. These are related largely to the cumbersome equipment, problems of interpretation and interference from other electrical equipment.

PROCESSED EEG TECHNIQUES

These offer no improvements in diagnostic sensitivity, but are simpler to use and clarify the display of information. Such techniques may be of limited value in evaluation of a complex situation, e.g. hypoxic changes occurring during hypothermia. There are numerous reports of the relationship between the processed EEG and anaesthetic depth, indicating that small changes are detectable which would be missed in the absence of processing.

Cerebral function monitor (CFM)

This compresses all frequency and amplitude information in the EEG into a single value. It uses two parietal electrodes, the signal from which is passed through a wide-band frequency filter to remove frequencies of less than 2 Hz and more than 15 Hz (to reduce artefacts and interference). The signal is amplified, rectified, integrated and compressed to produce a slow-running chart recording as a line, the height (above baseline) of which indicates total power (Fig. 12.16). Undulations reflect fluctuations in power from one moment to the next; upward movement indicates increased activity. The machine also monitors electrode impedance to detect artefacts from incorrect function of the electrodes.

Such a monitor requires supplementing at regular intervals by a full EEG because of the loss of information by processing. The main objection to the CFM is that the record is neither one of frequency nor amplitude but a mixture of the two. However, it does permit continuous monitoring of electrical activity.

The cerebral function analysing monitor (CFAM) produces a more detailed analysis of the EEG waveform and its frequency distribution (Fig. 12.17). The percentage of weighted activity of the α, β, θ and δ bands is displayed; this overcomes some of the objections to the loss of information which occurs with the standard CFM. Both muscle activity and electrode impedance are displayed continuously. Anaesthetics such as nitrous oxide produce a significant reduction in amplitude and a tendency towards lower frequencies on the CFAM.

Power spectrum analysis

This technique retains all information from the original EEG. Analysis of the EEG occurs as follows:

1. The EEG is digitized at frequent intervals, known as epochs (2–16 s).
2. The epoch of data is subjected to Fourier analysis, separating the total EEG waveform into a number of component sine waves of different amplitudes, the sum of which is equal to the original waveform, i.e. conversion into a number of standard waves for easy comparison.
3. The power spectrum is calculated by squaring the amplitudes of each individual frequency component, and displayed for each epoch graphically, so that patterns may be identified by examination of a number of epochs in succes-

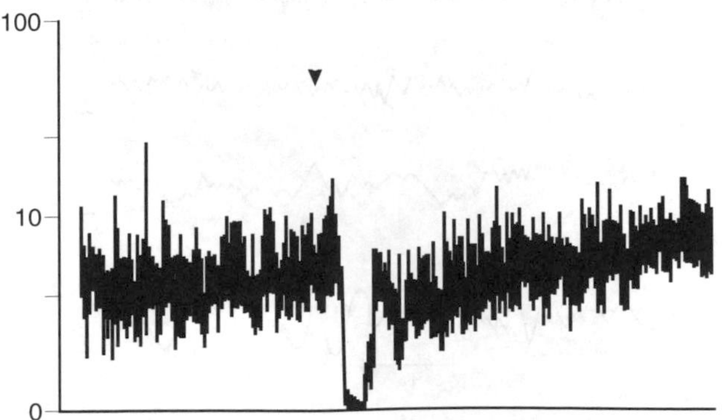

Fig. 12.16
Cerebral function monitor. This trace shows interruption of the circulation at the arrow, causing a transient absence of cerebral activity.

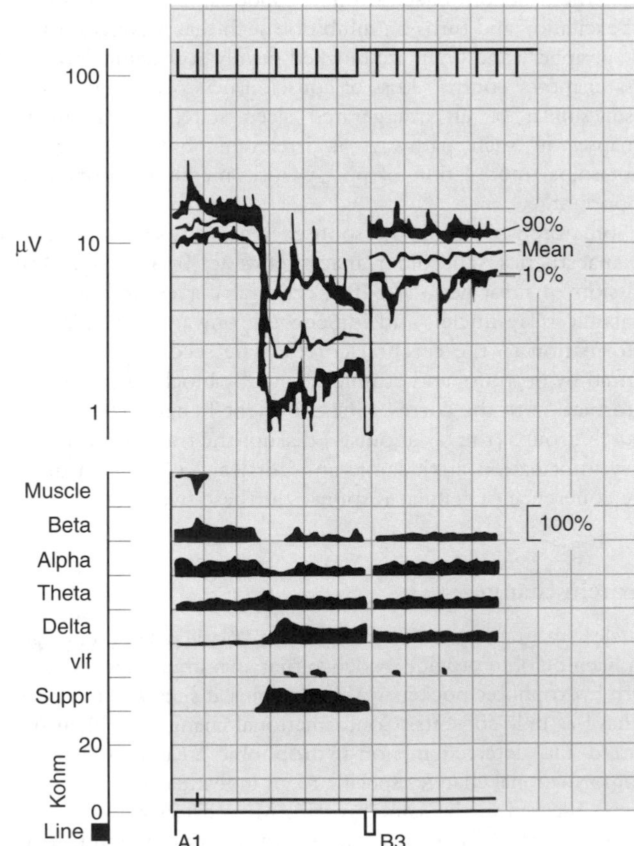

Fig. 12.17
Simulated trace from cerebral function analysing monitor, showing mean, 10th and 90th centiles of overall electroencephalogram amplitude distribution, and a display of relative distribution of activity in the β, α, θ and δ frequencies.

sion. If epochs are short (2–4 s), this constitutes almost a continuous monitor.

Advantages

- All information is retained and small changes may be identified readily.
- Each frequency band may be considered separately so that changes in one part of the spectrum cannot balance out changes elsewhere, as occurs with the CFM.
- Generation of the power spectrum minimizes baseline drift by converting all low-frequency components (0.05–0.50 Hz) to a single point.
- Predictable changes may be detected; for example, during halothane anaesthesia, there is less power at high frequencies and increased low-frequency activity.

A rapid-response graphical display is essential because one of the main advantages of this technique is the vast amount of data generated (2000 data points per minute for each EEG channel processed). The output consists of a graph of relative power versus frequency at each epoch of the analysis (Fig. 12.18). Time is presented vertically to produce a three-dimensional graph, with a hill-and-valley appearance. Hills constitute those frequencies making a large contribution and valleys occur at frequencies containing less power. The points behind the hill are not printed.

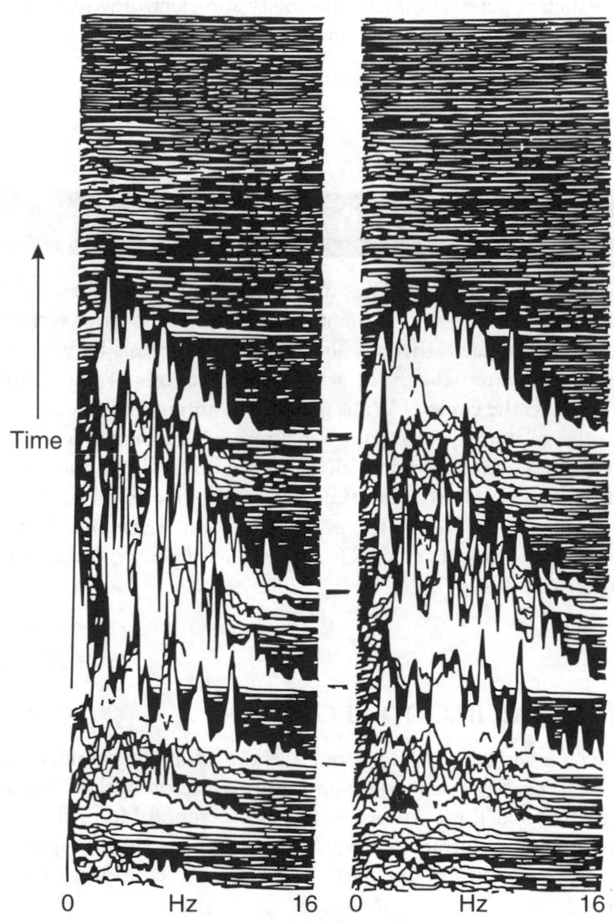

Fig. 12.18
Compressed spectral array. This trace shows fitting followed by electrical silence in a patient with meningoencephalitis.

Disadvantages

- High-amplitude activity obscures subsequent lower-amplitude activity at the same frequency.
- Both time and power are displayed vertically and therefore output requires a two-dimensional *XY* plotter. Another technique for displaying power spectrum of the EEG uses density modulation, which produces a grey-scale display.

Power spectrum techniques can detect differences between the two hemispheres and monitor changes during sedation techniques. Such therapy may require reduction in EEG activity to the level of burst suppression or reduction of activity in the CFM to 5 μV.

The CFM is the simplest automated EEG processor for intraoperative use, but it is less sensitive than the multilead EEG for detection of focal ischaemia. The CFM can discriminate between severe global cerebral ischaemia and hypoxia or hypotension, and to some extent indicates depth of anaesthesia. Gross anaesthetic overdose and severe global hypoperfusion are detectable. The CFM has proved useful in predicting the outcome of severe coma; patients with activity greater than 10 μV have survived, whereas all those with less than 3 μV died.

EVOKED POTENTIALS

Electrical events occurring in the cortex after stimulation of the sense organs may be detected by an exploring electrode over primary receiving areas for that sense. Evoked potential recordings constitute a non-invasive, objective and repeatable supplement to clinical examination. Uses include assessment of functional integrity of specific cortical areas and pathways within the CNS. Visual, auditory and somatosensory evoked potentials are widely used in diagnosis. In order to detect the low amplitudes involved, an electronic averaging technique must be used to exclude the larger amplitude background electrical noise, composed mainly of EEG activity, with some non-neuronal electrical activity.

The signal varies with body size, position of the applied stimulus, conduction velocity of axons, number of synapses, location of neural generators of the evoked potential (EP) component (i.e. either cortex or brain stem) and the presence of pathology.

Clinical applications of evoked potentials

Multiple sclerosis. As demyelination increases, complete conduction block occurs at lower temperatures. Subclinical lesions can be detected by the combined use of auditory, visual and somatosensory EPs, which show an abnormality in 80% of patients with a definite history.

Other demyelinating diseases. In demyelination, dissociation may occur of the EP peak latency and amplitude abnormalities. Latency prolongation with preservation of amplitude results from axon demyelination, but a reduction in peak amplitude occurs as more fibres die.

Intracranial tumours. EPs may be used in intraoperative monitoring of involvement of specific neural pathways. Auditory brain stem EPs have been used in the early diagnosis of posterior fossa tumours.

Head injury. Somatosensory EPs are sensitive to hypoxia and ischaemia. With a reduction in cerebral blood flow, there is a reduction in amplitude of somatosensory EPs, but the waveform is unchanged. Compressive lesions, e.g. subdural haematoma, increase the latency of the waveform. The number of wave peaks recognized in a finite period of time correlates well with outcome, but not with computed tomographic scan findings (i.e. gives information on functional rather than anatomical lesions).

Disease of, and surgery to, the spinal cord and brachial plexus. During surgery to the spinal cord, epidural motor EPs may be monitored and are relatively unaffected by anaesthetic drugs.

Investigation of apnoea in preterm infants. Auditory brain stem EP conduction time is longer in babies with apnoea than in those without, at similar postconception ages, suggesting that apnoea may be related to neural function in the brain stem.

Central conduction time (CCT)

This is the time delay between an action potential generated in the brain stem and the first cortical potential recordable (normally less than 6.4 ms). Other times are also described, e.g. the dorsal column to cortex conduction time. CCT is independent of body size and peripheral nerve conduction velocity and is probably also independent of body temperature and barbiturate concentrations. Changes result from cortical dysfunction, abnormal synaptic delay in the thalamus or cortex (or both) and slowed axonal conduction. CCT at 10 and 35 days correlates well with outcome in head injury. Changes in brain electrical activity vary with cerebral blood flow, and CCT has been used as an index of reduction of cerebral blood flow in subarachnoid haemorrhage. It may also be used as a monitor of developing ischaemia in association with surgery for subarachnoid haemorrhage.

For prediction of outcome in severe head injury, multimodality EPs are more accurate than clinical neurological signs, or the Glasgow Coma Scale.

NUCLEAR MAGNETIC RESONANCE (NMR)

Nuclei of atoms with an odd number of protons or neutrons absorb or emit electromagnetic radiation when placed in a magnetic field. Hydrogen (protons), phosphorus ^{31}P, sodium ^{23}Na and carbon ^{13}C nuclei have been studied; ^{31}P spectroscopy is used to measure concentrations of adenosine triphosphate, phosphocreatine (PCr) and intracellular pH in muscle, and neonatal brain metabolism. Repeated examinations, e.g. of tumour PCr, may indicate progression or remission of disease.

NMR imaging uses information on differences in relaxation times of nuclei. The contrast between grey and white matter in the brain is readily apparent, and excellent delineation is provided of pathologies such as demyelination and tumours in inaccessible sites. In the evaluation of lesions produced by multiple sclerosis or vascular lesions, findings are not pathognomonic but must be assessed, as with all ancillary investigation techniques, together with clinical signs. As with computed tomographic (CT) scanning, contrast enhancement may be used. The hazards associated with anaesthesia for NMR are discussed on (p. 607)

NEAR-INFRARED SPECTROPHOTOMETRY

Indices of cerebral oxygenation and haemodynamics may be quantified by this technique. Concentrations of oxygenated and reduced haemoglobin, oxidized cytochromes and total haemoglobin, together with cerebral blood volume and changes in cerebral blood flow, may be measured and displayed instantaneously. Striking changes have been observed in babies with cerebral oedema after birth trauma.

Some clinical aspects of neurophysiology may be investigated quantitatively, e.g. Glasgow Coma Scale. The increasing sophistication of peripheral nerve stimulators now makes it possible to monitor nerve conduction during neuromuscular blockade; this technique is discussed in Chapter 19. Electrodiagnostic procedures such as nerve conduction velocity and electromyography are useful investigations for neuromuscular disorders, but are beyond the scope of this chapter.

CEREBRAL CIRCULATION

The circle of Willis comprises an arterial circle at the base of the brain, supplied by the two internal carotid and two vertebral arteries. In humans, there is almost no anastomosis between the internal and external carotid arteries, but stenosis of one supplying vessel to the circle of Willis may be accommodated by an anastomotic collateral flow from other supplies. The branches of these four arteries communicate with each other over the surface of the cortex. Watershed areas between areas of major vessel supply are those most likely to suffer in hypoxia and ischaemia. Venous drainage is into sinuses which also receive CSF from arachnoid villi (see Ch. 11).

CEREBRAL BLOOD FLOW

In dealing with the damaged brain, there are many circumstances in which it is important to obtain information on both global and regional blood flow. Autoregulation of cerebral blood flow and manipulation of intracranial pressure are discussed in Chapter 57. These two important aspects are therefore not considered further here.

FURTHER READING

Angel A 1993 How do anaesthetics work? Current Anaesthesia and Critical Care 4: 37–45

Dahl J B, Kehlet H 1993 The value of pre-emptive analgesia in the treatment of postoperative pain. British Journal of Anaesthesia 70: 434–439

Department of Health A code of practice for the diagnosis of brain stem death. Health Service Circular, NHSE 1998; HSC 1998/035. HMSO, London

Franks N P, Lieb W R 1993 Selective actions of volatile general anaesthetics at molecular and cellular levels. British Journal Anaesthesia 71: 65–76

Franks N P, Lieb W R 1994 Molecular and cellular mechanisms of general anaesthesia. Nature 367: 607–614

Halsey M J, Prys-Roberts C, Strunin L 1993 (eds) Symposium on cellular and molecular aspects of anaesthesia. British Journal of Anaesthesia 71: 1–163

Insel P A 1996 Adrenergic receptors – evolving concepts and clinical implications. New England Journal of Medicine 334: 580–585

Maze M, Tranquilli W 1991 Alpha-2 adrenoreceptor agonists. Defining the role in clinical anesthesia. Anesthesiology 74: 581–605

Pallis C, Harley D H 1995 ABC of brainstem death, 2nd edn. BMJ Publishing Group, London

Violet J M, Downie D L, Nakisa R C, Lieb W R, Franks N P 1997 Differential sensitivities of mammalian neuronal and muscle nicotinic acetylcholine receptors to general anesthetics. Anesthesiology 86: 866–874

13 Inhalation anaesthetic agents

Volatile and gaseous anaesthetic agents remain popular for maintenance of anaesthesia and, under some circumstances, for induction of anaesthesia. In many situations, it is appropriate to use a mixture of 66% N_2O in oxygen and a small concentration of a volatile agent to maintain anaesthesia, although for reasons discussed below there are occasions when an anaesthetist might wish actively to avoid the use of nitrous oxide.

PROPERTIES OF THE IDEAL INHALATION ANAESTHETIC AGENT

- It should have a pleasant odour, be non-irritant to the respiratory tract and allow pleasant and rapid induction of anaesthesia.
- It should possess a low blood/gas solubility, which permits rapid induction of and rapid recovery from anaesthesia.
- It should be chemically stable in storage and should not interact with the material of anaesthetic circuits or with soda lime.
- It should be neither flammable nor explosive.
- It should be capable of producing unconsciousness with analgesia and preferably some degree of muscle relaxation.
- It should be sufficiently potent to allow the use of high inspired oxygen concentrations when necessary.
- It should not be metabolized in the body, be non-toxic and not provoke allergic reactions.
- It should produce minimal depression of the cardiovascular and respiratory systems and should not interact with other drugs used commonly during anaesthesia, e.g. pressor agents or catecholamines.
- It should be completely inert and eliminated completely and rapidly in an unchanged form via the lungs.
- It should be easy to administer using standard vaporizers.
- It should not be epileptogenic or raise intracranial pressure.

None of the inhalation anaesthetic agents approaches the standards required of the ideal agent.

MINIMUM ALVEOLAR CONCENTRATION (MAC)

MAC is the minimum alveolar concentration (in volumes per cent) of an anaesthetic at 1 atmosphere absolute (ata) that prevents movement of 50% of the population to a standard stimulus. Anaesthesia is related to the partial pressure of an inhalation agent in the brain rather than its percentage concentration in alveoli, but the term MAC has gained widespread acceptance as an index of anaesthetic potency because this can be measured. It can be applied to all inhalation anaesthetics and it permits comparison of different agents. However, it represents only one point on a dose–response curve; 1 MAC of one agent is equivalent in anaesthetic potency to 1 MAC of another, but it does not follow that the agents are equipotent at 2 MAC. Nevertheless, in general terms, 0.5 MAC of one agent in combination with 0.5 MAC of another approximates to 1 MAC in total.

The MAC values for the anaesthetic agents quoted in Table 13.1 (p. 163) were determined experimentally in humans (volunteers) breathing a mixture of the agent in oxygen. MAC values vary under the following circumstances.

Factors which lead to a reduction in MAC

- sedative drugs such as premedication agents, analgesics
- nitrous oxide
- increasing age
- drugs which affect neurotransmitter release such as methyldopa, pancuronium and clonidine
- higher atmospheric pressure, as anaesthetic potency is related to partial pressure – for example, MAC for enflurane is 1.68% (1.66 kPa) at a pressure of 1 ata, but 0.84% (still 1.66 kPa) at 2 ata
- hypotension
- hypothermia
- myxoedema
- pregnancy
- hypocapnia.

Factors which increase MAC

- decreasing age
- pyrexia
- induced sympathoadrenal stimulation, e.g. hypercapnia
- the presence of ephedrine, or amphetamine
- thyrotoxicosis
- chronic alcohol ingestion.

INDIVIDUAL ANAESTHETIC AGENTS

Physical properties of the inhalation anaesthetic agents are summarized in Appendix II p. 766. The structural formulae of the agents discussed in this chapter are shown in Figure 13.1.

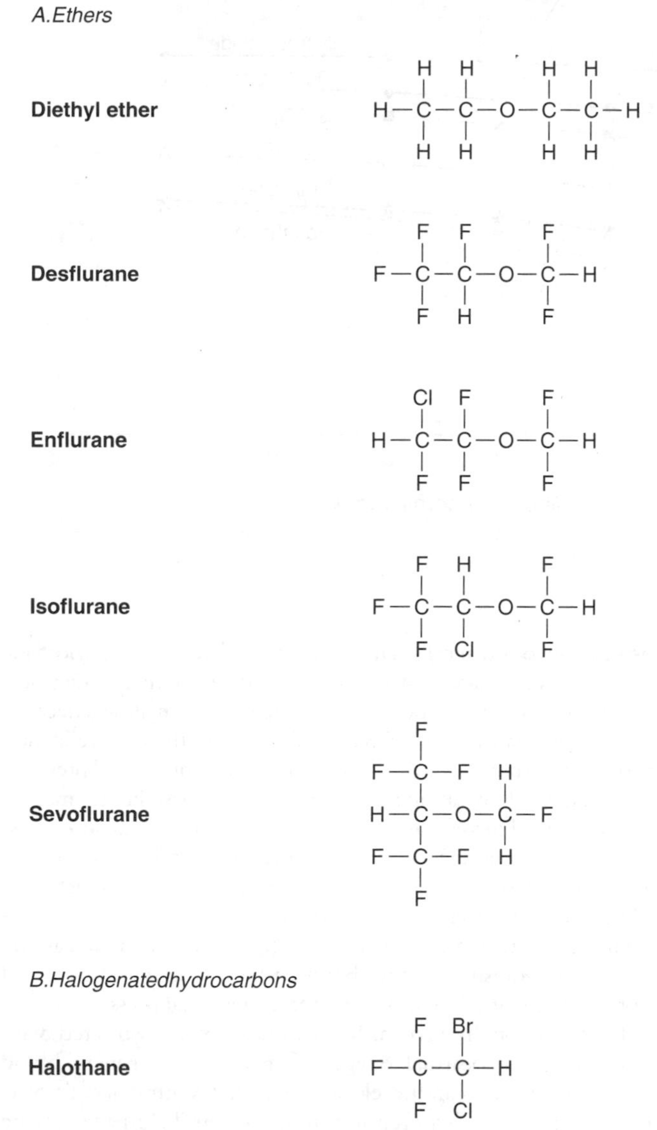

A. Ethers

Diethyl ether

```
    H   H       H   H
    |   |       |   |
H — C — C — O — C — C — H
    |   |       |   |
    H   H       H   H
```

Desflurane

```
    F   F       F
    |   |       |
F — C — C — O — C — H
    |   |       |
    F   H       F
```

Enflurane

```
    Cl  F       F
    |   |       |
H — C — C — O — C — H
    |   |       |
    F   F       F
```

Isoflurane

```
    F   H       F
    |   |       |
F — C — C — O — C — H
    |   |       |
    F   Cl      F
```

Sevoflurane

```
        F
        |
    F — C — F   H
        |       |
    H — C — O — C — F
        |       |
    F — C — F   H
        |
        F
```

B. Halogenated hydrocarbons

Halothane

```
    F   Br
    |   |
F — C — C — H
    |   |
    F   Cl
```

Fig. 13.1
Structural formulae of inhalation anaesthetic agents.

AGENTS IN COMMON CLINICAL USE

In Western countries, it is customary to use one of the five modern volatile anaesthetic agents – halothane, enflurane, isoflurane, sevoflurane and desflurane – vaporized in a mixture of nitrous oxide in oxygen. In recent years, the use of halothane has declined because of medicolegal pressure relating to the very rare occurrence of hepatotoxicity. Whilst this concern is less acute in Europe there is a clear trend to avoidance of repeated halothane anaesthesia. The use of sevoflurane is growing rapidly, particularly in paediatric anaesthesia because of its superior quality as an inhalation induction agent. Desflurane produces rapid recovery from anaesthesia, but it is very irritant to the airway and is therefore not used as an inhalation induction agent.

The following account of these agents, with a comparison of their pharmacological properties, may tend to exaggerate the differences between them. However, an equally satisfactory anaesthetic may be administered in the majority of patients with any of the five agents.

HALOTHANE

Halothane (2-bromo-2-chloro-1,1,1-trifluoroethane) was synthesized in 1951 and introduced into clinical practice in the UK in 1956. It is a colourless liquid with a relatively pleasant smell. It is decomposed by light. The addition of 0.01% thymol and storage in amber-coloured bottles renders it stable. Although it is decomposed by soda lime, it may be used safely with this mixture. It corrodes metals in vaporizers and breathing systems. In the presence of moisture, it corrodes aluminium, tin, lead, magnesium and alloys. It should be stored in a closed container away from light and heat.

Uptake and distribution

Halothane has a blood/gas solubility coefficient of 2.5, which is the highest of all the modern agents. It is not irritant to the airway and therefore inhalation induction with halothane is relatively fast when compared with either desflurane or isoflurane. However, it may take at least 30 min for the alveolar inspired concentration to reach 50% of the inspired concentration (Fig. 13.2); this is slower than for the other agents. As with all the volatile agents, it is customary to use the technique of 'over-pressure' and induce halothane anaesthesia with concentrations two to three times higher than the MAC value; the inspired concentration is reduced when a stable level of anaesthesia has been achieved. The MAC of halothane in oxygen is approximately 1.1% in the neonate, 0.95% in the infant, 0.9% at 1–2 years, 0.75% at 40 years (0.29 in 70% nitrous oxide) and 0.65% at 80 years.

Recovery from halothane anaesthesia is slower than with the other agents (Fig. 13.3) because of its high blood/gas solubility, and recovery is prolonged with increasing duration of anaesthesia.

Metabolism

Approximately 20% of halothane is metabolized in the liver, usually by oxidative pathways. The end-products are excreted in the urine. The major metabolites are bromine, chlorine, trifluoroacetic acid and trifluoroacetylethanol amide.

A small proportion of halothane may undergo reductive metabolism, particularly in the presence of hypoxaemia and when the hepatic microsomal enzymes have been stimulated by enzyme-inducing agents such as phenobarbital. Reductive metabolism may result in the formation of reactive metabolites and fluoride, although normally serum fluoride ion concentrations are considerably lower than those likely to induce renal dysfunction.

Respiratory system

Halothane is non-irritant and pleasant to breathe during induction of anaesthesia. There is rapid loss of pharyngeal and laryngeal reflexes and inhibition of salivary and bronchial secretions. In the unpremedicated subject, halothane anaesthesia is associated with an increase in ventilatory rate and reduction in tidal volume. $P_{a}CO_2$ increases as the depth of halothane anaesthesia increases (Fig. 13.4).

Halothane causes a dose-dependent decrease in mucociliary function, which may persist for several hours after anaesthesia. This may contribute to postoperative sputum retention.

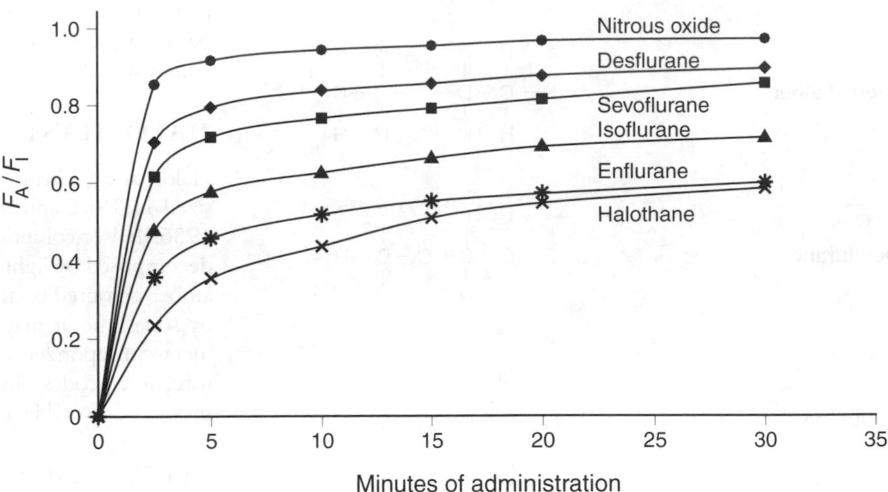

Fig. 13.2
Ratio of alveolar (F_A) to inspired (F_I) fractional concentration of nitrous oxide, desflurane, sevoflurane, isoflurane, enflurane and halothane in the first 30 min of anaesthesia. The plot of F_A/F_I expresses the rapidity with which alveolar concentration equilibrates with inspired concentration. It is most rapid for agents with a low blood/gas partition coefficient. (Adapted from Eger 1994, with permission.)

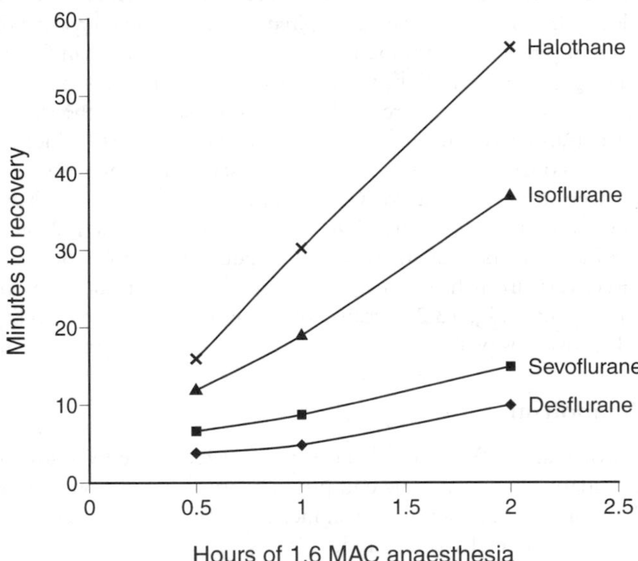

Fig. 13.3
Rapidity of recovery from anaesthesia is inversely proportional to the solubility of the anaesthetic: the most rapid recovery is with the least soluble anaesthetic (desflurane). The difference is amplified by duration of anaesthesia (note that the difference in time of recovery between the least (desflurane) and most soluble anaesthetic (halothane) is greater after 2 h of anaesthesia than after 0.5 h of anaesthesia). (From Weiskopf 1995 with permission.)

Halothane antagonizes bronchospasm and reduces airway resistance in patients with bronchoconstriction, possibly by central inhibition of reflex bronchoconstriction and relaxation of bronchial smooth muscle. It has been suggested that halothane exerts a β-mimetic effect on bronchial muscle.

Cardiovascular system

Halothane is a potent depressant of myocardial contractility and myocardial metabolic activity as a result of inhibition of glucose uptake by myocardial cells. During controlled ventilation, halothane anaesthesia is associated with dose-related depression of cardiac output (by decrease in myocardial contractility) with little effect on peripheral resistance (Figs 13.5 and 13.6). Thus, there is a reduction in arterial pressure (Fig. 13.7) and an increase in right atrial pressure. In spontaneously breathing patients, some of these effects may be offset by a small increase in P_aCO_2 which leads to a reduction in systemic vascular resistance and a shift in cardiac output back towards baseline values as a result of indirect sympathoadrenal stimulation.

The hypotensive effect of halothane is augmented by a reduction in heart rate, which commonly accompanies halothane anaesthesia. Antagonism of the bradycardia by administration of atropine frequently leads to an increase in arterial pressure.

The reduction in myocardial contractility is associated with reductions in myocardial oxygen demand and coronary blood flow. Provided that undue elevations in left ventricular diastolic pressure and undue hypotension do not occur, halothane may be advantageous in patients with coronary artery disease because of the reduced oxygen demand caused by a low heart rate and decreased contractility.

The depressant effects of halothane on cardiac output are augmented in the presence of β-blockade.

Arrhythmias are very common during halothane anaesthesia and far more frequent than with any of the other agents. Arrhythmias are produced by:

- increased myocardial excitability augmented by the presence of hypercapnia, hypoxaemia or increased circulating catecholamines
- bradycardia caused by central vagal stimulation.

During local infiltration with local anaesthetic solutions containing epinephrine, multifocal ventricular extrasystoles and sinus tachycardia have been observed and cardiac arrest has been reported. Thus, caution should be exercised when these solutions are used. The following recommendations have been made:

- Avoid hypoxaemia and hypercapnia.
- Avoid concentrations of epinephrine greater than 1 in 100 000.

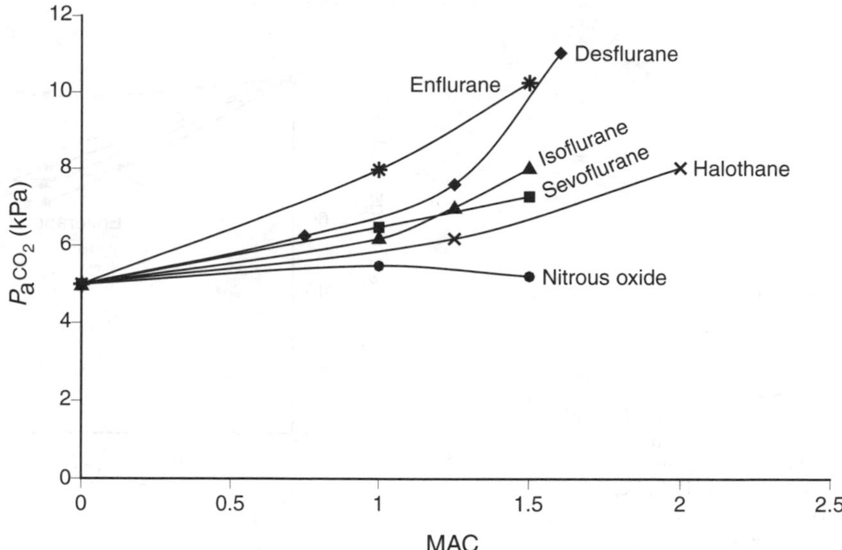

Fig. 13.4
Effects on P_aCO_2 of halothane, enflurane, isoflurane, sevoflurane, desflurane and nitrous oxide at equivalent MAC during spontaneous ventilation by healthy volunteers. (Nitrous oxide was administered in a hyperbaric chamber.)

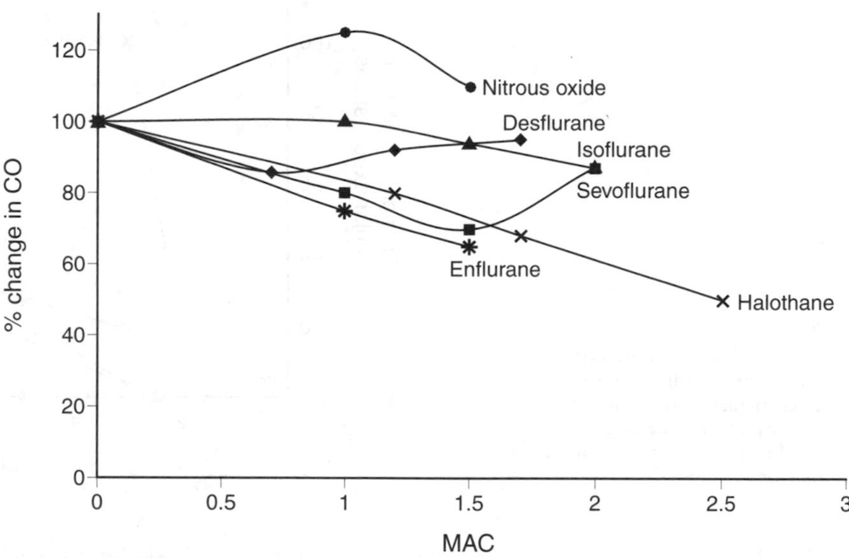

Fig. 13.5
Comparative effects of nitrous oxide, isoflurane, halothane, enflurane, desflurane and sevoflurane on cardiac output (CO) in healthy volunteers.

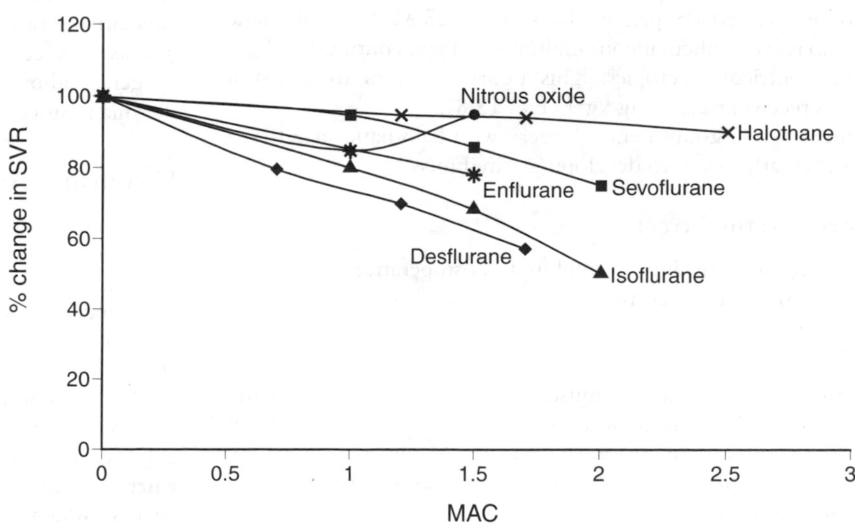

Fig.13.6
Comparative effects of nitrous oxide, halothane, enflurane, isoflurane, sevoflurane and desflurane on systemic vascular resistance (SVR) in healthy volunteers.

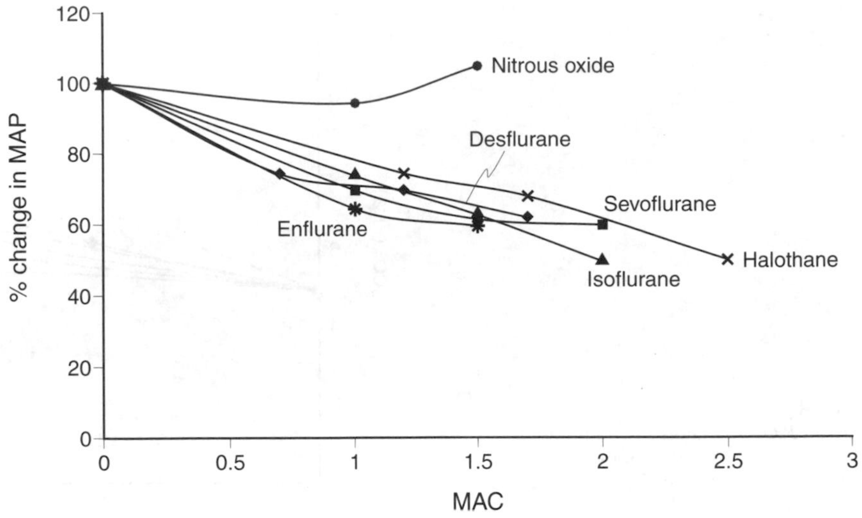

Fig. 13.7
Comparative effects of nitrous oxide, halothane, enflurane, isoflurane, sevoflurane and desflurane on mean arterial pressure (MAP) in healthy volunteers.

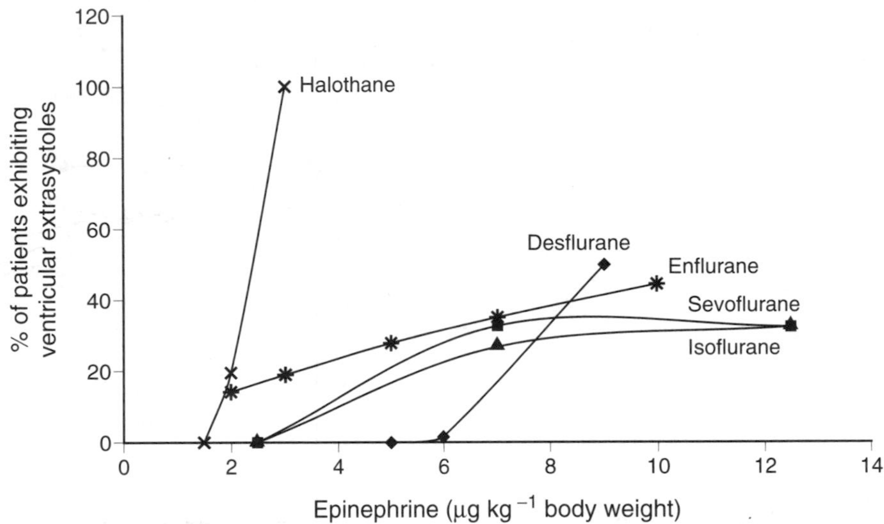

Fig. 13.8
Cumulative plots representing dose of subcutaneous epinephrine required to produce ventricular extrasystoles in normocapnic patients receiving 1.25 MAC of halothane, enflurane, isoflurane, sevoflurane or desflurane.

- Avoid a dosage in adults exceeding 10 ml of 1 in 100 000 epinephrine in 10 min (i.e. 100 μg) or 30 ml h^{-1} (300 μg).

Approximately 20% of patients breathing 1.25 MAC of halothane and who receive subcutaneous infiltration of epinephrine 2 μg kg^{-1} exhibit ventricular ectopics. This figure increases to 100% of patients receiving 2.5–3 μg kg^{-1} (Fig. 13.8).

Patients undergoing dental surgery with halothane anaesthesia are particularly prone to developing arhythmias.

Gastrointestinal tract

Gastrointestinal motility is inhibited. Postoperative nausea and vomiting are seldom severe.

Uterus

Halothane relaxes uterine muscle and may cause postpartum haemorrhage. It is said that a concentration of less than 0.5% is not associated with increased blood loss during anaesthesia for Caesarean section, but this concentration causes increased blood loss during therapeutic abortion.

Skeletal muscle

Halothane causes skeletal muscle relaxation and potentiates non-depolarizing relaxants. Postoperatively, shivering is common; this increases oxygen requirements and results in hypoxaemia unless oxygen is administered. Halothane can trigger malignant hyperthermia in susceptible patients.

Halothane-associated hepatic dysfunction

There are two types of dysfunction, which may take place after halothane anaesthesia. The first is mild and is associated with derangement in liver function tests. These changes are transient and generally resolve within a few days. Similar changes in liver function tests have also been reported after enflurane anaesthesia and, to a lesser extent, isoflurane anaesthesia.

This subclinical type of hepatic dysfunction, evidenced by an increase in glutathione-S-transferase (GST) concentrations, probably occurs as a result of metabolism of halothane in the liver where it reacts with hepatic macromolecules resulting in tissue necrosis which is worsened by hypoxaemia.

The second type of hepatic dysfunction is extremely uncommon and takes the form of severe jaundice, progressing to fulminating hepatic necrosis. The mortality of this condition varies between 30 and 70%. The likelihood of this type of hepatic dysfunction is increased by repeated exposure to the drug. The mechanism of these changes is probably the formation of a hapten–protein complex. The hapten is probably one of the metabolites of halothane, notably trifluoroacetyl (TFA)-halide as antibodies to TFA proteins have now been detected in patients who develop jaundice after halothane anaesthesia.

The incidence of type 2 liver dysfunction after halothane anaesthesia is extremely low – so low that it is extremely difficult to mount well controlled studies of the condition, and consequently this whole subject has been an area of great controversy over the last 10–15 years. Nonetheless, as a result of this concern, the Committee on Safety of Medicines has made the following recommendations in respect of halothane anaesthesia:

- A careful anaesthetic history should be taken to determine previous exposure and any previous reaction to halothane.
- Repeated exposure to halothane within a period of 3 months should be avoided unless there are overriding clinical circumstances.
- A history of unexplained jaundice or pyrexia after previous exposure to halothane is an absolute contraindication to its future use in that patient.

The incidence of halothane hepatotoxicity in paediatric practice is extremely low, although there have been case reports in children. Nevertheless, halothane is still widely used in paediatric anaesthesia

In summary, halothane is a very useful inhalation anaesthetic agent. Its main advantages are:

- smooth induction
- minimal stimulation of salivary and bronchial secretions; prior administration of atropine is unnecessary.
- bronchodilatation.

The disadvantages are:

- arrhythmias
- possibility of liver toxicity, especially with repeated administrations
- slow recovery compared with other new agents (Fig. 13.3).

ENFLURANE

Enflurane (2-chloro-1,1,2-trifluoroethyl difluoro-methyl ether) was synthesized in 1963 and first evaluated clinically in 1966. It was introduced into clinical practice in the USA in 1971.

Physical properties

Enflurane is a clear, colourless, volatile anaesthetic agent with a pleasant ethereal smell. It is non-flammable in clinical concentrations, stable with soda lime and metals and does not require preservatives. The MAC of enflurane is 1.68% in oxygen and 0.57% in 70% nitrous oxide.

Uptake and distribution

Enflurane has a blood/gas solubility coefficient of 1.9, which is between that of halothane and isoflurane. Thus, induction of and recovery from anaesthesia are faster than halothane but slower than isoflurane, desflurane and sevoflurane (Figs 13.2 and 13.3).

Metabolism

Approximately 2.5% of the absorbed dose is metabolized, predominantly to fluoride. In common with other ether anaesthetic agents, the presence of the ether bond imparts stability to the molecule.

Defluorination of enflurane is increased in patients treated with isoniazid, but not with a classic enzyme-inducing agent such as phenobarbital. Serum fluoride ion concentrations are greater after administration of enflurane to obese patients. To date, extensive studies have failed to demonstrate that the serum concentrations of fluoride ion reach toxic levels after enflurane anaesthesia. The plasma fluoride ion concentrations attained after enflurane anaesthesia are approximately 20 μmol L^{-1} (which is below the 50 μmol L^{-1} thought to be associated with renal damage after anaesthesia with methoxyflurane).

Respiratory system

Enflurane is non-irritant and does not increase salivary or bronchial secretions; thus inhalation induction is relatively pleasant and rapid.

In common with all other volatile anaesthetic agents, enflurane causes a dose-dependent depression of alveolar ventilation with a reduction in tidal volume and an increase in ventilatory rate in the unpremedicated subject. This results in an increase in arterial CO_2 concentration (Fig. 13.4).

Cardiovascular system

Enflurane causes dose-dependent depression of myocardial contractility, leading to a reduction in cardiac output (Fig. 13.5). In association with a small reduction in systemic vascular resistance, this leads to a dose-dependent reduction in arterial pressure (Figs 13.6 and 13.7). Because enflurane (unlike halothane) has no central vagal effects, hypotension leads to reflex tachycardia.

Enflurane anaesthesia is associated with a much smaller incidence of arrhythmias than halothane and much less sensitization of the myocardium to catecholamines, either endogenous or exogenous. Twenty per cent of patients receiving subcutaneous infiltration of epinephrine 3 μg kg^{-1} at 1.25 MAC of enflurane exhibit ventricular ectopics (Fig. 13.8).

Uterus

Enflurane relaxes uterine muscle in a dose-related manner.

Central nervous system

Enflurane produces a dose-dependent depression of EEG activity, but at moderate to high concentrations (more than 3%) it produces epileptiform paroxysmal spike activity and burst suppression. These are accentuated by hypocapnia. Twitching of the face and arm muscles may occur occasionally. Enflurane should be avoided in the epileptic patient.

Muscle relaxation

Enflurane produces dose-dependent muscle relaxation with potentiation of non-depolarizing neuromuscular blocking drugs to a greater extent than that produced by halothane. It can trigger malignant hyperthermia.

Hepatotoxicity

There have been several case reports of jaundice attributable to the use of enflurane, and derangement of liver enzymes also occurs after enflurane anaesthesia, although to a lesser extent than after halothane.

Cross-sensitization has been reported between halothane and enflurane, and therefore multiple administrations of halothane and enflurane should be avoided within short periods.

In summary, enflurane is a useful alternative agent to halothane. Its main advantages are:

- low risk of hepatic dysfunction
- low incidence of arrhythmias.

Its disadvantages are:

- seizure activity on EEG
- its use in patients with pre-existing renal disease or in those taking enzyme-inducing drugs may be unwise.

ISOFLURANE

Isoflurane (1-chloro-2,2,2-trifluoroethyl difluoro-methyl ether) is an isomer of enflurane and was synthesized in 1965. Clinical studies were undertaken in 1970, but because of early laboratory reports of carcinogenesis (which were not confirmed subsequently) it was not approved by the Food and Drug Administration in the United States until 1980.

Physical properties

Isoflurane is a colourless, volatile liquid with a slightly pungent odour. It is stable and does not react with metal or other substances. It does not require preservatives. Isoflurane is non-flammable in clinical concentrations. The MAC of isoflurane is 1.15% in oxygen and 0.56% in 70% nitrous oxide.

Uptake and distribution

Isoflurane has a low blood/gas solubility of 1.4 and thus alveolar concentrations equilibrate rapidly with inspired concentrations. The alveolar (or arterial) partial pressure of isoflurane increases to 50% of the inspired partial pressure within 4–8 min, and to 60% by 15 min (Fig. 13.2). However, the rate of induction is limited by the pungency of the vapour and clinically may be no faster than that which can be achieved with halothane. The incidence of coughing or breath-holding on induction is significantly greater with isoflurane than with halothane. It is not an ideal agent to use for inhalation induction.

Metabolism

Approximately 0.17% of the absorbed dose is metabolized. Metabolism takes place predominantly in the form of oxidation to produce difluoromethanol and trifluoroacetic acid; the former breaks down to formic acid and fluoride. Because of the minimal metabolism, only very small concentrations of serum fluoride ions are found, even after prolonged administration. The minimal metabolism renders hepatic and renal toxicity most unlikely.

Respiratory system

In common with other modern volatile agents, it causes dose-dependent depression of ventilation; there is a decrease in tidal volume but an increase in ventilatory rate in the absence of opioid drugs.

Cardiovascular system

In vitro, isoflurane is a myocardial depressant, but in clinical use there is less depression of cardiac output than with halothane or enflurane. Systemic hypotension occurs predominantly as a result of reduction in systemic vascular resistance (Figs 13.6 and 13.7). Arrhythmias are uncommon and there is little sensitization of the myocardium to catecholamines. Approximately 20% of patients breathing 1.25 MAC of isoflurane and who receive subcutaneous infiltration of epinephrine 6μg kg^{-1} exhibit ventricular ectopics (Fig 13.8).

In addition to dilating systemic arterioles, isoflurane causes coronary vasodilatation. There has been some controversy regarding the safety of isoflurane in patients with coronary artery disease because of the possibility that the coronary steal syndrome may be induced; dilatation in normal coronary arteries offers a low resistance to flow and may reduce perfusion through stenosed vessels. It has been shown that isoflurane affects small arterioles (which makes coronary steal a theoretical possibility), but the effect seems to occur only in end-tidal concentrations in excess of 0.5%. Production of myocardial ischaemia in clinical practice may be produced by a large number of factors in addition to coronary vasodilatation, including tachycardia, hypotension, increase in left ventricular end-diastolic pressure and reduced ventricular compliance. Attention should be directed to these factors before a diagnosis of isoflurane-induced coronary steal is considered.

Uterus

Isoflurane has an effect on the pregnant uterus similar to that of halothane and enflurane.

Central nervous system

Low concentrations of isoflurane do not cause any change in cerebral blood flow at normocapnia. In this respect, the drug is superior to enflurane and halothane, both of which cause cerebral vasodilatation. However, higher inspired concentrations of isoflurane cause vasodilatation and increase cerebral blood flow. It does not cause seizure activity on the EEG.

Muscle relaxation

Isoflurane causes dose-dependent depression of neuromuscular transmission with potentiation of non-depolarizing neuromuscular blocking drugs.

In summary, the advantages of isoflurane are:

- rapid recovery
- minimal biotransformation with little risk of hepatic or renal toxicity
- very low risk of arrhythmias
- muscle relaxation.

Its disadvantages are:

- a pungent odour which makes inhalation induction relatively unpleasant, particularly in children
- coronary vasodilatation with the possibility of coronary steal syndrome at high inspired concentrations.

SEVOFLURANE

Sevoflurane is a methyl propyl ether which was first synthesized in 1968 and reported in 1971. The initial development was slow because of some apparent toxic effects, which were later found to be caused by flawed experimental design. After its first use in volunteers in 1981, further work was delayed again because of the problems of biotransformation and stability with soda lime. The drug has been available for general clinical use in Japan since 1990, and by the end of 1993, 1 million patients had received sevoflurane. It has been introduced more recently in the UK.

Physical properties

It is non-flammable and has a pleasant smell. The blood/gas partition coefficient of sevoflurane is 0.69, which is about half of that of isoflurane (1.43) and closer to that of desflurane (0.42) and nitrous oxide (0.44). The MAC value of sevoflurane in adults is between 1.7 and 2% in oxygen and 0.66% in 60% nitrous oxide. The MAC, in common with other volatile agents, is higher in children (2.6% in oxygen and 2.0% in nitrous oxide) and neonates (3.3%) and it is reduced in the elderly (1.48%). It is stable and is stored in amber-coloured bottles. In the presence of water, it undergoes some hydrolysis and this reaction also occurs with soda lime.

Uptake and distribution

It has a low blood/gas partition coefficient and therefore the rate of equilibration between alveolar and inspired concentrations is faster than that for halothane, enflurane or isoflurane but slower than that for desflurane (Fig. 13.2). It is non-irritant to the upper respiratory tract and therefore the rate of induction of anaesthesia should be faster than that with any of the other agents.

Because of its higher partition coefficients in vessel-rich tissues, muscle and fat than corresponding values for desflurane, the rate of recovery is slower than that after desflurane anaesthesia (Fig. 13.3).

Metabolism

Approximately 5% of the absorbed dose is metabolized in the liver to two main metabolites. The major breakdown product is hexafluoroisopropanol, an organic fluoride molecule which is excreted in the urine as a glucuronide conjugate. Although this molecule is potentially hepatotoxic, conjugation of hexafluoroisopropanol occurs so rapidly that clinically significant liver damage seems theoretically impossible. The second breakdown product is inorganic fluoride ion. The mean peak fluoride ion concentration after 60 min of anaesthesia at 1 MAC is 22 μmol L^{-1}, which is similar to that produced after enflurane anaesthesia and significantly higher than that after an equivalent dose of isoflurane. The metabolism of sevoflurane is catalysed by the 2E1 isoform of cytochrome P450 which can be induced by phenobarbital, isoniazid and ethanol and inhibited by disulfiram.

Respiratory system

The drug is non-irritant to the upper respiratory tract. It produces dose-dependent ventilatory depression, reduces respiratory drive in response to hypoxia and increases carbon dioxide partial pressure comparable with levels achieved with other volatile agents (Fig. 13.4). The ventilatory depression associated with sevoflurane may result from a combination of central depression of medullary respiratory neurones and depression of diaphragmatic function and contractility. It relaxes bronchial smooth muscle but not as effectively as halothane.

Cardiovascular system

The properties of sevoflurane are similar to those of isoflurane with slightly smaller effects on heart rate (Fig. 13.9) and less coronary vasodilatation. It decreases arterial pressure (Fig. 13.7) mainly by reducing peripheral vascular resistance (Fig. 13.6), but cardiac output is well maintained over the normal anaesthetic maintenance doses (Fig. 13.5). There is mild myocardial depression resulting from its effect on calcium channels. Sevoflurane does not differ from isoflurane in its sensitization of the myocardium to exogenous catecholamines (Fig. 13.8). It is a less potent coronary arteriolar dilator and therefore does not appear to cause 'coronary steal'. Sevoflurane is associated with lower heart rate and therefore helps to reduce myocardial oxygen consumption.

Central nervous system

Its effects are similar to those of halothane, isoflurane and desflurane. Intracranial pressure increases at high inspired concentrations of sevoflurane but this effect is minimal over the 0.5–1.0 MAC range. It decreases cerebral vascular resistance and cerebral metabolic rate. It does not cause excitatory effects on the EEG.

Renal system

The peak concentration of inorganic fluoride after sevoflurane is similar to that after enflurane anaesthesia and there is a positive correlation between duration of exposure and the peak concentration of fluoride ions. Serum fluoride concentrations of greater than 50 μmol L^{-1} have been reported. However, renal toxicity does not appear to be related to inorganic fluoride concentrations following anaesthesia with sevoflurane as opposed to that associated with methoxyflurane. The apparent lack of renal toxicity with sevoflurane may be related to its rapid elimination from the body. This reduces the total amount of drug available for in vivo metabolism.

Renal blood flow is well preserved with sevoflurane.

Musculoskeletal system

In common with isoflurane, the drug potentiates non-depolarizing muscle relaxants to a similar extent. Sevoflurane can trigger malignant hyperthermia in susceptible patients and there have been cases reported in the literature.

Obstetric use

There are limited data on the use of sevoflurane in the obstetric population.

Interaction with carbon dioxide absorbers

Sevoflurane is absorbed and degraded by both soda lime and Baralyme. When mixed with soda lime in artificial situations, five breakdown products are identified, which are termed compounds A, B, C, D and E. These products are thought to be toxic in rats, primarily involving renal, hepatic and cerebral damage. However, in clinical situations, it is mainly compound A and, to a lesser extent, compound B that are produced. The evidence suggests that the concentration of compound A produced is well below the level that is toxic to animals. The use of Baralyme is associated with production of higher concentrations of compound A and this may be related to the higher temperature which is attained when Baralyme is used. The presence of moisture reduces compound A formation. The concentration of compound A is highest during low-flow anaesthesia (<2 L min $^{-1}$) and is reduced by increasing fresh gas flow rate. The toxicity of sevoflurane in combination with carbon dioxide absorbers is possibly more theoretical than a clinical problem but it may be wise to avoid its use with very low fresh gas flows and in patients with poor renal function.

In summary, sevoflurane is a newer inhalation anaesthetic agent which offers many advantages over other volatile agents. These are:

- smooth, fast induction
- rapid recovery
- ease of use, requiring conventional vaporizers (particularly when compared with desflurane).

Its disadvantages are:

- production of potentially toxic metabolites in the body
- instability with carbon dioxide absorbers
- still relatively expensive.

DESFLURANE

Between 1959 and 1966, Terrell and his associates at Ohio Medical Products synthesized more than 700 compounds to try to produce better inhalation anaesthetic agents. Two of these products were the halogenated methyl ethyl ethers, isoflurane and enflurane which have now been widely used. Some of the original 700 products were re-examined many years later. Many were discarded for a variety of reasons. One of these (the 653rd) was difficult to synthesize because of a potentially explosive step using elemental fluorine and it had a vapour pressure close to 1 atm. However, because it was predicted to have a low solubility in blood and hence would allow rapid recovery, it was re-examined with heightened interest. This product became known as desflurane. Desflurane was first used in humans in 1988 and it became available for general clinical use in the UK in 1993. Its structure (CHF_2-O-CHF-CF_3) differs from that of isoflurane (CHF_2-O-CHCl-CF_3) only in the substitution of fluorine for chlorine.

Physical properties

It is a colourless agent, which is stored in amber-coloured bottles without preservative. It is not broken down by soda lime, light or metals. It is non-flammable.

Desflurane has a boiling point of 23.5°C and a vapour pressure of 664 mmHg at 20°C and therefore it cannot be used in a standard vaporizer. A special vaporizer (the TEC 6) has been developed which requires a source of electric power to heat and pressurize it.

The MAC of desflurane is approximately 6% in oxygen (3% in 60% nitrous oxide). As with all volatile agents, its MAC is higher in children (9–10% in the neonate in oxygen, 7% in 60% nitrous oxide)

It has an ethereal but less pungent odour than isoflurane.

Uptake and distribution

Desflurane has a blood/gas partition coefficient of 0.42, almost the same as that of nitrous oxide. The rate of equilibration of alveolar with inspired concentrations of desflurane is virtually identical to that for nitrous oxide (Fig. 13.2). Induction of anaesthesia is therefore extremely rapid in theory but limited somewhat by a pungent nature. However, it is possible to alter the depth of anaesthesia very rapidly and the rate of recovery of anaesthesia is faster than that following any other volatile anaesthetic agent (Fig. 13.3).

Metabolism

There is very little defluorination of desflurane, and after prolonged anaesthesia there is only a very small increase in serum and urine trifluoroacetic acid levels. Approximately 0.02% of inhaled desflurane is metabolized in the body.

Respiratory system

Desflurane causes respiratory depression to a degree similar to that of isoflurane up to a MAC of 1.5. It increases P_aCO_2 (Fig. 13.4) and decreases the ventilatory response to imposed increases in P_aCO_2. It is irritant to the upper respiratory tract, particularly at concentrations greater than 6%. It is therefore not recommended for gaseous induction of anaesthesia because it causes coughing, breath-holding and laryngospasm.

Cardiovascular effects

Desflurane appears to have two distinct actions on the cardiovascular system. Firstly, its main actions are those which are similar to isoflurane: dose-related decreases in systemic vascular resistance, myocardial contractility and mean arterial pressure (Figs 13.5–13.7). Heart rate is unchanged at lower steady-state concentrations, but increases with higher concentrations (Fig. 13.9). Addition of nitrous oxide maintains heart rate unchanged. Cardiac output tends to be maintained as with isoflurane. The second cardiovascular action occurs when its inspired concentration is increased rapidly to greater than 1 MAC. In the absence of premedication drugs, this increases sympathetic activity, leading to increased heart rate and mean arterial pressure. Preliminary experimental studies in animals have not detected a coronary steal phenomenon similar to that produced by isoflurane. Desflurane, in common with isoflurane and sevoflurane, does not sensitize the myocardium to catecholamines (Fig. 13.8).

Central nervous system

The effects of desflurane are very similar to those of isoflurane. It depresses the EEG in a dose-related manner. It does not cause seizure activity at any level of anaesthesia, with or without hypocapnia. Desflurane decreases cerebrovascular resistance and can increase intracranial pressure in a dose-related manner. In dogs, it increases cerebral blood flow at deep levels of anaesthesia if systemic arterial pressure is maintained.

Musculoskeletal system

Desflurane causes muscle relaxation in a dose-related manner. Concentrations exceeding 1 MAC produce fade in response to tetanic stimulation of the ulnar nerve. It enhances the effect of muscle relaxants. Studies in susceptible swine indicate that desflurane can trigger malignant hyperthermia.

Therefore, in summary, desflurane offers some advantages over other agents:

- It has a low blood solubility; therefore it offers more precise control of maintenance of anaesthesia and rapid recovery.
- It is minimally biodegradable and therefore non-toxic to the liver and kidney.
- It does not cause convulsive activity on EEG.

However, it has some significant drawbacks:

- It cannot be used for inhalation induction because of its irritant effects on the airway.
- It causes a tachycardia at higher concentrations.
- It requires a special vaporizer. Although the TEC-6 vaporizer is reasonably easy to use, it is more complex than the more conventional vaporizers and the potential for failure may be higher.
- It is expensive.

COMPARISON OF HALOTHANE, ENFLURANE, ISOFLURANE, SEVOFLURANE AND DESFLURANE

Pharmacokinetics

The rate of equilibration of alveolar with inspired concentrations is related to blood/gas solubility. The rate of uptake of desflurane is faster than that of any of the other volatile agents and similar to that of nitrous oxide (Fig. 13.2). Despite its low blood/gas solubility, the rate of induction of anaesthesia with desflurane (and isoflurane) may be reduced because of the pungent odour compared with the more pleasant odours of sevoflurane, halothane and enflurane. Sevoflurane gives a smooth rapid induction and it is rapidly replacing halothane for induction in children. Potency, on the other hand, is related to the lower oil/water solubility. Sevoflurane and desflurane are less potent than the older agents as reflected by their higher MAC values.

On recovery from anaesthesia, the rate of elimination of desflurane is faster than that of the other agents (Fig. 13.3).

Respiratory system

All inhalation agents cause dose-related respiratory depression. This results in reduced tidal volume, increased respiratory rate and reduced minute ventilation. P_aCO_2 increases (Fig. 13.4). In unstimulated volunteers, enflurane and desflurane cause greater ventilatory depression than isoflurane, halothane or sevoflurane. Nitrous oxide does not cause hypercapnia. Thus the reduction in inspired volatile anaesthetic concentration permitted by addition of nitrous oxide is associated with less ventilatory depression. In addition, surgical stimulation is responsible for considerable antagonism of ventilatory depression during anaesthesia and P_aCO_2 does not normally reach the values shown in Figure 13.4 during surgery.

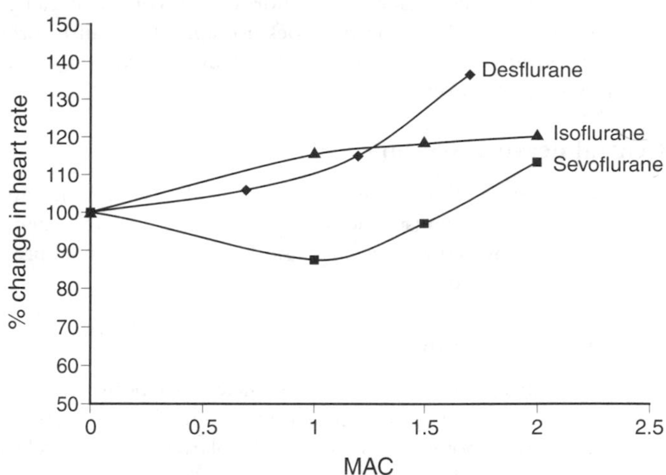

Fig. 13.9
Comparative effects of isoflurane, sevoflurane and desflurane on heart rate in healthy volunteers.

With all agents, depression of ventilation is associated with depression of whole body oxygen consumption and carbon dioxide production.

Halothane and, to a lesser extent, sevoflurane and enflurane cause bronchodilatation.

Cardiovascular system

All the agents reduce arterial pressure because of reduced systemic vascular resistance and myocardial depression to varying degrees. Desflurane and isoflurane tend to maintain cardiac output, decreasing arterial pressure by decreasing systemic vascular resistance. Halothane reduces arterial pressure by decreasing cardiac output with little effect on systemic vascular resistance.

Isoflurane, enflurane and desflurane increase heart rate as a result of sympathetic stimulation, whereas halothane and sevoflurane reduce heart rate.

The data in Figures 13.5–13.7 and 13.9 were derived from studies in volunteers who were not subjected to surgical stimulation and in whom artificial ventilation was used to achieve normocapnia.

Some of the cardiovascular effects of these volatile agents are antagonized by the addition of nitrous oxide. In addition, during spontaneous ventilation, the modest hypercapnia which occurs with all agents also offsets some of the changes. With enflurane and isoflurane, for example, cardiac output may be increased compared with pre-anaesthesia levels, although there is little effect on systemic arterial pressure.

Desflurane, isoflurane and sevoflurane do not sensitize the myocardium to exogenous catecholamines, but halothane and, to a lesser extent, enflurane predispose to arrhythmias.

Isoflurane causes coronary vasodilatation and it has been thought to cause coronary steal syndrome. Sevoflurane causes some coronary vasodilatation but does not appear to cause coronary steal syndrome. The other three agents do not cause any coronary vasodilatation.

Central nervous system

All agents cause dose-related depression of cerebral activity. Enflurane causes convulsive activity on the EEG. All the agents decrease cerebrovascular resistance and increase intracranial pressure in a dose-related manner.

Neuromuscular junction

All agents cause muscle relaxation sufficient to perform lower abdominal surgery in spontaneously breathing thin subjects. In addition, there is potentiation of non-depolarizing muscle relaxants. In this respect, isoflurane, sevoflurane and desflurane are similar and cause markedly greater potentiation than that produced by halothane or enflurane.

Metabolism

Halothane, enflurane and sevoflurane are metabolized to potentially toxic metabolites and desflurane is the most resistant to metabolism. Halothane is associated with liver toxicity, while sevoflurane and enflurane are associated with inorganic fluoride ion production.

Carbon dioxide absorbers

Sevoflurane and halothane react with soda lime, while the other three do not.

A comparison of other characteristics of the five agents is shown in Tables 13.1 and 13.2.

AGENTS IN OCCASIONAL USE

DIETHYL ETHER

Because of its flammability, the use of ether has been abandoned in Western countries, but it remains an agent of widespread use in underdeveloped countries. It therefore warrants a brief description in this text.

It is a colourless, highly volatile liquid with a characteristic smell. It is flammable in air and explosive in oxygen. Ether is decomposed by air, light and heat, the most important products being acetaldehyde and ether peroxide. It should be stored in a cool environment in opaque containers.

Uptake and distribution

Ether has a high blood/gas solubility coefficient of 12 and thus the rate of equilibration of alveolar with inspired concentrations is slow. Therefore induction and recovery with ether are slow.

Central nervous system

In common with all general anaesthetic agents, there is depression of the cortex, resulting in loss of higher inhibitions initially, followed by depression. Because induction of anaesthesia with ether is so slow, the classical stages of anaesthesia are seen; these are described in detail on p. 463 and in Figure 37.2.

Depression of the respiratory centre precedes that of the vasomotor centre. Ether anaesthesia is associated with stimulation of the sympathoadrenal system and increased levels of circulating catecholamines, which offset the direct myocardial depressant effect of the drug.

Respiratory system

Ether is irritant to the respiratory tract and provokes coughing, breath-holding and profuse secretions from all mucus-secreting glands, including the salivary glands and the respiratory tracts. Premedication with atropine or hyoscine is therefore essential.

Ether stimulates ventilation and minute volume is maintained with increasing depth of anaesthesia until surgical anaesthesia is achieved; thereafter, there is a gradual diminution in alveolar ventilation as plane 4 of stage 3 is approached (Fig. 37.2).

Because ether is irritant to the respiratory tract, laryngeal spasm is not uncommon during induction with ether, but during established anaesthesia there is dilatation of the bronchi and bronchioles; at one time, the drug was recommended for treatment of bronchospasm.

Cardiovascular system

In vitro, ether is a direct myocardial depressant. However, during light planes of clinical anaesthesia, there is sympathetic stimulation and this often results in little change in cardiac output, arterial pressure or peripheral resistance. In deep planes of anaesthesia, cardiac output decreases as a result of myocardial depression.

Cardiac arrhythmias occur rarely with ether and there is no sensitization of the myocardium to circulating catecholamines.

Alimentary system

Salivary and gastric secretions are increased during light anaesthesia but decreased during deep anaesthesia. Ether causes a very high incidence of postoperative nausea and vomiting.

Skeletal muscle

Ether relaxes skeletal muscle by depressing spinal reflexes and blocking motor end-plates. It therefore potentiates the effects of non-depolarizing muscle relaxants.

Uterus and placenta

The pregnant uterus is not affected during light anaesthesia, but relaxation occurs during deep anaesthesia. Placental transmission causes depression of the fetus.

Metabolism

At least 15% of ether is metabolized to carbon dioxide and water; approximately 4% is metabolized in the liver to acetaldehyde and ethanol.

Ether stimulates gluconeogenesis and therefore causes hyperglycaemia.

Table 13.1 Comparison of modern volatile anaesthetic agents

	Halothane	Enflurane	Isoflurane	Desflurane	Sevoflurane
Molecular weight	197.4	184.5	184.5	168	200.1
Boiling point (°C)	50	56	49	23.5	58.9
Blood/gas partition coefficient	2.5	1.9	1.4	0.42	0.69
Oil/gas partition coefficient	220	98	97	18.7	55
MAC (in oxygen)	0.75	1.68	1.15	7.3	1.7–2.0
Preservative	Thymol	None	None	None	None
Stability in CO_2 absorbers	?Unstable	Stable	Stable	Stable	Unstable

Table 13.2 Systemic effects of volatile agents

	Halothane	Enflurane	Isoflurane	Desflurane	Sevoflurane
Alveolar equilibration	Slow	Moderate	Moderate	Fast	Fast
Recovery	Slow	Moderate	Fast	Very fast	Fast
Cardiovascular system					
Heart rate	Reduced	Increased	Increased	Increased	Stable
Cardiac output	Reduced	Reduced	Slightly reduced	Stable	Slightly reduced
SVR	Stable	Slightly reduced	Reduced	Reduced	Reduced
MAP	Reduced	Reduced	Reduced	Reduced	Reduced
Coronary vasodilatation	Nil	Nil	Marked	Nill	Moderate
Sensitization of myocardium	Yes	Slight	No	No	No
Respiratory system					
Respiratory irritation	Nil	Nil	Significant	Significant	Nil
Respiratory depression	Yes	Marked	Yes	Marked	Yes
Central nervous system					
Seizure activity on EEG	No	Yes	No	No	No
Renal system					
Renal toxic metabolites	No	Yes	No	No	Yes
Liver					
Hepatotoxicity	Yes	No	No	No	Yes
Metabolism (%)	20	2.5	0.2	0.02	3–5
Musculoskeletal system					
Muscle weakness	Moderate	Moderate	Significant	Significant	Significant

SVR, systemic vascular resistance; MAP, mean arterial pressure.

Clinical use of ether

Ether has a much higher therapeutic ratio than halothane, enflurane or isoflurane and is therefore safer for administration in the hands of unskilled individuals or from an uncalibrated vaporizer. Because of its high blood/gas solubility coefficient and irritant properties to the respiratory tract, induction of anaesthesia is very slow.

Administration of ether may be undertaken using an anaesthetic breathing system with a non-calibrated vaporizer (Boyle's bottle) or calibrated vaporizer (the EMO, which may be used as a draw-over or as a plenum vaporizer). It may be used safely in a closed circuit with soda lime absorption.

Vapour strengths of up to 20% are required for induction; light anaesthesia can be maintained with 3–5% and deep anaesthesia with 5–6% inspired concentrations.

ANAESTHETIC GASES

NITROUS OXIDE (N_2O)

Manufacture

Nitrous oxide is prepared commercially by heating ammonium nitrate to a temperature of 245–270°C. Various impurities are produced in this process, including ammonia, nitric acid, nitrogen, nitric oxide and nitrogen dioxide.

After cooling, ammonia and nitric acid are reconstituted to ammonium nitrate, which is returned to the beginning of the process. The remaining gases then pass through a series of scrubbers. The purified gases are compressed and dried in an aluminium dryer. The resultant gases are expanded in a liquefier, with the nitrogen escaping as gas. Nitrous oxide is then evaporated, compressed and passed through another aluminium dryer before being stored in cylinders.

The higher oxides of nitrogen dissolve in water to form nitrous and nitric acids. These substances are toxic and produce methaemoglobinaemia and pulmonary oedema if inhaled. In the past, there have been several reports of death occurring during anaesthesia as a result of the inhalation of nitrous oxide contaminated with higher oxides of nitrogen.

Storage

Nitrous oxide is stored in compressed form as a liquid in cylinders at a pressure of 50 bar (5000 kPa; 750 lb in^{-2}). In the UK, the cylinders are painted blue.

Because the cylinder contains liquid and vapour, the total quantity of nitrous oxide contained in a cylinder can be ascertained only by weighing. Thus, the cylinder weights, full and empty, are stamped on the shoulder. Nitrous oxide cylinders should be kept in a vertical position during use so that the liquid phase remains at the bottom of the cylinder. During continuous use, the cylinder may cool as a result of the latent heat of vaporization of liquid anaesthetic and ice may form on the lower part of the cylinder.

Physical properties

Nitrous oxide is a sweet-smelling, non-irritant colourless gas, with a molecular weight of 44, boiling point –88°C, critical temperature 36.5°C and critical pressure 72.6 bar.

Nitrous oxide is not flammable but it supports combustion of fuels in the absence of oxygen.

Pharmacology

Nitrous oxide is frequently said to be a good analgesic but a weak anaesthetic. The latter refers to the fact that its MAC value is 105%. This value was calculated theoretically from its low oil/water solubility coefficient of 3.2 and has been confirmed experimentally in volunteers anaesthetized in a pressure chamber compressed to 2 ata, where the MAC value was found to be 52.5% N_2O.

As it is essential to administer a minimum F_IO_2 of 0.3, nitrous oxide alone is insufficient to produce an adequate depth of anaesthesia in all but the most seriously ill patients; therefore, nitrous oxide is used usually in combination with other agents. When using nitrous oxide in a relaxant technique, the inspired gas mixture should be supplemented with a low concentration of a volatile agent to eliminate the risk of awareness, which may occur if nitrous oxide anaesthesia is supplemented only by the administration of opioids.

Nitrous oxide has a low blood/gas solubility coefficient (0.47 at 37°C) and therefore the rate of equilibration of alveolar with inspired concentrations is very fast (Fig. 13.2).

Because of the low solubility, a change in alveolar ventilation has less effect on the rate of uptake than occurs with the more soluble agents such as halothane and ether (Fig. 13.10). Similarly, changes in cardiac output have less effect with nitrous oxide (Fig. 13.11). Nitrous oxide does not undergo metabolism in the body and is excreted unchanged.

The concentration effect

The inspired concentration of nitrous oxide affects its rate of equilibration; the higher the inspired concentration, the faster is the rate of equilibration between alveolar and inspired concentrations. Nitrous oxide is more soluble in blood than is nitrogen. Thus, the volume of nitrous oxide entering pulmonary capillary blood from the alveolus is greater than the volume of nitrogen moving in the opposite direction. As a result, the total volume of gas in the alveolus diminishes and the fractional concentrations of the remaining gases increase. This has two consequences:

- The higher the inspired concentration of nitrous oxide, the greater is the concentrating effect on the nitrous oxide remaining in the alveolus.
- At high inspired concentrations of nitrous oxide, the reduction in alveolar gas volume causes an increase in P_ACO_2. Equilibration with pulmonary capillary blood results in an increase in P_aCO_2.

The result of the concentration effect on equilibration of nitrous oxide is illustrated in Figure 13.12.

The second gas effect

When nitrous oxide is administered in a high concentration with a second anaesthetic agent, e.g. halothane, the reduction in gas volume in the alveoli caused by absorption of nitrous oxide increases the alveolar concentration of halothane, thereby augmenting the rate of equilibration with inspired gas. This is illustrated in the lower part of Figure 13.12. The second gas effect results also in small increases in P_AO_2 and P_aO_2.

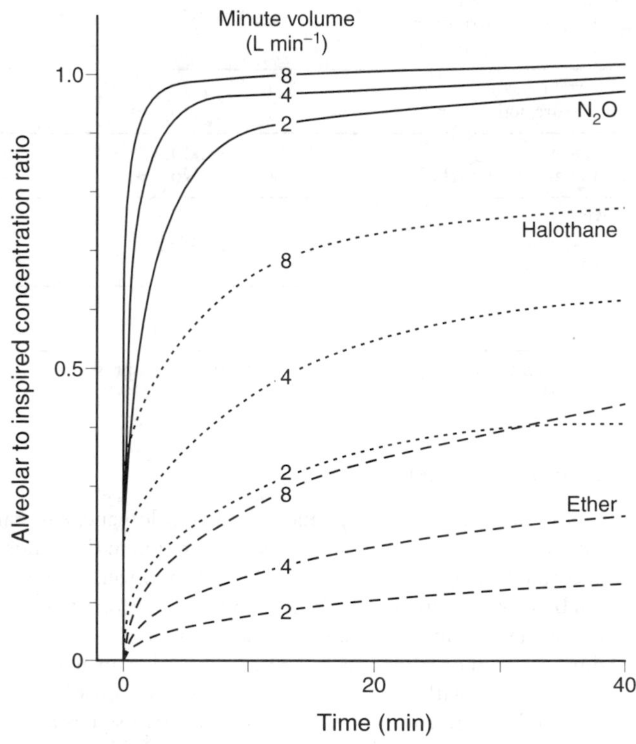

Fig. 13.10
Influence of minute volume on the rate of equilibration between alveolar and inspired concentrations of nitrous oxide, halothane and ether.
The effects of ventilation are more marked on the agents with higher blood/gas solubility coefficients.

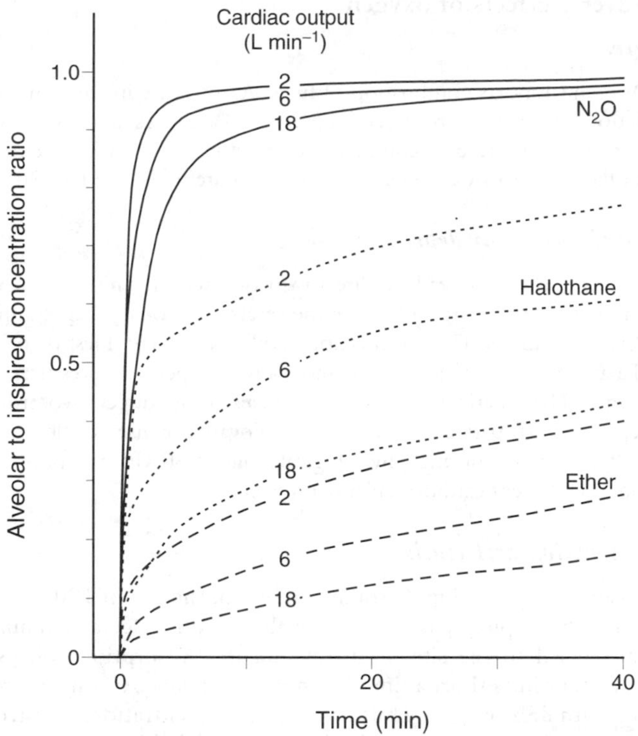

Fig. 13.11
Influence of cardiac output on the rate of equilibration between alveolar and inspired concentrations of nitrous oxide, halothane and ether. The effects of cardiac output are more marked on the agents with higher blood/gas solubility coefficients.

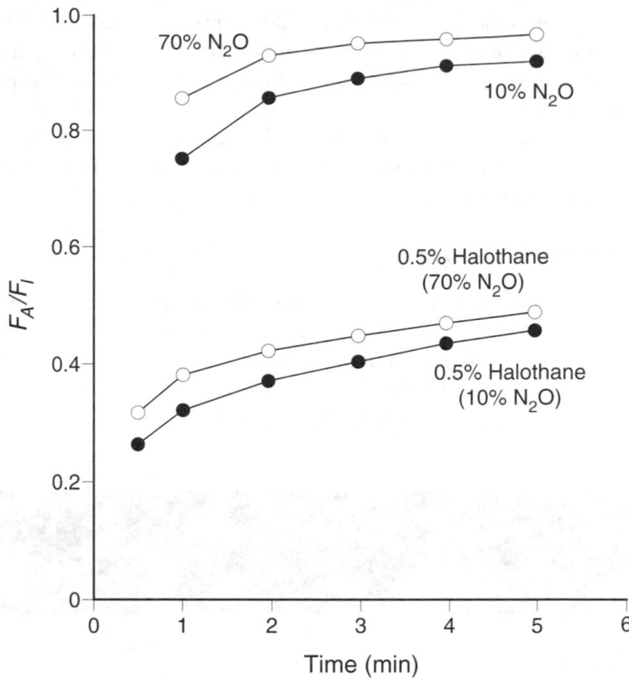

Fig. 13.12
The concentration and second gas effects. High concentrations of nitrous oxide increase the F_A/F_I ratio for nitrous oxide (the concentration effect) and for a volatile agent administered with nitrous oxide (the second gas effect). See text for details.

Side-effects of nitrous oxide

Diffusion hypoxia

At the end of an anaesthetic, when the inspired gas mixture is changed from nitrous oxide/oxygen to nitrogen/oxygen, hypoxaemia may occur as the volume of nitrous oxide diffusing from mixed venous blood into the alveolus is greater than the volume of nitrogen taken up from the alveolus into pulmonary capillary blood (the opposite of the concentration effect). Thus, the concentration of gases in the alveolus is diluted by nitrous oxide, leading to a reduction in P_aO_2 and P_aCO_2. In the healthy individual, diffusion hypoxia is relatively transient, but may last for up to 10 min at the end of anaesthesia; the extent of reduction in P_aO_2 may be of the order of 0.5–1.5 kPa. Administration of oxygen during this period is essential in order to avoid desaturation.

Effect on closed gas spaces

When blood containing nitrous oxide equilibrates with closed air-containing spaces inside the body, the volume of nitrous oxide that diffuses into the cavity exceeds the volume of nitrogen diffusing out. Thus, in compliant spaces, such as the bowel lumen or the pleural or peritoneal cavities, there is an increase in volume of the space. If the space cannot expand (e.g. sinuses, middle ear) there is an increase in pressure. In the middle ear, this may cause problems with surgery on the tympanic membrane. When nitrous oxide is administered in a concentration of 75%, the volume of a cavity may increase to as much as three to four times the original volume within 30 min. If an air embolus occurs in a patient who is breathing nitrous oxide, equilibration with the gas bubble leads to expansion of the embolus within seconds; the volume of the embolus may double within a very short period of time. A similar problem arises during prolonged procedures where nitrous oxide diffuses into the cuff of the tracheal tube and can increase the pressure exerted on the tracheal mucosa. Either avoiding the use of nitrous oxide or inflating the cuff with saline or nitrous oxide may prevent this.

Cardiovascular depression

Nitrous oxide is a direct myocardial depressant, but in the normal individual this effect is antagonized by indirectly mediated sympathoadrenal stimulation (effects similar to those produced by carbon dioxide). Thus, healthy patients exhibit little change in the cardiovascular system during nitrous oxide anaesthesia. However, in patients with pre-existing high levels of sympathoadrenal activity and poor myocardial contractility, the administration of nitrous oxide may cause reductions in cardiac output and arterial pressure. For this reason (in addition to avoidance of the risk of doubling the size of air emboli), nitrous oxide is avoided in some centres during anaesthesia for cardiac surgery.

Toxicity

Nitrous oxide affects vitamin B_{12} synthesis by inhibiting the enzyme methionine synthetase. This effect is important if the duration of nitrous oxide anaesthesia exceeds 8 h. Nitrous oxide also interferes with folic acid metabolism and impairs synthesis of DNA; prolonged exposure may cause agranulocytosis and bone marrow aplasia. Exposure of patients to nitrous oxide for 6 h or longer may result in megaloblastic anaemia. Occupational exposure to nitrous oxide may result in myeloneuropathy. This condition is similar to subacute combined degeneration of the spinal cord and has been reported in some dentists and also in individuals addicted to inhalation of nitrous oxide.

Teratogenic changes

Teratogenic changes have been observed in pregnant rats exposed to nitrous oxide for prolonged periods. There is no evidence that similar effects occur in humans, but it has been suggested that nitrous oxide should be avoided in early pregnancy; however, this is not a generally held view at the present time.

OTHER GASES USED DURING ANAESTHESIA

OXYGEN

Manufacture

Oxygen is manufactured commercially by fractional distillation of liquid air. Before liquefaction of air, carbon dioxide is removed and liquid oxygen and nitrogen separated by means of their different boiling points (oxygen, −183°C; nitrogen, −195°C).

Oxygen is supplied in cylinders at a pressure of 137 bar (approximately 2000 lb in^{-2}) at 15°C. The cylinders are painted black with a white shoulder.

Many institutions use piped oxygen and this is supplied either by a bank of oxygen cylinders, ensuring a continuous supply, or from liquid oxygen. Premises using in excess of 150 000 L of oxygen per week find the latter more economical. The pressure of oxygen in a hospital pipeline is approximately 4 bar (60 lb in^{-2}), which is the same as the pressure distal to the reducing valves of gas cylinders attached to anaesthetic machines.

Oxygen is tasteless, colourless and odourless, with a specific gravity of 1.105 and a molecular weight of 32. At atmospheric pressure, it liquefies at −183°C, but at 50 atm the liquefaction temperature increases to −119°C.

Oxygen supports combustion, although the gas itself is not flammable.

Oxygen concentrators

Oxygen concentrators produce oxygen from ambient air by absorption of nitrogen onto some types of alumina silicates. Oxygen concentrators are useful both in hospitals and in long-term domestic use in remote areas, in developing countries and in military surgery. The gas produced by oxygen concentrators contains small quantities of inert gases (e.g. argon) which are harmless.

Physiological effects

The physiological aspects of oxygen are discussed in Chapter 9 and the clinical uses in Chapter 41.

Adverse effects of oxygen

Fire

Oxygen supports combustion of fuels. An increase in the concentration of oxygen from 21% up to 100% causes a progressive increase in the rate of combustion with the production of either conflagrations or explosions with appropriate fuels (see Ch. 30).

Cardiovascular depression

An increase in P_aO_2 leads to direct vasoconstriction, which occurs in peripheral vasculature and also in the cerebral, coronary, hepatic and renal circulations. This effect is not manifest at a P_aO_2 of less than 30 kPa and assumes clinical importance only at hyperbaric pressures of oxygen. Hyperbaric pressures of oxygen also cause direct myocardial depression. In patients with severe cardiovascular disease, elevation of P_aO_2 from the normal physiological range to 80 kPa may produce clinically evident cardiovascular depression.

Absorption atelectasis

Because oxygen is highly soluble in blood, the use of 100% oxygen as the inspired gas may lead to absorption atelectasis in lung units distal to the site of airway closure. Absorption collapse may occur in as short a time as 6 min with 100% oxygen, and 60 min with 85% oxygen. Thus, even small concentrations of nitrogen exert an important splinting effect and this accounts for current avoidance of 100% oxygen in estimation of pulmonary shunt ratio ($\dot{Q}_s/\dot{Q}_t$) in patients with lung pathology, in whom a greater degree of airway closure would result in greater areas of alveolar atelectasis. Absorption atelectasis has been demonstrated in volunteers breathing 100% oxygen at FRC; atelectasis is evident on chest radiography for a period of at least 24 h after exposure.

CO_2 narcosis

In patients with chronic bronchitis and chronic CO_2 retention, there may be loss of sensitivity of the central chemoreceptors and some dependence of ventilation on drive from the peripheral chemoreceptors that respond to oxygen. Administration of a high F_IO_2 to such a patient may cause loss of peripheral chemoreceptor drive with the subsequent development of ventilatory failure.

Pulmonary oxygen toxicity

Chronic inhalation of a high inspired concentration of oxygen may result in the condition termed pulmonary oxygen toxicity (Lorrain–Smith effect), which is manifest by hyaline membranes, thickening of the interlobular and alveolar septa by oedema and fibroplastic proliferation. The clinical and radiological appearance of these changes is almost identical to that of the acute respiratory distress syndrome. The biochemical mechanisms underlying pulmonary oxygen toxicity probably include:

- oxidation of SH groups on essential enzymes such as coenzyme A
- peroxidation of lipids; the resulting lipid peroxides inhibit the function of the cell
- inhibition of the pathway of reversed electron transport, possibly by inhibition of iron and SH-containing flavoproteins.

These changes lead to loss of synthesis of pulmonary surfactant, encouraging the development of absorption collapse and alveolar oedema. The onset of oxygen-induced lung pathology occurs after approximately 30 h exposure to a P_IO_2 of 100 kPa.

Central nervous system oxygen toxicity

Convulsions, similar to those of grand mal epilepsy, occur during exposure to hyperbaric pressures of oxygen.

Retrolental fibroplasia

Retrolental fibroplasia (RLF) is the result of oxygen-induced retinal vasoconstriction, with obliteration of the most immature retinal vessels and subsequent new vessel formation at the site of damage in the form of a proliferative retinopathy. Leakage of intravascular fluid leads to vitreoretinal adhesions and even retinal detachment. Retrolental fibroplasia occurs in infants exposed to hyperoxia in the paediatric intensive care unit and is related not to the F_IO_2 *per se*, but to an elevated retinal artery PO_2. It is not known what the threshold of P_aO_2 is for the development of retinal damage, but an umbilical arterial PO_2 of 8–12 kPa (60–90 mmHg) is associated with a very low incidence of RLF and no signs of systemic hypoxia. It should be stressed, however, that there are many factors involved in the development of RLF in addition to arterial hyperoxia.

Depressed haemopoiesis

Long-term exposure to elevated F_IO_2 leads to depression of haemopoiesis and anaemia.

CARBON DIOXIDE

Carbon dioxide is a colourless gas with a pungent odour. It has a molecular weight of 44, a critical temperature of −31°C and a critical pressure of 73.8 bar.

Carbon dioxide is obtained commercially from four sources:

- as a by-product of fermentation in brewing of beer
- as a by-product of the manufacture of hydrogen
- by heating magnesium and calcium carbonate in the presence of their oxides
- as a combustion gas from burning fuel.

Carbon dioxide is supplied in a liquid state in grey cylinders at a pressure of 50 bar. The filling ratio (see p. 338) is 0.75 and the liquid phase occupies approximately 90–95% of the cylinder capacity.

Physiological data

The physiological aspects of CO_2 are dealt with predominantly in Chapter 9. Variations in cardiovascular state induced by alterations in P_aCO_2 may be similar to those induced by pain or lightness of anaesthesia and the differential diagnosis is described in Table 41.3. The cardiovascular effects of CO_2 are summarized in Table 13.3.

Table 13.3 Cardiovascular effects of CO_2

Arterial pressure Cardiac output Heart rate	Biphasic response. Progressive increase in these variables with increase in P_aCO_2 up to approximately 10 kPa as a result of indirect sympathetic stimulation. At very high P_aCO_2, these variables decrease as a result of myocardial depression
Skin Coronary circulation Cerebral circulation Gastrointestinal circulation	Dilatation with hypercapnia Constriction with hypocapnia

Uses of carbon dioxide in anaesthesia

The use of carbon dioxide in anaesthetic practice has declined as appreciation of its disadvantages has increased. Because of reports of accidental administration of high concentrations of CO_2, it is not available on most modern anaesthetic machines. Therefore, the uses of carbon dioxide are now mainly historical and included:

- provocation of hyperventilation in order to facilitate blind nasal intubation
- stimulation of spontaneous ventilation after a period of artificial hyperventilation.

MEDICAL AIR

Nitrous oxide is still commonly used in combination with a volatile agent to maintain anaesthesia. However, there is growing concern regarding its toxic effects and its cost. With the growing popularity of total intravenous anaesthesia, medical air is being used more frequently in combination with oxygen to maintain anaesthesia.

Medical air is obtained from the atmosphere near to the site of compression. Great care is taken to position the air intake in order to avoid contamination with pollutants such as carbon monoxide from car exhausts. Air is compressed to 137 bar and then passed through columns of activated alumina to remove water.

Air for medical purposes is supplied in cylinders (grey body and black and white shoulders in the UK) or as a piped system. A pressure of 4 bar is available for attachment to anaesthetic machines, and 7 bar for orthopaedic tools. Its composition varies slightly depending on location of compression and moisture content.

Uses of medical air

- driving gas for ventilators
- to operate power tools, e.g. orthopaedic drills
- together with oxygen and a volatile agent to maintain anaesthesia.

Advantages of air

- readily available
- non-toxic.

Disadvantages

- no analgesic properties.

XENON

Inert gases such as argon, krypton and xenon, which form crystalline hydrates, have been reported to exert anaesthetic actions. Cullen and Gross first reported the anaesthetic properties of xenon in humans in 1951. Xenon offers many advantages over nitrous oxide, for which it could theoretically be a suitable replacement. The reasons that it is not routinely available are that it is expensive, there are no commercially available anaesthetic machines in which to use xenon, its concentration in inspired gas cannot be measured with conventional anaesthetic gas analysers, and there is still limited clinical experience with its use.

Physical properties

Xenon is a non-explosive, colourless, and odourless gas. Its oil/gas partition coefficient of 0.14–0.2 is lower than that of nitrous oxide (0.47). It therefore provides rapid induction of and recovery from anaesthesia. Xenon is more potent than nitrous oxide, with a MAC of 70%. It does not undergo biotransformation and it is harmless to the ozone layer.

Systemic effects

Studies so far have shown no cardiorespiratory side-effects and lack of reduction in local organ perfusion. However, in common with nitrous oxide, xenon appears to be associated with postoperative nausea and vomiting.

FURTHER READING

Eger E I II 1994. New inhaled anaesthetic agents. Review article. Anesthesiology 80: 906–922

Jones R M 1994 Volatile anaesthetic agents. In: Nimmo W S, Rowbotham D J, Smith G (eds) Anaesthesia, 2nd edn. Blackwell Scientific Publications, Oxford, p 43–74

Jones R M, Eger E I II 1994 Desflurane, the third generation inhalation anaesthetic agent. Anaesthesia 50(suppl): 1–51

Smith I, Nathanson M, White P F 1996 Sevoflurane – a long awaited volatile agent. Review article. British Journal of Anaesthesia 76: 435–445

Weiskopf R B 1995 Anaesthesia 50 (suppl)

14 Intravenous anaesthetic agents

General anaesthesia may be produced by many drugs which depress the central nervous system (CNS), including sedatives, tranquillizers and hypnotic agents. However, for some drugs the doses required to produce surgical anaesthesia are so large that cardiovascular and respiratory depression commonly occur, and recovery is delayed for hours or even days. Only a few drugs are suitable for use routinely to produce anaesthesia after intravenous (i.v.) injection.

Intravenous anaesthetic agents are used commonly to induce anaesthesia, as induction is usually smoother and more rapid than that associated with most of the inhalation agents. Intravenous anaesthetics may also be used for maintenance, either alone or in combination with nitrous oxide; they may be administered as repeated bolus doses or by continuous i.v. infusion. Other uses include sedation during regional anaesthesia, sedation in the intensive therapy unit (ITU) and treatment of status epilepticus.

PROPERTIES OF THE IDEAL INTRAVENOUS ANAESTHETIC AGENT

- Rapid onset – this is achieved by an agent which is mainly un-ionized at blood pH and which is highly soluble in lipid; these properties permit penetration of the blood–brain barrier
- Rapid recovery – early recovery of consciousness is usually produced by rapid redistribution of the drug from the brain into other well-perfused tissues, particularly muscle. The plasma concentration of the drug decreases, and the drug diffuses out of the brain along a concentration gradient. The quality of the later recovery period is related more to the rate of metabolism of the drug; drugs with slow metabolism are associated with a more prolonged 'hangover' effect and accumulate if used in repeated doses or by infusion for maintenance of anaesthesia
- Analgesia at subanaesthetic concentrations
- Minimal cardiovascular and respiratory depression
- No emetic effects
- No excitatory phenomena (e.g. coughing, hiccup, involuntary movement) on induction
- No emergence phenomena (e.g. nightmares)
- No interaction with neuromuscular blocking drugs
- No pain on injection
- No venous sequelae
- Safe if injected inadvertently into an artery
- No toxic effects on other organs
- No release of histamine
- No hypersensitivity reactions
- Water-soluble formulation
- Long shelf-life
- No stimulation of porphyria.

None of the agents available at present meets all these requirements. Features of the commonly used i.v. anaesthetic agents are compared in Table 14.1, and a classification of i.v. anaesthetic drugs is shown in Table 14.2.

PHARMACOKINETICS OF INTRAVENOUS ANAESTHETIC DRUGS

After i.v. administration of a drug, there is an immediate rapid increase in plasma concentration followed by a slower decline. Anaesthesia is produced by diffusion of drug from arterial blood across the blood–brain barrier into the brain. The rate of transfer into the brain, and therefore the anaesthetic effect, is regulated by the following factors:

Protein binding. Only unbound drug is free to cross the blood–brain barrier. Protein binding may be reduced by low plasma protein concentrations or displacement by other drugs, resulting in higher concentrations of free drug and an exaggerated anaesthetic effect. Protein binding is also affected by changes in blood pH. Hyperventilation decreases protein binding and increases the anaesthetic effect.

Blood flow to the brain. Reduced cerebral blood flow (CBF), e.g. carotid artery stenosis, results in reduced delivery of drug to the brain. However, if CBF is reduced because of low cardiac output, initial blood concentrations are higher than normal after i.v. administration, and the anaesthetic effect may be delayed but enhanced.

Extracellular pH and pK_a of the drug. Only the non-ionized fraction of the drug penetrates the lipid blood–brain barrier; thus, the potency of the drug depends on the degree of ionization at the pH of extracellular fluid and the pK_a of the drug.

The relative solubilities of the drug in lipid and water. High lipid solubility enhances transfer into the brain.

Speed of injection. Rapid i.v. administration results in high initial concentrations of drug. This increases the speed of induction, but also the extent of cardiovascular and respiratory side-effects.

In general, any factor which increases the blood concentration of free drug, e.g. reduced protein binding or low cardiac output, also increases the intensity of side-effects.

Table 14.1 Main properties of intravenous anaesthetics

	Thiopental	Methohexital	Propofol	Ketamine	Etomidate
Physical properties					
Water-soluble	+	+	–	+	+[a]
Stable in solution	–	–	+	+	+
Long shelf-life	–	–	+	+	+
Pain on i.v. injection	–	+	++	–	++
Non-irritant on s.c. injection	–	±	+	+	
Painful on arterial injection	+	+	–		
No sequelae from intra-arterial injection	–	±	+		
Low incidence of venous thrombosis	+	+	+	+	–
Effects on body					
Rapid onset	+	+	+	+	+
Recovery due to:					
Redistribution	+	+	+	+	
Detoxification		+	+		
Cumulation	++	+	–	–	–
Induction					
Excitatory effects	–	++	+	+	+++
Respiratory complications	–	+	+	–	–
Cardiovascular					
Hypotension	+	+	++	–	+
Analgesic	–	–	–	++	–
Antanalgesic	+	+	–	–	?
Interaction with relaxants	–	–	–	–	–
Postoperative vomiting	–	–	–	++	+
Emergence delirium	–	–	–	++	–
Safe in porphyria	–	–	+	+	–

[a]Aqueous solution not commercially available.

Distribution to other tissues

The anaesthetic effect of all i.v. anaesthetic drugs in current use is terminated predominantly by distribution to other tissues. Figure 14.1 shows this distribution for thiopental. The percentage of the injected dose in each of four body compartments as time elapses is shown after i.v. injection. A large proportion of the drug is distributed initially into well-perfused organs (termed the vessel-rich group, or viscera – predominantly brain, liver and kidneys). Distribution into muscle (lean) is slower because of its low lipid content, but it is quantitatively important because of its relatively good blood supply and large mass. Despite their high lipid-solubility, i.v. anaesthetic drugs distribute slowly to adipose tissue (fat) because of its poor blood supply. Fat contributes little to the initial redistribution or termination of action of i.v. anaesthetic agents, but fat depots contain a large proportion of the injected dose of thiopental at 90 min, and 65–75% of the total remaining in the body at 24 h. There is also a small amount of redistribution

Table 14.2 Classification of intravenous anaesthetics

Rapidly acting (primary induction) agents
Barbiturates
Methohexital
Thiobarbiturates – thiopental, thiamylal
Imidazole compounds – etomidate[a]
Sterically hindered alkyl phenols – propofol
Steroids – eltanolone, Althesin, minaxolone (none currently available)
Eugenols – propanidid (not currently available)
Slower-acting (basal narcotic) agents
Ketamine
Benzodiazepines – diazepam, flunitrazepam, midazolam
Large-dose opioids – fentanyl, alfentanil, sufentanil, remifentanil
Neurolept combination – opioid + neuroleptic

[a]Limited use as infusion.

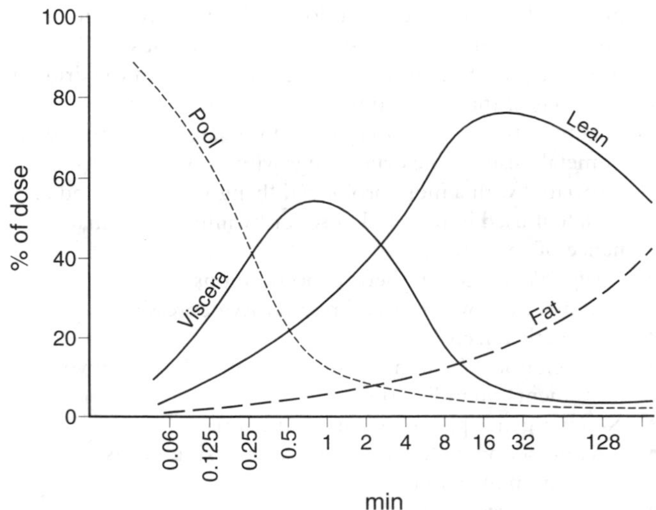

Fig. 14.1
Distribution of thiopental after intravenous bolus administration.

Table 14.3 Factors influencing the distribution of thiopental in the body

	Viscera	Muscle	Fat	Others
Relative blood flow	Rich	Good	Poor	Very poor
Blood flow (L min^{-1})	4.5	1.1	0.32	0.08
Tissue volume (L; *A*)	6	33	15	13
Tissue/blood partition coefficient (*B*)	1.5	1.5	11.0	1.5
Potential capacity (L; *A* × *B*)	9	50	160	20
Time constant (capacity/flow; min)	2	45	500	250

to areas with a very poor blood supply, e.g. bone. Table 14.3 indicates some of the properties of the body compartments in respect of the distribution of i.v. anaesthetic agents.

After a single i.v. dose, the concentration of drug in blood decreases as distribution occurs into viscera, and particularly muscle. Drug diffuses from the brain into blood along the changing concentration gradient, and recovery of consciousness occurs. Metabolism of most i.v. anaesthetic drugs occurs predominantly in the liver. If metabolism is rapid (indicated by a short elimination half-life), it may contribute to some extent to the recovery of consciousness. However, because of the large distribution volume of i.v. anaesthetic drugs, total elimination takes many hours, or, in some instances, days. A small proportion of drug may be excreted unchanged in the urine; the amount depends on the degree of ionization and the pH of urine.

BARBITURATES

Amobarbital and pentobarbital were used i.v. to induce anaesthesia in the late 1920s, but their actions were unpredictable and recovery was prolonged. Manipulation of the barbituric acid ring (Fig. 14.2) enabled a short duration of action to be achieved by:

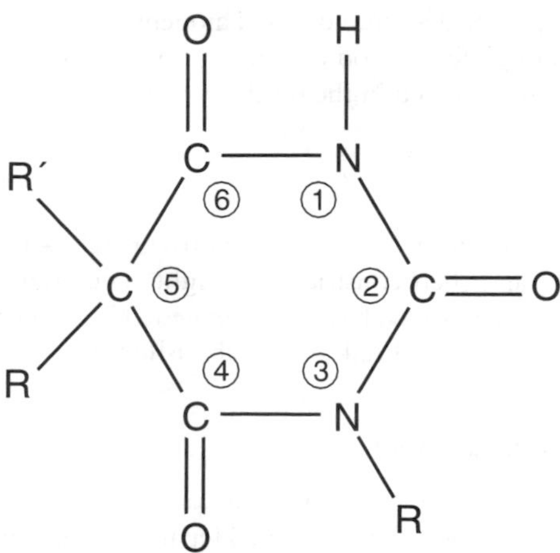

Fig. 14.2
Structure of barbiturate ring.

- substitution of a sulphur atom for oxygen at position 2
- substitution of a methyl group at position 1; this also confers potential convulsive activity and increases the incidence of excitatory phenomena.

An increased number of carbon atoms in the side chains at position 5 increases the potency of the agent. The presence of an aromatic nucleus in an alkyl group at position 5 produces compounds with convulsant properties; direct substitution with a phenyl group confers anticonvulsant activity.

The anaesthetically active barbiturates are classified chemically into four groups (Table 14.4). The methylated oxybarbiturate hexobarbital was moderately successful as an i.v. anaesthetic agent, but was superseded by the development in 1932 of thiopental. Thiopental remains one of the most commonly used i.v. anaesthetic agents throughout the world. Its pharmacology is therefore described fully in this chapter. Many of its effects are shared by other i.v. anaesthetic agents and consequently the pharmacology of these drugs is described more briefly.

THIOPENTAL SODIUM

Chemical structure

Sodium 5-ethyl-5-(1-methylbutyl)-2-thiobarbiturate.

Physical properties and presentation

Thiopental sodium, the sulphur analogue of pentobarbital, is a yellowish powder with a bitter taste and a faint smell of garlic. It is stored in nitrogen to prevent chemical reaction with atmospheric carbon dioxide, and mixed with 6% anhydrous sodium carbonate to increase its solubility in water. It is available in single-dose ampoules of 500 mg and is dissolved in distilled water to produce 2.5% (25 mg ml^{-1}) solution with a pH of 10.8; this solution is slightly hypotonic. Freshly prepared solution may be kept for 24 h. The oil/water partition coefficient of thiopental is 4.7, and the pK_a 7.6.

Central nervous system

Thiopental produces anaesthesia usually less than 30 s after i.v. injection, although there may be some delay in patients with a low cardiac output. There is progressive depression of the CNS, including spinal cord reflexes. The hypnotic action of thiopental is potent, but its analgesic effect is poor, and surgical anaesthesia is difficult to achieve unless large doses are used; these are associated with cardiorespiratory depression. The cerebral metabolic rate is reduced and there are secondary decreases in CBF, cerebral blood volume and intracranial pressure. Recovery of consciousness occurs at a higher blood concentration if a large dose is given, or if the drug is injected rapidly; this has been attributed to acute tolerance, but may represent only altered redistribution. Consciousness is usually regained in 5–10 min. At subanaesthetic blood concentrations (i.e. at low doses or during recovery), thiopental has an antanalgesic effect and reduces the pain threshold; this may result in restlessness in the postoperative period. Thiopental is a very potent anticonvulsant.

Sympathetic nervous system activity is depressed to a greater extent than parasympathetic; this may occasionally result in bradycardia. However, it is more usual for tachycardia to develop after induction of anaesthesia, partly because of baroreceptor inhibition

Table 14.4 Relation of chemical grouping to clinical action of barbiturates

Group	Substituents: Position 1	Substituents: Position 2	Group characteristics when given intravenously
Oxybarbiturates	H	O	Delay in onset of action depending on 5 and 5′ side chain. Useful as basal hypnotics. Prolonged action
Methyl barbiturates	CH_3	O	Usually rapid-acting with fairly rapid recovery. High incidence of excitatory phenomena
Thiobarbiturates	H	S	Rapid-acting, usually smooth onset of sleep and fairly prompt recovery
Methyl thiobarbiturates	CH_3	S	Rapid onset of action and very rapid recovery but with so high an incidence of excitatory phenomena as to preclude use in clinical practice

Table 14.5 Percentage incidences of pain on injection and thrombophlebitis after intravenous administration of anaesthetic drugs into a large vein in the antecubital fossa or a small vein in the dorsum of the hand or wrist

Agent	Pain: Large	Pain: Small	Thrombophlebitis: Large	Thrombophlebitis: Small
Saline 0.9%	0	0	0	0
Thiopental 2.5%	0	12	1	0
Methohexital 1%	8	21	0	0
Propofol	10	40	0	0
Etomidate	8	80	15	20

caused by modest hypotension and partly because of loss of vagal tone which may predominate normally in young healthy adults.

Cardiovascular system

Myocardial contractility is depressed and peripheral vasodilatation occurs, particularly when large doses are administered or if injection is rapid. Arterial pressure decreases, and profound hypotension may occur in the patient with hypovolaemia or cardiac disease. Heart rate may decrease, but there is often a reflex tachycardia (see above).

Respiratory system

Ventilatory drive is decreased by thiopental as a result of reduced sensitivity of the respiratory centre to carbon dioxide. A short period of apnoea is common, frequently preceded by a few deep breaths. Respiratory depression is influenced by premedication and is more pronounced if opioids have been administered; assisted or controlled ventilation may be required. When spontaneous ventilation is resumed, ventilatory rate and tidal volume are usually lower than normal, but they increase in response to surgical stimulation. There is an increase in bronchial muscle tone, although frank bronchospasm is uncommon.

Laryngeal spasm may be precipitated by surgical stimulation or the presence of secretions, blood or foreign bodies (e.g. an oropharyngeal or laryngeal mask airway) in the region of the pharynx or larynx. Thiopental is less satisfactory in this respect than propofol, and appears to depress the parasympathetic laryngeal reflex arc to a lesser extent than other areas of the CNS.

Skeletal muscle

Skeletal muscle tone is reduced at high blood concentrations, partly as a result of suppression of spinal cord reflexes. There is no significant direct effect on the neuromuscular junction. When thiopental is used as the sole anaesthetic agent, there is poor muscle relaxation, and movement in response to surgical stimulation is common.

Uterus and placenta

There is little effect on resting uterine tone, but uterine contractions are suppressed at high doses. Thiopental crosses the placenta readily, although fetal blood concentrations do not reach the same levels as those observed in the mother.

Eye

Intraocular pressure is reduced by approximately 40%. The pupil dilates first, and then constricts; the light reflex remains present until surgical anaesthesia has been attained. The corneal, conjunctival, eyelash and eyelid reflexes are abolished.

Hepatorenal function

The functions of the liver and kidneys are impaired transiently after administration of thiopental. Hepatic microsomal enzymes are induced and this may increase the metabolism and elimination of other drugs.

Pharmacokinetics

Blood concentrations of thiopental increase rapidly after i.v. administration. Between 75 and 85% of the drug is bound to protein, mostly albumin; thus, more free drug is available if plasma protein concentrations are reduced by malnutrition or disease. Protein binding is affected by pH and is decreased by alkalaemia; thus the concentration of free drug is increased during hyperventilation. Some drugs, e.g. phenylbutazone, occupy the same binding sites, and protein binding of thiopental may be reduced in their presence.

Thiopental diffuses readily into the CNS because of its lipid solubility and predominantly un-ionized state (61%) at body pH. Consciousness returns when the brain concentration decreases to a threshold value, dependent on the individual patient, the dose of drug and its rate of administration, but at this time nearly all of the injected dose is still present in the body.

Metabolism of thiopental occurs predominantly in the liver, and the metabolites are excreted by the kidneys; a small proportion is excreted unchanged in the urine. The terminal elimination half-life is approximately 11.5 h. Metabolism is a zero-order process; 10–15% of the remaining drug is metabolized each hour. Thus, up to 30% of the original dose may remain in the body at 24 h. Consequently, a 'hangover' effect is common; in addition, further doses of thiopental administered within 1–2 days may result in cumulation. Elimination is impaired in the elderly. In obese patients, dosage should be based on an estimate of lean body mass, as distribution to fat is slow. However, elimination may be delayed in obese patients because of increased retention of the drug by adipose tissue.

Dosage and administration

Thiopental is administered i.v. as a 2.5% solution; the use of a 5% solution increases the likelihood of serious complications and is *not* recommended. A small volume, e.g. 1–2 ml in adults, should be administered initially; the patient should be asked if any pain is experienced in case of inadvertent intra-arterial injection (see below) before the remainder of the induction dose is given.

The dose required to produce anaesthesia varies, and the response of each patient must be assessed carefully; cardiovascular depression is exaggerated if excessive doses are given. In healthy adults, an initial dose of 4 mg kg^{-1} should be administered over 15–20 s; if loss of the eyelash reflex does not occur within 30 s, supplementary doses of 50–100 mg should be given slowly until consciousness is lost. In young children, a dose of 6 mg kg^{-1} is usually necessary. Elderly patients often require smaller doses (e.g. 2.5–3 mg kg^{-1}) than young adults.

Induction is usually smooth and may be preceded by a taste of garlic. Side-effects are related to peak blood concentrations, and in patients in whom cardiovascular depression may occur the drug should be administered more slowly; in very frail patients, as little as 50 mg may be sufficient to induce sleep.

No other drug should be mixed with thiopental. Muscle relaxants should *not* be given until it is certain that anaesthesia has been induced. The i.v. cannula should be flushed with saline before vecuronium or atracurium is administered, to obviate precipitation.

Supplementary doses of 25–100 mg may be given to augment nitrous oxide/oxygen anaesthesia during short surgical procedures. However, recovery may be prolonged considerably if large total doses are used (> 10 mg kg^{-1}).

Adverse effects

Hypotension. The risk is increased if excessive doses are used, or if thiopental is administered to hypovolaemic, shocked or previously hypertensive patients. Hypotension is minimized by administering the drug slowly. Thiopental should not be administered to patients in the sitting position.

Respiratory depression. The risk is increased if excessive doses are used, or if opioid drugs have been administered. Facilities must be available to provide artificial ventilation.

Tissue necrosis. Local necrosis may follow perivenous injection. Median nerve damage may occur after extravasation in the antecubital fossa, and this site is *not* recommended. If perivenous injection occurs, the needle should be left in place and hyaluronidase injected.

Intra-arterial injection. This is usually the result of inadvertent injection into the brachial artery or an aberrant ulnar artery in the antecubital fossa but has occurred occasionally into aberrant arteries at the wrist. The patient usually complains of intense, burning pain, and this is an indication to stop injecting the drug immediately. The forearm and hand may become blanched and blisters may appear distally. Intra-arterial thiopental causes profound constriction of the artery accompanied by local release of norepinephrine. In addition, crystals of thiopental form in arterioles. In combination with thrombosis caused by endarteritis, adenosine triphosphate release from damaged red cells and aggregation of platelets, these result in emboli and may cause ischaemia or gangrene in parts of the forearm, hand or fingers.

The needle should be left in the artery and a vasodilator (e.g. papaverine 20 mg) administered. Stellate ganglion or brachial plexus block may reduce arterial spasm. Heparin should be given i.v. and oral anticoagulants should be prescribed after operation.

The risk of ischaemic damage after intra-arterial injection is much greater if a 5% solution of thiopental is used.

Laryngeal spasm. The causes have been discussed above.

Bronchospasm. This is unusual, but may be precipitated in asthmatic patients.

Allergic reactions. These range from cutaneous rashes to severe or fatal anaphylactic or anaphylactoid reactions with cardiovascular collapse. Severe reactions are rare (approximately 1 in 14 000–20 000). Hypersensitivity reactions to drugs administered during anaesthesia are discussed on page 518.

Thrombophlebitis. This is uncommon (Table 14.5) when the 2.5% solution is used.

Indications

- induction of anaesthesia
- maintenance of anaesthesia – thiopental is suitable only for short procedures because cumulation occurs with repeated doses
- treatment of status epilepticus
- reduction of intracranial pressure (see Ch. 57).

Absolute contraindications

- Airway obstruction – intravenous anaesthesia should not be used if there is anticipated difficulty in maintaining an adequate airway, e.g. epiglottitis, oral or pharyngeal tumours.

- Porphyria – barbiturates may precipitate lower motor neurone paralysis or severe cardiovascular collapse in patients with porphyria.
- Previous hypersensitivity reaction to a barbiturate.

Precautions

Special care is needed when thiopental is administered in the following circumstances:

Cardiovascular disease. Patients with hypovolaemia, myocardial disease, cardiac valvular stenosis or constrictive pericarditis are particularly sensitive to the hypotensive effects of thiopental. However, if the drug is administered with extreme caution, it is probably no more hazardous than other i.v. anaesthetic agents. Myocardial depression may be severe in patients with right-to-left intracardiac shunt because of high coronary artery concentrations of thiopental.

Severe hepatic disease. Reduced protein binding results in higher concentrations of free drug. Metabolism may be impaired, but this has little effect on early recovery. A normal dose may be administered, but very slowly.

Renal disease. In chronic renal failure, protein binding is reduced, but elimination is unaltered. A normal dose may be administered, but very slowly.

Muscle disease. Respiratory depression is exaggerated in patients with myasthenia gravis or dystrophia myotonica.

Reduced metabolic rate. Patients with myxoedema are exquisitely sensitive to the effects of thiopental.

Obstetrics. An adequate dose must be given to ensure that the mother is anaesthetized. However, excessive doses may result in respiratory or cardiovascular depression in the fetus, particularly if the interval between induction and delivery is short.

Outpatient anaesthesia. Early recovery is slow in comparison with other agents. This is seldom important unless rapid return of airway reflexes is essential, e.g. after oral or dental surgery. However, slow elimination of thiopental may result in persistent drowsiness for 24–36 h, and this impairs the ability to drive or use machinery. There is also potentiation of the effect of alcohol or sedative drugs ingested during that period. It is preferable to use a drug with more rapid elimination for patients who are ambulant within a few hours.

Adrenocortical insufficiency.

Extremes of age.

Asthma.

METHOHEXITAL SODIUM

Chemical structure

Sodium α-*dl*-5-allyl-1-methyl-5-(1-methyl-2-pentynyl) barbiturate.

Physical properties and presentation

Methohexital has two asymmetrical carbon atoms, and therefore four isomers. The α-*dl* isomers are clinically useful. The drug is presented as a white powder mixed with 6% anhydrous sodium carbonate and is readily soluble in distilled water. The resulting 1% (10 mg ml^{-1}) solution has a pH of 11.1 and pK_a of 7.9. Single-dose vials of 100 mg and multidose bottles containing 500 mg or 2.5 g are available in some countries. Although the solution is chemically stable for up to 6 weeks, the manufacturers recommend that it should not be stored for longer than 24 h because it does not contain antibacterial preservative.

Pharmacology

Central nervous system

Unconsciousness is usually induced in 15–30 s. Recovery is more rapid with methohexital than with thiopental, and occurs after 2–3 min; it is caused predominantly by redistribution. Drowsiness may persist for several hours until blood concentrations are decreased further by metabolism. Epileptiform activity has been demonstrated by electroencephalogram (EEG) in epileptic patients. However, in sufficient doses, methohexital acts as an anticonvulsant.

Cardiovascular system

In general, there is less hypotension in otherwise healthy patients than occurs after thiopental; the decrease in arterial pressure is mediated predominantly by vasodilatation. Heart rate may increase slightly because of a decrease in baroreceptor activity. The cardiovascular effects are more pronounced in patients with cardiac disease or hypovolaemia.

Respiratory system

Moderate hypoventilation occurs. There may be a short period of apnoea after i.v. injection.

Pharmacokinetics

A greater proportion of methohexital than thiopental is in the non-ionized state at body pH (approximately 75%), although the drug is less lipid-soluble than the thiobarbiturate. Binding to plasma protein occurs to a similar degree. Clearance from plasma is higher than that of thiopental, and the elimination half-life is considerably shorter (approximately 4 h). Thus, cumulation is less likely to occur after repeated doses.

Dosage and administration

Methohexital is administered i.v. in a dose of 1–1.5 mg kg^{-1} to induce anaesthesia in healthy young adult patients; smaller doses are required in the elderly and infirm.

Adverse effects

Cardiovascular and respiratory depression. This is probably less than that associated with thiopental.

Excitatory phenomena during induction, including dyskinetic muscle movements, coughing and hiccups. Muscle movements are reduced by administration of an opioid; the incidence of cough and hiccups is reduced by premedication with an anticholinergic agent. The incidence of excitatory effects is dose-related.

Epileptiform activity on EEG in epileptic subjects.

Pain on injection (Table 14.5).

Tissue damage after perivenous injection is rare with 1% solution.

Intra-arterial injection may cause gangrene, but the risk with 1% solution is considerably less than with 2.5% thiopental.

Allergic reactions occur, but are uncommon.

Thrombophlebitis is a rare complication.

Indications

Induction of anaesthesia, particularly when a rapid recovery is desirable. Methohexital has been used commonly as the anaesthetic agent for electroconvulsive therapy (ECT) and for induction of anaesthesia for outpatient dental and other minor procedures.

Absolute contraindications

These are the same as for thiopental.

Precautions

These are similar to the precautions listed for thiopental. However, methohexital is a suitable agent for outpatients. It should not be used to induce anaesthesia in patients who are known to be epileptic.

THIAMYLAL SODIUM

This is a sulphur analogue of quinalbarbital. It is slightly more potent than thiopental, but otherwise almost identical in its properties. It is not available in the UK, but is used in some other countries.

NON-BARBITURATE INTRAVENOUS ANAESTHETIC AGENTS

PROPOFOL

This phenol derivative was identified as a potentially useful intravenous anaesthetic agent in 1980, and became available commercially in 1986. It is more expensive than thiopental or methohexital, but has achieved great popularity because of its favourable recovery characteristics and its antiemetic effect.

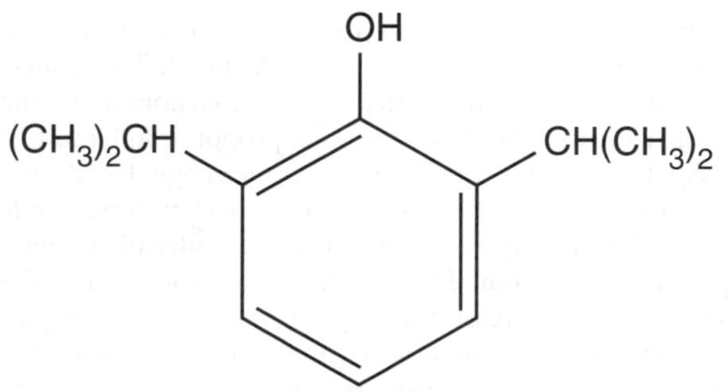

OH

$(CH_3)_2CH$ $CH(CH_3)_2$

Fig. 14.3
Chemical structure of propofol (2,6-di-isopropylphenol).

Chemical structure

2,6–Di-isopropylphenol (Fig. 14.3).

Physical properties and presentation

Propofol is extremely lipid-soluble, but almost insoluble in water. The drug was formulated initially in Cremophor EL. However, several other drugs formulated in this solubilizing agent were associated with release of histamine and an unacceptably high incidence of anaphylactoid reactions, and similar reactions occurred with this formulation of propofol. Consequently, the drug was reformulated in a white, aqueous emulsion containing soyabean oil and purified egg phosphatide. Ampoules of the drug contain 200 mg of propofol in 20 ml (10 mg ml^{-1}), and 50 ml bottles containing 1% (10 mg kg^{-1}) or 2% (20 mg kg^{-1}) solution, and 100 ml bottles containing 1% solution, are available for infusion. In addition, 50 ml pre-filled syringes of 1 and 2% solution are available and are designed principally for use in target-controlled infusion techniques (see below).

Pharmacology

Central nervous system

Anaesthesia is induced within 20–40 s after i.v. administration in otherwise healthy young adults. Transfer from blood to the sites of action in the brain is slower than with thiopental, and there is a delay in disappearance of the eyelash reflex, normally used as a sign of unconsciousness after administration of barbiturate anaesthetic agents. Overdosage of propofol, with exaggerated side-effects, may result if this clinical sign is used; loss of verbal contact is a better end-point. EEG frequency decreases, and amplitude increases. Propofol reduces the duration of seizures induced by ECT in humans. However, there have been reports of convulsions following the use of propofol and it is recommended that caution be exercised in administration of propofol to epileptic patients. Normally cerebral metabolic rate, CBF and intracranial pressure are reduced.

Recovery of consciousness is rapid and there is a minimal 'hangover' effect even in the immediate postanaesthetic period.

Cardiovascular system

In healthy patients, arterial pressure decreases to a greater degree after induction of anaesthesia with propofol than with thiopental; the reduction results predominantly from vasodilatation although there is a slight negative inotropic effect. In some patients, large decreases (> 40%) occur. The degree of hypotension is substantially reduced by decreasing the rate of administration of the drug and by appreciation of the kinetics of transfer from blood to brain (see above). The pressor response to tracheal intubation is attenuated to a greater degree by propofol than thiopental. Heart rate may increase slightly after induction of anaesthesia with propofol. However, there have been occasional reports of severe bradycardia and asystole during or shortly after administration of propofol, and it is recommended that a vagolytic agent (e.g. glycopyrronium or atropine) should be considered in patients with a pre-existing bradycardia or when propofol is used in conjunction with other drugs which are likely to cause bradycardia.

Respiratory system

After induction, apnoea occurs more commonly, and for a longer duration, than after thiopental. During infusion of propofol, tidal volume is lower and respiratory rate higher than in the conscious state. There is decreased ventilatory response to carbon dioxide. As with other agents, ventilatory depression is more marked if opioids are administered.

Propofol has no effect on bronchial muscle tone and laryngospasm is particularly uncommon. The suppression of laryngeal reflexes results in a low incidence of coughing or laryngospasm when a laryngeal mask airway (LMA) is introduced, and propofol is regarded by most anaesthetists as the drug of choice for induction of anaesthesia when the LMA is to be used.

Skeletal muscle

Tone is reduced, but movements may occur in response to surgical stimulation.

Gastrointestinal system

Propofol has no effect on gastrointestinal motility in animals. Its use is associated with a low incidence of postoperative nausea and vomiting.

Uterus and placenta

Propofol has been used extensively in patients undergoing gynaecological surgery, and it does not appear to have any clinically significant effect on uterine tone. Propofol crosses the placenta. Its safety to the neonate has not been established and its use in pregnancy (except for termination), in obstetric practice and in breast-feeding mothers is not recommended by the manufacturers.

Hepatorenal

There is a transient decrease in renal function, but the impairment is less than that associated with thiopental. Hepatic blood flow is decreased by the reductions in arterial pressure and cardiac output. Liver function tests are not deranged after infusion of propofol for 24 h.

Endocrine

Plasma concentrations of cortisol are decreased after administration of propofol, but a normal response occurs to administration of Synacthen.

Pharmacokinetics

In common with other i.v. anaesthetic drugs, propofol is distributed rapidly, and blood concentrations decline exponentially. Clearance of the drug from plasma is greater than would be expected if the drug was metabolized only in the liver, and it is believed that extrahepatic sites of metabolism exist. The kidneys excrete the metabolites of propofol (mainly glucuronides); only 0.3% of the administered dose of propofol is excreted unchanged. The terminal elimination half-life of propofol is 3–4.8 h, although its effective half-life is much shorter (30–60 min). The distribution and clearance of propofol are altered by concomitant administration of fentanyl. Elimination of propofol remains relatively constant even after infusions lasting for several days.

Dosage and administration

In healthy, unpremedicated adults, a dose of 1.5–2.5 mg kg^{-1} is required to induce anaesthesia. The dose should be reduced in the elderly; an initial dose of 1.25 mg kg^{-1} is appropriate, with subsequent additional doses of 10 mg until consciousness is lost. In children, a dose of 3–3.5 mg kg^{-1} is usually required; the drug is not recommended for use in children less than 1 month of age. Cardiovascular side-effects are reduced if the drug is injected slowly. Lower doses are required for induction in premedicated patients. Sedation during regional analgesia or endoscopy can be achieved with infusion rates of 1.5–4.5 mg kg^{-1} h^{-1}. Infusion rates of up to 15 mg kg^{-1} h^{-1} are required to supplement nitrous oxide/oxygen for surgical anaesthesia, although these may be reduced substantially if an opioid drug is administered. The average infusion rate is approximately 2 mg kg^{-1} h^{-1} in conjunction with a slow infusion of morphine (2 mg h^{-1}) for sedation of patients in ICU.

Adverse effects

Cardiovascular depression. Unless the drug is given very slowly, cardiovascular depression following a bolus dose of propofol is greater than that associated with a bolus dose of a barbiturate and is likely to cause profound hypotension in hypovolaemic or untreated hypertensive patients and in those with cardiac disease. Cardiovascular depression is modest if the drug is administered slowly or by infusion.

Respiratory depression. Apnoea is more common and of longer duration than after barbiturate administration.

Excitatory phenomena. These are more frequent on induction than with thiopental, but less than with methohexital. There have been occasional reports of convulsions and myoclonus during recovery from anaesthesia in which propofol has been used. Some of these reactions are delayed.

Pain on injection. This occurs in up to 40% of patients (Table 14.5). The incidence is greatly reduced if a large vein is used, if a small dose (10 mg) of lidocaine is injected shortly before propofol, or if lidocaine is mixed with propofol in the syringe (up to 1 ml of 0.5 or 1% lidocaine per 20 ml of propofol). Accidental extravasation or intra-arterial injection does not appear to result in adverse effects.

Allergic reactions. Skin rashes occur occasionally. Anaphylactic reactions have also been reported, but appear to be no more common than with thiopental.

Indications

Induction of anaesthesia. Propofol is indicated particularly when rapid early recovery of consciousness is required. Two hours after anaesthesia, there is no difference in psychomotor function between patients who have received propofol and those given thiopental or methohexital, but the former enjoy less drowsiness in the ensuing 12 h. The rapid recovery characteristics are lost if induction is followed by maintenance with inhalation agents for longer than 10–15 min. The rapid redistribution and metabolism of propofol may increase the risks of awareness during tracheal intubation after the administration of non-depolarizing muscle relaxants, or at the start of surgery, unless the lungs are ventilated with an appropriate mixture of inhaled anaesthetics, or additional doses or an infusion of propofol administered.

Sedation during surgery. Propofol has been used successfully for sedation during regional analgesic techniques and during endoscopy. Control of the airway may be lost at any time, and patients must be supervised continuously by an anaesthetist.

Total i.v. anaesthesia (see below). Propofol is the most suitable of the agents currently available. Recovery time is increased after infusion of propofol compared with that after a single bolus dose, but cumulation is significantly less than with the barbiturates.

Sedation in ICU. Propofol has been used successfully by infusion to sedate adult patients for several days in ICU. The level of sedation is controlled easily, and recovery is rapid (usually < 30 min).

Absolute contraindications

Airway obstruction and known hypersensitivity to the drug are probably the only absolute contraindications. Propofol appears to be safe in porphyric patients. Propofol should not be used for long-term sedation of children in the ICU because of a number of reports of adverse outcome.

Precautions

These are similar to those listed for thiopental. The side-effects of propofol make it less suitable than thiopental or methohexital for patients with existing cardiovascular compromise unless it is administered with great care. Propofol is more suitable than thiopental for outpatient anaesthesia, but its use does not obviate the need for an adequate period of recovery before discharge.

Solutions of propofol do not possess any antibacterial properties, and they support the growth of microorganisms. The drug must be drawn aseptically into a syringe and any unused solution should be discarded if not administered promptly. Propofol must not be administered via a microbiological filter.

ETOMIDATE

This carboxylated imidazole compound was introduced in 1972.

Chemical structure

D-Ethyl-1-(α-methylbenzyl)-imidazole-5-carboxylate.

Physical characteristics and presentation

Etomidate is soluble but unstable in water. It is presented as a clear aqueous solution containing 35% propylene glycol. Ampoules contain 20 mg of etomidate in 10 ml (2 mg kg^{-1}). The pH of the solution is 8.1.

Pharmacology

Etomidate is a rapidly acting general anaesthetic agent with a short duration of action (2–3 min) resulting predominantly from redistribution, although it is also eliminated rapidly from the body. In healthy patients, it produces less cardiovascular depression than does thiopental; however, there is little evidence that this benefit is retained if the cardiovascular system is compromised. Large doses may produce tachycardia. Respiratory depression is less than with other agents.

Etomidate depresses the synthesis of cortisol by the adrenal gland and impairs the response to adrenocorticotrophic hormone. Long-term infusions of the drug in ICU have been associated with increased infection and mortality, probably related to reduced immunological competence. Its effects on the adrenal gland occur also after a single bolus, and last for several hours.

Pharmacokinetics

Etomidate redistributes rapidly in the body. Approximately 76% is bound to protein. It is metabolized in the plasma and liver, mainly by esterase hydrolysis, and the metabolites are excreted in the urine; 2% is excreted unchanged. The terminal elimination half-life is approximately 75 min. There is little cumulation when repeated doses are given. The distribution and clearance of etomidate may be altered by concomitant administration of fentanyl.

Dosage and administration

An average dose of 0.3 mg kg^{-1} i.v. induces anaesthesia. The drug should be administered into a large vein to reduce the incidence of pain on injection.

Adverse effects

Suppression of synthesis of cortisol. See above.

Excitatory phenomena. Moderate or severe involuntary movements occur in up to 40% of patients during induction of anaesthesia. This incidence is reduced in patients premedicated with an opioid. Cough and hiccups occur in up to 10% of patients.

Pain on injection. This occurs in up to 80% of patients if a small vein is used, but in less than 10% when the drug is injected into a large vein in the antecubital fossa (Table 14.5). The incidence is reduced by prior injection of lidocaine 10 mg.

Nausea and vomiting. The incidence of nausea and vomiting is approximately 30%. This is very much higher than after propofol.

Emergence phenomena. The incidence of severe restlessness and delirium during recovery is greater with etomidate than barbiturates or propofol.

Venous thrombosis is more common than with other agents.

Indications

There are few positive indications for etomidate, although it is used by many anaesthetists in patients with a compromised cardiovascular system. It is suitable for outpatient anaesthesia, but has been superseded by propofol.

Absolute contraindications

- airway obstruction
- porphyria
- adrenal insufficiency
- long-term infusion.

Precautions

These are similar to the precautions listed for thiopental. Etomidate is suitable for outpatient anaesthesia. However, the incidence of excitatory phenomena is unacceptably high unless an opioid is administered; this delays recovery and is unsuitable for most outpatients.

KETAMINE HYDROCHLORIDE

This is a phencyclidine derivative and was introduced in 1965. It differs from other i.v. anaesthetic agents in many respects, and produces dissociative anaesthesia rather than generalized depression of the CNS.

Chemical structure

2-(*o*-Chlorophenyl)-2-(methylamino)-cyclo-hexanone hydrochloride.

Physical characteristics and presentation

Ketamine is soluble in water and is presented as solutions of 10 mg kg^{-1} containing sodium chloride to produce isotonicity, and 50 or 100 mg kg^{-1} in multidose vials which contain benzethonium chloride 0.1 mg kg^{-1} as preservative. The pH of the solutions is 3.5–5.5. The pK_a of ketamine is 7.5.

Pharmacology

Central nervous system

Ketamine is extremely lipid-soluble. After i.v. injection, it induces anaesthesia in 30–60 s. A single i.v. dose produces unconsciousness for 10–15 min. Ketamine is also effective within 3–4 min after i.m. injection and has a duration of action of 15–25 min. It is a potent somatic analgesic at subanaesthetic blood concentrations. Amnesia often persists for up to 1 h after recovery of consciousness. Induction of anaesthesia is smooth, but emergence delirium may occur, with restlessness, disorientation and agitation. Vivid and often unpleasant nightmares or hallucinations may occur during recovery and for up to 24 h. The incidences of emergence delirium and hallucinations are reduced by avoidance of verbal and tactile stimulation during the recovery period, or by concomitant administration of opioids, butyrophenones, benzodiazepines or physostigmine; however, unpleasant dreams may persist. Nightmares are reported less commonly by children and elderly patients.

The EEG changes associated with ketamine are unlike those seen with other i.v. anaesthetics, and consist of loss of alpha rhythm and predominant theta activity. Cerebral metabolic rate is increased in several regions of the brain, and CBF, cerebral blood volume and intracranial pressure increase.

Cardiovascular system

Arterial pressure increases by up to 25% and heart rate by approximately 20%. Cardiac output may increase, and myocardial oxygen consumption increases; the positive inotropic effect may be related to increased calcium influx mediated by cyclic adenosine monophosphate. There is increased myocardial sensitivity to epinephrine. Sympathetic stimulation of the peripheral circulation is decreased, resulting in vasodilatation in tissues innervated predominantly by α-adrenergic receptors, and vasoconstriction in those with β-receptors.

Respiratory system

Transient apnoea may occur after i.v. injection, but ventilation is well maintained thereafter and may increase slightly unless high doses are given. Pharyngeal and laryngeal reflexes and a patent airway are maintained well in comparison with other i.v. agents; however, their presence cannot be guaranteed, and normal precautions must be taken to protect the airway and prevent aspiration. Bronchial muscle is dilated.

Skeletal muscle

Muscle tone is usually increased. Spontaneous movements may occur, but reflex movement in response to surgery is uncommon.

Gastrointestinal system

Salivation is increased.

Uterus and placenta

Ketamine crosses the placenta readily. Fetal concentrations are approximately equal to those in the mother.

The eye

Intraocular pressure increases, although this effect is often transient. Eye movements often persist during surgical anaesthesia.

Pharmacokinetics

Only approximately 12% of ketamine is bound to protein. The initial peak concentration after i.v. injection decreases as the drug is distributed, but this occurs more slowly than with other i.v. anaesthetic agents. Metabolism occurs predominantly in the liver by demethylation and hydroxylation of the cyclohexanone ring; among the metabolites is norketamine, which is pharmacologically active. Approximately 80% of the injected dose is excreted renally as glucuronides; only 2.5% is excreted unchanged. The elimination half-life is approximately 2.5 h. Distribution and elimination are slower if halothane, benzodiazepines or barbiturates are administered concurrently.

After i.m. injection, peak concentrations are achieved after approximately 20 min.

Dosage and administration

Induction of anaesthesia is achieved with an average dose of 2 mg kg^{-1} i.v.; larger doses may be required in some patients, and smaller doses in the elderly or shocked patient. In all cases, the drug should be administered slowly. Additional doses of 1–1.5 mg kg^{-1} are required every 5–10 min. Between 8 and 10 mg kg^{-1} is used i.m. A dose of 0.25–0.5 mg kg^{-1} or an infusion of 50 μg kg^{-1} min^{-1} may be used to produce analgesia without loss of consciousness.

Adverse effects

- emergence delirium, nightmares and hallucinations
- hypertension and tachycardia – this may be harmful in previously hypertensive patients and in those with ischaemic heart disease
- prolonged recovery
- salivation – anticholinergic premedication is essential
- increased intracranial pressure
- allergic reactions – skin rashes have been reported.

Indications

The high-risk patient. Ketamine is useful in the shocked patient. Arterial pressure may decrease if hypovolaemia is present, and the drug must be given cautiously. These patients are usually heavily sedated in the postoperative period, and the risk of nightmares is therefore minimized.

Paediatric anaesthesia. Children undergoing minor surgery, investigations (e.g. cardiac catheterization), ophthalmic examinations or radiotherapy may be managed successfully with ketamine administered either i.m. or i.v.

Difficult locations. Ketamine has been used successfully at the site of accidents, and for analgesia and anaesthesia in casualties of war.

Analgesia and sedation. The analgesic action of ketamine may be used when wound dressings are changed, or while positioning patients with pain before performing regional anaesthesia (e.g. fractured neck of femur). Ketamine has been used to sedate asthmatic patients in the ICU.

Developing countries. Ketamine is used extensively in countries where anaesthetic equipment and trained staff are in short supply.

Absolute contraindications

- Airway obstruction – although the airway is maintained better with ketamine than with other agents, its patency cannot be guaranteed. Inhalation agents should be used for induction of anaesthesia if airway obstruction is anticipated.
- Raised intracranial pressure.

Precautions

Cardiovascular disease. Ketamine is unsuitable for patients with pre-existing hypertension, ischaemic heart disease or severe cardiac decompensation.

Repeated administration. Because of the prolonged recovery period, ketamine is not the most suitable drug for frequent procedures, e.g. prolonged courses of radiotherapy, as it disrupts sleep and eating patterns.

Visceral stimulation. Ketamine suppresses poorly the response to visceral stimulation; supplementation, e.g. with an opioid, is indicated if visceral stimulation is anticipated.

Outpatient anaesthesia. The prolonged recovery period and emergence phenomena make ketamine unsuitable for adult outpatients.

OTHER DRUGS

Benzodiazepines and opioids may also be used to induce general anaesthesia. However, very large doses are required, and recovery is prolonged. Their use is confined to specialist areas, e.g. cardiac anaesthesia. The pharmacology of these drugs is described in Chapters 16 and 17.

INTRAVENOUS MAINTENANCE OF ANAESTHESIA

INDICATIONS FOR INTRAVENOUS MAINTENANCE OF ANAESTHESIA

There are several situations in which i.v. anaesthesia (IVA; the use of an i.v. anaesthetic to supplement nitrous oxide) or total i.v. anaesthesia (TIVA) may offer advantages over the traditional inhalation techniques. In the doses required to maintain clinical anaesthesia, i.v. agents cause minimal cardiovascular depression. In comparison with the most commonly used volatile anaesthetic agents, IVA with propofol (the only currently available i.v. anaesthetic with an appropriate pharmacokinetic profile) offers rapid recovery of consciousness and good recovery of psychomotor function, although the newer volatile anaesthetics desflurane and sevoflurane are also associated with rapid recovery and minimal hangover effects.

The use of TIVA allows a high inspired oxygen concentration in situations where hypoxaemia may otherwise occur, such as one-lung anaesthesia or in severely ill or traumatized patients, and has obvious advantages in procedures such as laryngoscopy or bronchoscopy, when delivery of inhaled anaesthetic agents to the lungs may be difficult. TIVA may also be used to provide anaesthesia in circumstances where there are clinical reasons to avoid nitrous oxide, such as middle-ear surgery, prolonged bowel surgery and in patients with raised intracranial pressure. There are few contraindications to the use of IVA, provided that the anaesthetist is aware of the wide variability in response (see below). For surgical anaesthesia, it is desirable either to use nitrous oxide supplemented by IVA or to infuse an opioid in addition to the i.v. anaesthetic.

PRINCIPLES OF IVA

The calibrated vaporizer allows the anaesthetist to establish stable conditions, usually with relatively few changes in delivered concentration of volatile anaesthetic agents during an operation. This is largely because the patient tends to come into equilibrium with the delivered concentration, irrespective of body size or physiological variations; the total dose of drug taken up by the body is variable, but is relatively unimportant, and is determined by the characteristics of the patient and the drug rather than by the anaesthetist. The task of achieving equilibrium with i.v. anaesthetic agents is more complex, as delivery must be matched to the size of the patient and also to the expected rates of distribution and metabolism of the drug. Conventional methods of delivering i.v. agents result in the total dose of drug being determined by the anaesthetist, and the concentration achieved in the brain depends on the volume and rate of distribution, the relative solubility of the agent in various tissues, and the rate of elimination of the drug in the individual patient. Consequently, there is considerably more variability between patients in the infusion rate of an i.v. anaesthetic required to produce satisfactory anaesthesia than there is in the inspired concentration of an inhaled agent. There is concern among some anaesthetists that the difficulty in predicting the correct infusion rate for an individual patient may result in a higher risk of awareness in the paralysed patient, although the risks appear in practice to be similar, and related to inadvertent failure of delivery of the drug or the use of inappropriate infusion schemes rather than to an inherent flaw in the technique.

TECHNIQUES OF ADMINISTRATION

Intermittent injection

Although some anaesthetists are skilled in the delivery of i.v. anaesthetic agents by intermittent bolus injection, the plasma concentrations of drug and the anaesthetic effect fluctuate widely, and the technique is acceptable only for procedures of short duration in unparalysed patients.

Manual infusion techniques

The infusion rate required to achieve a predetermined concentration of an i.v. drug can be calculated if the clearance of the drug from plasma is known [infusion rate (μg min^{-1}) = steady-state plasma concentration (μg ml^{-1}) × clearance (ml min^{-1})]. One of the difficulties is that clearance is variable, and it is possible only to estimate the value by using population kinetics; depending on the patient's clearance in relation to the average, the actual plasma concentration achieved may be higher or lower than the intended concentration.

A fixed-rate infusion is inappropriate because the serum concentration of the drug increases only slowly, taking four to five times the elimination half-life of the drug to reach steady state (Fig. 14.4). A bolus injection followed by a continuous infusion results initially in achievement of an excessive concentration (with an increased incidence of side-effects), and this is followed by a prolonged dip below the intended plasma concentration (Fig. 14.5). In order to achieve a reasonably constant plasma concentration (other than in very long procedures), it is necessary to use a multistep infusion regimen, a concept similar to that of overpressure for inhaled agents. A commonly used scheme for propofol is injection of a bolus dose of 1 mg kg^{-1} followed by infusion initially at a rate of 10 mg kg^{-1} h^{-1} for 10 min, then 8 mg kg^{-1} h^{-1} for the next 10 min, and a maintenance infusion rate of 6 mg kg^{-1} h^{-1} thereafter. This achieves, on average, a plasma concentration of propofol of 3 μg ml^{-1}, and this is effective in achieving satisfactory anaesthesia in unparalysed patients who *also* receive nitrous oxide and fentanyl; higher infusion rates are required if nitrous oxide and fentanyl are not administered. These infusion rates must be regarded only as a guide and must be adjusted as necessary according to clinical signs of anaesthesia.

Target-controlled infusion (TCI) techniques

By programming a computer with appropriate pharmacokinetic data and equations, it is possible at frequent intervals (several times a minute) to calculate the appropriate infusion rate required to produce a preset target plasma concentration of drug. The drug is infused by a syringe driver. To produce a step increase in plasma concentration, the syringe driver infuses drug very rapidly (a slow bolus) and then delivers drug at a progressively decreasing infusion rate (Fig. 14.6). To decrease the plasma concentration, the syringe driver stops infusing until the computer calculates that the target concentration has been achieved, and then infuses drug at an appropriate rate to maintain a constant level. The anaesthetist is required only to enter the desired target concentration and to change it when clinically indicated, in the same way as a vaporizer might be manipulated according to clinical signs of anaesthesia.

The potential advantages of such a system are its simplicity, the rapidity with which plasma concentration can be changed (particularly upwards) and avoidance of the need for the anaesthetist to undertake any calculations (resulting in less potential for error). The actual concentration achieved may be > 50% greater than or less than the predicted concentration, although this is not a major practical disadvantage provided that the anaesthetist adjusts the target concentration according to clinical signs relating to adequacy of anaesthesia, rather than assuming that a specific target concentration always results in the desired effect.

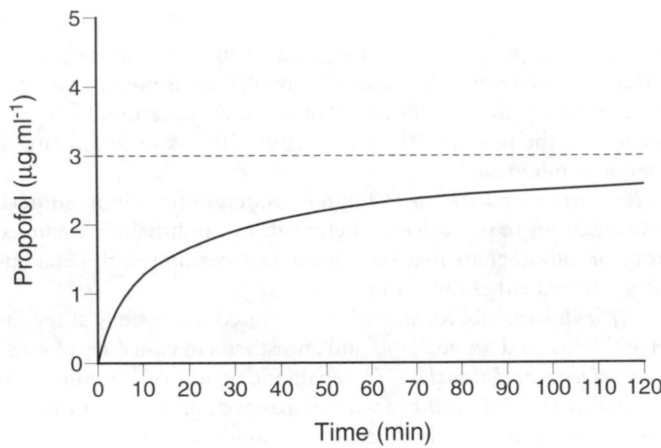

Fig. 14.4
Average blood concentration during the first 2 h of a continuous infusion of propofol at a rate of 6 mg kg^{-1} h^{-1}. Note that, even after 2 h, the equilibrium concentration of 3 μg.ml^{-1} has not been achieved.

Using a TCI system in female patients, the target concentration of propofol required to prevent movement in response to surgical incision in 50% of subjects (the equivalent of minimum alveolar concentration; MAC) was 6 μg ml^{-1} when patients breathed oxygen, and 4.5 μg ml^{-1} when 67% nitrous oxide was administered simultaneously.

A TCI system for administration of propofol is available in many countries. The anaesthetist is required to input the weight and age of the patient, and then to select the desired target concentration. These devices can be used only with pre-filled syringes, which contain an electronic tag which is recognized by the infusion pump. These TCI systems are currently suitable for use only

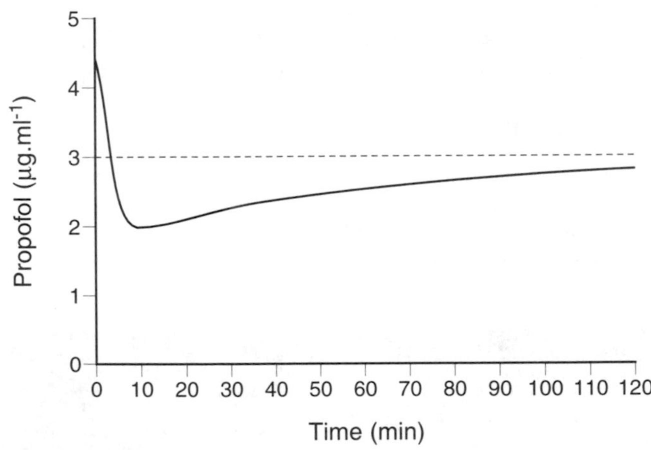

Fig. 14.5
Average blood propofol concentration following a bolus dose of propofol followed by a continuous infusion of 6 mg kg^{-1} h^{-1}. Note that the target concentration is initially exceeded, but that the blood concentration then falls below the target concentration, which is not achieved within 2 h.

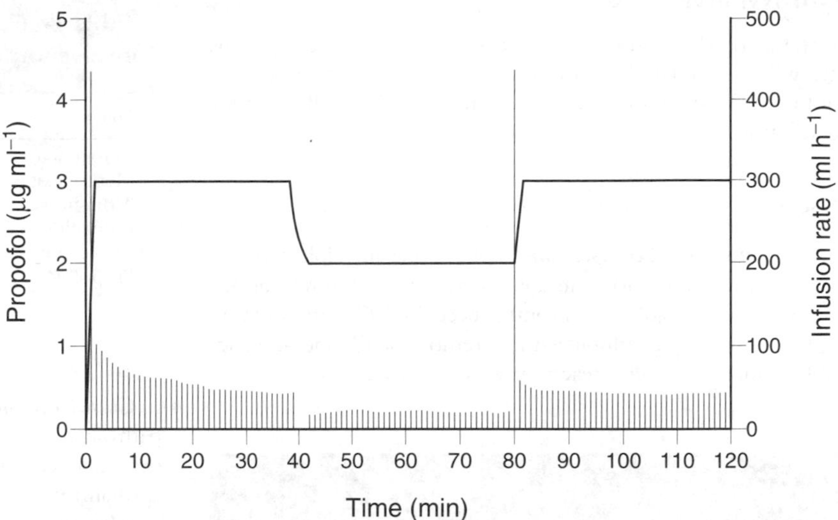

Fig. 14.6
Average blood concentrations of propofol achieved using a target-controlled infusion system. The narrow vertical lines represent the infusion rate calculated by the computer to achieve, and then to maintain, the target concentration in blood. A target concentration of 3 μg ml^{-1} was programmed initially. When the target concentration is reset to 2 μg ml^{-1}, the infusion is stopped and then restarted at a rate calculated to maintain that concentration. The target concentration is then increased to 3 μg ml^{-1}; the infusion pump delivers a rapid infusion rate to achieve the target concentration, and then gradually decreases the infusion rate to maintain a constant blood concentration.

in patients over the age of 16 years; the pharmacokinetic profile in children is different, and the use of adult pharmacokinetics may result in unstable plasma concentrations of propofol during prolonged infusion.

Target concentrations selected for elderly patients should be lower than those for younger adults, in order to minimize the risk of side-effects.

The TCI infusion pumps assume that the patient is conscious when the infusion is started. Consequently, it is inappropriate to connect and start a TCI system in a patient who is already unconscious, as this results in an initial overdose.

In adult patients under 55 years of age, anaesthesia can usually be induced with a target propofol concentration of 4–8 μg ml^{-1}. An initial target concentration at the lower end of that range is suitable for premedicated patients. Induction time is usually between 1 and 2 min. The brain concentration of propofol increases more slowly than the blood concentration, and following induction it is usually appropriate to reduce the target concentration; target propofol concentrations in the range of 3–6 μg ml^{-1} usually maintain satisfactory anaesthesia in patients who are also receiving an analgesic drug.

Later versions of the TCI infusion pumps show the predicted brain concentration, which can be used as a guide to the timing of alterations in the blood target concentration.

CLOSED-LOOP SYSTEMS

Target-controlled infusion systems may be used as part of a closed-loop system to control depth of anaesthesia. Because there is no method of measuring blood concentrations of i.v. anaesthetics online, it is necessary to use some form of monitor of depth of anaesthesia (such as the auditory evoked response; see Ch. 12) on the input side of the system.

DRUGS OF HISTORICAL INTEREST

Eltanolone

Eltanolone (3α-hydroxy-5β-pregnan-20-one; also known as 5β-pregnanolone) underwent clinical trials as an i.v. Induction agent in the 1990s. In common with propofol, eltanolone is poorly soluble in water, and it was formulated in an emulsion with 10% Intralipid. Induction and recovery were slower with eltanolone than with propofol. There was a very low incidence of excitatory activity or involuntary movements. Administration of eltanolone was associated with a significant increase in heart rate but little or no decrease in arterial pressure in volunteers and healthy patients. However, the drug reduces cardiac output to a greater extent than does propofol.

Propanidid

This agent was derived from eugenol (oil of cloves), and was first used in 1964. Its duration of action was exceedingly short, as it was metabolized very rapidly by plasma cholinesterase. There were high incidences of nausea, vomiting and muscle movements. It was solubilized in Cremophor EL (polyoxylated castor oil) and was associated with an unacceptable incidence of severe anaphylactoid reactions.

γ-Hydroxybutyric acid

Anaesthesia of slow onset and recovery was produced by this agent, which is related chemically to the neurotransmitter γ-aminobutyric acid. It was introduced in 1962. It is still used for basal sedation in some European countries.

Althesin

This drug, a mixture of two steroids (alphaxalone and alphadolone), was very similar to propofol in its anaesthetic profile, but was metabolized even more rapidly. It was introduced in 1972. In common with propanidid, it was solubilized in Cremophor EL and an unacceptable number of adverse reactions were reported.

ADVERSE REACTIONS TO INTRAVENOUS ANAESTHETIC AGENTS

These may take the form of pain on injection, venous thrombosis, involuntary muscle movement, hiccup, hypotension and postoperative delirium. All of these reactions may be modified by the anaesthetic technique.

Hypersensitivity reactions, which resemble the effects of histamine release, are more rare and less predictable. Other vasoactive agents may also be released. Reactions to i.v. anaesthetic agents are usually caused by one of the following mechanisms:

Type I hypersensitivity response. The drug interacts with specific immunoglobulin E (IgE) antibodies, which are often bound to the surface of mast cells; these become granulated and release histamine and other vasoactive amines.

Table 14.6 Incidences of adverse reactions to intravenous anaesthetic agents

Drug	Incidence
Thiopental	1:14000–1:20 000
Methohexital	1:1600–1:7000
Althesin	1:400–1:11 000
Propanidid	1:500–1:1700
Etomidate	1:450 000
Propofol	1:50 000–100 000 (estimated)

Classic complement-mediated reaction. The classic complement pathway may be activated by type II (cell surface antigen) or type III (immune complex formation) hypersensitivity reactions. IgG or IgM antibodies are involved.

Alternate complement pathway activation. Pre-formed antibodies to an antigen are not necessary for activation of this pathway; these reactions may therefore occur without prior exposure to the drug.

Direct pharmacological effects of the drug. These anaphylactoid reactions result from a direct effect on mast cells and basophils. There may be local cutaneous signs only. In more severe reactions, there are signs of systemic release of histamine.

Clinical features

In a severe hypersensitivity reaction, a flush may develop over the upper part of the body. There is usually hypotension, which may be profound. Cutaneous and glottic oedema may develop and may result in hypovolaemia because of loss of fluid from the circu-

Table 14.7 Management of allergic reactions

Aims • Correct arterial hypoxaemia • Restore intravascular fluid volume • Inhibit further release of chemical mediators
Routine *Airway* 100% oxygen
Epinephrine (either i.v. or i.m., depending on the severity of the reaction) 0.5 ml of 1:1000, repeated until circulation improves
Fluids: both crystalloids (saline 0.9% or Hartmann's solution) and colloids. The former may be ineffective in some cases
Bronchodilators if there is bronchospasm (e.g. aminophylline, 250–500 mg i.v.). If adverse reaction occurs during anaesthesia, consider use of halothane or ketamine for the relief of bronchoconstriction
Intermittent positive-pressure ventilation (IPPV): continue after resuscitation if there is pulmonary oedema
Use of inotropes to support the circulation, and antiarrhythmic drugs if necessary No data to show a beneficial effect of steroids in acute allergic anaphylactic reactions No agent affects the gastrointestinal symptoms Isoproterenol (isoprenaline) may worsen arterial hypoxaemia, by increasing dead space Antihistamines may be useful in angioneurotic oedema
Consider cerebral resuscitation if there is a prolonged period of cardiac arrest, hypotension or arterial hypoxaemia (e.g. mannitol, IPPV with mild hypocapnia)

lation. Very severe bronchospasm may also occur, although it is a feature in less than 50% of reactions. Diarrhoea often occurs some hours after the initial reaction.

Predisposing factors

Age. In general, adverse reactions are less common in children than in adults.

Pregnancy. There is an increased incidence of adverse reactions in pregnancy.

Gender. Anaphylactic reactions are more common in women.

Atopy. There may be an increased incidence of type IV (delayed hypersensitivity) reactions in non-atopic individuals, and a higher incidence of type I reactions in those with a history of extrinsic asthma, hay fever or penicillin allergy.

Previous exposure. Previous exposure to the drug, or to a drug with similar constituents, exerts a much greater influence on the incidence of reactions than does a history of atopy.

Solvents. Cremophor EL, which was used as a solvent for several i.v. anaesthetic agents, was associated with a high incidence of hypersensitivity reactions.

Incidence

The incidences of hypersensitivity reactions associated with i.v. anaesthetic agents are shown in Table 14.6.

Treatment

This is summarized in Table 14.7. Appropriate investigations should be undertaken after recovery to identify the drug responsible for the reaction.

FURTHER READING

Nimmo W S, Rowbotham D J, Smith G (eds) 1994 Anaesthesia, 2nd edn. Blackwell Scientific Publications. Oxford

McCaughey W, Clarke R S J, Fee J P H, Wallace W F M 1997 Anaesthetic physiology and pharmacology. Churchill Livingstone, Edinburgh

Sear J W 1994 Adverse effects of drugs given by injection. In: Taylor T H, Major E (eds) Hazards and complications of anaesthesia, 2nd edn. Churchill Livingstone, Edinburgh, pp. 273–306

15 Local anaesthetic agents

Local anaesthetic drugs act by producing a reversible block to the transmission of peripheral nerve impulses. A reversible block may also be produced by physical factors, including pressure and cold. Although nerve compression is of purely historical interest, cold (produced by the evaporation of ethyl chloride, the application of ice packs or use of a cryoprobe) still has a limited use.

Many types of drug have local anaesthetic actions (e.g. β-blockers and antihistamines), but all those known and used as local anaesthetics have originated from cocaine, the alkaloid found in the leaves of the South American bush *Erythroxylum coca*. Its local anaesthetic action was demonstrated first by Koller, an ophthalmic surgeon working in Vienna. Although most of the major local anaesthetic techniques were described within a few years of that discovery, the drug was not used widely other than as a topical agent because of its systemic toxicity, central nervous stimulant and addictive properties and tendency to produce allergic reactions.

The demonstration of the physical structure of cocaine as an ester of benzoic acid permitted the production of safer agents, all with the same general structure of an aromatic group joined to an amine by an intermediate chain containing either an ester or an amide link (Fig. 15.1). Procaine, an ester synthesized in 1904, was the first significant advance and it allowed wider use of local anaesthetic techniques. Many other drugs were introduced, but none displaced procaine as the standard until the synthesis of the standard amide, lidocaine, in the 1940s. The intermediate chain in lidocaine contains an amide bond and this obviated many of the problems associated with the ester group present in the older drugs. The subsequent production of other amide agents with varying clinical profiles has greatly extended the scope of modern local anaesthesia.

The mode of action of local anaesthetics is by blocking membrane depolarization in all excitable tissues. As local anaesthetics are injected at their site of action, only peripheral nerve is usually exposed to concentrations high enough to have a significant effect. However, when sufficient drug reaches other organs via the circulation, more widespread effects occur.

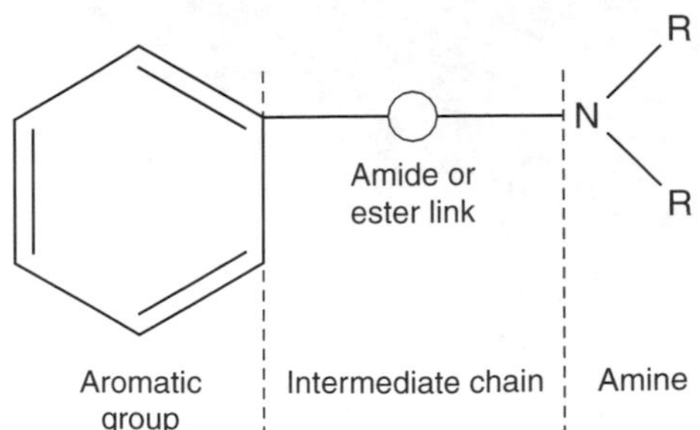

Fig. 15.1
General formula for local anaesthetic drugs.

MODE OF ACTION

NEURAL TRANSMISSION (Fig. 15.2)

During the resting phase, the interior of a peripheral nerve fibre has a potential difference of about –70 mV relative to the outside. When the nerve is stimulated, there is a rapid increase in the membrane potential to approximately +20 mV, followed by an immediate restoration to the resting level. This depolarization/repolarization sequence lasts 1–2 ms and produces the familiar action potential associated with the passage of a nerve impulse.

The resting potential is the net result of several factors affecting the distribution of ions across the cell membrane. Electrochemical and concentration gradients modify ionic diffusion, which is adjusted further by the semipermeable nature of the membrane and the action of the sodium/potassium pump. The resulting balance of these factors is a slight excess of anions in intracellular fluid.

Depolarization of the fibre is the result of a sudden increase in membrane permeability to sodium, which can thus diffuse down both electrochemical and concentration gradients. Sodium ions enter the cell through large protein molecules in the membrane (known as channels), which are closed during the resting phase. Stimulation of the nerve changes the configuration of these protein molecules so that the channels open and allow positively charged sodium ions to enter the cell. This increases the membrane potential to approximately +20 mV, when the electrochemical and concentration gradients for sodium balance each other and the channels close. Both concentration and electrochemical gradients then favour movement of potassium out through the membrane until the resting potential is restored. This outward movement of potassium is also facilitated by the opening of specific channels in the membrane. Relative to the total amounts present, only small numbers of ions take part in this exchange and the sodium/potassium pump restores their distribution during the resting phase.

At sensory nerve endings, the initial opening of sodium channels is produced by the appropriate physiological stimulus, which may be chemically mediated in some instances. When these sodium channels open, the potential at the nerve ending increases and results in a voltage gradient along the axon. This causes a current (known as a local current) to flow between the depolarized

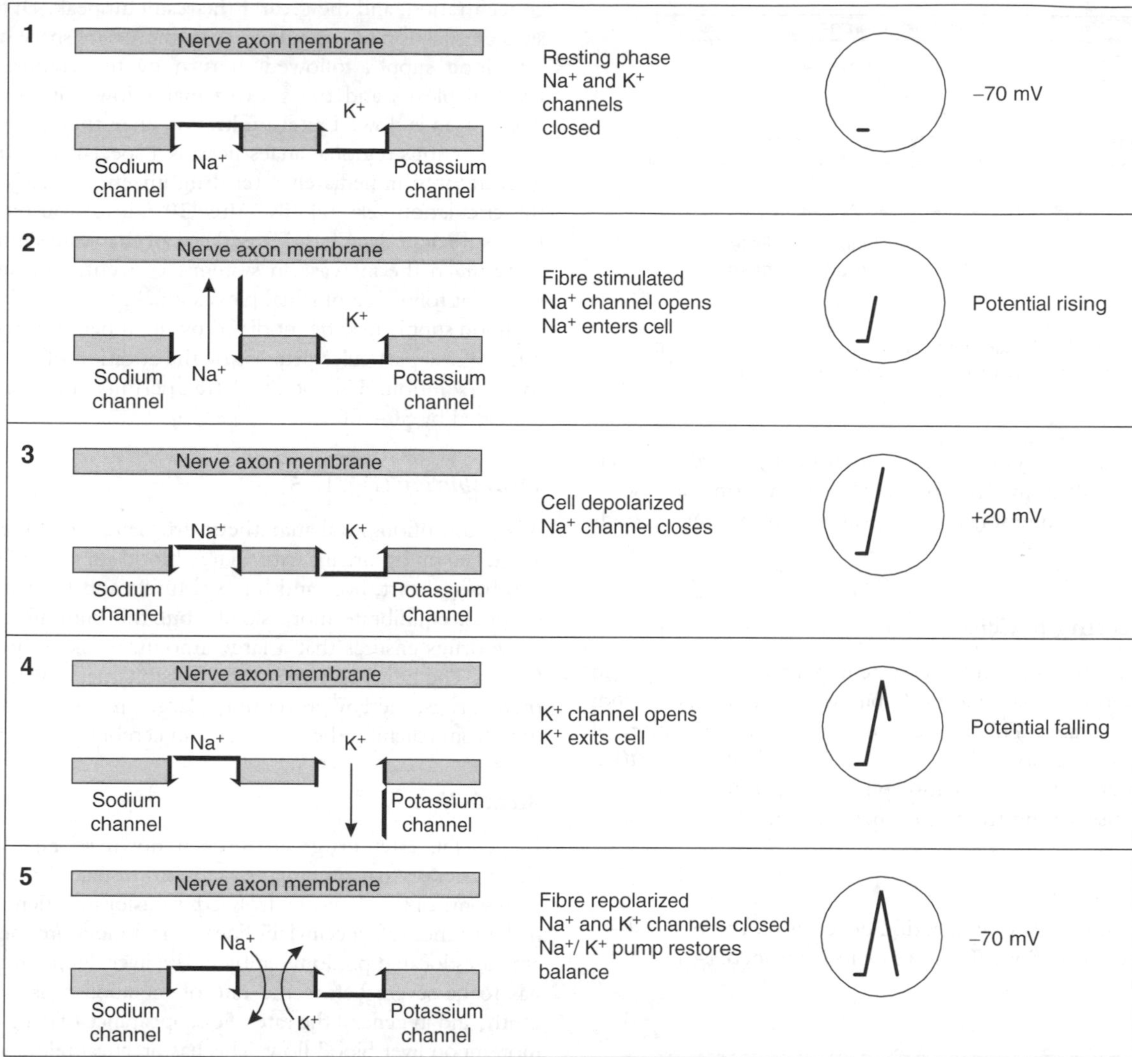

Fig. 15.2
Events occurring during transmission of a nerve impulse along an axon.

segment of nerve (which has a positive charge) and the next segment (which has a negative charge). The voltage change associated with this current causes the configurational change in the sodium channels in the next segment, so that the action potential is propagated along the nerve. A similar sequence is induced when transmitter substances act on specific receptors on the postjunctional membrane at synapses between nerves.

EFFECT OF LOCAL ANAESTHETIC DRUGS
(Fig. 15.3)

Local anaesthetics are usually injected in an acid solution as the hydrochloride salt (pH approximately 5). In such conditions, the tertiary amine group becomes quaternary and the molecules are thus soluble in water and suitable for injection. After injection, the pH increases as a result of buffering in the tissues and a proportion of the drug, determined by the pK_a, dissociates to release free base. Because it is lipid-soluble, the free base is able to pass through the lipid cell membrane to the interior of the axon, where re-ionization takes place. It is the re-ionized portion that enters and blocks the sodium channels, and prevents influx of sodium ions. As a result, no action potential is generated or transmitted, and conduction blockade occurs.

In addition to diffusing into nerves at the site of injection, the drug also enters capillaries and is removed by the circulation. Eventually, tissue concentration decreases below that in the nerves and the drug diffuses out, so allowing restoration of normal function.

SYSTEMIC TOXICITY

If significant amounts of local anaesthetic drug reach the tissues of heart and brain, they exert the same membrane-stabilizing effect as on peripheral nerve, resulting in progressive depression of function. The earliest feature of systemic toxicity is numbness or tingling of the tongue and circumoral area; this is the result of a rich blood supply depositing enough drug to have an effect on the nerve endings. The patient may become light-headed, anxious, drowsy and/or complain of tinnitus. If concentrations continue to increase, consciousness is lost and this may be preceded or followed by convulsions.

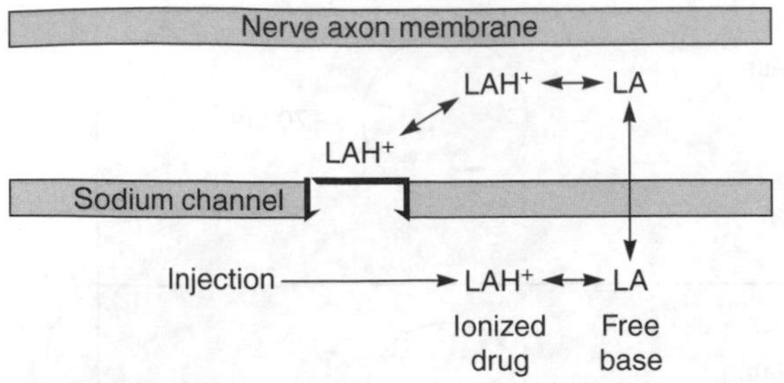

Fig. 15.3
Mode of action of a local anaesthetic (LA) drug. In order to penetrate the lipid cell membrane, the drug must be in free base form, while to effect a block, re-ionization must occur.

Coma and apnoea may develop subsequently. Cardiovascular collapse may result from direct myocardial depression and vasodilatation, but more commonly it is a result of hypoxaemia secondary to apnoea.

Factors affecting toxicity

The most common cause of life-threatening systemic toxicity is an inadvertent intravascular injection, but it may also result from absolute overdosage. The changes in plasma concentration of drug following injection (Fig. 15.4) are dependent on the total dose administered, the rate of absorption, the pattern of distribution to other tissues and the rate of metabolism.

Absorption

Absorption from the site of injection depends on the blood flow; the higher the blood flow, the more rapid is the increase in plasma concentration, and the greater the resultant peak. Of the common sites of injection of large doses, the intercostal space has the highest blood supply, followed in turn by the epidural space, the brachial plexus and the sites of major lower limb nerve block. Absorption is slowest after infiltration anaesthesia.

Intravenous regional anaesthesia is a special case. If the tourniquet deflates immediately after drug injection, a large dose enters the circulation very rapidly. After 20 min of tourniquet application, sufficient drug has diffused out of the vessels into the tissues to result in the increase in systemic concentration being smaller than that following brachial plexus block.

Blood supply may be modified by the inherent vasoactive properties of the particular drug or by the addition of vasoconstrictors to the solution. Use of the latter permits the safe dose to be increased by 50–100%.

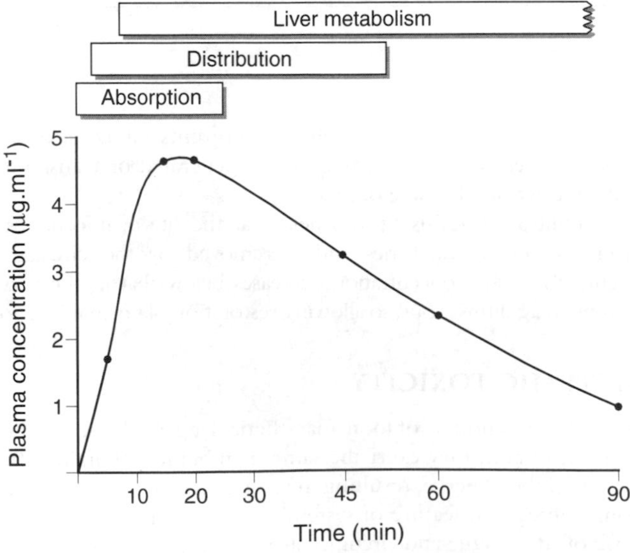

Fig. 15.4
Plasma concentration of lidocaine. Concentrations are shown after the injection into the lumbar epidural space of 400mg of lidocaine without epinephrine. The injection was made at time zero and the phases of absorption, distribution and metabolism are indicated.

Distribution (Fig. 15.5)

After absorption, local anaesthetic drugs are distributed rapidly to, and taken up by, organs with a large blood supply and high affinity, e.g. brain, heart, liver and lungs. Muscle and fat, with low blood supplies, equilibrate more slowly, but the high affinity of fat for these drugs ensures that a large amount is taken up into adipose tissues. The lungs sequester (and possibly metabolize) local anaesthetic drugs, thereby preventing a large proportion of the injected dose from reaching the coronary and cerebral circulations.

Metabolism

In general, ester drugs are broken down so rapidly by plasma cholinesterase that systemic toxicity is unusual. Toxicity may occur with some of the slowly hydrolysed drugs or in patients with abnormal enzymes (cf. succinylcholine). The amides are metabolized by amidases located predominantly in the liver. Hepatocellular disease has to be severe before the rate of metabolism is slowed significantly, and in general the rate of disappearance of drug is dependent more upon liver blood flow. This has practical relevance to the use of lidocaine as an antiarrhythmic in cardiogenic shock, where liver blood flow is diminished.

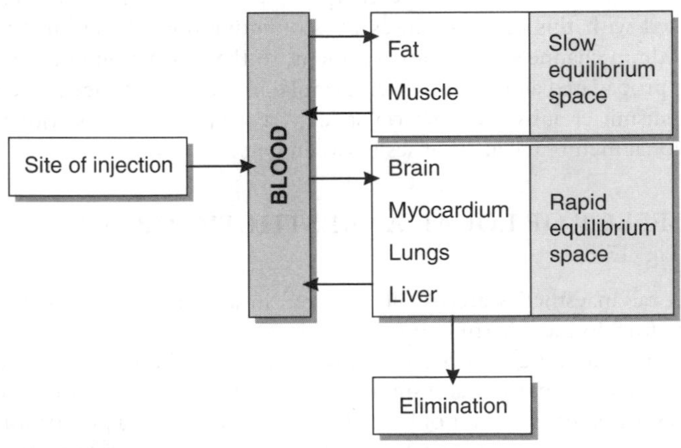

Fig. 15.5
Distribution of local anaesthetic drug after absorption from the site of injection.

Protein binding

Local anaesthetics are bound to plasma proteins to varying degrees. It is assumed sometimes that drugs with the greatest degrees of protein binding are less toxic because only a small fraction of the total amount in plasma is free to diffuse into the tissues and produce toxic effects. However, values for protein binding are obtained under laboratory conditions and probably bear little relationship to the dynamic situation that exists during the phase of rapid absorption. Furthermore, even if a drug is bound to protein, it is still available to diffuse into the tissues down a concentration gradient, as the bound portion is in equilibrium with that in solution in plasma. Thus, values for protein binding do not relate to acute toxicity of a drug.

Placental transfer

Much theoretical concern has been expressed about the mechanisms and effects of placental transfer of local anaesthetics administered to the mother during labour. Local anaesthetics cross the placenta as readily as other membranes, but their effects are of minimal significance when compared with those of conventional methods of analgesia and anaesthesia.

Fetal plasma protein may bind some drugs to a lesser extent than maternal protein so that *total* plasma concentration may be lower in the baby. It is claimed that such drugs are safer for the fetus. However, the concentration of *free* drug on each side of the placental membrane is the same, and as a result tissue concentrations are more similar in mother and fetus than total plasma concentrations. The neonatal liver metabolizes drugs slowly, but provided that delivery does not occur immediately after a toxic reaction, there should be little concern about effects on the baby.

Prevention of toxicity

The single most important factor in the prevention of toxicity is the avoidance of accidental intravascular injection. Careful aspiration tests are vital and should be repeated each time the needle is moved. However, a negative test is not an absolute guarantee, especially when a catheter technique is used. The initial injection of 2–3 ml of a solution that contains epinephrine (1:200 000) has been advocated; an increase in heart rate during the succeeding 1–2 min should indicate intravascular injection. However, epinephrine is not the safest of drugs and this method is no guarantee against subsequent migration of needle or cannula into a vessel.

An alternative is to repeat the aspiration test after each 5–10 ml of solution and to inject slowly. The patient should be watched for early signs of toxicity so that the injection may be stopped before there are major sequelae. Particular care should be taken when performing head and neck blocks because a very small dose may produce a major reaction if injected into a carotid or vertebral artery.

Overdosage may be avoided by consideration of the behaviour of the various drugs after injection at the particular site. Most practical manuals indicate the appropriate drug and dosage for each block, and these recommendations should be followed. Maximum safe dosages (for use in any situation) are often quoted for local anaesthetics with and without vasoconstrictor, but such recommendations are not really helpful as they ignore variations caused by factors such as the site of injection, the patient's general condition and the concomitant use of a general anaesthetic. If the same total dose is used, variations in drug concentration have no effect on toxicity. In adults, body weight correlates poorly with the risk of toxicity and it is better to modify the dose on the basis of an informed assessment of the patient's general condition.

Treatment of toxicity

No matter how careful the anaesthetist is with regard to prevention, facilities for treatment must always be available. The airway is maintained and oxygen administered by face mask, using artificial ventilation if apnoea occurs. Convulsions may be controlled with small increments of either midazolam (2 mg) or thiopental (50 mg). The latter may be more readily available and acts more rapidly. Excessive doses should not be given to control convulsions, as cardiorespiratory depression may be exacerbated. If cardiovascular collapse occurs despite adequate oxygenation (and this is rare), it should be treated with an adrenergic drug with α- and β-agonist properties, e.g. ephedrine in 3–5 mg increments.

ADDITIONAL SIDE-EFFECTS

Local anaesthetics are remarkably free from side-effects other than systemic toxicity which is an extension of pharmacological action. Complications of specific drugs are discussed later, but there are two general features – allergic reactions and drug interactions.

Allergic reactions

Allergy to the esters was relatively common, particularly with procaine, and was caused by *para*-aminobenzoic acid produced on hydrolysis. Most reactions were dermal in personnel handling the drugs, but fatal anaphylaxis has been recorded. Allergy to the amides is extremely rare and most reactions result from systemic toxicity, overdosage with vasoconstrictors, or are manifestations of anxiety. The occasional genuine allergic reaction is usually to a preservative in the solution rather than the drug itself.

Drug interactions

Interactions with other drugs do occur, although they rarely cause clinical problems. Therapy with anticholinesterases for myasthenia, or the concomitant administration of other drugs hydrolysed by plasma cholinesterase, increases the toxicity of the ester drugs, and competition for plasma protein binding sites may occur with the amides. Of more practical importance is that heavy sedation with anticonvulsants (e.g. benzodiazepines) may mask the early signs of toxicity. These drugs may even prevent convulsions, so that if a severe reaction does occur the patient may suddenly become deeply unconscious.

PHARMACOLOGY OF INDIVIDUAL DRUGS

The local anaesthetic drugs in current use vary in their clinical profile (stability, potency, duration, toxicity, etc.). These differences may be related to variations in physicochemical properties.

LOCAL ANAESTHETIC DRUG CHEMISTRY

As indicated above (Fig. 15.1), all the local anaesthetic drugs have a three-part structure, with either an ester or an amide bond at the centre. The important effects of the nature of this linkage on the route of metabolism and allergenicity have been discussed. The ester drugs also have short shelf-lives because they tend to hydrolyse spontaneously, especially on warming. The amides may be stored for long periods without loss of potency and are not heat-sensitive unless mixed with glucose to produce hyperbaric spinal solutions. As a general rule, solutions of amides in glucose and solutions of any ester may be heat-sterilized once, and should be used soon after autoclaving.

The clinical properties of an agent are primarily determined by its physicochemical properties. The important factors are the pK_a, lipid solubility (normally expressed as a partition coefficient) and degree of binding to protein. All these are influenced by the basic chemical structure (ester or amide) of the compound, and the addition of side chains to the basic molecule. A low pK_a favours rapid onset because more of the drug is in the lipid permeant, unionized form at physiological pH. The more lipid-soluble the agent is, the more potent it is likely to be, and duration of action relates to degree of protein binding. Higher pK_a and lower lipid solubility favour a greater degree of differential block of sensory and motor nerve functions (see below). The effects of differences in molecular structure often interact in complex ways, but a simple example of a structure–activity relationship is the addition of a butyl group to mepivacaine to produce bupivacaine, which is four times as potent and significantly longer-acting. Alterations in structure also affect the rate and the products of metabolism.

The effects of a local anaesthetic drug on blood vessels also modify its profile. Cocaine is a potent vasoconstrictor, but most of the other agents produce some degree of vasodilatation, which tends to shorten duration of action and increase toxicity. However, prilocaine and ropivacaine are exceptions and probably have slight vasoconstrictor properties at clinically used concentrations.

A final important chemical consideration is that several local anaesthetics, including bupivacaine and ropivacaine, exhibit optical isomerism because they contain an asymmetric carbon atom. Bupivacaine is usually presented as a racemic mixture of 'S' and 'R' enantiomers, but interest in the clinical use of single enantiomeric forms has been generated by evidence that the R-enantiomer has greater cardiotoxicity. Ropivacaine was the first local anaesthetic to be commercially available as a single S-isomer preparation, and chirocaine (S-bupivacaine) is being investigated for clinical use also.

Differential sensory and motor blockade

It is often stated that small diameter axons, such as C fibres, are more susceptible to local anaesthetic block than are larger diameter fibres. In terms of absolute sensitivity, the reverse is true; large diameter fibres are more sensitive than small ones. However, large diameter fibres are usually more heavily myelinated than small fibres and the myelin sheath presents a significant barrier to drug diffusion. As a result, small, unmyelinated fibres are blocked more rapidly by most local anaesthetic drugs. This difference in rate of blockade may be manipulated clinically with the aim of producing analgesia with relatively little motor blockade because skeletal muscle is innervated by larger, heavily myelinated fibres. Thus weak solutions (e.g. bupivacaine 0.125%) are employed with this aim. The newer agent, ropivacaine, appears to produce even greater separation of sensory and motor blockade and may become the agent of choice for epidural use in obstetrics and the postoperative period.

CLINICAL FACTORS AFFECTING DRUG PROFILE

Increasing the dose of a drug shortens its onset time and increases the duration of block. Dose may be increased by using either a higher concentration or a larger volume; a large volume of a dilute solution is usually more effective.

The site of injection also affects onset time and duration (in addition to potential toxicity). Onset is almost immediate after infiltration and is progressively delayed with subarachnoid, peripheral nerve and epidural blocks, respectively. The slowest onset follows brachial plexus block. The dose required and the likely duration of action tend to increase in much the same order as for onset time.

Pregnancy and age are said to increase segmental spread of epidurals. For many blocks, young, fit, tall patients seem to require more drug, as do obese, alcoholic or anxious patients, the last perhaps because they react to any sensation from the operative area.

INDIVIDUAL DRUG PROPERTIES

Only when all the above factors are taken into account may the properties of various drugs be compared. It is doubtful if, at equipotent concentrations, there are any real differences in speed of onset, but there are certainly variations in potency, duration and toxicity. The features of individual drugs are described below and in Table 15.1. Appropriate volumes and concentrations of local anaesthetic agents used commonly for specific blocks are detailed in Chapter 43.

Cocaine

Cocaine has no role in modern anaesthetic practice, although it is used in ear, nose and throat surgery for its vasoconstrictor action. Because of its use as a drug of addiction, it is increasingly difficult to obtain cocaine legitimately at a reasonable price.

Benzocaine

This is an excellent topical agent of low toxicity. It does not ionize and therefore its use is limited to topical application. In addition, its mode of action cannot be explained according to the theory outlined above. Instead, it is thought that benzocaine diffuses into the cell membrane, but not into the cytoplasm, and either causes the membrane to expand in the same way as is suggested for general anaesthetics (see Ch. 5) or enters the sodium channel from the lipid phase of the membrane. Whichever is the case, the mechanism may also be relevant to the action of the other agents.

Procaine

The incidence of allergic problems, short shelf-life and brief duration of action of procaine have resulted in its infrequent use at the present time.

Chloroprocaine

This is an ester which is widely used in the USA. Its profile is very similar to that of procaine, from which it differs only by the addition of a chlorine atom (Table 15.1). As a result, it is hydrolysed four times as quickly by cholinesterase and seems to be less allergenic. It is claimed to have a more rapid onset than any other agent but this may relate to its very low toxicity, which permits the use of relatively larger doses. There has been some concern that

Table 15.1 The features of individual local anaesthetic drugs

Proper name/ formula	% equivalent concentration[a]	Relative duration[a]	Toxicity	pK_a	Partition coefficient	% protein bound	Main use by anaesthetists in the UK
Cocaine 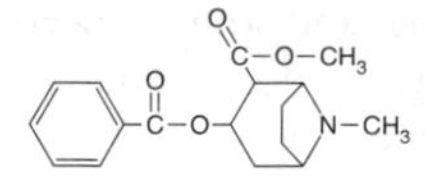	1	0.5	Very high	8.7	?	?	Nil.
Benzocaine 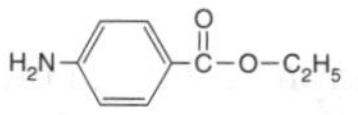	NA	2	Low	NA	132	?	Topical
Procaine 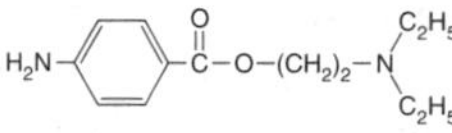	2	0.75	Low	8.9	3.1	5.8	Nil
Chloroprocaine 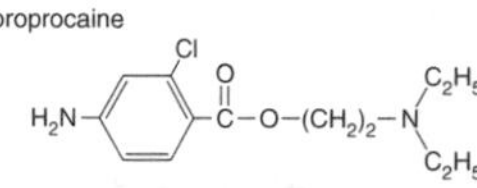	1	0.75	Low	9.1	17	?	Not available
Tetracaine 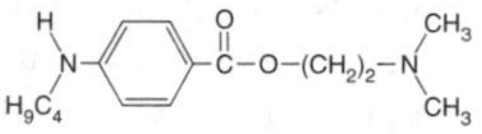	0.25	2	High	8.4	541	76	Topical
Lidocaine 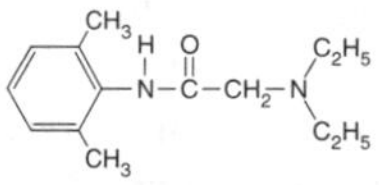	1	1	Medium	7.8	110	64	Infiltration Nerve block Epidural
Mepivacaine 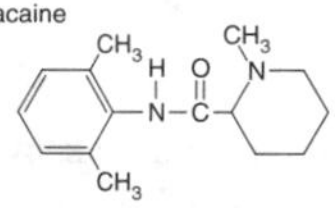	1	1	Medium	7.7	42	77	Not available
Prilocaine 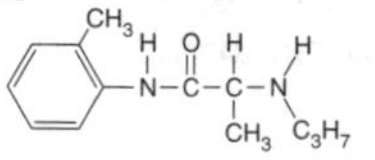	1	1.5	Low	7.7	50	55	Infiltration Nerve block IVRA
Cinchocaine 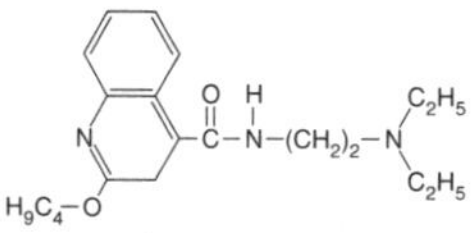	0.25	2	High	7.9	?	?	Not available
Ropivacaine 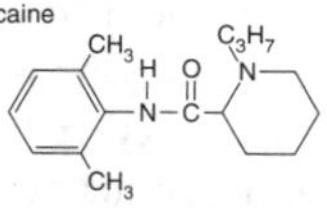	0.25	2–4	Medium	8.1	230	94	Epidural Nerve block
Bupivacaine 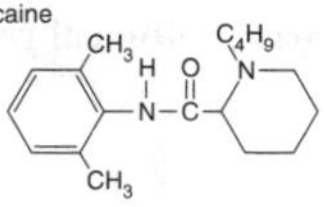	0.25	2–4	Medium	8.1	560	95	Epidural Spinal Nerve block
Etidocaine 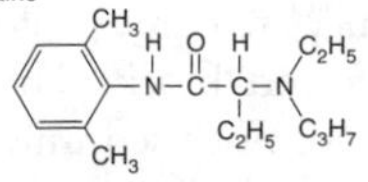	0.5	2–4	Medium	7.9	1853	94	Not available

[a]Lidocaine = 1. NA, not applicable (not used in solution); ?, information not available. NB: Published figures vary. See Strichartz et al (1990) for more details.

chloroprocaine might be neurotoxic, because of several reports of paraplegia after accidental intrathecal injection. However, the evidence suggests that it was the preservative in the solution that caused the problems and not the drug itself.

Tetracaine

This drug (also known as amethocaine) is relatively toxic for an ester because it is hydrolysed very slowly by cholinesterase. It is also very potent and is the standard drug in North America for subarachnoid anaesthesia. It has a prolonged duration of action, but also a slow onset time. It can be used intrathecally in hyperbaric or isobaric solutions. Its use in the UK is restricted to topical anaesthesia.

Lidocaine (previously lignocaine)

Having been used safely and effectively for every possible type of local anaesthetic procedure, lidocaine is currently the standard agent. It has no unusual features and is also a standard antiarrhythmic. Lidocaine is used commonly for infiltration in concentrations of 0.5–1.0% and for peripheral nerve blocks if an intermediate duration is required. It can be used for intravenous regional anaesthesia, although prilocaine is preferred. Lidocaine 5% has been used for subarachnoid anaesthesia, although the degree of spread is unpredictable, the duration of action is relatively short. However there are relatively new concerns about its neurotoxicity in such high concentrations. In a concentration of 1–2%, lidocaine produces epidural anaesthesia with a short onset time. Lidocaine 2–4% is used by many anaesthetists as a topical solution for anaesthesia of the upper airway before awake fibreoptic intubation.

Mepivacaine

This agent is very similar to lidocaine and seems to have neither advantages nor disadvantages in comparison.

Prilocaine

This is an underrated agent. It is equipotent to lidocaine, but has virtually no vasodilator action, is either metabolized or sequestered to a greater degree by the lungs, and is more rapidly metabolized by the liver. As a result, it is slightly longer-acting, considerably less toxic and is the drug of choice when the risk of toxicity is high. Metabolism produces *o*-toluidine, which reduces haemoglobin; thus, methaemoglobinaemia may occur but is rare unless the dose is considerably in excess of 600 mg. Cyanosis appears when 1.5 g dl^{-1} of haemoglobin is converted, and treatment with methylene blue (1 mg kg^{-1}) is effective immediately. Fetal haemoglobin is more sensitive, and prilocaine should not be used for epidural block during labour. Prilocaine is used mostly for infiltration and for intravenous regional anaesthesia.

Cinchocaine

Cinchocaine was the first amide agent to be produced (two decades before lidocaine). It is very potent and toxic. In common with tetracaine, it was used mainly for subarachnoid anaesthesia, but the drug is no longer available for clinical use.

Bupivacaine

The introduction of bupivacaine represented a significant advance in anaesthesia. Relative to potency, its acute central nervous system toxicity is only slightly lower than that of lidocaine, but its longer duration of action reduces the need for repeated doses, and thus the risks of cumulative toxicity.

Several deaths have occurred after accidental intravenous administration of large doses of bupivacaine, and some concern has been expressed that this drug might have a more toxic effect on the myocardium than other local anaesthetic agents. There is evidence that this is due to the R-enantiomer (see above), but relatively large doses must be given rapidly and intravenously for the effect to be clinically apparent.

Bupivacaine may be used for infiltration, although only in small doses because of its toxicity. It is used frequently for peripheral nerve blockade and for subarachnoid and epidural anaesthesia because of its prolonged duration of action.

Bupivacaine 0.5% is the most commonly used drug for subarachnoid anaesthesia in the UK. It may be used in a plain solution or in a hyperbaric formulation (see Ch. 43).

Ropivacaine

The cardiovascular toxicity of bupivacaine stimulated interest in finding other long-acting agents which do not possess this effect. Ropivacaine is similar chemically to bupivacaine (the butyl group attached to the amine is replaced by a propyl group), but it is presented as a single S-enantiomer. It is marginally less potent than bupivacaine, and produces a block of slightly shorter duration, but a greater degree of differential block in dilute solutions. At equipotent concentrations, ropivacaine appears to be less likely than bupivacaine to cause cardiac arrhythmias and collapse; resuscitation is more likely to be successful if toxicity does occur.

Etidocaine

This is an amide derived from lidocaine. It may be even longer-acting than bupivacaine and is of particular interest because it seems to produce a more profound effect on motor than sensory nerves; the reverse is probably true with other agents.

Chirocaine

This is the single S-enantiomer of bupivacaine. It has only recently become available for clinical use.

ADDITIVES

Many substances are added to local anaesthetics for pharmaceutical purposes. Sodium hydroxide and hydrochloric acid are used to adjust the pH, sodium chloride the tonicity, and glucose and water the baricity of solutions. Preservatives, e.g. methyl hydroxybenzoate, are added to multidose bottles and manufacturers recommend that these should not be used for subarachnoid or epidural block. Other additions are made for pharmacological reasons.

Vasoconstrictors

The addition of a vasoconstrictor to a solution of local anaesthetic drug slows the rate of absorption, reduces toxicity, prolongs duration and may result in a more profound block. These are all desirable effects, but vasoconstrictors are not used universally for several reasons. They are absolutely contraindicated for injection close to end-arteries (ring blocks of digits and penis) and in intravenous regional anaesthesia because of the risk of ischaemia.

There is also a theoretical risk that the use of vasoconstrictors may increase the risk of permanent neurological deficit by rendering nerve tissue ischaemic. While evidence is inconclusive, many anaesthetists feel that vasoconstrictors should not be used unless there is no alternative method of prolonging duration or reducing toxicity in the specific clinical situation.

Epinephrine is the most potent agent. It produces its own systemic toxicity and should be used with particular care, if at all, in patients with cardiac disease. Even in healthy patients, concentrations greater than 1:200 000 should not be used, and the maximum dose administered should not exceed 0.5 mg. Interactions with other sympathomimetic drugs, including tricyclic antidepressants, may occur, especially when adrenergic drugs are used systemically to treat hypotension.

Felypressin is a safer drug, although it causes pallor and may constrict the coronary circulation. It is usually available for dental use only.

Carbon dioxide

In order to speed the onset of blockade, some local anaesthetics have been produced as the carbonated salt, with carbon dioxide dissolved under pressure in the solution. The rationale for the use of these solutions is that after injection the carbon dioxide lowers intracellular pH and favours formation of more of the ionized active form of the drug. With blocks of slower onset, there is good evidence that a significant improvement is obtained.

Dextrans

There have been many attempts to prolong duration of action by mixing local anaesthetics with high-molecular-weight dextrans. The results are inconclusive, but the very large dextrans may be effective, especially in combination with epinephrine. 'Macromolecules' may be formed between dextran and local anaesthetic so that the latter is held in the tissues for longer periods.

Hyaluronidase

For many years, the enzyme hyaluronidase was added to local anaesthetics to aid spread by breaking down tissue barriers. There was little evidence that it had a significant effect and this practice has been abandoned, except perhaps in ophthalmic practice.

Mixtures

Some practitioners deliberately mix different local anaesthetics together in an attempt to obtain the advantages of both. One such combination (sometimes referred to as compounding) is lidocaine and bupivacaine; the aim is to achieve the rapid onset of the former and the long duration of the latter with a single injection. Another advantage claimed for compounding two drugs is a decrease in toxicity. However, local anaesthetic drug toxicity is additive, so that the use of 'half a dose' of each of two drugs is of no benefit. If an ester is combined with an amide, toxicity may increase because the amide slows hydrolysis of the ester by inhibiting plasma cholinesterase. It is more appropriate to use a catheter technique, to initiate the block with a dose of lidocaine and to maintain it with a dose of bupivacaine as the effect of lidocaine starts to regress.

A more effective combination is the eutectic mixture of local anaesthetics (EMLA). This is a mixture of the base (un-ionized) forms of lidocaine and prilocaine in a cream formulation. It is a local anaesthetic preparation which penetrates intact skin with some reliability. It takes up to 1 h to become effective but is very useful in paediatric practice, especially in children who need repeated venepuncture. It may also be of value for poor-risk patients undergoing skin grafting.

CHOICE OF LOCAL ANAESTHETIC AGENT

When using a local technique, the anaesthetist has to decide upon the concentration, volume and nature of the agent to be used. For lidocaine (the relative potencies of other agents are shown in Table 15.1), concentrations required are:

skin infiltration IVRA	0.5%
minor nerve block	1.0%
brachial plexus sciatic/femoral	1.0–1.5%
epidural	1.5–2.0%
subarachnoid	2.0–5.0%

Higher concentrations than these may be used to produce more profound peripheral blocks of faster onset. The volumes required for specific techniques are described in Chapter 43 and the interrelationships that exist between patient status and the required amount of drug are discussed above.

Ideally, several drugs of different potency, duration and toxicity should be available to permit a rational choice based upon the required dose, the particular risk of toxicity in that block and patient, and the likely duration of surgery. Often this is not possible, mainly for commercial reasons. For example, in the UK, lidocaine and bupivacaine are marketed in a full range of concentrations, but little else is available apart from the more dilute solutions of prilocaine. The availability of spinal anaesthetic solutions is particularly poor. For more peripheral blocks, lidocaine and bupivacaine may be used safely unless the risk of toxicity is relatively high (e.g. intravenous regional anaesthesia) when prilocaine is the drug of choice. When large volumes of more concentrated solutions are needed and the higher concentrations of prilocaine are not available, one of the other agents should be used in combination with epinephrine.

FURTHER READING

Covino B G, Wildsmith J A W 1998 Clinical pharmacology of local anesthetic agents. In: Cousins M J, Bridenbaugh P O (eds) Neural blockade in clinical anesthesia and management of pain, 3rd edn. Lippincott-Raven, Philadelphia, p 97–128

McClure J H 1996 Ropivacaine. British Journal of Anaesthesia 76: 300–307

Strichartz G R 1998 Neural physiology and local anesthetic action. In: Cousins M J, Bridenbaugh P O (eds) Neural blockade in clinical anesthesia and management of pain, 3rd edn. Lippincott-Raven, Philadelphia, p 25–54

Strichartz G R, Sanchez V, Arthur G R, Chafetz R, Martin D 1990 Fundamental properties of local anaesthetics. II. Measured octanol: buffer partition coefficients and pKa values of clinically used drugs. Anesthesia and Analgesia 71: 158–170

Tucker G T, Mather L E 1998 Properties, absorption, and disposition of local anesthetic agents. In: Cousins M J, Bridenbaugh P O (eds) Neural blockade in clinical anesthesia and management of pain, 3rd edn. Lippincott-Raven, Philadelphia, p 55–96

Wildsmith J A W, McClure J H, Armitage E N 2001 Principles and practice of regional anaesthesia, 3rd edn. Churchill Livingstone, Edinburgh

16 Sedative and anticonvulsant drugs

SEDATIVES

Sedation may be defined as the use of pharmacological agents to produce depression of the level of consciousness sufficient to result in drowsiness and anxiolysis without loss of verbal communication. The difference between sedative and anaesthetic drugs is largely one of usage. Many anaesthetic drugs may be used at reduced dosage to produce sedation. Drugs more usually used as sedatives produce a form of anaesthesia if given in high enough doses. There exists a seamless progression from so-called 'conscious' sedation to deep sedation where verbal contact and protective reflexes are lost, a state indistinguishable from general anaesthesia. The ability of the patient to maintain a patent airway independently is one characteristic of conscious sedation, but even at this level of sedation it cannot be assumed that protective reflexes are intact.

Indications for the use of sedative drugs

Premedication

'Sedo-analgesia'. This term describes the use of a combination of a sedative drug with local anaesthesia, e.g. in dental surgery or surgical procedures performed under regional blockade. The recent expansion in the development of minimally invasive surgery makes this technique more widely applicable.

Radiological procedures. Some patients, particularly children and anxious individuals, are unable to tolerate long and uncomfortable imaging procedures without sedation. Developments in the use and scope of interventional radiology have further increased the demand for sedation in the radiology department.

Endoscopy. Sedative drugs are commonly used to provide anxiolysis and sedation during endoscopic examinations and interventions. In gastrointestinal endoscopy, local analgesia is usually inappropriate, necessitating co-administration of systemic opioids. This significantly increases the risks of airway obstruction and ventilatory depression.

Intensive therapy. Most patients require sedation to facilitate mechanical ventilation and other therapeutic interventions. With the increasing sophistication of mechanical ventilators, the modern approach is to combine adequate analgesia with sufficient sedation to maintain the patient in a tranquil but rousable state. A system of sedation scoring should be used and the pharmacokinetic profiles of individual drugs considered, as sedatives are inevitably given by infusion for prolonged periods in patients with potential organ dysfunction and impaired ability to metabolize or excrete drugs.

Supplementation of general anaesthesia. Use is made of the synergy between sedative drugs and intravenous induction agents in the technique of co-induction. The administration of a small dose of sedative may result in a significant reduction in the dose of induction agent required, and therefore in the frequency of side-effects.

Recent developments

The administration of sedative drugs requires skill and vigilance, not least because of the seamless progression from light sedation to general anaesthesia. Traditionally, sedative drugs have been administered by intermittent intravenous bolus doses titrated to effect. There is considerable variability in the individual response to a given dose and there are many circumstances in which medical practitioners without anaesthetic training administer sedatives. Recent technological advances in microprocessor-controlled infusion pumps have improved the safety of administration of sedatives. Patient-controlled analgesia systems have been programmed for *patient-controlled sedation*, usually to maintain sedation after an initial bolus dose administered by the physician. When the system is wholly patient-controlled, the mean dose of sedative decreases while the range increases.

In *target-controlled infusion*, machines are programmed with the pharmacokinetic model of a drug and designed to achieve a given 'target' plasma concentration based on the patient's weight. To allow for variability in the pharmacodynamic effect of the drug, the operator may vary the target level.

Most sedative drugs may be categorized into one of three main groups: benzodiazepines, neuroleptics and $\alpha_2$adrenoceptor agonists. Drugs more usually classified as intravenous anaesthetic agents, particularly propofol and ketamine, are also used as sedatives in subanaesthetic doses; the pharmacology of these drugs is discussed in Chapter 14. Inhaled anaesthetics (Ch. 13) are also used occasionally as sedatives, in subanaesthetic concentrations.

BENZODIAZEPINES

These drugs were developed initially for their anxiolytic and hypnotic properties and largely replaced oral barbiturates in the 1960s. As parenteral preparations became available, they rapidly became established in anaesthesia and intensive care. All benzodiazepines have similar pharmacological effects; their therapeutic use is determined largely by their potency and the available pharmaceutical preparations. Benzodiazepines are often classified by their duration of action as long-acting (e.g. diazepam), medium-acting (e.g. temazepam) or short-acting (e.g. midazolam).

Table 16.1 Relationship between the effects seen with benzodiazepines and receptor occupancy

Midazolam dose	Effect	Receptor occupancy %	Flumazenil dose to reverse
Low dose	Anticonvulsant	20–25%	Low dose
	Anxiolysis	20–30%	
	Slight sedation		
	Reduced attention	25–50%	
	Amnesia		
	Intense sedation	60–90%	
	Muscle relaxation		
High dose	Anaesthesia		High dose

Pharmacology

Mechanism of action

Benzodiazepines exert their actions by specific high-affinity binding to the benzodiazepine receptor, which is part of the γ-aminobutyric acid (GABA) receptor complex. GABA is the major inhibitory neurotransmitter in the central nervous system (CNS), with most neurones undergoing GABAergic modulation. The benzodiazepine receptor is an integral binding site on the $GABA_A$ receptor subtype. Binding of the agonist facilitates the entry of chloride ions into the cell, resulting in hyperpolarization of the postsynaptic membrane, which makes the neurone resistant to excitation. Benzodiazepine receptors are found throughout the brain and spinal cord, with the highest density in the cerebral cortex, hippocampus and cerebellum.

The clinical CNS effects of benzodiazepines have been shown to correlate with receptor occupancy (see Table 16.1). The binding of other compounds to the benzodiazepine receptor explains the synergism seen with some other drugs, including propofol. The benzodiazepine antagonist flumazenil occupies the receptor but produces no activity. Benzodiazepine compounds have been developed which are ligands at the receptor but have inverse agonist activity, resulting in cerebral excitement. These compounds are also antagonized by flumazenil. This mirrors the way in which paradoxical reactions to benzodiazepines in the elderly are reversed by flumazenil and exacerbated by increasing the dose of the original drug. Other more sinister causes of restlessness, such as hypoxaemia and local anaesthetic toxicity, should always be excluded first. Chronic administration of benzodiazepines results in receptor downregulation, with decreased receptor binding and function, explaining, at least in part, the development of tolerance.

CNS effects

The characteristic CNS effects seen with all benzodiazepines are as follows.

Anxiolysis occurs at low dosage and these drugs are used extensively for the treatment of acute and chronic anxiety states. Longer-acting oral drugs such as diazepam and chlordiazepoxide have a place in the management of acute alcohol withdrawal states. Anxiolysis is very useful in premedication and during unfamiliar or unpleasant procedures.

Sedation occurs as a dose-dependent depression of cerebral activity, with mild sedation at low receptor occupancy progressing to a state similar to general anaesthesia when most receptor sites are occupied. Midazolam is firmly established as a safe intravenous sedative. Benzodiazepines have a high therapeutic index (ratio of effective to lethal dose) because, in overdosage, differences in receptor density result in greater sensitivity to cortical than to medullary depression. However, upper airway obstruction and loss of protective reflexes occur before profound sedation ensues, and are a major hazard to the patient following inadvertent oversedation and self-poisoning.

Amnesia is a common sequel to intravenous administration of benzodiazepines and is useful for patients undergoing unpleasant or repeated procedures. Retrograde amnesia has not been demonstrated. Prolonged periods of amnesia have been reported in association with the use of oral lorazepam, making it potentially dangerous in the day-case setting.

Anticonvulsant activity is the result of prevention of the subcortical spread of seizure activity. Intravenous diazepam is used to terminate seizures and clonazepam is used as an adjunct in chronic anticonvulsant therapy. Benzodiazepines increase the threshold to seizure activity in local anaesthetic toxicity but may also mask the early signs.

Muscle relaxation

Benzodiazepines produce a mild reduction in muscle tone, which can be advantageous, e.g. during mechanical ventilation in the intensive care unit, when reducing articular dislocations or during endoscopy. However, muscle relaxation is partly responsible for the airway obstruction which may occur during intravenous sedation. The muscle relaxation is not related to any effect at the neuromuscular junction, but results from suppression of the internuncial neurones of the spinal cord and depression of polysynaptic transmission in the brain.

Respiratory effects

Benzodiazepines produce dose-related central depression of ventilation. The ventilatory response to carbon dioxide is impaired and hypoxic ventilatory responses are markedly depressed. It follows that patients with hypoventilation syndromes and type 2 respiratory failure are particularly sensitive to the respiratory depressant effects of benzodiazepines. Ventilatory depression is exacerbated by airway obstruction and is more common in the elderly. Synergism occurs when both opioids and benzodiazepines are administered. If both types of drug are to be given intravenously, the opioid should be given first and its effect assessed. A dose reduction of benzodiazepine of up to 75% should be anticipated. It should be standard practice to provide supplemental oxygen and to monitor oxygen saturation by pulse oximetry during intravenous sedation.

Cardiovascular effects

Benzodiazepines produce modest haemodynamic effects, with good preservation of homeostatic reflex mechanisms and a much wider margin of safety than intravenous anaesthetic agents. A decrease in systemic vascular resistance results in a small decrease in arterial pressure. Significant hypotension may occur in hypovolaemic or vasoconstricted patients.

Pharmacokinetics

Benzodiazepines are relatively small lipid-soluble molecules, which are readily absorbed orally and which pass rapidly into the CNS. After intravenous bolus administration, termination of action occurs largely by redistribution. Elimination takes place by hepatic metabolism followed by renal excretion of the metabolites. There are two main pathways of metabolism involving either microsomal oxidation or glucuronide conjugation. The significance of this is that oxidation is much more likely to be affected by age, hepatic disease, drug interactions and other factors which alter cytochrome P450. Some of the benzodiazepines, including diazepam, have active metabolites, which greatly prolong their effect. Renal dysfunction results in the accumulation of metabolites, and this is an important factor in delayed recovery from prolonged sedation in the intensive therapy unit (ITU).

Diazepam

Diazepam was the first benzodiazepine available for parenteral use. It is insoluble in water and was formulated initially in propylene glycol, which is very irritant to veins and which is associated with a high incidence of thrombophlebitis. A lipid emulsion (Diazemuls) was developed later. Both formulations are presented in 2 ml ampoules of 5 mg ml^{-1}. Diazepam is also available orally as tablets or a syrup with a bioavailability of 100% and as a rectal solution and suppositories. The elimination half-life is 20–50 h, but active metabolites are produced, including desmethyldiazepam, which has a half-life of 36–200 h. Clearance is reduced in hepatic dysfunction.

Dosage

- *Premedication* – 10–15 mg orally 1–1.5 h preoperatively
- *Sedation* – 7–15 mg i.v. slowly; incremental bolus of 1–2 mg
- *Status epilepticus* – 2 mg, repeated every minute until seizure ends; maximum dose 20 mg
- *Intensive therapy* – not suitable for infusion; i.v. bolus dose 5–10 mg 4-hourly.

Midazolam

Midazolam is an imidazo-benzodiazepine derivative and it is the imidazole ring which imparts water solubility at pH less than 4. At blood pH, the drug becomes highly lipid-soluble and penetrates the brain rapidly with onset of sedation in 90 s and peak effect at 2–5 min. It is available in 2 ml (5 mg ml^{-1}) and 5 ml (2 mg ml^{-1}) ampoules and, unlike diazepam, may be diluted. It is also available as a 15 mg tablet with an oral bioavailability of 44%. Midazolam undergoes hepatic oxidative metabolism and has an elimination half-life of 2 h. The major metabolite, hydroxy-midazolam, has a half-life of around 1 h, and although it is biologically active, it is only clinically important after prolonged infusion in patients with renal impairment. Midazolam is 1.5–2 times more potent than diazepam and has much more favourable pharmacokinetics for use as a short-term intravenous sedative.

Dosage

- *Premedication* – 15 mg orally or 5 mg i.m.
- *Sedation* – 2–7 mg i.v. (elderly less than 4 mg); incremental bolus of 0.5–1 mg
- *Status epilepticus* – not recommended
- *Intensive therapy* – i.v. infusion 0.03–0.2 mg kg^{-1} h^{-1}.

Temazepam

This benzodiazepine is only available orally but is used widely as a premedicant because of its anxiolytic properties. It has an elimination half-life of 8 h and no active metabolites. A dose of 20 mg is effective within 1 h and lasts for a period of around 2 h, after which time there is little residual drowsiness.

Lorazepam

This drug is available for parenteral and oral administration but is not used routinely as an intravenous sedative. Metabolism is by glucuronidation, with an elimination half-life of 15 h and much longer duration of action than temazepam. When used for premedication, a dose of 2–4 mg is given the night before or early on the day of surgery, and amnesia is a marked feature.

Intravenous lorazepam may rarely be used in the management of status epilepticus and is indicated for severe acute panic attacks. The intramuscular route should be used only when no other route is available.

Adverse reactions

Adverse reactions to benzodiazepines are dose-related and predictable from their pharmacodynamic effects. Oversedation, ventilatory depression, haemodynamic instability and airway obstruction may all follow inadvertent overdosage and are more likely in elderly or debilitated patients.

Flumazenil

Flumazenil is a very high-affinity competitive antagonist for all other ligands at the benzodiazepine receptor. It rapidly reverses all the CNS effects of benzodiazepines and also the other potentially dangerous adverse physiological effects, including respiratory and cardiovascular depression and airway obstruction.

Flumazenil has only very slight intrinsic activity at high dose and is very well tolerated, with minimal adverse effects.

Flumazenil is rapidly cleared from plasma and metabolized by the liver. It has a very short elimination half-life of less than 1 h. Its duration of action depends on the dose administered and the identity and dose of the agonist. It ranges from 20 min to 2 h and the potential exists for resedation, necessitating a period of close observation. Repeated administration may be necessary.

Dosage and administration

Flumazenil is presented for intravenous use in ampoules containing 500 µg in 5 ml. The usual clinically effective dose is 0.2–1 mg given as 0.1–0.2 mg boluses and repeated at 1 min intervals. The dose in diagnosis of coma should not exceed 3 mg.

Indications

Reversal of sedation. It has been suggested that sedation be reversed electively to speed the throughput of day-case patients or to minimize the period of sedation in sick or debilitated patients. The risks of resedation make this undesirable as a routine. The reversal of inadvertent oversedation is uncontroversial and an important indication for the use of flumazenil.

In self-poisoning. Treatment of benzodiazepine overdosage in cases of unconsciousness and respiratory depression may avoid the need for artificial ventilation. Repeated doses or a continuous infusion are required until plasma concentrations of the agonist have decreased. In coma of unknown aetiology, flumazenil may be given as a diagnostic tool.

In the ITU. Prolonged sedation, resulting usually from the accumulation of midazolam in patients with renal failure, may be treated with an infusion of flumazenil. Occasionally, the drug is given as a bolus to reverse sedation and permit neurological assessment.

Precautions

Epileptic patients. There is a risk of seizures, especially if a benzodiazepine has been prescribed as anticonvulsant therapy.

Benzodiazepine dependence. Withdrawal symptoms may be precipitated.

Anxiety reactions. These may occur after rapid reversal of heavy sedation.

Patients with severe head injury. Flumazenil may precipitate a sudden increase in intracranial pressure.

NEUROLEPTICS

These groups of sedative drugs include the phenothiazines and the butyrophenones, and are also used as antipsychotics.

Neurolepsis describes a characteristic drug-induced change in behaviour. There is an altered state of awareness with suppression of spontaneous movement and a placid compliant affect. Loss of consciousness does not occur, and spinal and central reflexes remain intact. The combination of a neuroleptic drug with an opioid, usually fentanyl, is termed neuroleptanalgesia. This was a popular means of providing sedation before the advent of intravenous benzodiazepines. There is no amnesia and the patient may subsequently report unpleasant mental agitation despite a calm demeanour. The opioid obtunds the unpleasant mental experience but may result in respiratory depression. The addition of nitrous oxide may be used to produce neuroleptanaesthesia, in which consciousness is lost.

Mechanism of action

Neuroleptics interfere with dopaminergic transmission in the brain by blocking dopamine receptors. At some synapses, dopamine is the stimulatory transmitter and GABA the inhibitory transmitter, so in common with other sedatives, neuroleptics enhance the effects of GABA. Dopamine blockade results in useful antiemetic activity but also carries the inevitable potential for extrapyramidal side-effects. Neuroleptic drugs also have actions at cholinergic, α-adrenergic, histaminergic and serotinergic receptors, and these properties influence their side-effects.

Droperidol

Droperidol is a butyrophenone, a class of drug with structural similarities to the phenothiazines. It is a powerful antiemetic, acting at the chemoreceptor trigger zone. Large doses may produce dystonic reactions. Droperidol has mild α-adrenoceptor blocking actions, which may cause vasodilatation after intravenous administration, resulting in hypotension.

Droperidol has an onset time of 3–10 min after intravenous injection, with a duration of action of 12 h or longer. It undergoes hepatic metabolism, but approximately 10% of the drug is excreted unchanged in the urine.

Indications

Premedication. Droperidol may be given orally or intramuscularly, and reliably produces sedation. It may result in delayed recovery, with sedation persisting well into the postoperative period because the effects of anaesthetic drugs are potentiated.

Antiemesis. The dose is often limited to 2.5 mg intravenously to provide antiemesis without unwanted sedation.

Neuroleptanalgesia/anaesthesia. Droperidol is administered intravenously in a dose of up to 10 mg in combination with an opioid, usually fentanyl.

Haloperidol

Haloperidol is also a butyrophenone and has an even longer duration of action than droperidol. It has almost no α-adrenoceptor blocking activity. It is a potent antiemetic but has a high incidence of extrapyramidal side-effects. It has been reported as a cause of the neuroleptic malignant syndrome, a rare but potentially fatal reaction.

Haloperidol may be used in the short-term management of the acutely agitated patient, after sinister causes of confusion such as hypoxia and sepsis have been excluded. It may be given orally in a dose of 1.5–3 mg two to three times daily. It may also be administered by i.m. or i.v. injection in a dose of 2–5 mg.

Chlorpromazine

Chlorpromazine is a phenothiazine which is commonly prescribed as an antipsychotic but no longer used as an adjunct in anaesthesia. It may be used in the same way as haloperidol in the acutely confused patient. It has pronounced sedative properties and potentiates the actions of anaesthetic drugs. There is marked antiemetic activity. A mild anticholinergic action moderates the incidence of extrapyramidal effects. α-Adrenoceptor blockade produces vasodilatation and may result in hypotension. Central temperature control mechanisms are affected by chlorpromazine, with a reduced shivering response. The neuroleptic malignant syndrome has been reported following its use.

The dose used to treat acute agitation is usually 25 mg i.m. or i.v. The drug must be diluted and given slowly when used intravenously.

α_2-ADRENOCEPTOR AGONISTS

α_2-Adrenoceptor agonists have been used widely in veterinary anaesthetic practice for many years. Their properties of sedation, anxiolysis and analgesia have been recognized as potentially beneficial in humans, but they have not found a place in routine clinical practice. The main disadvantage is the risk of excessive cardiovascular depression.

Mechanism of action

α_2-Adrenergic receptors are involved in the regulation of the release of the neurotransmitter norepinephrine. These receptors were initially classified anatomically as presynaptic, but α_2-adrenoceptors are also found postsynaptically and extrasynaptically. The more correct pharmacological classification is based on the predominantly α_2 -selectivity of the antagonist yohimbine. α_2-Adrenoceptors are located peripherally and centrally, with the centrally mediated effects of particular relevance in anaesthesia.

The characteristic central effects of α_2-adrenoceptor agonists are sedation, anxiolysis and hypnosis. The locus caeruleus is a small neuronal nucleus in the upper brain stem that contains the major noradrenergic cell group in the brain. This nucleus is an important modulator of wakefulness. Activation of α_2-adrenoceptors results in inhibition of transmitter release. The locus caeruleus also has connections to the cortex, thalamus and vasomotor centre.

α_2-Adrenoceptor agonists have analgesic properties. Descending fibres from the locus caeruleus decrease nociceptive transmission at the spinal level. In addition, α_2-adrenoceptors occur in primary sensory neurones and the dorsal horn of the spinal cord.

Many ligands at α_2-adrenoceptors are substituted imidazoles. It has been demonstrated recently that in some tissues, including brain, non-adrenergic imidazole binding sites exist: the imidazoline (I) receptors. Imidazoline receptors are found in the medulla and are involved in the regulation of arterial pressure. First-generation, centrally acting antihypertensives such as clonidine were originally thought to act via α_2 actions alone, reducing sympathetic outflow. The main disadvantage of the perioperative use of clonidine is the potential for cardiovascular depression, with bradycardia and hypotension. Recent work suggests that the hypotensive effects are also mediated via I receptors. The new centrally acting antihypertensive moxonidine has activity primarily at I receptors and is much less sedative than clonidine. A sedative agent lacking adverse haemodynamic effects remains a hope for the future.

Clonidine

Clonidine is an imidazoline compound and a selective α_2-adrenoceptor agonist with an α_2:α_1 ratio of 200:1. It is currently the only drug in this group available for use in anaesthetic practice. Clonidine is lipid-soluble and is absorbed rapidly and almost completely after oral administration, with peak plasma concentrations occurring in 60–90 min. It may be administered transdermally and is also available as a solution for intravenous, intramuscular, epidural, intrathecal and local use. The elimination half-life is 9–13 h; 50% is excreted unchanged by the kidneys and 50% is metabolized in the liver.

Pharmacological effects

Clonidine produces sedation and anxiolysis. It also results in a reduction in requirements for both intravenous and volatile anaesthetic agents. There is a ceiling to the reduction of MAC effect, because of the potential for activity at α_1-receptors at high dose. More selective α_2-adrenoceptors agonists reduce MAC to a much greater extent.

Clonidine is a potent anolgesic, acting centrally and on the α_2-adrenoceptors of the dorsal horn. It may be administered intravenously, intrathecally or epidurally to produce an analgesic response. Synergism exists with opioids, and the actions of local anaesthetics are also potentiated. Clonidine is used to provide analgesia in the perioperative period and also in chronic pain syndromes.

The cardiovascular effects of clonidine probably involve both α_2-adrenoceptors and imidazoline receptors. Administration leads to a decrease in heart rate and arterial pressure. Clonidine is known to lower the 'set point' around which arterial pressure is regulated. The α_2-agonist effects are a reduction in sympathetic tone and an increase in parasympathetic tone. The resulting decreases in heart rate, myocardial contractility and systemic vascular resistance lead to a reduction in myocardial oxygen requirements. This may be used to advantage in attenuating stress-induced haemodynamic responses. However, undesirable cardiovascular depression has been the major limiting factor in developing the use of clonidine as a sedative.

Clonidine has minor respiratory effects, causing only a small reduction in minute ventilation.

Dosage and indications

Premedication. The oral dose is 200–300 μg given 1 h preoperatively.

Analgesia. Epidural clonidine is safe and effective in the management of acute postoperative pain. The epidural dose is 1–2 $\mu g\ kg^{-1}$.

Anaesthesia. Intravenous clonidine in a dose of 150–300 μg has been used as an adjunct to general anaesthesia and to attenuate haemodynamic responses. There may be a risk of awareness if haemodynamic variables alone are used to monitor the depth of anaesthesia. Prolonged duration of action and cardiovascular depression make clonidine unsuitable for use as a sedative for short procedures.

Withdrawal of drugs in dependence. Clonidine has been used to facilitate drug withdrawal in states of opioid, benzodiazepine and alcohol dependence.

Dexmedetomidine and medetomidine

Medetomidine is the prototype of the newer selective α_2-agonists. Its active ingredient, the D stereoisomer dexmedetomidine, is used routinely as an adjunct in veterinary anaesthesia. It has much greater efficacy than clonidine and is shorter-acting. The α_2:α_1 selectivity ratio is 1600:1 and the lack of α_1 activity leads to a MAC-sparing effect of up to 90%. Dexmedetomidine is an imidazole and so also binds to I receptors. In common with clonidine, this drug produces sedation, anxiolysis, analgesia and haemodynamic depression.

The selective α_2-adrenoreceptor antagonist atipamezole has been used in veterinary practice and reverses the sedation caused by dexmedetomidine.

ANTICONVULSANTS

Epilepsy is a common condition, affecting 350 000 people in the UK. Most patients with recurrent seizures require anticonvulsant therapy. In 30% of patients, there is an identifiable neurological or systemic disorder leading to the seizure. In the event of seizures occurring unexpectedly, treatable causes should be excluded. In the perioperative period, precipitating factors such as hypoglycaemia, electrolyte abnormalities and metabolic disturbance must be considered.

General principles of anticonvulsant therapy

Epileptic seizures have many manifestations. Seizure classification is based on clinical description and EEG pattern and is important in selecting the most effective therapy. Monotherapy is preferred for most patients. The best drug for the specific seizure type and individual patient is selected and administered in a dose high enough to bring the plasma concentration into the therapeutic range without unacceptable side-effects. For most of the established anticonvulsants, the complexity of their pharmacokinetic profiles makes therapeutic drug level monitoring necessary. Initial dosing schedules are complicated, because for many anticonvulsant drugs it is important to increase the dose slowly to avoid toxic side-effects. If seizure control remains poor, a second drug is added or substituted while the original choice is withdrawn slowly. Up to 70% of patients may be managed successfully with a single drug, but a substantial minority report seizures despite combination therapy.

There are several problems associated with the established anticonvulsants. These include sedation and cognitive impairment, long-term side-effects, pharmacokinetic interactions and teratogenesis. In the last decade, several new anticonvulsants have become available. Some of these appear to offer greater efficacy with fewer disadvantages, although at a higher cost.

Mechanisms of action

Anticonvulsant drugs act by inhibiting the abnormal cerebral discharge leading to the seizure or inhibiting its propagation through the brain. There is no class action for this group of drugs; they act by several different single or multiple mechanisms. The most important of these include enhancement of the effects of GABA and limiting sustained repetitive neuronal firing through voltage and use-dependent blockade of sodium channels. The indications for use and mechanisms of action of new and established anticonvulsants are shown in Table 16.2.

Pharmacokinetics

The pharmacokinetic profiles of many anticonvulsant drugs determine dosing schedules and important drug interactions leading to potential adverse effects. Some of the older drugs, including phenytoin and sodium valproate, have a high degree of protein binding. Bioactivity may be affected by changes in the availability of binding sites. Factors which may decrease protein binding, such as competition with other drugs or a decrease in serum albumin concentration, may lead to toxicity.

Hepatic metabolism is important in the elimination of most anticonvulsants. Plasma drug concentrations may be altered by changes in the activity of oxidative enzymes. Induction of microsomal enzymes accelerates the metabolism of both the inducer and other drugs. Some drugs inhibit metabolism and may interact with anticonvulsants to produce higher serum drug concentrations. Hepatic dysfunction may also result in decreased metabolism. Significant renal excretion of phenobarbital and ethosuximide leads to accumulation of these drugs in patients with impairment of renal function.

Table 16.2 Anticonvulsants: mechanisms of action and indications for use

Drug	Mechanism of action	Indications
Phenytoin	Voltage-dependent block of sodium channels	Partial and generalized tonic-clonic seizures
Pentobarbital	Increases chloride channel conductance and so enhances GABA-induced effects	Partial and generalized tonic-clonic seizures
Carbamazepine	Voltage-dependent block of sodium channels	Partial and generalized tonic-clonic seizures
Sodium valproate	Voltage-dependent block of sodium channels Increases calcium-dependent potassium conductance Other mechanisms also	All seizure types, especially idiopathic generalized epilepsy
Ethosuximide	Reduces slow calcium conductance in thalamic neurones	Uncomplicated absence seizures
Clonazepam, clobazam	Enhancement of GABA effects	All seizure types
Vigabatrin	Irreversible inhibition of the enzyme GABA transaminase	Add on for partial seizures +/− secondary generalizations. Mono-infantile spasms
Lamotrigine	Prolongs inactivated state of voltage-dependent sodium channels	Adjunct or monotherapy for partial and tonic-clonic seizures
Gabapentin	Unclear. May bind to a calcium channel	Add on for partial seizures +/− secondary generalizations
Topiramate	Blockade of sodium channels. Attenuation of neuronal excitation. Enhancement of GABA	Add on for refractory partial seizures +/− secondary generalizations
Tiagabine	Inhibits uptake of GABA into neurones	Add on for partial seizures +/− secondary generalizations

INDIVIDUAL DRUGS

Phenytoin

Phenytoin is a hydantoin, similar in structure to barbiturates. The usual oral dose is 250–500 mg daily. It is also available for intravenous use and has an important place in the management of status epilepticus (see below). Phenytoin has membrane-stabilizing actions and as a result has the potential to cause profound cardiovascular depression when administered too rapidly by the intravenous route. As it is formulated in propylene glycol, it is very irritant, with a high incidence of thrombophlebitis after intravenous administration. It is unsuitable for admixture with concurrent infusions. A new preparation, the pro-drug fos-phenytoin, is water-soluble and much less irritant. Phenytoin is 90% protein-bound and undergoes hepatic metabolism. Phenytoin has several important interactions with other drugs. It is an enzyme inducer and so may accelerate the metabolism of other drugs. It is noteworthy that the elimination half-life of phenytoin is concentration-dependent. At high plasma concentrations, the metabolism changes from first-order to saturation kinetics, with the risk of a large increase in plasma concentration from a small increase in dose. Other drugs, including cimetidine and amiodarone, which inhibit the metabolism of phenytoin, are likely to lead to neurotoxic effects because of the saturatable metabolism.

Phenytoin has a range of dose-related and idiosyncratic adverse effects. Reversible cosmetic changes are a problem. Neurotoxic symptoms at high plasma concentrations include drowsiness, dysarthria, ataxia, tremor and cognitive difficulties.

Phenobarbital

Phenobarbital is a barbiturate with a long half-life of 70–140 h. The usual dose is 60–180 mg orally at night. It is 50% protein-bound and largely undergoes hepatic metabolism, with 25% excreted unchanged in the urine. Phenobarbital is an enzyme inducer and so accelerates the metabolism of other drugs. The main disadvantage with this drug is sedation and other CNS effects, including depression of mood, cognition and memory. Children may develop hyperactivity and aggression. As with all barbiturates, toxic levels may lead to respiratory depression and death.

Primidone

Primidone is essentially a pro-drug and is metabolized to phenobarbital. It is less well tolerated than phenobarbital and is no longer recommended routinely in the management of epilepsy.

Carbamazepine

Carbamazepine is structurally related to tricyclic antidepressants. The usual daily dose is 0.8–1.2 g in divided doses. Carbamazepine is 70–80% protein-bound and undergoes hepatic metabolism. This produces an active metabolite, and with multiple doses the pharmacodynamic half-life is 8–24 h. Carbamazepine is an enzyme inducer and the eventual maintenance dose for each patient depends on the degree of autoinduction of its own metabolism. Carbamazepine accelerates hepatic oxidation and conjugation of other lipid-soluble drugs and has an important interaction with the oral contraceptive pill. Other drugs, including cimetidine, erythromycin and propoxyphene, inhibit the metabolism of carbamazepine and may lead to toxicity. Carbamazepine has a wider therapeutic index and fewer adverse effects than phenytoin or phenobarbital. The most common side-effects are diplopia, headache and nausea. A mild reversible leucopenia is not uncommon, but there are also reports of agranulocytosis and aplastic anaemia following its use. At high doses, it has an ADH-like effect, with retention of water and the development of hyponatraemia.

Sodium valproate

Sodium valproate is a derivative of carboxylic acid. The usual maintenance dose is 1–2 g daily in divided doses. It is also available as an intravenous solution when oral administration is not possible.

Sodium valproate is approximately 90% protein-bound. It undergoes hepatic metabolism with production of active metabolites and has an elimination half-life of 7–17 h. Sodium valproate is an enzyme inhibitor and may inhibit the metabolism of other drugs, including other anticonvulsants. Common side-effects include gastrointestinal disturbance, weight gain, menstrual irregularities and dose-related tremor. Mild hepatic dysfunction is common but there is also a risk of hepatotoxicity. Monitoring of liver function tests is recommended and the drug should be discontinued if the prothrombin time is prolonged.

Ethosuximide

Ethosuximide is the drug of choice for simple absence seizures. The usual dose is 1–1.5 g daily in divided doses. Ethosuximide is not protein-bound. It undergoes hepatic metabolism, with 25% excreted unchanged. It has an elimination half-life of 20–60 h, with more rapid clearance in children. Enzyme inhibitors and inducers may affect its metabolism. Common side-effects include gastrointestinal disturbance and adverse CNS effects, usually lethargy, dizziness and ataxia.

Clonazepam

Clonazepam is a benzodiazepine. The usual maintenance dose is 4–8 mg daily in divided doses. It is also available as an intravenous preparation which has a place in the management of status epilepticus.

Clonazepam is 90% protein-bound and undergoes hepatic metabolism with an elimination half-life of 30–40 h. The main disadvantage of clonazepam is its sedative effect. There is also a tendency to develop tolerance to its anti-epileptic activity, with an unfortunate rebound increase in seizure frequency when it is withdrawn.

Vigabatrin

This is the first of the newer anticonvulsants. The usual oral maintenance dose is 2–4 g daily. Vigabatrin is not protein-bound and is excreted unchanged in the urine. It has a short elimination half-life but its duration of action is longer, as it takes several days for the enzyme GABA transaminase to regenerate after treatment is stopped. It has few interactions with other drugs. Vigabatrin is usually well tolerated but CNS side-effects, including sedation and dizziness, may occur. The drug should be avoided if there is a psychiatric history because depression and psychosis have been reported.

Lamotrigine

The usual maintenance dose is 150–200 mg daily. Lamotrigine is metabolized in the liver and has an elimination half-life of 22–36 h. Its metabolism is accelerated by enzyme-inducing anticonvulsants such as phenytoin, and its action is prolonged by the enzyme inhibition of sodium valproate. Lamotrigine does not influence the metabolism of other drugs. Adverse effects are confined largely to the CNS, and include headache, diplopia, sedation, ataxia and tremor. These develop more commonly when lamotrigine is used in combination with carbamazepine.

Gabapentin

The usual maintenance dose is 1.2 g daily in three divided doses. Gabapentin is excreted unchanged by the kidneys and has a short half-life of 5–7 h. It does not interact significantly with other drugs. This drug is generally well tolerated, with a side-effect profile similar to that of lamotrigine.

Topiramate

The usual maintenance dose range is 200–400 mg daily in two doses. Topiramate undergoes hepatic metabolism which is accelerated by the enzyme inducers. Topiramate selectively reduces the clearance of phenytoin in some patients and may accelerate metabolism of the oral contraceptive pill. It has a wide range of adverse effects, the commonest being neurological symptoms, anorexia and weight loss. It also has the potential to cause nephrolithiasis as a result of inhibition of carbonic anhydrase. It is the only newer anticonvulsant which shows evidence of possible teratogenicity. These disadvantages are offset by its high efficacy.

Tiagabine

The usual maintenance dose range is 30–45 mg daily in three divided doses. Tiagabine undergoes hepatic metabolism which is accelerated by enzyme inducers. It has a short half-life of 5–9 h and does not affect the metabolism of other drugs. Side-effects include gastrointestinal upset and CNS effects, particularly dizziness.

ANAESTHETIC CONSIDERATIONS

Patients receiving long-term anticonvulsant therapy should receive their usual treatment regimens as far as possible, with the aim of maintaining therapeutic drug concentrations. The propensity for adverse interactions with many different drugs is particularly high with the established anticonvulsants. Changes in protein binding may result from disturbances of acid–base balance or hypoalbuminaemia. The development of renal or hepatic dysfunction in the perioperative period may reduce the elimination of anticonvulsants, leading to toxicity.

STATUS EPILEPTICUS

Status epilepticus may be defined as prolonged or repeated seizures without recovery between fits. Tonic-clonic status is a medical emergency requiring urgent control of seizures. Status lasting longer than 60 min results in permanent brain damage even if oxygenation is maintained, as excessive metabolic demands result in cell death.

Treatment of status epilepticus

1. Maintain the airway and oxygenate the lungs.
2. Give i.v. diazepam (Diazemuls) 2 mg min^{-1} until the seizure stops, up to a maximum dose of 20 mg. *Beware of respiratory depression.* Redistribution of diazepam may lead to a recurrence of seizures after about 20 min.
3. Load with phenytoin to prevent seizure recurrence; the loading dose is 15 mg kg^{-1}. Give intravenously at a rate not exceeding 50 mg min^{-1}. *Beware of cardiovascular depression.*
4. Ensure correctable causes of seizure have been treated, particularly hypoglycaemia.
5. In the event of failure to control seizures, options include:
   - — diazepam infusion: up to 8 mg h^{-1}
   - — thiopental infusion: loading dose 3–5 mg kg^{-1}
infusion: 1–3 mg kg^{-1} h^{-1}
   - — non-barbiturate anaesthesia.

This management should be undertaken only in an intensive care unit. Artificial ventilation of the lungs is required because of the risk of profound respiratory depression. Paralysis with neuromuscular blocking agents facilitates ventilation and decreases oxygen consumption, but masks continued seizure activity. It is therefore necessary to monitor the EEG, usually with the cerebral function analysing monitor.

When facilities for resuscitation are not available, rectal paraldehyde 5–10 ml may be used.

Clomethiazole

Clomethiazole is an anticonvulsant with a limited place in the management of status epilepticus. It was used extensively in the past to manage acute alcohol withdrawal states.

In addition to its anticonvulsant properties, it is a powerful sedative. Respiratory depression, airway obstruction and hypotension may follow rapid infusion. Prolonged infusion may be associated with a decreasing level of consciousness. Clomethiazole has a short half-life, but although the rate of infusion may theoretically be titrated against clinical effect, accumulation of the drug may lead to delayed recovery after prolonged administration.

Dosage and administration. Clomethiazole is available as a 0.8% solution for intravenous infusion. This solution contains only 32 mmol L^{-1} of sodium and no other electrolytes. Administration of large volumes carries a risk of water intoxication and fluid overload.

The solution is usually administered initially at a rate of 5–15 ml min^{-1} for about 6–8 min and then reduced to 0.5–1 ml min^{-1}.

FURTHER READING

Brodie M J, Dichter M A 1996 Antiepileptic drugs. New England Journal of Medicine 334: 168–175

Dichter M A, Brodie M J 1996 New antiepileptic drugs. New England Journal of Medicine 334: 1583–1590

Khan Z P, Ferguson C N, Jones R M 1999 Alpha 2 and imidazoline receptor antagonists. Anaesthesia 54: 146–165

Vickers M D, Morgan M, Spencer P S J, Read MS 1999 Drugs in anaesthetic and intensive care practice, 8th edn. Butterworths, London

Whitwam J G, McCloy R F (eds) 1998 Principles and practice of sedation, 2nd edn. Blackwell Science, Oxford

Wood M, Wood A J J (eds) 1990 Drugs and anaesthesia, 2nd edn. Williams & Wilkins, Baltimore

17 Physiology and measurement of pain

BASIC PRINCIPLES

ACUTE PAIN

Acute pain following trauma or surgery, with which all anaesthetists are familiar, is self-limiting and reduces as tissue damage resolves. By and large, the severity of pain reflects the degree of injury, particularly with injury to somatic structures such as bone and muscle; a broken leg hurts more than a simple sprain. However, the 'pain pathway', from the pain receptor ('nociceptor') to pain awareness in the brain, is not a simple relay system but a much more complex one in which the 'pain message' may be magnified or diminished depending on inputs from other neuronal systems.

It is not only the degree of tissue damage that determines pain intensity. For example, it is not infrequent that anaesthetists meet patients in whom the amount of postoperative pain appears to be disproportionate to the surgery. A postoperative patient may have so much pain that relief comes only with such doses of opioids that render the patient unconscious, while another patient who has had the same surgery may require no strong opioids at all. Most patients fall between these two extremes, but it is clear that good postoperative pain management requires not only a balanced pharmacological and technical approach, but also attention to the psychological and emotional state of the patient. Fear and anxiety increase pain and produce a poor response to drugs. However, they may be averted to a great extent by appropriate preparation, explanation and reassurance.

Pain, then, not only has a sensory component, such as sharp, stabbing or aching sensations, but also has an affective one, because it makes an individual feel miserable, irritable, anxious and afraid. Furthermore, these emotions may feed back and exacerbate suffering. In addition, past experience of pain may have an important impact on current pain. For example, a history of poor postoperative pain control may be associated with anxiety and fear following subsequent surgery, and good pain control may be particularly difficult to achieve. 'Pain' has sensory and emotional dimensions, and they interact together to produce what has been termed the 'overall pain experience'. The contribution of each of these dimensions may vary with time but the patient refers to all these experiences as 'pain'. In other words, 'pain is what the patient says it is', and this applies equally to both acute and chronic pain.

CHRONIC PAIN

Chronic pain is often defined in simple temporal terms as pain present for more than 6 months. This is oversimplistic, and in many ways chronic pain is different from acute pain. Acute pain has a useful physiological role, in that it serves to protect the injury from further damage until healing is complete. Chronic pain often has no useful physiological role. The impact of chronic pain on function and quality of life is often disproportionately greater than may be explained by the underlying pathology. Chronic pain is always associated with mood changes, and depression and anxiety are very common. Anger and guilt are emotions frequently observed. Chronic pain often impairs employment,

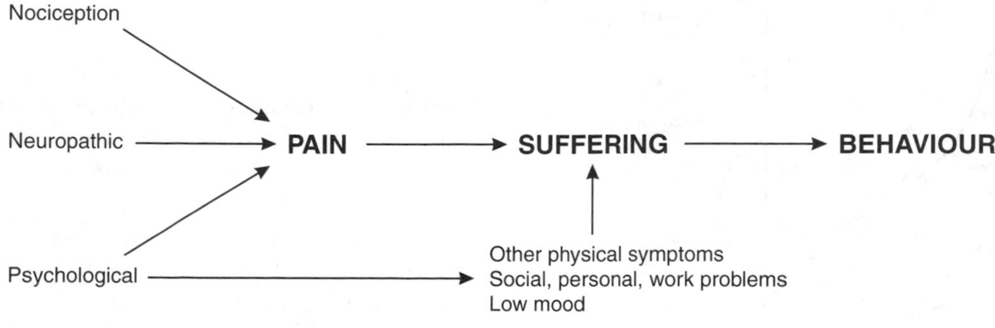

Fig. 17.1
The relationship between pain, suffering and behaviour.

social activity and personal relationships – and, indeed, every facet of life to a greater or lesser extent.

To understand chronic pain, it is particularly helpful to break down the 'overall pain experience' in terms of the pain and suffering that it causes (Fig. 17.1). Pain may be considered as the conscious *perception* of nociception, where nociception is the stimulation of nociceptors and generation of an afferent discharge to the spinal cord. Pain contributes to suffering, as do other unpleasant physical or emotional states. The behaviour of the patient is a visible representation of suffering. Behaviour may be 'appropriate' for the nociceptive stimulus (crying out following a fracture) or 'inappropriate' (grimacing and wincing in the absence of a clear nociceptive cause of pain). Some texts give the misleading impression that chronic pain rarely if ever has a significant sensory component, but instead the 'pain' is an expression of emotional distress. Whilst this scenario is observed occasionally, it does not apply to the great majority of chronic pain patients, who do have an ongoing sensory component from somatic, visceral or neurological structures. The challenge to the chronic pain team is to determine the balance between the nociceptive and other components that lead to the suffering and subsequent behaviour. This is best done in a multidisciplinary team consisting of medical doctors, psychologists, physiotherapists, nurses and psychiatrists.

BASIC ANATOMY AND PHYSIOLOGY

An overview of the basic anatomy of the pain pathway is shown in Figure 17.2

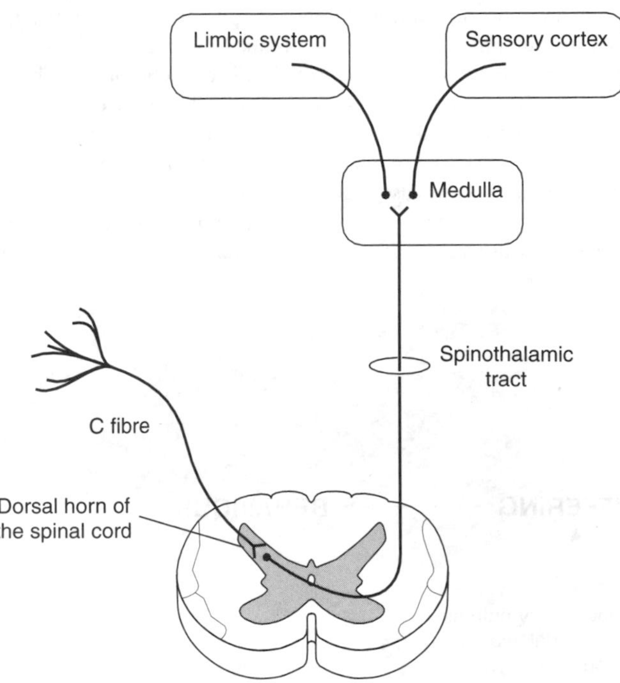

Fig. 17.2
Basic anatomy of the pain pathway.

NOCICEPTORS

Acute pain begins when a mechanical, chemical or thermal stimulus activates specific sensory nerve terminals, termed nociceptors. Providing the stimulus is of sufficient intensity, nociceptor activation occurs whether or not tissue damage has occurred, although the latter is usually the case. Nociceptors require a high stimulus threshold before they are activated. The initial stimulus for activation is probably mechanical distortion of the nerve terminal, followed by increase in local concentrations of K^+ and H^+. Tissue damage and inflammation lead to a reduction in the threshold for stimulation, a process termed 'peripheral sensitization' (see below).

PRIMARY AFFERENT FIBRES

Nociceptors are served by two types of afferent nerve fibres, Aδ and C. They may be distinguished by:

- the speed of conduction of nerve impulses
- the presence of myelin around the nerve
- the stimulus threshold required to activate the receptor (high or low)
- the nature of the stimulus that activates it.

Aδ fibres may be stimulated by mechanical or thermal, high- or low-threshold, stimuli. Most C fibres are stimulated by high-threshold chemical, mechanical and heat stimuli (CMH nociceptors), and are termed C polymodal fibres (Table 17.1).

The presence of two distinct groups of nerve fibres responding to noxious stimuli may be readily demonstrated. Following a noxious stimulus, an immediate sharp pain is experienced which reduces in intensity after a few seconds and is replaced by a persistent burning pain. The first and second pain sensations follow activation of Aδ and C fibres, respectively. The first pain allows rapid reflex and behavioural mechanisms to remove the individual from the source of pain (and injury). The second pain persists to prevent further injury and tissue damage when immediate danger has been averted.

THE SPINAL CORD

Dorsal horn neurones

The cell bodies of afferent fibres lie in the dorsal root ganglion, and the fibres synapse with cells in the dorsal horn of the spinal cord. The output from the dorsal horn neurone is dependent not only on the input from the afferent nerves, but also on the activity of other neuronal systems on the synapse. Some afferent neurones

Table 17.1 Characteristics of primary afferent fibres. Aβ is included for comparison

	C	Aδ	Aβ
Conduction velocity	IV (<2 ms^{-1})	III (10–40 ms^{-1})	II (>40 ms^{-1})
Myelination	No	Yes	Yes
Receptors	High threshold	High and low threshold	Low threshold

arriving at the spinal cord divide before entering the cord and send branches several spinal segments caudad and cephalad in the longitudinal tract of Lissauer before synapsing with a dorsal horn neurone. As a result, several dorsal horn neurones may be innervated by a single C-fibre afferent.

Neurotransmitters

The cell bodies of afferent neurones produce excitatory neurotransmitters which are transported to the nerve terminal in the spinal cord (Table 17.2).

Rexed laminae

A cross-section of the spinal cord shows 10 anatomically and physiologically distinct layers, termed Rexed laminae (Fig. 17.3). Laminae 1 to 6 and lamina 10 are the sites at which sensory afferents synapse with dorsal horn cells. Laminae 7–9 represent the motor horn. Aδ and C fibres terminate in several layers, including the outer marginal zone (lamina 1) and, in particular, the substantia gelatinosa (lamina 2). The dorsal horn cells in the substantia gelatinosa respond to noxious stimuli only.

Wide dynamic range neurones

Some of the dorsal horn cells in layers 3, 4 and 5 are able to respond to a wide range of inputs, including light touch and pain, and so are termed 'wide dynamic range' (WDR) neurones. A characteristic feature of WDR cells is *wind-up*, in which the output increases in the presence of a continuous, low-frequency, C-fibre input (see below). Another important feature is the *convergence* of neurones from both somatic and visceral structures onto the same WDR cell. This arrangement accounts for the phenomenon of referred pain, in which pain from a visceral source is experienced in part of the body innervated by cells that converge on the same dorsal horn neurone.

Expansion of the receptive field

The more intense the painful stimulus, the greater the number of activated C-fibre afferents. Therefore, intense stimulation leads to activation of dorsal horn neurones beyond the spinal segment containing the nociceptive source and so the receptive field expands.

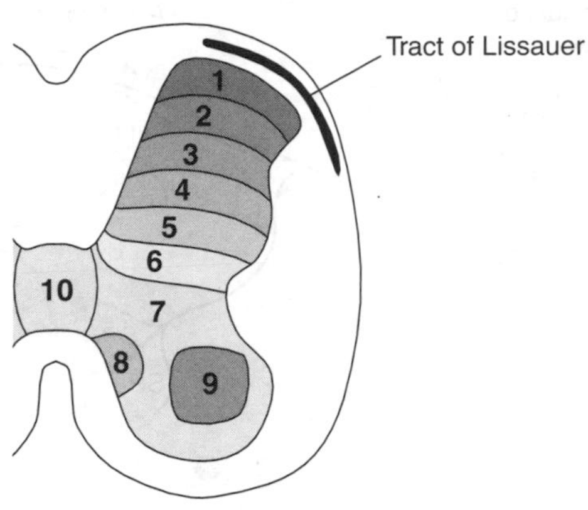

Fig. 17.3
Rexed laminae.

ASCENDING TRACTS AND SUPRASPINAL SYSTEMS

Most dorsal horn neurones project to higher centres in the brain by ascending several segments in the spinal cord before crossing over to the opposite ventrolateral side. They then join one of three major spinal systems:

- *Spinothalamic tract* – probably the most important for pain transmission, this tract projects to several nuclei in the thalamus. The spinothalamic tract is the target for treating intractable cancer pain by cordotomy.
- *Spinoreticular tract* – terminates in the reticular nuclei in the brain stem.
- *Spinomesencephalic tract* – terminates in the mesencephalic reticular formation and periaqueductal grey.

All the terminal sites of spinal tracts project to:

- somatosensory cortex, associated with the sensory aspect of pain
- limbic system, associated with the affective aspect of pain.

The 'pain pathway', from nociceptor to supraspinal sites, describes the anatomical layout. It must be remembered that the 'pain message' may undergo profound modulation at any synapse, which may lead to enhancement or diminution of the 'message' reaching the brain.

Table 17.2 Excitatory neurotransmitters released by pain afferent fibres in the dorsal horn of the spinal cord

Neuropeptides	Amino Acids
Substance P	Glutamate
Neurokinins (NKA, 1 and 2)	*N*-methyl D-aspartate (NMDA)
Calcitonin gene-related peptide (CGRP)	AMPA (derivative of aspartate)
Cholecystokinin (CCK)	
Vasoactive intestinal polypeptide	
Somatostatin	

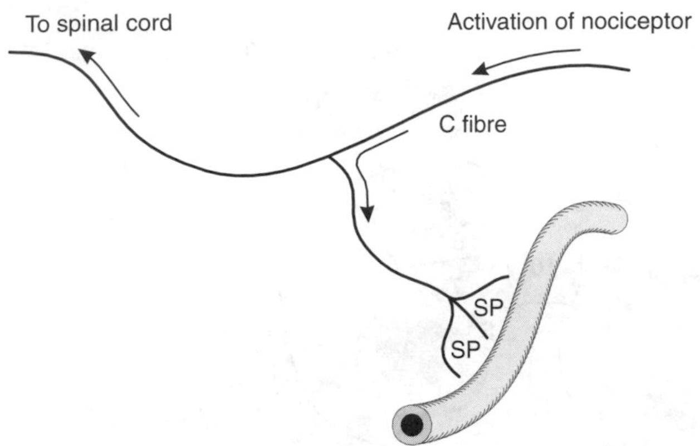

Fig. 17.4
Antidromic conduction.

PHYSIOLOGICAL CHANGES IN RESPONSE TO TISSUE DAMAGE

Tissue damage, whether from trauma or surgery, initiates changes in the pain pathway that maintain and even increase the pain experienced by the individual. These changes occur at:

- the site of tissue damage (peripheral sensitization)
- the dorsal horn of the spinal cord (central sensitization).

It is important to remember that these mechanisms are normal physiological events and serve to encourage the individual to protect the injury from further damage.

Both peripheral and central sensitization contribute towards hyperalgesia and allodynia. Hyperalgesia is increased pain in response to a painful stimulus, and allodynia is pain following a previously non-painful stimulus.

PERIPHERAL SENSITIZATION

The triple response

Minor injury produces the familiar 'triple response' of redness (capillary dilatation), wheal (oedema) and flare (arteriolar dilatation). Histamine is one of the first substances to be released into the surrounding tissue and is responsible for the wheal. Antidromic conduction in the C neurone releases substance P from nerve endings in the skin, which in turn causes arteriolar dilatation (Fig. 17.4).

The inflammatory soup

Depending on the magnitude of the injury, additional inflammatory mediators are released, including:

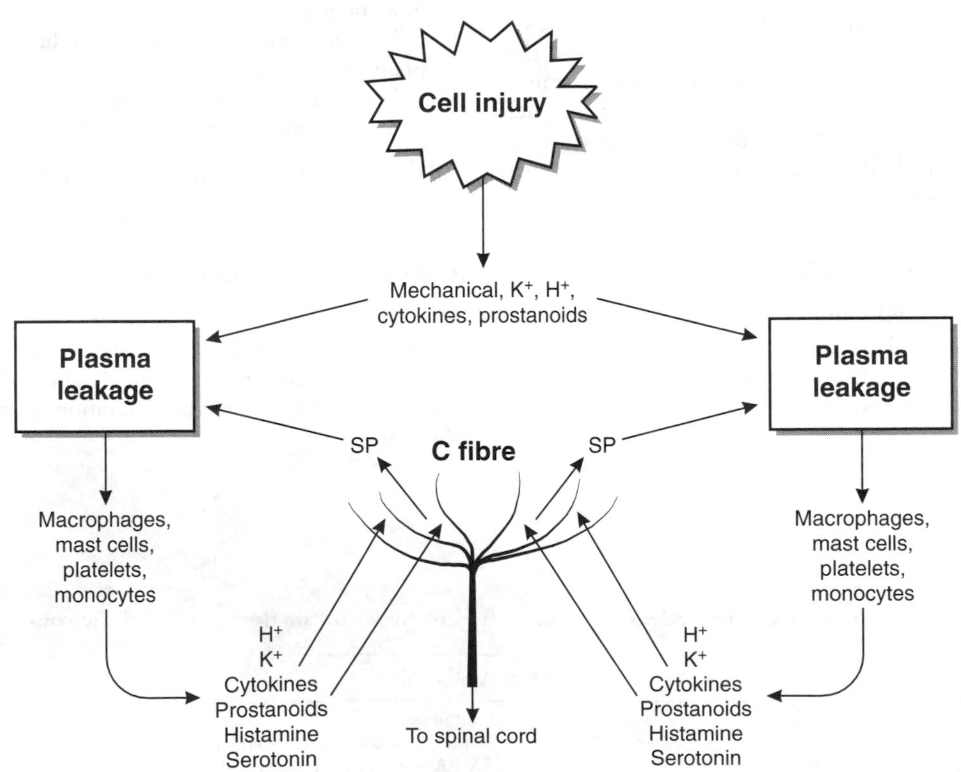

Fig. 17.5
Peripheral sensitization. SP; substance P.

Before sensitization

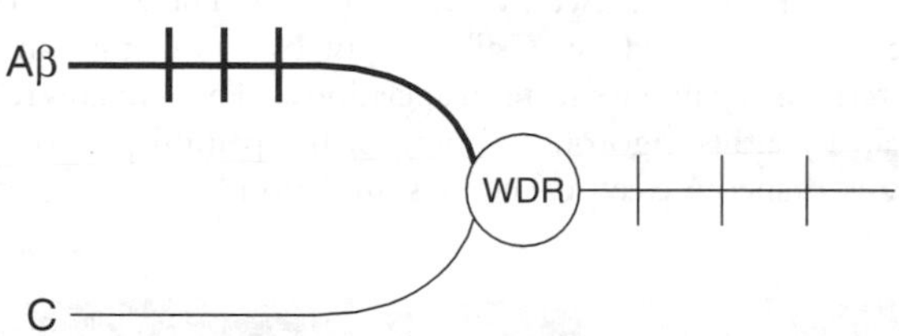

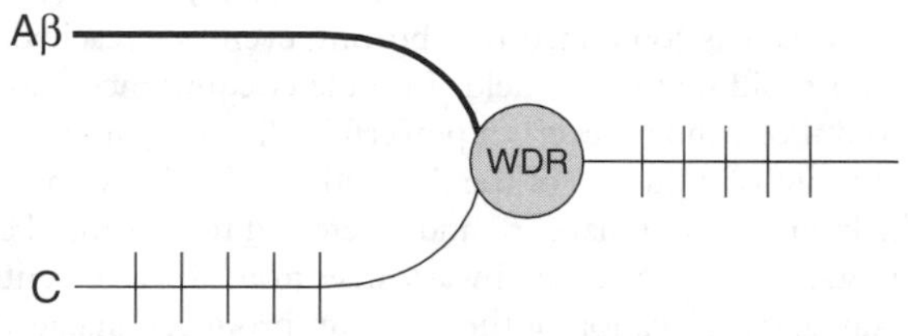

After sensitization

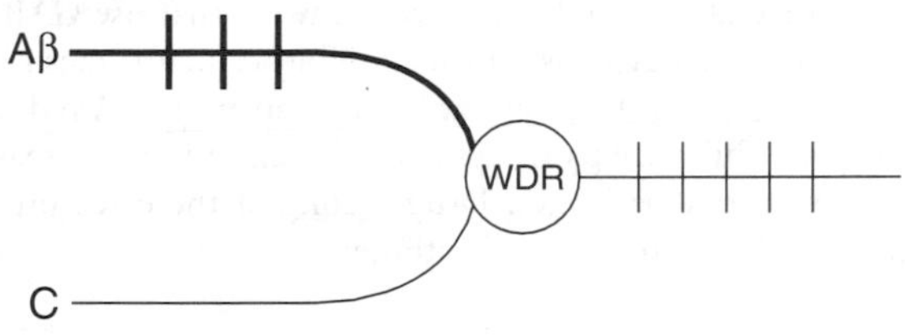

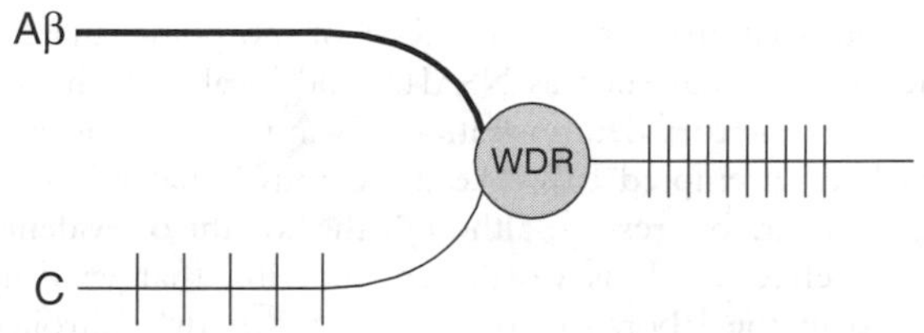

Fig 17.6
Central sensitization.

- bradykinin, formed from the precursor kallidin – bradykinin sensitizes nociceptors and induces them to release excitatory peptides, including substance P
- monoamines: serotonin (5HT) and norepinephrine – norepinephrine is released from sympathetic nerve terminals at the site of injury
- prostaglandins and leukotrienes, formed from arachidonic acid, which itself is produced following activation of phospholipase A_2 by bradykinin.

The effect on the C-afferent terminal of this 'inflammatory soup' is one of *sensitization* (Fig. 17.5). Now, the magnitude of the stimulus required to generate impulses in the C fibre is greatly reduced. Put another way, the threshold for stimulation is lowered. A stimulus of insufficient intensity to activate nociceptors prior to injury may do so following sensitization.

Not only are nociceptors sensitized following injury, but the number of nociceptors is increased. This is a reflection of the fact that perhaps one-third to one-half of the population of nociceptors are in a 'dormant' state and are not stimulated unless tissue damage occurs.

CENTRAL SENSITIZATION

The synapse between the C-afferent neurone and the dorsal horn cell is not simply a relay site of information from one cell to another. It allows modulation of the afferent input, so that the activity in the dorsal horn cell may be increased or decreased depending on the activity of other systems acting on the synapse.

Sensitization in the dorsal horn results in an exaggerated response in the dorsal horn cell not only to C-fibre input, but also for Aβ input (Fig. 17.6).

Wind-up

Sensitization increases the dorsal horn cell output for a given C-fibre input. In addition, within a narrow frequency range of C-fibre input, animal studies have demonstrated that WDR neurones respond to a repetitive C-fibre stimulation at a fixed frequency, not with a fixed frequency output, but rather by producing an output whose frequency progressively increases. This frequency-dependent, exaggerated response is termed 'wind-up' (Fig. 17.7).

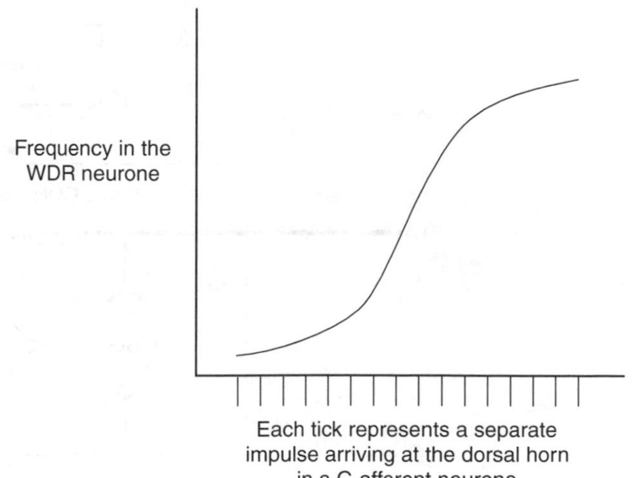

Fig. 17.7
Wind-up.

Mechanisms of central sensitization

Wind-up is caused by NMDA receptor activation, and experimentally induced wind-up may be inhibited by NMDA receptor antagonists, such as ketamine. On the other hand, it appears that Aβ sensitization is mediated via inhibition of pathways that use GABA (γ-aminobutyric acid). GABA is a major inhibitory neurotransmitter in the CNS, and NMDA is an excitatory transmitter. A reduction in activity in inhibitory pathways produces an indirect increase of activity in excitatory pathways. Drugs acting at these receptors may be a potentially useful site for treating pain.

PRE-EMPTIVE ANALGESIA

Pre-emptive analgesia implies analgesia directly as a result of reducing peripheral and/or central sensitization. Although studies have demonstrated pre-emptive effects of morphine, there is little evidence for drugs such as NSAIDs and local anaesthetics. Following the laboratory demonstration of wind-up, several clinical studies have attempted to evoke pre-emptive analgesia with ketamine, with variable results, although the weight of evidence suggests it is effective. It is worth remembering that wind-up demonstrated in the laboratory occurs under strictly controlled conditions, not least the frequency range at which the afferent fibres are stimulated.

GATE THEORY OF PAIN

Up until the 1960s, pain was considered to arise from peripheral nerves and reach the brain cortex via a direct route with no modulation on the way. It was clear to many workers that this theory did not explain many clinical cases such as phantom pain, hyperalgesia and allodynia, and the effect of past experience. The gate theory of pain, proposed by Ronald Melzack and Patrick Wall in 1965, was a major shift in thinking about pain mechanisms, and forms the basis of our current understanding. Central to the theory is the principle that inputs to the spinal cord (Aβ and C fibres) may be modulated by systems in the spinal cord (substantia gelatinosa, SG) and by descending systems from the brain (central control) (Fig. 17.8). The gate refers to the interaction of different systems on the dorsal horn cell, and is opened by C-fibre activity. The gate is closed by Aβ activity, which reduces C-fibre input by stimulating an inhibitory interneurone in the substantia gelatinosa. This explains reduction in pain by either vigorous rubbing of the painful part or the use of transcutaneous electrical nerve stimulation.

DESCENDING SYSTEMS

Injuries sustained during sporting events or even on the battlefield are often reported as being relatively painless, at least until the individual has completed the sporting event, or reached the safety of a first aid unit in the field. In these circumstances, attention on survival or winning exerts a powerful effect on pain intensity. This is a result of influence of the descending inhibitory pathways from the brain to the spinal cord and is referred to as 'central control' in the gate theory. Such pathways arise from discrete centres in the brain, and stimulation of these centres produces analgesia.

Two of the most important areas in the brain associated with descending inhibitory pathways are the periaqueductal grey (PAG) in the midbrain and the rostral ventromedial medulla (RVM). These have inputs from many areas of the brain in addition to each other. Both centres contain high concentrations of endogenous opioids and opioid receptors, and activation of these receptors increases activity in descending monoamine pathways (serotonin and norepinephrine) that project to the dorsal horn. This appears to conflict with what we know about opioid receptor activation in the dorsal horn of the spinal cord, which:

- inhibits neurotransmitter release from the presynaptic site of C-fibre afferent
- hyperpolarizes the postsynaptic cell membrane of the dorsal horn cell.

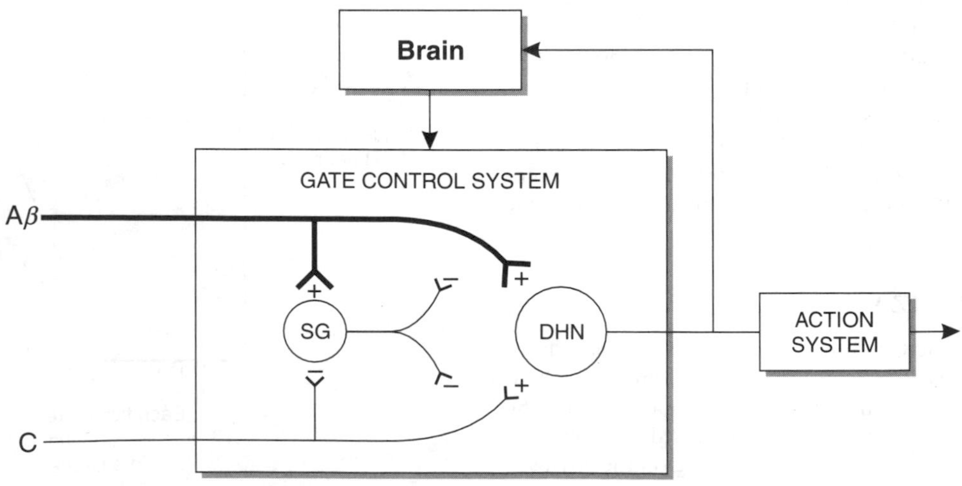

Fig. 17.8
Gate control theory of pain. SG; substantia gelatinosa. DHN; dorsal horn neurone.

This conflict is explained by the fact that activity in descending pathways is under the control of inhibitory interneurones. Inhibition of inhibitory interneurones increases activity in descending pathways.

OTHER MODULATORY SYSTEMS

It is clear that several different receptor systems may exert a profound influence on pain neurotransmission. So far, we have discussed the role of NMDA, GABA and endogenous opioid agonists (endorphins, enkephalins and dynorphins). Other systems in the spinal cord that modulate the dorsal horn neurone response include those using dopamine and cholecystokinin (CCK) as transmitters, and our understanding of these systems may provide clues to better analgesics.

VISCERAL PAIN

Unlike pain from superficial somatic structures, pain from the viscera is usually vague, poorly localized and felt to arise from 'inside' rather than near the body surface. Only when parietal structures are directly involved is the pain localized (appendicitis presents as a dull central abdominal pain until irritation of the parietal peritoneum, when it becomes localized to the right iliac fossa). Frequently, it is referred to structures distant from the source, e.g. pain from myocardial ischaemia may be referred to the left arm.

The viscera are innervated mainly by C fibres and they are activated by distension of hollow viscera, with increased activation in the presence of inflammation. The afferent neurones travel in autonomic nerves, mainly those of the sympathetic system. Indeed, sympathetic denervation is an effective means of intractable pain control of visceral origin, e.g. coeliac plexus block for pain from pancreatic carcinoma. However, there is good evidence that the parasympathetic system carries some afferent fibres, e.g. the pelvic nerve carries fibres from pelvic viscera, particularly bladder. Afferents arriving in the dorsal horn synapse with dorsal horn cells that synapse with somatic pain afferents, and there appears to be no distinct spinothalamic tract that transmits visceral pain sensation alone.

REFERRED PAIN

Referred pain is pain experienced in a site distant from the nociceptive stimulation. It occurs within the distribution of the spinal nerve innervating the source of pain, whether the source is visceral or somatic. Although many well known examples of referred pain exist (e.g. diaphragm irritation to the shoulder, cardiac pain to the left arm), it is important to remember that virtually any deep somatic or visceral pain may be referred. The size of referred pain may be considerable and the location surprisingly distant from the source. For example, pain from the lower cervical spine may be referred as far as the hand. This is quite different from neuropathic hand pain resulting from nerve root entrapment.

The site of referred pain may become tender and hyperalgesic and may account for some instances of 'trigger points' or even superficial tenderness which may otherwise be difficult to explain. This, and the fact that the onset of referred pain is slower than simple nociceptive stimulation, indicates that referred pain arises from mechanisms within the spinal cord. It is caused by convergence of different pain afferents onto common dorsal horn neurones. In addition, segmental embryological innervation remains throughout growth and explains the distance between, for instance, referred pain in the groin arising from the kidney.

Referred pain is usually described as an ache and is not associated with any other sensory abnormality. In this, it may be differentiated easily from neuropathic pain.

NEUROPATHIC PAIN

Patients often have difficulty describing neuropathic pain, but they are quite clear that it is qualitatively different from nociceptive pain (ask them to compare it with pain following surgery). Aching, squeezing, burning, shooting, uncomfortable paraesthesiae, profound hypersensitivity (frequently observed in trigeminal and postherpetic neuralgias, and peripheral nerve injuries) and numbness may all coexist. If the motor supply has been affected by the same disease process, weakness may be present.

Neuropathic pain may be defined as pain arising from an abnormality in a nerve(s) and may arise from a peripheral nerve or from within the CNS. At this point, it is useful to remember that pain may be *any* unpleasant sensation and not necessarily one evoked solely by nociceptor activation. Intense and persistent stimulation of Aβ neurones may produce 'painful' paraesthesia, and the same may occur for neurones conducting heat and cold. Note that stimulation of C-fibre afferents alone produces a burning sensation, a fact readily appreciated by the application of capsaicin cream.

NEUROMA

Neuropathic pain may be caused by the formation of a neuroma following trauma or surgery (amputation) to a peripheral nerve. The neuroma consists of outgrowths of the neurones from the proximal section of the cut nerve and may take days or weeks to develop. Both spontaneous and evoked firing are greatly increased and this may be attributed to the increase in concentration of sodium channels within the neuroma. Sodium channel blockers such as carbamazepine and mexiletine may be helpful.

POSTHERPETIC NEURALGIA

Postherpetic neuralgia is associated with marked pathological abnormalities in the dorsal root ganglion, peripheral nerve and dorsal horn. At the cellular level, demyelination, axonal degeneration and inflammatory cell infiltration may be observed, and extend to several spinal segments. The latter may account for the occasional patient who has an impressive response to epidural steroids. An interesting observation in many patients suffering neuralgias is that the symptoms may be relieved by local anaesthetic infiltration of the skin innervated by the affected nerve, clearly distal to the lesion. This indicates that in some cases a sensory input is required for abnormal sensation to be experienced, rather than arising spontaneously only from the pathology itself.

RADICULAR PAIN

Radicular pain is a neuropathic pain that arises in the distribution of a spinal nerve; it is caused by compression of either the cord itself or

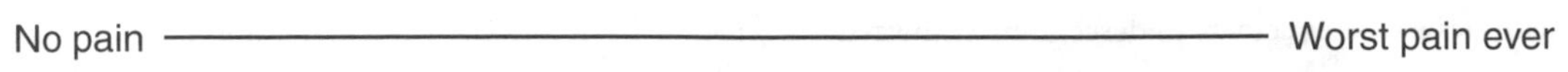

No pain ———————————————————— Worst pain ever

Fig. 17.9
Visual analogue scale.

a spinal nerve root. It may be caused by a prolapsed intervertebral disc, pressure from a collapsed vertebral body or even an osteophyte in the root canal. Symptoms reflect the degree of compression and may include paraesthesiae, numbness and weakness. Severe compression within the spinal canal may cause irreversible damage secondary to ischaemia and require urgent surgical decompression.

PAIN AND THE SYMPATHETIC NERVOUS SYSTEM

PERIPHERAL NERVE INJURY

Pain following peripheral nerve injury may be exacerbated by sympathetic activity. In these cases, the structures distal to the injury (almost invariably in a limb) are cold, discoloured, demonstrate marked allodynia and have worse pain in a cold environment. Symptoms are improved with a sympathetic block. In these cases, α-adrenoceptors are expressed on the damaged nerve and, in the presence of norepinephrine from local sympathetic nerves or circulating epinephrine, induce peripheral sensitization of nociceptors and even Aβ terminals. Stimulation of the latter may, in the presence of central sensitization, cause pain. However, many patients with persistent pain following trauma, with or without a peripheral nerve injury, do not have these symptoms, do not have sympathetically mediated pain, and so do not respond to a sympathetic block.

REFLEX SYMPATHETIC DYSTROPHY

Reflex sympathetic dystrophy (RSD) is a term given to a collection of symptoms following an injury, usually to a distal part of a limb. Symptoms are similar to those following nerve damage, although RSD is not associated with overt neurological damage; indeed, trauma preceding RSD is said to be 'mild', and symptoms 'disproportionate to the inciting event'. Symptoms include burning pain, allodynia, oedema, discoloration and abnormal sweating. Despite the clinical impression of pain secondary to overactivity of the sympathetic system, there is little scientific evidence that intravenous guanethidine (an α-adrenoreceptor antagonist) is effective. A diagnosis of RSD can be made despite a lack of response to a sympathetic block; RSD is simply a collection of symptoms of unknown pathology.

COMPLEX REGIONAL PAIN SYNDROME

The International Association for the Study of Pain recognized the confusion over terminology with RSD and a poor response to sympathectomy. The collection of symptoms that constituted RSD are now encompassed in 'complex regional pain syndrome type 1' (CRPS type 1). CRPS type 2 is the name given to the syndrome that occurs following overt nerve injury, which was previously known as causalgia. Note that pain relief following sympathectomy is not a prerequisite for making either diagnosis.

ISCHAEMIC PAIN

Patients with rest pain from peripheral vascular disease often respond well to a chemical lumbar sympathectomy. Pain is reduced because blood flow to ischaemic tissue is increased. Patients with severe Raynaud's disease may have dramatic improvement for the same reasons.

MEASUREMENT OF PAIN

The measurement of pain is important to provide information about its severity and cause, and to determine and evaluate treatment. In deciding upon a suitable measure of pain, it is important to remember that pain has sensory and affective qualities. Pain is not the same experience to each individual; if this were the case, it would allow it to be conveniently measured along a single scale.

THE VISUAL ANALOGUE SCALE

The visual analogue scale (VAS) is one of the most widely used measures of pain intensity. It consists of a 10 cm line marked at one end with 'no pain' and at the other with 'worst pain ever', or similar phrases (Fig. 17.9).

The patient is asked to indicate where on the line he or she rates the pain, and a numerical value is then given to it simply by measuring the length between 'no pain' and the patient's mark. The VAS is presented most conveniently as a slide rule with one side used by the patient and the other by the assessor.

Several modifications have been recommended to improve patient acceptability and understanding. For instance, to avoid grouping towards the centre of the scale, the written statements should not overlap the line. The scale may be represented like a thermometer, with the 'hot' end representing more severe pain. Providing the patient understands fully how to use the VAS (judged by asking the patient to demonstrate its use at the time of explanation), it provides a useful measure of the effectiveness of treatment.

VAS to record average pain over time

The VAS is used frequently to measure pain at the time of measurement, but in some cases, particularly patients with chronic pain, they may be asked to indicate the 'average' pain over a period of time. However, this may introduce bias because it is

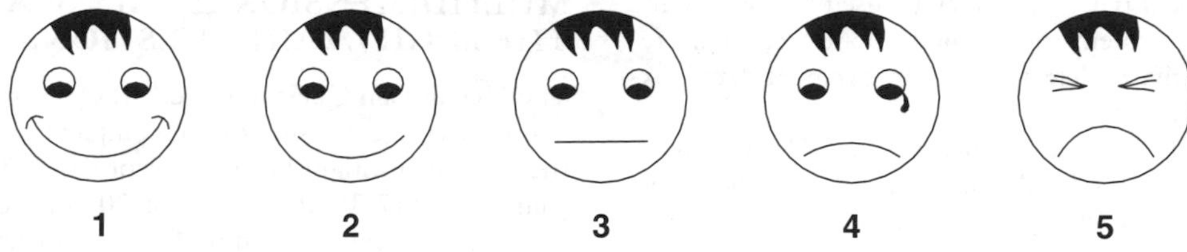

Fig. 17.10
The faces scale.

dependent on memory. It has been suggested that a more accurate measure of average pain over a period of time may be achieved by measuring the VAS at three different times of the day (e.g. 09.00, 13.00 and 18.00 h) for four consecutive days, and taking the average of the sum.

Advantages and disadvantages of the VAS

The main advantages of the VAS are ease of use and simplicity. Furthermore, it is independent of language. However, the main disadvantage is that it assumes that pain is a unidimensional experience, and does not differentiate between sensory and affective components. However, the VAS may be used to measure these factors independently of each other. Indeed, the 'Brief Pain Inventory' uses nine VASs to assess not only pain, but also the effect of pain on certain aspects of the patient's life, such as activity, mood, sleep and relationships with other people.

VERBAL AND NUMERICAL RATING SCALES

Verbal pain rating scales (such as none, mild, moderate, severe) have been used for many years and provide a simple tool to measure

Table 17.3 The McGill Pain Questionnaire

1	Flickering Quivering Pulsing Throbbing Beating Pounding	2	Jumping Flashing Shooting	3	Pricking Boring Drilling Stabbing Lancinating	4	Sharp Cutting Lacerating	5	Pinching Pressing Gnawing Cramping Crushing
6	Tugging Pulling Wrenching	7	Hot Burning Scalding Searing	8	Tingling Itchy Smarting Stinging	9	Dull Sore Hurting Aching Heavy	10	Tender Taut Rasping Splitting
11	Tiring Exhausting	12	Sickening Suffocating	13	Fearful Frightful Terrifying	14	Punishing Gruelling Cruel Vicious Killing	15	Wretched Blinding
16	Annoying Troublesome Miserable Intense Unbearable	17	Spreading Radiating Penetrating Piercing	18	Tight Numb Drawing Squeezing Tearing	19	Cool Cold Freezing	20	Nagging Nauseating Agonizing Dreadful Torturing

Present Pain Intensity
0 No pain
1 Mild
2 Discomforting
3 Distressing
4 Horrible
5 Excruciating

pain intensity. Verbal pain relief scales may be used to measure the effect of a particular treatment (none, mild, moderate, complete) and may be more sensitive at detecting an improvement than looking for a change in pain scores.

Numerical pain rating scales are similar to the VAS but replace the line with the numbers 0–10. Measurements of pain using verbal and numerical rating scales correlate with pain measured by the VAS. They have similar advantages and disadvantages.

PAIN MEASUREMENT IN CHILDREN

A measure of the severity of pain in children may be derived from the child, parents, carers and nursing staff. Ideally, a self-reported measure of pain is the most useful and scales similar to those in adults have been used. Although the VAS or category scales are suitable for most children over the age of 7–8 years old, younger children find the concept difficult to grasp, and some older children may not have the reading or cognitive skills to use it. The 'faces' scale is suitable for a wide age group in children and is simple to use (Fig. 17.10). Several variations of the faces scale have been developed and validated, including the 'Oucher scale', which has a vertical numerical scale on one side and six photographs of childrens' faces representing increasing amounts of pain, starting at no pain (0) and increasing to maximum possible pain (100). It is likely that all the face scales are as effective as each other.

An alternative approach to assessing pain in children is measuring their pain behaviour, such as crying. One obvious difficulty is that behavioural changes associated with pain may be associated with hunger, separation from parent, etc. Despite this problem, several behavioural scales have been introduced and are particularly useful in assessing postoperative pain. One of these is the CHEOPS (The Childrens' Hospital of Eastern Ontario Pain Scale), which measures crying, facial expression, body position, verbal expression, touch position and leg position. This scale is suitable for a wide range of ages, including children too young to be able to use the faces scale.

MULTIDIMENSIONAL PAIN SCALES: THE McGILL PAIN QUESTIONNAIRE

The McGill Pain Questionnaire (MPQ) was developed to provide a more accurate measure of the complete pain experience. Unlike the VAS, it distinguishes the sensory and affective nature of the pain (Table 17.3). It consists of 20 subgroups, with each subgroup containing between two and six adjectives that are qualitatively similar but which increase in intensity. Subgroups 1–10 measure the sensory component, and 11–15 the affective component. Subgroup 16 provides a measure of the intensity of the overall pain experience. During the development of the questionnaire, an additional three subgroups were added as they include descriptors used frequently by patients but not included in the 16 subgroups described. These are contained in subgroups 17–20 and are termed miscellaneous.

The patient is asked to indicate which words best describe the pain. One word only from each subgroup may be chosen, although if there are no adjectives from a subgroup that the patient feels describe the pain, then none is chosen.

The MPQ provides three quantitative measures, the pain rating index (PRI), the number of words used and the present pain intensity (PPI), which is a measure of the pain at the time of completion of the MPQ. The PRI is the sum of the rank values of the descriptors chosen by the patient.

The MPQ has proven to be a valid and reliable tool and is very widely used for both clinical and research work.

FURTHER READING

Bonica J J 1990 The management of pain, 3rd edn. Churchill Livingstone, Edinburgh

Patt R B 1992 Cancer pain, 2nd edn. Lippincott, Philadelphia

Waldman S D, Winnie A P 1996 Interventional pain management. Saunders, Philadelphia

Wall P D, Melzack R 1994 Textbook of pain, 3rd edn. Churchill Livingstone, Edinburgh

18 Analgesic drugs

An ideal analgesic is a drug which suppresses pain of all types and all severities but does not inhibit other sensations, motor activity or sensorimotor association, or have toxic effects on other tissues or organs. It should be lipophilic, mainly undissociated at body pH to enable absorption, have no active metabolites and be metabolized by ubiquitous enzymes or be easily antagonized. The ideal duration of action depends on the clinical context. It should be available, therefore, in fast-acting and slow-release forms. The opioids and the cyclooxygenase inhibitors are, so far, the closest to this ideal.

OPIOIDS

NOMENCLATURE

Opium is obtained from the juice of the oriental poppy, *Papaver somniferum*. The term opioid was used for all those drugs, natural or synthetic, that had actions similar to those of morphine. With the advent of the antagonists and partial agonists, it became the term for those drugs that bind to an opioid receptor. The term opiate is used for an opioid drug derived from opium and also for morphine-like drugs which are not peptides.

OPIOID RECEPTORS

There are three principal opioid receptors:

- the mu (μ) receptor – so termed because it appeared to be responsible for the actions of ***m***orphine
- the delta (δ) receptor – so termed because the mouse vas ***d***eferens was less responsive to morphine than to other, otherwise less potent, opioids.
- the kappa (κ) receptor – so termed because it was responsible for the range of actions of the opioid ***k***etazocine.

The sigma (σ) receptor (after *SKF* 10047) is now no longer classed as an opioid receptor. It binds to ligands which also bind to the phencyclidine site of the *N*-methyl-D-aspartate (NMDA) receptor-linked channel.

Since 1992 and the cloning of the genes which encode these receptors, they have also been known as MOR (μ), DOR (δ) and KOR (κ) receptors. In 1997, the International Union of Pharmacology reclassified them in order of cloning: OP_1 (δ), OP_2 (κ) and OP_3 (μ).

The opioid receptors are similar to each other. They all couple through pertussis toxin-sensitive G-proteins. They have the same actions at the membrane (see below) and they have the same general structure of an extracellular N-terminal structure, seven transmembrane domains and an intracellular C-terminal structure.

A new receptor has been cloned which is responsible for analgesia. Because this receptor appeared to have no endogenous ligand and because opioids which have a high affinity for other opioid receptors have a low affinity to the new receptor, it was termed the orphan opioid receptor or the opioid receptor-like receptor (ORL-1). Later, an endogenous peptide was found to react with this receptor. This peptide is known both as 'orphanin FQ' and 'nociceptin'.

Receptor subtypes

There is less agreement about receptor subtypes. Receptors may vary in the amino acids in the C fragment, for example, but this may be related to an alteration of the receptor after formation in the membrane rather than being expressed by different genes.

MECHANISM OF ACTION

There are three principal effects of an opioid binding to a μ, δ or κ opioid receptor via inhibitory G-protein-mediated events:

- inhibition of calcium entry into the cell via N, P, Q, R calcium channels
- facilitation of potassium efflux
- inhibition of adenylyl cyclase.

Calcium entry into an afferent nociceptive neurone causes excitatory neurotransmitter (such as substance P) release, prolonged depolarization, long-term potentiation and increased expression of the proto-oncogenes, which causes increased sensitivity of the neurone. Potassium efflux causes hyperpolarization so that a greater voltage change is required to reach the threshold for depolarization.

Adenylyl cyclase is necessary for the generation of cyclic adenosine monophosphate, which is associated with the phosphorylation of membrane proteins and alteration of ion channels.

Opioids also activate L-type and inhibit T-type voltage-operated calcium channels. In addition, opioids produce facilitatory effects by stimulating cyclic AMP formation and converting PIP_2 to IP_3 and diacyl glycerol. These effects are more likely to occur at low concentrations (i.e. nanomolar rather than micromolar). They may, however, be part of the process that leads to tolerance.

SITES OF ACTION

Opioids have three principal sites of action in the normal nociceptive pathway:

- On the presynaptic terminal of the primary nociceptive afferent, inhibition of calcium influx prevents excitatory neurotransmitter release.
- On the postsynaptic terminal, increased potassium efflux causes hyperpolarization, making it less excitable. Inhibition of calcium influx also reduces the prolonged phase of depolarization.
- Activation of descending inhibition, by stimulating the cells in the periaqueductal grey matter (PAG) which relay to the raphe nuclei of the medulla and thence to the dorsal horn, reduces nociceptive input.

The stimulation of PAG by opioids is indirect. The inhibitory neurones are inhibited by continuous release of γ-aminobutyric acid (GABA). Opioids inhibit this spontaneous release by increasing potassium conductance.

Peripheral receptors

Under some circumstances, opioids appear to be able to reduce nociception by a peripheral mechanism. N-methylmorphine and N-methylnalorphine may reduce nociception, although neither can significantly cross the blood–brain barrier or enter the spinal cord.

In inflammation, there are changes in sensitivity such that the background nociceptive impulse generation approaches threshold levels for onward transmission. Wind-up and central sensitization occur and silent nociceptors in some joints and tissues become active. Opioid receptors are found on primary afferent peripheral nerve terminals. In humans, the efficacy of opioids applied peripherally in post-traumatic and inflammatory states is not uniform. Opioids applied to the pleural cavity, or in some cases perineurally, have shown little effect, whereas morphine applied to inflamed joints, especially the knee, has shown more antinociception than would be expected from the dose given systemically.

AGONISTS, PARTIAL AGONISTS AND ANTAGONISTS

If a ligand (drug or endogenous substance) binds to a receptor and causes a change in the effector mechanism associated with the receptor to produce a physiological change, it is said to be an agonist. If the ligand binds to the receptor but has no effect, and if it can block an agonist binding to that site, it is said to be an antagonist. If the resultant effect of receptor binding increases with the amount of ligand present to produce a maximal effect, it is said to be a full agonist. If the effect increases with the amount of ligand but the maximal effect is not achieved, the ligand is said to be a partial agonist. Partial agonism may occur because the effect requires binding of a large proportion of receptors or because the ligand binds in more than one way so that one form of binding produces an effect and the other is ineffective. It follows that when a full agonist causes tolerance by reducing the numbers of potentially effective receptors, either by inactivation or endocytosis or by reduced expression, the maximal effect may not be achievable and the full agonist becomes a partial agonist. A weak partial agonist with moderate to high affinity might be considered primarily an antagonist. The type, selectivity and effects of opioid receptor binding are shown in Tables 18.1 and 18.2.

The effect of adding a partial agonist (e.g. buprenorphine) to an agonist (e.g. morphine) depends on the doses used. If both drugs are used in low concentrations, there are plenty of unoccupied receptors and the effects of the two drugs are additive. As the proportion of the occupied receptors approaches the total, binding to the available receptors by drug becomes increasingly unlikely and greater amounts of drug are required to achieve an incremental increase in effect. As the partial agonist requires proportionately more receptors to produce a given effect, it acts as a competitive antagonist, reducing the effect which is achieved by the agonist alone.

BIOAVAILABILITY

Morphine undergoes extensive first-pass metabolism such that approximately 30% reaches the systemic circulation. However, with repeated prolonged administration and the cumulation of the active metabolite, morphine-6-glucuronide, the oral formulation achieves 30–50% of the efficacy of systemic administration. Morphine has a longer duration of action than its plasma half-life suggests because morphine is slow to diffuse out of the brain and the concentrations in the brain and spinal cord lag behind those in plasma.

METABOLISM AND EXCRETION

The opioids are converted mainly to polar metabolites which are excreted by the kidneys. Those with free hydroxyl groups (e.g. morphine) are conjugated with glucuronide; 70% of morphine is converted to the inactive morphine-3-glucuronide. Esters, e.g. pethidine and diacetylmorphine, are hydrolysed by tissue esterases. N-demethylation also occurs; for example, methadone undergoes demethylation and cyclization. Pethidine is converted mainly to pethidinic acid but is partly demethylated to norpethidine.

ENTEROHEPATIC AND GASTROENTERIC RECIRCULATION

Morphine and other opioids are excreted partly in the bile as water-soluble glucuronides. These are excreted into the gut where they are metabolized by the normal gut flora to the parent opioid and reabsorbed. The more lipid-soluble opioids may diffuse into the stomach mucosa and lumen, where they are ionized and concentrated because of the low pH. Later, gastric emptying and reabsorption from the small intestine may produce a secondary peak effect.

ACTIONS OF MORPHINE AND OTHER TYPICAL OPIOIDS

Analgesia

Morphine is effective in most kinds of pain, acute and chronic, inflammatory and non-inflammatory, from visceral and parietal structures. It is less effective for neurogenic pain, such as phantom limb pain or trigeminal neuralgia, or for the sharp pain of move-

Table 18.1 Selectivity of opioids for and effect on opioid receptors

Opioid	μ (OP3) receptor	δ (OP1) receptor	κ (OP2) receptor
Endogenous peptides			
β-endorphin	AAA	AAA	AAA
Leu-enkephalin	A	AAA	
Met-enkephalin	AA	AAA	
Dynorphin 8	AA	A	AAA
Endomorphin-1, -2	AAAA		
Opioid drugs			
Morphine, codeine, oxymorphone	AAA	A	A
Pethidine	AA	A	A
Fentanyl, alfentanil, sufentanil	AAA	A	
Methadone	AAA		
Buprenorphine	aaa		Ant
Mixed agonists			
Pentazocine	a/Ant	A	AA
Nalbuphine	Ant	A	aa
Nalorphine	Ant		aa
Antagonists			
Naloxone	Ant!!	Ant	Ant!
Naltrexone	Ant!!	Ant	Ant!

A, agonist; a, partial agonist; Ant, antagonist.
AA is a stronger agonist than A.
Ant! has more affinity for receptor than Ant.

ment such as that from an unsupported fracture. It increases pain tolerance in addition to raising pain thresholds. κ Agonists such as nalorphine, pentazocine or nalbuphine have not yet been demonstrated to be as effective as the μ agonists.

Respiratory system

Opioids depress ventilation by reducing carbon dioxide sensitivity and hypoxic drive and causing disorder in the rhythmicity of the ventilatory pattern. Ventilatory depression causing an increase in P_aCO_2 or reducing the ventilatory response to P_aCO_2 occurs even with small doses of μ agonists (Fig. 18.1). The decrease in sensitivity of the respiratory centre to P_aCO_2 is associated with depression of sensitivity of the neurones on the ventral surface of the medulla rather than of the medullary respiratory centre itself. It is not associated with depression of other medullary vital centres such as the vasomotor centre. Endogenous opioids are involved in

Table 18.2 The effects of opioid receptor activation

	μ (OP3) receptor	δ (OP1) receptor	κ (OP2) receptor
Analgesia			
Supraspinal	✓✓✓		
Spinal	✓✓	✓	✓
Peripheral	✓✓		✓✓
Ventilatory depression	✓✓✓	✓✓	
Miosis	✓✓		
Constipation	✓✓✓	✓✓	✓
Euphoria	✓✓✓	?	
Dysphoria, hallucinations			✓✓✓
Somnolence	✓✓		✓✓
Physical dependence	✓✓✓		✓
Tolerance	✓✓✓	✓✓	✓

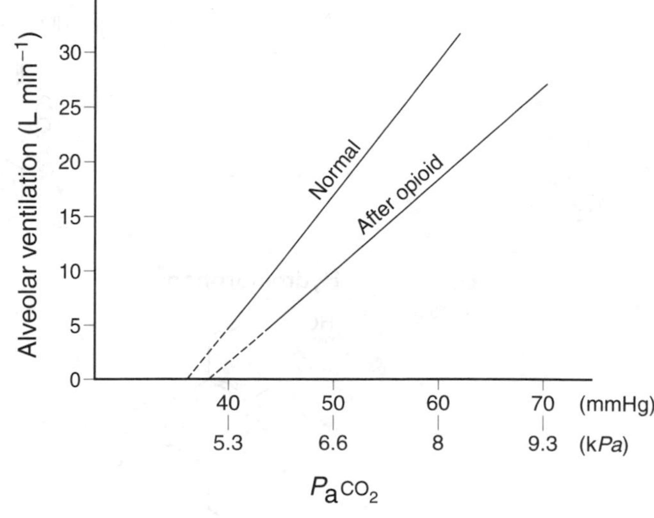

Fig. 18.1
The ventilatory response to P_aCO_2 in the normal individual and after administration of morphine. Note that the response curve is not only shifted to the right but that its slope is decreased also.

the control of ventilation as naloxone increases CO_2 sensitivity during resistive airway loading.

Sleep may intensify the depressant effect of the opioids. During normal inspiration, the subatmospheric pressure in the pharynx approximates the tongue to the soft palate, narrowing the airway. This is opposed by the muscle tone of the tongue and pharynx. Sleep and opioids depress the tone of genioglossus and the pharyngeal muscles. Opioid depression of ventilation is more common between midnight and 6 o'clock in the morning. Opioids also suppress rapid eye movement (REM) sleep. After days of drug-induced sleep or sleep deprivation, rebound of REM sleep leads to reduced airway tone and a tendency to obstruction.

Cough suppression

Opioids suppress cough but this activity does not parallel their effect as analgesics. Codeine and pholcodine suppress cough to a degree similar to that of morphine but have much less analgesic or respiratory depressant activity.

Nausea and vomiting

All opioids cause nausea and vomiting. They stimulate the chemoreceptor trigger zone in the area postrema which is influenced by chemicals in both blood and cerebrospinal fluid.

Gastrointestinal tract

Opioids increase the tone and decrease the motility of the gastrointestinal tract. Initial stimulation of the small intestine is followed by hypotonia or atony. Sphincter tone is increased and the gall bladder contracts. Morphine may cause a 10-fold increase in biliary pressure.

Miosis or pupillary constriction

This is caused by μ and κ receptor-mediated 'stimulation' of the Edinger–Westphal nucleus of the oculomotor nerve. It persists even after severe overdosage; most other forms of coma are associated with pupillary dilatation.

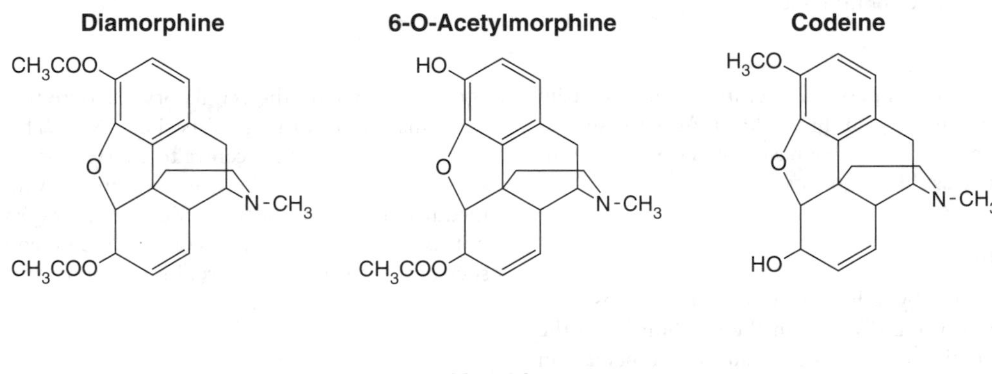

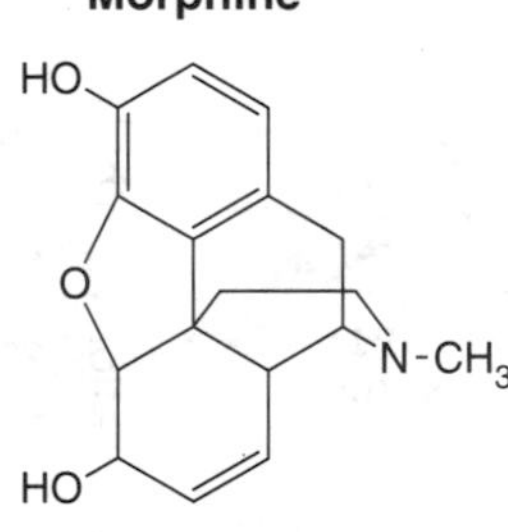

Hydromorphone

HO

O

N-CH3

O

Naloxone

HO

O

N-CH2CH=CH2

OH

O

Fig. 18.2
The structure of morphine and the phenanthrenes.

Cardiovascular system

In the absence of hypercapnia, most opioids have no significant direct effect on the force of contraction of the heart or, apart from the effect of histamine release by morphine, on arterial pressure. They cause bradycardia but no other arrhythmias. If the arterial pressure is maintained or raised because of nociception or because of catecholamine release in the presence of hypovolaemia, it may decrease after opioids. Without hypercapnia, cerebral blood flow is reduced minimally because of reduced cerebral activity. Respiratory depression and hypercapnia are associated with a decrease in cerebral vascular resistance, increase in cerebral blood flow and an increase in intracranial pressure.

Hormone response

The hormone response to nociception – increases in epinephrine, norepinephrine, cortisol and glucagon – is reduced by relatively high doses of opioids.

Histamine release and pruritus

Morphine releases histamine from mast cells, unrelated to the action on opioid receptors. It is related to speed of injection and concentration. Local effects include urticaria and itching and systemic effects include bronchoconstriction and hypotension. Pethidine and other phenylpiperidino opioids are unlikely to produce this effect.

Pruritus after spinal administration is caused by all μ opioid agonists and may usually be reversed by naloxone. It occurs most often after intrathecal opioids and is most pronounced on the face, nose and torso. The mechanism is centrally mediated and evidence exists to support suppression of inhibitory pathways, facilitation of excitatory pathways and glycine antagonism.

Immunity

After long-term opioid abuse, there is frequently depression of the immune system which appears to be independent of self-neglect.

Hallucinations

These are most common with κ agonists, but morphine, pethidine and other μ agonists also cause hallucinations.

Dependence and tolerance

Tolerance is the decreasing effect of a fixed concentration of drug. Physical dependence is the increasing effect of the antagonist or of the withdrawal of the drug. These two phenomena usually occur synchronously. In some individuals, opioids may produce strong psychological dependence, expressed as a craving for the drug, which is usually more socially destructive and may last for months or years. Craving may be defined as a compulsive need to take the substance which overrides other needs and behaviour such as eating, drinking, responsibilities and fears of exposure or punishment.

Cross-tolerance and dependence occur between agonists acting on the same receptor but not between those acting on different receptors, so that a κ agonist may be effective against the pain in a morphine- or fentanyl-tolerant patient.

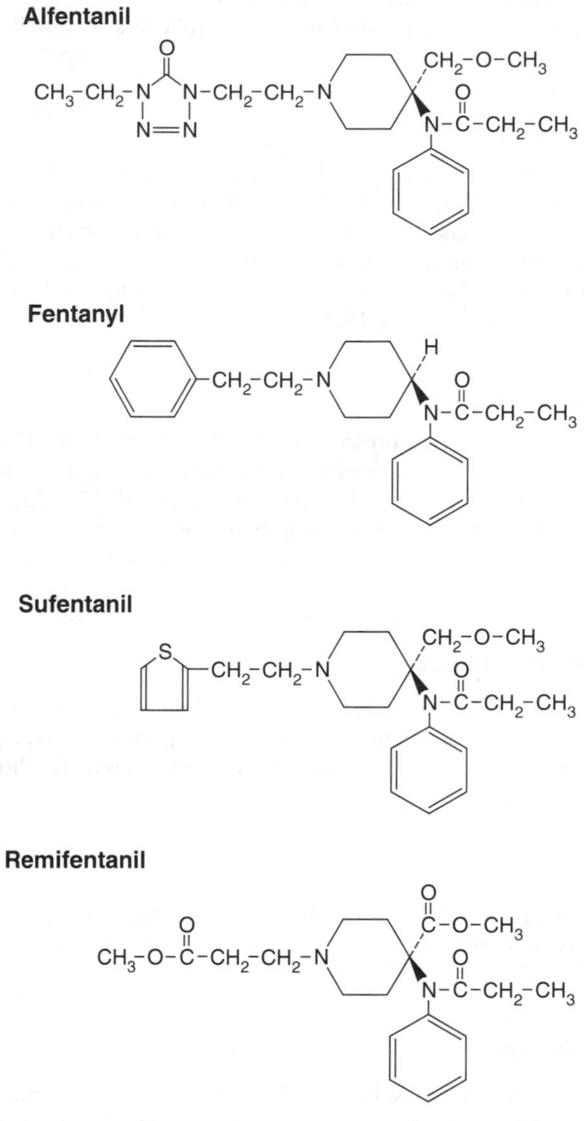

Alfentanil

Fentanyl

Sufentanil

Remifentanil

Fig. 18.3
The structures of phenylpiperidine opioids.

OTHER OPIOIDS

Structure–function relationships

The structures of some common opioids are shown in Figures 18.2 and 18.3.

Morphine is a phenanthrene and has a phenyl ring, and a 6-carbon ring in the same plane, and two ring structures at right angles to those. There is a phenol group (OH) at the 3 position and an alcoholic group (OH) at the 6 position. These are hydrophilic and substitution tends to increase lipid solubility and oral bioavailability. Diamorphine has acetyl groups (CH_3CO) replacing the hydrogen at both the 3 and 6 positions. Monoacetyl morphine has an acetyl group at the 6 position. Codeine has a methyl group at the 3 position. Diamorphine (diacetylmorphine) is both more water-soluble and more lipid-soluble than morphine. Unsaturated substitutions of the methyl group attached to the nitrogen tend to be associated with antagonist activity (nalorphine and naloxone: $CH_2CH{=}CH_2$)

Pethidine, fentanyl, alfentanil and sufentanil are phenylpiperidines, and methadone and propoxyphene are phenylheptylamines.

Diamorphine

Diamorphine was introduced into medicine in 1898, but is not available in many countries because it is associated with an increased tendency to cause euphoria and dependency. It is metabolized principally to monoacetyl morphine and morphine. Its pK_a is similar to that of morphine but its lipid solubility is much greater (see Table 18.3).

Papaveretum

Once the commonest prescribed form of morphine in the UK, the use of papaveretum has waned since its withdrawal and reformulation without noscapine. Papaveretum contained 47.5–52.2% of morphine base. Papaveretum injection now contains 7.7 or 15.4 mg ml^{-1} of papaveretum and is equivalent to 5 or 10 mg of anhydrous morphine, respectively.

Hydromorphone

This has similar actions to those of morphine. It is seven to eight times more potent than morphine but its principal advantage is that it has no active metabolites and is therefore useful for those in renal failure.

Codeine

This is a weak opioid with a very low affinity for opioid receptors. Its action is thought to result mainly from metabolism to morphine (10%).

Methadone

Methadone has a long but variable half-life (see Table 18.3) and achievement of steady state with regular dosing takes several days. During the first 2–3 days, it should be administered 4–6 hourly. As accumulation occurs, it may be given 12-hourly, then every 24 h. It is absorbed well and has good bioavailablity. Because the onset and offset of effect are slow, the potential for dependence is reduced and it is commonly used in addiction rehabilitation programmes. There are reports which state that it has an action at the NMDA receptor-linked channel.

Pethidine

Pethidine has opioid and atropine-like effects and may have less effect than morphine on the biliary sphincter and the renal tract. Its duration of action is shorter than that of morphine and its intrinsic efficacy is lower. It has a negative inotropic effect on the heart even after only 2–2.5 mg kg^{-1}. Pethidine does not inhibit the contractions of the uterus, but it readily passes across the placental barrier.

Pethidine is metabolized to desmethylpethidine (norpethidine) and either directly or thence to pethidinic acid (see Fig. 18.4).

Norpethidine has an elimination half-life four to five times that of pethidine, half the analgesic potency and twice the stimulant effect on the central nervous system. After excessive or repeated dosing, or during renal failure, norpethidine accumulates and causes adverse mood effects, tremulousness, myoclonus and seizures. Monoamine oxidase inhibitors (MAOIs) increase the metabolism to norpethidine and, given in combination with MAOIs, pethidine may cause muscle rigidity, hyperthermia, hypertension, seizures and death.

Fentanyl

Fentanyl is very lipid-soluble, passes easily across lipid membranes and acts much more quickly than morphine. After a single dose, the duration of action is short and the offset of effect is almost entirely due to redistribution. However, the elimination half-life is similar to that of morphine. It is metabolized predominantly in the liver and the metabolites are inactive. For single doses or acute intravenous infusions, the potency is 75–125 times that of morphine, but in chronic administration, as in fentanyl patches, it is 30–40 times that of morphine. It has little effect on the heart or arterial pressure.

Table 18.3 Pharmacokinetic variables of some opioids

Opioid	Terminal half-life (h)	Distribution half-life (min)	Volume of distribution (L kg^{-1})	Clearance (L min^{-1})	Octanol: water partition coefficient	Relative lipid solubility	pK_a	% ionized at pH 7.4	Protein binding (%)
Morphine	2–3.5	2–10	1.5–4	1–1.2	1.4	1	7.9	76	25–35
Diamorphine	2–3.5[a]	1.7–5.3	0.6–0.8	31	52	200	7.8		Not recorded
Pethidine	1.8 –5	4–17	4.2	0.8–1.2	40	30	8.7	95	40–50
Fentanyl	1.5–5.5	5–28	3.1–5	0.8–1.3	810–955	580	8.4	91	80
Alfentanil	1.5–2	10	0.5	0.3–4.5	145	90	6.5	11	90
Sufentanil	2.5	1	2.9	0.75	1750	1285	8		92
Remifentanil	0.15		0.4	3			7.07		
Methadone	13–47[b]	10	51	0.15	28–57	83	8.3	89	
Hydromorphone	2.1–4	14	1.3–4	0.4–1.7	1.28		8.1		60–90

[a]As morphine.
[b]The first dose of methadone has a plasma half-life of 6–8 h.

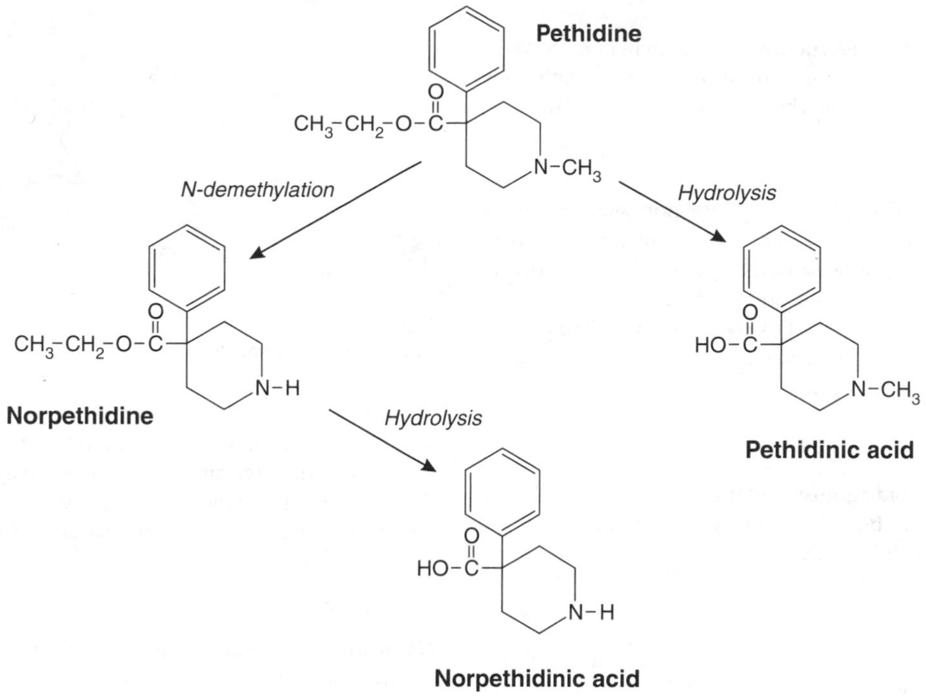

Fig. 18.4
The metabolism of pethidine.

It has a high first-pass metabolism (70%) and is not administered orally, but it is administered via a wide range of routes (see Table 18.4, p. 219).

The transdermal controlled-release patch is made possible by the high lipid solubility of fentanyl. A large drug reservoir of fentanyl (2.5–10 mg) is placed in a shallow depression in an impermeable laminate. The open surface of this laminate is closed by a rate-limiting microporous membrane covered with an adhesive, which is attached to the skin. The large concentration gradient provides the driving force for diffusion. Different infusion rates are achieved by varying the surface area of the patch; these are available at 25–100 μg h^{-1} over 3 days. After 3 days, the patch is removed and another placed on a different skin site. The dermis also acts as a depot site so that the plasma concentration does not achieve 90% of steady-state concentration until about 15 h after application. Similarly, after the patch is removed, the plasma concentration declines slowly with a half-life of about 15–20 h.

Alfentanil

Alfentanil has a more rapid onset of action and a shorter duration of effect than fentanyl. Although less lipid-soluble than fentanyl, it is nine times more un-ionized at normal plasma pH, in which form the drug crosses the lipid membrane of the blood–brain barrier. It is ninety times more lipid-soluble than morphine. Although the clearance of alfentanil is half that of fentanyl, the volume of distribution is one-fifth and the elimination half-life is less than half that of fentanyl. It is approximately one-third as potent as fentanyl and lasts approximately one-third as long, so that the requirement is about nine times that of fentanyl to maintain a steady analgesic concentration. Sedation, cardiovascular stability and ventilatory depression are similar to those of fentanyl.

Remifentanil

Remifentanil is formulated as lyophilized white crystalline powder for reconstitution with water. The vials contain glycine and are unsuitable for epidural or intrathecal administration. The solution, when diluted to 20 μg ml^{-1} with dextrose 5%, is stable for 24 h. Remifentanil is an ultrashort-acting opioid with μ-opioid activity. It is context-insensitive, in that the half-life, clearance and distribution are independent of the duration and strength of the infusion. It is metabolized by non-specific blood and tissue esterases and the capacity of the body to metabolize it is nearly limitless. Those who have abnormal plasma cholinesterases may metabolize remifentanil normally. The terminal elimination half-life is approximately 10 min and the primary reason for offset of action is metabolism and elimination rather than redistribution. It is 70% protein-bound and the volume of distribution at steady state is small: 0.3–0.4 L kg^{-1}. The only active metabolite is nearly as short-lived and is 600 times less potent. From the time the infusion is switched off, the duration of action of the usual plasma concentrations is about 3–6 min with no residual effects. Any postoperative analgesia must be given as or before the remifentanil is discontinued.

The adverse effects are those of all opioids. In the absence of muscle relaxation and in high-dose regimens, truncal muscle rigidity may present as apnoea and manual inflation of the lungs may be difficult. Truncal rigidity may usually be avoided if incremental doses are given as slow infusions rather than boluses or if increases in infusion rates are made in small increments or at intervals of more than 10 min. Using a concentration of 100 μg ml^{-1} and an infusion rate of 0.2–0.5 μg kg^{-1} min^{-1}, this problem is unlikely to occur. Bradycardia may occur especially when associated with abdominal or external ocular muscle traction. Remifentanil is not associated with histamine release.

Sufentanil

Sufentanil is closely related in structure to fentanyl (Fig. 18.3). It is five to 10 times as potent and slightly shorter-acting. Although used widely, it does not have a marketing licence in the UK.

Buprenorphine

Buprenorphine is a semi-synthetic, highly lipophilic base with affinity at the μ receptor but relatively low intrinsic activity. It is classed as a partial agonist. Because of its high affinity, it is difficult to reverse the effects with naloxone and because of the stability of the binding, the onset and offset of effect are slower than plasma concentrations would suggest. Its terminal plasma half-life is about 4 h, but its action lasts about 8 h.

Phenazocine

Phenazocine is a full opioid agonist, suitable for severe pain. It has less tendency to increase biliary pressures and to cause somnolence. It may be given sublingually.

Pentazocine

Pentazocine is an agonist at the κ and σ receptors, but it is also a partial agonist or antagonist at the μ receptor. It may cause ventilatory depression which requires higher-than-normal doses of naloxone to reverse. The ceiling analgesic effect is achieved in the adult at approximately 60 mg when approximately 80% of subjects experience some psychotomimetic effects. The hallucinations associated with pentazocine are typically more vivid and unpleasant than those associated with morphine. It is not recommended for prescription, except for those who have come to rely on it. Dependence is unusual but not rare.

Meptazinol

Meptazinol is a partial agonist of the opioid receptors but its mechanism of action may also involve the cholinergic receptors. It is bound mainly in the cortex and spinal cord, and less than other opioids in the mid-brain and ileum. Its main disadvantage is the higher incidence of nausea and vomiting associated with its use. It has good cardiovascular stability, does not inhibit uterine contraction and causes less respiratory depression than pethidine in equianalgesic doses. It crosses the placenta, but the half-life in the neonate is not prolonged (approximately 3 h).

Nalbuphine

A partial agonist at the κ receptor, nalbuphine is an antagonist or weak partial agonist at the μ receptor. The effect of 10 mg in an adult is similar to that of 10 mg of morphine. Maximal analgesic and respiratory depressant effects occur at a dose of about 0.45 mg kg^{-1}. Dysphoria is less common than with other κ agonists or opioid agonist-antagonists. Somnolence is common. Its advantages are that it may be effective in morphine-tolerant subjects and that it antagonizes the effects of morphine while still preserving some analgesic effect.

Naloxone

Naloxone is used as a short-acting opioid antagonist. It is relatively selective for the μ opioid receptor. Because of its short duration of action, opioid terminated depression may return when the effects of naloxone have terminated. Naloxone may precipitate the sympathetic drive of unrelieved pain, e.g. tachycardia, hypertension, arrhythmias etc. It has an oral bioavailability of < 3%.

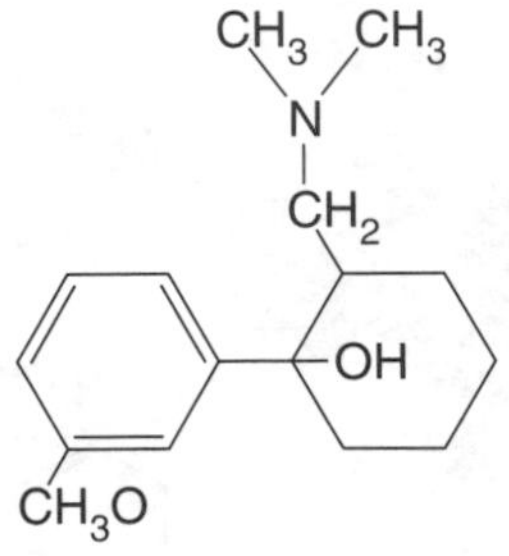

Fig. 18.5
The structure of tramadol.

Naltrexone

Naltrexone has a much longer half-life than that of naloxone and is effective orally for as long as 24 h. It has been used to treat opioid addiction and compulsive eating and morbid obesity.

Tramadol

Tramadol is formulated as a racemic mixture of two enantiomers . It is the phenylpiperidine analogue of codeine (Fig. 18.5).

Oral tramadol is absorbed rapidly and has a bioavailablity of 70% after a single dose, and 90–100% after multiple dosing due to a reduction in first-pass metabolism. It reaches peak plasma concentrations after 2–4 h. It is 20% bound to plasma proteins. About 85% of the absorbed dose is metabolized in the liver by demethylation and conjugation; 90% is excreted through the kidneys. About 10% is metabolized to O-desmethyltramadol which is an active metabolite having greater affinity for the μ opioid receptor and a half-life of 9 h.

Its mode of action is threefold. It binds to and activates the opioid receptors with a 20-fold preference for μ receptor. This action is weak but is that of a full agonist. It also inhibits the neuronal re-uptake of norepinephrine, potentiates the release of serotonin and causes descending inhibition of nociception.

The symptoms of overdose are those of the opioids but include cardiovascular collapse, confusion, coma and convulsions.

In therapeutic doses, the effects on ventilation and the cardiovascular system are clinically insignificant. Side-effects seen in clinical use include nausea, dry mouth, sweating, vomiting and urinary retention. Constipation is less common than with other opioids.

Tramadol and MAOIs potentiate each other to cause excitation and hypertension.

ROUTES OF OPIOID ADMINISTRATION

The routes by which opioids may be given are shown in Table 18.4.

Opioids administered to the spinal canal, either epidurally or intrathecally, are more potent and last longer than when applied

Table 18.4 Routes of administration for opioids

Available route of administration	IV	IM	SC	SL/OT	O	Sp	TD	N	I
Morphine	✓	✓	✓		✓	✓			✓
Diamorphine	✓	✓	✓		✓	✓		✓	✓
Pethidine	✓	✓	✓		✓	✓			
Fentanyl	✓	✓	✓	✓		✓	✓	✓	✓
Alfentanil	✓	✓	✓						
Remifentanil	✓					×		✓	
Methadone	✓	✓	✓		✓	✓			
Codeine	✓	✓	✓		✓				
Buprenorphine	✓	✓	✓	✓		✓			

IV, intravenous; IM, intramuscular; SC, subcutaneous; SL, sublingual; OT, oral transmucosal; O, oral; Sp, spinal, intrathecal or epidural; TD, transdermal; N, nasal; I, inhalation.
✓, has been used by this route although not necessarily with a marketing authorization
×, should not be used by this route

systemically. The epidural dose of highly lipid-soluble opioids such as fentanyl tends to be of the same order as that given systemically because, systemically, these opioids are distributed to the richly perfused lipid tissues such as the brain and spinal cord. From the epidural space, the drugs diffuse either into the spinal cerebrospinal fluid or mainly (96–98%) into the fat and the epidural blood vessels.

Transfer from the epidural space to the cord requires the passage across a fibrous membrane and lipid membranes. The rate of transfer depends on the size of the molecule, lipid solubility and degree of ionization. Pethidine and fentanyl have a relatively fast onset (peak concentrations of fentanyl within the cerebrospinal fluid occur within 15 min compared with 1–2 h for morphine).

Respiratory depression may occur after spinal administration and cephalad spread of any opioid but is more likely to occur without warning and after a longer time interval with water-soluble opioids such as morphine. Delayed, sudden cessation of ventilation is also more probable if the opioid is given as a bolus rather than as a slow infusion, if it is dissolved in a large volume of solvent and if it is administered into the cervical or thoracic spine rather than the lumbar or sacral spine.

PARACETAMOL

Paracetamol (Fig. 18.6) was first used in medicine in 1893, but it was not prescribed extensively until after 1949 when it was recognized as the main and less toxic metabolite of phenacetin.

PHARMACOKINETICS

Absorption

After oral administration, peak plasma concentrations are achieved after 30–60 min, absorption taking place by passive transport mostly from the jejunum and ileum. Paracetamol is absorbed unchanged from the gastrointestinal tract (bioavailability, 70–90%).

Absorption from the rectum is variable; bioavailability is 70–90% of that obtained after oral administration and the time required to reach peak blood concentrations is longer than with oral tablets.

Absorption in neonates may be reduced or delayed compared with older children.

Paracetamol is not bound significantly to plasma proteins after therapeutic doses. In neonates, the plasma protein binding is slightly higher than in adults. Unconjugated paracetamol may pass from the maternal circulation to the fetus.

Metabolism

Paracetamol is partially metabolized by hepatic microsomal enzymes to the sulphate (26%), glucuronide (49%) and cysteine (3%) conjugates which are pharmacologically inactive. Less than 5% is excreted unchanged in the urine and faeces. A minor metabolite in normal circumstances is N-acetyl-p-amino-benzoquinoneimine which is formed by N-hydroxylation and is usually conjugated with glutathione and made harmless. If glutathione is lacking, this reactive metabolite accumulates and binds covalently with (alkylates) macromolecules in the hepatocyte causing necrosis. The formation of this metabolite is increased if the cytochrome P450 mixed function oxidase is induced by drugs such as barbiturates or carbamazepine.

The plasma half-life of paracetamol is 2–3 h after usual doses (2–5 h in the neonate). After hepatotoxic doses, conjugation with glucuronide is impaired and the half-life is increased proportionately to the liver damage.

Pharmacodynamics

Paracetamol is analgesic and antipyretic but has no anti-inflammatory actions. It is effective in concentrations of 10–20 mg L^{-1}.

Interactions

Paracetamol metabolism is enhanced by anticonvulsants and oral contraceptive agents. There is both a synergistic and an additive analgesic effect when given with opioids. There are few interactions with other drugs, as paracetamol does not alter regional blood flow, or compete for enzyme systems or plasma protein binding sites to any significant degree.

Clinical use

Paracetamol is used for mild to moderate pain. It is as effective as aspirin and most non-steroidal anti-inflammatory drugs for

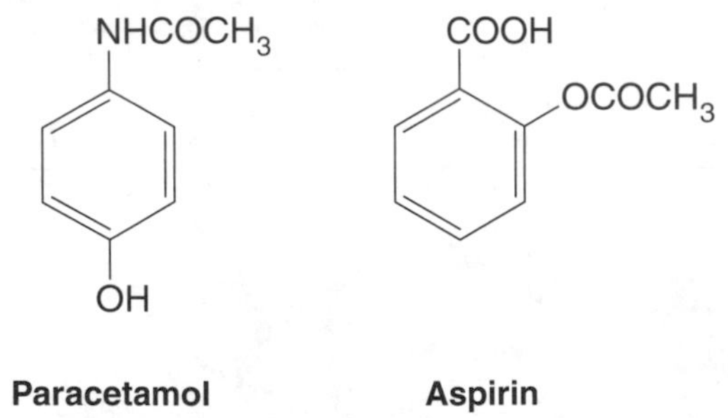

Fig. 18.6
The structures of paracetamol and aspirin.

non-inflammatory pain. It is available alone or in combination with weak opioids or as an aspirin–paracetamol ester (benorylate).

Adverse effects

These relate mainly to poisoning but paracetamol may also, in chronic usage, cause headaches. Occasionally, skin rashes, methaemoglobinaemia and haemolytic anaemia occur.

PARACETAMOL POISONING

Hepatotoxicity is produced by a toxic reactive metabolite (see above). The threshold dose in an adult has been estimated to be 10–15 g, but lower doses have been associated with liver toxicity when combined with alcohol abuse or fasting. In very high doses, acute proximal tubular necrosis of the kidney occurs and is, as in the liver, associated with depletion of glutathione and covalent binding.

Treatment of overdose

Liver damage is always associated with glutathione depletion. Unfortunately, glutathione itself does not enter cells readily and is only effective in extremely high doses. Glutathione precursors and related compounds, such as cysteine, acetylcysteine, cysteamine and methionine, prevent liver damage following paracetamol overdosage. Intravenous N-acetylcysteine is the treatment of choice but must be given within 10 h of ingestion of the overdose and is completely effective if given within 8 h. Oral acetylcysteine and oral methionine are less effective, probably because of the unreliability of oral absorption in the presence of nausea and vomiting (or before gastric aspiration). Transient allergic reactions have been reported rarely, but otherwise acetylcysteine appears devoid of serious side-effects.

NON-STEROIDAL ANTI-INFLAMMATORY DRUGS (NSAIDs)

The efficacy of salicylates (as willow bark) was reported by Stone in 1763. Aspirin was first synthesized by Bayer in 1853. The clinical use of acetylsalicylic acid (aspirin) was described independently by Witthauer and Wohlgemuth in 1899, the latter advocating acetylsalicylic acid because salicylic acid caused stomach pains. The mechanism of action of aspirin was first described by John Vane in 1971.

ACTIONS

NSAIDs reduce nociception which is related to inflammation and inflammatory mediators whether from trauma, infection, immune reactions or neural transmitter release. They also modify the inflammatory reaction and lower a raised temperature towards normal.

The relative extent to which these effects are achieved are not necessarily interrelated, although they all inhibit the production of the prostaglandins. For example, ketorolac in usual analgesic doses has little anti-inflammatory effect. Aspirin is anti-inflammatory only in doses which are higher than those required for analgesia. Indomethacin is powerfully anti-inflammatory in usual analgesic doses.

All NSAIDs inhibit prostaglandin synthesis by inhibiting the enzyme cyclooxygenase (COX). There are two types of COX: COX-1 and COX-2. The structures of COX-1 and COX-2 have been described, purified and cloned. COX-1 is called a constitutive enzyme because it is present in almost all tissues for most of the time and is instrumental in maintaining functions such as regional blood flow and gastric mucus secretion. COX-2 is present in the brain, spinal cord and macula densa of the glomerulus, and intermittently present in the ovary and uterus. It can be induced in inflammatory cells when they are activated by, say, interleukin-1 and tumour necrosing factor. Induction of COX-2 is transient, reaching a maximum after 4–6 h after stimulation and returning to baseline after 24 h. It is inhibited by the glucocorticosteroids. Many NSAIDs are more selective for COX-1 than for COX-2 (Table 18.5).

UNWANTED ACTIONS

Because of the widespread use of NSAIDs, especially in the elderly, the number of patients suffering from serious side-effects is high. Most side-effects are thought to be the result of inhibiting COX-1.

Gastrointestinal tract

Gastrointestinal disorders are the commonest of these unwanted effects. They include dyspepsia (or oesophageal irritation) and gastric erosions, which may present with bleeding or perforation. Piroxicam reportedly causes most symptomatic bleeding perhaps because of its long half-life and cumulation in the elderly. Naproxen and diclofenac are less often implicated and ibuprofen is said to be the safest in this respect, although when equi-anti-inflammatory doses are used, endoscopic evidence of increased safety is absent. Erosions or ulcers are caused by uninhibited acid secretion, reduced mucus and bicarbonate secretion, reduced mucosal blood flow and biochemical bridging of the mucus barrier allowing the hydrogen ions to enter the mucosal cells.

Less common intestinal side-effects are leakage of fluid through the ileum and the formation of tight mucosal folds which may be intermittent or persistent and may cause intestinal obstruction (pseudodiaphragmatic disease). Nausea and vomiting, diarrhoea or constipation may also occur.

These problems may be reduced by misoprostol, a prostaglandin E_1 analogue, H_2- receptor antagonists such as cimetidine or ranitidine, or proton pump inhibitors such as omeprazole or lansoprazole. Misoprostol causes abdominal or retrosternal discomfort, diarrhoea and uterine contractions.

Renal

When the renal blood flow is normal or high, little prostaglandin is released by the kidney. Where renal blood flow is reduced, when endogenous vasoconstrictors such as angiotensin and norepinephrine are released, or when cyclosporin has been given, prostaglandins are released (PGE_2 in the medulla and PGI_2 in the glomerulus) causing compensatory vasodilatation. NSAIDs may cause acute renal failure when given during blood loss or hypotension, cardiac failure, cirrhosis of the liver, nephrotic syndrome or glomerulonephritis and also during some forms of chemotherapy.

Prostaglandins also cause natriuresis and NSAIDs may cause salt and water retention and therefore exacerbate heart failure. NSAIDs indirectly suppress renin and aldosterone secretion and may lead to hyperkalaemia.

Rarely NSAIDs may cause an allergic interstitial nephritis which may present as acute renal failure or as the nephrotic syndrome up to 1 year after starting NSAIDs. Fenoprofen, which binds irreversibly to albumin, is most often implicated.

Also rarely, chronic NSAID consumption may cause an analgesic nephropathy of chronic nephritis and renal papillary necrosis.

COX-2 enzymes are expressed in the macula densa of the juxtaglomerular apparatus in contact with the granular cells of the afferent and efferent arterioles which synthesize, store and release renin. It is possible that the COX-2 inhibitors will not be free of the renal side-effects of the other NSAIDs.

Clotting

Vascular damage, thrombin and bradykinin cause platelets to aggregate and release thromboxane, which causes further aggregation. Aggregation is inhibited by prostacyclin (PGI_2).

Aspirin inhibits COX-1 irreversibly and therefore diminishes both prostacyclin in the endothelial cells and thromboxane in the platelets. However, the endothelial cells produce more enzyme and prostacyclin, but the platelets, which are without nuclei, cannot produce more thromboxane. Low-dose aspirin progressively alters the balance in favour of prostacyclin, whereas high-dose aspirin reduces both prostacyclin and thromboxane.

Asthma and bronchospasm

Bronchospasm may occur after NSAID administration as part of an anaphylactic reaction because of the release of histamine and bradykinin. It may also be the result of cyclooxygenase inhibition, accumulation of arachidonic acid and increased conversion to leukotrienes in the lung.

Skin reactions

Skin reactions most commonly occur with mefenamic acid and sulindac and include mild rashes, urticaria, photosensitivity and dermolysis.

Central nervous system

Regular high-dose aspirin may cause VIIIth nerve damage, i.e. tinnitus, reduced hearing and vertigo. Overdosage causes medullary stimulation and hyperventilation. Higher doses or prolonged exposure lead to acidosis and respiratory depression.

Reye's syndrome, a rare form of encephalopathy associated with fatty change in the liver, appears to be peculiar to aspirin and occurs almost entirely in those less than 12 years old in association with a viral infection and pyrexia.

Reproductive system

NSAIDs inhibit uterine contractions and prolong labour. It has also been shown that, in subfertile males, the concentration of prostaglandin in the seminal fluid correlates with fertility.

Ductus arteriosus

PGE_2 is a potent dilator of the ductus arteriosus and indomethacin, for example, may cause closure, even premature closure, of a patent ductus arteriosus and may be used for this purpose in a premature newborn.

PHARMACOKINETICS

Absorption

All active NSAIDs are weak acids and mainly un-ionized in the acid medium of the stomach where absorption is facilitated. However, most absorption occurs in the small intestine because the un-ionized form may be very insoluble (e.g. aspirin) and the

Table 18.5 Examples of selectivity of NSAID for cyclooxygenase-1 and cyclooxygenase-2

More effective on COX-1 than on COX-2	Similarly effective on COX-1 and COX-2	More effective on COX-2 than on COX-1
Aspirin (166:1)	Diclofenac	Celecoxib
Indomethacin (60:1)	Naproxen	Rofecoxib
Ibuprofen (15:1)	Etodolac	Meloxicam
Piroxicam (250:1)	Ketorolac	
	Nabumetone	

absorptive area of the microvilli of the small intestine is much more extensive. Most have pK_a values less than 5 and are therefore 99% ionized above a pH of 7. Most are almost insoluble in water at body pH, although the sodium salt (diclofenac sodium, naproxen sodium) is more soluble. Ketorolac trometamol is most soluble and can be given intravenously as a bolus and intramuscularly without causing significant irritation. Tenoxicam and ketoprofen may be given intravenously as a slow bolus, and diclofenac as a 30 min infusion. Ketorolac and tenoxicam may be given intramuscularly. Ketoprofen and diclofenac may be given intramuscularly also, but only deeply into a large muscle, and even then diclofenac can cause chemical abscesses.

Protein binding and distribution

Most NSAIDs are extensively protein-bound (90–99%). At low doses, aspirin is highly protein-bound but as the concentration increases, relatively less is bound and more is available for action in the tissues and transfer across the blood–brain barrier. Ketoprofen is also variably bound. Aspirin is bound to the same site on albumin as warfarin, giving rise to interactions.

The volume of distribution is therefore low (approximately 0.1–0.2 L kg^{-1}) with the exception of indomethacin which has protein binding of 90% and V_d of 0.3–1.6 L kg^{-1}.

Metabolism and excretion

Many NSAIDs are oxidized or hydroxylated and then conjugated and excreted in the urine. Some metabolites have activity. Nabumetone is a prodrug and the metabolite (6-methoxy-2-naphthyl acetic acid) is more active than the parent drug.

Diclofenac and its metabolites are conjugated to glucuronides and sulphates; 65% is excreted in the urine and 35% in the bile. The metabolites are less active than the parent compound. The terminal half-life is 1–2 h. Ketorolac trometamol has a terminal half-life of 5 h and is excreted almost entirely through the kidney (> 90%).

Naproxen has a terminal half-life of 12–15 h and is excreted almost entirely through the kidney as the conjugate.

Tenoxicam is cleared mainly through the urine as the inactive hydroxypyridyl metabolite, but a third is through the bile as the glucuronide.

CHOICE OF NSAID

NSAIDs have the potential to reduce pain, especially late post-inflammatory pain, and are usually more effective for dental- and orthopaedic-generated pain than are the weak opioids. Ibuprofen is recommended as the first-line NSAID for simple analgesia because it has the lowest number of adverse reactions reported per unit number of prescriptions. Diclofenac is popular because it is available in several formulations. Ketorolac is the first choice for intravenous administration because of its relatively high solubility.

The selective COX-2 inhibitors have been shown to have similar analgesic efficacy as diclofenac. They have shown little or no gastric irritation in trials. Platelet inhibition does not occur with a dose more than 50 times that used clinically. Their effects on renal function and asthma are, as yet, unclear.

FURTHER READING

Dollery C 1999 (ed) Therapeutic drugs. Churchill Livingstone, Edinburgh

Fields H L, Liebeskind J C 1994 (ed) Pharmacological approaches to the treatment of chronic pain: new concepts and critical issues. Progress in Pain Research and Management 1. IASP Press, Seattle

McQuay H J, Moore R A 1998 An evidence-based resource for pain relief. Oxford University Press, Oxford

Rang H P, Dale M M, Ritter J M (eds) 1999 Pharmacology. Churchill Livingstone, Edinburgh

Rowbotham D J 1998 (ed) Guidelines for the use of non-steroidal anti-inflammmatory drugs in the perioperative period. Royal College of Anaesthetists, London

19 Muscle function and neuromuscular blockade

In the last 60 years, neuromuscular blocking drugs have become an established part of anaesthetic practice. They were first administered in 1942, when Griffith and Johnson in Montreal used Intocostrin, a biologically standardized mixture of the alkaloids of the plant *Chondrodendron tomentosum*, to facilitate relaxation during cyclopropane anaesthesia. Previously, only inhalation agents (nitrous oxide, ether, cyclopropane and chloroform) had been used during general anaesthesia, making surgical access for some procedures difficult because of lack of muscle relaxation. To achieve significant muscle relaxation, it was necessary to deepen anaesthesia, which often had adverse cardiac and respiratory effects. Local analgesia was the only alternative.

At first, muscle relaxants were used only occasionally, in small doses, as an adjuvant to aid in the management of a difficult case; they were not used routinely. A tracheal tube was not necessarily passed, artificial ventilation was not used and the residual block was not routinely reversed; all of these caused significant morbidity and mortality, as demonstrated in the famous retrospective study by Beecher & Todd (1954). By 1946, however, it was appreciated that using drugs such as curare in larger doses allowed the depth of anaesthesia to be lightened, and it was suggested that incremental doses should also be used during prolonged surgery, rather than deepening anaesthesia – an entirely new concept at that time. The use of routine tracheal intubation and artificial ventilation then evolved.

Gray & Halton (1946) in Liverpool reported their experience of using the pure alkaloid, tubocurarine, in over 1000 patients receiving various anaesthetic agents. Over the following 6 years, they developed a concise description of the necessary ingredients of any anaesthetic technique; narcosis, analgesia and muscle relaxation were essential – the *triad* of anaesthesia. A fourth ingredient, controlled apnoea, was added at a later stage to emphasize the need for fully controlled ventilation, reducing the amount of relaxant required. This concept is the basis of the use of neuromuscular blocking drugs in modern anaesthetic practice. In particular, it has allowed seriously ill patients undergoing complex surgery to be anaesthetized safely and to be cared for postoperatively in the intensive therapy unit.

PHYSIOLOGY OF NEUROMUSCULAR TRANSMISSION

Acetylcholine, the neurotransmitter at the neuromuscular junction, is released from presynaptic nerve endings on the passage of a nerve impulse (an action potential) down the axon to the nerve terminal. The neurotransmitter is synthesized from choline and acetylcoenzyme A by the enzyme *choline acetyltransferase* and stored in vesicles in the nerve terminal. The action potential depolarizes the nerve terminal to release the neurotransmitter; entry of Ca^{2+} ions into the nerve terminal is a necessary part of the process. On the arrival of an action potential, the storage vesicles are transferred to the active zones on the edge of the axonal membrane, where they fuse with the terminal wall to release the acetylcholine (Fig. 19.1). There are about 1000 active sites at each nerve ending and any one nerve action potential leads to the release of 200–300 vesicles. In addition, small *quanta* of acetylcholine, presumably equivalent to the contents of one vesicle, are released at the neuromuscular junction spontaneously, causing miniature end-plate potentials (MEPPs) on the postsynaptic membrane, but these are insufficient to generate a muscle action potential.

The active sites of release are aligned directly opposite the acetylcholine receptors on the junctional folds of the postsynaptic membrane, lying on the muscle surface. The junctional cleft, the gap between the nerve terminal and the muscle membrane, has a width of only 60 nm. It contains the enzyme *acetylcholinesterase,* which is responsible for the ultimate breakdown of acetylcholine. This enzyme is also present, in higher concentrations, in the junctional folds in the postsynaptic membrane (Fig. 19.1). The choline produced by the breakdown of acetylcholine is taken up across the nerve membrane to be reused in the synthesis of the transmitter.

The nicotinic acetylcholine receptors on the postsynaptic membrane are organized in discrete clusters on the shoulders of the junctional folds (Fig. 19.1). Each cluster is about 0.1 μm in diameter and contains a few hundred receptors. Each receptor consists of five subunits, two of which, the alpha (α; MW = 40 000 Da), are identical. The other three, slightly larger subunits, are the beta (β), delta (δ) and epsilon (ε). In fetal muscle, the epsilon is replaced by a gamma (γ) subunit. Each subunit of the receptor is a glycosated protein – a chain of amino acids – coded by a different gene.

The receptors are arranged as a cylinder which spans the membrane, with a central, normally closed, channel – the ionophore (Fig. 19.2). Each of the α subunits carries a single acetylcholine binding region on its extracellular surface. They also bind neuromuscular blocking drugs.

Activation of the receptor requires both α sites to be occupied, producing a structural change in the receptor complex that opens the central channel running between the receptors for a very short period, about 1 ms (Fig. 19.2). This allows the movement of cations such as Na^+, K^+, Ca^{2+} and Mg^{2+} along their concentration gradients. The main change is an influx of Na^+ ions, the *end-plate*

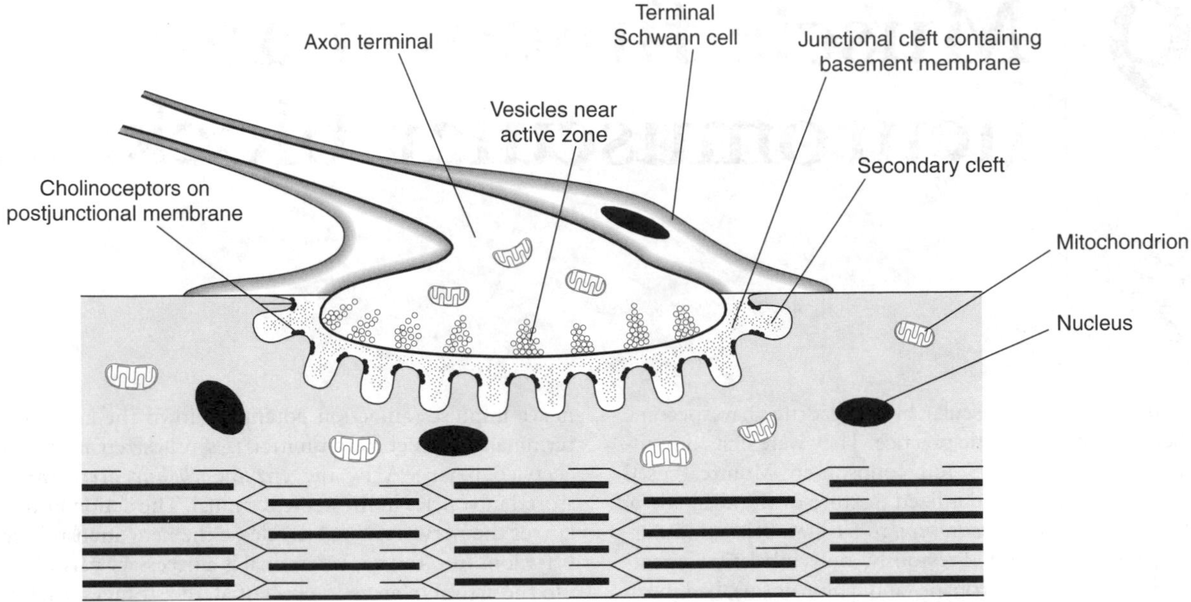

Fig. 19.1
The neuromuscular junction with an axon terminal, containing vesicles of acetylcholine. The neurotransmitter is released on arrival of an action potential and crosses the junctional cleft to stimulate the postjunctional receptors on the shoulders of the secondary clefts. (Reproduced with kind permission of Professor WC Bowman.)

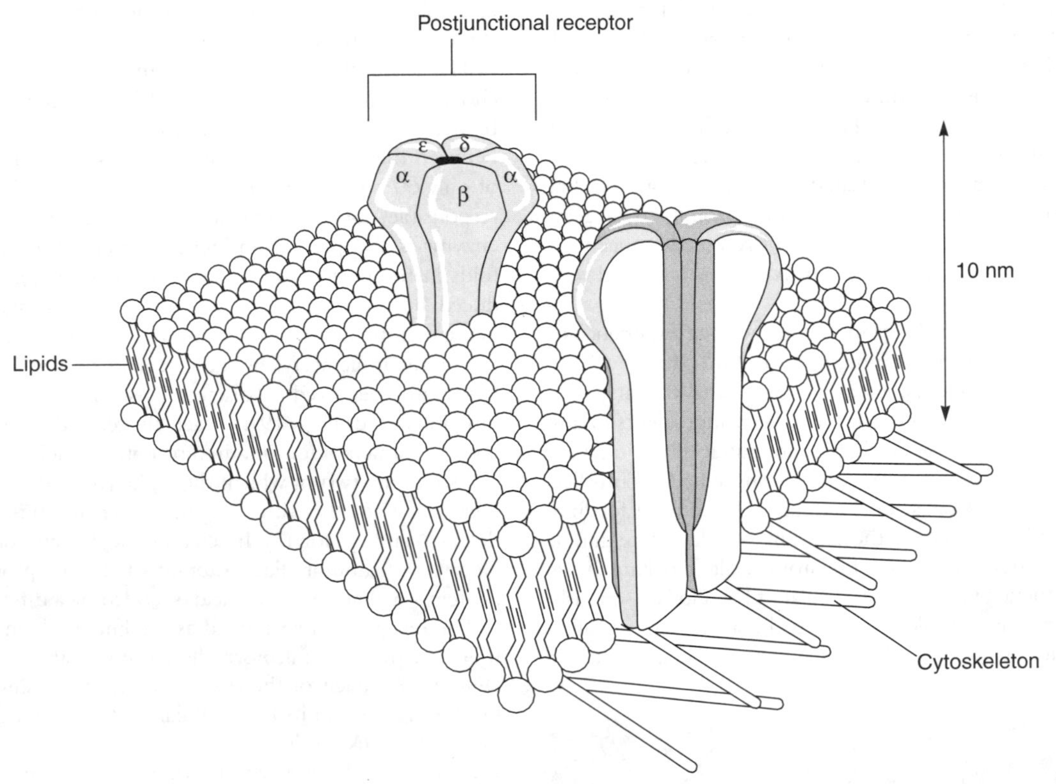

Fig. 19.2
Two postjunctional receptors, embedded in the lipid layer of the postsynaptic muscle membrane. The α, β, ε and δ subunits are demonstrated on the surface of one receptor and the ionophore is seen in cross-section on the other receptor. On stimulation of the two α subunits by two molecules of acetylcholine, the ionophore opens to allow the passage of the end-plate current. (Reproduced with kind permission of Professor WC Bowman.)

current, followed by an efflux of K^+ ions. The summation of this current through a large number of receptor channels lowers the transmembrane potential of the end-plate region sufficiently to depolarize it and generate a muscle action potential sufficient to allow muscle contraction.

At rest, the transmembrane potential is about –90 mV (inside negative). Under normal physiological conditions, a depolarization of about 40 mV occurs, lowering the potential from –90 to –50 mV. When the *end-plate potential* reaches this critical threshold, it triggers an *all-or-nothing* action potential that passes around the sarcolemma to activate muscle contraction via a mechanism involving Ca^{2+} release from the sarcoplasmic reticulum.

Each acetylcholine molecule is involved in opening one ion channel only before it is broken down rapidly by acetylcholinesterase; it does not interact with any of the other receptors. There is a large safety factor in the transmission process, in respect of both the amount of acetylcholine released and the number of postsynaptic receptors. Much more acetylcholine is released than is necessary to trigger the action potential. The end-plate region is depolarized for only a very short period (a few ms) before it rapidly repolarizes and is ready to transmit another impulse.

Acetylcholine receptors are also present on the presynaptic area of the nerve terminal. It is thought that a positive feedback mechanism exists for the further release of acetylcholine, such that some of the released molecules of acetylcholine stimulate these presynaptic receptors, producing further mobilization of the neurotransmitter to the readily releasable sites, ready for the arrival of the next nerve stimulus (Fig. 19.3).

In health, postsynaptic acetylcholine receptors are restricted to the neuromuscular junction by a mechanism involving the presence of an active nerve terminal. In many disease states affecting the neuromuscular junction, this control is lost and acetylcholine receptors develop on the adjacent muscle surface. The excessive release of K^+ ions from diseased or swollen muscle on administration of succinylcholine is probably the result of stimulation of these *extrajunctional receptors.* They develop in many conditions, including polyneuropathies, severe burns and muscle disorders.

The physiology of neuromuscular transmission has been described in detail by Bowman (1992).

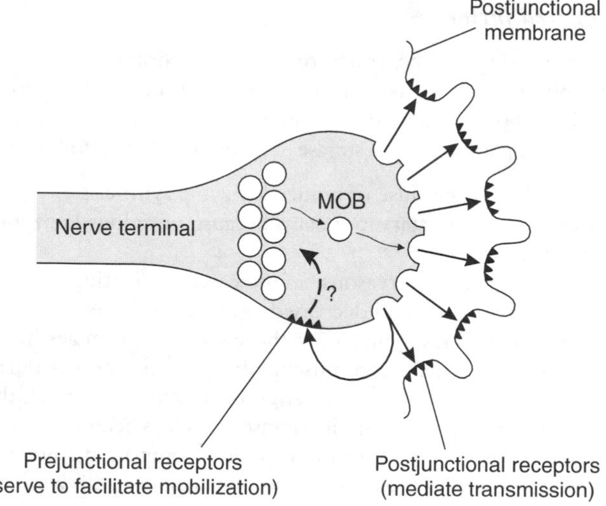

Fig. 19.3
Acetylcholine receptors are present on the shoulders of the axon terminal, as well as on the postjunctional membrane. Stimulation of the prejunctional receptors mobilizes (MOB) the vesicles of acetylcholine to move into the active zone, ready for release on arrival of another nerve impulse. The exact mechanism is unknown. (Reproduced with kind permission of Professor WC Bowman.)

PHARMACOLOGY OF NEUROMUSCULAR TRANSMISSION

Neuromuscular blocking agents used regularly by anaesthetists are classified into *depolarizing* (or *non-competitive*) and *non-depolarizing* (or *competitive)* agents.

DEPOLARIZING NEUROMUSCULAR BLOCKING AGENTS

The only depolarizing relaxant now available in clinical practice is succinylcholine. Decamethonium was used clinically in the UK for many years, but it is now available only for research purposes.

Succinylcholine chloride

This quaternary ammonium compound is comparable to two molecules of acetylcholine linked together (Fig. 19.4). The two quaternary ammonium radicals $N^+(CH_3)_3$ have the capacity to cling to each of the α units of the postsynaptic acetylcholine receptor, altering its structural conformation and opening the ion channel, but for a longer period than does a molecule of acetylcholine. Administration of succinylcholine therefore results in an initial depolarization and muscle contraction, termed *fasciculation*. As this effect persists, however, further action potentials cannot pass down the ion channels and the muscle becomes flaccid; repolarization does not occur.

The dose of succinylcholine necessary for tracheal intubation in adults is about 1.0–1.5 mg kg^{-1}. This dose has the most rapid onset of action of any of the muscle relaxants presently available, producing profound block within 1 min. Succinylcholine is therefore of particular benefit when it is essential to achieve tracheal intubation rapidly, as in a patient with a full stomach or an obstetric patient. It is also indicated if tracheal intubation is expected to be difficult for anatomical reasons, as it produces optimal intubating conditions.

The drug is metabolized predominantly in the plasma by the enzyme *plasma cholinesterase,* once known as pseudocholinesterase, at a very rapid rate. Recovery from neuromuscular block may start to occur within 3 min and is complete within 12–15 min. The use of an anticholinesterase such as neostigmine, which would inhibit such enzyme activity, is contraindicated (see below). About 10% of the drug is excreted in the urine; there is very little metabolism in the liver although some breakdown by non-specific esterases occurs in the plasma.

If plasma cholinesterase is structurally abnormal because of inherited factors, or if its concentration is reduced by acquired factors, then the duration of action of the drug may be altered significantly.

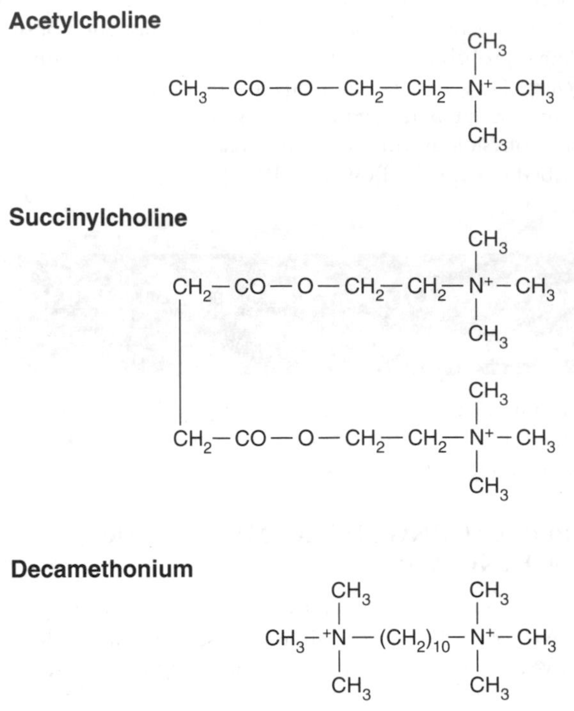

Acetylcholine

$$CH_3{-}CO{-}O{-}CH_2{-}CH_2{-}N^{+}(CH_3)_3$$

Succinylcholine

$$\begin{array}{l} CH_2{-}CO{-}O{-}CH_2{-}CH_2{-}N^{+}(CH_3)_3 \\ | \\ CH_2{-}CO{-}O{-}CH_2{-}CH_2{-}N^{+}(CH_3)_3 \end{array}$$

Decamethonium

$$(CH_3)_3{-}{}^{+}N{-}(CH_2)_{10}{-}N^{+}(CH_3)_3$$

Fig. 19.4
The chemical structures of acetylcholine and succinylcholine. The similarity between the structure of succinylcholine and two molecules of acetylcholine can be seen. The structure of decamethonium is also shown. The quaternary ammonium radicals $N^{+}(CH_3)_3$, cling to the α subunits of the postsynaptic receptor.

Inherited factors

The exact structure of plasma cholinesterase is determined genetically, by autosomal genes, and has now been completely defined. Several abnormalities in the amino acid sequence of the normal enzyme, usually designated $E_1{}^{u}$, are recognized. The most common is produced by the atypical gene, $E_1{}^{a}$, which occurs in about 4% of the Caucasian population. Thus a patient who is a *heterozygote* for the atypical gene ($E_1{}^{u}$, $E_1{}^{a}$) will have a longer effect from a standard dose of succinylcholine (about 30 min). If the individual is a *homozygote* for the atypical gene ($E_1{}^{a}$, $E_1{}^{a}$), succinylcholine may have an effect for over 2 h, which may be inconvenient to the anaesthetist during an operating list. Other, rarer, abnormalities in the structure of plasma cholinesterase are also recognized, e.g. the fluoride ($E_1{}^{f}$) and silent ($E_1{}^{s}$) genes. The latter has very little capacity to metabolize succinylcholine and thus neuromuscular block in the homozygous state lasts for at least 3 h. In such patients, non-specific esterases gradually clear the drug from plasma.

It has been suggested that a source of cholinesterase, such as fresh frozen plasma, should be administered in such cases, or an anticholinesterase such as neostigmine used to reverse what has usually developed into a *dual block* (see below). However, it is wiser to:

- Keep the patient anaesthetized and the lungs ventilated artificially.
- Monitor neuromuscular transmission accurately until full recovery from residual neuromuscular block.

It is possible that in the near future, genetically engineered plasma cholinesterase will become available, albeit at a high cost; this may be useful to treat prolonged block.

This condition is not life-threatening, but the risk of awareness is considerable, especially after the end of surgery, when the anaesthetist, who may not yet have made the diagnosis, is attempting to waken the patient. Anaesthesia must be continued until full recovery from neuromuscular block.

As plasma cholinesterase activity is reduced by the presence of succinylcholine, a plasma sample to measure the patient's cholinesterase activity should not be taken for several days after prolonged block has been experienced, by which time new enzyme will have been synthesized. A patient who is found to have reduced enzyme activity and structurally abnormal enzyme should be given a warning card or alarm bracelet, detailing his or her genetic status. Detailing the genetic status of the patient's immediate relatives should be considered.

Kalow & Genest (1957) first described a method for detecting structurally abnormal cholinesterase. If plasma from a patient of normal genotype is added to a water bath containing a substrate such as benzoylcholine, a chemical reaction occurs with plasma cholinesterase, emitting light of a given wavelength, which may be detected spectrophotometrically. If dibucaine is also added to the water bath, this reaction is inhibited; no light is produced. The percentage inhibition is referred to as the ***dibucaine number***. A patient with normal plasma cholinesterase has a high dibucaine number of 77–83. A heterozygote for the atypical gene has a dibucaine number of 45–68; in a homozygote, the dibucaine number is less than 30.

If fluoride is added to the solution instead of dibucaine, the fluoride gene may be detected. If there is no reaction in the presence of the substrate only, the silent gene is present.

Acquired factors

In these instances, the structure of plasma cholinesterase is normal, but its activity is reduced. Thus neuromuscular block is lengthened by only a matter of minutes, rather than hours. Causes of reduced plasma cholinesterase activity include the following:

- Liver disease, because of reduced enzyme synthesis.
- Carcinomatosis, starvation, also because of reduced enzyme synthesis.
- Pregnancy, for two reasons: an increased circulating volume (dilutional effect) and decreased enzyme synthesis.
- Anticholinesterases, including those used by the anaesthetist to reverse residual neuromuscular block after a non-depolarizing muscle relaxant (e.g. neostigmine or edrophonium); these drugs inhibit plasma cholinesterase as well as acetylcholinesterase. The organophosphorus compound *ecothiopate*, once used topically as a miotic in ophthalmology, is also an anticholinesterase.
- Other drugs which are metabolized by plasma cholinesterase, and which therefore decrease its availability, include etomidate, propanidid, ester local analgesics, anti-cancer drugs such as methotrexate, monoamine oxidase inhibitors and esmolol (the short-acting β-blocker).
- Hypothyroidism.

- Cardiopulmonary bypass, plasmapheresis.
- Renal disease.

Side-effects of succinylcholine

Although succinylcholine is a very useful drug for achieving tracheal intubation rapidly, it has several undesirable side-effects which may limit its use:

Muscle pains

These occur especially in the patient who is ambulant soon after surgery, such as the day-case patient. The pains, thought possibly to be due to the initial fasciculations, are more common in young, fit people with a large muscle mass. They occur in unusual sites, such as the diaphragm and between the scapulae, and are not relieved easily by conventional analgesics. They may be reduced by the use of a small dose of a non-depolarizing muscle relaxant given immediately prior to the administration of succinylcholine, e.g. gallamine 10 mg (which is thought to be most efficacious in this respect), or atracurium 2.5 mg. However, this technique, termed *pre-curarization* or *pretreatment*, reduces the potency of succinylcholine, necessitating administration of a larger dose to produce the same effect. Many other drugs have been used in an attempt to reduce the muscle pains, including lidocaine, calcium, magnesium and repeated doses of thiopental, but none is completely reliable.

Increased intraocular pressure

This is thought to be due in part to the initial contraction of the external ocular muscles and contracture of the internal ocular muscles on administration of succinylcholine. It is not reduced by pre-curarization. The effect lasts for as long as the neuromuscular block and concern has been expressed that it may be sufficient to cause expulsion of the vitreal contents in the patient with an open eye injury. This is probably unlikely. Protection of the airway from gastric contents must take priority in the patient with a full stomach in addition to an eye injury, as inhalation of gastric contents may threaten life.

It is also possible that succinylcholine may increase intracranial pressure, although this is less certain.

Increased intragastric pressure

In the presence of a normal lower oesophageal sphincter, the increase in intragastric pressure produced by succinylcholine should be insufficient to produce regurgitation of gastric contents. However, in the patient with incompetence of this sphincter from, for example, a hiatus hernia, regurgitation may occur.

Hyperkalaemia

It has long been recognized that administration of succinylcholine during halothane anaesthesia increases the serum potassium concentration by 0.5 mmol L^{-1} (Paton 1959). This effect is thought to be due to muscle fasciculation. It is probable that the effect is less marked with the newer potent inhalation agents, e.g. isoflurane. A similar increase occurs in patients with renal failure, but as these patients may already have an elevated serum potassium concentration, such an increase may precipitate cardiac irregularities and even cardiac arrest.

In some conditions in which the muscle cells are swollen or damaged, or in which there is proliferation of extrajunctional receptors, this release of potassium may be exaggerated. This is most marked in the burned patient, in whom potassium levels up to 13 mmol L^{-1} have been reported. In such patients, pre-curarization is of no benefit. Succinylcholine is best avoided in this condition. In diseases of the muscle cell, or its nerve supply, hyperkalaemia after succinylcholine may also be exaggerated. These include the muscular dystrophies, dystrophia myotonica and paraplegia. Hyperkalaemia has been reported to cause death in such patients. Succinylcholine may also precipitate a prolonged contracture of the masseter muscles in patients with these disorders, making tracheal intubation impossible. The drug is best avoided in any patient with a neuromuscular disorder, including the patient with *malignant hyperthermia*, in whom the drug is a recognized trigger factor (see p. 521).

Hyperkalaemia after succinylcholine has also been reported, albeit rarely, in patients with widespread intra-abdominal infection, severe trauma and closed head injury.

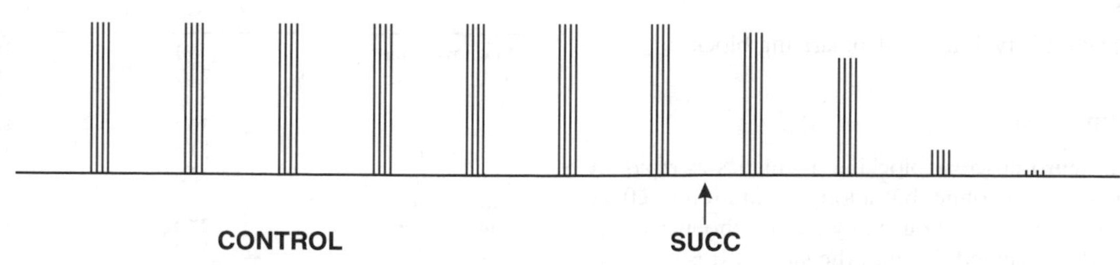

Fig. 19.5
The train-of-four twitch response recorded before (CONTROL) and after a dose of succinylcholine. Before administration of succinycholine 1 mg kg^{-1}, four twitches of equal height are visible. After giving the drug (SUCC), the height of all four twitches decreases equally; no 'fade' of the train-of-four is seen. Within one minute, the trace has been ablated.

Cardiovascular effects

Succinylcholine has muscarinic in addition to nicotinic effects, as does acetylcholine. The direct vagal effect (muscarinic) produces a sinus bradycardia, especially in patients with a high vagal tone, such as children and the physically fit. It is also more common in the patient who has not received an anticholinergic agent such as atropine, or who is given repeated increments of succinylcholine. It is advisable to use an anticholinergic routinely if more than one dose of succinylcholine is planned. Nodal or ventricular escape beats may develop in extreme circumstances.

Anaphylactic reactions

Anaphylactic reactions to succinylcholine are rare, but may occur, especially after repeated exposure to the drug. They are more common after succinylcholine than any other neuromuscular blocking agent.

Characteristics of depolarizing neuromuscular block

If neuromuscular block is monitored (see below), several differences between depolarizing and non-depolarizing block may be defined. In the presence of a small dose of succinylcholine:

- A decreased response to a single, low-voltage (1 Hz) twitch stimulus applied to a peripheral nerve is detected. Tetanic stimulation (e.g. at 50 Hz) produces a small, but sustained, response.
- If four twitch stimuli are applied at 2 Hz over 2 s (train-of-four stimulus), followed by a 10 s interval before the next train-of-four, no decrease in the height of successive stimuli is noted (Fig. 19.5).
- The application of a 5 s burst of tetanic stimulation after the application of a single twitch, followed 3 s later by a further twitch stimulus, produces no potentiation of the twitch height; there is no *post-tetanic potentiation* (sometimes termed *facilitation*).
- Neuromuscular block is *potentiated* by the administration of an anticholinesterase such as neostigmine or edrophonium.
- If repeated doses of succinylcholine are given, the characteristics of this depolarizing block alter; signs typical of a non-depolarizing block develop (see below). Initially, such changes are demonstrable only at fast rates of stimulation, but with further increments of succinylcholine they may occur at slower rates. This phenomenon is termed 'dual block'.
- Muscle fasciculation is typical of a depolarizing block.

Decamethonium

This depolarizing neuromuscular blocking agent has as rapid an onset of action as succinylcholine, but a longer duration of effect (about 20 min), as it is not metabolized by plasma cholinesterase, but mainly excreted unchanged through the kidney. It is prone to produce *tachyphylaxis* – a rapid increase in the dose required incrementally to produce the same effect – which, together with its route of excretion, limit its use. It is no longer available for clinical use.

NON-DEPOLARIZING NEUROMUSCULAR BLOCKING AGENTS

Unlike succinylcholine, these drugs do not alter the structural conformity of the postsynaptic acetylcholine receptor and therefore do not produce an initial contraction. Instead, they compete with the neurotransmitter at this site, reversibly binding to one or two of the α-receptors, whenever these are not occupied by acetylcholine. The end-plate potential produced in the presence of a non-depolarizing agent is therefore smaller; it does not reach the threshold necessary to fire off a propagating action potential to activate the sarcolemma and produce an initial muscle contraction. Over 75% of the postsynaptic receptors have to be blocked in this way before there is a failure of muscle contraction – a large safety factor. However, in large doses, non-depolarizing muscle relaxants impair neuromuscular transmission sufficiently to produce profound neuromuscular block.

No metabolism of any neuromuscular blocking agent is thought to occur at the neuromuscular junction. By the end of surgery, the end-plate concentration of the relaxant is decreasing as the drug diffuses down a concentration gradient into the plasma, from which it is cleared. Thus more receptors are stimulated by the neurotransmitter, allowing recovery from block. An anticholinesterase given at this time increases the half-life of acetylcholine at the neuromuscular junction, facilitating recovery.

Non-depolarizing muscle relaxants are highly ionized, water-soluble drugs, which are distributed mainly in plasma and extracellular fluid. Thus they have a relatively small volume of distribution. They are of two main types of chemical structure: either *benzylisoquinolinium compounds*, such as tubocurarine, alcuronium, atracurium, mivacurium and cisatracurium, or *aminosteroid compounds*, such as pancuronium, vecuronium, pipecuronium, rocuronium and rapacuronium (Org 9487). All

Table 19.1 Time to 95% depression of the twitch response, after a dose of 2 × ED_{95} of a neuromuscular blocking drug (when tracheal intubation should be possible), and time to 20–25% recovery, when an anticholinesterase can be used reliably to reverse residual block produced by a non-depolarizing drug

	95% twitch depression (s)	20–25% recovery (min)
Succinylcholine	60	10
Tubocurarine	220	80+
Alcuronium	420	70
Gallamine	300	80
Atracurium	110	43
Doxacurium	250	83
Mivacurium	170	16
Pancuronium	220	75
Vecuronium	180	33
Pipecuronium	300	95
Rocuronium	75	33
Cisatracurium	150	45
Rapacuronium	<75	15

these drugs possess at least one quaternary ammonium group $N^+(CH_3)_3$, to bind to an α subunit on the postsynaptic receptor. Their structural type determines many of their chemical properties. Some benzylisoquinolinium compounds consist of quaternary ammonium groups joined by a thin chain of methyl groups. They are therefore more liable to some breakdown in the plasma than are the aminosteroids. They are also more likely to release histamine.

Non-depolarizing muscle relaxants are usually administered in multiples of the effective dose (ED) required to produce 95% neuromuscular block (ED_{95}). A dose of at least 2 × ED_{95} is required to produce adequate conditions for reliable tracheal intubation in all patients.

Benzylisoquinolinium compounds

Tubocurarine chloride

This is the only naturally occurring muscle relaxant. It is derived from the bark of the South American plant *Chondrodendron tomentosum* and has been used for centuries by South American Indians as an arrow poison. It was the first non-depolarizing neuromuscular blocking agent to be used in humans, by Griffith and Johnson in Montreal, Canada, in 1942. An intubating dose is of the order of 0.5–0.6 mg kg^{-1}. It is a drug with a long onset of action and a prolonged duration of effect (Table 19.1), and its effects are potentiated by inhalation agents and prior administration of succinylcholine. It has a marked propensity to produce histamine release and thus hypotension, with possibly a compensatory tachycardia. In large doses, it may also produce ganglion blockade, which potentiates these cardiovascular effects. It is excreted unchanged through the kidney, with some biliary excretion. It is no longer available in the UK.

Alcuronium chloride

This drug is a semi-synthetic derivative of toxiferin, an alkaloid of calabash curare. It has less histamine-releasing properties, and therefore cardiovascular effect, than tubocurarine, although it may have some vagolytic effect, producing a mild tachycardia. It also has a long onset time and nearly as long a duration of effect as tubocurarine (Table 19.1). It is almost entirely excreted unchanged through the kidney. An intubating dose is of the order of 0.2–0.25 mg kg^{-1}. Before the advent of atracurium and vecuronium, this cheap agent was widely used, but now its popularity has declined and it is no longer commercially available in the UK.

Gallamine triethiodide

This synthetic substance is a trisquaternary amine. It was first used in France in 1948. An intubating dose in adults is of the order of 160 mg. It has a similar onset to, but slightly shorter duration of action than, tubocurarine, and is almost entirely excreted by the kidney. Consequently, it should not be used in patients with renal impairment. Being more lipid-soluble than bisquaternary amines, it crosses the placenta to a significant degree and should not be used in obstetric practice. Gallamine has potent vagolytic properties and produces some direct sympathomimetic stimulation. Thus, it frequently increases pulse rate and arterial pressure.

The only regular use of gallamine in the UK is as a small pretreatment dose (10 mg) prior to succinylcholine, when it seems to be more efficacious than any other non-depolarizing muscle relaxant in minimizing muscle pains.

Atracurium besylate

This drug, introduced into clinical practice in 1982, was developed by Stenlake at Strathclyde University. He recognized that quaternary ammonium compounds break down spontaneously at varying temperature and pH, a phenomenon known for over 100 years as *Hofmann degradation*. Many such substances also have neuromuscular blocking properties, and in the search for such an agent that broke down at body temperature and pH, atracurium was developed. Hofmann degradation may be considered as a 'safety net' in the sick patient with impaired liver or renal function, as atracurium will still be cleared from the body. Some renal excretion occurs in the healthy patient (10%), as does ester hydrolysis in the plasma; probably only about 45% of the drug is eliminated by Hofmann degradation in the normal patient.

Atracurium (and vecuronium) was developed in an attempt to obtain a non-depolarizing agent which had a more rapid onset, was shorter-acting and had less cardiovascular effects than did the older agents. Atracurium (0.5 mg kg^{-1}) does not produce neuromuscular block as rapidly as succinylcholine; onset time is 2.0–2.5 min, depending on the dose used (Table 19.1). However, it produces more rapid recovery than the older non-depolarizing agents and may easily be reversed 20–25 min after administration of a dose of 2 × ED_{95} (0.45 mg kg^{-1}). The drug does not have any direct cardiovascular effect, but may release histamine (about a third of that released by tubocurarine) and may therefore produce a local wheal and flare around the injection site, especially if a small vein is used. This may be accompanied by a slight fall in arterial pressure.

A metabolite of Hofmann degradation, *laudanosine*, has epileptogenic properties, although this complication has never been reported in humans. The plasma levels of laudanosine required to make animals convulse are much higher than those reached during general anaesthesia, even if large doses of atracurium are given during a prolonged procedure, and there is little cause for concern about this metabolite in clinical practice. In patients in the ITU with multiple organ failure, who may receive atracurium for several days, laudanosine levels are higher, but as yet no reports have occurred of cerebral toxicity.

Cisatracurium

This is the most recently introduced benzylisoquinolinium neuromuscular blocker. It is of particular interest because it is an example of the development of a specific isomer of a drug to produce a 'clean' substance with the desired clinical actions but with reduced side-effects. Cisatracurium is the 1R-*cis* 1′R-*cis* isomer of atracurium, and one of the 10 possible isomers of the parent compound. It is three to four times more potent than atracurium (ED_{95} = 0.05 mg kg^{-1}) and has a slightly longer onset and duration of action. Its main advantage is that it does not release histamine and therefore is associated with greater cardiovascular stability. It undergoes even more Hofmann degradation than atracurium. As a lower dose of this more potent drug is given, it produces less laudanosine than an equipotent dose of atracurium.

It is therefore particularly useful in the critically ill patient requiring prolonged infusion of a neuromuscular blocking drug.

Doxacurium chloride

This bisquaternary ammonium compound is available in the USA, but it is doubtful if it will be launched in the UK. It undergoes a small amount of metabolism in the plasma by cholinesterase (6%), but is excreted mainly through the kidney. It is the most potent non-depolarizing neuromuscular blocking agent available; an intubating dose is only 0.05 mg kg^{-1}. It has a very long onset of action (Table 19.1) and a prolonged and unpredictable duration of effect. However, it has no cardiovascular effects and may therefore be of use during long surgical procedures in which cardiovascular stability is required, e.g. cardiac surgery.

Mivacurium chloride

This drug is metabolized by plasma cholinesterase at 88% of the rate of succinylcholine. An intubating dose ($2 \times ED_{95} = 0.15$ mg kg^{-1}) has a similar onset of action to an equipotent dose of atracurium, but in the presence of normal plasma cholinesterase, recovery after mivacurium is much faster (Table 19.1) and administration of an anticholinesterase may not be necessary (if neuromuscular function is being monitored and good recovery can be demonstrated). Full recovery in such circumstances takes about 20–25 min, but the drug may be antagonized easily within 15 min. Mivacurium is useful particularly for surgical procedures requiring muscle relaxation in which even atracurium and vecuronium seem too long-acting, and when it is desirable to avoid the side-effects of succinylcholine, e.g. for bronchoscopy, oesophagoscopy, laparoscopy or tonsillectomy. The drug produces a similar amount of histamine release as does atracurium.

In the presence of reduced plasma cholinesterase activity, because of either inherited or acquired factors, the duration of action of mivacurium may be increased. In patients heterozygous for the atypical cholinesterase gene, the duration of action of mivacurium is comparable to that of atracurium, negating its advantages. The action of the drug may also be prolonged in patients with hepatic and renal disease.

Aminosteroid compounds

This group of non-depolarizing neuromuscular blocking agents all possess at least one quaternary ammonium group, attached to a steroid nucleus. They produce fewer adverse cardiovascular effects than do the benzylisoquinolinium compounds and do not stimulate histamine release from mast cells to the same degree. They are excreted unchanged through the kidney and also undergo deacetylation in the liver. The deacetylated metabolites may possess weak neuromuscular blocking properties. The parent compound may also be excreted unchanged in the bile.

Pancuronium bromide

This bisquaternary amine, the first steroid muscle relaxant used clinically, was developed by Savege and Hewitt in the Organon laboratories and marketed in 1964. The intubating dose is 0.1 mg kg^{-1}, which takes 3–4 min to reach its maximum effect (Table 19.1). The clinical duration of action of the drug is long, especially in the presence of potent inhalation agents or renal dysfunction, as 60% of a dose of the drug is excreted unchanged through the kidney. It is also deacetylated in the liver; some of the metabolites have neuromuscular blocking properties.

Pancuronium does not stimulate histamine release and is therefore of use in patients with a history of allergy. However, it has direct vagolytic and sympathomimetic effects which may cause tachycardia and hypertension. It slightly inhibits plasma cholinesterase and therefore potentiates any drug metabolized by this enzyme, e.g. succinylcholine and mivacurium.

Vecuronium bromide

This steroidal agent was developed in an attempt to reduce the cardiovascular effects of pancuronium. It is very similar in structure to the older drug, differing only in the loss of a methyl group from one quaternary ammonium radical. Thus it is a monoquaternary amine. An intubating dose of 0.1 mg kg^{-1} produces profound neuromuscular block within 3 min, which is slightly longer than the onset time of atracurium, but shorter than tubocurarine and pancuronium. This dose produces clinical block for about 30 min. Vecuronium rarely produces histamine release, nor does it have any direct cardiovascular effects, although it allows the cardiac effects of other anaesthetic agents, such as bradycardia produced by the opioids, to go unchallenged. Vecuronium is excreted through the kidney (30%), although to a lesser extent than pancuronium, and undergoes hepatic deacetylation; repeated doses should be used with care in patients with renal or hepatic disease.

Pipecuronium bromide

This analogue of pancuronium was developed in Hungary in 1980 and is now marketed in Eastern Europe and the USA. An intubating dose is 0.07 mg kg^{-1}. The onset time and time to recovery from block are similar to those of pancuronium (Table 19.1), and excretion of the drug through the kidney is significant (66%). In contrast to pancuronium, pipecuronium produces marked cardiovascular stability, having no vagolytic or sympathomimetic effects. It may therefore be of use during major surgery in patients with cardiac disease.

Rocuronium bromide

This monoquaternary amine has a very rapid onset of action for a non-depolarizing muscle relaxant. It is six to eight times less potent than vecuronium but has approximately the same molecular weight; consequently, a greater number of drug molecules may reach the postjunctional receptors within the first few circulations, enabling faster development of neuromuscular block. In a dose of 0.6 mg kg^{-1}, good or excellent intubating conditions are usually achieved within 60–90 s; this is only slightly slower than the onset time of succinylcholine. The clinical duration is 30–45 min.

In most other respects, rocuronium resembles vecuronium. The drug stimulates little histamine release or cardiovascular disturbance, although in high doses it has a mild vagolytic property which sometimes results in an increase in heart rate. The drug is excreted unchanged in the urine and in the bile, and thus the duration of action may be increased by severe renal or hepatic dysfunction.

Rapacuronium bromide (Org 9487)

This is the latest aminosteroid to become available. It is even less potent than rocuronium ($2 \times ED_{90} = 1.15$ mg kg^{-1}) and in equipotent doses may have an even more rapid onset of action (<75 s). It is rapidly cleared from the plasma by hepatic uptake and deacetylation and thus has a shorter duration of effect than rocuronium of 12–15 min (Table 19.1). As with the deacetylation of vecuronium, a metabolite of rapacuronium has neuromuscular blocking properties (Org 9488). This may prolong the effect of incremental doses of the drug.

Rapacuronium has similar cardiovascular effects to rocuronium but it may also produce bronchospasm, possibly because of the release of histamine or leukotrienes. It is supplied as a powder to be made up into a solution immediately before use.

Factors affecting duration of non-depolarizing neuromuscular block

The duration of action of non-depolarizing muscle relaxants is affected by a number of factors. Effects are most marked with the longer-acting agents, such as tubocurarine and pancuronium.

Prior administration of succinylcholine potentiates the effect and lengthens the duration of action of non-depolarizing drugs.

Concomitant administration of a potent inhalation agent increases the duration of block. This is most marked with the ether anaesthetic agents such as isoflurane, enflurane and sevoflurane, but occurs to a lesser extent with halothane.

pH changes. Metabolic and, to a lesser extent, respiratory acidosis extend the duration of block. With monoquaternary amines such as tubocurarine and vecuronium, this effect is produced probably by the ionization, under acidic conditions, of a second nitrogen atom in the molecule, making the drug more potent.

Body temperature. Hypothermia potentiates block as impairment of organ function delays metabolism and excretion of these drugs. This may occur in patients undergoing cardiac surgery; reduced doses of muscle relaxants are required during cardiopulmonary bypass.

Age. Non-depolarizing muscle relaxants which depend on organ metabolism and excretion may be expected to have a prolonged effect in old age, as organ function deteriorates. In healthy neonates, who have a higher extracellular volume than adults, resistance may occur, but if the baby is sick or immature then, because of underdevelopment of the neuromuscular junction and other organ function, increased sensitivity may be encountered. Children of school age tend to be relatively resistant to non-depolarizing muscle relaxants, when given on a weight basis.

Electrolyte changes. A low serum potassium concentration potentiates neuromuscular block by changing the value of the resting membrane potential of the postsynaptic membrane. A reduced ionized calcium concentration also potentiates block by impairing presynaptic acetylcholine release.

Myasthenia gravis. In this disease, the number and half-life of the postsynaptic receptors are reduced by autoantibodies produced in the thymus gland. Thus, the patient is more sensitive to the effects of non-depolarizing muscle relaxants. Resistance to succinylcholine may be encountered.

Other disease states. Because of the altered pharmacokinetics of muscle relaxants in hepatic and renal disease, prolongation of action may be found in these conditions, especially if excretion of the drug is dependent upon these organs.

Characteristics of non-depolarizing neuromuscular block

If a small, subparalysing dose of a non-depolarizing neuromuscular blocking drug is administered, the following characteristics are recognized:

- A decreased response to a low-voltage twitch stimulus (e.g. 1 Hz) which, if repeated, decreases further in amplitude. This effect, which is in contrast to that produced by a depolarizing drug, also occurs to a greater degree when the train-of-four twitch response is applied, and with higher, tetanic rates of stimulation. It is often referred to as 'fade' or decrement.
- Post-tetanic potentiation (PTP) or facilitation (PTF) of the twitch response may be demonstrated (see Fig. 19.6).
- Neuromuscular block is reversed by the administration of an anticholinesterase.
- No muscle fasciculation is visible.

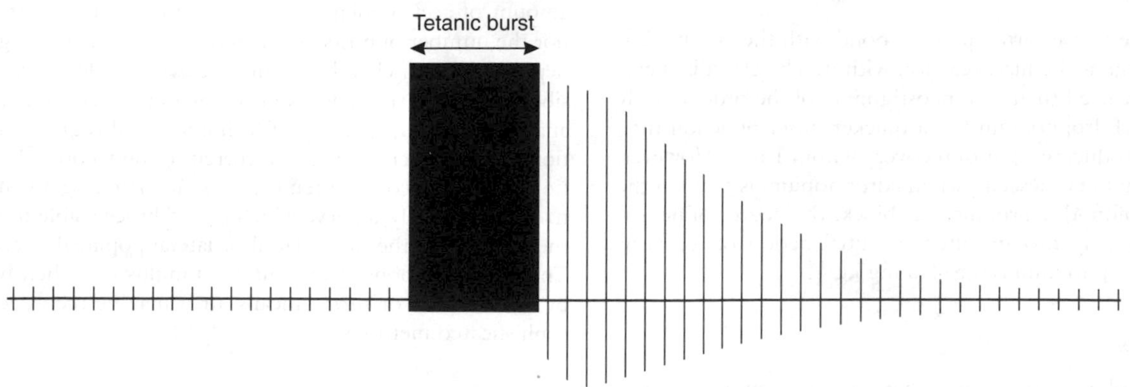

Fig. 19.6
A 5-s burst of tetanus (50 Hz), applied after a run of single twitch stimuli, causes a transient increase in the height of subsequent twitches, although they gradually decrease to their former height; this is post-tetanic potentiation (PTP) or facilitation (PTF).

ANTICHOLINESTERASES

These agents are used in clinical practice to inhibit the action of acetylcholinesterase at the neuromuscular junction, thus prolonging the half-life of acetylcholine and potentiating its effect, especially in the presence of residual amounts of non-depolarizing muscle relaxant at the end of surgery. The most commonly used anticholinesterase during anaesthesia is neostigmine, but edrophonium and pyridostigmine are also available. These carbamate esters are water-soluble, quaternary ammonium compounds which are poorly absorbed from the gastrointestinal tract. The more lipid-soluble tertiary amine, physostigmine, has a similar effect and is more suitable for oral administration, but crosses the blood–brain barrier.

Organophosphorus compounds also inhibit acetylcholinesterase, but unlike other agents, their effect is irreversible; recovery occurs only on generation of more enzyme, which takes some weeks.

Anticholinesterases are also given orally to patients with *myasthenia gravis*. In this disease, the patient possesses antibodies to the postsynaptic nicotinic receptor, reducing the efficacy of acetylcholine. The use of these drugs is thought to increase the amount and duration of action of acetylcholine at the neuromuscular junction, thus enhancing neuromuscular transmission.

Neostigmine

This drug combines reversibly with acetylcholinesterase by the formation of an ester linkage, which lasts about 30 min. Neostigmine is excreted largely unchanged through the kidney and has a half-life of about 45 min. It is presented in brown vials, as it breaks down on exposure to light. Neostigmine potentiates the action of acetylcholine wherever it is a neurotransmitter, including all cholinergic nerve endings; thus it produces bradycardia, salivation, sweating, bronchospasm, increased intestinal motility and blurred vision. These cholinergic effects may be reduced by the simultaneous administration of an anticholinergic agent such as atropine or glycopyrrolate. The usual dose of neostigmine is of the order of 0.035 mg kg^{-1}, in combination with either atropine 0.015 mg kg^{-1} or glycopyrrolate 0.01 mg kg^{-1}. Neostigmine takes at least 2 min to have an initial effect, and recovery from neuromuscular block is maximally enhanced by 5–7 min.

Edrophonium

This anticholinesterase forms an ionic bond with the enzyme but does not undergo a chemical reaction with it. The effect is therefore more short-lived than with neostigmine, of the order of only a few minutes. Edrophonium has a quicker onset of action than neostigmine, producing signs of recovery within 1 min. However, its effects are more evanescent; when edrophonium is given in the presence of profound neuromuscular block, the degree of neuromuscular block may *increase* after an initial period of recovery. The dose of edrophonium is 0.5–1.0 mg kg^{-1}.

Pyridostigmine

This drug has a longer onset time than neostigmine or edrophonium, and also a longer duration of action. It is used more frequently as oral therapy in patients with myasthenia gravis than in anaesthesia.

Physostigmine

This anticholinesterase, also known as *eserine*, is a tertiary amine and is more lipid-soluble than the other carbamate esters. It is therefore more easily absorbed from the gastrointestinal tract, and also crosses the blood–brain barrier.

Organophosphorus compounds

These substances are considered to be irreversible inhibitors of acetylcholinesterase, as by phosphorylation of the enzyme they produce a very stable complex which is resistant to reactivation or hydrolysis. Synthesis of new enzyme must occur before recovery. These agents, which include di-isopropylfluorophosphonate (DFP) and tetraethylpyrophosphate (TEPP), are used as insecticides and chemical warfare agents. They are readily absorbed through the lungs and skin. Poisoning is not uncommon among farm workers. Muscarinic effects, such as salivation, sweating and bronchospasm, are combined with nicotinic effects, such as muscle weakness. Central nervous effects such as tremor and convulsions may occur, as may unconsciousness and respiratory failure. Reactivators of acetylcholinesterase are used to treat this form of poisoning; they include *pralidoxime* and *obidoxime*. Atropine, anticonvulsants and artificial ventilation may be necessary. Chronic exposure may produce a polyneuritis. Carbamates such as pyridostigmine are used prophylactically in those threatened by chemical warfare with these compounds.

Ecothiopate is an organophosphorus compound with a quaternary amine group; it was used as an eye drop preparation in ophthalmology to produce miosis in narrow-angle glaucoma. It inhibits cholinesterase by phosphorylation and thus potentiates all esters metabolized by this enzyme. It has now been withdrawn from the UK market.

A new generation of organophosphorus compounds may be beneficial in Alzheimer's disease, and clinical trials are in progress. Neuromuscular blockers must be used with caution if such patients require anaesthesia.

NEUROMUSCULAR MONITORING

There is no clinical tool available to measure accurately neuromuscular transmission in a muscle group. Thus, neither the amount of acetylcholine released in response to a given stimulus nor the number of postsynaptic receptors blocked by a given non-depolarizing muscle relaxant may be assessed. However, it is possible to obtain a crude estimate of muscle contraction during anaesthesia using a variety of techniques. All require the application to a peripheral nerve of a current of up to 60 mA, for a fraction of a millisecond (often 0.2 ms), necessitating a voltage of up to 300 V. Usually, a nerve which is readily accessible to the anaesthetist, such as the ulnar, facial or lateral popliteal nerve, is used. The muscle response to the nerve stimulus may then be assessed by either *visual* or *tactile* means, or it may be recorded by more sophisticated methods.

Mechanomyography

A strain-gauge transducer may be used to measure the force of contraction of, for instance, the thumb, in response to stimulation

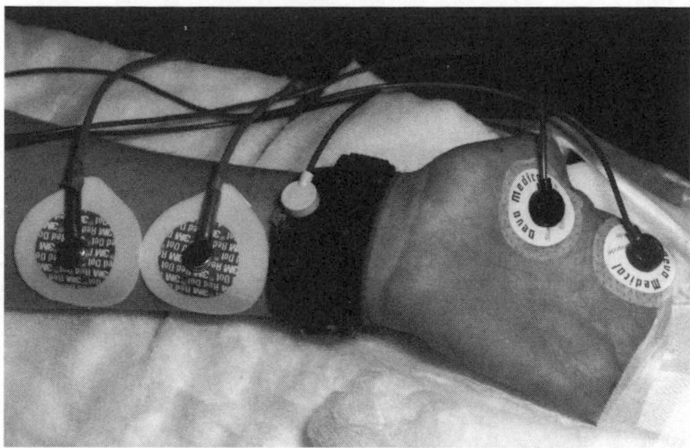

Fig. 19.7
The necessary positioning of the hand to obtain an electromyographic recording of the response of the adductor pollicis muscle to stimulation of the ulnar nerve is demonstrated. An earth electrode is placed round the wrist. Two recording electrodes are placed over the muscle on the hand; the distal one lies over the motor point.

of the ulnar nerve at the wrist. This measurement may then be charted using a recording device. Accurate measurements of the twitch or tetanic response may be made, although the hand must be splinted firmly for reproducible results. This technique is primarily a research tool.

Electromyography

The electromyographic response of a muscle is measured in response to the same electrical stimulus, using recording electrodes similar to ECG pads placed over the motor point of the stimulated muscle. For instance, if the ulnar nerve is stimulated, the recording electrodes are placed over the motor point of adductor pollicis in the thumb (Fig. 19.7). A compound muscle action potential may be recorded. Although primarily a research tool, there are now several simple clinical instruments, such as the Datex Relaxograph, which give a less accurate, but similar recording. Maintaining the exact position of the hand is not as essential with electromyography as with mechanomyography.

Accelerography

With this technique, the acceleration of the thumb is measured in response to the nerve stimulus and the force of contraction may be derived (force = mass × acceleration). Clinical equipment is available (e.g. the accelerograph) which provides a quantitative assessment of, for instance, the twitch height in comparison with a control reading.

MODES OF STIMULATION

Several different rates of stimulation can be applied to the nerve in an attempt to produce a sensitive index of neuromuscular function. It is considered essential always to apply a *supramaximal* stimulus to the nerve, i.e. the strength of the electrical stimulus (V) should be increased until the response no longer increases. It is then increased by a further 25%.

Twitch

A square-wave stimulus of short duration (0.1–0.2 ms) is applied to a peripheral nerve. In isolation, such a stimulus is of limited value, although if applied repeatedly, perhaps before and after a dose of a muscle relaxant, it may be possible to assess crudely the effects of the drug. Such rates of stimulation have the benefit of being less painful, with no untoward effects after recovery from anaesthesia.

Train-of-four twitch response

In an attempt to assess the degree of neuromuscular block clinically, Ali et al (1971) described a development of the twitch response which, it was hoped, would be more sensitive than repeated single twitches. Four stimuli, (at 2 Hz), are applied over 2 s, with a 10-s gap between each train-of-four. On administration of a small dose of a non-depolarizing muscle relaxant, *fade* of the amplitude of the train-of-four may be visible. The ratio of the amplitude of the fourth to the first twitch is called the *train-of-four ratio*. In the presence of a larger dose of such a drug, the fourth twitch disappears first, then the third, followed by the second and, finally, the first twitch (Fig. 19.8A). On recovery from neuromuscular block, the first twitch appears first, then the second (when the first twitch has recovered to about 20% control), then the third, and finally the fourth (Fig. 19.8B).

It is generally thought that at least three of the four twitches must be absent to obtain adequate surgical access for upper abdominal surgery. It is also preferable to reverse residual block with an anticholinesterase only when the second twitch is visible, if good recovery is to be relied upon. After reversal, good muscle tone – as assessed clinically by the patient being able to cough, raise his or her head from the pillow for at least 5 s, protrude the tongue and have good grip strength – may be anticipated when the train-of-four ratio has reached at least 0.7.

It is recognized that, although the number of twitches present in the train-of-four during profound neuromuscular block is easily counted by visual or tactile means, it is impossible, even for the expert, to assess the value of the train-of-four ratio by these methods. In addition, visual or tactile evaluation fails to detect any fade of the train-of-four when the ratio is in excess of 50%. Thus, failure to detect fade with a nerve stimulator does not always guarantee adequate reversal. A recording of the response is preferable.

Tetanic stimulation

This is the most sensitive form of neuromuscular stimulation. Frequencies of 50–100 Hz are applied to a peripheral nerve to detect even minor degrees of residual neuromuscular block; thus, tetanic fade may be present when the twitch response is normal. Tetanic rates of stimulation may be applied under anaesthesia, but in the awake patient they are intolerable. Indeed, on recovery from anaesthesia in which tetanic stimulation has been applied, the patient may be aware of some discomfort in the area of application.

Post-tetanic potentiation or facilitation

This method of monitoring was developed in an attempt to assess more profound degrees of neuromuscular block produced by non-depolarizing neuromuscular blocking agents. If a single

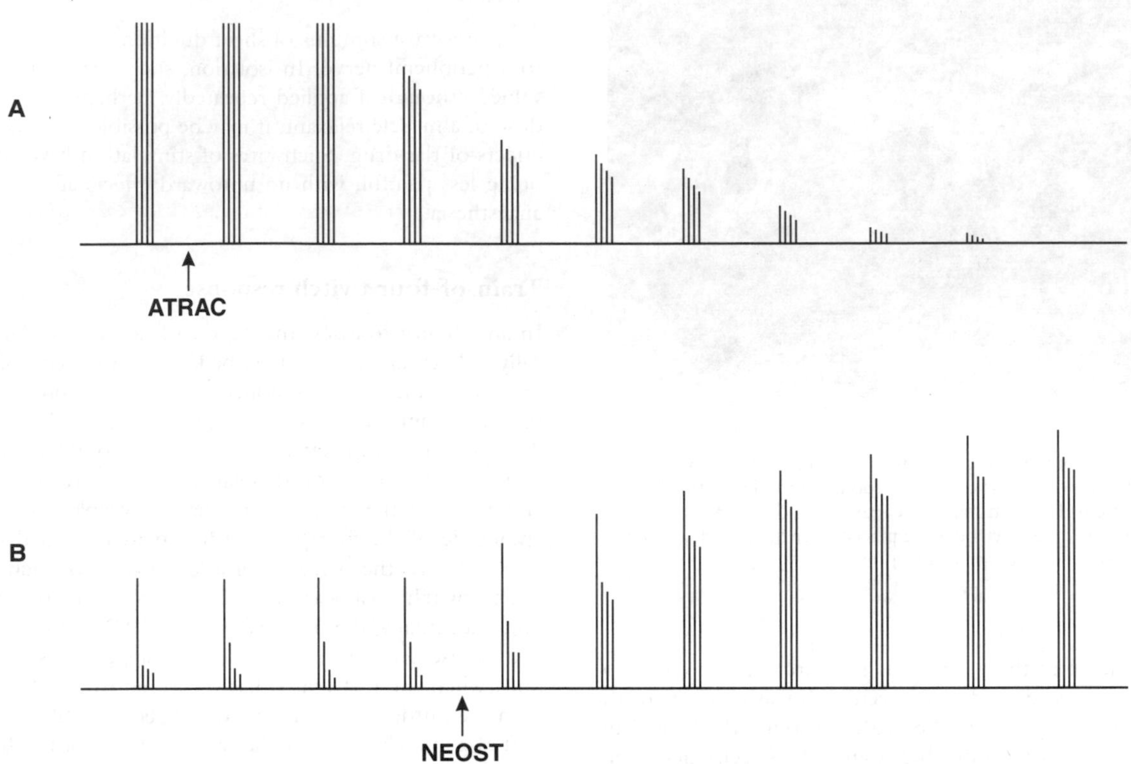

Fig. 19.8
A. After the administration of a non-depolarizing muscle relaxant (in this instance atracurium 0.5 mg kg^{-1}), the decrease in height of the fourth twitch of the train-of-four response is more marked than the decrease in height of the third twitch, which is more marked than the decrease in the second, which is greater than the decrease in the first. The effect is known as 'fade'. Within 2 min, the train-of-four response has been ablated completely. **B.** On recovery, the first twitch response appears first, then the second, the third and finally the fourth. Marked fade is present, but on adminisration of an anticholinesterase, (neostigmine, NEOST recovery) of all four twitches occurs rapidly.

twitch stimulus is applied to the nerve with little or no neuromuscular response, but after a 5 s delay a burst of 50 Hz tetanus is given for 5 s, the effect of a further twitch stimulus 3 s later produces an enhanced effect (Fig. 19.6). In the presence of profound block, repeated single twitches applied after the tetanus until the response disappears can be counted; this is termed the *post-tetanic count.* The augmentation of the twitch is thought to be due to presynaptic mobilization of acetylcholine, as a result of the positive feedback effect of the run of tetanus.

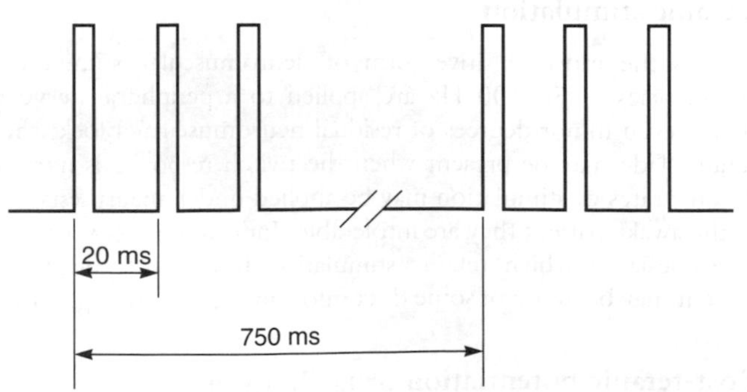

Fig. 19.9
The pattern of double-burst stimulation. Three bursts of 50 Hz tetanus, at 20 ms intervals, every 750 ms are shown.

Double-burst stimulation (DBS)

In an attempt to develop a clinical tool which would allow more accurate assessment by visual or tactile means of the fade of the twitch response after administration of a non-depolarizing drug, Viby-Mogensen suggested the application of two or three short bursts of 50 Hz tetanus, each comprising two or three impulses separated by a 750 ms interval. Each square wave impulse lasts for 0.2 ms (Fig. 19.9). If records of the fade of the DBS and the train-of-four response are compared, they are very similar, but there is evidence to suggest that visual assessment of the DBS is more accurate.

INDICATIONS FOR NEUROMUSCULAR MONITORING

It is preferable always to monitor neuromuscular function when a muscle relaxant is used during anaesthesia, but it is especially indicated in the following circumstances:

- during prolonged anaesthesia, when repeated increments of neuromuscular blocking agents are required
- when infusions of muscle relaxants are given (including in the ITU)
- in the presence of renal or hepatic dysfunction
- in patients with neuromuscular disorders
- in patients with a history of sensitivity to a muscle relaxant or poor recovery from block
- when poor reversal of neuromuscular block is encountered unexpectedly.

FURTHER READING

Ali H H, Utting J E, Gray T C 1971 Quantitative assessment of residual antidepolarising block (Part II). British Journal of Anaesthesia 43: 478–484

Beecher H K, Todd D P 1954 A study of the deaths associated with anaesthesia and surgery. Annals of Surgery 140: 2–34

Bevan D R, Bevan J C, Donati F 1988 Muscle relaxants in clinical anesthesia. Year Book Medical Publishers, Chicago

Bowman W C 1992 Pharmacology of neuromuscular function. John Wright, Bristol

Gray T C, Halton J 1946 A milestone in anaesthesia? (d-tubocurarine chloride). Proceedings of the Royal Society of Medicine 39: 400–410

Hunter J M 1995 New neuromuscular blocking drugs. New England Journal of Medicine 332: 1691–1699

Kalow W, Genest K 1957 A method of detection of atypical forms of human pseudocholinesterase. Canadian Journal of Biochemistry and Physiology 35: 339–346

Paton W D M 1959 The effects of muscle relaxants other than muscle relaxation. Anesthesiology 29: 453–463

Viby-Mogensen J 1982 Clinical assessment of neuromuscular transmission. British Journal of Anaesthesia 54: 209–223

20 Gastrointestinal physiology

The extraction of water and nutrients from food and its absorption comprise the primary function of the gastrointestinal (GI) tract. This depends upon a variety of mechanisms that soften the food, propel it through the GI tract and expose it to bile and digestive enzymes. The digested contents of the GI tract are absorbed by the intestinal mucosa into the portal circulation. Both chemical and physical factors are important in digestion. Prior to swallowing, food is chewed and mixed with salivary amylase. It is softened further and broken down by muscular contractions of the stomach wall and by the action of gastric acid and enzymes to produce a liquefied residue termed chyme which is ejected through the pylorus into the duodenum where it is mixed thoroughly with biliary and pancreatic secretions, aided again by gut wall contractions. Eventually, the products of digestion are exposed to the enormous absorptivesurface area of the small intestine. Undigested matter is passed on to the colon and expelled by defaecation. This complex process is controlled by neural and hormonal processes.

ANATOMY

The GI tract extends from the posterior pharynx to the anus and is basically a muscular tube of three layers (two longitudinal, one circular) lined with epithelial mucosa. The mesentery contains nerves, lymphatics and blood vessels (Fig. 20.1).

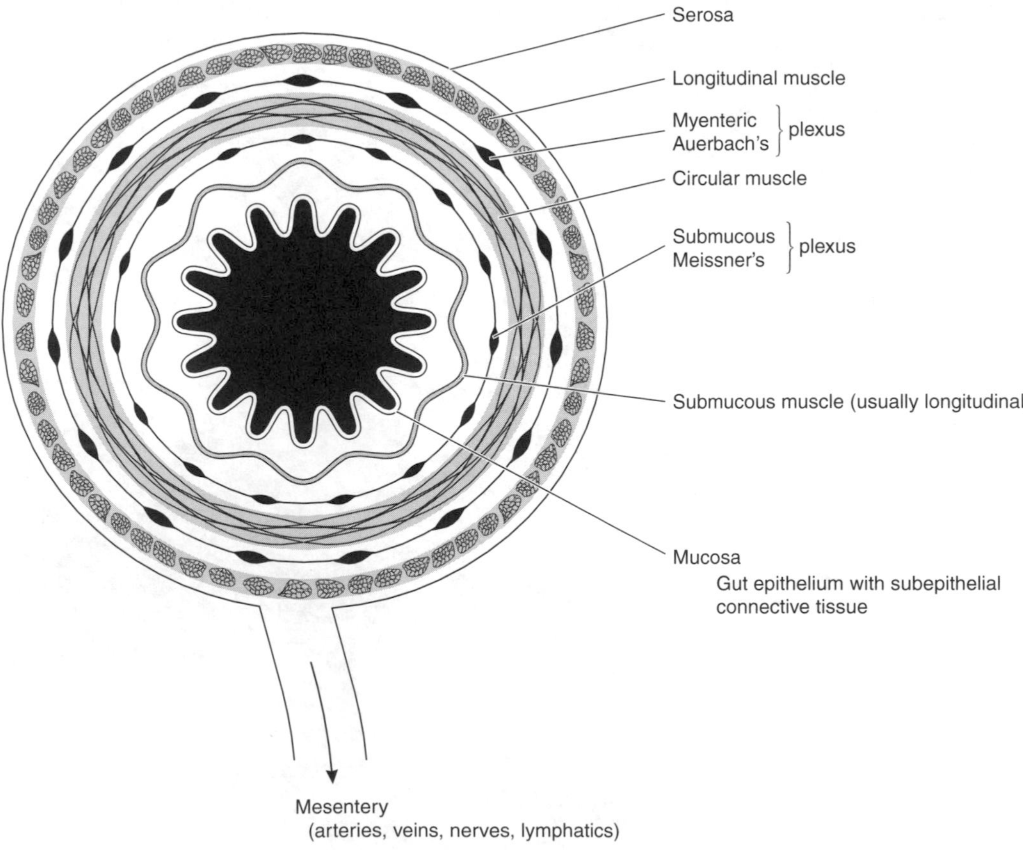

Fig. 20.1
Layers of the gastrointestinal tract.

The GI tract is divided into four distinct regions: oesophagus, stomach, small intestine (duodenum, jejunum, ileum) and large intestine (caecum, colon, rectum). Blood from the GI tract drains via the portal vein to the liver.

REGULATION OF GI FUNCTION

The function of the GI tract is coordinated by a complex interplay between the autonomic nervous system (neurocrine secretion), paracrine secretion and endocrine (hormonal) activity.

INNERVATION

Autonomic nervous system

The GI tract is innervated by the sympathetic and parasympathetic nervous systems. Preganglionic parasympathetic cholinergic activity generally increases activity of intestinal smooth muscle. Postganglionic noradrenergic sympathetic fibres decrease activity but enhance sphincter contraction.

Enteric nervous system

Two major intrinsic networks of nerve fibres constitute the enteric nervous system (ENS) of the GI tract. The myenteric (Auerbach's) plexus lies between the outer longitudinal and middle circular muscle layers and the submucous (Meissner's) plexus between the middle circular layer and the mucosa (Fig. 20.1). The ENS is concerned with the regulation of GI function and is linked to the central nervous system by the autonomic nervous system. However, the ENS may function without external innervation. The myenteric plexus innervates the longitudinal and circular smooth muscle layers and is concerned primarily with motor control. The submucosal plexus innervates the glandular epithelium, intestinal endocrine cells and submucosal blood vessels. It is most developed in the small intestine where it is involved in secretory control.

Activity in the ENS results in the release of neurotransmitters (neurocrines) which have effects on other nerve, smooth muscle, paracrine and endocrine cells. More than 20 neurotransmitters have been identified in the ENS (Table 20.1). Acetylcholine (ACh) and tachykinins (e.g. substance P) cause smooth muscle contraction. Vasoactive intestinal peptide (VIP), nitric oxide (NO) and adenosine triphosphate (ATP) relax smooth muscle. Stimulation of the mucosa releases 5-hydroxytryptamine (5-HT) which is involved in the initiation of the peristaltic reflex. Other neuropeptides found in the ENS include somatostatin, histamine, cholecystokinin and gastrin-releasing peptide. Some of these peptides also act in a paracrine fashion and some enter the bloodstream as hormones.

PARACRINES

Paracrines are chemicals that diffuse through interstitial fluid, exerting an effect close to their site of release (Table 20.1). Although paracrines have local direct actions only, the overall effect may be widespread because of the extensive distribution of cells from which they are produced or because they influence the release of gut hormones from endocrine cells. Histamine and somatostatin are

Table 20.1 Physiological actions of neurotransmitters, paracrines and hormones in the GI tract

	Physiological functions
Neurotransmitters	
5-Hydroxytryptamine	Peristalsis, emesis
Acetylcholine	Peristalsis, smooth muscle contraction
Adenosine triphosphate	Peristalsis, smooth muscle relaxation
Gastrin-releasing peptide	Gastrin secretion
Nitric oxide	Peristalsis, smooth muscle relaxation
Somatostatin	Inhibition of GI hormone release and gland secretions
Substance P	Peristalsis, smooth muscle contraction
Vasoactive intestinal peptide (VIP)	Peristalsis, smooth muscle relaxation Relaxation of sphincters
Paracrines	
Histamine	Gastric acid secretion
Somatostatin	Inhibition of GI hormone release and gland secretions
GI hormones	
Gastrin	Gastric acid and pepsin secretion Mucosal trophic action
Cholecystokinin (CCK)	Pancreatic and gall bladder secretion Inhibition of gastric emptying Pancreatic trophic action
Secretin	Stimulation of pepsin, pancreatic and biliary alkali Exocrine pancreatic trophic action Inhibition of gastric acid
Gastric inhibitory peptide (GIP)	Insulin release Inhibition of gastric acid
Motilin	Migrating motor complex

important gut paracrines. Enterochromaffin-like (ECL) cells secrete histamine which is involved in the control of gastric acid secretion. Somatostatin is found throughout the gastric and duodenal mucosa and in the pancreas. It reduces secretions by exerting an inhibitory effect on GI hormones and parietal cells.

HORMONES

Gastrointestinal hormones are released from endocrine cells into the bloodstream and exert their actions at remote sites by means of receptor interaction in a target tissue. On the basis of structure and function, many hormones may be classified into one of two groups: gastrin family (e.g. gastrin, cholecystokinin [CCK]) or secretin family (e.g. secretin, glucagon, VIP, gastric inhibitory peptide [GIP]). Endocrine cells are distributed widely throughout the GI mucosa.

Gastrin

Gastrin is produced by G cells located in the gastric antral mucosa. G cells contain gastrin granules and are flask-shaped with a broad base and a narrow apex that reaches the mucosal surface. Receptors are present on the microvilli which project from the apex into the lumen. Other hormone-secreting cells in the GI tract have a similar morphology. Gastrin-secreting tumours (gastrinomas) occur in the pancreas, but it is uncertain if any gastrin is present in the pancreas in normal adults, although it is present in the fetus.

Stimulation of gastric acid and pepsin secretion is the primary purpose of gastrin. Gastric distension, intragastric products of protein digestion and vagal stimulation cause gastrin release (Table 20.2). Luminal acid inhibits gastrin release, thus providing a negative feedback system. Vagal innervation of the G cell is unusual in that it is not cholinergic, but involves gastrin-releasing peptide (GRP).

Cholecystokinin

CCK-secreting cells are located in the small intestine, particularly the duodenum and jejunum. CCK is also present in nerves in the distal ileum and colon. It causes contraction of the gall bladder and stimulates secretions of enzymes and alkaline fluid by the exocrine pancreas. It augments the action of secretin by stimulating secretion of an alkaline pancreatic juice. CCK inhibits gastric emptying.

The main stimulus for the secretion of CCK is the presence of peptides, amino acids and fatty acids in the duodenal lumen. Bile and pancreatic juice entering the duodenum in response to CCK enhance digestion of protein and fat, thus stimulating further secretion of CCK. This positive feedback mechanism is terminated when the products of digestion move further down the GI tract.

Table 20.2 Factors affecting secretion of gastrin

Enhanced	Inhibited
Vagus nerve	Intraluminal acid
Intraluminal peptides	Somatostatin
Gastric distension	Secretin
Epinephrine	GIP
Calcium	VIP
	Calcitonin
	Glucagon

Secretin

Secretin is secreted by cells located deep in the glands of the mucosa of the proximal small intestine. It is released when the duodenal pH is < 4–5 and enhances secretion of bicarbonate by the cells of the pancreatic duct and biliary tract and augments the action of CCK (release of pancreatic enzymes). It also inhibits gastric acid secretion and may cause contraction of the pyloric sphincter. Secretion is enhanced also by the presence of intraluminal products of protein digestion and acid on the mucosa of the upper small intestine.

Gastric inhibitory peptide

Gastric inhibitory peptide is produced by cells in the mucosa of the duodenum and jejunum and its release is stimulated by carbohydrate and fat in the duodenum. It stimulates the release of insulin in preparation for absorption of carbohydrates. The name reflects the fact that, when it was discovered, it was found to inhibit gastric secretions. However, this effect is less important at physiological concentrations.

Motilin

Motilin is secreted by cells in the duodenal mucosa. It is involved in the regulation of interdigestive gut motility, preparing the intestine for the next meal. It is released in a cyclical manner during fasting with a periodicity of 1–2 h. It stimulates a burst of peristalsis (migrating motor complex) which starts in the stomach and sweeps through the small intestine, clearing it of undigested matter and other debris in preparation for the next meal.

Vasoactive intestinal peptide

Vasoactive intestinal peptide is found in GI tract nervous tissue and stimulates the intestinal secretion of electrolytes and water. Other actions include relaxation of intestinal smooth muscle (including sphincters), dilatation of peripheral blood vessels and inhibition of gastric acid secretion. Fat causes its release from the jejunum and it is an effective inhibitor of gastrin-stimulated acid secretion.

Trophic effects of GI hormones

In addition to their effects on gut motility and secretions, some GI hormones also exert important trophic effects. Gastrin is an essential factor in maintaining gastrointestinal mucosal integrity, and CCK and secretin are involved in growth of the exocrine pancreas.

PERISTALSIS

Peristalsis is a reflex response, independent of extrinsic innervation, initiated when the gut wall is stretched by intraluminal contents, resulting in a wave of muscular contraction. It occurs throughout the GI tract and allows the contents to be propelled in an anterograde manner at various rates (2–25 cm min^{-1}). The ENS (especially the myenteric plexus) is responsible for the generation of the peristaltic waves, but the autonomic nervous system modulates this activity (parasympathetic increases, sympathetic activity decreases).

Distension of the gut wall and release of 5-HT initiate the peristaltic reflex. Activity in sensory afferents stimulates cholinergic interneurones that pass both proximally and distally in the myenteric plexus. Proximally, the release of ACh and substance P from excitatory motor neurones causes contraction of circular smooth muscle. At the same time, distal smooth muscle relaxation is brought about by release of VIP, NO and ATP from inhibitory interneurones. A ring of contraction develops behind the food bolus to propel it along the lumen. The same pattern of reflex activity is then activated in a more distal segment, thus propagating the movement.

BASIC ELECTRICAL RHYTHM

Smooth muscle of the GI tract, except the oesophagus and proximal stomach, exhibits spontaneous rhythmic fluctuations in membrane potential (–65 to –45 mV). This basic electrical rhythm (BER) is initiated by stellate muscle which has similar properties to pacemaker cells. The BER rarely causes muscle contraction, but spike potentials superimposed on the most depolarizing phases of the BER waves do increase muscle tension. ACh increases spike frequency and muscle tension and epinephrine has the opposite effect. The function of the BER is to coordinate peristaltic and other motor activity, i.e. contractions occur only during the depolarizing phase of the waves.

MIGRATING MOTOR COMPLEX

During fasting, the electrical and motor activity of GI smooth muscle becomes modified so that cycles of motor activity migrate from the stomach to the distal ileum at intervals of approximately 90 min and at a speed of 5 cm min^{-1}. Each cycle, or migrating motor complex (MMC), starts with a quiescent phase (phase I), continues with a period of irregular electrical and mechanical activity (phase II) and ends with a burst of regular activity (phase III). Gastric, bile and pancreatic secretion increase during each MMC, but their precise function in this context is not known. Ingestion of food stops the generation of MMCs immediately.

MOUTH AND OESOPHAGUS

SALIVA

Salivary enzymes are contained in the secretory (zymogen) granules of the acinar cells and discharged into the ducts. Approximately 1.5 L of saliva (pH 7–8) are secreted per day. Saliva contains two digestive enzymes: lingual lipase secreted by glands on the tongue, and salivary α-amylase, secreted by the salivary glands. Saliva also contains mucins (lubrication, protection of oral mucosa), IgA, lysozyme, lactoferrin and proline-rich proteins.

Saliva performs several important functions. It facilitates swallowing, lubricates and cleans the mouth, dissolves substances which stimulate taste buds and aids speech. Buffers maintain oral pH at about 7.0 and help to neutralize regurgitated gastric acid. Saliva also has an antibacterial action and initiates carbohydrate digestion (salivary amylase).

Stimulation of the parasympathetic nerve supply causes secretion of dilute saliva. Sympathetic stimulation causes secretion of small amounts of saliva rich in organic constituents from the submandibular glands.

ANATOMY OF THE OESOPHAGUS

The oesophagus is a continuation of the pharynx. In its proximal third, it comprises striated muscle innervated by efferents from the myenteric plexus. Striated muscle is replaced gradually by smooth muscle, and at the distal third of the oesophagus, all muscle is smooth. The typical arrangement of outer longitudinal and inner circular muscle layers is present. At the pharyngo-oesophageal junction, the muscle forms the upper oesophageal sphincter (UOS). The lower oesophageal sphincter (LOS) is located at the gastro-oesophageal junction. In the resting state, both the UOS and LOS are closed, with a resting tone considerably higher than in the adjacent oesophagus.

SWALLOWING REFLEX

Swallowing is initiated by the voluntary action of collecting the contents of the mouth on the tongue and propelling them backwards into the pharynx when the reflex becomes involuntary. It is triggered by afferent impulses in the trigeminal, glossopharyngeal and vagus nerves. Integration of the reflex takes place in the nucleus ambiguus and the nucleus of the tractus solitarius with efferents via the trigeminal, facial, vagus and hypoglossal nerves. Food in the pharynx stimulates a wave of involuntary contraction in the pharyngeal muscles and relaxation of the UOS; permitting the swallowed material to enter the oesophagus. A peristaltic ring of oesophageal muscle forms behind the material, which is then swept down the oesophagus at a speed of 2–4 cm s^{-1}. Therefore, it takes approximately 10–15 s to pass through the oesophagus (length 30 cm) and enter the stomach. However, in the upright position, liquids and semisolid foods fall by gravity to the lower oesophagus ahead of the peristaltic wave. Coordinated relaxation of the UOS and LOS occurs as the food bolus passes. Any remaining food or regurgitated gastric contents stimulates secondary peristalsis.

LOWER OESOPHAGEAL SPHINCTER

Unlike the rest of the oesophagus, the musculature of the gastro-oesophageal junction or LOS has a high resting tone which relaxes upon swallowing. The tonic activity of the LOS between meals prevents reflux of gastric contents into the oesophagus. The LOS is made up of three components: oesophageal smooth muscle (intrinsic sphincter), crural skeletal muscle fibres of the diaphragm (extrinsic sphincter) and oblique fibres of the stomach wall ('flap valve' helping to close off the oesophagogastric junction when intragastric pressure increases).

Release of ACh from vagal endings causes the intrinsic sphincter to contract, and release of NO and VIP from interneurones innervated by other vagal fibres causes it to relax. Contraction of the crural portion of the diaphragm (extrinsic sphincter), which is innervated by the phrenic nerve, is coordinated with respiration and contractions of chest and abdominal muscles.

THE STOMACH

Acid, enzymes and gastric contractions liquefy food in the stomach into gastric chyme.

GASTRIC EMPTYING

The circular, longitudinal and oblique arrangement of muscle in the stomach wall is more complex than in other parts of the GI tract. Three types of motility patterns can be detected in the stomach: receptive relaxation and contraction, peristaltic propulsion and mixing, and the migrating motor complex.

During feeding, smooth muscle in the wall of the proximal stomach relaxes to accommodate the food with little increase in intragastric pressure (receptive relaxation). This is followed by contractions of low amplitude and long duration which reduce the size of the stomach as gastric emptying occurs. In the proximal stomach, food may remain undisturbed for up to an hour, enabling carbohydrate digestion to take place by salivary amylase. In the mid and distal parts of the stomach, peristalsis is more vigorous. Contractions are generated in the mid-stomach and pass distally towards the pylorus at a rate of three per minute. Propagation speed increases as the pylorus is approached when the peristaltic wave overtakes the gastric contents. This causes forward propulsion of some contents through the pylorus and backwards movement of the remainder into the body of the stomach. Vagal stimulation and gastrin increase gastric peristalsis, whereas sympathetic stimulation, secretin, GIP and somatostatin depress activity.

The speed at which substances empty from the stomach depends on their physical state and chemical composition. Liquids empty more rapidly than solids. Nutrients in the duodenum activate chemoreceptors which reflexly inhibit gastric emptying, allowing time for further digestion and absorption in the small intestine. Hypertonicity, fatty acids and hydrogen ions activate the secretion of CCK, secretin and GIP, which inhibit gastric emptying.

Factors affecting the rate of gastric emptying

Several physiological, pathological and pharmacological factors occurring in the perioperative period may delay gastric emptying and increase the risk of inhalation of gastric contents (Table 20.3). Obstruction of the GI tract, electrolyte imbalance and opioids are common causes.

Metoclopramide and domperidone are antidopaminergics and enhance gastric emptying. However, at therapeutic doses, they do not reverse opioid-induced delay. Cisapride is a 5-HT_4 agonist and causes release of ACh at the myenteric plexus. It is an effective gastric prokinetic. Erythromycin promotes motility of the GI tract directly, unrelated to its action on bacterial flora.

GASTRIC SECRETIONS

Gastric glands secrete approximately 2 L day^{-1}. Gastric secretions contain four main components: hydrochloric acid, pepsin, mucus and intrinsic factor. Hydrochloric acid is necessary to release pepsin from its proenzyme pepsinogen. Many ingested bacteria are killed by the acidic environment of the stomach, and hydrochloric acid also aids protein digestion and stimulates the flow of bile and pancreatic juice. Pepsin initiates protein digestion. Mucus is essential for protection of the mucosal cells. Intrinsic factor is required for the efficient absorption of vitamin B_{12} in the terminal ileum.

Glands are located in the body and fundus of the stomach and are of several types: parietal, peptic and mucus-secreting cells. Parietal (oxyntic) cells secrete hydrochloric acid and intrinsic factor, and chief (peptic, zymogen) cells secrete pepsinogen (Fig. 20.2).

Control of gastric acid secretion

Plasma gastrin concentrations (from G cells), ACh (from vagal efferents) and histamine (from ECL cells) are important in the control of gastric acid secretion. Gastrin has two actions: it stimulates parietal cells directly to secrete acid and it stimulates the release of histamine from ECL cells. Histamine diffuses to H_2-receptors on parietal cells (paracrine effect) causing acid secretion (Fig. 20.3).

Increased vagal tone causes acid secretion by stimulation of G, ECL and parietal cells. The neurotransmitter at the ECL and parietal cell is ACh (muscarinic receptor) and that at the G cell is GRP. Therefore, vagally mediated acid secretion results from direct stimulation of the parietal cell and indirectly by gastrin and histamine release.

Two second-messenger systems are activated in the parietal cell to bring about the synthesis and release of hydrogen ion. Gastrin and ACh activate the phospholipase C–inositol triphosphate system, whereas histamine activates adenyl cyclase via H_2-receptors and excitatory G-protein. The prostaglandin PGE_2 inhibits adenyl cyclase via receptor-linked inhibitory G-protein. The final common pathway is activation of H^+/K^+ -ATPase (proton pump) which transports H^+ ions into the gastric lumen in exchange for extracellular K^+ ions (Fig. 20.3). Generation of H^+ ions within the parietal cell starts with the formation of carbonic acid from carbon dioxide and water catalysed by carbonic anhydrase.

Table 20.3 Perioperative causes of delayed gastric emptying

Physiological
Pain
In some patients:
Anxiety
Pregnancy
Pathological
GI obstruction
Diabetes
Gastritis
Electrolyte abnormalities
Raised intracranial pressure
Migraine
Pharmacological
Opioids (all routes of administration)
Anticholinergics
Dopaminergics
Sympathomimetics
Ethanol
Ganglion blockers

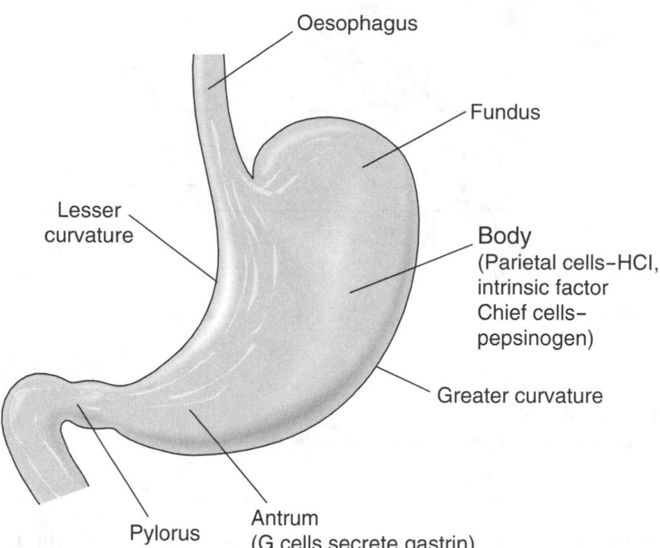

Fig. 20.2
Anatomy of the stomach.

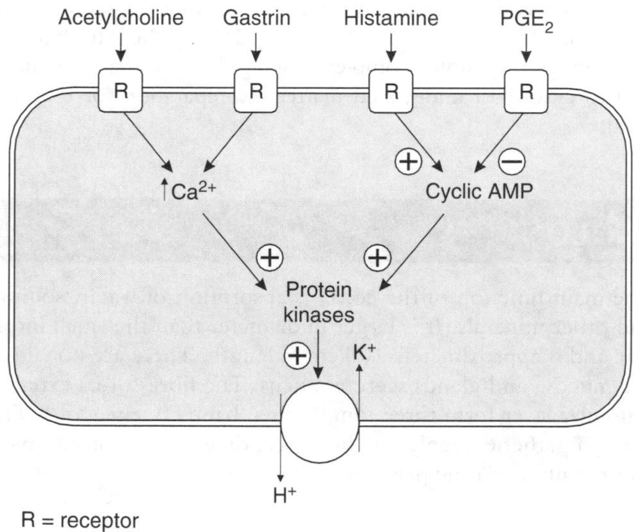

Fig. 20.3
Control of gastric acid production in the parietal cell. (Adapted from Ganong 1995.)

Physiological control of gastric acid production may be considered in terms of cephalic, gastric and intestinal factors. Cephalic factors (anticipation, sight, smell, taste) via vagal efferents are responsible for the secretion of gastric acid before food ingestion. Arrival of food in the stomach (gastric phase) stimulates acid secretion in several ways. When the stomach is empty, a gastric pH < 3 inhibits directly gastrin release from G cells, but food increases the pH and removes this inhibition. Distension of the stomach activates mechanoreceptors resulting in acid secretion via vagal afferents and efferents, gastrin release from G cells and acid secretion from parietal cells. Finally, peptides and amino acids from protein digestion stimulate gastric antral and duodenal G cells to secrete gastrin (intestinal factors). This is of minor importance compared with cephalic and gastric factors.

As the stomach empties, gastric acid secretion returns to baseline levels. Cephalic and gastric factors diminish and somatostatin (primary paracrine inhibitor of acid secretion) is released when gastric pH becomes < 3. Somatostatin-secreting cells are located in close proximity to gastrin cells and exert a continuous inhibitory restraint on the secretion of gastrin. Secretin and, to a lesser extent, GIP reduce acid secretion by inhibition of parietal and G cells. Secretin release occurs in response to the acidification of duodenal chyme. It also stimulates pancreatic and biliary alkaline secretion.

Drugs inhibiting gastric acid production

These drugs include the H_2-receptor antagonists (e.g. cimetidine, ranitidine), proton pump inhibitors (PPIs, e.g. omeprazole, lansoprazole) and prostaglandin analogues (e.g. misoprostol). The last also increase mucosal blood flow and enhance mucus and bicarbonate production. They are often prescribed in association with non-steroidal anti-inflammatory drugs.

H_2-receptor antagonists inhibit acid secretion by competitive and reversible inhibition of H_2-receptors on the parietal cell surface, blocking the action of histamine on acid secretion. Indirectly, they inhibit the synergistic influences of gastrin and cholinergic vagal stimulation on acid secretion also. The final common pathway of acid secretion is blocked by PPIs through inhibition of H^+/K^+-ATPase in the apical membrane of the parietal cell. They have a greater potential to achieve absolute inhibition of acid secretion compared with H_2-receptor antagonists. Also, PPIs inactivate the enzyme by irreversible covalent binding, and synthesis of new enzyme is required for further acid secretion.

Pepsinogen and pepsin

Pepsinogen is a pro-enzyme secreted from peptic (chief) cells. Some pepsinogen is also secreted from mucosal cells in the gastric antrum and the duodenum. It is converted into pepsin in the presence of gastric acid. The main stimulus for its release is increased vagal activity during the cephalic and gastric phases of acid secretion. Entry of acidic gastric chyme into the duodenum stimulates release of secretin and this, in addition to gastrin, causes further secretion of pepsinogen.

Mucus

The gastric mucosa secretes soluble and insoluble mucus consisting of glycoproteins (mucins). Surface mucus cells secrete insoluble mucus and bicarbonate which, together with sloughed mucosal cells, form a protective barrier over the mucosal surface. Secretion of this type of mucus is stimulated by prostaglandins. Soluble mucus is secreted in response to vagal stimulation and functions mainly as a lubricant.

Intrinsic factor

Intrinsic factor is a glycoprotein secreted by parietal cells and is necessary for the absorption of vitamin B_{12} (cyanocobalamin) from the small intestine. It forms a complex with vitamin B_{12} and binds to specific receptors in the ileum where it is absorbed by endocytosis.

EXOCRINE PANCREATIC SECRETIONS

Pancreatic secretions contain enzymes of major digestive importance. The pancreas is under the influence of neuronal reflex mechanisms and hormones (e.g. secretin and CCK).

Pancreatic juice is alkaline (high bicarbonate concentration) and approximately 1.5 L is secreted per day. Bile and intestinal juices are also neutral or alkaline and, consequently, the pH of duodenal contents is 6–7. Pancreatic enzymes are secreted as inactive proenzymes. Trypsinogen is converted to trypsin on entering the duodenum by the brush border enzyme enteropeptidase. Trypsin converts chymotrypsinogen into chymotrypsin, proelastase into elastase and procarboxypeptidase into carboxypeptidase. Another enzyme produced by the pancreas and activated by trypsin is phospholipase A_2. This enzyme cleaves a fatty acid off lecithin to form lysolecithin. The pancreas protects itself from trypsin-induced damage by secreting a trypsin inhibitor.

The most influential factor controlling pancreatic secretion is hormonal. Secretin acts on the pancreatic ducts to cause copious secretion of an alkaline juice rich in bicarbonate but poor in enzymes. Secretin also stimulates bile secretion. CCK acts on acinar cells, causing the release of pancreatic enzymes. In addition, ACh and vagal stimulation cause secretion of a small amount of enzyme-rich pancreatic juice.

SMALL INTESTINE

Digestion continues in the small intestine where the products are absorbed together with most vitamins and fluid. Nine litres of fluid enter the small intestine per day (diet 2 L, secretions 7 L) but only 1–2 L pass into the colon.

At the ligament of Treitz, the duodenum becomes the jejunum. The proximal 40% of the small intestine represents the jejunum and the distal 60% is termed the ileum. The mucous membrane is covered by villi (20–40 per mm^2) throughout the length of the small intestine (approximately 285 cm). The luminal aspects of the villi cells form minute microvilli, which are covered by a sugar-rich layer (glycocalyx). The microvilli and the glycocalyx make up the brush border upon which reside digestive enzymes (e.g. disaccharidases, peptidases).

Mucus (complex high-molecular-weight glycoproteins) is secreted by Brunner's glands in the duodenum and by goblet cells in the mucosa of the small and large intestine. Secretion is accelerated by cholinergic stimulation and by chemical and physical irritation.

The frequency of BERs in the proximal jejunum is 12 min^{-1}, declining to 8 min^{-1} in the distal ileum. Three types of smooth muscle contractions occur: peristaltic waves, segmentation contractions and tonic contractions. Peristalsis propels the chyme towards the large intestine. Stationary segmenting contractions divide the small intestine into segments at regular intervals (Fig. 20.4). After a short period, relaxation occurs followed by further contractions in adjacent parts of the gut wall forming new segments. These contractions do not advance contents along the GI tract but allow maximal exposure to the mucosal surface. Tonic contractions are relatively prolonged and isolate one part of the intestine from another. Both these contractions slow transit time and enhance efficiency of absorption.

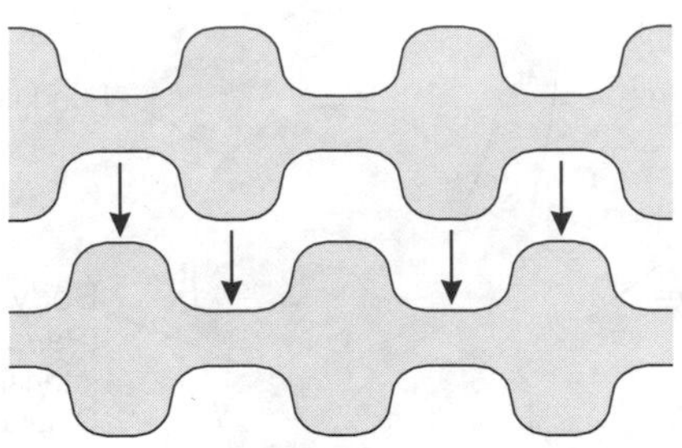

Fig. 20.4
Stationary segmenting contraction in the small intestine.

Increased vagal activity stimulates intestinal motility, as do gastrin, CCK and insulin. Sympathetic stimulation, secretin and glucagon inhibit smooth muscle activity. During the interdigestive phase, migrating motor complexes sweep through the small intestine to clear it of undigested matter in preparation for the next meal.

COLON

The main function of the colon is absorption of water, sodium and other minerals. It is larger in diameter than the small intestine and is approximately 100 cm in length. There are no villi in the mucosa and glands secrete mucus. The fibres of its external muscular layer form three longitudinal bands (taenia coli). The parasympathetic supply to the descending and sigmoid colon and rectum is via the pelvic nerves (S2, 3, 4).

COLONIC MOTILITY

The ileocaecal valve is normally closed and prevents reflux of colonic contents into the ileum. It opens when a peristaltic wave arrives, allowing ileal contents to enter the caecum. Passage into the caecum also increases when it relaxes in response to chyme leaving the stomach (gastroileal reflex).

Colonic motility patterns include stationary segmental contractions, mass movement and defaection. Stationary segmental contractions are of longer duration than those in the small intestine but their function is similar. They are more frequent in the descending and sigmoid colon and rectum. Mass movement contractions occur about three times per day and move material down the colon into the rectum, the distension of which initiates the defaecation reflex. These are coordinated by BERs (9 min^{-1} ileocaecal valve, 16 min^{-1} sigmoid colon).

Distension of the rectum has two effects: it causes the urge to defaecate and relaxation of the internal sphincter (rectosphincteric reflex). The sympathetic supply to the internal (involuntary) sphincter is excitatory, whereas the parasympathetic supply is inhibitory. The pudendal nerve innervates the external anal sphincter. Defaecation is a spinal reflex that may be inhibited voluntarily by contracting the external sphincter or facilitated by relaxing the sphincter and contracting the abdominal muscles. Distension of the stomach initiates contractions of the rectum and frequently a desire to defaecate (gastrocolic reflex) and this may be initiated by gastrin.

ABSORPTION IN THE COLON

The large intestine has a very large absorptive capacity and is often used for administration of drugs. Sodium is absorbed actively, creating an osmotic gradient along which follows water. There is a net secretion of K^+ and HCO_3^- ions into the colon. Stools contain inorganic material, undigested plant fibres, bacteria and water.

COLONIC BACTERIA

The are few bacteria in the jejunum, more in the ileum, but large numbers in the colon. Colonic bacteria include not only bacilli, such as *Escherichia coli* and *Enterobacter aerogenes*, but also pleomorphic organisms such as *Bacteroides fragilis* and cocci of various types. They have beneficial and potentially harmful effects. Some microorganisms synthesize vitamin K and several of the B complex vitamins. Folic acid produced by bacteria is absorbed in significant amounts. Furthermore, short-chain fatty acids produced by bacterial action have beneficial effects on the colonic mucosa.

Adequate nutrition in herbivores depends upon breakdown of cellulose and related plant carbohydrates by GI microorganisms. This does not occur in humans. Dietary cellulose, hemicellulose and lignin are important components of the dietary fibre.

DIGESTION

Ingested large and complex molecules (carbohydrates, proteins, triglycerides) are degraded for absorption into simple sugars, small peptides, amino acids, free fatty acids (FFAs) and monoglycerides. Some are absorbed by active transport mechanisms and others by passive diffusion along concentration gradients.

Salivary glands secrete amylase in response to parasympathetic stimuli, which digests starch into maltose and oligosaccharides. Salivary amylase activity continues for some time in the stomach. Hydrochloric acid converts pepsinogen (secreted by the chief cells) into pepsin and contributes to the breakdown of ingested connective tissue by denaturing protein. Pepsin is a protease that hydrolyses protein into amino acids and short-chain peptides.

Pancreatic bicarbonate neutralizes acid in the duodenum, providing an optimum pH for pancreatic digestive enzymes. These include trypsinogen and chymotrypsinogen (proteolytic, cleaved to trypsin and chymotrypsin by trypsin), enterokinase (cleaves trypsin from trypsinogen) and procarboxypeptidase (cleaves terminal amino acids from proteins, activated by trypsin to carboxypeptidase). Lipids are digested by lipase (hydrolyses triglycerides into FFAs and monoglycerides), phospholipase and cholesterol esterase. Pancreatic amylase degrades starch into oligosaccharides (mostly maltose), and ribonuclease and deoxyribonuclease hydrolyse nucleic acids.

Bile salts are involved in both the digestion and absorption of fat. They convert large lipid droplets into micelles (approximately 20 lipid molecules) to form a lipid emulsion. Micelles suspended in this aqueous emulsion are more susceptible to the action of lipase which breaks them down into FFAs and monoglycerides which are then absorbed in the small intestine. Cholesterol and fat-soluble vitamins are also absorbed by the same mechanism.

Monosaccharides are absorbed by a variety of mechanisms, including facilitated diffusion (e.g. fructose) and active carrier-mediated Na^+-coupled transport mechanisms (e.g. glucose, galactose). Amino acids are absorbed by carrier-mediated transport systems which are specific for different groups of amino acids.

FURTHER READING

Ganong W F 1999 Review of medical physiology, 19th edn. Appleton & Lange, CT

Oglivy A J, Smith G 1995 The gastrointestinal tract and anaesthesia. European Journal of Anaesthesiology 12(Suppl 10): 35–42

Thompson H M, Rowbotham D J 2000 Gut motility and secretions. In: Hemmings H, Hopkins P (eds) Foundations of anaesthesia. Mosby, London

21 Nausea, vomiting and their treatment

Death or serious morbidity resulting directly from anaesthesia is now extremely rare. However, postoperative nausea and vomiting (PONV) is still very common. Surveys have confirmed that PONV is feared considerably by patients undergoing surgery. Indeed, it often comes before postoperative pain when patients are asked to rank their concerns. Therefore, every anaesthetist must be aware of the physiology of PONV and its consequences, causes, associated factors and management.

VOMITING REFLEX

All reflexes, including the vomiting reflex, consist of afferent inputs, a degree of central processing and motor afferents. The vomiting reflex is summarized in Fig. 21.1.

VOMITING CENTRE

The vomiting centre is not an anatomical entity but represents several nuclei in the brain stem (e.g. nucleus tractus solitarius, respiratory neural networks) which are responsible for the coordination of the efferent limb of the vomiting reflex. It receives input from the afferent limbs of the reflex and the chemoreceptor trigger zone (CTZ).

CHEMORECEPTOR TRIGGER ZONE

The CTZ is situated in the area postrema in the floor of the fourth ventricle. Evidence from ablation studies by Borison and Wang in the 1950s and the fact that the blood– brain barrier is defective in this area suggest that the CTZ is responsible for detecting toxins circulating in the blood and cerebrospinal fluid. However, it may be that a more precise area for this function is the nearby nucleus tractus solitarius where dopamine and opioid receptors are abundant.

AFFERENT LIMBS OF VOMITING REFLEX

Gastrointestinal tract

Information from mechano- and chemoreceptors in the gastrointestinal tract is relayed via the vagus nerve to the nucleus tractus solitarius in the brain stem. Abnormal gastric or intestinal distension, increased smooth muscle contraction and abnormal or toxic gastrointestinal contents can trigger the vomiting reflex. Peripheral 5-HT_3 receptors are intimately involved in this system. Radiation, chemotherapy and other toxins release 5-HT from chromaffin cells in the gut, which stimulates vagal afferents – a process inhibited by the 5-HT_3 antagonist antiemetics (see below). Dopamine receptors are also abundant in the upper gastrointestinal tract.

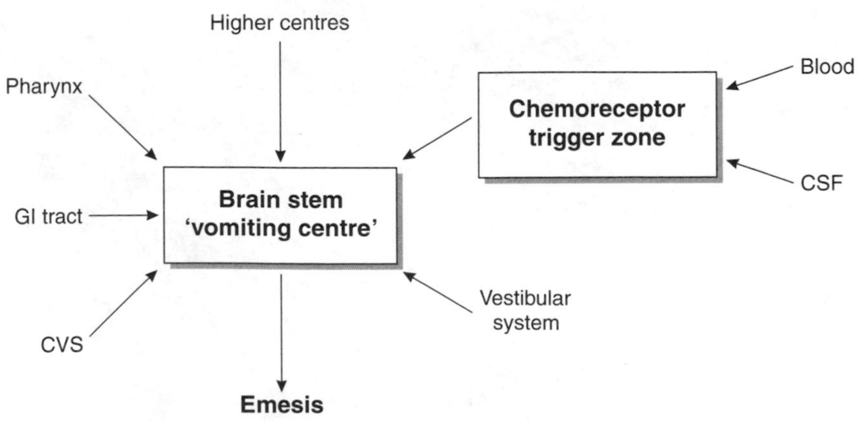

Fig. 21.1
The vomiting reflex.

Vestibular system

Input from the vestibular system is responsible for motion sickness, particularly when vestibular and visual signals conflict. Patients with a history of motion sickness and those who are moved excessively in the early postoperative period are more likely to suffer from PONV.

Cardiovascular system

Stimulation of afferents from both cardiac ventricles and blood vessels may lead to vomiting. For example, hypotension and myocardial infarction are often associated with nausea and vomiting.

Higher centres

Input from higher centres often plays a vital role in the genesis of PONV. A calm, well informed patient who is denied unpleasant sights, sounds and smells is less likely to experience nausea or vomiting.

Miscellaneous inputs

Nausea and vomiting are frequently induced by stimulation of pharyngeal afferents, e.g. nasopharyngeal tube, endoscopy. Stimulation of the auricular branch of the vagus nerve on examination of the ear with an auroscope may induce sudden vomiting, especially in children. It is advisable to examine the ear from behind.

The role of sympathetic innervation of the gastrointestinal tract in PONV is not clear. However, pain pathways from the viscera reside in the splanchnic nerves and visceral pain is a frequent cause of nausea and vomiting.

EFFERENT LIMB OF THE VOMITING REFLEX

Nausea

Nausea is not an inevitable consequence of vomiting but it is often the most troublesome symptom after surgery and anaesthesia. It is thought to be caused by the same stimuli that are responsible for vomiting, but the nature of the higher centres involved in this sensation are unknown. As a symptom, it is difficult to investigate because it is entirely objective and cannot be measured in animals. However, a consistent finding is that antiemetic therapy is often very effective in reducing the incidence of vomiting or retching, but less so for nausea.

Vomiting

The processes involved in vomiting are summarized in Figure 21.2. In the prodromal or pre-ejection phase, there is a relaxation of the gastric muscles followed by small intestinal retrograde peristalsis. The latter forces intestinal contents into the relaxed stomach. At the beginning of the ejection phase, the anterior abdominal muscles and the diaphragm contract together, accompanied by retrograde contraction of the striated musculature of the oesophagus. At the same time, the upper oesophageal sphincter becomes widely dilated. During vomiting, the oesophagus is not obstructed by diaphragmatic contraction, as the crural (peri-oesophageal) muscles of the diaphragm are relaxed. This autonomic and somatic activity is coordinated in the brain stem ('vomiting centre' – see above).

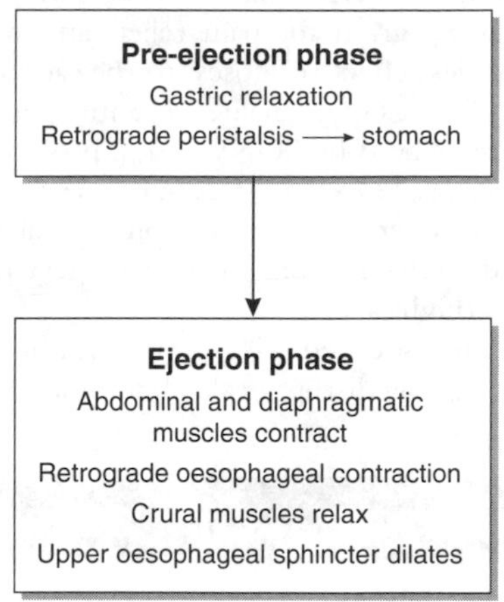

Fig. 21.2
Vomiting.

Retching

Retching (i.e. unproductive vomiting) often occurs before vomiting and when the retrograde intestinal peristalsis reaches the stomach. During retching, the abdominal muscles and diaphragm contract less intensely and there is no retrograde oesophageal contraction or crural relaxation. Clinically, retching is a frequent and distressing symptom, often associated with intense nausea.

ADVERSE EFFECTS OF PONV

The potential adverse effects of PONV are summarized in Table 21.1. The most important and frequent adverse effect is the profound distress of most patients when they experience nausea and vomiting.

Aspiration of stomach contents is an important cause of anaesthetic mortality and morbidity and can occur in the postoperative period, particularly if the patient is drowsy. Nausea and vomiting

Table 21.1 Adverse effects of PONV
Patient distress
Aspiration of stomach contents
Limitation of analgesia
Poor surgical outcome
Eyes
Head and neck
Oesophageal
Abdominal wound
Dehydration and/or requirement for intravenous fluids
Delayed oral input
Drugs
Nutrition
Fluids
Delayed mobilization
Delayed discharge from day-care unit

make this more likely. PONV may limit significantly the dose of opioid that may be given for pain relief, and prevention with antiemetics enables effective doses to be administered. Oral administration of drugs (e.g. analgesics, antihypertensives), fluids and nutrients are delayed by PONV and, if prolonged, may cause significant problems. PONV is often more severe on movement and may delay postoperative mobilization. It is also an important cause of delayed discharge from day-care surgery units, including unscheduled overnight stay.

PONV may be associated with poor surgical outcome – for example, vomiting may disrupt neck, abdominal and eye sutures.

FACTORS ASSOCIATED WITH PONV

Many studies have investigated the relative importance of patient, surgical and anaesthetic factors in the incidence of PONV. Some factors have been associated with an increased risk, but presently the likelihood of PONV in individual patients cannot be predicted with any certainty.

PATIENT FACTORS

Studies have revealed several patient factors which are associated with a relatively high risk of PONV. A previous history of PONV is a strong association. Children and females are at greater risk but there is no difference between the sexes in childhood or old age. The influence of the menstrual cycle and obesity has been investigated but there is no consistent evidence that they are an important factors. However, it is likely that a predisposition to travel sickness is important.

SURGICAL FACTORS

The surgical factors associated with an increased risk of PONV are summarized in Table 21.2. Major and minor gynaecological procedures are associated consistently with PONV. Indeed, gynaecological surgery is often used in studies investigating the efficacy of new antiemetics. PONV after ENT surgery may be more frequent because of stimulation of pharyngeal afferents, blood in the gastrointestinal tract and the fact that it is a common procedure in children. In abdominal surgery, almost all the efferent limbs of the vomiting reflex are stimulated. Duration of surgery and anaesthesia may also be important.

Table 21.2 Surgical factors associated with an increased risk of PONV

Type of surgery
Gynaecological
ENT
Gastrointestinal
Head and neck
Squint correction
Duration of surgery
Postoperative antibiotics

Table 21.3 Anaesthetic factors associated with an increased risk of PONV

Opioids
Volatile agents
Intravenous induction agents (c.f. propofol)
Thiopental
Etomidate
Methohexital
Experience of anaesthetist
Postoperative pain
Hypotension during epidural/spinal anaesthesia
?N_2O
?Neostigmine

ANAESTHETIC FACTORS (see Table 21.3)

Choice of induction agent may influence the incidence of PONV; etomidate and methohexital are comparatively more emetogenic. The incidence of PONV associated with induction and/or maintenance of anaesthesia with propofol is lower than that with other intravenous and volatile agents. Indeed, it has been suggested that propofol has antiemetic properties, but the evidence for this is not yet convincing.

Nitrous oxide when used alone, e.g. Entonox, may cause nausea and vomiting, but its effect is uncertain when used as part of a balanced anaesthetic technique. Modern volatile agents are less emetogenic compared with older agents, e.g. ether, trichlorothylene, methoxyflurane, but still contribute to the overall likelihood of PONV.

It is clear that the perioperative use of opioids (oral, i.m., i.v., epidural, spinal) is associated with an increased incidence of PONV and many anaesthetic techniques aim to avoid opioids for this reason. Paradoxically, postoperative pain may cause PONV, which may be alleviated by judicious use of opioids.

Antagonism of neuromuscular blockade with neostigmine has been blamed for PONV but recent data have not confirmed this. Episodes of hypotension during spinal or epidural anaesthesia are a common cause of nausea and vomiting. Indeed, nausea is often the first sign of this problem. In addition, there is a lower incidence of PONV in patients anaesthetized by experienced anaesthetists compared with those managed by novices. The inexperienced tend to maintain anaesthesia at a deeper plane and are more likely to inflate the stomach with air during manual ventilation.

MANAGEMENT OF PONV

PREVENTION OF PONV

Prevention rather than treatment of PONV should be the anaesthetist's aim. However, there is no agreed protocol as to which patients should receive preventive antiemetic therapy, but the relative indication for prophylaxis increases as the number of risk factors increase.

There is an important organizational factor in the incidence of PONV. Antiemetics are often prescribed but not given. The overall incidence of PONV in a hospital is reduced if all professionals involved in the care of the patient understand the importance and

Table 21.4 Important causes of PONV

Hypotension
Hypoxaemia
Drugs
Opioids
Antibiotics
Intra-abdominal pathology
Psychological factors
Mobilization
Fluid intake
Nasogastric tube
Pain

Table 21.5 Types of antiemetic

Antagonists
Dopaminergic
Cholinergic
Histaminergic
5-HT3
NK-1
Agonists
Dexamethasone
Cannabinoids

nature of antiemetic therapy and an agreed management protocol is in place.

TREATMENT OF PONV

Treat the cause

An important principle in the management of any symptom is to seek and treat the cause before treating the symptom itself. This is relevant when dealing with a patient with PONV. There are many important causes of PONV and these are summarized in Table 21.4.

PONV may indicate postoperative hypotension; simply administering an antiemetic does not help and may mask an important sign. Hypoxaemia should be treated with oxygen and investigated further if necessary. Early fluid intake or mobilization, particularly after day-case surgery is a common cause. Psychological factors, e.g. anxiety, loss of control and illness beliefs, play an important role and may respond to appropriate non-pharmacological management. Occasionally, PONV may herald significant intra-abdominal or other pathology resulting from a surgical complication. This should be borne in mind constantly, particularly before discharge from the day-care unit.

Opioids are a common cause of PONV, particularly if they are administered injudiciously. Changing to a local anaesthetic technique or adopting a more balanced approach to analgesia may solve the problem. It should be remembered that many other drugs are emetogenic. Antibiotics are a common culprit and their use should be reassessed if PONV is a severe problem.

Antiemetic therapy

In practice, many patients with PONV require parenteral antiemetic therapy. If an antiemetic has been given previously, there are several factors to consider when choosing the appropriate drug. If the previous drug was effective for some time and it is likely that its plasma concentrations are now low, it is probably appropriate to administer the same drug. However, if the drug was administered relatively recently, a different antiemetic is required. It makes pharmacological sense to choose a drug which acts at a different receptor (see below).

PHARMACOLOGY OF ANTIEMETICS

TYPES OF ANTIEMETIC

The agonists and antagonists available for use as antiemetics are summarized in Table 21.5. Antiemetics may be antagonists at the dopamine (D_2 – e.g. metoclopramide, droperidol, prochlorperazine), 5-HT_3 (e.g. ondansetron, dolasetron) and cholinergic (e.g. cyclizine) receptors.

Dexamethasone and cannabinoids (e.g. nabilone, dronabinol) are effective against chemotherapy-induced emesis. The efficacy of cannabinoids for PONV is uncertain but there is increasing evidence that dexamethasone is effective. Antagonists at the NK-1 receptor are antiemetic also and their site of action is probably in the brain stem where there is an abundance of these receptors. They are presently undergoing clinical trials.

Metoclopramide

Metoclopramide acts at the dopamine receptors in the stomach, upper intestine and CTZ. It enhances gastric emptying, intestinal transit and lower oesophageal sphincter pressure. It is still prescribed frequently as an antiemetic, but at the recommended dose (10 mg) it is no better than placebo in many situations.

Table 21.6 Approximate pharmacokinetic values of the commonly used antiemetics

	Bioavailability (%)	t_{max} (h)	$t_{1/2}$ (h)
Metoclopramide	80 (range 32–97)	1–2.5	4
Prochlorperazine	14	2.8	6 (range 1–15)
Droperidol			2
Cyclizine			13–20
Ondansetron	60	0.5–2	4
Granesitron	60		3–6
Dolasetron		1[a]	7–9[a]

[a]Active metabolite

The bioavailability of metoclopramide after oral administration is unpredictable (Table 21.6) and time to maximum concentration (t_{max}) is 1–2.5 h. Its elimination half-life is approximately 4 h but its redistribution half-life after intravenous administration is short (approximately 5 min).

Side-effects include extrapyramidal reactions, usually dystonia (e.g. facial muscle spasm, trismus, abnormal tongue movements, oculogyric crises, opisthotonus). They occur more commonly in young females (approximately 1 in 5000). Agitation has been reported after metoclopramide premedication. Hypotension, sinus tachycardia, supraventricular tachycardia and sinus bradycardia have been described after intravenous injection. It is recommended that an intravenous dose should be given over a period of 1–2 min.

Phenothiazines

Phenothiazines are antiemetics because of their dopamine receptor antagonist activity. They were synthesized originally by dye chemists in the late 19th century, but it was only in the 1930s that the sedative and antiemetic effects of promethazine were discovered. Promethazine is used occasionally as premedication for children but its sedative effect restricts its use as an antiemetic. Perphenazine was used extensively as an antiemetic but was associated with a high incidence of extrapyramidal side-effects and is now used rarely. Prochlorperazine is prescribed very frequently for PONV.

Prochlorperazine

Prochlorperazine was synthesized in 1949 and introduced for the prevention of PONV in the 1950s. Although relatively few controlled studies are available, it is likely that prochlorperazine is an effective antiemetic. Elimination half-life is approximately 6 h and oral bioavailability is poor (Table 21.6).

Extrapyramidal side-effects are similar in nature to those associated with metoclopramide but less frequent. Sedation is not usually a problem in doses used for PONV. Rare side-effects include cholestatic jaundice, skin sensitization and haematological abnormalities.

Butyrophenones

Butyrophenones are used as major tranquillizers and neuroleptics. They are dopamine antagonists. Only droperidol is administered perioperatively but haloperidol is prescribed occasionally as an antiemetic in palliative medicine.

Droperidol

Droperidol is administered intravenously and was developed originally for use in neuroleptic anaesthetic regimens. This technique, which involved the combination of high-dose opioids and droperidol with no volatile agent, has now been abandoned because of concerns regarding awareness. The redistribution half-life of droperidol is approximately 10 min and elimination half-life 2 h (Table 21.6).

Many studies have confirmed the efficacy of droperidol against placebo, but sedation is often reported. Side-effects are similar to those of the phenothiazines. Extrapyramidal reactions are less frequent compared with metoclopramide. Feelings of apprehension, restlessness and even nightmares are less obvious but occur more frequently. In addition to antagonistic effects at the dopamine receptor, droperidol is also an α-adrenergic antagonist and may cause vasodilatation and hypotension. It has been recently withdrawn from use in the UK.

Anticholinergics

Hyoscine (scopolamine) and atropine are anticholinergics with antiemetic actions. Cyclizine is also anticholinergic but also an antagonist at the histamine type-1 receptor. Cyclizine is administered most frequently for PONV.

Cyclizine

In recent years, cyclizine has become more popular for the prevention and treatment of PONV. Although there are relatively few well controlled studies, its popularity probably reflects reasonable efficacy combined with a low incidence of side-effects. Its elimination half-life is 13–20 h.

Extrapyramidal side-effects are not associated with cyclizine, but sedation and dry mouth (anticholinergic action) may occur. Other complications include urinary retention, blurred vision, restlessness and hallucinations when given in large doses. In patients with severe cardiac failure, it may increase arterial pressure, heart rate and pulmonary wedge pressure, leading to a reduction in cardiac output.

5-HT_3 receptor antagonists

5-HT_3 receptor antagonists were developed as antiemetics when it was realized that the efficacy of high-dose metoclopramide (i.e. 10 mg kg^{-1}) in chemotherapy-induced emesis was the result of some degree of antagonism at the 5-HT_3 receptor. Ondansetron was the first available specific potent 5-HT_3 receptor antagonist.

Ondansetron

Several studies have confirmed the efficacy of ondansetron for PONV. It may be given orally or intravenously. Oral bioavailability is approximately 60% and elimination half-life is 4 h (Table 21.6).

A major advantage of ondansetron is its wide therapeutic index. The most common side-effects are mild headache and constipation; it is not associated with extrapyramidal side-effects, sedation or prolongation of recovery from anaesthesia

Other 5-HT_3 antagonists

Granesitron has similar pharmacological properties to those of ondansetron. It is available for oral and intravenous administration. Dolasetron relies upon an active metabolite for its activity.

Dexamethasone

The efficacy of dexamethasone for the prevention of chemotherapy-induced nausea and vomiting is well established. Its mode of action is unclear and the plasma half-life is approximately 3 h. There is increasing evidence that the efficacy of a single intravenous dose (8 mg) of dexamethasone for the prevention of PONV is comparable with that of standard antiemetics. It may be useful particularly when used in combination with 5-HT_3 antagonists. Classic steroid side-effects do not occur with a single dose and, to date, no adverse effects have been reported. However, further work is required before dexamethasone may be considered for routine prophylaxis of PONV.

COMBINATION THERAPY

The efficacy of antiemetic therapy for the prevention or treatment of PONV may be enhanced by combination therapy. It makes pharmacological sense to administer drugs which act at different receptors. Presently, there is considerable interest in this and most studies have found combinations to be significantly more efficacious than a single drug.

The most commonly investigated combinations are droperidol–ondansetron and ondansetron–dexamethasone, but combinations of cyclizine and prochlorperazine are also possible.

ACUPUNCTURE AND PONV

The use of acupuncture was championed in the 1980s by the late Professor Dundee. Acupuncture for nausea is performed at the P6 (Neiguan) point which is situated between the tendons of the flexor carpi radialis and palmaris longus, 2 Chinese inches from the distal skin crease. A Chinese inch is the width of the interphalangeal joint of the thumb. Studies using meta-analysis have confirmed that stimulation of the P6 point is indeed effective if applied before or after anaesthesia. It is less effective if applied during anaesthesia. There are no significant side-effects of this therapy and it should be considered as a serious option if personnel are available to administer it.

FURTHER READING

Rose J B, Watcha M F 1999 Postoperative nausea and vomiting in paediatric patients. British Journal of Anaesthesia 83: 104–117

Rowbotham D J 1992 Current management of postoperative nausea and vomiting. British Journal of Anaesthesia 69: 46–59S

Strunin L, Rowbotham DJ, Miles L (eds) 1999 The effective management of post-operative nausea and vomiting. Aesculapius Medical Press, London

Watcha M F, White P F 1992 Postoperative nausea and vomiting – its etiology, treatment, and prevention. Anesthesiology 77: 162–184

Woodhouse A, Mather L E 1997 Nausea and vomiting in the postoperative patient-controlled analgesia environment. Anaesthesia 52: 770–775

22 The liver

ANATOMY AND FUNCTION: OVERVIEW

The normal adult liver weighs approximately 1.5 kg and is situated in the right upper quadrant of the abdomen. The liver is divided into four lobes – the right, left, caudate and quadrate lobes – which are marked by various tendinous attachments to the liver surface. The liver is unique in that it has a dual blood supply from the hepatic artery and the portal vein. Hepatic venous blood drains into three hepatic veins which join the inferior vena cava. Bile is secreted into bile canaliculi which coalesce to form the right and left bile ducts and then the hepatic and common bile ducts.

The liver receives the total venous outflow of the gastrointestinal tract. It is therefore the first organ to be exposed to a multitude of substances absorbed from the gastrointestinal tract, including nutrients, drugs, microorganisms and toxins.

The function of the liver may be classified as:

- metabolic
- synthetic
- detoxification
- storage.

However, the role of the liver in handling some substances may fit into more than one of these categories.

Substances synthesized by the liver include bile, plasma proteins and amino acids, urea from ammonia, glycogen from carbohydrates and cholecalciferol. In the fetus, it is a site of red blood cell production. The liver is the site of metabolism of carbohydrate, fat and protein and is also important for the metabolism of drugs and hormones. It has a major immunological role as it is the primary site of detoxification of gut-derived bacteria and toxins. Finally, the liver is a reservoir of blood which may be redistributed into the central circulation during hypovolaemic shock.

Hepatocytes perform most of these functions and account for 60% of the mass of the liver. Hepatocyte intracellular organelles include mitochondria (oxidative phosphorylation and Krebs cycle), rough and smooth endoplasmic reticulum (protein, triglyceride and drug metabolism, conjugation of bilirubin and steroid synthesis) and lysosomes (storage of ferritin, copper, bile pigments and lipofuscin).

LIVER BLOOD SUPPLY

The liver has a dual blood supply from the hepatic artery and the portal vein. Total liver blood flow in the adult is between 1100 and 1800 ml min^{-1}. Blood from the hepatic artery is highly saturated with oxygen (98%) and, although only 30% of total liver blood flow, it is responsible for 40–55% of liver oxygen supply. The portal vein is formed by the union of the splenic and superior mesenteric veins. It consists of the venous effluent of the gut and therefore has a lower oxygen saturation (75%). It has a relatively smaller contribution to hepatic oxygen supply compared with the hepatic artery, despite its greater flow. The mean arterial pressure in the hepatic arterioles is 4.7 kPa (35 mmHg), compared with 1.7 kPa (13 mmHg) in the portal vein. The portal circulation is valveless, and therefore retrograde flow is possible in some conditions, e.g. portal hypertension.

Terminal branches of the hepatic artery and portal vein run throughout the liver in portal tracts (portal triads). On histological slides, these tracts form roughly hexagonal-shaped units of hepatocytes termed hepatic lobules (Fig. 22.1). At each corner of the lobule is a portal tract and in the middle a central hepatic vein. Blood from the arteriole and venule in the portal tract flows through an extensive capillary network into the central vein. This capillary network (hepatic sinusoids) has a highly fenestrated epithelium which is separated from the hepatocytes by the space of Disse. Plasma from the small bowel flows from the sinusoids through the fenestrae and into the space of Disse, which is in contact with the highly villous surface of the hepatocytes (Fig. 22.2).

Plasma from the space of Disse flows retrogradely into lymphatic channels in the portal tracts and is a major source of production of lymph. Kupffer cells, which represent 80–90% of the body's macrophages and 20–30% of the mass of the liver, line the space of Disse. They phagocytose gut-derived bacteria, denature foreign proteins and scavenge ferritin and haemosiderin.

The pressure in the sinusoids is about 0.4 kPa (3 mmHg) higher than that in the hepatic veins. Therefore blood from the sinusoids drains into the central hepatic vein of each hepatic lobule. These veins join sublobular veins which coalesce to form the three major hepatic veins.

Bile produced by hepatocytes is excreted into bile canaliculi, which are essentially intracellular spaces between hepatocytes. These transport bile in the opposite direction to sinusoidal blood flow, to epithelialized bile ducts in the portal triads. From here, bile flows into the larger biliary system which becomes the right and left hepatic ducts.

LIVER ACINI (Fig. 22.1)

The functional unit of the liver is termed the hepatic acinus and is based on the relative perfusion of hepatocytes within a hepatic lobule. Liver cells close to a terminal blood vessel are supplied preferentially with oxygenated blood compared with cells furthest

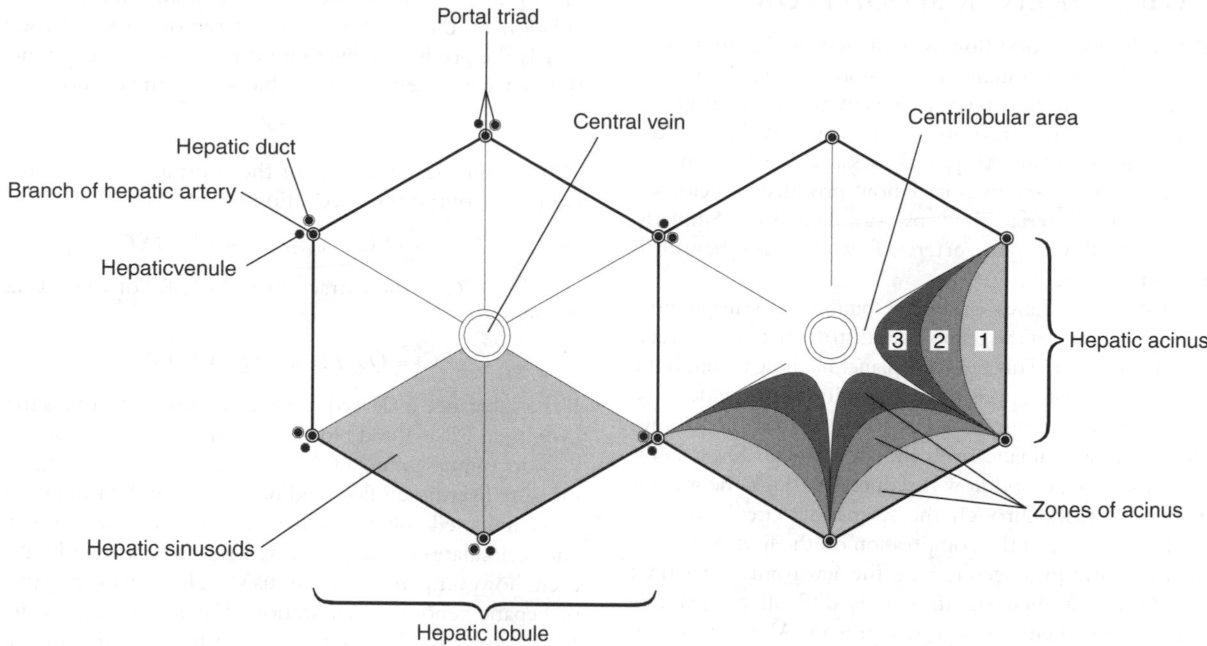

Fig. 22.1
Hepatic lobule and acinus.

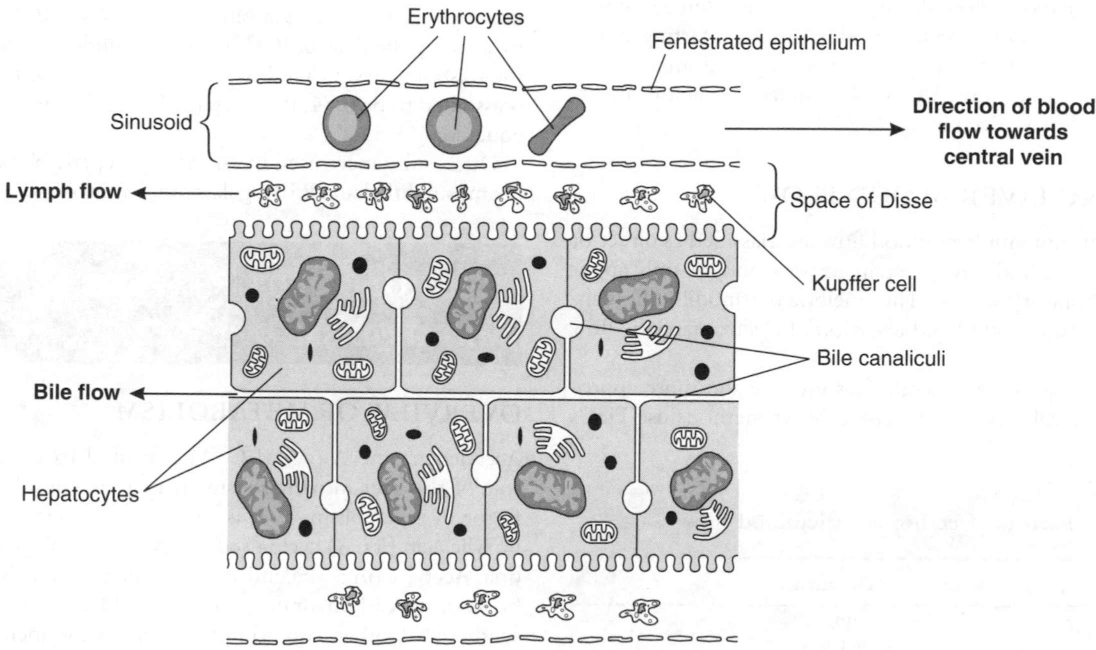

Fig. 22.2
The hepatic sinusoid.

away. Because of the roughly hexagonal arrangement of the portal triads, perfusion within an acinus is divided into three zones.

Zone 1 is the periportal hepatocytes which have the highest metabolic activity. These cells contain high concentrations of transaminases used in protein metabolism. Zone 3 is the centrilobular hepatocytes around the central vein. These are perfused with relatively low saturated blood and are the site of drug biotransformation. They have a high cytochrome P450 concentration. Zone 2 cells are intermediate in terms of oxygen tension and enzyme activities compared with the other two zones. Because of this distribution, the centrilobular hepatocytes are most prone to hypoxic injury during periods of low perfusion or poisoning.

REGULATION OF LIVER BLOOD FLOW

In normal health, liver blood flow is regulated by the interaction of the arterial and venous systems. Below systolic arterial pressures of 80 mmHg, basal hepatic arterial tone is minimal, but at higher pressures vasoconstriction prevents excessive arterial blood flow. Portal flow is linearly related to portal pressure and resistance in the hepatic bed. Decreases in portal flow produce a reciprocal increase in hepatic arterial flow by vasodilatation. Similarly, increases in portal flow reduce arterial flow. This mechanism is regulated by adenosine.

Hepatic blood flow varies during respiration. In inspiration, downward displacement of the diaphragm distorts the hepatic veins causing partial occlusion. This reduces splanchnic flow through the liver because of increased venous resistance. However, the decrease in intrathoracic pressure augments inferior vena cava blood flow, and therefore venous drainage from the kidneys and lower limbs increases. In expiration, blood flow is reduced through the inferior vena cava, but increases through the splanchnic circulation and liver, because of a release of the compression on the liver bed.

Many of the hormones secreted by the gastrointestinal tract affect blood flow, but their significance is difficult to quantify. However, from a therapeutic aspect, vasopressin (ADH) is used in the treatment of bleeding oesophageal varices as it reduces splanchnic and hepatic blood flow.

Hepatic blood blow is also altered by many drugs (including anaesthetic agents), surgery and disease states. Increases or decreases in liver blood flow during surgery are often caused by the combined effects of several opposing factors affecting blood flow. Hypotension due to any cause (e.g. regional anaesthesia) reduces hepatic blood flow. A general summary of factors affecting liver blood flow is given in Table 22.1.

MEASURING LIVER BLOOD FLOW

Methods of determining liver blood flow are classified as direct or indirect. Direct methods are generally invasive and are only applicable in the laboratory setting. They include thermodilution techniques, Doppler ultrasound and insertion of electromagnetic flow probes.

Indirect techniques are generally less invasive and more appropriate in the clinical setting. The commonest methods use Fick's principle of measuring the clearance of an indicator from the circulation by the liver. The rate of removal (R) of the indicator equals the product of liver blood flow (Q) and the concentration difference between the inflow blood and the outflow:

$$R = Q(C_i - C_o)$$

R/C_i is the clearance (Cl) of the substance. Therefore, dividing either side of the above equation by C_i gives:

$$R/C_i = Q(C_i - C_o)/C_i \text{ or } Cl = Q(C_i - C_o)/C_i$$

$(C_i - C_o)/C_i$ is the extraction ratio (ER) of the substance, and therefore:

$$Cl = Q \times ER \text{ and } Q = Cl/ER \qquad (1)$$

If the substance is cleared completely during first pass through the liver, then ER = 1 and blood flow equals the clearance.

Indocyanine green (ICG) is the commonest agent used to measure liver blood flow and has an ER of 0.74 in healthy adults. It is eliminated only by the liver and does not undergo enterohepatic recirculation. For accuracy, hepatic vein sampling should be used, however peripheral venous sampling gives an approximation of hepatic venous concentration. Usually, a constant infusion of ICG is given for 20 min following a bolus. Simultaneous samples of arterial and venous blood are taken, and the clearance and extraction ratios determined. Hepatic blood flow is then calculated using equation (1).

A single bolus technique may be used to estimate hepatic blood flow by repeat venous sampling. Clearance of ICG is determined by dividing the dose of ICG by the area under the curve (AUC) of the washout curve: Cl = dose/AUC. If the extraction ratio of ICG is assumed to be 0.74, then hepatic blood flow is determined from equation (1).

Other substances used in estimating hepatic blood flow include bromosulphthalein (BSP), galactose, sorbitol and lidocaine.

Table 22.1 Factors affecting hepatic blood flow

Increase	Decrease
Postprandial	IPPV
Acute hepatitis	PEEP
Hypercapnia	Hypocapnia
Pentagastrin	Hypoxaemia
Cholecystokinin	Cirrhosis
Vasoactive intestinal peptide	α-stimulation
Glucagon	β-blockade
β-stimulation	Ganglion blockers
	Epidural anaesthesia
	Intravenous and inhalation anaesthetics
	Acidosis
	ADH
	Laparotomy/laparoscopy

THE ROLE OF THE LIVER IN METABOLISM

OVERVIEW OF METABOLISM

Acetylcoenzyme A (acetyl-CoA) is central to understanding the role of the liver in metabolism. It may be considered as a major factor in metabolism, as it is the primary substrate in the tricarboxylic acid (TCA) cycle used to produce ATP by cell mitochondria. Acetyl-CoA is the end-point of the catabolic pathways which break down carbohydrates, proteins and fats. It is also used in the synthesis of other compounds in the body, including ketones, fatty acids and steroids. Therefore, in the sections below, one should appreciate the pivotal role of acetyl-CoA, as it is often the link between many diverse metabolic pathways (Fig. 22.3).

PROTEIN METABOLISM

The liver is a site for protein anabolism and catabolism. However, protein metabolism occurs also in skeletal muscle, intestines, kidneys and fat. Amino acids are the building blocks of all proteins and are derived from dietary proteins or muscle breakdown, or are synthesized in the liver. Together, these contribute to the amino acid

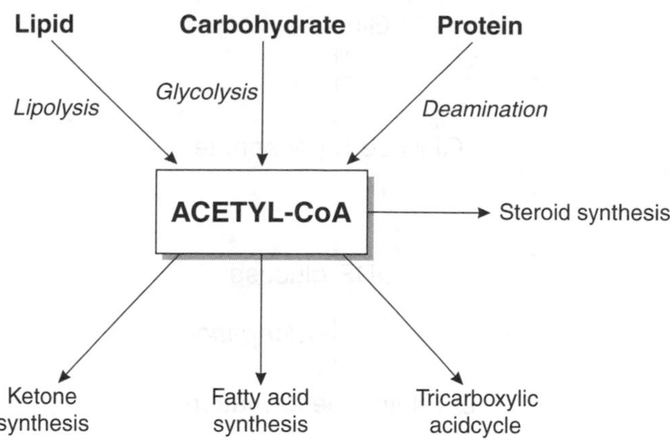

Fig. 22.3
The role of acetyl-CoA in liver metabolism.

pool within the liver, which represents about 300 g of protein continually used as substrate for amino acid synthesis, which is replenished by amino acids from muscle breakdown and dietary sources. Normally, about 35–55 g of protein is lost per day and this must be replaced by dietary protein to maintain a neutral nitrogen balance.

The key reactions involved in protein metabolism are transamination and oxidative deamination. Transamination converts one amino acid into another by catalysing the transfer of an amino group of an α-amino acid (e.g. alanine) to an α-keto acid (e.g. α-ketoglutarate), to produce a new amino acid and keto acid. Alanine transaminase (ALT) and aspartate transaminase (AST) are the commonest transaminases in the liver and are used in the synthesis or breakdown of amino acids. Using these reactions, new amino acids are synthesized from unwanted ones.

Oxidative deamination is used in the catabolism of amino acids. It is the mechanism by which excess amino acids are removed from the body and involves the removal of the amino group, leaving ammonia and a keto acid. Ammonia, a toxic product, is converted into urea by the liver and the keto acids are used as intermediates of the TCA and glycolytic cycles. Urea is an economical way of excreting ammonia, as it has a high nitrogen content and is water-soluble. It is therefore excreted in the urine, making it an efficient way to excrete excess nitrogen. In liver failure, urea synthesis is impaired and ammonia accumulates. This is thought to be a major chemical responsible for the development of hepatic encephalopathy in these situations.

Prealbumin and albumin

The liver is the only source of albumin and produces about 10 g day^{-1} in the healthy adult to replace losses. Albumin is important for the maintenance of plasma oncotic pressure and as a carrier of drugs, hormones and bilirubin.

Globulins

These are serum proteins which are classified into α-globulins, β-globulins and γ-globulins. The γ-globulins are immunoglobulins synthesized by plasma cells, but the liver synthesizes many α- and β-globulins. Serum globulins may be separated by serum electrophoresis.

α-1-globulins include α-1-antitrypsin and α-1-acid glycoprotein. α-1-antitrypsin is a protease inhibitor and inherited disorders in its synthesis lead to cirrhosis and panacinar emphysema. α-1-acid glycoprotein is important for binding basic drugs.

α-2-globulins include haptoglobulin (HPT), α-2-macroglobulin and caeruloplasmin. HPT binds to free haemoglobin released from lysed blood cells. The HPT–haem complex is taken up by the liver for metabolism of the haem molecule. α-2-macromolecule is a protease inhibitor and caeruloplasmin is a carrier protein for copper. It is deficient in Wilson's disease.

β-globulins secreted by the liver include transferrin (iron transport), low-density lipoprotein (see below) and complement proteins. The complement proteins are a group of more than 20 glycoproteins, synthesized mainly by the liver. They are synthesized as inactive pro-enzymes which, when activated, form the cascade reactions of the complement system.

Clotting factors

All the clotting factors, except factor VIII, are synthesized by the liver, in addition to antithrombin III, a natural anticoagulant.

Acute-phase reaction proteins

During tissue injury, infection or inflammation, the liver synthesizes a heterogeneous group of plasma proteins termed the acute-phase reaction proteins. These include complement proteins, fibrinogen, α-1-antitrypsin, caeruloplasmin and HPT. In addition, hepatic production of C-reactive protein (CRP) and serum amyloid A increases. The function of these two proteins is unknown but may involve modulation of complement and other immunological functions. C-reactive protein may be used as a marker of acute inflammation in acute illness.

CARBOHYDRATE METABOLISM

The liver is essential for the maintenance of normal blood glucose. The hepatic metabolic processes involved in carbohydrate metabolism are gluconeogenesis, glycogenesis and glycogenolysis. The liver is also a site of metabolism of fructose, sorbitol and ethanol.

Gluconeogenesis (Fig. 22.4)

Gluconeogenesis is defined as the production of glucose from non-carbohydrate sources. Maintenance of blood glucose is important, as it is the main fuel for the brain and red blood cells. In the fasted state, carbohydrate stores (in the form of liver glycogen) are depleted in 12–24 h. Therefore, alternative substrates are required for glucose synthesis by gluconeogenesis. The main substrates are amino acids (muscle breakdown), glycerol (triacylglycerol) and lactate (anaerobic metabolism in skeletal muscle and red blood cells). The liver is the main site of gluconeogenesis, but it also occurs in the renal cortex during prolonged starvation. Fat cannot be converted into glucose, but instead is used for ketone production, which the brain utilizes as an energy source in prolonged starvation.

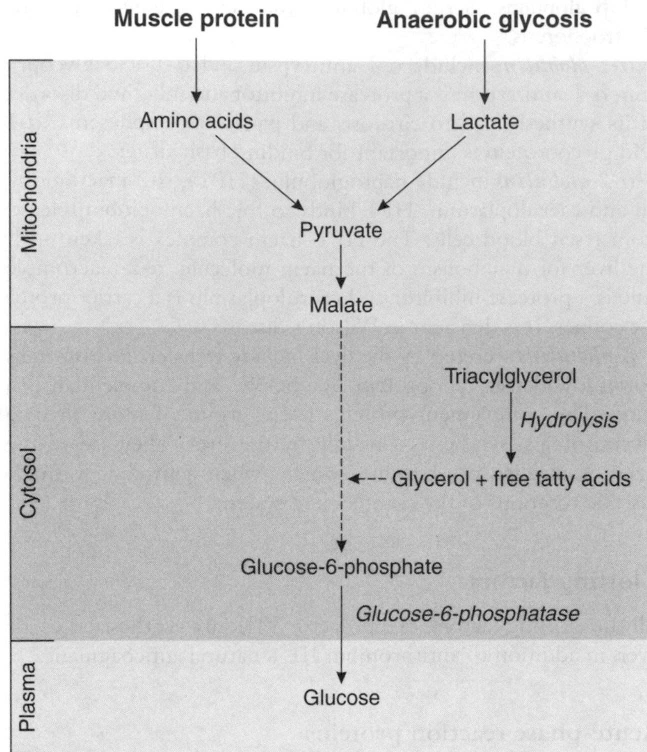

Fig. 22.4
Summary of gluconeogenesis.

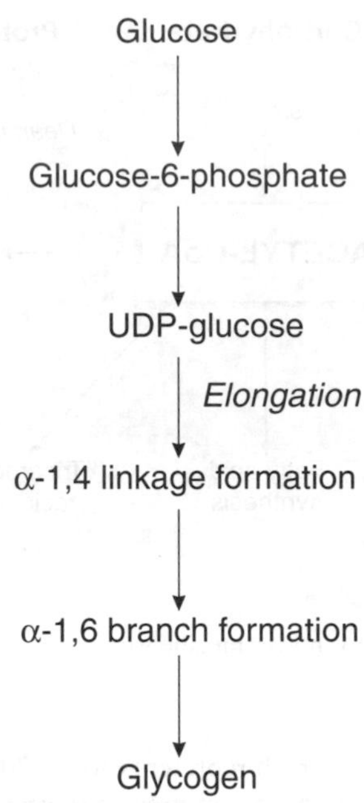

Fig. 22.5
Glycogenesis.

Gluconeogenesis is not a simple reversal of glycolysis, but is a series of reactions which occur in the cytoplasm and mitochondria. Amino acids, lactate and triacylglycerol may enter the series of reactions as several intermediates. Gluconeogenesis starts with pyruvate entering mitochondria for conversion into oxaloacetate. Both lactate and several amino acids may be converted into pyruvate and therefore enter the pathway by this route. Triacylglycerol enters the pathway later by conversion into fructose-1,6-diphosphate. The final reaction in gluconeogenesis is the conversion of glucose-6-phosphate into glucose catalysed by glucose-6-phosphatase. This enzyme is unique to the liver and allows the release of free glucose from the liver into the circulation. Gluconeogenesis is stimulated by increases in circulating glucagon, cortisol and adrenocorticotrophic hormone (ACTH). These hormones play a significant role in the stress response after surgery, trauma or during starvation when gluconeogenesis is most prevalent. The net effect is an increase in substrates for glucose synthesis and a stimulus for pyruvate to be used in gluconeogenesis rather than enter the TCA cycle.

Glycogenesis (Fig. 22.5)

Excess dietary glucose is converted into a readily accessible carbohydrate store in the liver and skeletal muscle termed glycogen. Glycogen is a highly branched polymer of glucose present in cell cytosol as granules. Because of its branched structure, it may be broken down rapidly by enzymes to glucose. Following a meal, liver and muscle glycogen stores increase, and are then used as a continual supply of glucose between meals. However, only liver glycogen may be used to increase blood glucose concentrations, as the muscle cells lack glucose-6-phosphatase. Therefore, glucose derived from muscle glycogen may only be used within the muscle cell.

Glycogenesis is stimulated by insulin and occurs in the cell cytosol. Glucose is phosphorylated to glucose-6-phosphate to maintain a low intracellular concentration of glucose. Uptake of glucose by the cell is aided by maintaining this concentration gradient. By a series of reactions, glucose-6-phosphate is converted to UDP-glucose which is then polymerized into a single chain of repeating molecules via α-1,4 bonds. Individual chains are then joined by α-1,6 bonds to form a highly branched molecule.

Glycogenolysis

Glycogen breakdown is stimulated by epinephrine and glucagon (liver glycogen only). Glycogen phosphorylase cleaves α-1,4 linkages to release glucose-1-phosphate. This is then converted to glucose-6-phosphate which may enter the glycolysis pathway or (in the liver) be converted to glucose and released into the circulation. α-1,6 linkages are cleaved by other enzymes to leave single chains for glycogen phosphorylase. Glycogen storage diseases are caused by deficiencies of the various enzymes used in the metabolism of glycogen.

Sucrose metabolism

Dietary sucrose is digested in the gut by sucrase to glucose and fructose. The liver is the principal organ for the metabolism of fructose (the muscle has a minor role). Fructose enters the liver and is phosphorylated by fructokinase to fructose-1-phosphate. This is then converted to glyceraldehyde-3-phosphate which may enter the glycolysis or gluconeogenesis pathways.

Ethanol metabolism

Ethanol is metabolized in the liver by several enzyme systems. The most important is the oxidation of ethanol to acetaldehyde by alcohol dehydrogenase using NAD^+ as a co-factor. Acetaldehyde is taken up by mitochondria and oxidized to acetate by aldehyde dehydrogenase. The acetate is released by the liver and used for metabolism by other tissues.

LIPID METABOLISM

Liver involvement in the metabolism of lipids includes synthesis and breakdown of fats, cholesterol metabolism, transport of lipids in the circulation and ketone body metabolism.

Lipid synthesis (Fig. 22.6)

Fatty acids are an important fuel derived from the breakdown of stored fat. However, the liver also synthesizes fatty acids from non-lipid substances using acetyl-CoA as the primary substrate. Excess dietary glucose not required for glycogen synthesis is converted to pyruvate via glycolysis. The pyruvate is converted to acetyl-CoA and, instead of entering the TCA cycle to produce further ATP, the acetyl-CoA is used for fatty acid synthesis (lipogenesis). This involves irreversible conversion of acetyl-CoA to malonyl-CoA in the cell cytosol by acetyl-CoA carboxylase. The final product is palmitate, a 16-carbon saturated fatty acid. This is formed by a series of reactions which sequentially add two carbon units, derived from malonyl-CoA, to a growing fatty acid chain. A small amount of stearate, an 18-carbon fatty acid, is also produced by this process. These fatty acids may be used for the synthesis of other fatty acids in other tissues.

Lipogenesis occurs in the liver, adipose tissue and mammary glands. Fatty acid synthesis is stimulated in energy-rich situations and by insulin. Increases in ATP produced by the TCA cycle inhibit the enzymes in this pathway. There is then an increase in available citrate which activates acetyl-CoA carboxylase. Acetyl-CoA is therefore used preferentially for fatty acid synthesis rather than entering the TCA cycle with further production of ATP.

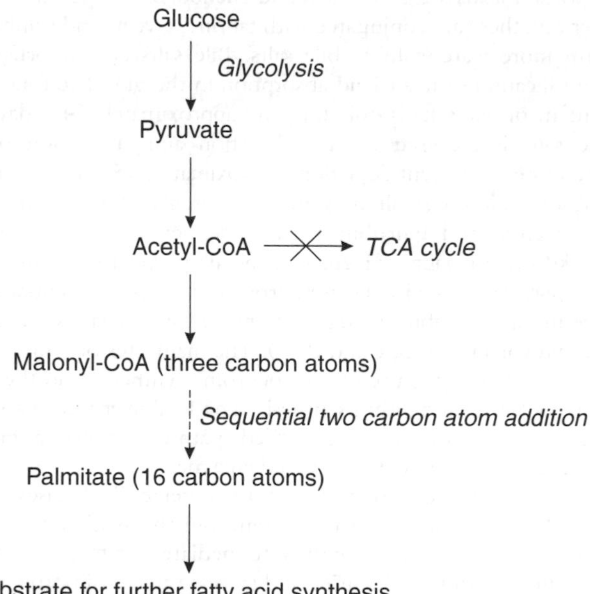

Fig. 22.6
Lipid synthesis.

Lipid breakdown (lipolysis) (Fig. 22.7)

Fat is stored in adipose tissue as triacylglycerol, a molecule consisting of three fatty acids attached to a molecule of glycerol. The first stage of lipolysis is the hydrolysis of triacylglycerol to glycerol and free fatty acids in the adipose tissue. The reaction is catalysed by lipase. The free fatty acids circulate in the plasma bound to albumin. They are taken up by the liver and skeletal muscle, where CoA is attached in the cytosol to form acyl-CoA. Acyl-CoA then enters the mitochondria and, in a series of repeated reactions (β oxidation), two carbon atoms are removed as acetyl-CoA, which may then enter the TCA cycle for ATP production.

Regulation of lipolysis depends on the activity of lipase in the adipose tissue. During prolonged exercise, epinephrine activates adenylate cyclase leading to an increase in cAMP. An increase in cAMP activates cAMP-dependent protein kinase which activates lipase in adipose tissue. The same enzyme also inhibits fatty acid synthesis. Glucagon and ACTH have the same effects in starvation, leading to a breakdown in body fat stores. Insulin has the opposite effects, inhibiting lipolysis and promoting fatty acid synthesis.

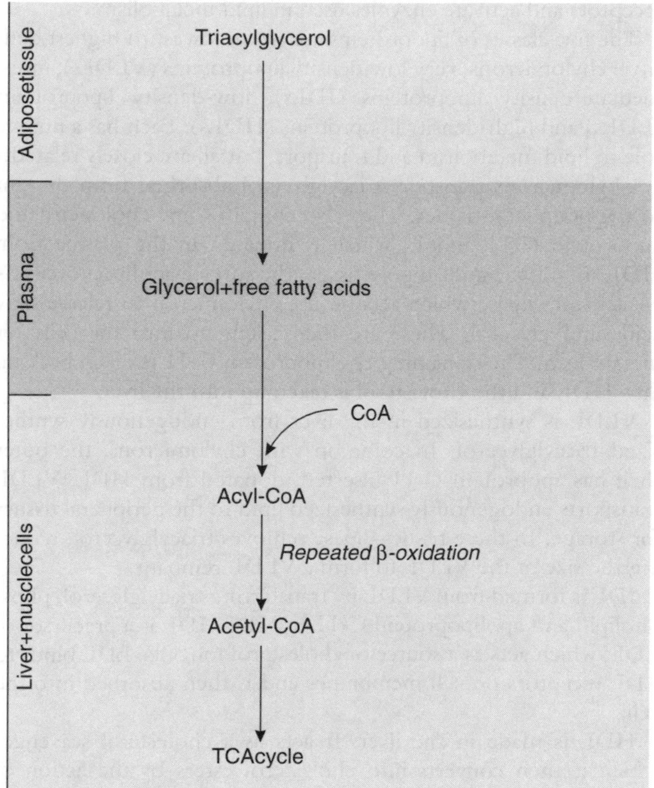

Fig. 22.7
Summary of lipid breakdown.

Cholesterol metabolism

Cholesterol is a 27-carbon steroid molecule used in the synthesis of cell membranes, steroid hormones, bile acids and vitamin D. Although most cholesterol is obtained from the diet, the liver is an important site of synthesis. In health, the synthesis and excretion of cholesterol is closely controlled to avoid cholesterol accumulation.

Cholesterol is synthesized in a series of reactions in the cell cytoplasm. Initially, three acetyl-CoA molecules are used to form a five-carbon isoprene unit and one molecule of carbon dioxide. The rate-limiting step in this process involves an enzyme termed HMG-CoA reductase. Next, six isoprene units are condensed to form cholesterol.

HMG-CoA reductase is the main site of regulation of cholesterol synthesis. It is inhibited by an increase in cholesterol concentrations and also by the cholesterol-lowering drugs simvastatin and pravastatin.

Most cholesterol is converted to cholesterol esters to make it less water-soluble and to aid storage. In the cell, esterification is catalysed by acyl-CoA cholesterol acyl transferase (ACAT). In the plasma, free cholesterol is converted to esters in high-density lipoproteins (HDLs) by the action of lecithin-cholesterol transferase (LCAT).

Transport of lipids in the plasma

Lipids are transported in the plasma as lipoproteins. Lipoproteins are a family of particles with a similar structure, consisting of a lipid core of triacylglycerol and cholesterol esters. This core is surrounded by a shell of phospholipid, free cholesterol and apolipoproteins. Apolipoproteins are a group of molecules which are vital to the transport of lipids, as they act as ligands for tissue receptors and activate enzymes used in lipid metabolism.

The five classes of lipoproteins are (from lowest to highest density): chylomicrons, very low-density lipoproteins (VLDLs), intermediate-density lipoproteins (IDLs), low-density lipoproteins (LDLs) and high-density lipoproteins (HDLs). Each has a unique role in lipid metabolism and transport, but all are closely related.

Chylomicrons transport triacylglycerol absorbed from the gut to the peripheral tissues. They also contain some cholesterol and apoprotein C-11 and E, which is donated in the plasma from HDL. In muscle and adipose tissue, the surface apolipoprotein C-11 activates lipase which acts on the chylomicron to release fatty acids and glycerol. These are then taken up into the cells for metabolism. The remaining apolipoprotein C-11 is taken back up into HDL and the cholesterol is taken up into the liver.

VLDL is synthesized in the liver from endogenously synthesized triacylglycerol. In common with chylomicrons, the outer shell has apoprotein C-11 inserted, donated from HDL. VLDL transports endogenously synthesized lipid to the peripheral tissues for storage. In these tissues, lipase removes triacylglycerol, reducing the size of the VLDL to form a VLDL remnant.

IDL is formed from VLDL by transferring triacylglycerol, phospholipid and apolipoprotein C-11 to HDL. IDL is a precursor of LDL, which acts as a source of cholesterol for cells. LDL binds to LDL receptors on cell membranes and is then absorbed into the cell.

HDL is made in the liver. It acts as a cholesterol scavenger which it then converts into cholesterol esters by the action of LCAT. These esters are then donated to VLDL or IDL to form LDL. HDL is also a source of apolipoproteins for other lipoproteins.

Ketone metabolism

The liver is the site of ketone production in the body. The three important ketones are acetoacetate, 3-hydroxybutyrate and acetone. All are acidic and are normally produced only in small quantities. However, during starvation or severe exercise, when glucose is in short supply as a fuel, they are an important source of energy for the brain, heart and skeletal muscle. The production of ketones normally equals the rate of utilization to prevent accumulation and acidosis. However, in diabetic ketoacidosis, production is uncontrolled, leading to life-threatening acidaemia.

Ketone synthesis occurs in hepatocyte mitochondria using acetyl-CoA (derived from β-oxidation of fatty acids or breakdown of ketogenic amino acids) as the precursor. In a series of steps, acetoacetate is produced which is then reduced to 3-hydroxybutyrate. Acetone is formed from the spontaneous decarboxylation of acetoacetic acid. The normal ratio of 3-hydroxybutyrate to acetoacetate is 3–6:1. In non-ketotic states, acetyl-CoA enters the TCA cycle by combining with oxaloacetate to produce citrate. During stress, oxaloacetate in the TCA cycle is used for gluconeogenesis and there is a reduction in the amount of oxaloacetate to combine with acetyl-CoA. The excess acetyl-CoA is therefore used for ketone production.

Ketones are released from the liver and are taken up by tissues (brain, heart and muscle) which may convert them back to acetyl-CoA in the mitochondria. This then enters the TCA cycle with the production of ATP. The liver is unable to use ketones for energy, as hepatocytes lack an essential enzyme used in this production of acetyl-CoA from ketones.

BILE SYNTHESIS

The liver synthesizes approximately 1 L of bile a day. Bile is a complex mixture of bile acids (salts), bile pigments, water and inorganic and organic compounds. The synthesis and metabolism of bile acids and bile pigments should not be confused.

Bile acids are synthesized in the liver from cholesterol. The two important acids are cholic acid and chenodeoxycholic acid. In the liver cell, these are conjugated with taurine, glycine and sulphate to form more water-soluble bile salts. Bile salts are important for emulsification of fats to aid absorption in the gut. The total body content of bile salts is only 6 g, and approximately 24 g day^{-1} of bile salts is required for the digestion and absorption of fat. Therefore, to prevent depletion, approximately 95% of bile salts are reabsorbed in the small intestine and recirculated back to the liver.

Biliverdin and bilirubin are bile pigments derived from the breakdown of haem. Haem is a metalloporphyrin consisting of four pyrrole rings with a central iron atom. It is an essential structure in haemoglobin, myoglobin and certain enzymes, including the cytochromes a, b, c and P450. The main sites of synthesis are the liver, where it is used for cytochrome synthesis, and the bone marrow for haemoglobin synthesis. The fetal liver is also a site of haemoglobin synthesis. The synthetic pathway involves a series of eight reactions catalysed by several enzymes.

Porphyria is a collection of six distinct metabolic diseases caused by a deficiency of one of the enzymes in the synthetic pathway. This leads to cumulation of the intermediate porphyrins with subsequent excretion in the urine and faeces. Attacks of porphyria are precipitated by several factors, including some drugs which activate the first enzyme in the synthetic pathway (δ-ALA synthetase). These drugs include barbiturates and steroids.

Haem is broken down in the liver, spleen and bone marrow by Kupffer cells and other macrophages to produce biliverdin (Fe_3^+). This is reduced to bilirubin (Fe_2^+) in the macrophage cytoplasm, which is then released into the plasma and transported to the liver bound to albumin. In the liver, it is taken up into the hepatocyte and conjugated with glucuronide in the rough endoplasmic reticulum. This is catalysed by UDP-glucuronyl transferase to produce mono- (20%) and di-glucuronides (80%). These water-soluble compounds are then secreted into the biliary canaliculi and subsequently excreted into the gut in bile. In the small intestine, bilirubin is further reduced to urobilinogen, which is then deconjugated by intestinal flora to urobilin and stercobilin. These are excreted in the faeces, although a proportion is reabsorbed to be taken up by the liver or excreted in the urine.

The composition of bile is altered in the biliary canaliculi by secretion of water and electrolytes, cholesterol, vitamins, fatty acids, phospholipids and mucin. In the gall bladder and larger bile ducts, bile is concentrated by the removal of water until it reaches the composition that is finally excreted into the gut.

ROLE OF THE LIVER IN DRUG METABOLISM

The liver is the main organ responsible for metabolism of exogenous (xenobiotic) and endogenous (endobiotic) compounds. The basic mechanism is the conversion of lipophilic compounds into hydrophilic compounds which can then be excreted. With drug metabolism, active compounds are usually converted into inactive or non-toxic metabolites. However some drugs may be converted to more active or toxic metabolites. Traditionally, drug metabolism is divided into two groups of reactions: phase 1 and phase 2.

Phase 1 reactions alter existing functional groups of drugs to increase the compound's water solubility. This is accomplished by reductase, hydrolase and oxidase enzymes (Table 22.2). Reduction and hydrolysis occur in the cytoplasm of the hepatocyte, whereas oxidation occurs in the smooth endoplasmic reticulum. Oxidation is the commonest type of reaction and involves several different reactions, including aliphatic and aromatic hydroxylation, O-dealkylation, N-oxidation, desulphuration and dehalogenation.

Table 22.2 Examples of phase 1 reactions

Oxidation	
N-dealkylation	Morphine, lidocaine
O-dealkylation	Codeine, pancuronium
Aliphatic hydroxylation	Ibuprofen, thiopental
Aromatic hydroxylation	Phenytoin, fentanyl
Deamination	Cimetidine
Dehalogenation	Halothane, enflurane
S-oxidation	Paracetamol
Reduction	
Azoreduction	Fazadinium
Nitroreduction	Nitrazepam
Hydrolysis	
Ester hydrolysis	Procaine, aspirin
Amide hydrolysis	Lidocaine, indomethacin

Oxidation reactions are catalysed by a group of haem-containing enzymes termed the cytochrome P450 system (mixed function oxidases). This is not a single enzyme, but a 'super family' of many isoenzymes, concentrated in the centrilobular region of the hepatic lobule. There is considerable variation between individuals in their P450 profile, which may affect rates of metabolism. This is a result of differences in genetic profile, health and exposure to toxins or drugs including alcohol.

Phase 2 reactions occur predominantly in the cell cytosol. The majority of drugs undergo phase 1 metabolism before proceeding on to phase 2 reactions. However, with some drugs, phase 1 is not necessary before conjugation. The commonest phase 2 reaction is conjugation with glucuronic acid, by attaching it to hydroxyl or carboxyl groups on the drug. This reaction is catalysed by UDP-glucuronosyl transferase, and the glucuronic acid is derived from a by-product of the pentose phosphate pathway, UDP-glucuronic acid. Other phase 2 reactions include sulphation and acetylation (Table 22.3).

TESTS OF LIVER FUNCTION

Liver function tests may be used to assess hepatocellular damage, cholestasis and synthetic capacity and to quantify overall liver function. No single test is diagnostic, but a logical approach using several specific tests may often identify the pathology of liver disease.

INDICATORS OF LIVER DAMAGE

Damaged cells release intracellular enzymes into the circulation which may be detected by plasma assays. The main enzymes which can be measured in the plasma and signify hepatocyte injury are aspartate transaminase (AST), alanine transaminase (ALT), lactate dehydrogenase (LDH) and glutamate dehydrogenase (GDH).

Aspartate transaminase is also found in other tissues, including heart, muscle, pancreas and kidney. It is therefore not specific for liver damage. Alanine transaminase is only produced in the liver and is specific for liver disease. Both enzymes are released by damaged hepatocytes following injury by hypoxia, infection or drugs. Aspartate transaminase is cleared more rapidly from the circulation than alanine transaminase. Following acute injury, there may be a dramatic increase in concentration in plasma AST and ALT. However, in chronic diseases, plasma concentrations may be normal or only slightly increased.

Lactate dehydrogenase is released from many tissues and is therefore not specific to liver injury. The enzyme exists as five isoenzymes, of which LDH 4 and 5 are found in the liver. Therefore, measurement of these isoenzymes is more appropriate in liver disease. It has a short half-life and plasma concentrations decrease early when regression of the disease occurs.

Table 22.3 Examples of phase 2 reactions

Glucuronidation	Paracetamol Morphine Diazepam
Sulphation	Steroids
Acetylation	Sulphonamides Procainamide

INDICATORS OF CHOLESTASIS

Bilirubin

Cholestasis is impaired excretion of bile into the duodenum. It may be caused by factors within the liver or extrahepatic causes (e.g. gallstones). Jaundice is present when the plasma bilirubin concentration is greater than 35 μmol L^{-1}, although it is often not clinically detected until it is greater than 50 μmol L^{-1}. Two forms of bilirubin may be measured in the plasma – conjugated (water-soluble) and unconjugated (lipid-soluble) – although most laboratories report only total bilirubin concentration.

In cholestatic jaundice, the hepatocytes still conjugate bilirubin and excrete it into the canaliculi. Because of failure to drain the canaliculi of bile, overspill of conjugated bilirubin occurs from the canaliculi into the sinusoids. Therefore, plasma concentrations of conjugated bilirubin increase. Cholestasis also has a detrimental effect on the hepatocytes and often some necrosis is inevitable, producing increases in plasma transaminases and unconjugated bilirubin. Similarly, hepatocyte necrosis secondary to any cause produces jaundice, because of blockage of the canaliculi by cell oedema or debris.

Increase in plasma unconjugated bilirubin alone suggests haemolysis or defective uptake and conjugation of bilirubin, e.g. Gilbert's disease.

Alkaline phosphatase

This is a membrane-bound enzyme found in the liver, bone, intestines and placenta. It is synthesized by bile canalicular membranes and plamsa concentrations are increased in cholestatic jaundice and, to a lesser extent, in hepatocellular disease. Simultaneous increases in plasma γ-glutamyl transferase (γ-GT) confirm the source of the alkaline phosphatase as hepatobiliary. Increased concentrations may also be found with hepatic tumours, infiltrations or abscesses.

γ-Glutamyl transferase

This enzyme is synthesized by hepatocytes and many other tissues. It is therefore not specific for liver disease as plasma concentrations are often raised after myocardial infarction and acute pancreatitis. However, it is often increased in very early alcoholic liver disease before other enzyme changes occur. Its use in confirming the source of a raised alkaline phosphatase concentration as hepatobiliary is described above.

INDICATORS OF IMPAIRED SYNTHETIC FUNCTION

Plasma proteins synthesized by the liver are reduced in liver disease. The rate at which their plasma concentrations decrease depends on their half-life in the circulation. Albumin has a relatively long half-life of 20 days and therefore is a poor prognostic indicator in acute liver disease. Following trauma or major surgery, plasma albumin concentration decreases rapidly because of catabolism and redistribution outside the vascular compartment. In chronic liver disease, albumin is reduced because of decreased synthesis and is a better prognostic indicator. Prealbumin has a shorter half-life of 1.5 days and can be useful in assessing acute liver disease.

Coagulation factors are better indicators of hepatic synthesis because they have short half-lives. Factor VII has the shortest half-life (1.5–6 h) and its activity may be monitored by measuring prothrombin time. Factor VIII is not synthesized in the liver and concentrations may actually be increased in liver disease. Similarly, concentrations of fibrinogen do not correlate with synthetic function.

Plasma cholinesterase is synthesized and released from the liver. Concentrations and activity are often reduced in severe liver disease, although they may be increased in some conditions, including alcoholic fatty liver.

QUANTITATIVE ASSESSMENTS OF LIVER FUNCTION

Several tests have been developed to assess the quantitative function of the liver by measuring hepatic clearance of specific drugs or compounds. Although these tests give an overall indication of hepatic function, they are limited in that they only assess one or two enzymatic functions. Consequently, they may correlate poorly with long-term prognosis. Indocyanine green and bromosulphthalein, which are used to measure hepatic blood flow, can also be used to assess function. Given the high extraction ratio of ICG, its metabolism is related to hepatic blood flow. Following a large dose, its metabolism is by zero-order kinetics because of enzyme saturation, and its elimination is dependent on the functional mass of liver.

Lidocaine is metabolized by liver cytochrome P450 to monoethylglycinexylidine (MEGX). The plasma concentration of this metabolite correlates with functioning hepatic mass, and consequently measurement of lidocaine metabolism is a relatively simple method to assess liver function. Finally, Kupffer cell function may be assessed by measuring the clearance of a radioactively labelled colloid, as 90% of colloids are eliminated in the liver.

FURTHER READING

Benyon S 1998 Mosby's crash course. Metabolism and nutrition. Mosby, London

Park G R, Kang Y (eds) 1995 Anesthesia and intensive care for patients with liver disease. Butterworth-Heinemann, Boston

Strunin L, Thomson S (eds) 1992 Baillière's clinical anaesthesiology. The liver and anaesthesia. Baillière Tindall, London, vol 6, no. 4

23 Haematology

Surgery and anaesthesia make heavy demands on departments of haematology and blood transfusion. Consultation between the anaesthetist and haematologist should be frequent both in the operating theatre and in the intensive therapy unit if the provision of, for example, appropriate blood components and the correct investigation of the bleeding patient are to proceed smoothly and expeditiously. The UK Department of Health's policy that hospital transfusion committees should now exist in every hospital should result in improved efficiency and appropriateness in the use of blood and blood products.

ANAEMIA

Anaemia is present when the red cell mass (the erythron) is reduced below the reference range for the patient's age and sex. There are many causes, which are classified conventionally as:

- *Blood loss* – may be acute or chronic.
- *Failure of erythropoiesis* – resulting from, for example, inadequate supplies to the bone marrow of nutrients: iron, vitamin B_{12}, folate, some hormones or protein. Erythropoiesis may be impaired by bone marrow infiltration in leukaemia or other malignant disease. Anaemia of chronic disease is the term used for the secondary anaemias of chronic inflammation, infection and malignancy (when the marrow is not infiltrated). Such anaemia is also seen in rheumatoid arthritis and chronic renal failure.
- *Shortened red cell lifespan*. The haemolytic anaemias are subdivided into:
  - —inherited, e.g. hereditary spherocytosis, sickle cell anaemia and some red cell enzyme defects
  - —acquired, e.g. autoimmune haemolytic anaemia, paroxysmal nocturnal haemoglobinuria and drug-induced haemolysis.

Alternative classifications are possible and forms of anaemia may be allocated to more than one category. Thus, chronic blood loss produces negative iron balance with eventual failure of erythropoiesis from iron deficiency. Pernicious anaemia is an erythropoietic failure resulting from lack of correct digestion of vitamin B_{12}, but red cell precursors and mature red cells in this disease have a shortened life span.

Anaemia is demonstrated by the measurement of the amount of haemoglobin in a known volume of blood. Haemoglobin concentration is reported as grams per decilitre (g dl^{-1}) or grams per litre (g L^{-1}). Anaemia is said to be present in an adult male if the haemoglobin concentration is less than 13.5 g dl^{-1} (135 g L^{-1}) and in an adult female if less than 11.5 g dl^{-1} (115 g L^{-1}). In the first year of life, the haemoglobin concentration decreases from 13.5–19.5 g dl^{-1} at birth to 9.5 g dl^{-1} at 1 month to attain levels at 12 months close to those of female adults. In pregnancy, haemoglobin levels should not decrease below 11.5 g dl^{-1} if iron and/or folate are not deficient.

Modern electronic blood counting equipment provides accurate red cell indices in addition to haemoglobin estimation and these provide guidance on the type of anaemia before resort to further investigation. It is worth noting that the commonest form of anaemia worldwide is that caused by iron deficiency.

With the notable exception of acute blood loss, reduction in red cell mass is accompanied by an increase in plasma volume, thus preserving blood volume. The mechanism for this is not clear but it is one of the compensatory mechanisms adopted during anaemia of any duration. Of equal importance is a shift of the oxygen dissociation curve to the right through increased synthesis of 2,3-diphosphoglycerate (2,3-DPG) in the red cell via the Embden–Meyerhof pathway of anaerobic glycolysis and the Rapaport–Luebering shunt. Increases in 2,3-DPG render the haemoglobin molecule less avid for oxygen at any given partial pressure and improve tissue oxygenation. Two remaining compensatory mechanisms in anaemia are an increase in cardiac stroke volume and an increase in heart rate.

In acute blood loss, red cells and plasma are lost together, such that in the first few hours haemoglobin and haematocrit measurements change little and cannot be used to estimate blood loss. Surgeons have always attributed much importance to the haematocrit, but in continued acute bleeding the haemoglobin and haematocrit move in parallel. Haemodilution is complete by 24–48 h if transfusion of red cells is not carried out.

GENETIC ABNORMALITIES OF HAEMOGLOBIN

The inherited abnormalities of haemoglobin include a complex and diverse series of genetic defects resulting from impaired production of normal globin chains (thalassaemias) or synthesis of an abnormal haemoglobin. The thalassaemias are characterized by absent or reduced production of the affected globin chain whilst the other chains which make up the haemoglobin molecule are structurally normal. In the haemoglobinopathies, the affected chain, usually the β or α chain, has an amino acid substitution which, if it affects the structure or function of the haemoglobin molecule as a whole, may produce clinical effects.

β-THALASSAEMIA

β-Thalassaemia, in which β-globin chain synthesis is impaired, is classified into three clinical grades.

β-Thalassaemia trait (thalassaemia minor) is the heterozygous state and produces little clinical effect. There may be slight anaemia and the condition may be mistaken for iron deficiency. In pregnancy, the haemoglobin may decrease below the reference range.

Thalassaemia intermedia, as the name implies, is associated with more marked anaemia than thalassaemia trait and is generally caused by double heterozygosity or homozygosity of less severe β-thalassaemia genes. Occasionally, patients may require transfusions of red cells.

Thalassaemia major (Cooley's anaemia) is the homozygous inheritance of severe β-thalassaemia genes; β-chain production is reduced (β^+) or absent (β^0), thus impairing the synthesis of adult haemoglobin. Without blood transfusion the condition is generally fatal in the early years of childhood, and even with regular transfusion support, patients may not live beyond their early 20s as a result of iron overload. Long-term iron chelation therapy may prevent transfusional iron overload and bone marrow transplantation may be considered.

α-THALASSAEMIA

α-Thalassaemia is a genetically variegate disorder which ranges in severity from fetal death in utero in the homozygous form to a mild hypochromic disorder in the heterozygous form. Patients with three of the four α-chain genes deleted suffer HbH disease of intermediate severity and some require transfusion with red cells.

SICKLE CELL DISEASE

More than 100 haemoglobin variants have been described, but only one has significant global clinical impact – haemoglobin S. Ten per cent of patients of African extraction carry the S gene. It is also seen in Italy, Greece, Arabia and the Indian subcontinent. Haemoglobin S has valine substituted for glutamine in position 6 of the β-globin chain and this confers physical differences on the haemoglobin molecule with profound clinical consequences in homozygotes. Haemoglobin S becomes insoluble at oxygen tensions in the venous range (5– 5.5 kPa) and crystallizes, imposing a sickle cell shape on the red cell. The sickled red cell is rigid and does not pass easily through capillaries, leading to occlusion, tissue infarction and the pain which is characteristic of clinical episodes known as crises. Red cell survival is reduced greatly and homozygous patients invariably have anaemia (6–10 g dl^{-1}) and jaundice. Heterozygotes are mostly asymptomatic but their red cells may sickle when oxygen tensions are unphysiologically low. Haemoglobin S may exist in combination with other genetic defects of haemoglobin, the most significant combinations being HbS/β^0-thalassaemia and HbSC disease. Symptoms may be similar to those of homozygous HbSS although HbSC has a particular tendency to thrombosis and retinopathies.

Patients with haemoglobinopathies are at risk of unique perioperative complications and increased mortality. Haemoglobin electrophoresis should therefore be performed in all patients of affected ethnic groups to establish the presence or absence of haemoglobin S before anaesthesia. In an emergency, sickle haemoglobin may be demonstrated rapidly in patients' blood using a commercial kit, e.g. Sickledex (Ortho Diagnostics). It may be necessary to pre-transfuse homozygotes electively or consider exchange transfusion to raise the percentage of haemoglobin A compared with haemoglobin S, particularly for surgery involving cardiopulmonary bypass. In all cases, it is essential to maintain good oxygenation pre-, intra- and postoperatively, and consideration should be given to oxygen therapy for 24 h after anaesthesia. Postoperative infarctive episodes may occur even with the most meticulous attention to detail. Acute chest syndrome is often underdiagnosed, and documentation of intraoperative temperature, hypoxia and volume status is vital. Sickling is enhanced by low blood pH, high red cell 2,3-DPG, stasis, dehydration and increased plasma osmolality. Avoidance of these factors is imperative.

HAEMOSTASIS AND THROMBOSIS

NORMAL MECHANISMS

Haemostasis involves an interaction between vascular endothelium, platelets and coagulation proteins to seal the point of injury of the vessel wall.

The vessel wall

Extracellular matrix proteins such as collagen in the blood vessel wall fulfil an essential role in haemostasis by promoting platelet adhesion at the site of vessel injury. The endothelial cell also has a powerful influence on haemostasis by virtue of the factors that it synthesizes. These include tissue factor, von Willebrand factor (VWF), prostacyclin, antithrombin, protein S, thrombomodulin and tissue plasminogen activator.

Platelets

The initial response of platelets to a break in the endothelial lining is adherence to subendothelial microfibrils and collagen through binding with VWF. Platelets then change shape from a disc to a sphere and extend long pseudopodia to enhance interaction between adjacent platelets. Reorganization of the internal constituents forces the granules to the plasma membrane where, triggered by exposed collagen and production of thrombin, they release their contents onto the surface of the platelet. These include proteins such as VWF, factor V, β-thromboglobulin and platelet factor 4 from α-granules, and ADP, ATP and serotonin from dense granules. The arachidonic acid pathway is also stimulated, resulting in thromboxane formation that further potentiates platelet aggregation and release. Together with serotonin, it also has a profound vasoconstrictive effect. ADP aids binding of fibrinogen to platelet receptors, allowing bound platelet aggregates to form.

Activated platelets also provide a phospholipid surface for many of the reactions involved in the coagulation pathway (Fig. 23.1).

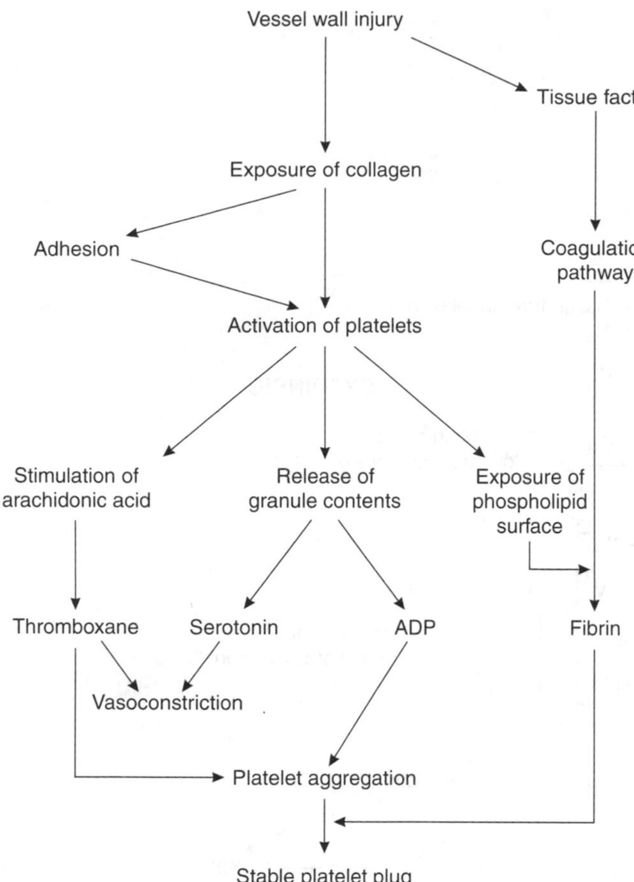

Fig. 23.1
The role of platelets in haemostasis.

The coagulation pathway

The role of the coagulation proteins in haemostasis has traditionally been described in terms of two distinct pathways that feed into a final common pathway, ultimately resulting in the formation of thrombin, the cleavage of fibrinogen to form fibrin, and stabilization of the platelet plug (Fig. 23.2). The activity of these pathways is measured routinely in the laboratory. The intrinsic pathway is tested by the activated partial thromboplastin time (APTT), which provides a good measure of the function of factors VIII, IX, XI and XII and contact factors, while the extrinsic pathway, involving factor VII and tissue factor, is measured using the prothrombin time (PT).

While this system remains invaluable for understanding in vitro tests of coagulation, it does not accurately reflect events in vivo. It is now hypothesized that there is a single pathway with several feedback loops (Fig. 23.3). The principal initiator of the pathway is tissue factor, an integral membrane glycoprotein present on cells beneath the endothelium. Tissue factor forms a complex with factor VII, which directly activates both factors X and IX. Factor Xa is responsible for the subsequent production of the first traces of thrombin. Through powerful positive feedback mechanisms, thrombin then amplifies its own production, thus accelerating the formation of fibrin. Activated by thrombin, factor XIII stabilizes the fibrin polymer by cross-linkages between adjacent strands. Strands of fibrin then truss platelets and red cells into the platelet plug.

Natural inhibitors to coagulation

Several protective mechanisms exist to inhibit the unbridled extension of thrombus and vessel occlusion. As the vessel relaxes, returning blood flow dilutes activated clotting proteins and mechanically discourages extension of the plug. Vascular endothelial cells secrete prostacyclin, a powerful inhibitor of platelet aggregation. Tissue factor pathway inhibitor (TFPI) complexes with factors VIIa and Xa to switch off tissue factor-mediated coagulation. Circulating inhibitors neutralize clotting intermediates, the most important being antithrombin (AT), which regulates factors Xa and thrombin. The binding of thrombin to thrombomodulin, an endothelial cell receptor, activates the vitamin K-dependent inhibitors protein C and its cofactor S. These cleave and inactivate factors VIIIa and Va. Thus thrombin is converted from a procoagulant to an anticoagulant. Inherited individual deficiencies of antithrombin, protein C and protein S present with thrombotic events.

The fibrinolytic pathway

The fibrinolytic system (Fig. 23.4) is also of great importance. It has similar triggers to those of coagulation and is regulated by controlled activation and inhibition. The active enzyme of fibrinolysis is plasmin, which degrades fibrin into soluble products. It is derived from an inactive precursor, plasminogen. The two activators of plasminogen are tissue plasminogen activator (tPA), which is concerned principally with dissolution of circulating fibrin and urokinase, involved in pericellular breakdown of fibrin. Both plasminogen and activator bind to fibrin. The resulting fibrin degradation products (FDPs) are both anticoagulant and interfere with fibrin polymerization.

Inhibition of the fibrinolytic system occurs at the level of plasmin itself, by α_2 antiplasmin, or plasminogen activator, with specific plasminogen activator inhibitors (PAIs). Deficiency of these proteins may result in bleeding tendency.

THE BLEEDING PATIENT

The anaesthetist and surgeon are confronted not infrequently by a patient who is known to have a pre-existing haemostatic defect and the haematologist is asked if the patient is either fit for surgery or may be rendered operable.

INHERITED COAGULATION ABNORMALITIES

These comprise classic haemophilia (haemophilia A) arising from coagulation factor VIII deficiency, Christmas disease (haemophilia B) from deficiency of factor IX (and clinically identical to classic haemophilia) and von Willebrand's disease from deficiency of von Willebrand factor (VWF), a protein responsible for platelet adhesion and stability of the factor VIII molecule in the circulation. Other inherited coagulation factor deficiencies occur but are uncommon.

The bleeding manifestations in the haemophilias are related directly to the degree of deficiency. Patients with severe haemophilia, with factor VIII or IX levels of < 1 U dl^{-1}, usually have frequent spontaneous haemorrhage into joints and muscles. In moderate haemophilia, with levels of 1–5 U dl^{-1}, spontaneous bleeding is less common, and in those mildly affected (levels > 5 U dl^{-1})

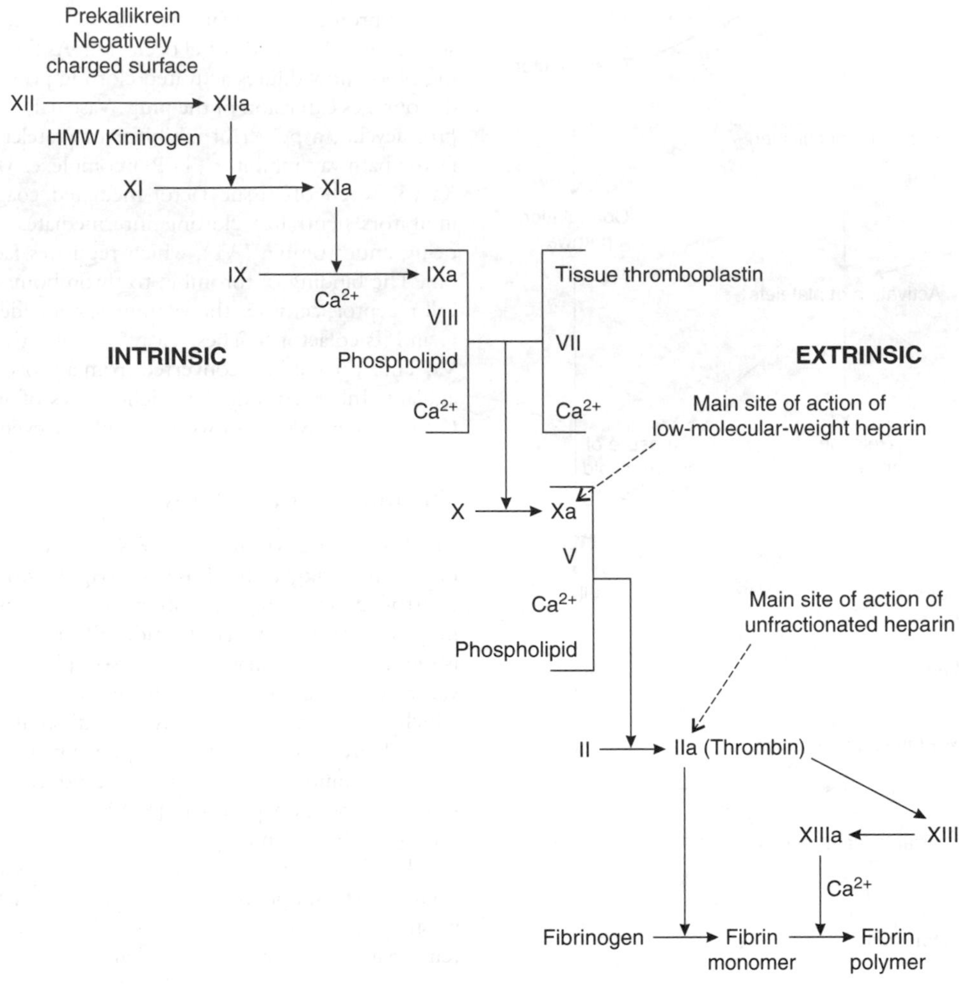

Fig. 23.2
Intrinsic and extrinsic coagulation pathways – 'a' indicates activation of the factor concerned. Phospholipid is provided by platelets and plasma. The actions of standard and low-molecular-weight heparin are indicated.

spontaneous bleeding is uncommon. These patients may remain undiagnosed until late in life. However, any haemophiliac patient, whatever grade of severity, may bleed excessively if challenged by trauma or by surgery, and an occasional patient is diagnosed initially under those circumstances.

For surgery to proceed safely, the concentration of the appropriate factor must be raised to, and maintained at, a haemostatic level. The manner in which this is achieved depends on the type of surgery envisaged, the native factor level in the plasma, the half-life of the factor concerned after infusion, the type of factor concentrate available and the number of days to healing (which in turn depends on the procedure that has been performed). Moderate and severe haemophiliacs require treatment with factor VIII or IX concentrates perioperatively and for bleeding episodes. Products used are either derived from pooled US plasma or manufactured by recombinant technology. Mild haemophilia and most types of von Willebrand's disease can often be treated with desmopressin (DDAVP), which may be given by intravenous, subcutaneous or intranasal routes. This increases plasma concentrations of factor VIII by 2–6 times and von Willebrand factor by 2–4 times after about 30 min. As DDAVP is an antidiuretic, care should be taken with fluid balance to avoid volume overload.

A percentage of haemophiliacs, particularly haemophilia A, develop inhibitory antibodies, making management much more difficult. Morbidity and mortality occur from inability to achieve adequate haemostasis. Surgery should be performed only if absolutely necessary and should be carried out in designated haemophilia centres which have the staff, technical facilities and experience to supervise the haemostatic management of such patients. Options for treatment include high-dose human factor VIII, porcine factor VIII or bypassing agents such as recombinant factor VIIa or activated prothrombin complex concentrate (aPCC) such as FEIBA (factor eight inhibitor bypassing activity).

Many haemophiliacs in the UK have become infected with HIV, hepatitis C and other viruses as a result of the previous use of contaminated blood products. Heat treatment and other biological and chemical manipulations of factor concentrates and the increasing use of recombinant products have improved the safety of treatment for the haemophiliac population.

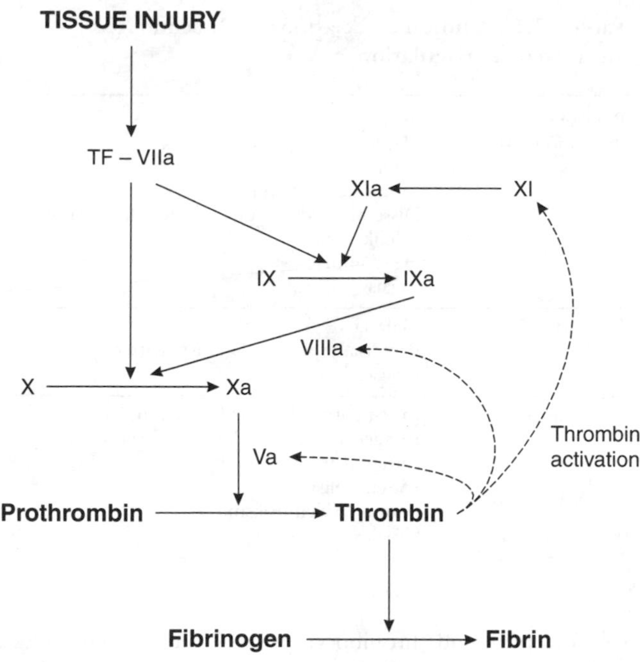

Fig. 23.3
The revised coagulation pathway.

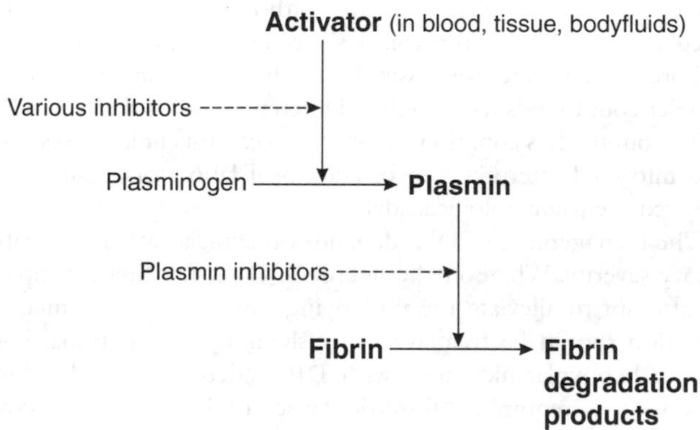

Fig. 23.4
The fibrinolytic system.

THROMBOCYTOPENIA

The normal whole-blood platelet count is 150–400 $\times 10^9$ L^{-1}. The lower limit of normal, or reference range, depends upon the method used for their quantitation, but a platelet count below 100×10^9 L^{-1} is considered to be thrombocytopenia. The risk of haemostatic failure increases as the platelet count decreases, and when levels below 30×10^9 L^{-1} are reached, spontaneous bleeding may occur. Bleeding is precipitated if there is local pathology, e.g. peptic ulcer, or if there is a surgical wound. Thrombocytopenic bleeding occurs less at a particular platelet count if the low platelet numbers result from peripheral destruction with a functional bone marrow (e.g. autoimmune thrombocytopenia) than if platelet production is impaired, e.g. in bone marrow disorders (e.g. leukaemia or myeloma).

For unexplained, new-onset thrombocytopenia, examination of the blood film may provide some clues to the cause. This may reveal platelet clumping, as in pseudothrombocytopenia, in which case the blood count should be repeated on a citrated sample, or the presence of schistocytes, suggestive of disseminated intravascular coagulation (DIC) or thrombotic thrombocytopenic purpura (TTP). Other laboratory tests should include a coagulation screen for DIC, and liver function and renal function tests. Consideration should also be given to the patient's medications, including heparin and the IIb/IIIa blockers used for cardiac procedures. In patients who have had a massive transfusion (replacement of blood volume in less than 24 h), platelet numbers decline progressively, although rarely to below 50×10^9 L^{-1}. Post-transfusion purpura is a rare delayed complication of blood transfusion in which recipient antiplatelet antibodies cause severe consumption of autologous and allogeneic platelets.

DISORDERS OF PLATELET FUNCTION

For adequate primary haemostasis, the platelets should also function normally. In comparison with the rare inherited disorders of platelet function, drug-induced platelet metabolic damage occurs more commonly. Aspirin (acetylsalicylic acid) is the prime example, causing inhibition of the enzyme cyclooxygenase with impaired thromboxane synthesis. Its effect on measured in vitro function of platelets lasts up to 10 days. Non-steroidal anti-inflammatory drugs (NSAIDs) and sulphinpyrazone have similar effects and degrees of platelet dysfunction are caused by many other therapeutic agents. Bleeding may occur in the face of adequate platelet numbers and patients should be encouraged to discontinue the drug, preferably 2 weeks before major surgery. Uraemia is accompanied by acquired platelet dysfunction, partly as a result of increased catabolism of VWF, and this may be corrected by dialysis or improved with DDAVP or cryoprecipitate, both of which enhance VWF levels. Correction of anaemia is also important to encourage platelets to marginate to the periphery of the blood vessel, increasing their contact with the vessel wall. Cardiopulmonary bypass affects both platelet number and function. This is mainly a result of platelet activation and consumption caused by heparin and the equipment itself. If post-pump microvascular bleeding occurs, platelets often need to be maintained above 10×10^9 L^{-1} to compensate for the functional defect. Platelets in the myeloproliferative disorders, including some leukaemias, may function poorly.

Careful examination of the patient reveals clues to deficient or defective platelets: petechial purpura particularly below the knee, blood-filled blisters in the mouth and fundal haemorrhages. For the patient in theatre, oozing at the operation and venepuncture sites acts as an indicator. Platelet function in vivo is measured best by the template bleeding time carried out by haematology staff according to strict methodology. This should not be undertaken unless platelet numbers have been shown to be normal or bleeding is out of proportion to platelet numbers and coagulation is demonstrably normal. The strategy of platelet transfusion is described below.

THE ANTICOAGULATED PATIENT

A commonly encountered problem is that of the patient receiving oral anticoagulants who presents as an emergency requiring surgical intervention within a short time. Surgeons are generally reluctant to proceed without at least partial reversal of anticoagulation.

Vitamin K may be given, by slow intravenous injection, to reverse the warfarin defect, although it should be noted that if excess is given, it might render the patient refractory to further warfarinization for days or weeks. The dose of vitamin K in warfarin-induced serious haemorrhage is 5 mg, but in the therapeutically anticoagulated patient about to undergo surgery, doses of 0.5–1.0 mg are usually sufficient. Reversal may take up to 12 h and cannot be hastened by a larger dose. If surgery cannot be delayed, partial reversal may be achieved with fresh frozen plasma (FFP). Up to 1 L may be needed and its effect should be determined by further measurement of international normalized ratio (INR). Full reversal of warfarin is better achieved with factor VII-rich prothrombin complex concentrate (PCC), also containing factors II, IX and X, at a dose of 50 U kg^{-1} body weight, but it must be remembered that this product could exacerbate an underlying hypercoagulable state.

For elective operations, warfarin should be stopped or adjusted at least 3 days beforehand to achieve an INR of approximately 2.0 on the day of surgery. Whether heparin needs to be substituted when the INR drops to the lower limit of the therapeutic range depends on the balance of risks of thrombosis and perioperative bleeding. In general, patients with a mechanical heart valve should be treated in the same way, as the short-term risk of thromboembolism when anticoagulation is discontinued for a few days is very small. The highest risk is seen in patients with a ball-and-cage valve in the mitral position and these patients might be considered for continuous heparin infusion.

The timing of reinstitution of warfarin depends on the risk of postoperative haemorrhage, but in general it can be restarted as soon as the patient has an oral intake.

DISSEMINATED INTRAVASCULAR COAGULATION

This is also referred to as *consumption coagulopathy*, which reflects the pathogenesis. Essentially, the process represents the inappropriate triggering of the coagulation cascade in flowing blood by specific disease processes. There is considerable variation in severity, ranging from the coagulopathy as the predominant clinical manifestation (with haemostatic failure) to merely a laboratory sign of the underlying disease with no clinical haemostatic lesion. Some possible causes are listed in Table 23.1.

Table 23.1 Clinical associations of disseminated intravascular coagulation

Release of tissue thromboplastin	Eclampsia Placental abruption Fetal death in utero Amniotic fluid embolism Disseminated malignancy including acute leukaemia Head injury Burns
Infection	Malaria Bacteria, especially Gram-negative Viruses
Miscellaneous	Incompatible blood transfusion Extracorporeal circulation Antigen–antibody complexes Fat embolism Pulmonary embolism Shock

The principal laboratory findings are produced by the consumption of platelets during intravascular coagulation with reduction of fibrinogen and elevation of FDP in the serum as secondary (physiological) fibrinolysis breaks down thrombus. Thrombocytopenia, hypofibrinogenaemia and elevation of serum FDP are thus the hallmarks of DIC. Scrutiny of the blood film may reveal red cell distortion or fragmentation if there is associated microangiopathy.

As the majority of clotting tests rely on the fibrinogen–fibrin reaction as the end-point, the PT, APTT and thrombin time are prolonged as a result of the anticoagulant effect of FDP and consumption of other coagulation factors (II, V, VIII). DIC that is associated with endotoxaemia and endothelial damage tends to have more profound thrombocytopenia. There is some suggestion that in severe DIC, there is, in addition, an induced platelet function defect. DIC is inevitable to some degree where there is tissue damage (particularly the brain), hypotension, shock and poor organ perfusion.

Variants of the syndrome (with similar laboratory findings) may occur with localized extravascular consumption (e.g. placental abruption) and localized intravascular consumption (e.g. aortic aneurysm). Occasionally, primary pathological fibrinolysis (PF) occurs without the microthrombosis seen in DIC, e.g. in neoplasia. Laboratory tests are not dissimilar to those used in DIC but the platelet count tends to be higher. Differentiation of the commoner DIC from the less common PF rests on a careful clinical assessment and informed interpretation of additional laboratory tests, which may require haematological advice.

The management of DIC depends on clinical rather than laboratory severity. Whatever the degree of DIC, the first principle is an attempt to alleviate the underlying cause. In septicaemia, the infection should be treated vigorously along conventional lines, and in hypovolaemic shock with DIC, adequate blood volume expansion is required. Obstetric causes of DIC usually recover promptly after evacuation of the uterus. After successful treatment, most patients with DIC settle spontaneously and only in those with significant and continuing coagulation failure is there a need to repair the haemostatic mechanism with blood components. This includes the administration of FFP, cryoprecipitate (which is rich in fibrinogen) and platelets. As a rough guide, platelets should be maintained above 50×10^{9} L^{-1}, fibrinogen > 1g L^{-1} and PT and APTT not greater than 1.5 times the control. Heparin may be required if thrombosis is the predominant feature. Clinical trials suggest that antithrombin and protein C concentrates may be of value for severe cases. Advice should be sought from the haematologist.

LIVER DISEASE

Hepatocellular disease (cirrhosis or acute liver failure) gives rise to a variety of abnormalities of coagulation. Diminished protein synthesis leads to low levels of vitamin K-dependent clotting factors (II, VII, IX and X), factor V, factor XIII and fibrinogen. Accumulation of fibrin degradation products results from increased fibrinolysis, as a result of increased plasminogen activator, and impaired clearance from the plasma. Platelets are often reduced in number, particularly in the presence of hypersplenism, alcoholism or folate deficiency and may be dysfunctional. These abnormalities produce a laboratory profile similar to that seen in DIC, although the latter usually gives rise to greater prolongation of the thrombin time. Recourse to vitamin K, FFP, cryoprecipitate and platelet support may be required for bleeding or proposed surgery. FFP and cryoprecipitate often need to be repeated at approximately 6 h in view of the short biological half-life of some of the factors, and care must be taken to avoid fluid overload in patients with an already expanded plasma volume.

THE THROMBOTIC PATIENT

The interaction of and balance between coagulation and fibrinolysis are essential in maintaining vessel integrity and patency after injury. Disturbance of normal mechanisms may give rise to venous thromboembolism. Risk factors are well-recognized (Table 23.2), but thrombosis usually results from interplay of both genetic and acquired factors. Important amongst these is the hypercoagulability that follows surgery and anaesthesia, and surgeons are increasingly using various prophylactic strategies to prevent this complication. The risk for thrombosis must be assessed on an individual basis, taking into account pre-existing patient variables and the nature of the illness, trauma or planned surgery. For low-risk patients, such as those having minor surgery and with no additional risk factors, early mobilization and adequate hydration are usually sufficient. Heparin should be considered for patients at higher risk. Subcutaneous low-dose unfractionated heparin or low-molecular-weight heparin (LMWH) are most widely used. The advantages of the latter are increased bioavailability, giving a more predictable response and longer duration of action, allowing for once-daily injections. Evidence shows that LMWHs are just as effective in preventing postoperative deep vein thrombosis and for some operations, such as orthopaedic surgery, they are more so. As the majority of venous thromboses begin to develop during surgery but present after discharge from hospital, prophylaxis is usually started just before the procedure and continued until the patient is ambulatory. Mechanical devices such as pneumatic compression or graduated stockings might be of additional benefit.

If a patient who is therapeutically heparinized requires emergency surgery, cessation of the infusion may suffice because of the short half-life of the drug. The laboratory test of choice to monitor adequacy of unfractionated heparin is the APTT, which should be 1.5–2.5 times the normal control value. This desired ratio may differ between laboratories. Prior to emergency surgery in the heparinized patient, recourse to the APTT may indicate that there is little risk of bleeding if the ratio is less than 1.5. Reversal of heparin in an emergency may be achieved using protamine sulphate given by slow intravenous injection at a dose of 1 mg per 100 units of heparin. Not more than 50 mg of protamine sulphate should be given because, in addition to side-effects of flushing, bradycardia and hypotension, it is itself an anticoagulant. Protamine only partially reverses the anti-Xa activity of LMWHs. The same dose should be given as for unfractionated heparin unless the LMWH was given more than 3 h previously, in which case the dose should be reduced by at least half. Additional protamine may be required (at approximately 60 min intervals) in view of its short half- life and continuous absorption of subcutaneous heparin.

Table 23.2 Risk factors for venous thrombosis

Hereditary thrombophilias
Factor V Leiden
Prothrombin mutation
Hyperhomocysteinaemia
Protein C deficiency
Protein S deficiency
Antithrombin III deficiency
Dysfibrinogenaemia
Hypercoagulable states due to physiological stimuli
Pregnancy
Oestrogen therapy
Surgery
Immobilization
Advancing age
Obesity
Hypercoagulable states associated with pathological conditions
Antiphospholipid antibodies
Hyperhomocysteinaemia
Previous venous thromboembolism
Congestive cardiac failure
Malignancy
Nephrotic syndrome
Heparin-induced thrombocytopenia
Paroxysmal nocturnal haemoglobinuria
Myeloproliferative disorders

HEPARIN-INDUCED THROMBOCYTOPENIA (HIT)

Approximately 2–3% of patients receiving unfractionated heparin for 5 or more days develop an immunologically mediated reaction, causing a relatively sudden decrease in platelet count to below 100×10^9 L^{-1}. It is caused by production of antibody to the heparin–platelet factor 4 complex on the surface of platelets (platelet factor 4 being a heparin-binding glycoprotein stored in platelet alpha granules). In a high proportion of cases, the resulting platelet activation leads to acute venous or arterial thrombosis and other events, including adrenal haemorrhagic infarction and skin necrosis at the sites of heparin injection. HIT also occurs in patients receiving prophylactic doses of heparin or LMWH but is much less common. The diagnosis should be suspected in a patient who has received heparin in any form for more than 4–5 days (or less if there has been previous exposure to heparin) and who has a relatively sudden decline in platelet count to less than 100×10^9 L^{-1} or to less than 50% of previous values. The diagnosis and management are made on clinical grounds, although they may be confirmed by laboratory tests, which are performed in some centres. All forms of heparin should be discontinued, and if anticoagulation is still required, alternatives should be used. Suitable substitutes are recombinant hirudin, a thrombin-specific inhibitor, or danaparoid sodium, a low-molecular-weight heparinoid.

BLOOD TRANSFUSION

PROCESSING OF BLOOD FOR TRANSFUSION

Strict medical selection of donors minimizes infection risks to the recipient in addition to ensuring donor safety. Furthermore, in the UK, all blood donations are screened for hepatitis B, hepatitis C, HIV-1 and HIV-2 and syphilis. These measures have resulted in an almost negligible risk of transfusion-transmitted disease, which will be reduced even further when donors are screened by polymerase chain reaction (PCR) assays, which should further shorten the window periods.

Blood is collected into sterile plastic bags containing CPD-A (citrate, phosphate, dextrose, adenine), which acts both as an anticoagulant and as a preservative. The packs are centrifuged to separate the different components, including red cells, plasma and platelets. The components are now leucodepleted to eliminate leucocyte-associated infections and white cell-mediated transfusion reactions. FFP is used either for direct transfusion or for the large-scale manufacture of products including albumin, coagulation factors and immunoglobulins. In view of a theoretical risk of transmission of CJD, plasma for large-scale processing is now being obtained from the USA, although there have been no cases reported to date. While red cells, platelets and FFP do not usually undergo further manufacturing procedures to reduce the risk of viral transmission, derivatives from pooled plasma are subjected to further purification and viral inactivation steps to destroy any infectious agents which might escape detection.

RED CELL PRODUCTS

Only a small proportion of units is issued as whole blood, the majority being red cell concentrates. Some red cell concentrates are suspended in plasma and are produced by the removal of 150–200 ml of plasma from the final donated volume. Most units have a much greater percentage of plasma removed and are re-suspended in a preservative solution. The additive used in the UK is SAGM (saline, adenine, glucose, mannitol). Red cell concentrates are more viscous than whole blood and have a higher haematocrit (Table 23.3). All preparations have a shelf-life of 35 days. Small-volume red cell split units may be prepared for paediatric transfusion. Preparations for neonatal exchange transfusions must meet specified criteria.

Storage of red cells should be at 2–6°C in blood bank refrigerators, with in-built alarm systems. Appropriate temperatures inhibit bacterial replication, slow red cell glycolysis with some preservation of 2,3-DPG and prevent freezing of blood with lysis of cells on warming. Resort to other domestic-type refrigerators is hazardous because of the risk of inadequate thermostatic control. Ministry of Health-type insulation boxes maintain pre-cooled red cells for transfusion at a satisfactory temperature, when used with ice inserts, for up to 8 h and are usually available upon request. Blood should be transfused cold except in certain situations such as large-volume transfusion or for patients with cold haemagglutinin disease when a blood warmer may be required. Units which have been out of storage for more than 30 min should be discarded. Protocols should always be in place to ensure that adequate checks are made before administration.

BLOOD GROUPS

The ABO blood groups first described in 1901 by Landsteiner and the Rhesus system (Rh) described by Landsteiner and Weiner in 1940 form the important blood group systems for those practising blood transfusion primarily at the bedside. However, there are many other clinically important blood group systems that are of more immediate concern to the blood transfusion laboratory staff. Problems relating to these groups are normally resolved by the laboratory before blood products are issued as compatible for use in the patient.

ABO groups

In the UK, 47% of persons are group O, 42% group A, 8% group B and 3% group AB. Patients, and thus donors, have these percentage distributions (Table 23.4). Proportions vary elsewhere in the world mainly from increased gene frequency of group B. ABO blood group substances may also be found on leucocytes and platelets, and 77% of persons secrete ABO blood group substances in body fluids. A and B antigens are present on red cells early in fetal development, but the corresponding antibodies appear only after birth at 3–6 months of age and are present in greatest strength at the age of 10 years. They are naturally occurring, i.e. they are a constant feature of the system in all persons and do not arise as a result of exposure to A or B blood group substances at some time during life. They are pres-

Table 23.3 Blood components

Component	Volume	Comments
Whole blood	450 ± 45 ml	HCT 0.35–0.45
Concentrated red cells	280 ± 60 ml	HCT 0.55–0.75
Red cells with additive (SAGM)	350 ± 70 ml	HCT 0.50–0.70
FFP (random donor)	150 – 300 ml	
Cryoprecipitate	15 – 25 ml	> 140 mg fibrinogen/unit
Platelets (adult therapeutic dose)	200 – 300 ml	> 240 × 10^9 platelets

HCT, haematocrit; FFP, fresh frozen plasma.

Table 23.4 Distribution of ABO blood groups in the UK, their red cell antigens and antibodies

	%	RBC antigen	Serum	
O	47	–	Anti-A Anti-B	'Universal donor'
A	42	A	Anti-B	
B	8	B	Anti-A	
AB	3	A + B	–	'Universal recipient'

Rhesus D positive 85%.
Rhesus D negative 15%.

ent invariably in the serum when the red cells lack the corresponding antigen. Table 23.4 shows the old rationale, now outmoded, for the designation of group O persons as 'universal donors', because they lack group A and B substances in their red cells, and persons of group AB as 'universal recipients' as their serum does not contain either anti-A or anti-B. ABO antibodies are predominantly IgM and thus do not cross the placenta. An occasional person, usually group O, may have immune anti-A (or less commonly, anti-B), an IgG molecule capable of crossing the placenta and active at 37°C. If pregnant with a group A (or B) fetus, ABO maternofetal incompatibility may ensue with haemolytic disease of the newborn.

Whenever possible, blood transfusion laboratories try to provide blood of the same ABO group as the recipient. If a patient of group AB requires an emergency transfusion of more than a few units, further AB units may be unavailable and group A or B blood is used. If ABO-compatible blood is unavailable for a group B patient, group O is used with suitable preceding compatibility tests.

ABO-incompatible transfusion accidents are the most serious, with complement activation resulting in significant morbidity and mortality. Usual symptoms of distress, chest or abdominal pain and breathlessness are masked during anaesthesia when hypotension and uncontrollable bleeding caused by DIC may be the only signs. Incompatible transfusions nearly always arise from incorrect labelling of the sample or request form, or inadequate checks before administration of the blood.

Rhesus antigens

Shortly after the discovery of the Rhesus antigens it was recognized that some haemolytic transfusion reactions and haemolytic disease of the newborn (erythroblastosis fetalis) resulted from incompatibilities in this system. In bedside blood transfusion practice, the Rh D antigen is the most important of the Rhesus system, although others also exist, namely C, c, E and e antigens. The Rhesus factors are inherited in a 'packet', one from each parent, each 'packet' containing one of each pair of alleles, C, D and E. The commonest genes are CDe (gene frequency 0.41) and cde (0.39) followed by cDE (0.14). The other genes are much less common.

Antibodies of clinical significance occur in the Rhesus system and these rarely occur naturally, i.e. they are formed as the result of exposure to Rhesus antigens that the patient does not possess naturally. The most common antibody is anti-D, usually as a result of the bearing of a Rh D-positive fetus by a Rh D-negative woman. The national (UK) programme for prevention of Rhesus immunization in pregnancy has reduced the incidence of this. Rhesus antibodies are detected readily in compatibility tests but, if undetected, may result in delayed haemolytic transfusion reactions, with impaired survival of the transfused cells. Fever, declining haemoglobin concentration, jaundice and haemoglobinuria may appear 5–10 days after transfusion.

Other blood groups

The known number of blood group antigens is increasing constantly, usually because of the discovery first of the corresponding antibody. Many are of little clinical significance, although some cause immediate or delayed haemolytic reactions. Specificity and ability to react at 37°C characterize those antibodies in recipient serum which necessitate the provision of red cells lacking the corresponding antigen. Of greatest importance are, in order of frequency, Kell, Duffy, Kidd, Ss and Lewis. Of all clinically significant alloantibodies, 83% are in the Rhesus system (Table 23.5).

BLOOD GROUPING AND PRE-TRANSFUSION COMPATIBILITY TESTS

The introduction of commercial gel-based technology has revolutionized compatibility testing, facilitating the use of automated apparatus for undertaking these tests in large batches. This process may take up to half a day, but in the emergency situation, if the patient's group is not known, it can be ascertained within 5–10 min.

A group and antibody screen is carried out ideally in advance of the requirement to provide blood for transfusion. It consists of:

- ABO and Rh D grouping of the patient
- detection, at 37°C, of Rhesus and other atypical antibodies in recipient serum which would result in a transfusion reaction and reduced red cell survival
- verification of results by a computer or manual check of previous records.

If these tests are done according to recommended and quality-assured techniques and the patient's antibody screen is negative, then the actual crossmatch need only consist of an immediate spin of donor cells and recipient serum at room temperature to exclude the important ABO incompatibilities. This significantly reduces the delay in supplying blood to most patients.

In emergency situations, the risks of delaying transfusion must be weighed against the risks of using units which have not been fully crossmatched. Blood of the recipient's ABO and Rh D group should be supplied, but if a sample from the patient is unavailable, group O blood may be used, which would also need to be Rh D-negative for women of childbearing age and female children.

Table 23.5 Percentage frequency of clinically important 37°C alloantibodies detected in recipients

Anti-D	61
Anti-C (± D)	11
Anti-E	7
Anti-Kell	6
Anti-c	4
Anti-Duffy	2.2
Anti-Kidd	0.9
Anti-e	0.5
Anti-Ss	0.04
Others (Lewis included)	7

TRANSFUSION REACTIONS

In addition to the immediate or delayed haemolytic transfusion reactions referred to above, there are other types of reaction which may interfere with completion of transfusion of blood or blood components. Non-haemolytic febrile reactions, caused by recipient HLA antibodies to donor white cells, occur in 1–2% of red cell or platelet transfusions. Fever and rigors usually occur 30–60 min after the start of the transfusion. Most reactions are managed by slowing or stopping the transfusion and giving paracetamol. As platelets also express HLA antigens, there is often a failure of the platelet count to increase unless HLA-compatible platelets are used. With the introduction of universal leucodepletion, these problems should become less prevalent.

Allergic reactions to donor plasma proteins may cause urticaria and itching. Anaphylaxis is rare but life-threatening and may result from reaction between IgA in the transfused blood and anti-IgA in the recipient.

Transfusion-associated acute lung injury (TRALI) is often under-recognized. Antibodies in donor plasma react with recipient white cells, causing capillary leak and non-cardiogenic pulmonary oedema.

Other reactions to stored blood include fluid overload, bacterial contamination and late complications such as iron overload, transmission of viruses, graft-versus-host disease and immunosuppression.

A national confidential reporting system known as SHOT (serious hazards of transfusion) has now been established and should raise awareness of adverse events and factors contributing to their occurrence. Some complications of blood transfusion are listed in Table 23.6.

TRANSFUSION AND SURGERY

Traditionally, anaemic patients have been transfused perioperatively to achieve a haemoglobin level of >10 g dl^{-1}. There is no evidence that this is beneficial, and in young patients, who can tolerate lower haemoglobins and in whom late sequelae of transfusions have greater consequences, it may be harmful. However, in older or fragile patients, especially those with cardiovascular disease, transfusion may be appropriate to avoid any contribution to the risk of myocardial ischaemia. So, while a specific level of haemoglobin cannot be endorsed as a universal threshold for transfusion, decisions should be made on an individual basis, taking into account factors such as age and co-morbidity.

Autologous transfusion, involving pre-deposit, acute normovolaemic haemodilution (ANH) or intraoperative cell salvage may be appropriate in some situations. Pre-deposit autologous transfusion entails collection and storage of blood in advance of a planned operation and is suitable for relatively healthy individuals requiring elective surgery where blood loss is inevitable. This is a costly exercise, with many prepared units being wasted, and is not usually recommended. For ANH, blood is withdrawn from the patient immediately before surgery and replaced with colloid or crystalloid solution. The resultant lower haematocrit may lead to less red cell loss during surgery and may improve oxygen delivery as a result of a reduction in whole blood viscosity. The blood is stored in the operating theatre for return to the patient postoperatively. It remains to be shown if ANH is effective in reducing transfusion requirements in the patient. Intraoperative cell salvage involves suction, anticoagulation, washing and return of red cells shed at operation. ANH and cell salvage are suitable for surgery where the expected loss is >20% total blood volume. Potential contamination of blood makes cell salvage techniques contraindicated where there is bacterial sepsis. For all forms of autologous transfusion, the patient must be fully informed of the procedure and the possibility that they may still require additional allogeneic blood. Jehovah's witnesses do not usually accept autologous blood, although some accept intraoperative cell salvage.

Table 23.6 Complications of blood transfusion

Transmission of disease, e.g. viral hepatitis, syphilis, malaria, HIV
Bacterial contamination
Pyrogenic reactions
Incompatibility reactions
Haemolytic reactions
Allergic reactions
Citrate toxicity
Hypothermia
Hyperkalaemia
Metabolic acidosis
Circulatory overload
Air embolism
Microaggregate embolism

PLASMA VOLUME EXPANDERS

In acute hypovolaemia, plasma volume expanders are frequently used while blood is being prepared. Transfusion is often started with electrolyte solutions but continued with volume expanders. Three non-human source materials are in use.

Gelatins

In these preparations, animal gelatin is modified to produce an average molecular weight of 30 000–35 000 Da. The two available products, polygeline (Haemaccel) and succinylated gelatin (Gelofusine), have a pH, colloid osmotic pressure and viscosity similar to those of plasma. Their half-lives are approximately 4 h. They have a shelf-life at ambient temperatures of up to 8 years. Occasionally, rapid infusion, particularly in a normovolaemic patient, may result in the release of vasoactive substances that cause rash, hypotension and tachycardia; these may be managed by antihistamines and/or hydrocortisone, and the infusion should be discontinued. Gelatin solutions do not interfere with blood grouping or compatibility testing and renal function is not impaired.

The two preparations differ in their electrolyte content. Polygeline has a high calcium content (6.25 mmol L^{-1}) and thus should not be allowed to mix with citrated blood components. Gelofusine contains only a little calcium (0.4 mmol L^{-1}) and may be mixed with bank blood. No more than 1–1.5 L of gelatin solution should be transfused before blood is available.

Etherified starch

This plasma volume expander is an artificial colloid derived from amylopectin and closely resembles glycogen. Its average molecular weight is 200 000–450 000 Da and its infusion results in an expansion of plasma volume slightly in excess of the volume infused. Plasma volume expansion is maintained for at least 24 h.

Contraindications and side-effects are similar to those of dextran 70. No more than 1 L should be given.

Dextrans

Dextran 70 injection BP (6% dextran) is used most frequently in 5% glucose or in 0.9% saline. The average molecular weight of the material is 70 000 Da. Dextrans should not be administered to patients with renal impairment, severe congestive heart failure or thrombocytopenia. The dextrans are believed to interfere with the haemostatic mechanism if transfused in large quantity and cause difficulty with grouping and compatibility tests in the laboratory by promotion of rouleaux. This is less of a problem with the introduction into blood transfusion laboratories of gel technology. No acutely bleeding patient should receive more than 1.5 L and, as unpredictable allergic reactions may occur with erythema, bronchospasm, urticaria and hypotension, the patient should be observed carefully during the first few minutes of the infusion. If such a reaction occurs, usually as a result of the presence of antidextran antibodies, the infusion should be stopped immediately and resuscitation measures undertaken.

Human albumin solution

This material, known previously as plasma protein fraction, is prepared from donor plasma both by the Bio-Products Laboratory of the National Blood Service and by the pharmaceutical industry. It contains protein (principally albumin), 45 g L^{-1} in saline. It is heat-treated and present evidence suggests that this inactivates hepatitis-producing agents. It has a 3-year shelf-life (away from light). Until now it has been free from obvious side-effects but its safety has recently been brought into question as a result of a meta-analysis performed by the Cochrane Injuries Group Albumin Reviewers. The Committee on Safety of Medicines now recommends that its use should focus only on replacement of lost fluids, rather than correction of hypoalbuminaemia or the underlying illness causing hypovolaemia, and that haemodynamic monitoring of patients should be undertaken. In general, albumin has little clinical advantage over other colloid plasma volume expanders and it is substantially more expensive. Human albumin solution is now made from plasma from non-UK donors.

Concentrated solutions containing 20% albumin are useful for albumin replacement, particularly in liver disease. As there is a high risk of fluid overload and pulmonary oedema, it should be infused carefully with consideration given to the concomitant use of diuretics.

PLATELET THERAPY

Unlike red cells, platelets have an inconveniently short shelf-life. Whereas red cells in CPD-A have a safe storage life of 35 days, platelets in the same anticoagulant are only satisfactory when given to the recipient within 5 days of donation. This places obvious constraints on the supply of viable platelets to hospitals by transfusion centres. Platelets are supplied usually as concentrates, i.e. platelet-rich plasma (PRP), produced by gentle centrifugation of freshly donated blood, spun down again and much of the supernatant plasma removed. Adult doses of platelets may also be collected by apheresis of single donors. Platelet concentrates are stored at 22°C with agitation. Currently, platelets are not cross-matched but should be ABO-compatible to avoid risk of haemolysis caused by donor anti-A or anti-B.

In surgical practice, as a general rule, significant bleeding should not occur if platelet numbers are greater than 100×10^9 L^{-1}. Below 30×10^9 L^{-1}, bleeding may be anticipated. Between 30 and 100×10^9 L^{-1}, operative and postoperative oozing depends on the nature of the surgical procedure and the aetiology of the thrombocytopenia.

If surgery is to be covered with platelet transfusions, they may need to be given twice on the day of surgery, the first dose at least 60 min preoperatively. Further platelets should be assessed on the patient's progress and laboratory results, but twice-daily doses on the first and succeeding postoperative days may be required. Satisfactory post-transfusion increments in the platelet count should be demonstrated if bleeding continues to be troublesome.

Patients with autoimmune thrombocytopenia in whom medical treatment has failed may be referred for splenectomy with very low platelet counts. They do not require platelet transfusion for two reasons. First, therapeutic platelets would be of short survival, being cleared by the same immune mechanism which is causing the patient's thrombocytopenia. Second, following the tying of the splenic pedicle, platelet counts may increase rapidly, ensuring adequate intra- and postoperative haemostasis. However, the local blood bank should be notified of the elective splenectomy in order that platelets might be provided at relatively short notice if required.

In DIC, from any cause, where consumption has been documented as severe and haemorrhage is a clinical problem, or in the massively transfused patient with haemostatic failure, platelet transfusions should be given to maintain a count above 50×10^9 L^{-1}. The effects of these and of any transfused FFP or cryoprecipitate should be monitored by repeat laboratory tests and clinical evidence of reduced bleeding.

FURTHER READING

Bloom A L, Thomas D P 1994 Haemostasis and thrombosis, 2nd edn. Churchill Livingstone, Edinburgh

Contreras M (ed) 1998 ABC of transfusion, 3rd edn. BMJ Publishing Group, London

Hoffbrand A V, Pettit J E 1997 Essential haematology, 3rd edn. Blackwell Science, Oxford

Mollison P L, Engelfriet C P, Contreras M 1997 Blood transfusion in clinical medicine, 10th edn. Blackwell Science, Oxford

Nagel R 1997 Sickle cell anemia. Blackwell Science, Oxford

Petz L D, Swisher S M N (eds) 1995 Clinical practice of transfusion medicine, 3rd edn. Churchill Livingstone, Edinburgh

Provan D 1998 ABC of clinical haematology. BMJ Publishing Group, London

24 Immunology and body defences

The immune system in humans is a very adaptable system which has evolved to provide protection against both pathogenic invading organisms and cancer cells. This extremely complex system is able to recognize and eliminate a huge variety of foreign cells and molecules. An immune response may be classified functionally into recognition and response. Immune recognition is extremely specific, enabling discrimination between the subtle chemical differences which distinguish foreign pathogens from each other. In addition, the immune system is able recognize the body's own cells and proteins from foreign ones. When a foreign molecule has been recognized, termed the recognition response, the immune system recruits the involvement of several other cells and molecules to elicit an appropriate response to enable the neutralization or elimination of the particular organism. This is termed the effector response. Exposure to the same organism again at a later date induces a memory response, with enhanced immune reactivity which eliminates the pathogen and prevents disease.

INNATE IMMUNITY

Immunity may be defined as the state of protection from infectious disease, and comprises both specific and non-specific components. Non-specific, or innate, immunity is the basic in-built resistance to disease which a species possesses. Innate immunity comprises four defensive barriers, which offer protection through anatomical, physiological, phagocytic/endocytic and inflammatory strategies.

ANATOMICAL BARRIERS

Anatomical barriers are the body's first line of defence, preventing entry of pathogens and hence infection. These include the skin and mucous membranes.

The skin

Intact skin prevents the penetration of most pathogens. Skin consists of two layers, the thinner outer layer, or epidermis, and the thicker dermis. The epidermis is renewed every 2–4 weeks and does not contain blood vessels. The dermis is composed of connective tissue and contains blood vessels, hair follicles, sebaceous glands and sweat glands. The sebaceous glands produce an oily substance termed sebum, made up of lactic acid and fatty acids, maintaining the pH of the skin at around 4. This low pH inhibits bacterial growth. Bacteria which metabolize sebum live on the skin and are responsible for a rare form of acne. Acne treatments such as isotretinoin inhibit sebum formation. Breaks in the skin such as small cuts and insect bites are obvious routes of infection, and diseases such as malaria and Lyme disease are spread via insect bites.

Mucous membranes

The conjunctivae and the alimentary, respiratory and urogenital tracts are covered by mucous membranes, instead of skin. Many pathogens enter the body by binding to and penetrating mucous membranes, but these are protected by saliva, tears and mucus, which wash away organisms and also contain antiviral and antibacterial substances. In the lower respiratory and gastrointestinal tracts, organisms trapped in mucus are propelled out of the body by ciliary action. Some organisms have evolved such that they can evade this defence mechanism. For example, the influenza virus has a surface molecule which enables it to attach to cells in the mucous membrane, preventing it from being washed away through the action of cilia. The adherence of bacteria to mucous membranes is dependent on the interaction of protrusions on the bacteria and specific glycoproteins on some mucous membrane epithelial cells, which explains why only some tissues are susceptible to bacterial invasion.

PHYSIOLOGICAL BARRIERS

If an organism manages to breach the anatomical barriers, other innate defences come into play. Physiological barriers include temperature, pH and a variety of soluble factors, including lysozyme, interferons and complement. Many species are resistant to some diseases because their body temperature inhibits pathogen growth; for example, hens have a high body temperature which inhibits the growth of anthrax. Gastric acidity prevents the growth of many organisms, and newborn infants are more prone to some diseases because their stomach contents are less acidic. Lysozyme, found in mucus, is an enzyme which cleaves the peptidoglycan layer of bacterial cell walls. Interferons are produced by virus-infected cells and bind to nearby cells causing a generalized antiviral state. Complement is a group of serum proteins which circulate in an inactive state. They may be activated by non-specific immune mechanisms which convert the inactive proenzymes to active enzymes through an enzyme cascade, which results in membrane damaging reactions, destroying pathogenic organisms and facilitating their clearance.

Complement

The complement system is activated via a sequential enzymatic cascade and has an important role in antigen clearance. There are two pathways of complement activation; the classic pathway, which involves activation by specific immunoglobulin molecules; and the alternative pathway in which activation is by a variety of microorganisms and immune complexes. Each pathway results in the activation of different complement proteins, but the end-point is the same – the generation of a membrane attack complex which is how complement is able to lyse foreign cells. This complex displaces phospholipids within cell membranes, making large holes, disrupting the membrane and resulting in cell lysis. Complement components also amplify reactions between antigens and antibodies, attract phagocytic cells to sites of infection and promote phagocytosis, and activate B lymphocytes. The complement system is non-specific and, in theory, attacks both its own body cells and foreign cells. To prevent host cell damage, there are regulatory mechanisms which restrict complement reactions to specific targets. This is achieved by spontaneous breakdown of active complement components and release of inactivating proteins.

ENDOCYTOSIS AND PHAGOCYTOSIS

Another important innate defence mechanism is the ingestion of extracellular macromolecules and particles by processes termed endocytosis and phagocytosis, respectively. In endocytosis, macromolecules in extracellular fluid are internalized by invagination of the plasma membrane to form endocytic vesicles. Endocytosis may take place via two mechanisms – pinocytosis and receptor-mediated endocytosis. Pinocytosis occurs through non-specific membrane invagination, whereas in receptor-mediated endocytosis, macromolecules are engulfed selectively after binding to specific membrane receptors. The ingested material is degraded by enzymes of the endocytic processing pathway.

Phagocytosis involves ingestion of particles, including whole microorganisms, via expansion of the plasma membrane to form phagosomes. Virtually all cells are able to endocytose but phagocytosis occurs in only a few specialized cells. Professional phagocytes are the polymorphonuclear neutrophils, mast cells and macrophages, and non-professional phagocytes include endothelial cells and hepatocytes. Cells infected with viruses and parasites are killed by large granular lymphocytes, termed natural killer (NK) cells, and eosinophils. When particles are ingested into phagosomes, the phagosomes fuse with lysosomes and the contents are digested in a similar way to endocytosis.

THE INFLAMMATORY RESPONSE

The inflammatory response to tissue damage or invasion by pathogenic organisms results in vasodilatation, increased capillary per-

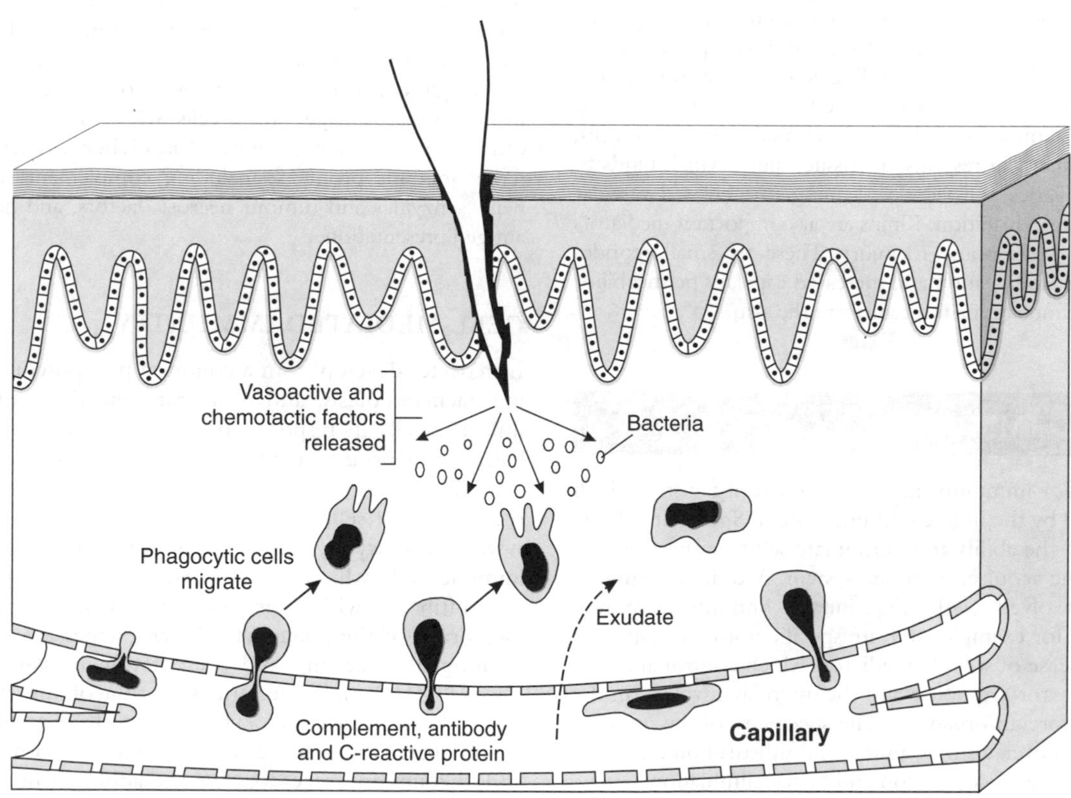

Fig. 24.1
Major events in the inflammatory response. A bacterial infection causes tissue damage with release of various vasoactive and chemotactic factors. These factors induce increased blood flow to the area, increased capillary permeability and influxes of leucocytes from the blood into the tissues. The serum proteins in the exudate have antibacterial properties and the phagocytes begin to engulf bacteria.

meability and influx of phagocytic cells (Fig. 24.1). Vasodilatation occurs as the vessels constrict, resulting in engorgement of the capillary network, causing tissue redness or erythema and increased tissue temperature, whilst increased capillary permeability enables influx of fluid and cells from the capillaries into the tissue. The accumulating fluid exudate has a high protein content and its accumulation contributes to the tissue swelling (oedema). The increased capillary permeability also helps migration of leucocytes into the tissues, particularly phagocytes. Movement of phagocytic cells involves a complex series of events, including margination or adherence of cells to the endothelial cell wall, extravasation or movement of the cells between the capillary cell walls into the tissue, and chemotaxis, the migration of the cells through the tissue to the site of inflammation. The process of white cell margination is a carefully regulated process involving molecules termed adhesion molecules. These comprise three structurally dissimilar groups of molecules which are located on the extracellular portion of the cell membrane of both endothelial cells and leucocytes. Examples include E-selectin, intercellular adhesion molecule (ICAM) and vascular cell adhesion molecule (VCAM). These molecules cause circulating white cells initially to slow down and then roll along the endothelium. Firm adherence and transmigration then occur.

The inflammatory response is initiated by a series of interactions which involve several chemical mediators, produced from the invading organisms, damaged cells, cells of the immune system and plasma enzyme systems. Among the chemical mediators released as a result of tissue damage are the acute-phase proteins. The circulating levels of these increase considerably during tissue damaging infections. C-reactive protein is a major acute-phase protein produced by the liver and which binds to the C-polysaccharide component found on many bacteria and fungi. This binding activates the complement system, resulting in both complement-mediated lysis and increased phagocytosis. Histamine is a chemical released from mast cells, basophils and platelets in response to tissue injury, which binds to receptors on capillaries and venules, leading to increased vascular permeability and vasodilatation. Kinins are also important mediators of the inflammatory response to injury. These are small peptides which also cause vasodilatation and increased capillary permeability. Bradykinin also stimulates pain receptors in the skin.

ACQUIRED IMMUNITY

Acquired (specific) immunity inactivates microorganisms which are not destroyed by the innate immune system. Specificity, diversity, memory and the ability to discriminate self from non-self are key features of the acquired immune system. Acquired immunity is intricately involved with the innate immune response. Phagocytic cells, for example, activate specific immune responses and stimulate release of soluble mediators which control and regulate the inflammatory response and the interplay involved in the elimination of a foreign organism. The specificity of the immune system is such that even a single amino acid substitution can mean that an antigen escapes recognition and hence elimination.

The acquired immune response may also be classified into humoral (from body fluid) and cell-mediated immunity. The humoral component involves interaction of B cells with antigen and their proliferation and differentiation into plasma cells, which secrete antibodies. Antibody is the effector of the humoral response via its binding to antigen, thereby neutralizing and facilitating its removal. This process also activates the complement system. Unlike B cells, where membrane-bound antibody enables direct recognition of antigen, T cells may only recognize antigen in the presence of cell membrane proteins termed the major histocompatibility complex (MHC) molecules. Effector T cells generated in response to antigen associated with MHC molecules are responsible for cell-mediated immunity. There are two types of T cells: T-helper (Th) cells and T-cytotoxic (Tc) cells. Th cells secrete cytokines, which are low-molecular-weight proteins and which activate various phagocytic cells, B cells, Tc cells, macrophages and various other cells. Under the influence of cytokines secreted by Th cells, Tc cells which recognize the antigen–MHC molecule complex differentiate into a type of effector cell termed a cytotoxic T lymphocyte. These cells do not secrete cytokines, but they have cytotoxic activities, including elimination of cells displaying antigen, i.e. altered self cells, such as virus-infected cells, foreign tissue grafts and tumour cells.

MAJOR HISTOCOMPATIBILITY COMPLEX

The MHC is a tightly linked cluster of genes located on chromosome 6 and required for antigen recognition. They also play major roles in the acceptance of self (histocompatible) or non-self (histoincompatible). MHC molecules play an important role in antigen recognition by T cells, and determine the response of an individual to infectious antigens and hence susceptibility to disease. The MHC genes are organized into those encoding three classes of molecules: class I, class II and class III. Class I genes encode glycoproteins expressed on the surface of most nucleated cells and present antigens for the activation of specific T cells. Class II genes encode glycoproteins expressed mainly on antigen-presenting cells, including macrophages and B cells, where they present antigen to other defined T-cell populations. Class III genes encode several different immune products, including complement system components, enzymes and tumour necrosis factors, and have no role in antigen presentation.

CELL-MEDIATED IMMUNITY

Leucocytes develop from a common pluripotent stem cell during haematopoiesis, and proliferate and differentiate into the different cells in response to haematopoietic growth factors, balanced by programmed cell death or apoptosis. The lymphocyte, the only cell to possess specificity, diversity, memory and recognition of self/non-self, is the central line of the immune system. Monocytes, macrophages and neutrophils are accessory immune cells which phagocytose, facilitated by complement and antibody, which increase attachment of antigen to the membrane of the phagocyte. Macrophages are also important in antigen processing and presentation in association with a class II MHC molecule, and secretion of the cytokine interleukin-1 (IL-1). Lymphocytes constantly recirculate via interaction between cell adhesion molecules on the vascular endothelium and receptors for the adhesion molecules on the circulating cells.

Different maturational stages of lymphocytes and other immune cells may be distinguished by their expression of specific molecules on the cell membranes, which are termed cluster of differentiation (CD) antigens.

Lymphocytes

Antibodies activate the complement system, stimulate phagocytic cells and specifically inactivate microorganisms. Lymphocytes, the basis of the acquired immune defence system, consist of antibody-producing plasma cells derived from B lymphocytes, and T lymphocytes which control intracellular infections. Binding of microorganisms to antibodies on the cell surface of B cells leads to preferential selection of these antibody-producing cells. This is termed priming, and subsequent responses are faster and amplified, and provide the basis of vaccination. T cells exploit two main strategies to combat intracellular infections – secretion of soluble mediators which activate other cells to enhance microbial defence mechanisms, and production of cytotoxic T lymphocytes which kill the target organism. NK cells have an important role in tumour cell destruction. They are large granular lymphocytes which do not exhibit immunological memory and are non-specific in their recognition of tumour cells.

CONTROL OF ADAPTIVE T-CELL SELECTION

Regulation of MHC gene expression, e.g. by cytokines, plays a fundamental role in the immune system, as alterations of cell surface expression of class I or II molecules may affect the efficiency of antigen presentation. T lymphocytes consist of two subsets:

- T-helper (Th) cells which are CD4+ and recognize class II MHC molecules and which produce γ-interferon (IFN-γ) and other macrophage-activating factors
- cytotoxic or killer T cells (Tc) which are CD8+ and recognize both specific antigens and class I MHC molecules on the surface of infected cells.

T-helper cells

Circulating Th cells are capable of unrestricted cytokine expression and are prompted into a more restricted and focused pattern of cytokine production depending on signals received at the outset of infection. The cells may be classified according to the pattern of cytokines they produce. Th1 category cells secrete a characteristic set of cytokines which push the system towards cellular immunity (cellular cytotoxicity). Th2 cells are associated with humoral or antibody-mediated immunity. Typically, Th1 cells secrete IL-2, interferon-γ (IFN-γ), tumour necrosis factor β (TNF-β) and transforming growth factor β (TGF-β), whereas Th2 cells secrete IL-4, IL-5, IL-6, IL-9, IL-10 and IL-13 and also help B-cell antibody production. Both cell types produce IL-3, TNFα and granulocyte-macrophage stimulating factor (GM-CSF). IL-12 and IL-4 have been identified as early inducers of Th1 and Th2 responses, respectively, and therefore the local balance of these cytokines is an important determinant of subsequent immune responses (Fig. 24.2).

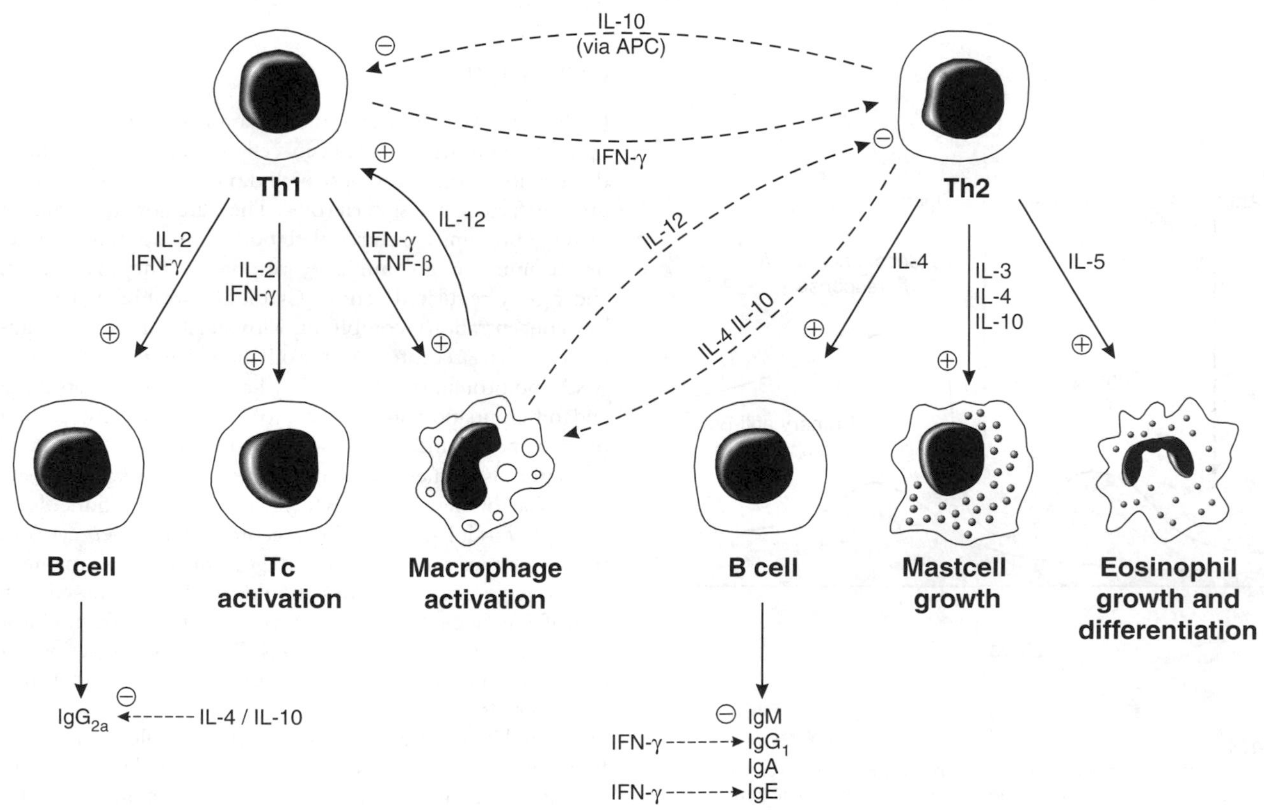

Fig. 24.2
Cross-regulation by cytokines secreted from Th1 and Th2 subsets. Solid arrows indicate stimulatory effects; dashed arrows indicate inhibitory effects (see text for abbreviations).

PROCESSING AND PRESENTATION OF ANTIGENS

Antigens are substances, including proteins, carbohydrates and glycoproteins, which are capable of interacting with the products of a specific immune response. An antigen which is capable of eliciting a specific immune response by itself is called an immunogen. Foreign protein antigens must be degraded into small peptides and complexed with class I or class II MHC molecules in order to be recognized by a T cell; this is termed antigen processing. Complexing with class I or II MHC molecules seems to be determined by the way in which the antigen enters the cell.

Mature immunocompetent animals possess large numbers of antigen-reactive T and B cells, and long before any contact with an antigen, each T and B lymphocyte already possesses specificity to antigens. This is achieved by random gene rearrangements in the bone marrow during maturation of lymphocytes. When antigen interacts with and activates mature, antigenically committed T and B cells, it causes expansion of the particular population of cells with that antigenic specificity – this is termed clonal selection and expansion. This process explains both specificity and memory attributes. Specificity is implicit because only those lymphocytes possessing appropriate receptors are clonally expanded. Memory occurs because there is a larger number of antigen-reactive lymphocytes present after clonal selection and many of these lymphocytes have a longer life span – these are called memory cells. The initial encounter of antigen-specific lymphocytes with an antigen induces a primary response, and later encounters are more rapid and heightened secondary responses (Fig. 24.3). Self/non-self recognition is achieved by elimination of lymphocytes which bear self-reactive receptors.

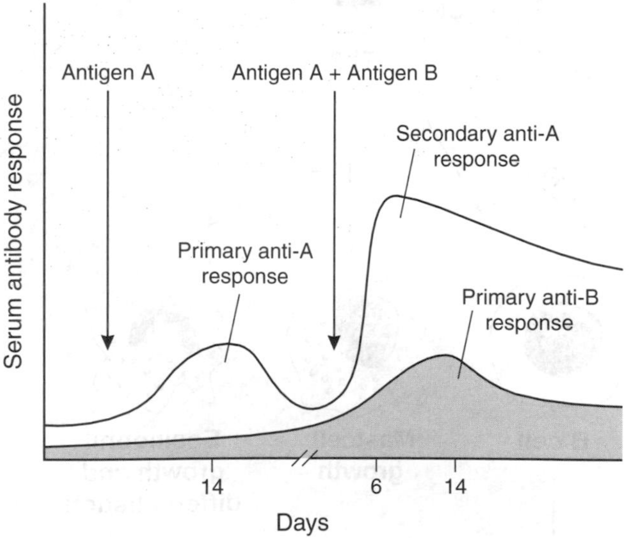

Fig. 24.3
Differences in the primary and secondary responses to injected antigen (humoral response) reflect the phenomenon of immunological memory. When an animal is injected with an antigen, it produces a primary serum antibody response of low magnitude and relatively short duration, peaking at around 10–17 days. A second immunization with the same antigen results in a secondary response that is greater in magnitude, peaks in 2–7 days, and lasts longer (months to years) than the primary response.

ANTIBODY STRUCTURE

The protein molecules which combine specifically with antigens are termed antibodies or immunoglobulins. Antibody molecules consist of two identical light chains and two identical heavy chains joined by disulphide bonds. Each heavy and light chain has a variable amino acid sequence region and a constant region. The unique heavy chain constant region sequences determine the five classes or isotypes of antibody – IgM, IgG, IgD, IgA and IgE. These isotypes vary in their effector function, serum concentration and half-life. IgG is the most common isotype and the only immunoglobulin to cross the placenta. IgM exists as a pentamer and is most effective in viral neutralization, bacterial agglutination and complement activation. IgA is the predominant isotype in external secretions, including breast milk and mucus. IgD and IgE are the least abundant isotypes; IgD and IgM are the major isotypes on mature B cells and IgE mediates mast cell degranulation.

Monoclonal antibodies are homogeneous antibodies with the same antigenic specificity. These antibodies are produced by a hybridoma, which is a group of identical cells termed a clone. These clones are manufactured by fusing normal lymphocytes with myeloma cells; the clone keeps its normal antibody functions and receptors of lymphocytes but has the immortal growth characteristics of myeloma cells. Monoclonal antibodies provide an indefinite supply of antibody with a highly defined antigenic specificity.

CYTOKINES

Orchestration of immune and inflammatory responses depends upon communication between cells by soluble molecules given the generic term cytokines, including chemokines, interleukins, growth factors and interferons. They are low-molecular-weight secreted proteins which regulate both the amplitude and duration of the immune/inflammatory responses. They have a transient and tightly regulated action. Cytokines are highly active at very low concentrations, combining with small numbers of high-affinity cell surface receptors and producing changes in the patterns of RNA and protein synthesis. They have multiple effects on growth and differentiation in a variety of cell types, with considerable overlap and redundancy between them, partially accounted for by induction of synthesis of common proteins. Interaction may occur in a type of network in which one cytokine induces another, through modulation of the receptor of another cytokine and through either synergism or antagonism of two cytokines acting on the same cell. Cytokines should not be considered as having identifying labels for being growth stimulators or inhibitors and pro- or anti-inflammatory actions. Their specific actions depend on the stimulus, the cell type and the presence of other mediators and receptors.

Chemokines are a family of small molecules characterized by four conserved cysteine residues. The α chemokines have two pairs of cysteine residues separated by a variable amino acid (C–X–C) and chemoattract neutrophils (e.g. IL-8, platelet basic protein, epithelial neutrophil-activating peptide), whereas β chemokines have two adjacent pairs of cysteine groups (C–C) and are chemotactic for monocytes/macrophages (e.g. platelet factor 4, monocyte chemotactic protein 1, macrophage inflammatory protein 1) and T cells (e.g. RANTES). Chemokines have been said to have more restricted actions than cytokines, but this is more likely to result from differential expression of receptors.

Interferons (IFN-α, -β, -γ) are a family of broad-spectrum antiviral agents which also modulate the activity of other cells, particularly IL-8 and platelet-activating factor (PAF) production, antibody production by B cells and activation of cytotoxic macrophages. Growth factors regulate the differentiation, proliferation, activity and function of specific cell types. The best known are colony-stimulating factors (CSFs), which cause colony formation by haematogenic progenitor cells (e.g. GM-CSF). Other examples include factors which regulate the growth of nerve cells, fibroblasts, epidermis and hepatocytes.

In addition to the low-molecular-weight protein mediators, there are also lipid mediators of inflammation which include PAF and arachidonic acid metabolites. PAF is a labile alkyl phospholipid released from a variety of cells in the presence of antigen and leucocytes in response to immune complexes. In addition to its actions on platelets, the effects of PAF include the priming of macrophages to other inflammatory mediators and alterations of microvascular permeability. Arachidonic acid metabolites include the prostaglandins, leukotrienes, HETEs and HPETEs, all of which have profound inflammatory and vascular actions, and may regulate and be regulated by other cytokines.

TNF-α and -β have a vast range of similar effects and are usually referred to as inflammatory cytokines. They have a central role in initiating the cascade of other cytokines and factors that comprise the immune response to infection. The wide variety of effects may be explained by the wide distribution of their receptors, their ability to activate multiple signal transduction pathways and their ability to induce or suppress many genes, including those for growth factors, cytokines, transcription factors, receptors and acute-phase proteins. Although both TNFs have similar biological activities, regulation of the expression and processing of the two are different.

RECEPTORS AND ANTAGONISTS

The biological activities of cytokines are regulated by specific cellular receptors. Often these receptors comprise multiple subunits providing phased stages of activation and biological action. For example, the IL-2 receptor complex consists of three subunits, IL-2Rα, IL-2Rβ and IL-2Rγ. Although the IL-2Rα/β combination can bind IL-2, IL-2Rγ is also required for high-affinity binding, ligand internalization and signalling, which are required for maximal effect. Other cellular receptors are present in more than one type which act alone but have different binding affinities for different forms of a cytokine protein (e.g. IL-1 receptor type I binds IL-1α better than IL-1β, and IL-1 receptor type II has more affinity for IL-1β). Binding of a cytokine to one type of receptor may result in interactions with another receptor; the two receptors for TNF, for example, use ligand passing in which TNF binds transiently to receptor type I, with full signal transduction, but may then move on to the type II receptor with activation of another signal for apoptosis or programmed cell killing.

Soluble cytokine receptors have been identified which compete with membrane-bound receptors, thus regulating cytokine signals. Exceptions to this are soluble receptors for IL-6 and ciliary neurotrophic factor, which act as agonists rather than antagonists. Such soluble receptors may be membrane-bound receptors which are shed into the circulation either intact or as truncated forms (e.g. soluble TNF receptors, sTNF-Rs), or may begin as related precursor molecules which are enzymatically cleaved (e.g. IL-1R). Soluble receptors may appear in response to stimuli as part of a naturally occurring independent regulatory process to limit the harmful effects of a mediator (e.g. sTNF-R), but some soluble receptors have little binding activity and may represent superficial and unimportant losses of cellular receptors (e.g. the soluble form of the IL-2Rα). Soluble cytokine receptors not only mediate biological activity, but also control desensitization to ligands by reduced availability, decreased signalling and by stimulating cellular mechanisms which may result in lack of activity.

The biological actions of some cytokines are also regulated by receptor antagonists. The receptor antagonist for IL-1 (IL-1ra) competes with cell receptors for IL-1, but when bound does not induce signalling. IL-1ra binds to cell receptors much more avidly than to soluble receptors, such that soluble receptors have little effect on the inhibitory action of the receptor antagonist. The soluble receptor also inhibits activation of the pro-IL-1β precursor. The appearance of IL-1ra is regulated independently by other cytokines as part of the inflammatory process.

HYPERSENSITIVITY REACTIONS

A localized inflammatory reaction termed delayed type hypersensitivity (DTH) may occur when some subpopulations of activated Th cells encounter some antigens. Tissue damage is usually limited and DTH plays an important role in defence against intracellular pathogens and contact antigens. Development of a DTH response requires a sensitization episode beforehand, when Th cells are activated and expanded clonally by antigen presented with the required class II MHC molecule. A second exposure to the antigen induces an effector response, where T cells produce a variety of cytokines leading to recruitment and activation of macrophages and other non-specific inflammatory cells. The activated T cells are generally Th1 subtype. A DTH response becomes apparent about 24 h following secondary antigen contact, peaking after about 48–72 h. The delay is a result of the time taken for cytokines to activate and recruit macrophages. A complex and amplified interaction of many non-specific cells then occurs, but only about 5% of the participating cells are antigen-specific. The macrophage is the primary effector cell of DTH responses and the influx and activation of these cells provide an effective host response against intracellular pathogens. Generally the pathogen is cleared with little tissue damage, but prolonged DTH responses themselves may be damaging, ultimately leading to tissue necrosis in extreme cases.

Immediate hypersensitivity reactions occur within 8 h of secondary allergen exposure and are not cell-mediated, but humoral in nature, resulting in generation of antibody-secreting plasma cells and memory cells. The hypersensitivity reactions may be classified into type I (IgE-dependent), type II (antibody-mediated cytotoxicity), type III (immune complex-mediated hypersensitivity) and type IV (delayed type hypersensitivity) and are shown in Table 24.1. Type I reactions are mediated by IgE antibodies which bind to receptors on mast cells or basophils, leading to degranulation and release of mediators. The principal effects are smooth muscle contraction and vasodilatation, and these may result in serious life-threatening systemic anaphylaxis, asthma, hay fever and eczema. Table 24.2 shows common antigens associated with type I reactions.

Type II hypersensitivity reactions occur when antibody reacts with antigenic markers on the cell surface leading to cell death

Table 24.1 Classification of hypersensitivity reactions

Type	Name	Time	Mechanisms	Manifestations
I	IgE-mediated	2–30 min	Antigen binding to IgE induces release of vasoactive mediators	Systemic and local anaphylaxis
II	Antibody-mediated cytotoxic	5–8 h	Antibody to cell surface antigens activates complement and antibody-dependent cytotoxicity	Blood transfusion reactions, autoimmune haemolytic anaemia
III	Immune complex-mediated	2–8 h	Immune complex deposition induces complement activation	Systemic lupus erythematosus, rheumatoid arthritis, glomerulonephritis
IV	(delayed reaction)	Cell-mediated	24–72 h	Sensitized Th cells release cytokines Contact dermatitis, graft rejection

through complement-mediated lysis or antibody-dependent cytotoxicity. Type II reactions include haemolytic disease of the newborn, and autoimmune diseases such as Goodpasture's syndrome and myasthenia gravis.

Type III reactions are mediated by formation of antigen–antibody or immune complexes and subsequent complement activation. Deposition of immune complexes near the site of antigen entry causes release of lytic enzymes by accumulated neutrophils and results in localized tissue damage. The formation of circulating immune complexes is involved in several conditions, including allergies to penicillin, infectious diseases such as hepatitis and autoimmune diseases such as rheumatoid arthritis.

TRANSPLANTATION IMMUNOLOGY

Transplantation is the transfer of cells, tissues or organs from one site to another. Tissues that are antigenically similar or histocompatible do not induce rejection, and the opposite is termed histoincompatible. Graft rejection is an immunological response involving cell-mediated responses, specifically T lymphocytes. The immune response is mounted against tissue antigens on the transplanted tissue that differ from those of the host. The most vigorous of these reactions involve the MHC. However, even with identical MHC antigens, differences in minor histocompatibility loci outside the MHC may contribute to graft rejection.

Graft rejection may be divided into the sensitization and effector stages. During sensitization, leucocytes derived from the donor migrate from the donor tissue into lymph nodes where they are recognized as foreign by Th cells, stimulating Th cell proliferation. This is followed by migration of the effector Th cells into the graft and rejection follows. Graft rejection can be suppressed by specific and non-specific immunosuppressive agents. Non-specific agents include purine analogues, corticosteroids, cyclosporin, total lymphoid X-irradiation and antilymphocyte serum. Specific approaches, such as blocking proliferation of activated T cells using monoclonal antibodies to the IL-2 receptor, or depletion of T-cell populations with anti-CD3 or -CD4 antibodies, have also been used.

BLOOD TRANSFUSION AND POSTOPERATIVE IMMUNOCOMPETENCE

It is well recognized that blood transfusion suppresses some aspects of the immune response, causing depressed delayed hypersensitivity reactions, decreased NK cell activity, decreased Th helper cells and decreased IL-2 production. Although there are several theories to explain these effects, the explanation is still not clear, nor is it clear which of the components of the blood transfusion are responsible for the changes. It does, however, appear that the donor leucocytes carrying foreign antigens are most likely to be responsible for the immunosuppression.

Table 24.2 Common antigens associated with type I hypersensitivity

Proteins Foreign serum Vaccines Latex
Plant pollens Rye grass Ragweed Timothy grass Birch trees
Drugs Penicillin Sulphonamides Local anaesthetics Salicylates
Foods Nuts Seafood Eggs Peas, beans
Insect venoms Bee Wasp Ant
Mould spores
Animal hair and dander

The immunosuppressive effects of transfusion are compounded in the patient undergoing surgery by the effects of anaesthesia and the stress response of the surgery itself. Three areas of concern have been highlighted as important:

- tumour recurrence rate
- postoperative infection rate
- the clinical course of pre-existing inflammatory disorders such as Crohn's disease.

CANCER IMMUNOLOGY

Tumour cells display surface structures which are recognized as antigenic and which promote an immune response. Macrophages mediate tumour destruction by lytic enzymes and production of TNF-α. NK cells recognize tumour cells by an unknown mechanism and either bind to antibody-coated tumour cells – this is termed antibody-dependent cell-mediated cytotoxicity – or secrete a cytotoxic factor which is apparently only cytotoxic for tumour cells. Tumour cell antigens may often elicit the generation of specific serum antibodies, which activate the complement system, producing the membrane attack complex. However, some tumours are able to endocytose the hole in the cell membrane produced by the membrane attack complex pore and repair the cell membrane before lysis occurs. Complement products may also induce chemotaxis of macrophages and neutrophils and release of toxic mediators. Ironically, antibodies to tumour cells may also enhance tumour growth, possibly by masking tumour antigens and preventing recognition by NK cells.

CANCER IMMUNOTHERAPY

Several experimental immunotherapy regimens have been used in the treatment of cancer. Injections of cytokines, including IFN and TNF-α, have been shown to be beneficial in some cancers. However, cytokine therapy may also result in unwanted side-effects, including fever, hypotension and decreased leucocyte counts. In vitro activation of lymphocytes with irradiated tumour cells in the presence of IL-2 has also been used. This approach results in induction of lymphokine-activated cells (LAK cells), comprising cytotoxic lymphocytes and NK cells, which may then be re-infused into the patient, providing enhanced tumour killing capacity. Monoclonal antibodies to CD3, which activate T lymphocytes in vitro and reduce non-specific T-cell activation in vivo, have been used successfully in reducing tumour growth in mice (Fig. 24.4), but human studies have not been performed. Gene therapy in which cells from patients with cancer are altered genetically to increase immune responses in some way are among recent developments in cancer immunotherapy. Specifically, trials in patients with melanoma, in whom melanoma cells are transfected to produce TNF-α and IFN-γ, are underway. In addition, patients with lung cancer are being given gene therapy to introduce two genes, one which suppresses tumour cell growth and another antisense gene which blocks activation of a gene that results in proliferation of tumour cells. Genetic therapy is likely to be the way forward in cancer immunotherapy.

HIV AND AIDS

Human immunodeficiency virus (HIV) is the causative agent for acquired immunodeficiency syndrome (AIDS). The virus infects host cells by binding to CD4 molecules on cell membranes. When the virus enters the cell, it copies its RNA into DNA. The DNA then integrates into the host DNA, forming a pro-virus which can remain in a dormant state for varying lengths of time. Activation of an HIV-infected Th cell also triggers activation of the pro-virus, leading to destruction of the host cell and to severe immune system depression. As only about 0.01% of the Th cells are infected by the virus in an HIV-infected individual, the extensive depletion of the Th-cell population implies that uninfected Th cells are also destroyed. Several mechanisms have been proposed for this, including complement-mediated lysis, apoptosis or antibody-mediated cytotoxicity. Early immunological changes include loss of in vitro proliferative responses of Th cells, reduced IgM synthesis, increased cytokine synthesis and reduced DTH responses. Later abnormalities include:

- loss of germinal centres in lymph nodes
- marked decreases in Th cell numbers and functions
- lack of proliferation of HIV-specific B cells and lack of anti-HIV antibodies
- shift in cytokine production from Th1 to Th2 subsets
- complete absence of DTH responses.

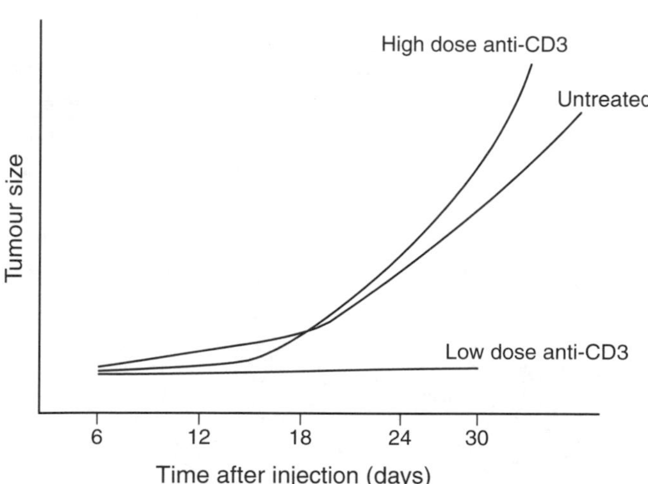

Fig. 24.4
Effect of anti-CD3 monoclonal antibody on tumour growth in mice. Animals were injected with live fibrosarcoma cells and simultaneously with high- or low-dose anti-CD3. The low dose inhibited tumour growth, whereas the high dose appeared to enhance tumour growth compared with untreated controls.

IMMUNE MODULATION BY ANAESTHETIC AGENTS

Increased susceptibility to infection is common in postoperative patients, and although trauma, surgical stress and endocrine responses modify the immune response, anaesthetic agents also modulate immune function, as shown by in vitro studies of the responses of immunologically important cells to clinically relevant concentrations of anaesthetic agents. Both volatile and intravenous anaesthetic agents, and opioids such as morphine and fentanyl have been shown to suppress a variety of functions essential to the recruitment and activity of neutrophils, lymphocyte function and NK-cell activity. Although many studies have shown marked effects of a variety of different anaesthetic and analgesic agents on neutrophil, monocyte and lymphocyte function, and also on cytokine responses to mediator stimulation, the clinical relevance of such degrees of immunosuppression in a previously healthy population is likely to be negligible. However, anaesthesia-induced effects on specific components of the immune system may be relevant in vulnerable patient populations, including the elderly, paediatric patients, the critically ill and those who are immunocompromised.

FURTHER READING

Farrar M A, Schreiber R D 1993 The molecular biology of interferon-gamma. Annual Reviews in Immunology 11: 571–611

Free S 1998 Latex allergy: what it could mean to you. Australian Critical Care 11: 40–43

Morisaki H, Suematsu M, Wakabayashi Y et al 1997 Leukocyte-endothelium interaction in the rat mesenteric microcirculation during halothane or sevoflurane anesthesia. Anesthesiology 87: 591–598

Rose-John S, Heinrich P C 1994 Soluble receptors for cytokines and growth factors: generation and biological function. Biochemical Journal 300: 281–290

Sheeran P, Hall G M 1997 Cytokines in anaesthesia. British Journal of Anaesthesia78: 201–219

Stevenson G W, Hall S C, Rudnick S, Seleny F L, Stevenson H C 1990 The effect of anesthetic agents on the human immune response. Anesthesiology 72: 542–552

Tami J A, Parr M D, Thompson J S 1986 The immune system. American Journal of Hospital Pharmacology 43: 2483–2493

Wheatley T, Veitch P S 1997 Effect of blood transfusion on postoperative immunocompetence. British Journal of Anaesthesia 78: 489–492

25 Renal physiology

The kidney plays a vital role in maintaining body homeostasis. It safeguards the stable internal environment necessary for each of the cellular components to function efficiently, despite a varying fluid and solute intake by the organism as a whole. Homeostasis is achieved by a combination of complex processes:

- excretion of the waste products of metabolism
- control of the extracellular fluid (ECF), which influences indirectly the intracellular composition in terms of volume, osmolarity and acid–base status
- production of hormones and vitamins which influence other organs and systems in the body.

Before discussing the various components and functions of the kidney, it is necessary to consider briefly the body fluids and their compartments.

Table 25.1 Composition and volume of body fluids according to compartment

	Intravascular (plasma) 3 L	Interstitial 11 L	Intracellular 28 L
Sodium (mmol) L^{-1}	142	142	10
Potassium (mmol L^{-1}	5	5	150
Chloride (mmol L^{-1})	103	113	10
Bicarbonate (mmol L^{-1})	25	26	10
Protein (g L^{-1})	60–80	0	25
Osmolality (mosmol kg^{-1})	285	285	285

BODY FLUIDS AND COMPARTMENTS

Total body water in males is approximately 60% of total body weight, i.e. 42 L for a 70 kg man. In females, total body water is approximately 10% less, because of the greater proportion of body fat compared with males; fat cells have a lower water content than other cells of the body. The water is distributed in various spaces or compartments:

- *Intracellular fluid.* This is the largest water compartment in the body, representing two-thirds of total body water (approximately 28 L).
- *Extracellular fluid.* This constitutes the remaining one-third of total body water (14 L) and may be subdivided further into two compartments:
    - —intravascular, i.e. within the plasma (3 L)
    - —interstitial: this fluid (approximately 11 L) is outside the intravascular compartment.

The composition of the various fluids differs with the requirements of each compartment (Table 25.1). Sodium is the main cation in the extracellular compartment, whereas potassium is the principal cation of the intracellular compartment. This is achieved by the different permeability of cell membranes for some cations; the cell membrane is approximately 50 times more permeable to potassium than to sodium. Intracellular protein carries a negative charge which attracts the positively charged potassium ions. Most importantly, however, the sodium pump extrudes sodium actively from the cell in exchange for potassium with the use of the enzyme Na/K-ATPase.

The water content of plasma is 93%; the remainder comprises proteins, lipids and other high-molecular-weight substances. Therefore, the actual value for sodium concentration in intravascular water should be approximately 153 mmol L^{-1}, which of course is higher than the normal plasma sodium value (135–140 mmol L^{-1}). In clinical practice, if the proportion of water is reduced, e.g. by substantial increases in protein, lipid or glucose concentration, the plasma sodium value is spuriously lowered and is termed 'pseudohyponatraemia'.

Cell membranes are permeable to water and there is a continual flux of fluid among the different body compartments at different rates of exchange. Two main mechanisms are responsible for these fluid shifts: osmotic pressure and hydrostatic pressure.

Osmotic pressure

Osmotic pressure is the pressure exerted by the number of particles in a solution. Osmolality, the usual term used in clinical practice, is defined as the number of milliosmoles per kg of water (mosmol kg^{-1}). It should not be confused with the term osmolarity which is defined as the number of milliosmoles per litre of water (mosmol L^{-1}). Osmolarity is affected by changes in temperature, whereas osmolality is not.

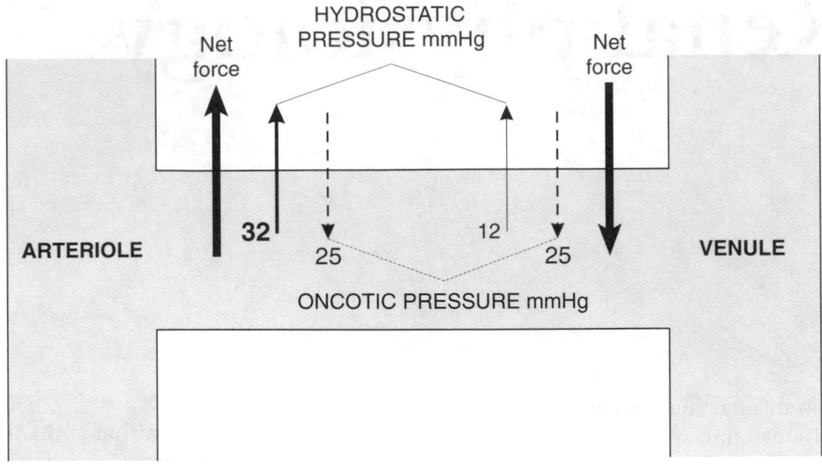

Fig. 25.1
Hydrostatic forces across a capillary wall (Starling's forces).

Ions, being in greater abundance, exert a greater osmotic pressure. For example, 1 mmol of sodium chloride exerts an osmotic pressure of 2 mosmol, as each molecule is composed of one sodium and one chloride ion. Although of a larger molecular mass, proteins exert less osmotic pressure. Water moves freely across a semipermeable membrane and does so from an area of low osmolality to one of higher osmolality, i.e. the increase in osmotic pressure attracts water. This movement continues until the osmotic pressure is equal on both sides of the membrane. This mechanism is, in effect, between the intracellular and interstitial compartments. As shown in Table 25.1, the osmolality in the compartments is identical. Any increase in intracellular osmolality increases water transport in the cell, thereby increasing its volume, and vice versa.

Hydrostatic pressure

This is the mechanism for fluid movement across a capillary bed from the intravascular to the interstitial compartment. Figure 25.1 shows the various pressures exerted as the hydrostatic pressure decreases from 32 mmHg at the arterial end to 12 mmHg at the venous end of the capillary. The oncotic pressure exerted by plasma proteins represents a constant 'negative' pressure that draws fluid into the capillary. Thus, fluid moves out of the arterial capillary and is withdrawn at the venous end. These hydrostatic pressures are known as Starling's forces. There is a small interstitial pressure, estimated to be approximately 2–5 mmHg, although it appears to have little or no effect on this mechanism unless the capillary is damaged by some pathological process and allows leakage of protein into the interstitium. If this occurs, the interstitial pressure is increased and the existing balance of forces is altered.

RENAL BLOOD FLOW

Before considering renal blood flow, it is necessary to understand the gross anatomy of the kidney.

There are two populations of nephrons in the kidney:

- *Cortical.* These nephrons (approximately 85%) lie within the cortex of the kidney and have short loops of Henle which dip only into the outer medulla.
- *Juxtamedullary.* These nephrons, which constitute the remaining 15%, lie in the juxtamedullary area of the cortex and are distinguished from their outer cortical neighbours by having long loops of Henle entering the inner medulla to participate in the diluting and concentrating mechanisms of the kidney.

The blood supply to the kidney is from the renal artery, which, having entered the renal pelvis, divides into a number of interlobar arteries. These further divide into the arcuate arteries and supply the small interlobular arteries from which the glomerular vessels arise. Each glomerulus is supplied by a single afferent arteriole which branches into a network throughout the glomerulus. It then reforms into a single vessel, the efferent arteriole. The efferent arteriole in turn forms branches around the proximal tubule (pars recta) and around the loop of Henle to form the vasa recta. It is possible for the efferent arteriole from one glomerulus to form the vasa recta of an adjacent tubule. The mesh of vessels then reforms into a single vessel, which drains into the interlobular vein and thence to the renal vein.

Each afferent artery has a region of renin-secreting granular cells which form part of the juxtaglomerular apparatus of the nephron. This specialized apparatus is involved with the renin–angiotensin system (see below) and also consists of extraglomerular mesangial cells and the macula densa region of the thick ascending limb.

Considering its size in relation to other organs of the body, the kidney receives a high blood flow (approximately 20–25% of cardiac output). This amounts to 500–600 ml min^{-1} to each kidney. Such a flow rate is necessary to carry sufficient oxygen for the high-energy requirements of tubular processes, especially sodium reabsorption.

Renal plasma flow (RPF) may be measured using the Fick principle:

$$\text{RPF} = \frac{U_X V}{\text{RA}_X - \text{RV}_X}$$

where U_x is the urine concentration of a substance x, V is the urine volume, RA_x is the renal artery concentration of the substance, and RV_x is the renal vein concentration of the substance.

The commonest substance used to measure RPF is para-aminohippuric acid (PAH), which is cleared almost completely in one passage through the kidney. It is both filtered by the glomerulus and secreted by the renal tubule. In this instance, RV should be negligible and, as there is no extrarenal clearance of PAH, the expression may be modified:

$$\text{RPF} = \frac{U_{\text{PAH}}V}{P_{\text{PAH}}} \text{ ml min}^{-1}$$

where V is the urine volume (ml min^{-1}), U_{PAH} is the urine PAH concentration (mg ml^{-1}) and P_{PAH} is the plasma PAH concentration (mg ml^{-1}).

Renal blood flow (RBF) may be calculated by adjusting the RPF for the haematocrit (Hct):

$$\text{RBF} = \frac{\text{RPF}}{1 - \text{Hct}} \text{ ml min}^{-1}$$

As only 90% of PAH is extracted by the human kidney, the clearance of PAH (C_{PAH}) underestimates RPF by approximately 10%. In order to improve the accuracy of measurement, it is possible to estimate RPF from the disappearance curve of intravenously injected ^{131}I-labelled PAH, eliminating the potential error introduced by timed urine collections. Using PAH to measure RBF is inaccurate if the renal extraction is impaired. This may occur in chronic renal failure or tubular disorders, or if the plasma concentration of PAH exceeds the maximum secretion capacity of the tubules.

Many other methods of measuring renal blood flow have been described. These include measuring the uptake of radiolabelled inert gases (krypton or xenon) by the kidneys following injection into the renal artery, or measuring the uptake of radioisotopes, e g. potassium (^{42}K) or rubidium (^{86}Rb). A particular advantage of these techniques is that they also allow the distribution of blood flow within the kidney to be studied.

From such studies, it has been shown that the cortex receives a blood supply of approximately 500 ml min^{-1} 100 g^{-1}, the outer medulla receives approximately 100 ml min^{-1}100 g^{-1} and the inner medulla only 20 ml min^{-1} 100g^{-1}. The lower medullary flow rate is necessary for the efficient working of the countercurrent mechanism in the loop of Henle (see below). The medullary region is relatively hypoxaemic, with a $P\text{O}_2$ of approximately 1.3–2.6 kPa compared with 6.5 kPa in the cortex, and therefore is prone to hypoxic injury if blood flow is reduced.

Total renal blood flow (RBF) is determined by Ohm's law:

$$\text{RBF} = \frac{P_{\text{art}} - P_{\text{ven}}}{\text{resistance}}$$

where P_{art} is the renal artery pressure, P_{ven} is the renal venous pressure, and resistance refers to resistance within the kidney.

Resistance is determined primarily by the tone in the afferent and efferent arterioles within the glomerulus. In the normal kidney, the control of renal blood flow and its distribution within the kidney are determined by a complex interaction of neurological factors and endocrine and locally released vasoactive substances. The afferent and efferent renal arterioles have sympathetic innervation from T4 to L2. Increasing sympathetic activity, e.g. in response to shock, preferentially causes vasoconstriction of the afferent artery, thereby reducing renal blood flow.

Substances which reduce renal blood flow by arteriolar vasoconstriction include angiotensin II and endothelin, a potent vasoconstrictor secreted by the renal vessel endothelium in response to sympathetic stimulation and angiotensin II.

Renal vessel vasodilators increase renal blood flow and include prostaglandins (PGI_2, PGE_2), nitric oxide, bradykinin and dopamine. Many of these vasoactive compounds are synthesized within the kidney and, in addition to their effects on total renal blood flow, many alter the distribution of blood flow between the cortex and the medulla. In normal health, many of these mediators probably have a minimal influence on the regulation of renal blood flow and its distribution. However, in disease or in states of stress (e.g. haemorrhage), they play a significant role in maintaining adequate renal perfusion. For example, administration of a non-steroidal anti-inflammatory drug (NSAID) to a hypotensive patient may have disastrous consequences on renal function due to inhibition of prostaglandin synthesis.

There are two other properties that confer distinguishing features on the renal circulation. First, the mean glomerular capillary pressure is maintained at 45 mmHg, which is approximately 20 mmHg more than other capillary networks in the body. This is necessary for glomerular filtration (see below). The mean peritubular capillary pressure is only 15 mmHg and lower than intratubular pressure, thereby enhancing tubular reabsorption.

The second feature is autoregulation, which occurs in the cortex but not in the medulla and allows constant blood flow when renal perfusion pressure is altered. It is an intrinsic property of the renal vasculature, i.e. it is independent of nerves or hormones, and occurs over a range of systolic arterial pressure from 90 to 180 mmHg. Over this range, glomerular filtration rate (GFR) parallels RBF, but glomerular filtration ceases when systolic arterial pressure falls below 60 mmHg. The effects of autoregulation are achieved by changes in resistance in the afferent and efferent arterioles. When arterial pressure decreases, there is relative vasodilatation of the afferent arteriole and vasoconstriction of the efferent arteriole. This results in an increase in the fraction of plasma filtered (filtration fraction) and glomerular filtration is maintained. If arterial pressure increases, vasoconstriction occurs in the afferent arteriole, with the opposite effects on filtration fraction.

The autoregulatory mechanism may be dampened by vasodilator drugs which act on smooth muscle vasculature, e.g. acetylcholine, dopamine, prostaglandins and the calcium channel blockers.

The exact mechanism of autoregulation is a matter of debate. Originally it was believed to result either from mechanical factors, i.e. skimming of red blood cells and an increase in blood viscosity within the renal vasculature, or as a response to an overall increase in intrarenal pressure generated by changes in systemic arterial pressure. Current evidence favours the 'myogenic theory' which states that the increase in smooth muscle contraction is produced by an increase in the intraluminal pressure or in the tangential tension of the vascular wall.

A second mechanism called tubuloglomerular feedback may also be involved. This states that increasing renal blood flow and glomerular filtration (see below) produce an increase in filtered sodium (or other substance) in the distal tubule of the nephron. This is detected by juxtaglomerular apparatus which secretes a substance from the macula densa that produces afferent arteriolar vasoconstriction and a reduction in renal blood flow. The exact mediator is unknown, but adenosine or ATP, which are selective afferent arteriolar vasoconstrictors, may be involved.

GLOMERULAR FILTRATION

The process of glomerular filtration allows 180 L per 24 h or 120 ml min^{-1} of fluid and solutes to pass through the glomerular capillaries via the endothelial fenestrations, the glomerular capillary basement membrane and the pedicles of the podocytes into Bowman's space. The fluid which enters the proximal tubule from Bowman's space is an ultrafiltrate of plasma, i.e. it is virtually protein-free. Small amounts of albumin pass through the glomerular basement membrane and are reabsorbed almost entirely in the early proximal tubule so that the final urinary concentration of albumin is less than 120 mg 24 h^{-1}. The ease with which solutes pass through the glomerular basement membrane depends on their size, charge and possibly shape.

The filtering process is extremely efficient for substances of low molecular weight, i.e. the ratio of solute concentration between the plasma within the glomerular capillary and the fluid in Bowman's capsule is 1. As molecular weight increases, the amount of filtered solute decreases until a cut-off point at a molecular weight of 70 000 is reached, above which no further molecules pass. It should be noted that this range allows for a small quantity of albumin (molecular weight 69 000) to be filtered. The constituents of the glomerular basement membrane are mainly negatively charged sialoproteins which repel negatively charged protein particles in plasma. It has been demonstrated that dextrans, with a molecular weight similar to some small proteins but with no charge, pass through the glomerular basement membrane 10–20% more efficiently. There is also evidence that changes in molecular shape may facilitate the passage of some molecules through the membrane.

The forces required to drive glomerular filtration are similar to the Starling forces across capillary networks elsewhere in the body, although of a greater magnitude. The mean arterial pressure in the glomerular capillary is 45 mmHg compared with 20 mmHg elsewhere. As discussed previously, this is a result of the presence of a second resistance vessel, namely the efferent arteriole. Also, this pressure remains relatively constant over a wide range of systolic arterial pressures as a result of the process of autoregulation. GFR is a product of the forces driving filtration minus the forces opposing filtration and may be expressed thus:

$$\text{GFR} \propto (P_{CAP} + \pi_{BC}) - (P_{BC} + \pi_{CAP})$$

where P_{CAP} is the hydrostatic pressure in the glomerular capillary, P_{BC} is the hydrostatic pressure in Bowman's capsule, π_{BC} is the oncotic pressure in Bowman's capsule, and π_{CAP} is the oncotic pressure in the glomerular capillary.

However, as π_{BC} is negligible, i.e. ultrafiltrate is virtually protein-free, the relationship may be rewritten:

$$\text{GFR} \propto P_{CAP} - P_{BC} - \pi_{CAP}$$

To convert this relationship into an equation, the sieving coefficient (K_f), i.e. the resistance to flow across the glomerular basement membrane, is introduced:

$$\text{GFR} = K_f (P_{CAP} - P_{BC} - \pi_{CAP})$$

Measurement of GFR

The measurement of GFR is one of the commonest assessments of renal function in clinical practice. It is measured by determining the clearance of a substance which is filtered by the glomerulus but not reabsorbed or secreted by the renal tubule. The polyfructose inulin (MW 5000) is such a substance. Using the standard clearance formula:

$$C_{in} = \frac{U_{in} V}{P_{in}} = 120 \text{ ml min}^{-1}$$

where C_{in} is the inulin clearance (ml min^{-1}), U_{in} is the inulin concentration in urine (mg ml^{-1}), P_{in} is the inulin concentration in plasma (mg ml^{-1}), and V is the urine volume (ml min^{-1}).

There are two major disadvantages to this technique. First, as inulin does not occur naturally in the body, it is necessary to infuse inulin intravenously to achieve a steady plasma level. To overcome this, it is customary to measure creatinine clearance using plasma creatinine, a product of muscle metabolism. There is a slight diurnal variation of plasma creatinine levels and creatinine is secreted by the renal tubules at very low GFR. However, creatinine clearance values are adequate for clinical practice and relate reasonably closely to inulin clearance.

The other disadvantage is the accuracy of timed urine collections. As with measurement of RPF, it is possible to use a radioactive-labelled substance to measure GFR. Chromium-labelled ethylene diamine tetracetic acid (^{51}Cr-EDTA) is injected intravenously and the disappearance rate calculated from blood samples obtained at 2 and 4 h after injection. This avoids urine collection, may be standardized for body surface area (as should all measurements of GFR) and may be used as an accurate reference method.

Filtration fraction

Although RPF is quite large, only a proportion is filtered and that proportion is called the filtration fraction (FF). It is derived as follows:

$$\text{FF} = \frac{\text{GFR}}{\text{RPF}} = \frac{\text{Cin}}{C_{PAH}} = \frac{120 \text{ ml min}^{-1}}{600} = 0.2\ (20\%)$$

FF may alter as a result of autoregulation. For example, if RBF decreases, there is an increase in efferent arteriolar vasoconstriction and FF increases in order to maintain glomerular filtration.

TUBULAR FUNCTION

The role of the renal tubule is to modify the volume and composition of the glomerular filtrate according to the needs of the organism. This is an enormous task – 180 L of filtrate are produced daily and it is necessary to reduce this volume by 99% to achieve a final 24 h urine volume of approximately 1.8 L. Similarly, approximately 25 000 mmol of sodium are filtered per day, the vast majority of this being reabsorbed to provide a urinary output of 100–200 mmol 24 h^{-1}. In addition, the kidney conserves other filtered substances that are essential for the maintenance of homoeostasis, e.g. glucose, bicarbonate, phosphate, etc. The renal tubule is also responsible for excretion of waste products of ingestion or metabolism, e.g. potassium, urea, creatinine, etc. The final regulation of acid–base status and of the concentration or dilution of the urine is also performed along the renal tubule.

Although each nephron acts as a single unit, it is possible, for ease of understanding, to divide tubular function into the individual portions of the tubule, i.e. proximal tubule, loop of Henle, distal tubule and collecting tubule. In simple terms, the proximal tubule may be considered the 'bulk reabsorber', and the remainder the 'fine regulator' (Fig. 25.2).

PROXIMAL TUBULE

In many ways, the proximal tubule is considered the bulk reabsorber as it is responsible for reducing the volume of glomerular filtrate by approximately 80%. Seventy per cent of sodium and chloride, 90% of calcium, bicarbonate and magnesium, and 100% of glucose, phosphate and amino acids are reabsorbed during their passage through the proximal tubule. The fluid entering the proximal tubule from Bowman's space has a composition similar to that of plasma, except for the absence of protein (see Table 25.1). As the reabsorptive process is isosmotic, the osmolality remains identical at the beginning and end of the proximal tubule (290 mosmol kg^{-1}). The main ion to be reabsorbed in terms of concentration, energy requirements and its effect on other reabsorptive processes is sodium.

Sodium reabsorption

Sodium is reabsorbed through the proximal tubular cell both passively and actively.

Passive reabsorption. There are two forms of passive reabsorption for sodium:

- *Chemical.* The intracellular sodium concentration in the proximal tubular cell is 30 mmol L^{-1}. This is considerably less than the concentration of 140 mmol L^{-1} in the tubular fluid and therefore sodium travels down the chemical gradient from the lumen to the cell.
- *Electrical.* The potential difference within the tubular cell is –70 mV. This creates an electrical gradient for the positively charged sodium ions to travel from the lumen into the cell. Chloride, although negatively charged, travels with sodium in linked transport.

Active transport. When sodium is within the cell, it is actively pumped in two directions. The first is into the intercellular space behind the so-called 'tight junction' (Fig. 25.3). This is an active energy-requiring pump which appears to be Na/K-ATPase-independent. The effect of increased sodium concentration in the intercellular space is to increase the osmolality, and thus water passes from the cell into that space. The sodium and water within the intercellular space are then available for reabsorption by the peritubular capillary. In conditions of extracellular fluid expansion, the tight junction may open and sodium flows together with water from the intercellular space into the tubular lumen (back flow).

There is a second sodium pump situated on the contraluminal surface of the tubular cell. This is an Na/K-ATPase-dependent pump which exchanges sodium for potassium. Potassium, however, is freely permeable through the cell wall and may diffuse passively out again into the peritubular space. Again, the sodium in the peritubular space is available for reabsorption into the peritubular capillary.

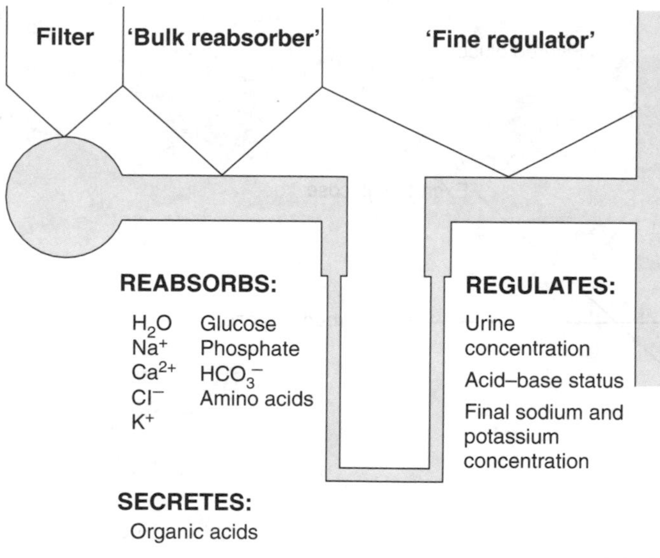

Fig. 25.2
Simple schema of tubular function.

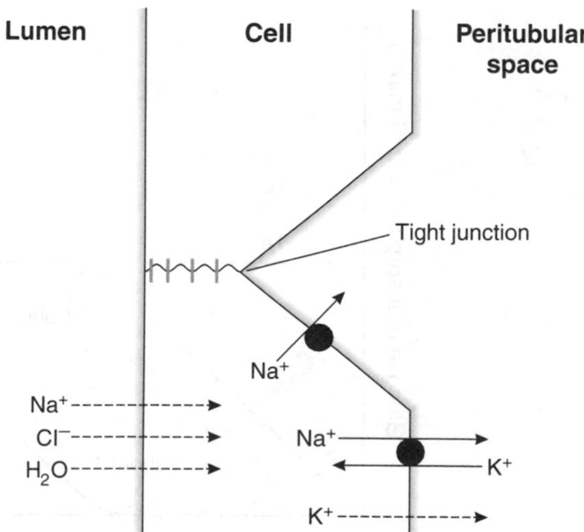

Fig. 25.3
Sodium transport through a proximal tubular cell.

The movement of sodium, chloride and water into the peritubular capillary is governed by Starling's forces. The driving forces are hydrostatic pressure in the peritubular space and capillary oncotic pressure; the opposing forces are capillary hydrostatic pressure and oncotic pressure in the peritubular space. However, as peritubular space oncotic pressure is negligible and the peritubular space hydrostatic pressure is small, the main controlling factor is peritubular oncotic pressure. The sodium, chloride and water which are not taken up into the peritubular capillary re-enter the tubular lumen via the tight junction, i.e. there is an increase in back flow.

Having described the mechanisms of sodium reabsorption within the proximal tubular cell, it is necessary also to consider sodium reabsorption and excretion by the kidney as a whole. As previously stated, the daily fractional excretion of sodium (the amount of sodium excreted in the final urine relative to the filtered load of sodium) remains relatively constant at approximately 1–2%. The filtered load (expressed in mmol min^{-1}) is the product of GFR and plasma sodium concentration. However, the sodium intake varies and various mechanisms are required to cope with states of relative hypo- and hypervolaemia. Three main mechanisms are responsible:

Glomerulotubular balance. Glomerular filtration rate remains relatively constant despite changes in systemic arterial pressure because of the autoregulatory mechanism. However, small changes in GFR produce large changes in the filtered load of sodium. When these occur, sodium reabsorption must alter in order to prevent large alterations in final sodium excretion. The anatomical arrangement of the peritubular capillaries, originating from the efferent arteriole, provides the ideal situation for a compensatory mechanism. When GFR decreases, there is a decrease in filtration fraction. This reduces the normally occurring increase in peritubular capillary oncotic pressure, which in turn decreases reabsorption of sodium, chloride and water from the peritubular space. Conversely, if GFR increases, there is an increase in filtration fraction, a greater increase in peritubular capillary oncotic pressure and enhanced reabsorption. This mechanism is known as 'glomerulotubular balance'.

Aldosterone. Aldosterone has its main site of action in the distal tubule and is considered later.

Atrial natriuretic factor. It has been known for over 20 years that when blood of a volume-expanded animal is perfused into a normal animal, avoiding volume expansion in the recipient, there is a modest increase in fractional sodium excretion, despite unchanged renal haemodynamics. This phenomenon has been demonstrated in both isolated perfused and denervated kidneys and has led to the postulate that during volume expansion there is secretion of a so-called 'natriuretic factor'. This is now known to be a 28-amino-acid peptide hormone secreted from the atria called atrial natriuretic peptide (ANP). Increasing circulating volume produces stretch of the atria and stimulates ANP release. Its main actions are on the kidney and it promotes salt and water excretion by inhibiting renin and aldosterone release, increasing GFR and sodium filtration by efferent arteriolar vasoconstriction and reducing sodium reabsorption in the proximal tubule. Other effects of ANP include increased excretion of phosphate, magnesium, calcium and, to a lesser extent, potassium.

The possibility that redistribution of intrarenal blood flow exerts an influence on overall sodium balance has yet to be fully evaluated. It is known that in cardiac failure, when a state of positive sodium balance occurs from increased sodium reabsorption, blood flow is directed away from the short outer cortical nephrons (salt-losing) and directed to the longer juxtamedullary nephrons (salt-retaining). It is not known if a similar modified mechanism plays a significant role in daily sodium balance.

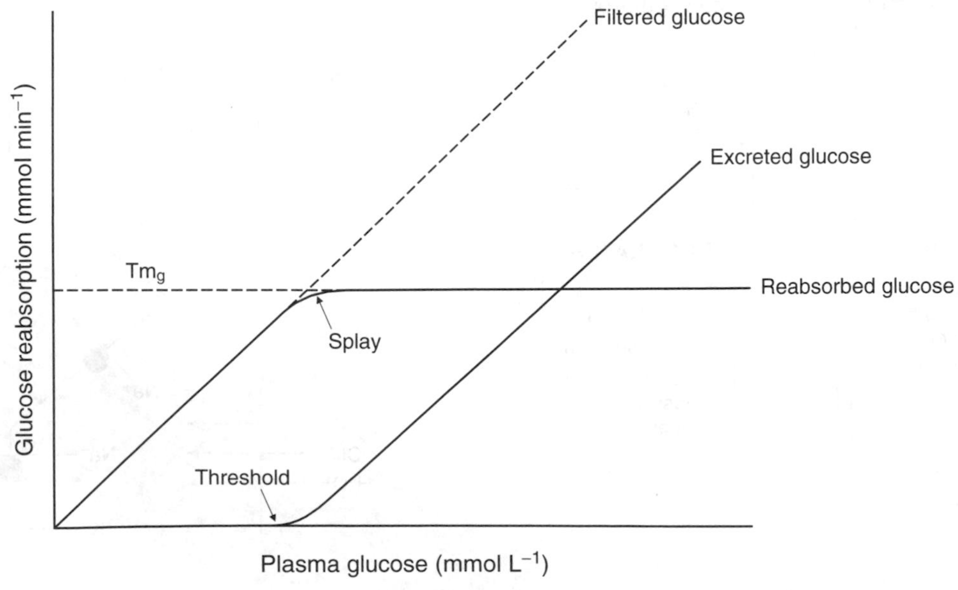

Fig. 25.4
The mechanism of glucose reabsorption in the proximal tubule.

Rate-limited tubular transport

As shown in Figure 25.2, glucose, phosphate, bicarbonate and amino acids are reabsorbed almost totally in the proximal renal tubule. The mode of reabsorption differs from that described for sodium, chloride and water. The basic mechanism, as obtained in a titration study, is shown in Figure 25.4 using glucose as the example. During such a study, plasma glucose concentration is slowly increased, avoiding extracellular fluid volume expansion. Plasma and urinary glucose concentrations and GFR are measured. As the plasma glucose concentration increases, glucose appears in the urine when the point of the renal threshold for glucose has been reached. This occurs when the plasma glucose concentration is approximately 10 mmol L^{-1} in humans. The tubular reabsorption of glucose continues to increase with increments in plasma glucose concentration until a plateau is reached when no further increase in glucose reabsorption rate can be achieved despite an increase in the filtered load of glucose. At that point, the transport mechanisms for glucose reabsorption by the tubular cells have been fully saturated. Thereafter, glucose excretion increases in parallel with the filtered load of glucose as plasma glucose concentration increases. The 'plateau' at which maximal glucose reabsorption occurs is termed 'the tubular maximal reabsorption for glucose' (Tm_g). In humans, the value is 20 mmol min^{-1}. It should be noted from Figure 25.4 that the point at which glucose reabsorption reaches its maximum is not a fine 'cut-off' but a small curve entitled 'splay'. Splay is caused by the heterogeneity of the nephron population in respect of glucose reabsorption. Some nephrons reabsorb maximally at a lower plasma glucose concentration than other nephrons within the kidney. A large splay is the cause of one type of renal glycosuria.

The same mechanism applies for phosphate reabsorption in the proximal tubule, although this differs slightly from glucose in that the excretion of phosphate follows the filtered load more closely and the Tm for phosphate is much lower (0.125 mmol min^{-1}). The Tm for bicarbonate is approximately 3–3.5 mmol min^{-1} but may be altered by hydrogen ion secretion. There are five identified individual transport processes for the different groups of amino acids but their reabsorptive kinetics are similar to that of glucose. The reabsorption of sulphate in the proximal tubule also follows a similar pattern. Many of the above substances share a co-transport system with sodium. It is known that when proximal tubular reabsorption of sodium decreases with an increased fractional excretion of sodium, Tm is decreased for glucose, phosphate and bicarbonate.

The mechanism of bicarbonate transport through the tubular cell (Fig. 25.5) is of particular importance because of its role in the renal regulation of acid–base balance. This mechanism may be summarized in three equations:

$$NaHCO_3 \Leftrightarrow Na^+ + HCO_3^- \quad (1)$$

$$HCO_3^- + H^+ \underset{\text{ANHYDRASE}}{\overset{\text{CARBONIC}}{\Leftrightarrow}} H_2CO_3 \Leftrightarrow H_2O + CO_2 \quad (2)$$

$$H_2O + CO_2 \underset{\text{ANHYDRASE}}{\overset{\text{CARBONIC}}{\Leftrightarrow}} H_2CO_3 \Leftrightarrow H^+ + HCO_3^- \quad (3)$$

Bicarbonate enters the tubular lumen as sodium bicarbonate and dissociates into bicarbonate (a relatively impermeable anion) and sodium (equation 1). The sodium passes into the cell in exchange for a hydrogen ion. The hydrogen ion combines with bicarbonate in the tubular lumen to form carbonic acid. The enzyme carbonic anhydrase, present on the brush border of the proximal tubular cell, splits carbonic acid into carbon dioxide and water (equation 2), both of which are freely permeable and enter the tubular cell. Here, intracellular carbonic anhydrase reforms carbonic acid, which in turn dissociates into free hydrogen and bicarbonate ions (equation 3). The bicarbonate ion passes through the basal cell membrane into the peritubular space and is available for reabsorption by the peritubular capillary. The hydrogen ion can be extruded from the cell in exchange for sodium and the cycle repeated. The enzyme carbonic anhydrase participates in both the dissociation and formation of carbonic acid depending on its site of action.

Another substance reabsorbed in the proximal tubule is uric acid. This is a small molecule which is filtered freely and over 90% is reabsorbed in the proximal tubule. However, uric acid homoeostasis is regulated by secretion of uric acid in the distal tubule. Anther small molecule which is filtered freely is urea, and approximately 50% of the filtered load is reabsorbed passively in the proximal tubule, the remainder passing down into the distal tubule to participate in the osmolar regulatory mechanisms of the inner medulla.

In addition to hydrogen ions, some other substances such as organic acids and bases are secreted (i.e. moved from the peritubular capillary into the tubular lumen) in the proximal tubule. These include a number of drugs, e.g. penicillin, PAH. The secretory processes may be either active or passive and some have tubular maximal secretory capacities.

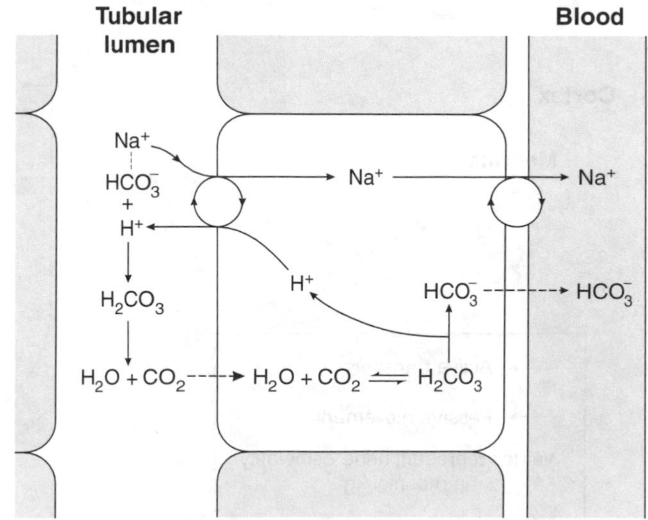

Fig. 25.5
Bicarbonate reabsorption in the proximal tubule.

THE LOOP OF HENLE, DISTAL TUBULE AND COLLECTING DUCT (Fig. 25.6)

These sections of the nephron are responsible for the regulation of urine volume and osmolality, acid–base balance and final adjustments to the sodium and potassium content of tubular fluid. The final composition of the urine leaving the collecting ducts will vary according to the needs of the body, but will be a result of changes that have occurred to the tubular fluid in these sections of the nephron.

Control of urine volume and osmolality

In health, plasma osmolality is maintained between 280 and 290 mosmol kg^{-1}, despite often large variations in daily fluid and electrolyte intake. In states of relative dehydration, the kidney minimizes water excretion, so small volumes of hyperosmolar urine are produced. Conversely, in overhydration, the kidney produces large volumes of dilute hypo-osmolar urine. The kidney is so efficient in this process that it can produce urine with an osmolality between varying 60 and 1200 mosmol kg^{-1}, depending on the state of hydration. This function of the kidney is dependent on the maintenance of an osmotic gradient between the interstitial fluid and the collecting ducts in the renal medulla. It is achieved by the loops of Henle in the juxtamedullary nephrons using a countercurrent mechanism. This increases the osmolality of the surrounding interstitium from 290 mosmol kg^{-1} in the outer cortex to 1200 mosmol kg^{-1} in the papillary medulla. This is achieved using two main mechanisms – sodium reabsorption from the ascending limb of the loop of Henle and urea accumulation in the medullary interstitium:

- *Sodium reabsorption.* The loop of Henle consists of a descending and an ascending limb. The thin descending limb is freely

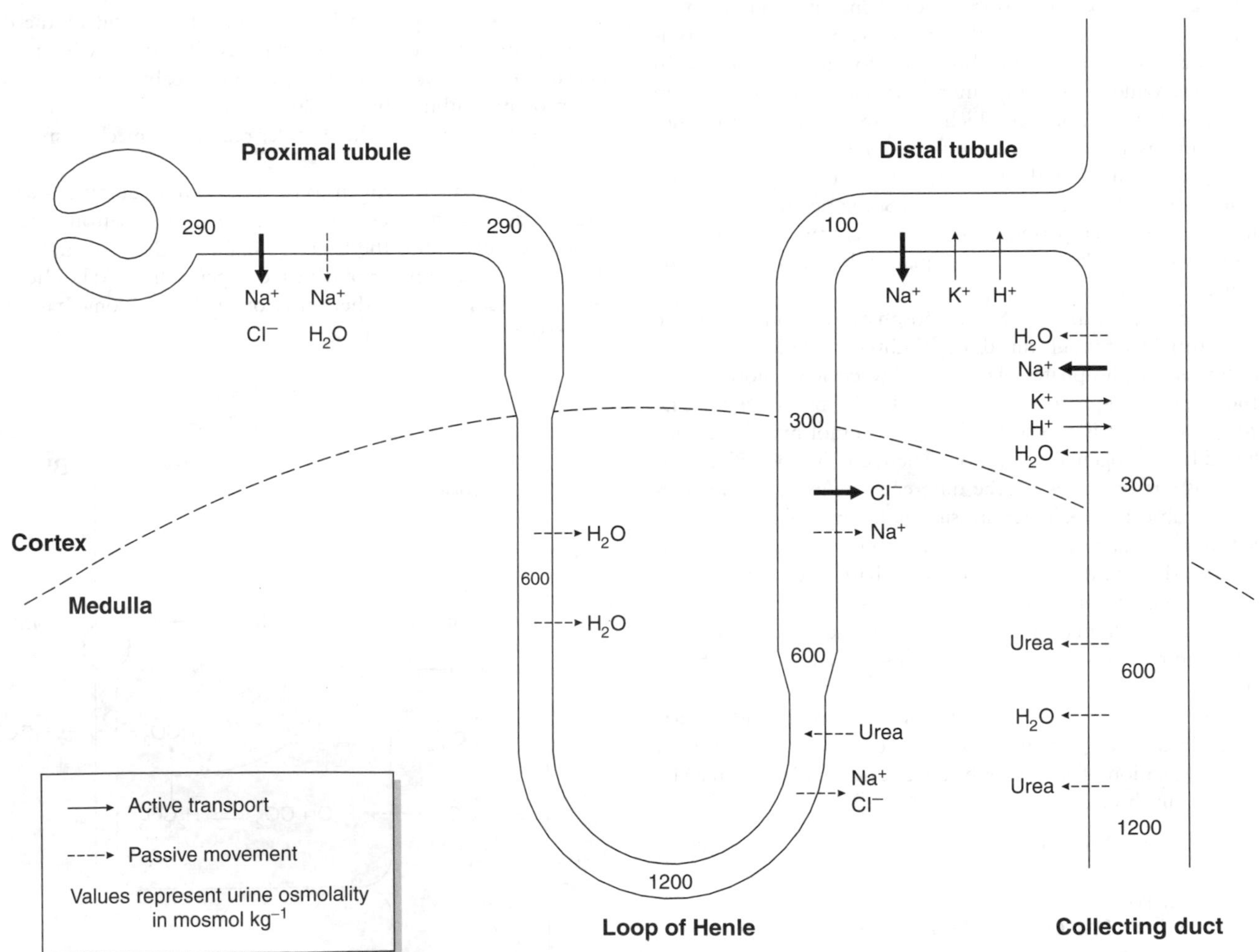

Fig. 25.6
Concentration of glomerular filtrate in the loop of Henle amd collecting tubule.

permeable to water but less so to sodium and chloride. The ascending limb consists of a thin first part and a thick second part, both of which are impermeable to water, but the thick part actively moves sodium and chloride into the interstitium. It is thought that chloride is actively transported out of the tubule with sodium moving by a co-transport mechanism (see above). Irrespective of the mechanism, the net result is an increase in the osmolality of the medullary interstitium and dilution of the tubular fluid within the thick part of the loop.

- *Urea recycling*. Urea contributes up to 50% of the interstitial osmolality in the medulla as a result of urea absorption from the collecting tubules. The cortical part of the collecting tubule is permeable to water but not to urea. Therefore, water is reabsorbed, increasing the osmolality of the fluid remaining in the tubule. However, the medullary part of the collecting tubule is permeable to urea, which passes out into the interstitium, thereby increasing the medullary osmolality. Antidiuretic hormone (ADH) further increases the permeability of the collecting duct to urea (see below). Some urea is absorbed by the descending limb and thin ascending limb of the loop of Henle and is then recycled through the medullary collecting tubule. This serves to concentrate urea in the medullary interstitium and maintain its high osmolality.

Tubular fluid entering the descending limb has an osmolality of 290 mosmol kg^{-1}. As it descends, water and, to a lesser extent, sodium and chloride move into the interstitium because of the osmotic gradient between the tubule and surrounding interstitium. Therefore, the osmolality of the tubular fluid increases as it descends into the medulla until it is equivalent to that at the tip of the loop (1200 mosmol kg^{-1}). On passing up the ascending limb, sodium and chloride are removed but water is retained so the osmolality decreases from 1200 to 100 mosmol kg^{-1}. For this reason, this region of the nephron is also known as the diluting segment.

The vasa recta play an important role in this osmolar transport. Although there is no active transport present in these vessels, water and solutes are freely permeable. The osmolality of blood entering the vasa recta is the same as that of the fluid entering the descending limb (i.e. 290 mosmol kg), and slowly increases to 1200 mosmol kg^{-1} as it passes down to the tip of the loop. This is achieved by the passage of water and solutes across its surface. As indicated previously, the blood flow is significantly slower in the lower parts of the vasa recta, thus improving the efficiency of this exchange. As the vasa recta move from the medullary tip back towards the cortex, the same process occurs and the osmolality is returned to 290 mosmol kg^{-1}. As a consequence of the low flow rate in these vessels, the oxygen content and energy requirements are reduced markedly.

By the time the glomerular filtrate enters the collecting tubule, its original volume has been reduced to 5%, and when it leaves the collecting tubule it is further reduced to 1%. Final urine volumes depend in part on the extracellular fluid volume and its regulation via sodium excretion and in part on the regulation of plasma osmolality. The osmolar regulation system has a detector (osmoreceptors), a messenger (antidiuretic hormone, ADH) and an effector (the collecting tubule).

Osmoreceptors situated in the hypothalamus detect changes in plasma osmolality, the major contribution being from plasma sodium. An increase in plasma osmolality stimulates the synthesis of ADH (vasopressin) in the supraoptic nuclei of the hypothalamus. This hormone is an octapeptide (8-arginine vasopressin) which passes along the nerve fibres to the posterior pituitary. After appropriate stimulation, the hormone is released from storage granules in the posterior pituitary and secreted into the systemic circulation. Its action on the peritubular cell membrane is to increase the permeability to water. This involves activation of the 3′,5′-cAMP system. Water is then reabsorbed from the collecting tubule and passes into the peritubular capillary to return the plasma osmolality to normal and reduce the urine volume. The reverse situation occurs if plasma osmolality decreases. ADH secretion ceases and the collecting tubule becomes impermeable to water; more water is excreted, urine volume increases and plasma osmolality increases towards normal levels. By this mechanism, it is possible that urine osmolality may vary from a hypotonic urine with a minimum value of approximately 60 mosmol kg^{-1} to a maximal value of 1200 mosmol kg^{-1}. It should be noted that the final osmolality of hypertonic urine is equivalent to the tonicity at the tip of the renal medulla. ADH also increases the amount of urea reabsorbed in the cortical part of the collecting tubule, thereby contributing to the counter-current mechanism by increasing medullary tip osmolality.

It is possible to estimate the action of ADH by determining the amount of water excreted or reabsorbed compared with the amount of solutes excreted. Osmolar clearance (C_{osm}), an expression of solute excretion, is determined by using the standard clearance formula:

$$C_{osm} = \frac{U_{osm}V}{P_{osm}}$$

where U_{osm} is the osmolar clearance (ml min^{-1}), P_{osm} is the plasma osmolality (mosmol kg^{-1}) and V is the urine excretion rate (ml min^{-1}).

If urine is dilute (i.e. hypotonic), V is greater than C_{osm}. The difference is termed free water clearance (C_{H_2O}) and may be expressed as follows:

$$C_{H_2O}\ (\text{ml min}^{-1}) = V - C_{osm}$$

Conversely, if urine is concentrated (i.e. hypertonic), more water is reabsorbed and C becomes greater than V. Free water clearance then becomes negative.

Another way of explaining negative free water clearance is to consider that water is being reabsorbed, i.e. solute-free water reabsorption, and this may be expressed as follows:

$$V = C_{osm} - T^{c}_{H_2O}$$

or

$$T^{c}_{H_2O} = C_{osm} - V$$

By varying the amount of water reabsorbed in the collecting tubule and influencing the plasma sodium concentration, it may be seen that osmolar regulation plays a vital part in controlling body fluid status. The two systems, i.e. osmolar regulation and volume regulation, are interrelated, and in considering overall fluid balance it is not possible to dissociate the two.

Sodium–potassium exchange

More than 90% of filtered potassium is reabsorbed in the proximal tubule, and potassium that appears in the final urine is secreted in the distal tubule by a transport process coupled loosely to active sodium transport. As sodium is reabsorbed from the tubular lumen, a negative potential is created within the lumen which allows potassium to move passively down an electrochemical gradient. In this region, hydrogen ions are also secreted and compete with potassium to a degree dependent on the acid–base status. The control of sodium reabsorption in the distal tubule is primarily hormonal and probably controlled via the renin–angiotensin system.

RENIN–ANGIOTENSIN SYSTEM

The renin–angiotensin system is an important part of the complex mechanism responsible for controlling extracellular fluid volume, the other 'effector' parts being plasma proteins (see above) and osmolar control. Renin is a proteolytic enzyme secreted from the juxtaglomerular apparatus situated in the afferent arteriole. The secretion of renin is a matter of some debate. It has been suggested that a baroreceptor mechanism situated in the afferent arteriole detects a decrease in renal blood flow and responds by increasing renin production. The alternative hypothesis is that changes in sodium concentration in the distal tubule are detected by the macula densa situated in the early part of the distal tubule, increases in sodium concentration causing an increase in renin secretion. Other stimuli for renin release may be important, including neural (e.g. β stimulation) and endocrine factors (e.g. ANP), although their significance is not fully known.

Renin acts on a plasma protein, angiotensinogen, and splits off a decapeptide, angiotensin I. A converting enzyme found in both plasma and various tissues of the body, including lung, converts angiotensin I to angiotensin II. This agent has many actions. It is a potent vasopressor which acts on the glomerular arterioles and thereby contributes to glomerulotubular balance. It also has a direct action on the brain, stimulating the thirst centre. Of most importance is its effect of stimulating secretion of aldosterone from the zona glomerulosa of the adrenal gland. Plasma aldosterone levels are also affected by the plasma potassium concentration, an increase in potassium reducing the aldosterone concentration. The converse occurs with plasma sodium concentration, i.e. a decrease in plasma sodium increases aldosterone. The main action of aldosterone is to increase sodium reabsorption in the distal tubule. Potassium and/or hydrogen ions are then secreted into the tubule in exchange for reabsorbed sodium. The renin–angiotensin system has its own feedback control, angiotensin II suppressing further secretion of renin.

RENAL REGULATION OF ACID–BASE BALANCE

The distal tubule participates both qualitatively and quantitatively in acid–base control. As described previously, the majority (up to 80%) of filtered bicarbonate is reabsorbed in the proximal tubule and the remainder by the distal tubule. The absorptive mechanism for bicarbonate reabsorption in the distal tubule is similar to that of the proximal tubule, namely the formation and dissociation of carbonic acid by the enzyme carbonic anhydrase. Conversely, although there is some hydrogen ion secretion in the proximal tubule, the bulk is secreted in the distal tubule.

Hydrogen ions are excreted in the final urine in combination with either ammonia or phosphates. Approximately 60 mmol of hydrogen ions are excreted per day, of which two-thirds are combined with ammonia (NH_3) to form ammonium ion (NH_4^+) and one-third with sodium phosphate salts, often referred to as titratable acids (TAs).

Ammonia (NH_3) is generated within the tubular cell mainly from the metabolism of the amino acid glutamine. When glutamine is converted to either glutamate or α-ketoglutarate, which enters the citric acid cycle, a free ammonia molecule is generated. This is freely permeable through the cell wall and passes down the concentration gradient into the tubular lumen, where it combines with free hydrogen ions to form NH_4^+. This hydrophilic anion is unable to re-enter tubular cells and so is excreted in the urine.

The remaining one-third of hydrogen ions are excreted when combined with phosphate. Disodium hydrophosphate enters the distal tubule and dissociates. One sodium ion is reabsorbed, leaving a negatively charged molecule. The positive hydrogen ion in the tubular lumen combines to form sodium dihydrophosphate which is excreted in the final urine.

Hydrogen ions for both ammonium and TA formation come from intracellular dissociation of carbonic acid, and the net effect is the intracellular generation of a bicarbonate ion which passes through the basal border of the cell into the peritubular capillary. The amount of hydrogen ion secretion and bicarbonate regeneration depends predominantly on the acid–base status. The total hydrogen ion secretion may be expressed by the following formula:

$$\text{Total } H^+ \text{ excretion} = NH_4^+ \text{ excretion} + \text{TA excretion} - HCO_3 \text{ excretion}$$

OTHER FUNCTIONS

Erythropoietin

Erythropoietin (EPO) is a glycoprotein produced by peritubular interstitial cells in the kidney. In the adult, the kidneys produce over 85% of the body's erythropoietin, whereas in the fetus the liver is an important source. EPO stimulates the production of erythrocyte stem cells in the bone marrow and has a relatively short half-life (5 h). Renal synthesis of EPO is stimulated by renal ischaemia, hypoxaemia or anaemia. In chronic renal failure, reduced or absent EPO production results in anaemia.

Vitamin D metabolism

The kidney is also involved in vitamin D metabolism. Cholecalciferol synthesized in the skin is hydroxylated to 25-hydroxycholecalciferol in the liver. Further hydroxylation to 1,25-dihydroxycholecalciferol occurs in the renal tubular cells by the enzyme 1α-hydroxylase. The activity of this enzyme is regulated by parathyroid hormone, serum phosphate concentrations and negative feedback.

FURTHER READING

Koeppen B M, Stanton B A 1996 Renal physiology, 2nd edn. Mosby, St Louis

26 Drugs used in renal disease

DRUG CONSIDERATIONS IN PATIENTS WITH RENAL DYSFUNCTION

INFLUENCE OF RENAL DISEASE ON PHARMACOKINETICS

Renal disease may affect drug pharmacokinetics through several mechanisms. Acidic drugs bind mainly to albumin. In renal failure, a decrease in serum albumin, an increase in serum urea, and the competition of endogenous substrates and drug metabolites for plasma protein binding sites lead to a decrease in the plasma protein binding of drugs. Highly protein-bound drugs have an increased unbound, active, free fraction. Under these circumstances, there may be an increase in the volume of distribution. Drugs are metabolized in the liver to water-soluble, inactive metabolites. Although uraemia has an effect on the intermediary metabolism of the liver, it does not seem to affect hepatic drug metabolism in humans.

The duration of action of most drugs administered by bolus or short-term infusion is dependent on redistribution and not elimination. It is usually not necessary to decrease the initial loading dose in patients with renal dysfunction, but subsequent maintenance doses may cause drug accumulation and should be reduced appropriately. The inactive water-soluble metabolites of drugs are eliminated by passive filtration at the glomerulus. A reduction in glomerular filtration in renal disease patients may lead to accumulation of these metabolites.

INFLUENCE OF DRUGS ON RENAL FUNCTION

All anaesthetic agents may cause a generalized depression of renal function which is transient and clinically insignificant. However, nephrotoxic drugs can impair renal function permanently (Table 26.1). For example, they may lead to severe sodium and water depletion, reduction in renal blood supply, direct renal damage or renal obstruction. Some drugs cause renal insufficiency by more than one mechanism.

Table 26.1 Mechanisms of drug-induced renal damage
Sodium and water depletion
Reduced renal perfusion
Direct renal toxicity
Urinary obstruction

Some of the fluorinated inhalation agents have a well recognized nephrotoxic effect, because they increase the serum inorganic fluoride concentration. Prolonged exposure of the renal tubules to fluoride ions causes polyuric renal dysfunction, leading to dehydration, hypernatraemia and increased plasma osmolarity. Experience with methoxyflurane (no longer in clinical use) has suggested that a plasma fluoride level of 50 μmol L^{-1} is potentially nephrotoxic. Although halothane and isoflurane do not seem to have a significant effect, prolonged administration of enflurane may lead to nephrotoxic fluoride ion concentrations.

Sevoflurane undergoes approximately 5% metabolism and one of the primary metabolites is fluoride. There were initial concerns that sevoflurane may be similar to methoxyflurane and impair the ability of the kidneys to concentrate urine. However, after sevoflurane administration is stopped, there is a rapid decrease in plasma fluoride concentration because of its insolubility and rapid pulmonary elimination. The intrarenal metabolic production of fluoride is also much less with sevoflurane than with methoxyflurane. Although after extensive use it would appear that sevoflurane renal toxicity is not a problem in clinical practice, its prolonged use is not recommended in patients with significantly impaired renal function.

Aprotinin is a serine-protease inhibitor and an antifibrinolytic agent occasionally administered during major surgery to improve haemostasis. It undergoes active reabsorption by the proximal tubules and is metabolized by enzymes in the kidney. There is some controversy about its effect on renal function. Although some studies have shown a low incidence of reversible renal dysfunction, others have shown changes in biochemical markers of tubular damage without evidence of renal impairment.

Other drugs with potential for impairing renal function include aminoglycosides and non-steroidal anti-inflammatory drugs (NSAIDs) in the presence of sepsis, radiocontrast agents and various chemotherapeutic drugs.

VASOACTIVE DRUGS USED DURING RENAL DYSFUNCTION

DOPAMINE

Dopamine is an important endogenous catecholamine, a precursor of norepinephrine and epinephrine, and a neurotransmitter in its own right. It can be administered pharmacologically and has complicated pharmacodynamic effects, including inotropy, chronotropy, vasoconstriction, and renal and splanchnic vasodilatation. Dopamine is inactive orally and has to be administered as an intravenous infusion, because it is metabolized within minutes by the enzymes dopamine β-hydroxylase and monoamine oxidase ($t_{1/2} < 2$ min). Dopamine must be diluted before infusion.

Mechanism of action

In common with all catecholamines, dopamine acts on different receptors in a diverse dose-related fashion. Dopamine receptors are present in various sites in the body and have been classified into five subtypes. The two most important receptors in the peripheral cardiovascular and renal systems are DA_1 and DA_2.

The infusion of relatively low concentrations of dopamine activates postsynaptic DA_1 receptors in blood vessels and the renal tubules. Stimulation leads to vasodilatation and improves some measures of renal function, such as cortical renal blood flow, glomerular filtration rate (GFR), sodium excretion and urine output. There is also an increase in mesenteric flow. Activation of presynaptic DA_2 receptors decreases intrarenal norepinephrine release, which leads to vasodilatation. It also causes inhibition of aldosterone secretion from the adrenal glands and a consequent decrease in sodium reabsorption. Theoretically, this should decrease renal oxygen consumption and improve the renal oxygen supply/demand relationship.

Dopamine stimulates its receptors in the renal and splanchnic beds at low infusion rates (0.1–2 μg kg^{-1} min^{-1}). This effect is accompanied by little change in cardiac output or heart rate. A reduction in arterial pressure may occur because of inhibition of the sympathetic nervous system by stimulation of the DA_2 receptors, and by DA_1-induced vasodilatation.

Increased infusion (2–5 μg kg^{-1} min^{-1}) stimulates β_1- and β_2-adrenergic receptors, which causes an increase in myocardial contractility, stroke volume and cardiac output. At this infusion rate, the heart rate usually does not change.

Higher doses of dopamine (> 10 μg kg^{-1} min^{-1}) lead to stimulation of the α-adrenergic receptors, causing vasoconstriction, an increase in peripheral vascular resistance and a decrease in renal and splanchnic blood flow.

The dopamine infusion rates given above are guidelines and there is considerable intra- and inter-patient variation. The maximum dose at which dopamine affects only dopamine receptors is debatable and must be individually determined. Because of the up- and downregulation of receptors, in any one patient, the appropriate dose for a required effect may vary from hour to hour.

Clinical uses

Dopamine is often used to preserve regional blood flow, but its perceived effectiveness is based largely on anecdotal reports and experimental data. Improved haemodynamics, renal vasodilatation and increase in renal blood flow do have diuretic and natriuretic effects. Because the urine output of the critically ill patient is considered a good marker of tissue perfusion by many clinicians, the diuretic properties of dopamine are valued. However, clinical studies have not demonstrated any benefit of 'low dose' dopamine for renal protection or for the prevention and treatment of acute renal failure in critically ill patients.

The use of higher doses of dopamine as an inotrope during cardiac failure, or a vasopressor during hypotension, is well established. Under these circumstances, it will have a beneficial effect on renal function, but it is important to ensure that there is an adequate circulating blood volume.

Side-effects

Side-effects of dopamine include tachyarrhythmias, vasoconstriction with acute hypertension, and nausea and vomiting because of a direct effect on receptors within the chemoreceptor trigger zone. Ideally, dopamine should be administered through a central venous catheter because extravasation may cause sloughing and necrosis of local surrounding tissues.

DOPEXAMINE

Dopexamine is a synthetic catecholamine with structural and pharmacological similarities to dopamine, and is used for its increase in cardiac output and renal and splanchnic vasodilator effects. It is inactive orally and, because of its short half-life (~ 6 min), it is administered intravenously as an infusion. Infusion rate starts at 0.5 μg kg^{-1} min^{-1} and is titrated to a therapeutic response (up to 6 μg kg^{-1} min^{-1}). Tolerance is usually associated with receptor downregulation. Its metabolism is by the recognized pathways for all the catecholamines.

Dopexamine is an agonist at vascular and renal dopaminergic DA_1 and DA_2 receptors. It also stimulates cardiac and vascular β_2-receptors, and has a limited indirect β_1 effect. It therefore combines vasodilator, chronotropic and mild inotropic activity and is used in low cardiac output states where specific renal and hepatosplanchnic vasodilatation is considered beneficial. The heart rate is increased in a dose-related manner and it produces a natriuresis and diuresis. The protective effect of dopexamine on the kidneys is theoretical and an effect on outcome still has to be proven.

The most common side-effect is a tachycardia and ventricular ectopic beats when higher doses are used. Nausea and vomiting, probably caused by stimulation of DA_2 receptors in the chemoreceptor trigger zone, have been reported.

FENOLDOPAM

Fenoldopam is a selective DA_1 agonist. It may be administered orally or intravenously and has been used for the management of congestive cardiac failure and hypertension.

ADENOSINE

Adenosine is a natural purine and is an important mediator in the control of renal blood flow and glomerular filtration. It causes peripheral vasodilatation and decreases arterial pressure when given intravenously. Adenosine-induced arterial hypotension inhibits renin release by the juxtaglomerular cells and has an interesting effect on the renal vasculature. It leads to transient vasoconstriction of the afferent arterioles, combined with vasodilatation of the efferent arterioles. This results in decreases in renal blood flow and glomerular filtration pressure and rate. There have been suggestions that this temporary decrease in renal function might play a protective role against an ischaemic insult. A decrease in GFR is usually associated with decreases in ultrafiltrate volume, reabsorption and oxygen demand. Whether adenosine changes the outcome of an ischaemic insult and acute renal injury in clinical practice has not been confirmed.

Adenosine also slows the heart rate and impairs atrioventricular conduction and is used in the treatment of supraventricular tachycardias.

CALCIUM CHANNEL BLOCKERS

Calcium antagonists (Ch. 7) act selectively on calcium channels in the cellular membrane of cardiac and vascular smooth muscle cells. Free calcium within the vascular smooth muscle enhances vascular tone and contributes to vasoconstriction. Calcium antagonists reduce the transmembrane calcium influx in these cells and via this mechanism are responsible for relaxation of the vascular smooth muscle and subsequent vasodilatation.

Apart from the vasodilatation, these drugs have a direct diuretic effect that contributes to their long-term antihypertensive action. Nifedipine increases the urine volume and sodium excretion, and may inhibit aldosterone release. This diuretic action is independent of any change in renal blood flow or GFR.

Because of the vasodilator effect on the vasculature, these drugs have been found to be useful in the management of conditions in which pathological vasoconstriction occurs, such as hypertension, Raynaud's disease, migraine and Prinzmetal's angina.

Calcium antagonists are often used as renovascular vasodilators in selected situations, e.g. renal transplantation. In kidney recipients, diltiazem has been shown to cause vasodilatation within the kidneys and improve intrarenal circulation. They also decrease calcium influx and production of oxygen free radicals on reperfusion after the ischaemic insult. In these patients, calcium antagonists significantly improve renal function and decrease the incidence of post-transplant acute tubular necrosis. Furthermore, they may reduce the vasoconstrictive action of cyclosporin. In spite of all the apparent beneficial effects, calcium antagonists have failed to improve graft survival.

Calcium antagonists may cause hypotension and thereby decrease renal perfusion. Therefore their use is not really justified in most cases of post-ischaemic acute renal failure. The effects of the depolarizing and non-depolarizing neuromuscular blocking agents might be enhanced by the calcium antagonists. Caution should always be exercised when this combination is used in patients with renal dysfunction.

ANGIOTENSIN-CONVERTING ENZYME (ACE) INHIBITORS

Many patients with hypertension or cardiac failure have an increased activity of the renin–angiotensin–aldosterone system. This leads to an elevated systemic vascular resistance, further decreases in cardiac output and renal perfusion, and more sodium and fluid retention. These patients are often receiving diuretic treatment, which in itself triggers renin activity. The ACE inhibitors (e.g. captopril, enalapril, lisinopril) are being used increasingly in this scenario, in place of, or in combination with, diuretics.

ACE inhibitors have a much greater affinity for the active site on the ACE than the natural substrate, angiotensin I. Consequently, the conversion of angiotensin I to angiotensin II is blocked. ACE is also responsible for the breakdown of bradykinin which is a potent vasodilator. Therefore, ACE inhibitors not only lead to vasodilatation but, because of the decreases in aldosterone formation and sodium re-uptake, also have an indirect potassium-retaining diuretic effect. The combination of ACE inhibitors and the potassium-saving diuretics should be avoided because of the risk of hyperkalaemia.

Angiotensin II is important for the maintenance of an adequate glomerular filtration pressure in patients with decreased renal perfusion. In the presence of renal artery stenosis, the use of ACE inhibitors may lead to an impairment of renal function by decreasing renal perfusion pressure, caused by the decrease in arterial pressure together with dilatation of the efferent arteriole of the glomerulus. Underlying renal impairment should therefore always be excluded before using ACE inhibitors, and patients receiving these agents should be monitored carefully.

NOREPINEPHRINE/EPINEPHRINE/PHENYLEPHRINE

Although norepinephrine and epinephrine also have β-receptor effects, all three of these drugs are very potent vasoconstrictors acting on the vascular α-receptors (Ch. 7). Their use is often accompanied by fear of inducing decreases in renal blood flow, GFR and renal function.

The efferent arterioles are the major sites of flow resistance in the kidney and determine renal blood flow, perfusion pressure and GFR. In cases of hypotension or septic shock, restoring the perfusion pressure of the kidney is of the utmost importance. An infusion of one of these vasoconstrictors may improve renal perfusion pressure provided fluid resuscitation has been adequate.

ANTIDIURETIC HORMONE/VASOPRESSIN/DESMOPRESSIN/DDAVP

Antidiuretic hormone (ADH) is a naturally occurring hormone, produced in the hypothalamus, transported by nerve axons down to the posterior pituitary gland and, from there, secreted into the blood. The release of ADH is regulated by the osmolarity of the extracellular body fluids, changes in arterial pressure and intravascular volume, and the sympathetic nervous system. An increase in blood osmolarity and hypovolaemia stimulate the hypothalamic osmoreceptors and arterial baroreceptors as part of the stress response. ADH is released and acts primarily on receptors in the distal convoluted tubule and collecting ducts of the nephron, to increase free water reabsorption and restore the plasma volume. The presence or absence of ADH determines to a large extent whether the kidney excretes a dilute or a concentrated urine (Ch. 25). ADH is also termed vasopressin, because it has a very potent vasoconstrictor effect, even more powerful than that of angiotensin.

Vasopressin decreases splanchnic and renal blood flow and is sometimes used to treat bleeding oesophageal varices. Desmopressin (DDAVP, 1-desamino-8-D-arginine vasopressin) is a synthetic form of vasopressin that does not cause vasoconstriction. It is used in cases of central diabetes insipidus (i.e. spontaneous diuresis with an urine osmolarity below 200 mosm L^{-1}).

DDAVP also has an influence on the coagulation system by increasing factor VIII von Willebrand (VIII:vWF), factor VIII coagulant (VIII:C), and factor VIII-related antigen (VIIIr:Ag) activity by stimulating its release from the storage sites. A dose of 0.3 μg kg^{-1} is often used in the treatment of haemorrhage in haemophiliacs.

Platelet dysfunction often occurs in renal disease when a high urea is present. The increase in bleeding time (> 15 min), despite a normal platelet count (> 100×10^9 L^{-1}), can be corrected before major surgery. The most appropriate treatment currently is the administration of DDAVP in the same dose as above. It has also been used prophylactically to reduce bleeding after cardiac surgery.

DDAVP cannot be used repeatedly because the endothelial storage sites of factor VIII:C become depleted, resulting in tachyphylaxis. Because it also seems to release tissue plasminogen activator, DDAVP can enhance fibrinolysis and the simultaneous use of an antifibrinolytic agent has to be considered. Although vasopressin is a vasoconstrictor, rapid injection of DDAVP may cause acute hypotension as a result of vasodilatation.

DIURETICS

Diuretics are probably among the most frequently prescribed groups of drugs in clinical practice. By definition, they cause a diuresis of water and sodium. When used on a long-term basis as antihypertensive agents, or for chronic cardiac failure, they not only change the body's sodium and fluid balance, but also act as mild vascular dilators. In the more acute perioperative and critical care scenario when a major diuretic effect is required, diuretics are used in higher doses. In acute cardiac failure, these drugs are very valuable because of their high benefit–risk ratio. Diuretics are often used to 'protect' the kidneys during ischaemic episodes such as aortic cross-clamping and cardiopulmonary bypass. However, human studies have failed to show the effectiveness of these agents in the prevention of ischaemic acute renal failure. There is also no clear evidence that polyuric renal dysfunction has a better outcome than oliguric renal failure, but it is generally accepted that the intensive care management of a critically ill patient is easier if there is a urine output.

Diuretics are classified according to their mechanism and site of action on the nephron (see Fig. 26.1):

- glomerulus and proximal renal tubule – e.g. osmotic diuretics, carbon anhydrase inhibitors
- ascending limb of the loop of Henle – e.g. loop diuretics
- distal tubule – e.g. thiazides, potassium-sparing diuretics
- collecting ducts – e.g. aldosterone antagonists.

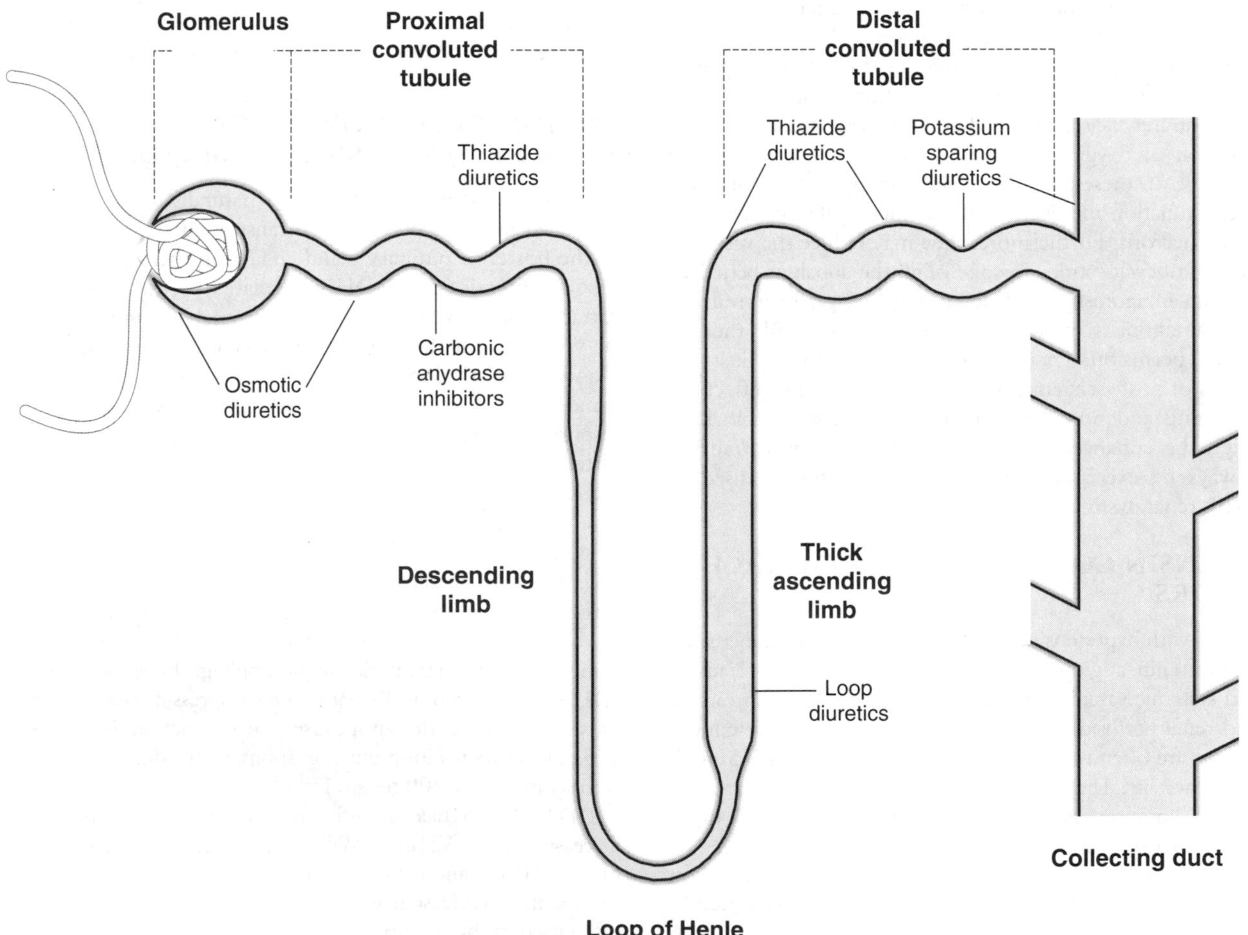

Fig. 26.1
Sites of action of diuretics.

CARBONIC ANHYDRASE INHIBITORS

Acetazolamide

Acetazolamide is well absorbed, not metabolized, but excreted almost unchanged by the kidney within 24 h. Toxicity is very rare.

Acetazolamide is a carbonic anhydrase inhibitor and acts in the proximal convoluted tubule of the nephron. Under normal physiological conditions, this enzyme is responsible for reabsorption of sodium and excretion of hydrogen ions in this part of the kidney. Inhibition of the carbonic anhydrase enzyme decreases the excretion of hydrogen ions, and therefore sodium and bicarbonate ions stay in the renal tubule. This results in the production of an alkaline urine with a high sodium bicarbonate content. This increased sodium excretion leads to a modest diuresis. Chloride ions are retained instead of bicarbonate to maintain an ionic balance. All these changes result in a hyperchloraemic metabolic acidosis.

Carbonic anhydrase inhibitors are seldom used as primary diuretics because of their weak diuretic effect. In the management of salicylate overdose, they may be used to start an alkaline diuresis to eliminate the weak organic acids. The most common use of acetazolamide is to reduce the intraocular pressure of glaucoma patients. The inhibition of carbonic anhydrase results in a decreased formation of ocular aqueous humour and cerebrospinal fluid. It is valuable in the prevention and management of acute mountain sickness. When used in patients with familial periodic paralysis, the metabolic acidosis increases the potassium concentration in the skeletal muscles and improves symptoms.

OSMOTIC DIURETICS

Mannitol

Mannitol is absorbed unreliably from the gastrointestinal tract and therefore has to be given by intravenous injection; doses of 0.25–1 g kg^{-1} are used. Initially it stays within the intravascular space but is then slowly redistributed into the extravascular compartment. Mannitol does not undergo metabolism and is excreted unchanged through the kidneys.

Mannitol expands the intravascular volume and then undergoes free glomerular filtration with almost no reabsorption in the proximal tubule. It also decreases the energy-consuming process of sodium and water reabsorption in the proximal tubule. This leads to an osmotic force that retains water and sodium in the tubule with a consequent osmotic diuresis, i.e. an increased urinary excretion of sodium, water, bicarbonate and chloride. Mannitol does not alter urinary pH. The raised renal blood flow reduces the rate of renin secretion which decreases the kidney's urine-concentrating effect.

Mannitol is often used prophylactically to protect the kidneys against an ischaemic incident (e.g. cardiopulmonary bypass, aortic cross-clamping or hypotensive episodes) and subsequent acute renal failure. It has been suggested that decreasing the oxygen demand in the proximal tubular cells preserves oxygen balance. By increasing tubular flow, it might also provide a flushing effect to remove necrotic cellular debris from the renal tubules after ischaemic injury. The hyperosmotic and oxygen radical scavenging effects of this drug might also reduce tubular endothelial cell swelling. However, although mannitol has been shown to be effective in animal experiments, studies have failed to show a renal protective effect in clinical practice. There is also little evidence that conversion from an oliguric to a non-oliguric renal failure decreases the mortality rate in critically ill patients. Nevertheless, mannitol is used regularly during renal transplantation to help 'preserve' the donor kidney.

Anaesthetists often administer mannitol to reduce intracranial (Ch. 57) and intraocular pressure.

In patients with a compromised cardiac function, mannitol may precipitate pulmonary oedema. Occasionally it may cause hypersensitivity reactions. If the blood–brain barrier is not intact after a head injury or neurosurgery, mannitol may enter the brain, draw water with it and cause rebound cerebral swelling.

LOOP DIURETICS

Furosemide, bumetanide and ethacrynic acid are classified as loop diuretics because of their common site of action. Furosemide is the most commonly used loop diuretic.

Furosemide

Furosemide is usually administered intravenously (0.1–1 mg kg^{-1}) or orally (0.75–3 mg kg^{-1}). It is well absorbed orally and about 60% of the dose reaches the central circulation within a short period, with the peak effect after 1–1.5 h. Intravenous furosemide is usually started as a slow 20–40 mg injection in adults, but higher doses or even an infusion may be required in the case of elderly patients with renal failure or severe congestive cardiac failure. Approximately 90% of the drug is bound to plasma proteins and its volume of distribution is relatively low. Metabolism and excretion into the gastrointestinal tract contribute to about 30% of the elimination of a dose of furosemide. The rest is excreted unchanged through glomerular filtration and tubular secretion. Impaired renal function affects the elimination process, but liver disease does not seem to influence this. The elimination half-life of furosemide is 1–1.5 h.

Loop diuretics act primarily on the medullary part of the ascending limb of the loop of Henle. After initial glomerular filtration and proximal tubular secretion, furosemide inhibits the active reabsorption of chloride in the thick portion of the ascending limb. This leads to chloride, sodium, potassium and hydrogen ions remaining in the tubule to maintain electrical neutrality, and their increased excretion in the urine. The extent of the following diuresis is determined by the concentration of furosemide active in this part of the tubule. Because the ascending limb plays an important role in the reabsorption of sodium chloride in the kidney, furosemide results in a marked diuretic response. The decrease in sodium chloride reabsorption leads to a reduced urine-concentrating ability of the normally hypertonic medullary interstitium.

Furosemide increases renal artery blood flow if the intravascular fluid volume is maintained. It causes redistribution so that flow to the outer part of the cortex remains unchanged while inner cortex and medullary flow is increased. It leads to an improved renal tissue oxygen tension. This effect, together with the increased release of renin and the activation of the angiotensin–aldosterone axis, is mediated via prostaglandins. A particular advantage of loop diuretics is the high ceiling effect (i.e. increasing doses lead to increasing diuresis).

In case of acute pulmonary oedema or other oedematous states of fluid overload due to cardiac, renal or liver failure, furosemide is the diuretic of choice. It reduces the intravascular fluid volume by promoting a rapid, powerful diuresis even in the presence of a low GFR. The pulmonary vascular bed and capacitance vessels are dilated by furosemide, and often a relief of dyspnoea and a reduction in pulmonary pressures may take place before the diuretic effect has occurred. In hypertensive patients, the vasodilatation and preload reduction lead to a decrease in arterial pressure.

The use of furosemide for prophylactic protection of the kidney against ischaemic injury and in the treatment of acute renal failure is controversial. In common with mannitol, furosemide has been shown in animal studies to help protect the kidney against ischaemic damage. Human studies, however, failed to support this. Loop diuretics, if administered early in the course of ischaemic acute renal failure, may change an oliguric into a non-oliguric state. Although non-oliguric acute renal failure is generally associated with a lower mortality rate, there is little evidence that this conversion changes the outcome. Furosemide should never be used, however, to treat oliguria caused by a decreased intravascular fluid volume or dehydration, because the following diuresis could exaggerate hypovolaemia and renal ischaemic injury. It is important to restore the intravascular volume status first before any pharmacological intervention.

A raised intracranial pressure is often treated with furosemide. It mobilizes the oedema fluid, decreases cerebrospinal fluid production and lowers the intracranial pressure without changing the plasma osmolarity. In contrast to mannitol, a disrupted blood–brain barrier does not influence the effect of furosemide on the intracranial pressure.

Excessive doses of furosemide often lead to fluid or electrolyte abnormalities. Severe hypokalaemia may precipitate dangerous cardiac arrhythmias, especially in the presence of high concentrations of digitalis. It may also enhance the effect of non-depolarizing muscle relaxants. Hypovolaemia, dehydration and the consequent haemoconcentration may lead to changes in blood viscosity. Hyperuricaemia and prerenal uraemia may develop and may precipitate an acute gout attack in a patient with pre-existing gout.

Furosemide may cause high concentrations of aminoglycosides and cephalosporins in the kidneys and this may enhance their nephrotoxic effect. Prolonged high blood concentrations of furosemide may cause transient or permanent deafness because of changes in the endolymph electrolyte composition. Patients allergic to other sulphonamide drugs may have a cross-sensitivity, although idiosyncratic reactions are rare.

Bumetanide

The mechanism of action of bumetanide and its effects are similar to those of furosemide. The difference between these two drugs is the greater potency and bioavailability of bumetanide; therefore, smaller doses are needed. The normal adult dose is 0.5–3 mg i.v. over 1–2 min. The onset of diuresis is within 30 min and this usually lasts for about 4 h. The pharmacokinetics are similar to those of furosemide, with the exception that bumetanide is absorbed completely after oral administration and its rate of elimination is less dependent on renal function. Potassium loss is also a problem with bumetanide. Ototoxicity may be slightly less frequent than with furosemide, but renal toxicity is more of a problem. In clinical practice, there is no clear advantage or disadvantage over furosemide, providing equivalent doses are administered.

Ethacrynic acid

Although the molecular structure of ethacrynic acid is very different from that of furosemide, it has almost identical pharmacological properties. After intravenous administration, it binds strongly to plasma proteins and the majority of the drug is eliminated by active secretion into the renal tubule. Almost one-third is excreted in the bile. The risk of toxicity and side effects is probably equivalent to that of furosemide.

THIAZIDE DIURETICS

Although thiazide diuretics are seldom used by anaesthetists, many patients scheduled for surgery are receiving these drugs for chronic hypertension or cardiac failure. There are a large number of thiazides available, all with a similar dose–response curve and diuretic effect. Bendroflumethiazide, chlorothiazide, hydrochlorothiazide and chlorthalidone are a few examples of the better known thiazide diuretics. The majority have a duration of action of 6–12 h. In comparison with loop diuretics, thiazides have a longer duration of action, act at a different site, have a low 'ceiling' effect and are less effective in renal failure.

Thiazide diuretics are administered orally, absorbed rapidly from the gastrointestinal tract and initiate a diuresis within 1–2 h. The major distinction between the available thiazides is their difference in elimination rate. They are distributed in the extracellular space and eliminated in the proximal tubule of the nephron by active secretion.

Thiazides inhibit the active pump for sodium and chloride reabsorption in the cortical ascending part of the loop of Henle and the distal convoluted tubule. Therefore, the urine-concentrating ability of the kidney is not impaired. as normally this area is responsible for less than 5% of sodium reabsorption. The diuresis achieved by the thiazides is therefore never as effective as that of the loop diuretics. It is mild but sustained. In contrast with loop diuretics, the excretion of calcium is decreased and hypercalcaemia may become a problem. In the presence of aldosterone activity, the increase in sodium delivery to the distal renal tubules is associated with increased potassium loss, similar to that of the loop diuretics. The reduced clearance of uric acid by thiazides may cause hyperuricaemia.

Thiazides are used extensively in low doses, and often combined with a low-sodium diet, for the management of essential hypertension. A reduction in extracellular fluid volume and mild peripheral vasodilatation are responsible for the sustained antihypertensive effect. The full antihypertensive effect may take up to 12 weeks to become established. Higher doses of thiazides are used for the management of congestive cardiac failure and other oedematous conditions such as nephrotic syndrome and liver cirrhosis.

The most common side-effects of the thiazides are probably dehydration and hypovolaemia. This may present as orthostatic hypotension. When administered chronically, these drugs lead typically to a diuretic-induced hypokalaemic, hypochloraemic, metabolic alkalosis. In combination with magnesium depletion, the hypokalaemia may trigger serious cardiac arrhythmias, in addition to digitalis toxicity, muscle weakness and the potentiation of non-depolarizing muscle relaxants.

Thiazides decrease the tubular secretion of urate, which may lead to a hyperuricaemia and gout. They are sulphonamide derivatives and may therefore cause inhibition of insulin release from the pancreas and blockade of peripheral glucose utilization. This may precipitate hyperglycaemia or an increase in insulin requirements in a patient with diabetes mellitus. They also lead to an increase in total blood cholesterol.

POTASSIUM-SPARING DIURETICS

Only a small part of sodium reabsorption into the renal cells takes place via the sodium–potassium exchange mechanism in the distal tubules. The potassium-retaining diuretics act on the distal convoluted tubules and the collecting ducts and therefore cause only a limited diuresis. There are two subgroups in this category: drugs acting independently of the aldosterone mechanism (e.g. triamterene and amiloride) and aldosterone antagonists (e.g. spironolactone).

These drugs increase the urinary excretion of sodium, chloride and bicarbonate and lead to an increase in urinary pH. They prevent excessive loss of potassium that occurs with the loop and thiazide diuretics by reducing the sodium–potassium exchange. Potassium-sparing drugs do, however, augment the diuretic response of these drugs when given in combination.

Amiloride and triamterene

Amiloride acts directly on the distal tubule and collecting duct. It causes potassium retention and an increase in sodium loss. After oral intake, up to 25% is absorbed, onset of its peak effect is within 6 h, and it is then excreted unchanged in the urine. Amiloride is almost always used in combination with thiazide or loop diuretics. It then has a synergistic action in terms of diuresis, although it opposes the potassium loss. Amiloride has few side-effects. Hyperkalaemia and acidosis may occur, and it is therefore contraindicated in patients with renal failure.

Triamterene has characteristics similar to those of amiloride.

Spironolactone

Aldosterone causes sodium reabsorption and potassium loss in the distal convoluted tubule. Spironolactone has a steroid molecular structure, acts as a competitive antagonist on the aldosterone receptors and inhibits sodium reabsorption and potassium loss. In the absence of aldosterone, it has no effect.

After oral absorption, spironolactone is immediately metabolized to a number of metabolites. Some of these are active and act for up to 15 h.

Spironolactone is the logical choice of diuretic in the management of cirrhosis of the liver, ascites and secondary hyperaldosteronism. Cardiac failure or hypertension in the presence of high mineralocorticoid levels (Conn's syndrome or prednisone therapy) is another indication. It is often combined with thiazides to maximize the diuretic effect and prevent potassium loss.

Hyperkalaemia may develop if spironolactone is used in the presence of renal dysfunction. If it is used in high doses, it may cause gynaecomastia and impotence.

When diuretics are prescribed in a patient with fluid retention and oedema, three important principles have to be kept in mind. First, although a dramatic diuretic response may be required in pulmonary oedema and acute cardiac failure, a mild sustained diuresis is more appropriate in the majority of patients with a need for diuretics. This approach will reduce the side-effects. Second, plasma potassium concentrations and hydration status must always be monitored when a diuretic is being used. Third, diuretic therapy only treats the symptoms and does not influence the underlying cause or change the outcome of a patient with oedema.

DRUGS AND RENAL TRANSPLANTATION

The optimal treatment for end-stage renal failure is renal transplantation. Apart from optimizing the recipient's general health (e.g. correction of anaemia, preoperative dialysis, etc.), immunosuppression plays an extremely important role in graft survival.

ERYTHROPOIETIN

Erythropoietin is a circulating hormone secreted by the kidneys. It stimulates the bone marrow to produce red blood cells. The ability of the kidney to secrete erythropoietin deteriorates as excretory function decreases. Patients with severe chronic renal failure are unable to produce adequate quantities of erythropoietin, which leads to diminished red blood cell production. The retention of toxic substances also contributes to bone marrow depression. In addition, red cell survival is reduced by 50% in advanced renal failure. Therefore these patients almost always develop a chronic anaemia.

Long-term administration of recombinant human erythropoietin (rHUEPO) in chronic renal failure patients results in global stimulation of the bone marrow, increasing red blood cell differentiation and maintaining cell viability, thereby improving anaemia. It also decreases bleeding by increasing platelet adhesion in haemodialysed uraemic patients. A side-effect of rHUEPO is the development of hypertension or exacerbation of existing hypertension.

IMMUNOSUPPRESSION

Prednisolone and azathioprine

Corticosteroids were the first drugs to be used as immunosuppressive agents. Initially, very high doses were used, producing the typical steroid side-effects, e.g. Cushingoid appearance, hypertension, hyperglycaemia and osteoporosis. Experience and research showed that large doses were not necessary and that better results and fewer side-effects were possible with lower doses.

The 'modern era' of immunosuppression started with the discovery of azathioprine. For a long period of time, the combination of azathioprine and corticosteroids was the 'gold standard' in transplant surgery. Azathioprine is a derivative of 6-mercaptopurine and is metabolized to its active form in the liver. It affects the synthesis of DNA and RNA and is broken down by the enzyme xanthine oxidase. Co-administration of allopurinol (xanthine oxidase inhibitor) is contraindicated because it may result in bone marrow suppression, agranulocytosis and leucopenia. Patients receiving azathioprine are prone to develop viral warts or malignancies of the skin and hepatic dysfunction.

Cyclosporin A and cyclosporin-neoral

The next major advance in transplant surgery was the discovery of cyclosporin A. This fungal peptide prevents the proliferation and clonal expansion of T lymphocytes. The chance of acute rejection is reduced significantly by administration of this drug. In spite of the large number of side-effects of cyclosporin A, it has been accepted as the new standard against which all other immunosuppressants are judged. Cyclosporin A is lipophilic and incompletely absorbed in the small bowel. Serious side-effects such as gingival hypertrophy, hepatotoxicity and nephrotoxicity make this a less than perfect drug. For a long time, classic triple therapy consisted of prednisolone, azathioprine and cyclosporin A.

Recently, cyclosporin was released in a new form: cyclosporin-neoral. Neoral is a microemulsion that enhances the bioavailability of cyclosporin through improved absorption. Cyclosporin-neoral is equipotent to the parent drug and most renal transplant patients are presently receiving this agent.

Rapamycin

Rapamycin is a macrolide with antifungal and potent immunosuppressant effects. It prevents proliferation of T cells and antagonizes the action of interleukin-2 on its receptor. This agent is 100 times more potent than cyclosporin A. It has no adverse effects on liver or renal function, but has the potential to enhance the nephrotoxicity and hepatotoxicity of cyclosporin.

FK506 (Tacrolimus)

FK506 is a new macrolide antibiotic with a similar structure to rapamycin. It is a very potent immunosuppressant drug that inhibits the activation of T cells and interleukin-2 generation. The principle side-effects are nephrotoxicity and neurotoxicity.

Mycophenolate mofetil

Mycophenolate mofetil (MMF) is the newest immunosuppressant licensed to be used in renal transplantation. It inhibits a key enzyme in the purine synthesis pathway and therefore has a specific effect on B and T lymphocytes. The synthesis of adhesion molecules is also inhibited by MMF. It seems as though MMF effectively prevents chronic rejection in renal transplant patients. MMF is neither nephrotoxic nor hepatotoxic.

The immunosuppressants are usually used in combination with each other. A typical perioperative regimen for renal transplantation is shown in Table 26.2.

Despite their powerful immunosuppressant effects, it is unlikely that any of the new or existing drugs may be used as monotherapy. The role of drugs inhibiting antigen presentation and the use of monoclonal antibodies are still being defined.

Table 26.2 A typical perioperative regimen for renal transplant

Preoperative
Induction immunosuppression (cyclosporin-neoral, FK506, rapamycin)
Heparin 5000 units subcutaneous
Ranitidine 150 mg orally (stress ulcer prophylaxis)
Nifedipine 20 mg orally (vasodilator, free radical scavenger)
At induction
Antibiotic prophylaxis–co-amoxiclav (augmentin) 1.2 g intravenous methylprednisolone 0.5 g i.v.
During vascular anastomosis
Mannitol 0.5 g kg^{-1} intravenous
± dopamine 3–5 μg kg^{-1} min^{-1}
Postoperative
Antibiotic prophylaxis
Heparin 5000 units subcutaneous, twice daily
Aspirin 150 mg orally
Ranitidine 150 mg orally, twice daily
Co-trimoxazole 480 mg orally, daily (protection against *Pneumocystis carinii*)
Immunosuppression ('triple therapy')

FURTHER READING

Aronson J K 1999 Drugs and renal insufficiency. Medicine: systemic aspects of renal disease

Aronson S, Blumenthal R 1998 Perioperative renal dysfunction and cardiovascular anaesthesia: concerns and controversies. Journal of Cardiothoracic and Vascular Anesthesia 12: 567–586

Bevan D R 1994 Renal function. In: Nimmo W S, Rowbotham D J, Smith G (eds) Anaesthesia, 2nd edn. Blackwell Scientific Publications, Oxford, p 272–290

Girbes A R J, Hoogenberg K 1998 The use of dopamine and norepinephrine in the ICU. In: Vincent J-L (ed) Yearbook of intensive care and emergency medicine. Springer-Verlag, p 178–187

Guyton A C, Hall J E 1997 The body fluids and the kidneys. In: Guyton A C, Hall J E (eds) Human physiology and mechanisms of disease, 6th edn. WB Saunders, Philadelphia, p 201–254

Sear J W, Holland D E 1994 Anaesthesia for patients with renal dysfunction. In: Nimmo W S, Rowbotham D J, Smith G (eds) Anaesthesia, 2nd edn. Blackwell Scientific Publications, Oxford, p 1277–1300

27 Metabolism, the stress response to surgery and perioperative thermoregulation

METABOLISM

Metabolism may be defined as the chemical processes which enable cells to function. Basal metabolic rate, i.e. the minimum amount of energy required to maintain basic autonomic function and normal homeostasis in a healthy resting person, is approximately 25–30 cal kg^{-1} day^{-1} (equivalent to 40 Kcal $m^{-2}h^{-1}$). For example, energy is required by the myocardium to maintain heart rate and stroke volume and by nerve and muscle membranes to maintain membrane potentials. Chemical reactions producing this energy are coupled with the relevant physiological process. In muscle cells, for instance, the release of energy from adenosine triphosphate (ATP) is coupled to mechanical interaction of actin and myosin fibres, producing muscle contraction.

It is beyond the scope of this chapter to describe all cellular biochemical reactions. Instead, it provides an overview of the chemical processes of the cell and their physiological importance.

ATP is the 'energy currency' of the body because it is present in all cells and most physiological processes acquire energy from it. Oxidation of nutrients in cells releases energy, which is used to regenerate ATP. Conversion of one molecule of ATP to ADP releases 8 kcal of energy (1 kcal is the amount of energy required to raise the temperature of 1 L of water through 1°C). Additional hydrolysis of the phosphate bond from ADP to AMP also releases 8 kcal, as shown in Fig. 27.1.

Because the majority of cellular activity is involved in rendering the energy in foods available for various physiological functions, metabolism may be classified into that of carbohydrate, protein and fat.

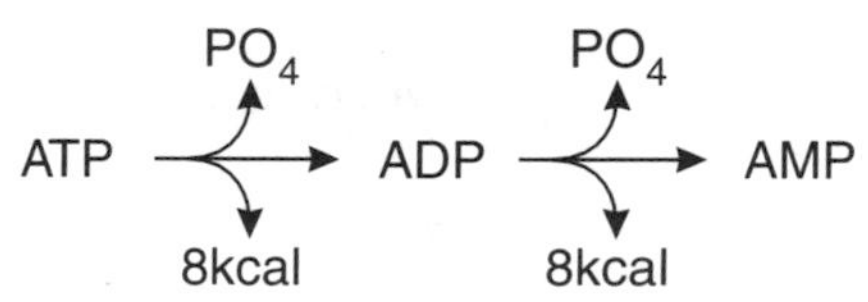

$$\text{ATP} \xrightarrow[\text{8kcal}]{PO_4} \text{ADP} \xrightarrow[\text{8kcal}]{PO_4} \text{AMP}$$

Fig. 27.1
Hydrolysis of adenosine triphosphate (ATP).

CARBOHYDRATE METABOLISM

Most of the final product of carbohydrate digestion is glucose, which is used to form ATP in cells. As the cellular membrane is impermeable to glucose, it is transported by a carrier protein across the membrane in a process termed *facilitated diffusion*. This is a passive process (i.e. it does not require energy expenditure by the cell), in contrast to glucose absorption in the gastrointestinal tract or reabsorption in the renal tubule, both of which are active (i.e. energy-consuming processes, involving co-transport with sodium ions). Facilitated diffusion of glucose into cells is increased 10-fold in the presence of insulin, without which the rate of uptake would be inadequate.

After absorption into cells, glucose may be used immediately or stored in the form of glycogen, particularly in liver and muscle. The process of releasing glucose molecules from the glycogen molecule in times of high metabolic demand is termed *glycogenolysis*. This process is initiated by an enzyme termed *phosphorylase*, which is activated in the presence of epinephrine and glucagon. Epinephrine is released by the sympathetic nervous system, while glucagon is released from the α cells of the pancreas in response to hypoglycaemia.

The mechanism of glucose catabolism involves an extensive series of enzyme-controlled steps, rather than a single reaction. This is because oxidation of 1 mol of glucose (180 g) releases almost 686 kcal of energy, but only 8 kcal is required to form one molecule of ATP (Fig. 27.1). Therefore, an elaborate series of reactions, termed the *glycolytic pathway*, releases small quantities of energy resulting in the synthesis of 38 mol of ATP from each mole of glucose. As each of these can release 8 kcal, a total of 304 kcal of energy in the form of ATP is synthesized. Hence, the efficiency of the glycolytic pathway is 44%, the rest of the energy being released as heat.

The glycolytic pathway may be summarized as:

1. Glycolysis, i.e. splitting the glucose molecule into two molecules of pyruvic acid; this results in the formation of two molecules of ATP.
2. Oxidation of the pyruvic acid molecules (involving the Krebs citric acid cycle), creating another two molecules of ATP from each pyruvic acid molecule.

3. Oxidative phosphorylation, i.e. the formation of ATP by the oxidation of hydrogen, created during glycolysis and oxidation of the end-products of glycolysis – 90% of ATP molecules are formed by this final process.

Anaerobic glycolysis

This is the process of ATP formation in the absence of oxygen and is possible because the first two steps of glycolysis do not require oxygen. In the absence of oxygen, pyruvic acid molecules and hydrogen ions accumulate, which would normally stop the reaction. However, pyruvic acid and hydrogen ions combine in the presence of the enzyme *lactic dehydrogenase* to form lactic acid, which easily diffuses out of cells, allowing anaerobic glycolysis to continue. This is a highly inefficient use of the energy within glucose. When oxygen is again available to the cells, lactic acid is reconverted to glucose or used directly for energy.

The glycolytic pathway metabolizes 70% of glucose. A second mechanism (the phosphogluconate pathway) is responsible for metabolism of the remaining 30%. The importance of this pathway is that ATP is formed independently of the enzymes needed in the glycolytic pathway, and hence an enzymatic abnormality in the glycolytic pathway does not completely inhibit energy metabolism.

Gluconeogenesis

This is the formation of glucose from amino acids, which are usually used for protein formation. It occurs when stores of glycogen are depleted. Prolonged hypoglycaemia is the main trigger for this process, but ACTH and thyroxine also have a role.

PROTEIN METABOLISM

Proteins are composed of amino acids, of which there are 20 different types in humans. All amino acids have a weak acid group (-COOH) and an amine group (-NH_2). They are joined by peptide linkages to form *peptide chains*, a reaction which releases a molecule of water in the process (Fig. 27.2). The blood concentration of amino acids is approximately 1–2 mmol L^{-1}. Entry into cells requires facilitated or active transport using carrier mechanisms. They are then conjugated into proteins by the formation of peptide linkages. Formation of the peptide link requires 0.5–4.0 kcal provided by ATP. Large proteins may be composed of several peptide chains wrapped around each other and bound by weaker links, e.g. hydrogen bonds, electrostatic forces and sulphydryl bonds.

There is a reversible equilibrium between the amino acids in plasma, plasma proteins and tissue proteins. Proteins may be synthesized from amino acids in all cells of the body, the type of protein depending on the genetic material in the DNA, which determines the sequence of amino acids formed and hence controls the nature of the synthesized proteins. Amino acids may be *essential* (i.e. must be ingested as they cannot be synthesized in the body) or *non-essential* (i.e. may be synthesized in the cells). Synthesis of the latter is by the process of *transamination*, whereby an amine radical (-NH_2) is transferred to the corresponding α-keto acid. Breakdown of excess amino acids are degraded into glucose (gluconeogenesis) for use as energy or storage as fat, both of which occur in the liver. The breakdown of amino acids occurs by the process of *deamination*, the removal of the amine group (Fig. 27.3). The amine radical may be recycled to other molecules or released as ammonia. In the liver, two molecules of ammonia are combined to form urea.

During starvation or when no protein is ingested (e.g. after major surgery), 20–30 g day^{-1} of protein is catabolized for energy purposes. This occurs despite the continuing availability of some

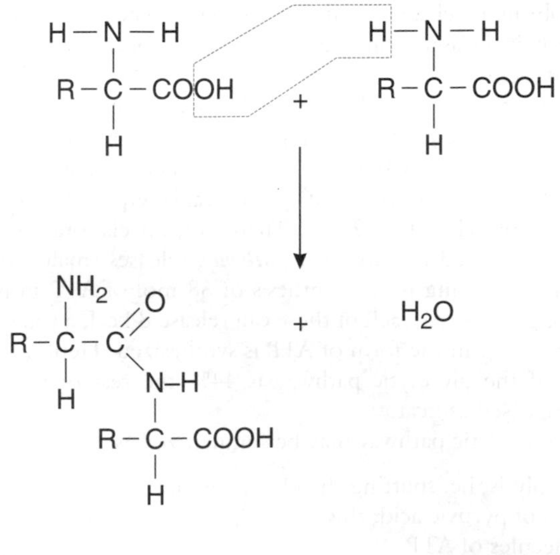

Fig. 27.2
Formation of peptide link. Note that the amine -NH_2 and weakly acidic -COOH groups combine to form the peptide link and a molecule of water.

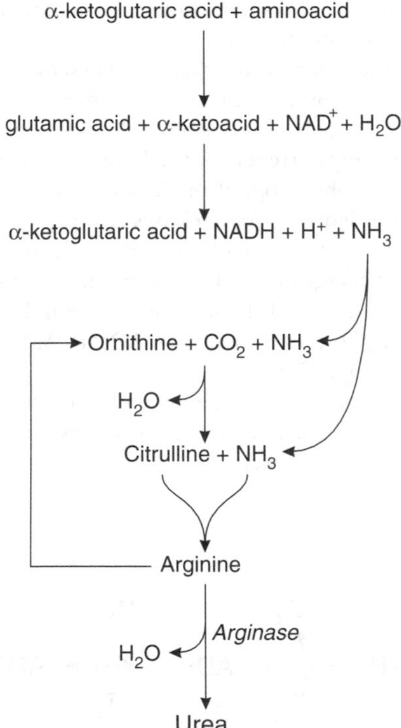

Fig. 27.3
Formation of urea.

stored carbohydrates and fats. When carbohydrate and fat stores are exhausted, the rate of protein catabolism is increased to > 100 g day^{-1}, resulting in a rapid decline in tissue function.

Several hormones influence protein metabolism. Growth hormone, insulin and testosterone are anabolic, i.e. they increase the rate of cellular protein synthesis. Glucocorticoids decrease the amount of protein in most tissues, except the liver. Thyroxine indirectly affects protein metabolism by affecting metabolic rate. If insufficient energy sources are available to cells, thyroxine may contribute to excess protein breakdown. Conversely, if adequate amino acid and energy sources are available, thyroxine may increase the rate of protein synthesis.

LIPID METABOLISM

Lipids are chemically distinct compounds which include triglycerides (TGs), cholesterol and phospholipids (PLs). The basic structure of TGs and PLs is the fatty acid, and although cholesterol does not contain fatty acid, its sterol nucleus is formed from fatty acid molecules. Fatty acid is simply a long-chain hydrocarbon organic acid. TGs are composed of three long-chain fatty acids bound with one molecule of glycerol (Fig. 27.4).

After absorption in the gastrointestinal tract, lipids are aggregated into droplets (0.1–0.5 μm), termed chylomicrons, which pass into the lymphatic system. These chylomicrons are removed as they pass through the liver and adipose capillaries by ***lipoprotein lipase***, which hydrolyses the TGs and PLs from the chylomicrons as they adhere to the endothelium of the cell wall. The fatty acids are highly lipid-soluble and diffuse through the liver or adipose cell membrane into these cells. Adipose cells are modified fibroblasts capable of storing TGs in quantities up to 95% of their volume. However, they are more than storage vessels and contain enzymes for synthesizing and breaking down TGs, PLs and cholesterol.

Transport of lipids from the liver or adipose cells to other tissues that need it as an energy source occurs by means of binding the fatty acids to plasma albumin. The fatty acids are then referred to as ***free fatty acids*** (FFAs), to distinguish them from other fatty acids in the plasma. After 12 h of fasting, all chylomicrons have been removed from the blood, and circulating lipids then occur in the form of ***lipoproteins***. These are smaller particles than chylomicrons but are also composed of TGs, PLs and cholesterol, together with protein. They are formed in the liver and may be classified as:

- very low-density lipoproteins (VLDLs), consisting mainly of TGs
- low-density lipoproteins (LDLs), consisting mainly of cholesterol
- high-density lipoproteins (HDLs), consisting mainly of protein.

Triglycerides as energy

Lipids are ingested in similar proportions to carbohydrates and may be used as an energy source immediately or stored in the liver or adipose cells for later use as an energy source. The stages in the use of TGs as an energy source are as follows (see also Fig. 27.5):

1. In this first stage, TG is hydrolysed to its constituent glycerol and three fatty acids; glycerol is then conjugated to glycerol-3-phosphate and enters the glycolytic pathway, which generates ATP as described above.

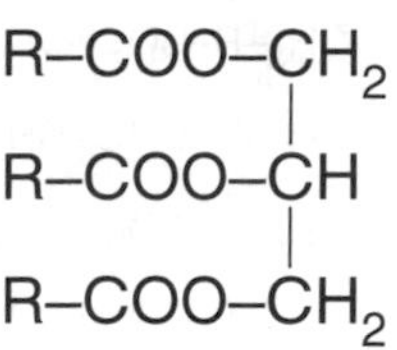

Fig. 27.4
Triglyceride structure.

2. Fatty acids must enter the cell mitochondria to be oxidized. This process requires ***carnitine*** as a carrier agent.
3. Each fatty acid is combined with coenzyme A (CoA), at a cost of two ATP molecules.
4. The fatty acid is degraded in two-carbon segments. The most important in this complex series of steps is the removal of two hydrogen atoms from the alpha and beta carbon atoms (the carbon atoms nearest the COOH end of the fatty acid molecule), which results in a double bond between the alpha and beta carbon atoms.
5. This compound splits between the alpha and beta carbon atoms, forming acetyl-CoA and another fatty acid combined with coenzyme A (fatty acyl-CoA), which is two carbon atoms shorter than the original.
6. The acetyl-CoA enters the citric acid cycle, generating ATP as described above. The new, shorter fatty acyl-CoA undergoes the same degradation steps until only acetyl-CoA remains. For example, stearic acid contains 18 carbon atoms, and hence this cycle is repeated nine times and nine molecules of acetyl-CoA are formed.

The precise number of ATP molecules formed from a molecule of TG depends on the length of the fatty acid chain, longer chains providing more two-carbon segments and hence more molecules of ATP. For example, stearic acid, with 16 carbon atoms in its chain, is metabolized to eight molecules of acetyl-CoA, which yields a total of 148 molecules of ATP. Two ATP molecules are consumed in the initial combination of the fatty acid with CoA, leaving a net gain of 146 molecules of ATP per oxidation of each molecule of this particular fatty acid.

Ketones

Initial degradation of fatty acids occurs in the liver, but the acetyl-CoA is not used immediately. ***Acetoacetic acid*** is formed from two molecules of acetyl-CoA, which is largely reduced by addition of two H atoms to form ***β-hydroxybutyric acid***. A smaller quantity of acetoacetic acid is decarboxylated to form ***acetone*** (Fig. 27.6). These three substances, collectively known as ketones, are organic acids, which diffuse freely out of the liver and are transported to the peripheral tissues, where they may be utilized for energy. Their importance is that they accumulate in diabetes and starvation, such as may occur in the perioperative period. In both circumstances, no carbohydrates are being metabolized. In diabetes, no insulin results in a reduction in intracellular glucose, and in starvation, carbohydrates are lacking simply because they are not being ingested. The ensuing breakdown of fat as described above results

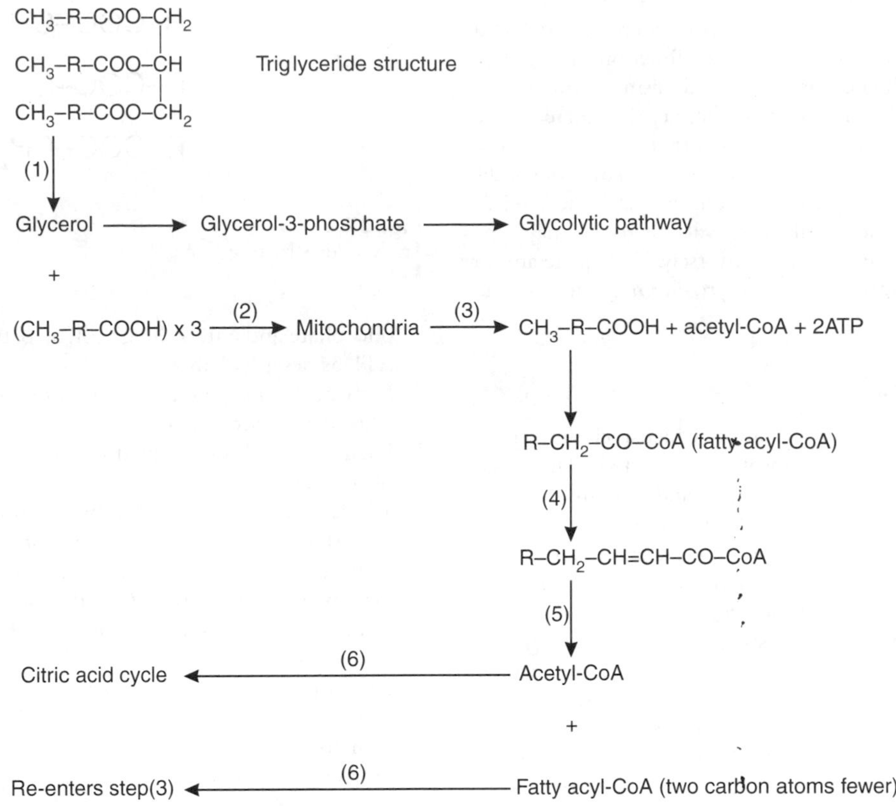

Fig. 27.5
Metabolism of triglycerides. The bracketed numbers refer to the stages described in the text.

in large quantities of ketones being released from the liver to the peripheral tissues. There is a limit to the rate at which ketones can be utilized by the tissues, because depletion of essential carbohydrate intermediate metabolites slows the rate at which acetyl-CoA can enter the Krebs cycle. Hence, blood ketone concentration may increase rapidly, causing metabolic acidosis and ketonuria.

Endocrine regulation of triglyceride metabolism

The effect of insulin has been described above. In addition, catecholamines released during stress or heavy exercise cause rapid breakdown of TGs and release of fatty acids. Stress also causes release of ACTH from the anterior pituitary, resulting in increased glucocorticoid secretion by the adrenal glands, with a similar effect on catecholamines and TG metabolism. Growth hormone has similar effects and thyroxine has an indirect effect by increasing the overall rate of energy metabolism.

Cholesterol

Cholesterol is a lipid with a sterol nucleus and is formed from acetyl-CoA. It may be absorbed from food or synthesized in the liver and, in small quantities, by all cells. Its function is predominantly (80%) the formation of bile salts in the liver, which promote the digestion and absorption of lipids. The remainder is used in the formation of adrenocortical and sex hormones and it is also deposited in the skin, where it resists the absorption of water-soluble chemicals. Factors affecting blood cholesterol concentrations are as follows (see also Fig. 27.7):

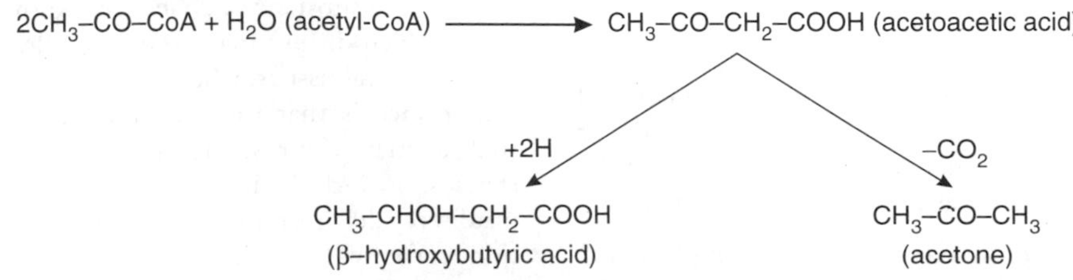

Fig. 27.6
Ketone formation.

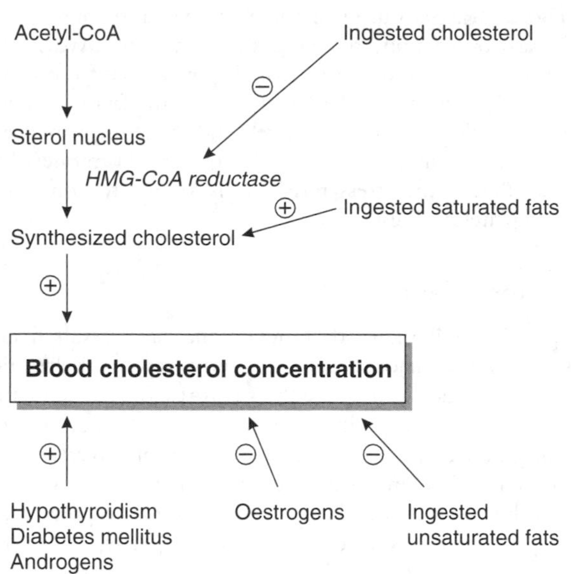

Fig. 27.7
Factors affecting blood cholesterol.

- There is a feedback mechanism whereby increased cholesterol absorption from the diet results in inhibition of the enzyme *HMG-CoA reductase*, which regulates synthesis of cholesterol.
- Saturated fats increase the amount of acetyl-CoA in the liver, causing increased endogenous cholesterol synthesis. Hence a cholesterol-lowering diet must also be low in saturated fats.
- Polyunsaturated fatty acids lower blood cholesterol by an unknown mechanism.
- There are many hormonal influences in cholesterol metabolism also, including increased plasma concentrations in response to abnormally low concentrations of thyroid hormone, insulin and androgens. Oestrogen reduces cholesterol by an unknown mechanism.

MEASURING METABOLIC RATE

Most of the energy expended within the body becomes heat, except when obvious external physical work is being done. Therefore, basal metabolic rate may be determined by measuring the quantity of heat given out by the body at rest. This may be achieved by placing the subject in a chamber termed a calorimeter. In addition, as more than 95% of the energy expended within the resting body derives from the reaction of oxygen with different substances, the rate of utilization of oxygen is also an accurate index of metabolic rate. Calculating oxygen consumption to estimate metabolic rate is termed *indirect calorimetry*. The quantity of energy liberated by a subject on an average diet is approximately 4.8 kcal L^{-1} of oxygen consumed. The factors influencing metabolic rate are shown in Table 27.1.

Table 27.1 Factors influencing metabolic rate
Malnutrition (if prolonged, by 20%).
Sleep (by 15%)
Exercise (up to 2000 x basal)
Protein ingestion.
Age: < 5 years × 2 rate of > 70
Thyroid hormone imbalance (increase or decrease by 50%)
Sympathetic stimulation
Testosterone (by 15%)
Temperature
Anaesthesia (20% reduction) (regional anaesthesia – no effect)

THE STRESS RESPONSE TO SURGERY

Surgery or trauma consistently elicits a characteristic neuroendocrine and cytokine response in proportion to the extent of injury or metabolic insult. Therefore, minor surgery on a limb has a negligible stress response, in contrast to major surgery such as a laparotomy or thoracotomy. There is an initial 'ebb' or shock phase, followed by a 'flow' or hyperdynamic phase. In surgery, the flow phase *is* the stress response for all practical purposes and its characteristics are shown in Table 27.2. There are two principal components to the stress response to surgery: the neuroendocrine response and the cytokine response.

The neuroendocrine response is stimulated initially by painful afferent neural stimuli reaching the CNS. It may be diminished and sometimes eliminated altogether by dense neural blockade from a regional anaesthetic.

The cytokine component of the stress response, on the other hand, is stimulated by local tissue damage at the site of the surgery itself and is independent of neural blockade. It is diminished by minimally invasive surgery, especially laparoscopic techniques.

Until the 1970s, the stress response was thought to be an adaptive homeostatic response to a physiological insult, enhancing resistance to stress. However, there is growing evidence that the stress response is actually detrimental and is associated with postoperative morbidity. It has adverse effects on several key physiological systems, including the cardiovascular, respiratory and gastroenterological systems.

Immediately after surgical incision under general anaesthesia, there is a marked increase in serum cortisol concentration. It continues to increase after surgery, peaking 6–12 h later, but remains elevated for up to 3 days afterwards. These changes are typical of those occurring after major surgery for all of the neuroendocrine hormones and mediators listed in Table 27.2.

CONSEQUENCES OF THE NEUROENDOCRINE ELEMENT OF THE STRESS RESPONSE

Protein catabolism

Major surgery results in a net excretion of nitrogen-containing compounds, referred to as negative nitrogen balance, reflecting catabolism of protein into amino acids for gluconeogenesis. This is partly because of perioperative starvation, but mainly because of the stress response, which causes decreased total protein synthesis, in addition to protein breakdown. Peripheral skeletal muscle is predominantly affected, but visceral protein may also be catabolized. Catecholamines, cortisol, glucagon and interleukins (IL-1 and IL-6) are all involved in proteolysis and gluconeogenesis. Protein catabolism contributes to weight loss, impaired wound healing and may delay overall postoperative recovery. Up to 0.5 kg day^{-1} of lean muscle mass may be lost postoperatively because of this aspect of the stress response.

Carbohydrate mobilization

Hyperglycaemia and insulin intolerance are major features of the stress response and may persist for several days postoperatively. They result from increased blood concentrations of catecholamines, cortisol and glucagon and also from sympathetic nervous system stimulation (by further increasing catecholamine release from the adrenal medulla). These hormones also inhibit insulin and therefore glucose uptake into muscle, fat and liver. Moreover, there is decreased sensitivity of muscle and liver to circulating insulin during the stress response. Blood glucose concentrations may increase by about 10 mmol L^{-1}, leading to glycosuria and osmotic diuresis.

Fat metabolism

The net effect of the hormonal alterations listed in Table 27.2 is lipolysis, stimulated by catecholamines acting at β_1-adrenoreceptors, with resultant increased concentrations of FFAs in the circulation. FFAs may be oxidized in the liver to form ketones (e.g. acetoacetate), which may be used as a source of energy by peripheral tissues.

Cardiovascular effects

The stress response to surgery and postoperative pain activates the sympathetic nervous system (SNS), which may increase myocardial oxygen demand by increasing heart rate and arterial pressure (see Fig. 27.8). Activation of the SNS may also cause coronary artery vasoconstriction, reducing the supply of oxygen to the myocardium, which in turn would predispose to myocardial ischaemia. This effect may be aggravated by the fact that there is a hypercoagulable state postoperatively and the stress response is an important factor in causing this. Antidiuretic hormone (ADH), increased during the stress response, is known to contribute to increased platelet adhesiveness.

Respiratory effects

Postoperative pulmonary dysfunction may also result from the stress response to major surgery. The most important alteration in respiratory function caused by the stress response is reduction in functional residual capacity (FRC). This is the amount of air remaining in the lungs at the end of a normal expiration. When FRC is reduced, it may become less than the closing capacity, which is the volume of air in the lungs required to prevent alveolar collapse. When FRC is less than closing capacity, airway closure occurs, with resultant ventilation–perfusion mismatch, shunting of blood and hypoxaemia.

Gastrointestinal effects

The stress response to surgery stimulates both afferent nociceptive input and efferent SNS output, resulting in ileus and excessive SNS stimulation relative to parasympathetic nervous system (PNS) stimulation. Postoperative ileus is a temporary impairment of gastrointestinal motility after major surgery. It delays resumption of an enteral diet, which in itself prolongs the stress response to surgery.

Table 27.2 Components of the stress response to surgery

Response	Consequence	Result
Neuroendocrine		
Hypothalamic–pituitary–adrenal	ACTH, GH, ADH (↑) β-endorphin, prolactin (↑)	Activation of adrenocortical hormones Mobilization of glucose reserves Water retention Protein catabolism and gluconeogenesis
Sympathetic nervous system stimulation	Catecholamines (↑)	↑ Heart rate and cardiac output ↑ SVR and arterial pressure
	Hypothalamic–pituitary–adrenal (↑)	Activation of adrenocortical hormones; mobilization of glucose reserves; water retention; protein catabolism and gluconeogenesis
	Renin–angiotensin–aldosterone (↑)	↑ SVR, retention Na^+ and H_2O, secretion K^+
	↑ Glucagon	↑ Glucose, lipolysis, insulin resistance
	↓ Insulin, testosterone	Hyperglycaemia, catabolic state
	↑ Acute-phase proteins (liver)	↓ Liver synthesis of albumin
Cytokine		
Cytokine and inflammatory mediator release	IL-1, IL-6, TNF (↑) Prostaglandins (↑)	↑ Platelet adhesion ↑ Coagulation ↑ Hypothalamic–pituitary–adrenal activity
	Neutrophils (↑) Lymphocytes (↓)	Local inflammation, pain
Pyrexia (due to ↑ IL-1)	↑ Metabolic rate	↑ Demand on cardiovascular system

ACTH, adrenocorticotrophic hormone; GH, growth hormone; ADH, antidiuretic hormone; SVR, systemic vascular resistance; TNF, tumour necrosis factor.

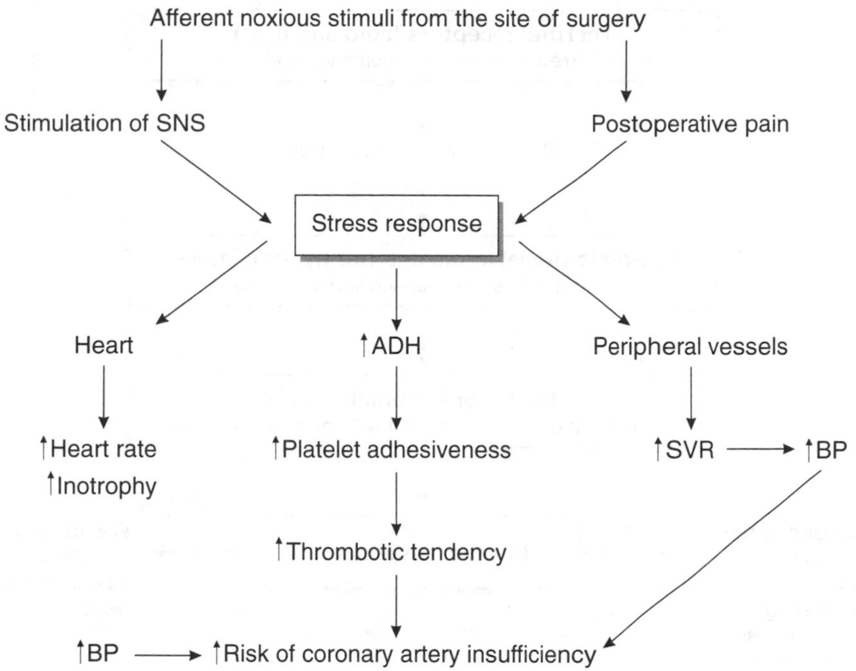

Fig. 27.8
Effect of the stress response to surgery on the cardiovascular system. SVR, systemic vascular resistance; SNS, sympathetic nervous system.

Immunological system effects

Many mediators of the stress response (cortisol, interleukins, prostaglandins etc.) are cellular and humoral immunosuppressants. It is not known if stress response-mediated immunosuppression, which occurs for several days after surgery, influences patient outcome.

TRIGGERING THE STRESS RESPONSE

Although there is detailed knowledge of the various components of the stress response, the relative importance of the various signals involved in eliciting it are unclear (Table 27.3).

Afferent neural stimuli

Afferent noxious stimuli (such as pain, pressure, burning, distension) are transmitted by Aδ and C nerve fibres. These pathways are discussed in detail in Chapter 17. They enter the spinal cord via the dorsal root and synapse in the dorsal horn.

Table 27.3 Triggers of the neuroendocrine and cytokine response in patients after surgery

Noxious afferent stimuli (especially pain)
Local inflammatory tissue factors, especially cytokines
Pain and anxiety
Starvation
Hypothermia and shivering
Haemorrhage
Acidosis
Hypoxaemia
Infection

Local factors and the immunological (cytokine) response

Afferent neural stimuli are not the sole means of eliciting the stress response to surgery. Severe injury in a denervated limb also elicits the response, suggesting a non-neural stimulus. Cytokines and mediators of inflammation are released in response to local tissue destruction or trauma, increasing peripheral nociceptive activity. The magnitude of this response is proportional to the extent of tissue damage.

EFFECT OF GENERAL ANAESTHESIA ON THE STRESS RESPONSE

Intravenous and inhalation anaesthetic agents have no appreciable effect on either the neuroendocrine or the cytokine elements of the stress response, irrespective of dose. However, high-dose opioid analgesia (e.g. morphine 4 mg kg^{-1} or fentanyl 50–100 μg kg^{-1}) may completely inhibit the neuroendocrine element. If the opioid is given *after* the surgical incision, it does not prevent the emergence of the stress response. These high doses of opioids are impractical for most operations.

EFFECT OF REGIONAL (EPIDURAL) ANAESTHESIA ON THE STRESS RESPONSE

Neuroendocrine element

While only very high-dose, opioid-based general anaesthesia completely inhibits the stress response to upper abdominal surgery,

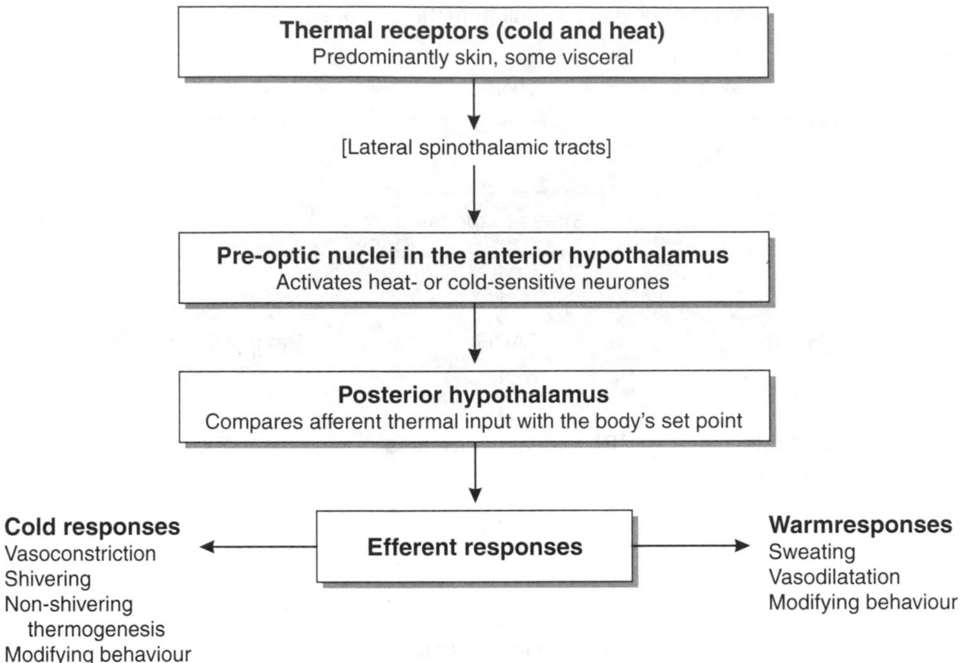

Fig. 27.9
Control of thermoregulation.

epidural anaesthesia, commenced before the surgical incision and continued postoperatively, can significantly reduce it. Epidural anaesthesia and analgesia for lower limb or pelvic surgery completely suppresses the response. Administration of local anaesthetic drugs into the epidural space is more effective than administration of opioids alone.

Cytokine element

The systemic release of cytokines in response to local tissue damage is not influenced by any anaesthetic technique, including epidural anaesthesia and analgesia. However, the cytokine element of the stress response is reduced by limiting the extent of the surgical incision, in particular, by use of laparoscopic techniques.

THERMOREGULATION AND ANAESTHESIA

Core body temperature is normally maintained within the narrow range of 36.7–37.1°C, even in the presence of widely varying environmental temperatures (i.e. –10 to 50°C).

HEAT BALANCE

Heat is lost from the body by four processes: convection, radiation, conduction and evaporation. Heat loss by radiation is related to the temperature difference between the patient and the ambient environment. Convective heat loss occurs when the layer of air next to the skin moves or is disturbed, thereby removing its insulative properties. Classic physiological teaching is that the proportion of the total heat loss caused by each mechanism is: radiation, 40%; convection, 30%; conduction, 5%; and evaporation, 25% – but these proportions may change markedly for patients anaesthetized in the theatre environment.

PHYSIOLOGY

Thermoregulation is achieved by a physiological control system consisting of peripheral and central thermoreceptors, an integrating control centre and efferent response systems (Fig. 27.9). Afferent thermal input comes from anatomically distinct cold and heat receptors, located predominantly in the skin, but also centrally. The central control mechanism, situated in the hypothalamus, determines mean body temperature by integrating thermal signals from peripheral and core structures and comparing mean body temperature with a predetermined 'set point' temperature. In humans, the efferent responses to effect change in body heat content may be classified as behavioural and autonomic.

Autonomic mechanisms involve control of cutaneous vascular smooth muscle tone, shivering and non-shivering thermogenesis and sweating.

Afferent thermal signals

The afferent thermal input may be central or peripheral. Thermally sensitive receptors located in the skin and mucous membranes mediate thermal sensation and contribute to thermoregulatory

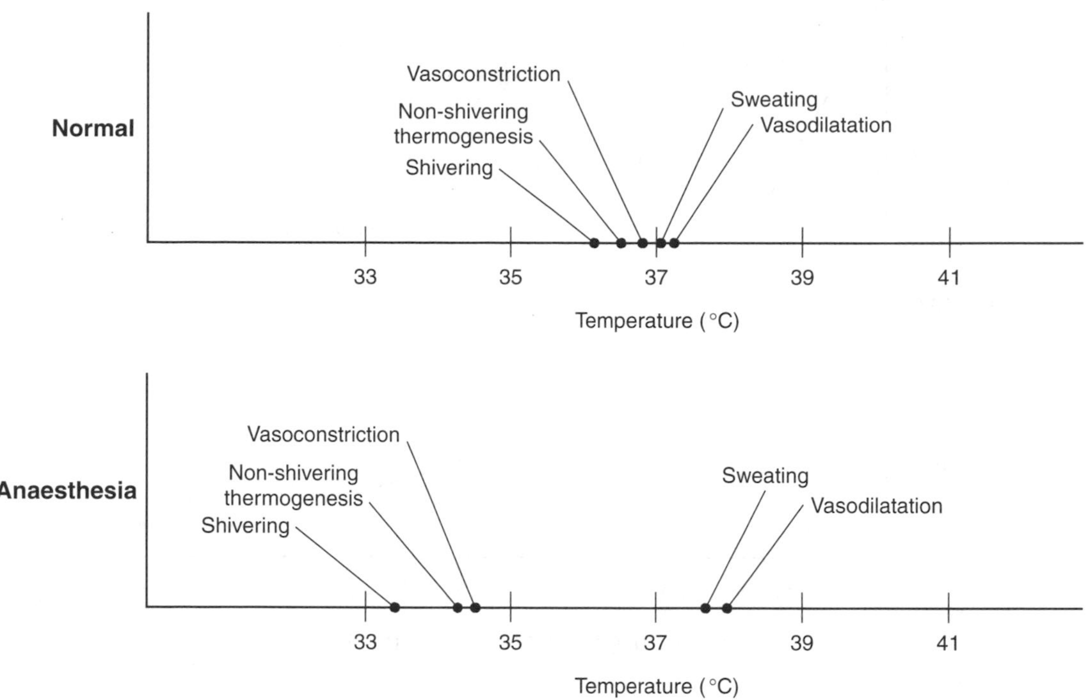

Fig. 27.10
Threshold temperatures for the thermoregulatory responses under normal conditions and under general anaesthesia. (Reproduced with permission from Sessler 1994).

reflexes. Cold-specific receptors are innervated by Aδ fibres. Heat receptors are innervated by C fibres. Cold receptors in the skin outnumber heat receptors 10-fold and are the major mechanism by which the body protects itself against cold temperatures. Afferent input from these cold receptors in the skin is transmitted to the posterior hypothalamus. In addition to the peripheral cold receptors, there is central cold reception in the hypothalamus, although its effects are masked by the predominant peripheral influence.

Central integration: the hypothalamus

The afferent mechanisms provide feedback to temperature-regulating centres in the hypothalamus (Fig. 27.9). The pre-optic area of the hypothalamus contains temperature-sensitive and temperature-insensitive neurones. The temperature-sensitive neurones, which predominate by 4:1, increase their discharge rate in response to increased local heat and this activates heat loss mechanisms. Conversely, cold-sensitive neurones increase their rate of discharge in response to cooling. Neurones sensitive to local thermal stimuli also exist in the posterior hypothalamus, reticular formation, medulla and spinal cord. Detection of cold differs from detection of heat, in that the principal mechanism of detection of cold is input from cutaneous cold receptors.

The posterior hypothalamus integrates cold afferent signals from the periphery with heat-sensitive stimulation from the pre-optic area of the hypothalamus and instigates the effector responses. The set point or physiological 'thermostat' of the thermoregulatory system is the temperature at which the system requires zero action to maintain that temperature (36.7–37.1°C). The limits of this range represent the thresholds at which cold or heat responses are instigated, and hence it has been termed the 'interthreshold range.' Normally it is no more than 0.4°C, but is increased to 4.0°C during general anaesthesia (Fig. 27.10).

Effector responses

The thermoregulatory responses are characterized by altered behaviour (quantitatively the most effective mechanism), a vasomotor response (consisting of vasoconstriction and piloerection or vasodilatation and sweating) and shivering with increased basal metabolic rate. In the conscious individual, behaviour modification is more powerful than the autonomic mechanisms. When the hypothalamic thermostat indicates an excessively cool body temperature, impulses pass from the hypothalamus to the cerebral cortex to give the individual the sensation of feeling cold. The result is modified behaviour, such as increased motor activity, moving to warmer surroundings or adding additional clothing. The control of behavioural responses to cold is based largely on cutaneous thermal signals. When the set point temperature range has been breached, autonomic effector responses are activated.

Shivering and non-shivering thermogenesis

Adjacent to the centre in the posterior hypothalamus on which the impulses from cold receptors impinge, there is a motor centre for shivering. It is normally inhibited by impulses from the heat-sensitive area in the anterior hypothalamus, but when cold

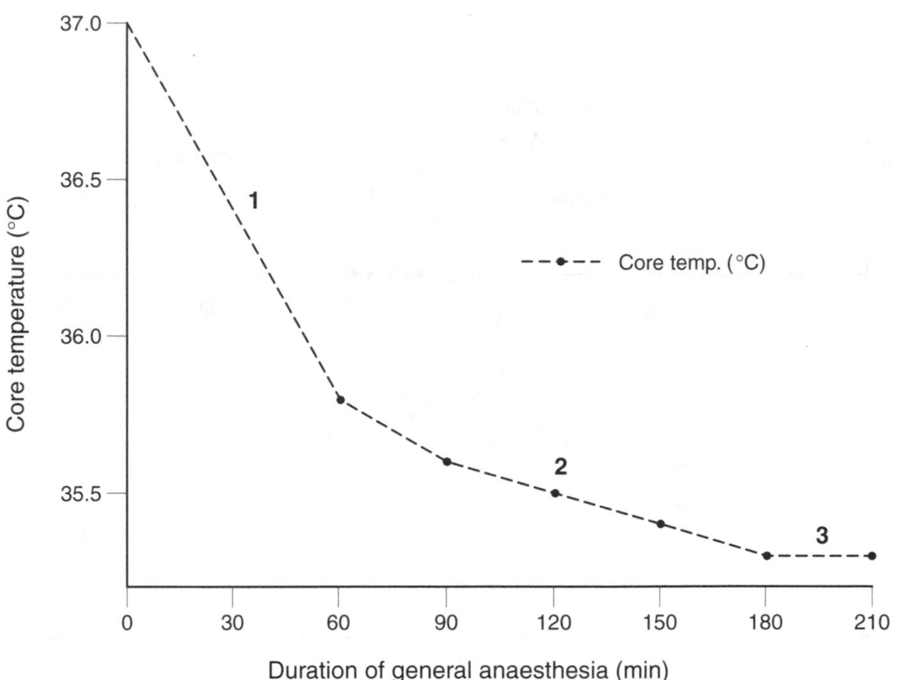

Fig. 27.11
Pattern of perioperative hypothermia. *Phase 1* – induction of general anaesthesia results in a core temperature reduction of approximately 1°C in the first hour, as a result of core-to-peripheral heat redistribution. *Phase 2* – following initial redistribution hypothermia, core temperature continues to decrease in a slower, linear fashion for approximately 2 h, as a result of cutaneous heat loss exceeding metabolic heat production. *Phase 3* – plateau: core temperature remains constant for the duration of surgery, where heat loss equals metabolic heat production.

impulses exceed a certain rate, the motor centre for shivering becomes activated by 'spillover' of signals and it sends impulses bilaterally into the spinal cord. Initially, this increases the tone of skeletal muscles throughout the body, but when this muscle tone increases above a specific level, shivering is observed.

Two patterns of muscular activity, seen in electromyography studies, contribute to the phenomenon of post-anaesthetic shivering; first, a tonic pattern (4–8 cycles min^{-1} characteristic of the response to hypothermia in awake patients) is observed, and then a phasic (6–7 Hz) pattern resembling clonus.

The elicitation of *non-shivering thermogenesis* is an important mechanism in increasing heat production, particularly in neonates. Non-shivering thermogenesis occurs mainly in brown adipose tissue (BAT). This subtype of adipose tissue contains large numbers of mitochondria in its cells and these are supplied by an extensive SNS innervation. When sympathetic stimulation occurs, oxidative metabolism of the mitochondria is stimulated. However, it is *uncoupled* to phosphorylation, so that heat is produced instead of generating ATP. In adults, the amount of BAT is small, and non-shivering thermogenesis increases the rate of heat production by less than 10–15%. In infants, it may double heat production.

MEASUREMENT OF TEMPERATURE

Core temperature may be evaluated reliably by an infrared thermometer at the tympanic membrane and by thermistors positioned in the distal oesophagus, nasopharynx or pulmonary artery. Skin surface temperature varies with ambient temperature and induction of anaesthesia and is usually also measured with a thermistor, or alternatively with a liquid crystal thermometer. Measurement of temperature at the skin surface has also been used to estimate the core temperature, by heating the sensor to eliminate the core–surface temperature gradient.

EFFECT OF GENERAL ANAESTHESIA ON THERMOREGULATION

General anaesthesia causes thermoregulatory impairment characterized by an increase in heat-response thresholds and a decrease in cold-response thresholds, such that the normal interthreshold range (between which no effector response occurs) is increased from approximately 0.4 to 4.0°C. Both heat-response and cold-response thresholds are affected (Fig. 27.10). All general anaesthetic agents impair thermoregulatory responses to a similar, but not identical, extent. All the currently used volatile anaesthetic agents decrease the vasoconstriction and shivering thresholds. Mild hypothermia during general anaesthesia follows a distinctive pattern and occurs in three phases: first, an initial rapid decrease in core temperature of approximately 1°C over the first hour; second, a slower linear decrease to 34–35°C; and third, a core temperature plateau (or thermal equilibrium) is then reached, where heat loss to the periphery equals heat gained from core metabolic heat production (Fig. 27.11).

The initial rapid reduction in core temperature is greater than that which would be explained by a lowering of metabolic rate and heat loss, and is in fact attributable to *core-to-peripheral redistribution* of body heat. Mean body temperature and body heat content remain constant during this first hour. The subsequent core temperature plateau largely results from thermoregulatory vasoconstriction, triggered by a core temperature of 33–35°C.

EFFECT OF REGIONAL ANAESTHESIA ON THERMOREGULATION

Both epidural and spinal anaesthesia decrease, to a similar extent, vasoconstriction and shivering thresholds, but not as much as general anaesthesia. Because local anaesthetics administered into the subarachnoid or epidural space do not obviously interact with the hypothalamic control centres, the mechanism of this thermal disturbance during regional anaesthesia is uncertain, However, it is consistent with thermoregulatory impairment caused by the effects of the regional block on *afferent* thermal information.

In contrast with general anaesthesia, where the heat produced by shivering is unchanged, heat produced by epidural anaesthesia is reduced by approximately 60%. This occurs because shivering above the upper limit of block does not compensate for the inability of muscles below the block to engage in shivering. As with general anaesthesia, core hypothermia (by 0.6–1.5°C) occurs during the first hour or so after epidural anaesthesia because of core-to-peripheral redistribution of body heat from the epidural-induced vasodilatation. However, with prolonged epidural anaesthesia, the degree of core hypothermia is less than after general anaesthesia, because of vasoconstriction above the level of the block. Shivering during regional anaesthesia, in common with that after general anaesthesia, is usually preceded by core hypothermia and vasoconstriction above the level of the block.

After the core-to-peripheral redistribution of body heat, the degree of subsequent hypothermia depends on the balance of cutaneous heat loss and rate of metabolic heat production. During epidural anaesthesia, heat loss may be accelerated by reduced vasoconstriction caused by the block. Hence, heat loss continues unabated during epidural anaesthesia despite the activation of the effector mechanisms above the level of the block. This is seen especially where general and epidural anaesthesia are combined.

CONSEQUENCES OF PERIOPERATIVE MILD HYPOTHERMIA (Table 27.4)

In particular circumstances, hypothermia may have a protective effect in terms of reducing basal metabolic rate. The use of moderate hypothermia is routine practice in many centres during cardiopulmonary bypass. It is generally agreed, however, that the deleterious consequences of mild hypothermia outweigh the potential benefits, with evidence emerging that hypothermia *per se* is responsible for adverse postoperative outcomes. In particular, hypothermic patients are more likely to have postoperative wound infections than normothermic patients. The initial 3–4 h after bacterial contamination are thought to be crucial in determining if clinical infection ensues. In vitro studies suggest that platelet function and coagulation are impaired by hypothermia, and mildly hypothermic patients lose > 25% more blood in the perioperative period than do normothermic patients. In addition, perioperative thermal discomfort is often remembered by patients as the worst aspect of their perioperative experience.

Table 27.4 Consequences of perioperative hypothermia
Increased wound infection
Increased surgical bleeding
Increased incidence of myocardial infarction and malignant arrhythmias
Delayed recovery from anaesthesia
Excessive SNS stimulation on waking
Prolonged drug metabolism
Negative nitrogen balance
Impaired immune function
Patient discomfort

POST-ANAESTHETIC SHIVERING

Post-anaesthetic shivering affects 5–65% of patients after general anaesthesia and 33% during epidural regional anaesthesia. It is usually defined as readily detectable fasciculation or tremor of the face, jaw, head, trunk or extremities lasting longer than 15 s. Apart from the obvious discomfort, post-anaesthetic shivering, in common with hypothermia, is associated with a number of potentially deleterious sequelae (Table 27.5). Post-anaesthetic shivering is usually preceded by core hypothermia and vasoconstriction.

While hypothermia is one factor in the aetiology of post-anaesthetic shivering, not all patients who shiver are hypothermic. Studies on postoperative patients have indicated that male gender, age (16–60 years) and anticholinergic premedication are risk factors for post-anaesthetic shivering, while the intraoperative use of pethidine virtually abolished it. The use of propofol reduces the incidence of postoperative shivering compared with thiopental.

PHYSICAL, ACTIVE AND PASSIVE STRATEGIES FOR AVOIDING PERIOPERATIVE HYPOTHERMIA

Preventing redistribution-induced hypothermia may be achieved by physical and pharmacological means (Table 27.6). Redistribution of heat results when anaesthetic-induced vasodilatation allows heat to flow from the core to the periphery down its concentration gradient. Pre-emptive skin surface warming does not increase core temperature but increases body heat content, particularly in the legs, and removes the gradient for heat loss via the skin. This approach is rarely used in clinical practice, however, because it requires 1 h of prewarming.

Passive insulation, including cotton drapes, has been used perioperatively to reduce heat loss to the environment. Because only 10% of metabolic heat production is lost in heating and humidifying inspired gases, this method is relatively ineffective at maintaining normothermia. Heat and moisture exchange filters retain significant amounts of moisture and heat within the respiratory system, but are

Table 27.5 Consequences of post-anaesthetic shivering
Increased O_2 consumption and CO_2 production
Catecholamine release and SNS stimulation
Increased cardiac output, heart rate, BP
Increased intraocular pressure
Decreased $S_{\bar{v}}O_2$
Lactic acidosis
Interference with monitoring
Patient discomfort

Table 27.6 Strategies for prevention and treatment of perioperative hypothermia and post-anaesthetic shivering

Prevention
Intraoperative use of forced air warming device
Reflective 'space' blankets
Heating and humidifying inspired gases
Increasing ambient temperature
Warmed i.v. fluids
Treatment
Pethidine 0.33 mg kg^{-1} i.v. or epidural (and other opioids to a lesser extent)
Doxapram 1.5 mg kg^{-1}
Clonidine 2 μg kg^{-1}
Methylphenidate 0.1 mg kg^{-1}
Physostigmine 0.04 mg kg^{-1}
Ondansetron 0.1 mg kg^{-1}

only 50% as effective as active mechanisms. Ambient temperature determines the rate of heat loss by radiation and convection and maintains normothermia if close to initial, pre-induction, core temperature (36°C). However, this is usually impractical, as operating room staff usually find this temperature uncomfortable. Water mattresses are demonstrably ineffective at preventing heat loss, possibly because relatively little heat is lost from the back. Moreover, decreased local tissue perfusion associated with local temperatures of 40°C may lead to skin necrosis. Conductive losses may be reduced if intravenous fluids are warmed before or during administration.

Forced air warming systems are undoubtedly the best way to maintain normothermia during long procedures and are particularly effective when used intraoperatively for vasodilated patients, allowing heat applied peripherally to be rapidly transferred to the core. Their use increases core temperature and reduces the incidence of post-anaesthetic shivering.

TREATMENT OF POSTOPERATIVE SHIVERING

Postoperative shivering should not be treated in isolation from perioperative hypothermia. Not all patients who shiver are hypothermic, but most are and successful treatment of shivering in these patients without concomitant management of hypothermia may result in deepening hypothermia. However, the mainstay of symptomatic treatment of postoperative shivering is pharmacological (Table 27.6)

A wide range of drugs is effective and it would be surprising if all worked on a single part of the thermoregulatory mechanism. Pethidine is remarkably effective in treating postoperative shivering, 25 mg being sufficient in the majority of adults. There is evidence suggesting this may be the result of an action at the κ opioid receptor.

One hypothesis for the mechanism of post-anaesthetic shivering is that, because the brain recovers later than the spinal cord, uninhibited spinal clonic tremor occurs, resulting in shivering. Consistent with this hypothesis, doxapram (a cerebral stimulant) has also been shown to be an effective treatment. It is not as effective as pethidine. Various drugs, the mechanism of action of which are unclear, are also effective. Physostigmine prevents the onset of post-anaesthetic shivering, implying that cholinergic pathways are involved in the thermoregulatory mechanisms that lead to shivering. Clonidine, an α_2-adrenergic agonist and ondansetron, a serotonergic antagonist are also effective.

FURTHER READING

Buggy D J, Crossley A W A 2000 Thermoregulation, perioperative hypothermia and post-anaesthetic shivering. British Journal of Anaesthesia 84: 615–628

Buggy D J, Smith G 1999 Epidural anaesthesia and analgesia – better outcome after major surgery? British Medical Journal 316: 530–531

Frank S M et al 1997 Perioperative maintenance of normothermia reduces the incidence of morbid cardiac events. JAMA 277: 1127–1134

Guyton A C, Hall J E 1996 Metabolism and temperature regulation. In: Guyton A C, Hall J E (eds) Textbook of medical physiology, 9th edn. W B Saunders, Philadelphia

Kehlet H 1998 Modification of responses to surgery by neural blockade. In: Cousins M J, Bridenbaugh P J (eds) Neural blockade in clinical anesthesia and management of pain, 3rd edn. Lippincott-Raven, Philadelphia, p 128–175

Kurz A, Sessler D I, Lenhardt R 1996 Perioperative normothermia to reduce the incidence of surgical wound infection and shorten hospitalisation. New England Journal of Medicine 334: 1209–1215

Schmied H, Kurz A, Sessler D I, Kosek S, Reiter A 1996 Mild hypothermia increases blood loss and transfusion requirements during total hip arthroplasty. Lancet 347: 289–292

Sessler D I 2000 Temperature monitoring. In: Miller R D (ed) Anesthesia, 5th edn. Churchill Livingstone, Philadelphia, p 1367–1389

28 Endocrine function

In unicellular organisms such as bacteria, fungi and protozoa, the entire cell may respond quickly to any stimulus within its environment. Any substances released within the cell need only travel minute distances to act. However, in complicated multicellular organisms, such as humans, comprising specialized organs and cell types, there needs to be some means to coordinate responses to the environment.

In mammals, this integration of responses is achieved by the nervous and endocrine systems, which transmit signals to distant sites in the body. These systems work in tandem with each other. The endocrine system is specialized to coordinate slow chronic transmission of signals via the circulatory system. This allows all areas of the body to be reached. The messengers for this system are the hormones. A hormone is a substance which is secreted into the bloodstream and exerts its effects on a target tissue distant to the site of release.

The effects of a hormone are brought about by its interaction with a specific receptor on the target tissue. These receptors may be on the surface of the cell membrane linked to G-proteins or tyrosine kinase, producing release of intracellular second messengers or phosphorylation of enzyme systems that may be activated or inhibited. Alternatively, the hormone may interact with a receptor in the cell nucleus to influence gene expression and ultimately protein transcription. Polypeptide hormones interact with cell surface receptors, whereas steroid and thyroid hormones interact with intranuclear receptors.

HORMONAL CONTROL

Control of the endocrine system relies on the process of feedback. This is the process by which the response of a cell to a signal influences the further output of the signal. In positive feedback, which occurs rarely in biological systems, the signal results in a response that causes an increase in the size of the signal. In negative feedback, the stimulus causes a response that reduces the magnitude of the stimulus. Hormonal regulation is subject mainly to negative feedback systems.

For the purposes of this chapter, the following endocrine systems are considered: hypothalamic–pituitary function, adrenal cortex and medulla, parathyroid and calcium homeostasis, thyroid and pancreas. The endocrine function of the gonads and the physiology of reproduction are not discussed, as these do not form part of the primary FRCA syllabus.

HYPOTHALAMIC AND PITUITARY FUNCTION

ANATOMY

The hypothalamus is at the anterior end of the diencephalon which lies below the hypothalamic sulcus and in front of the

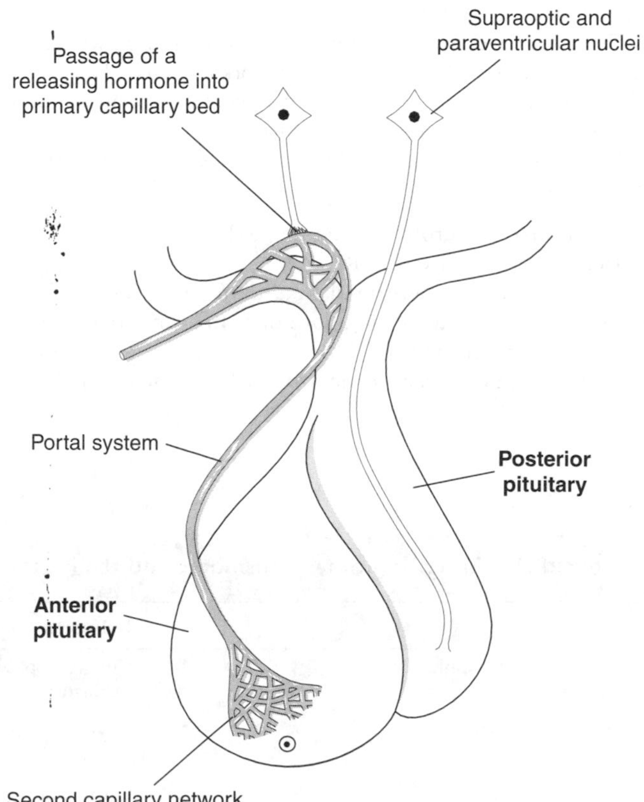

Fig. 28.1
Anatomy of pituitary showing the hypophyseal portal system.

interpenduncular nuclei. The pituitary is connected to the underside of the hypothalamus by the pituitary stalk and there are neural connections between the hypothalamus and the posterior lobe of the pituitary.

The pituitary consists of an anterior and a posterior lobe, together with a median eminence (which has little function in humans) and sits in the pituitary fossa.

Embryologically, the posterior lobe is derived from an invagination of the floor of the third ventricle, and the anterior lobe from an invagination of the roof of the pharynx termed Rathke's pouch. This explains the two distinct lobes of the pituitary (Fig. 28.1).

Sympathetic nerve fibres connect to the anterior lobe via its capsule, and parasympathetic fibres via the petrosal nerves. The portal hypophyseal vessels form a vascular link between the hypothalamus and the anterior lobe. This system (a true portal system) begins with a primary capillary plexus within the hypothalamus and drains to another capillary plexus within the anterior lobe of the pituitary, without passing through the heart. This is the route by which the hypothalamic releasing and inhibiting factors reach the anterior pituitary. The portal system lies outside the blood–brain barrier.

HISTOLOGY

The posterior lobe contains nerve terminals and axons that arise from the supraoptic and paraventricular nuclei in the hypothalamus. The nerve endings are seen in close approximation with blood vessels. These nerve endings contain oxytocin and antidiuretic hormone (ADH).

The anterior lobe is made up of many cell types in which cords of cells interlace with an extensive network of sinusoidal capillaries with fenestrated endothelium. The cells contain granules of stored hormone that are excreted by exocytosis.

The cells are divided by their immunocytochemical staining into five types:

- somatotropes – growth hormone (GH)
- lactotropes – prolactin (PRL)
- thyrotropes – thyroid-stimulating hormone (TSH)
- gonadotropes – luteinizing hormone (LH) and follicle-stimulating hormone (FSH)
- corticotropes – adrenocorticotrophic hormone (ACTH).

POSTERIOR PITUITARY FUNCTION

The hormones of the posterior pituitary are synthesized in the neuronal cell bodies of the supraoptic and paraventricular nuclei of the hypothalamus and consist of the nonapeptides, oxytocin and ADH (vasopressin). The synthesized hormones travel down the axons of the nerve cells in granules to their endings which lie in close approximation to blood vessels. The hormones are then secreted by exocytosis in response to an action potential travelling down the nerve cell. Oxytocin is not discussed further in this chapter.

Effects of ADH

Antidiuretic hormone increases the permeability of the collecting ducts in the kidney to water. This allows water to enter the hyperosmolar interstitium of the renal medulla. Consequently, the urine is concentrated and water is conserved. In large doses, ADH causes an increase in systemic arterial pressure (and is therefore also termed vasopressin).

Three subtypes of ADH receptors have been found, all linked to G-proteins. Binding to the V_{1A} or V_{1B} subtypes leads to activation of phospholipase C to form inositol triphosphate, which in turn increases intracellular calcium. Binding to the V_2 subtype (found in nephrons) leads to an increase in cAMP via a stimulatory G-protein (G_s). ADH is metabolized rapidly by the kidney and liver with a half-life of approximately 18 min.

Control of ADH secretion

The main stimuli to ADH release are changes in plasma osmotic pressure and extracellular fluid volume. The rate of neuronal firing from cells within the supraoptic and paraventricular nuclei increases when the plasma osmolality exceeds 285 mosmol kg^{-1}, and ADH is released into the blood stream. The osmoreceptors are outside the blood–brain barrier. Low-pressure receptors in the large veins, the atria and pulmonary vessels sense a reduction in the extracellular fluid volume and cause an increase in the secretion of ADH. This occurs before any hypotension caused by hypovolaemia, which in itself is a potent stimulus to the release of ADH.

Table 28.1 Anterior pituitary hormones and their releasing/inhibiting hormones

Hormone	Releasing hormone	Release-inhibiting hormone
Adrenocorticotrophic hormone	Corticotrophin releasing hormone	–
Thyroid-stimulating hormone	Thyrotrophin releasing hormone	–
Growth hormone	Growth hormone releasing hormone	Growth hormone inhibiting hormone (somatostatin)
Luteinizing hormone/ follicle-stimulating hormone	Gonadotrophin releasing hormone	–
Prolactin	–	Dopamine

ANTERIOR PITUITARY HORMONES

The anterior pituitary secretes six hormones (mentioned above) under the control of hypothalamic releasing and inhibiting hormones which are secreted into the hypophyseal portal system. ACTH, TSH, GH, LH and FSH have releasing hormones, and GH and PRL have release-inhibiting hormones (Table 28.1).

All the pituitary hormones are proteins. TSH, LH and FSH are glycoproteins with two subunits α and β, the α subunit being common to all three. ACTH, PRL and GH are simple polypeptides. With the exception of GH, all the hormones act on other endocrine glands to influence their secretion. They are discussed later in the relevant sections.

Growth hormone

This is a single-chain polypeptide of molecular weight 22 kDa and half-life 6 min which is metabolized rapidly by the liver. Approximately 50% of GH in the blood is bound to plasma proteins, forming a reservoir of hormone.

Growth hormone receptors are found on the cell membrane and are part of the cytokine receptor superfamily. These receptors have a large extracellular portion which contains two GH binding sites. GH binds to two receptors, causing them to form a dimer, and this results in the secretion of somatomedin (insulin-like growth factor I, IGF-I).

Control of GH secretion

Growth hormone is under the control of the hypothalamus, which secretes GH releasing hormone (GHRH) and GH inhibiting hormone (GHIH). GHRH secretion is episodic, whereas GHIH secretion is more tonic. Both are secreted into the hypothalamic–pituitary portal system. GH is under negative feedback control, in common with all the other pituitary hormones. There are three main stimuli for GH release: threatened or actual substrate deficiency (fasting or hypoglycaemia), raised circulating amino acids and stressful stimuli (pyrogens).

Effects of GH

Growth. If the epiphyses have not fused, there is an increase in the rate of chondrogenesis and a widening of the growth plate. After epiphyseal fusion, linear growth is no longer possible and, if GH is secreted in excess, the clinical features of acromegaly develop (this takes many years). GH increases body protein content and reduces fat content. GH is also synergistic with ACTH and causes an increase in adrenal cortical mass.

Protein and electrolyte metabolism. GH is an anabolic hormone and causes a positive nitrogen and phosphate balance. This results in an increased synthesis of soluble collagen, an elevated plasma phosphate and reduced urea, amino acids and cholesterol. GH also increases the rate of calcium absorption from the gut and increases 4-hydroxyprolene excretion in the urine.

Urinary Na^+ and K^+ excretion is reduced by a mechanism that is independent of the adrenals.

Carbohydrate metabolism. GH is diabetogenic and ketogenic. It increases hepatic glucose production, has an anti-insulin effect on muscle and increases the level of circulating free fatty acids (FFAs).

GH does not stimulate the B cells of the pancreas directly, but increases the ability of the pancreas to respond to an insulinogenic stimulus.

Somatomedins

All of the effects of GH are mediated by the interaction between GH and somatomedins such as IGF-I. Somatomedins are released by the liver and other tissues in response to GH. IGF-I inhibits the release of GHRH and GH in a negative feedback fashion

ADRENAL CORTEX AND MEDULLA

ANATOMY

The adrenal glands are situated at the superior poles of each kidney and may be thought of as two separate glands: an outer cortex and the inner medulla. Medullary tissue may also be found at extra-adrenal sites along the course of the abdominal aorta.

The cortex and medulla have different embryological origins, the cortex from mesoderm and the medulla from the neural crest.

In keeping with all the other endocrine glands, the adrenals are richly vascularized. The adrenal gland derives its blood supply from three blood vessels: a direct branch from the aorta, one from a branch of the phrenic artery and one from the renal artery. These arteries form a plexus on the capsule of the gland and blood flows through sinusoids to the medulla. Blood is drained through a single adrenal vein that leaves at the hilum of the gland to join the inferior vena cava. Preganglionic sympathetic nerve fibres that release acetylcholine richly innervate the adrenal medulla.

The medulla comprises 30% of the gland. It consists of interlacing cords of densely innervated cells which contain granules. There are numerous venous sinuses separating the cells. Two cell types are found: larger cells with fewer granules that secrete epinephrine, and smaller cells with numerous dense vesicles that secrete norepinephrine. Ninety per cent of the cells are of the epinephrine-secreting type.

The cortex consists of three distinct zones. The outer zona glomerulosa, which is made up of whorls of cells, merges into the zona fasciculata formed of columns of cells with prominent venous sinuses. This layer merges into the inner zona reticularis made up of a network of cells (Fig. 28.2). These cells are abundant in lipid, which reflects the fact that they synthesize and secrete lipid hormones. All the cells secrete corticosterone, but the enzymes responsible for aldosterone synthesis are found only in the zona glomerulosa. The enzymes for cortisol and sex hormone synthesis are found in the zona fasciculata and zona reticularis. The zona glomerulosa also forms the new cortical cells, which allows regeneration. The adrenal medulla cannot regenerate.

ADRENAL CORTEX

All the hormones from this part of the gland are based on the cyclopentanoperhydrophenanthrene nucleus (Fig. 28.3). Gonadal and adrenocortical steroids (mineralocorticoids and glucocorticoids) are of three types, classified according to the number of carbon atoms in the molecule. C21 steroids comprise progesterone and the corticoids, C19 steroids are the androgens, and C18 steroids are the oestrogens (see Table 28.2).

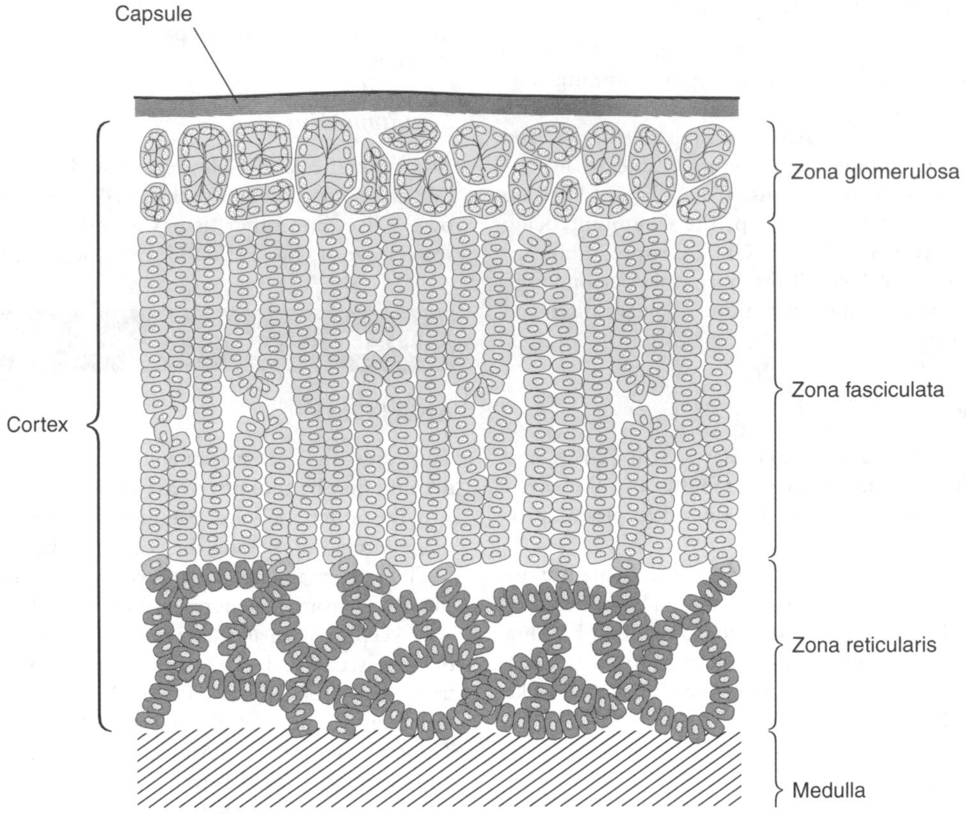

Fig. 28.2
Adrenocortical histology.

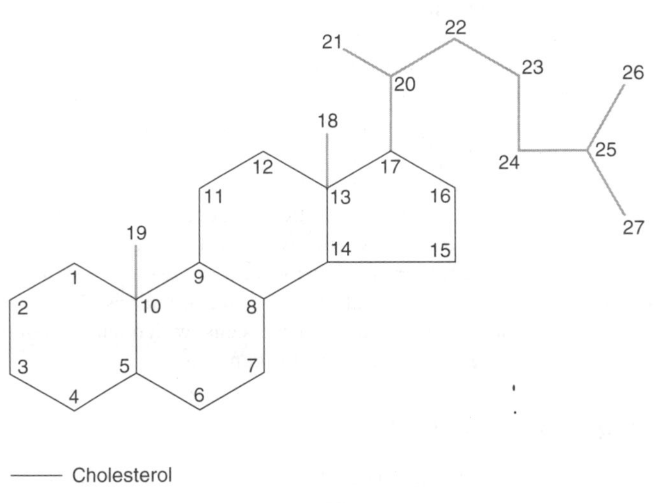

Fig. 28.3
The cyclopentanoperhydrophenanthrene nucleus. It is the basic structure of all steroid hormones.

All the steroids are secreted as the free steroid, except for dehydroepiandosterone (DHEA) which is conjugated to sulphate. Cortisol and corticosterone are the main glucocorticoids secreted, with a ratio of 7:1. The principal mineralocorticoid secreted is aldosterone and although deoxycorticosterone is secreted in appreciable quantities, it has only 3% of the activity of aldosterone.

Synthetic steroids

By modifying the side chains, it is possible to alter the steroid receptor affinity, modify its half-life or alter its mineralocorticoid or glucocorticoid effects (Table 28.3).

Table 28.2 Adrenocortical hormones

Steroid group	Steroid
Glucocorticoids	Cortisol Corticosterone
Mineralocorticoids	Aldosterone Deoxycorticosterone
Androgens	Dehydroepiandosterone (DHEA) Androstenedione
Oestrogens	Oestradiol

Table 28.3 Glucocorticoid and mineralocorticoid activity (relative to cortisol) of some naturally occurring and synthetic steroids

Steroid	Glucocorticoid activity	Mineralocorticoid activity
Cortisol	1	1
Corticosterone	0.3	15
Aldosterone	0.3	3000
Deoxycorticosterone	0.2	100
Cortisone	0.7	1
Prednisolone	4	0.8
Fludrocortisone	10	125
Dexamethasone	25	0

Hormone synthesis

Cholesterol is the precursor for all steroid hormones. Some cholesterol is made within the adrenal gland from acetate, but the majority comes from the circulating low-density lipoproteins (LDLs). LDL receptors are abundant on adrenocortical cells. Cholesterol is esterified upon entry into the cell and stored in lipid droplets (this gives the adrenal cortex a yellowish appearance when cut). It is then transported to the mitochondria by a sterol carrier protein and converted to pregnanelone by cholesterol desmolase (part of the P450 cytochrome family) (Fig. 28.4). Pregnanelone then moves to the smooth endoplasmic reticulum (SER) where it is dehydrogenated to form progesterone by 3β-hydroxysteroid dehydrogenase (not P450). In the zona fasciculata and zona reticularis, some of the pregnanelone and progesterone is hydroxylated in the SER by 17α-hydroxylase (P450) to form 17-hydroxypregnanelone and 17-hydroxyprogesterone. 21β-Hydroxylase (SER) then converts these to 11-deoxycorticosterone and 11-deoxycortisol. Cortisol and corticosterone are subsequently formed by the action of 11β-hydroxylase (P450).

In the zona fasciculata and reticularis, corticosterone and cortisol diffuse out into the circulation, but in the zona glomerulosa, corticosterone is converted into 18-hydroxycorticosterone and then aldosterone by the action of aldosterone synthetase. Its activity is stimulated by angiotensin II. The zona glomerulosa also lacks the enzyme 17α-hydroxylase and cannot make 17-hydroxysteroids such as DHEA or sex steroids.

Hormone transport

Cortisol is bound to transcortin and cortisol-binding globulin (CBG), with minimal amounts bound to albumin. Corticosterone is less avidly bound. In the bound phase, the steroids are physiologically inactive, and only the free unbound form can exert its effect. The bound portion functions as a reservoir (similar to T_4). Aldosterone has minimal protein binding.

Metabolism

Cortisol is metabolized in the liver and conjugated with glucuronide to render it water-soluble so it can be excreted in the urine. Aldosterone is also metabolized by the liver and conjugated with glucuronide.

Actions of glucocorticoids

The physiological actions of glucocorticoids are mediated via an intranuclear receptor that promotes the transcription of various genes, which leads to the synthesis of new enzymes and proteins that alter cell function. Glucocorticoids are essential to life. Their actions are far-reaching, affecting intermediary metabolism, vascular reactivity, central nervous system function and the stress response.

Intermediary metabolism

Glucocorticoids are catabolic, causing protein breakdown, increased hepatic gluconeogenesis and glycogenolysis, raised plasma glucose concentration and increased glucose-6-phosphatase activity. They have an anti-insulin effect and worsen diabetes when given in therapeutic doses.

Glucocorticoids are said to have a permissive action. This implies that they are necessary to allow catecholamines to exert their calorigenic and lipolytic effects. They also enable inotropy and bronchodilatation mediated by β-adrenergic receptors. Without glucocorticoids, the vascular system is unreactive to epinephrine and norepinephrine. Additionally, the vascular endothelium becomes more permeable. In the stress response, ACTH stimulates the release of glucocorticoids, which permit optimal functioning of the sympathetic nervous system. Glucocorticoids also allow the excretion of a water load, deficiency leading to the risk of water intoxication.

Control of glucocorticoid function

The hypothalamus, anterior lobe of the pituitary and the adrenal cortex are involved in a negative feedback system for glucocorticoid regulation. Basal and reactive release of glucocorticoids are dependent upon ACTH release.

ACTH

ACTH is a linear polypeptide chain of 39 amino acids and originates from the much larger pro-opiomelanocortin molecule. The first 23 amino acids are conserved in all mammalian species. Its plasma half-life is 10 min.

ACTH secretion has a well defined circadian rhythm, with irregular bursts through the day, and cortisol levels mirror this. The

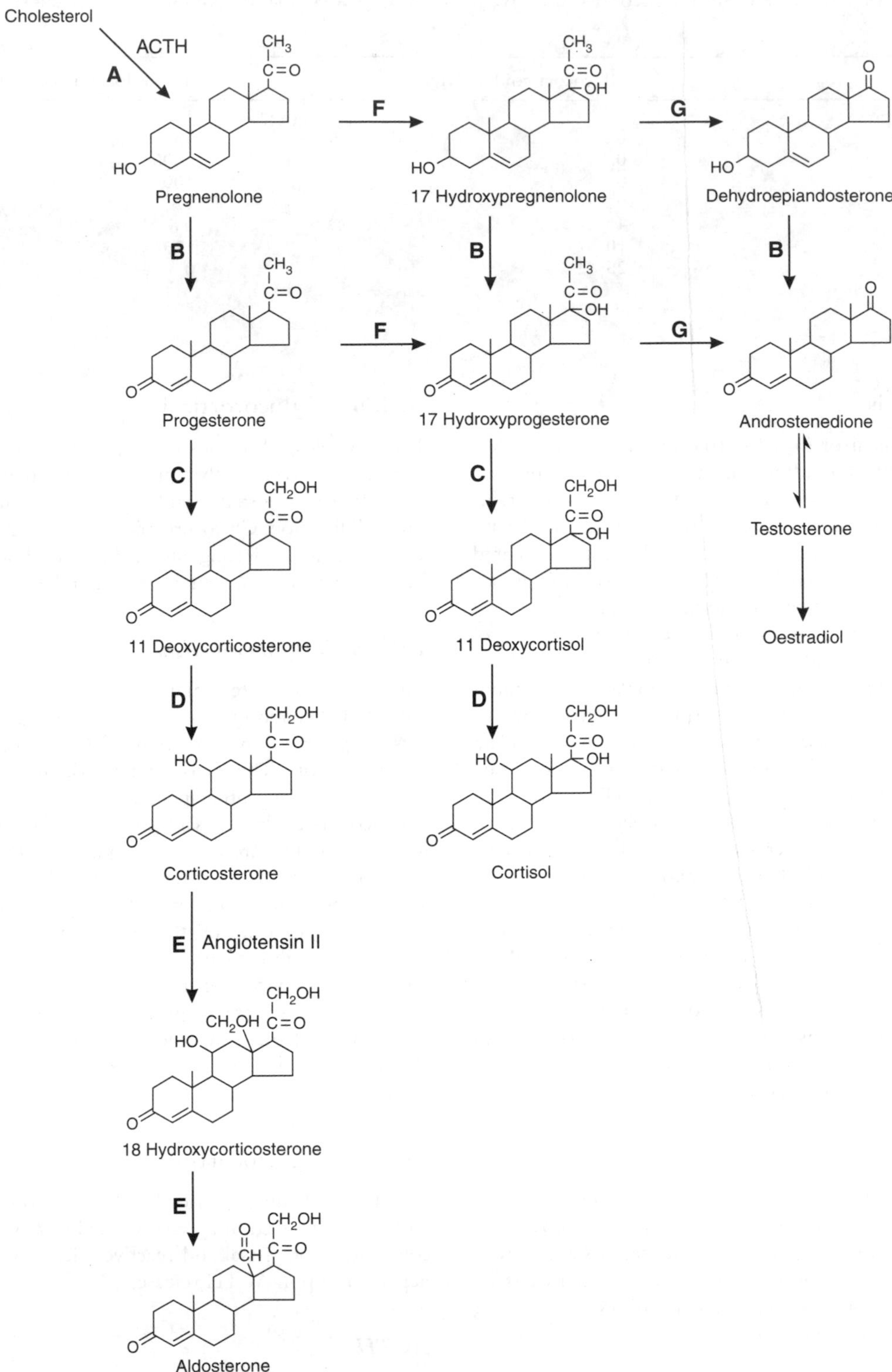

Fig. 28.4
Steroid hormone synthetic pathway. Enzymes – **A**, cholesterol desmolase (cytochrome P450); **B**, 3β-hydroxysteroid dehydrogenase; **C**, 21β-hydroxylase (cytochrome P450); **D**, 11β-hydroxylase (cytochrome P450); **E**, aldosterone synthetase; **F**, 17α-hydroxylase (cytochrome P450); **G**, 17,20-lyase (cytochrome P450). (Adapted with permission from Ganong 1999.)

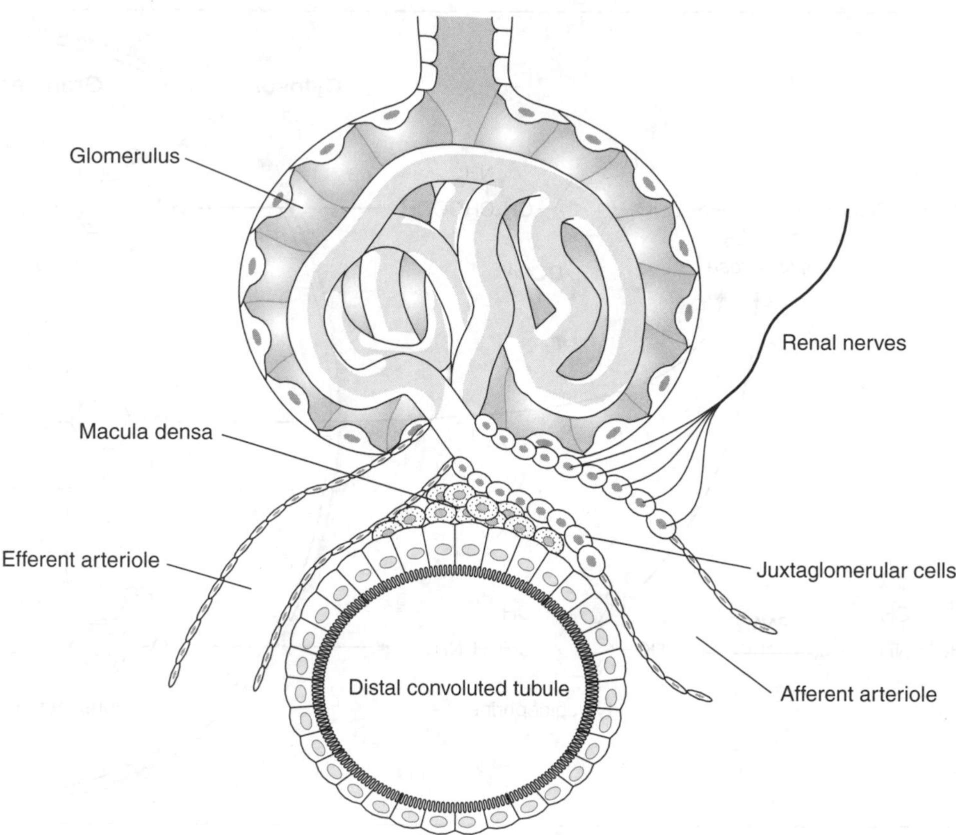

Fig. 28.5
The relationship between the distal convoluted tubule, macula densa and afferent arteriole, which comprise the juxtaglomerular apparatus. (Adapted with permission from Ganong 1999.)

bursts are more frequent in the early morning, and approximately 75% of cortisol secretion occurs between 04.00 and 10.00 h. The bursts are least frequent in the evening. During stressful stimuli, ACTH is released far in excess of that required to produce a maximal response in the adrenals. This is caused by corticotrophin releasing hormone (CRH) release from the hypothalamus. ACTH and cortisol have an inhibitory effect on CRH release. Cortisol inhibits ACTH release.

ACTH acts via a G-protein-linked receptor to stimulate adenylyl cyclase. This results in an increase in intracellular cAMP that stimulates protein kinase A to phosphorylate cholesterol ester hydrolase. This increases the conversion of free cholesterol to its ester, which prompts the formation to pregnanelone. ACTH also stimulates the synthesis of all the P450 enzymes involved in the formation of the adrenocortical hormones

Actions of mineralocorticoids

In keeping with all steroid hormones, aldosterone acts via an intranuclear receptor. The main effect seems to be to increase the number of Na^+/K^+-ATPase proteins on the distal tubule of the nephron. Aldosterone may also bind to the Na^+ channel to increase its activity. The net effect is to increase the amount of Na^+ reabsorbed from the urine, sweat, saliva and gastric juice at the expense of K^+ and H^+ ions. This results in expansion of the extracellular fluid.

In vitro, the mineralocorticoid receptor (MCR) has a higher affinity than the glucocorticoid receptor (GCR) for glucocorticoids. However, glucocorticoids do not bind to the MCRs in renal cells because the renal cell cytoplasm contains 11β-hydroxysteroid dehydrogenase which hydrolyses cortisol and corticosterone, but not aldosterone.

Regulation of aldosterone secretion

The pituitary (via ACTH), the renin–angiotensin system and the plasma K^+ concentration influence mineralocorticoid secretion. ACTH stimulates aldosterone production in the same way as glucocorticoid production, although aldosterone production is much less sensitive than glucocorticoid production. A change in Na^+ concentration is the major factor in aldosterone release, a decrease of only 20 mmol L^{-1} being required. K^+ concentration needs to increase by only 1 mmol L^{-1} to stimulate a response.

Renin–angiotensin system

The juxtaglomerular apparatus is formed where the distal convoluted tubule passes between the afferent and efferent arterioles.

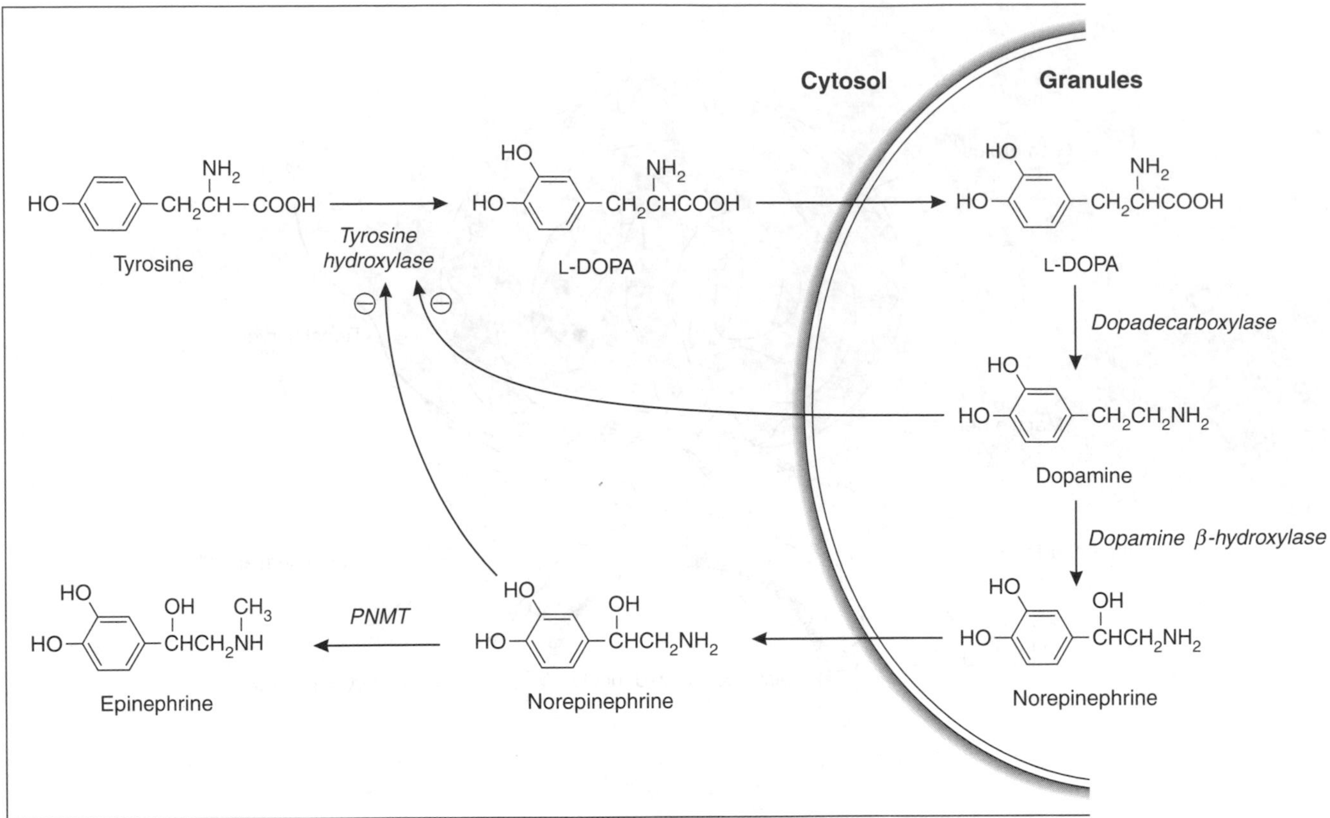

Fig. 28.6
Pathway for catecholamine synthesis.

Where the cells of the tubule are in contact with the afferent arteriole, the epithelium becomes modified to form the macula densa. The cells in the media of the afferent arteriole also change to become juxtaglomerular cells. These cells contain granules of renin (Fig. 28.5).

Renin is secreted into the lumen of the afferent arteriole in response to increased sympathetic renal nerve stimulation, catecholamines, reduced extracellular fluid volume and prostaglandins. The reduced extracellular fluid volume causes a reduction in the Na^+ load to the distal tubule and this is detected by the macula densa. Renin release is inhibited by an increased flux of Na^+ and K^+ ions across the macula densa, increased afferent arteriolar pressure, angiotensin II and ADH.

Renin is an aspartyl protease of molecular weight 37 kDa and half-life 80 min. Its only known function is to cleave the decapeptide angiotensin I from angiotensinogen. In the lungs, under the influence of angiotensin-converting enzyme (ACE), angiotensin I is converted to angiotensin II (octapeptide).

Angiotensin II has a half-life of 2 min. It is rapidly destroyed to form angiotensin III, which has some biological activity. Red blood cells and other tissues have angiotensinase activity. Angiotensin II stimulates mineralocorticoid release in two ways. First, it stimulates the conversion of cholesterol to pregnanelone. Second, it facilitates the conversion of corticosterone to aldosterone. It does not affect the production of other steroid hormones, which require ACTH.

The main role of the renin–angiotensin–aldosterone system is in the preservation of the extracellular fluid volume. It takes time for aldosterone to act, yet there is reduced sodium excretion within minutes of an appropriate stimulus. Other factors that are involved include variations in the glomerular filtration rate (GFR), atrial natriuretic peptide (ANP), the presence or absence of osmotically active substances and changes in tubular Na^+ reabsorption.

ADRENAL MEDULLA

The medulla secretes the catecholamines epinephrine, norepinephrine and dopamine. In humans, the vast majority of output is epinephrine (this reflects the fact that 90% of the cells produce epinephrine).

Catecholamine synthesis

Tyrosine is actively transported into the cells and converted to dihydroxyphenylalanine (DOPA) and dopamine by cytosolic enzymes (Fig. 28.6). Dopamine is then transported into granulated vesicles where it is converted to norepinephrine by dopamine β-hydroxylase. The rate-limiting step in this pathway is the conversion of tyrosine to DOPA by tyrosine hydroxylase. Dopamine and norepinephrine provide control over the enzyme pathway by inhibiting this enzyme. Norepinephrine is then converted to epinephrine by the enzyme phenylethanolamine-N-methyltransferase (PNMT), which is situated in the cytosol. PNMT is only found in the brain and adrenal medulla, not in sympathetic ganglia. Medullary PNMT may be induced by high-dose glucocorticoids (note that the adrenal medulla is already bathed by blood rich in steroids from the adrenal cortex). After hypophysectomy, ACTH and glucocorticoid levels are low, resulting in a low level of epinephrine secretion.

The synthesized epinephrine and norepinephrine are stored in vesicles with ATP and chromogranin A. The transport mechanism that concentrates the catecholamines in the vesicles is inhibited by reserpine. The vesicles are released by calcium-dependent exocytosis into the medullary venous sinuses. ATP, chromogranin A and dopamine β-hydroxylase are released at the same time. Levels of chromogranin A provide an index of sympathetic activity.

Catecholamines have a half-life of 2 min, with up to 70% of epinephrine and norepinephrine conjugated in the plasma. The remainder is metabolized by the liver.

Actions of catecholamines

Catecholamines exert their effects via stimulation of α- and β-adrenoreceptors and so mimic the sympathetic nervous system. They also have effects on metabolism.

Metabolic effects

Catecholamines cause an increase in liver and muscle glycogenolysis, FFA mobilization and plasma lactate. They also cause an increase in the basal metabolic rate.

Cardiovascular effects

Epinephrine and norepinephrine have inotropic effects, increasing the rate and force of contraction in the isolated heart. They also increase myocardial excitability.

In vivo, norepinephrine causes an increase in the systolic and diastolic arterial pressures, with a reduction in heart rate brought about by the baroreceptor reflex that leads to a reduction in cardiac output. Epinephrine, on the other hand, causes a widening of the pulse pressure by decreasing the diastolic arterial pressure and increasing systolic. This has less effect on the baroreceptors and epinephrine is more chronotropic on the heart, leading to an increase in cardiac output.

Regulation of adrenal medullary function

Epinephrine concentration may increase by 100% on standing from the supine position.

Increased medullary secretion is part of the diffuse sympathetic discharge seen in emergency situations. The calorigenic effects of catecholamines are seen in response to cold. Animals with denervated adrenals shiver sooner and more vigorously. Hypoglycaemia is a potent stimulus.

THYROID FUNCTION

ANATOMY

The gland consists of two lobes connected by an isthmus situated in front of the larynx at the level of C6. It derives its blood supply from the superior and inferior thyroid arteries and is drained by the corresponding veins. The gland is composed of multiple follicles that contain colloid. A single layer of epithelial cells, the appearance of which depends on the gland's activity, surrounds each follicle. During the inactive phase, the epithelium is flat, the colloid abundant and the follicles are large. When active, the epithelium is cuboidal or columnar, the colloid is reduced with scalloped edges and the follicles are small (Fig. 28.7). Microvilli project into the colloid to increase the resorptive surface area. The cells sit on a basal lamina that separates them from the capillaries and have a prominent endoplasmic reticulum. In keeping with the other endocrine glands, the capillaries are fenestrated and abundant. This allows easy passage of secreted hormones into the bloodstream.

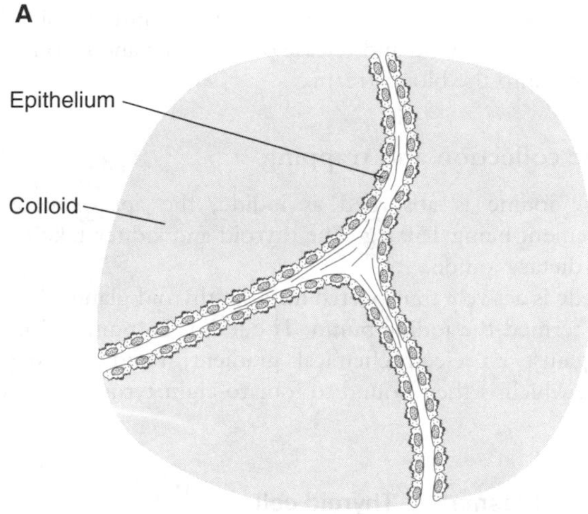

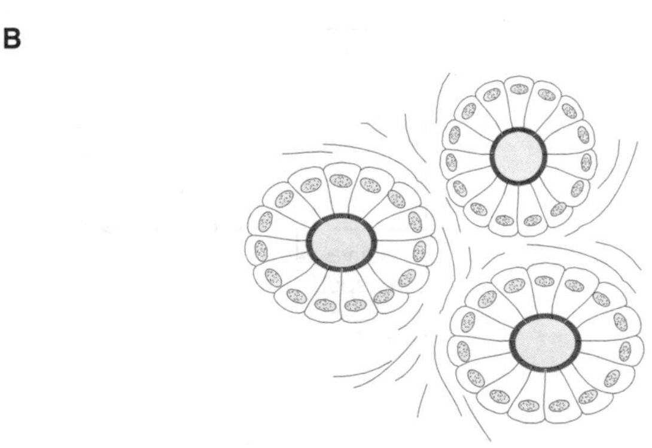

Fig. 28.7
Thyroid gland histology with different levels of activity. **A.** Inactive thyroid gland – note the flattened epithelium and abundant colloid. **B.** Active thyroid gland – note the larger epithelial cells and the reduced volume of colloid. Colloid has punched out lacunae next to the cells. (Adapted with permission from Ganong 1999.)

HORMONE SYNTHESIS AND STORAGE

The thyroid cells have three main functions (Fig. 28.8):

- collection and transport of iodine into the cell
- synthesis of thyroglobulin and its secretion into colloid
- ingestion of colloid and release of thyroxine and triiodothyronine into the bloodstream.

Iodine collection and trapping

Dietary iodine is absorbed as iodide, the approximate daily requirement being 150 µg. The thyroid and kidney take up most of the dietary iodide.

Iodide is actively transported into the thyroid gland by a mechanism termed the iodide pump. The iodide is 'pumped' into the cell against an electrochemical gradient, rapidly oxidized to iodine, which is then bound to four to eight tyrosine residues in thyroglobulin. Iodide transport can be blocked competitively by the perchlorate ion. Iodine binding to tyrosine is blocked by the antithyroid drugs carbimazole and propylthiouracil. Thyroid-stimulating hormone (TSH) stimulates iodide transport, which is also dependent on Na^+/K^+-ATPase and hence can be blocked by oubain.

Thyroid hormone synthesis

Thyroglobulin is a glycoprotein of molecular weight 660 kDa and is 10% carbohydrate. It contains 123 tyrosine residues but only four to eight are involved in hormone synthesis. Thyroglobulin is synthesized by the thyroid cells and secreted into the colloid by exocytosis. Synthesis of thyroid hormones takes place in the colloid. When iodide is oxidized to iodine, it is attached to tyrosine in the 3 position to make 3-monoiodotyrosine (MIT). MIT is then iodinated at the 5 position to make 3,5-diiodotyrosine

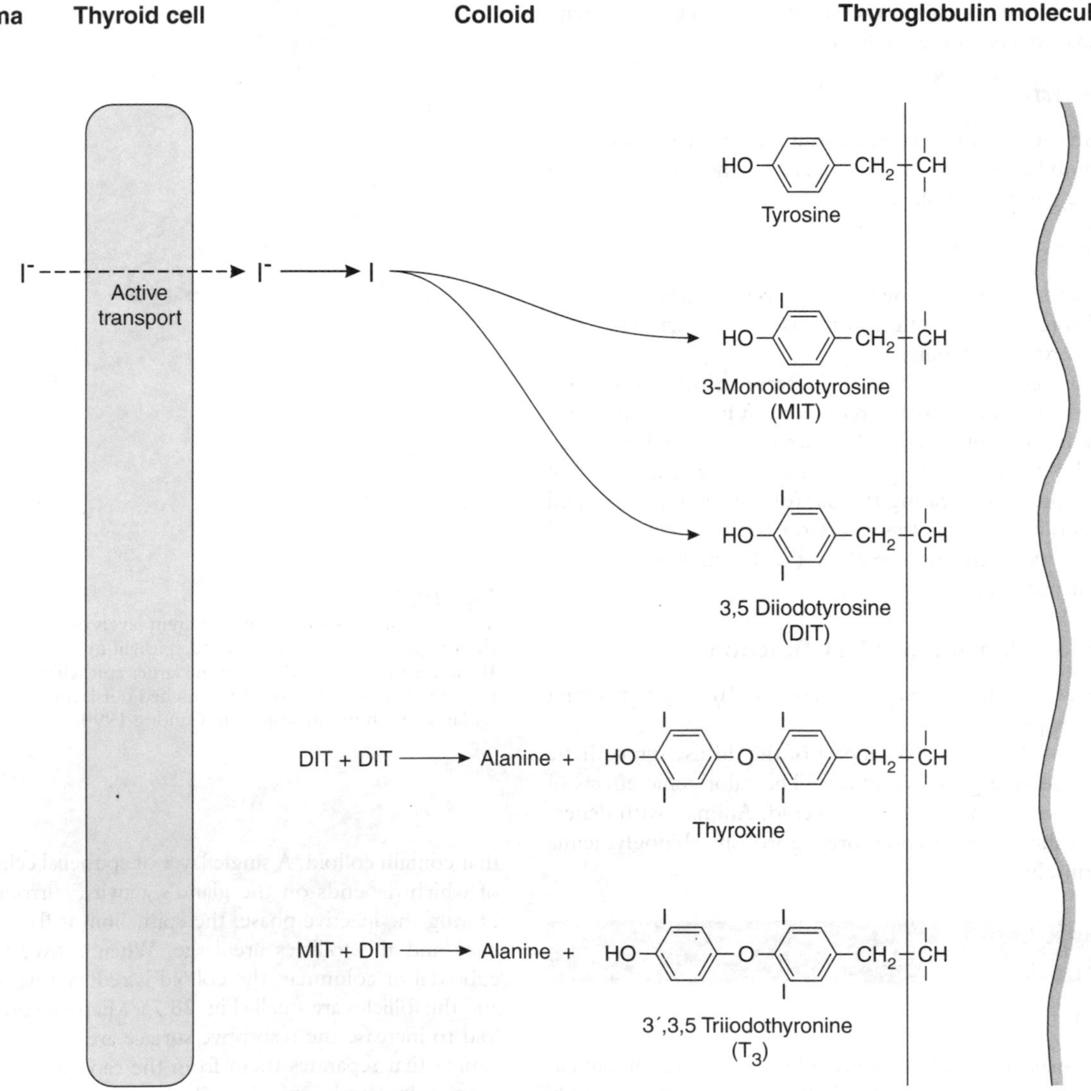

Fig. 28.8
Functions of the thyroid cells. (Adapted with permission from Ganong 1999.)

(DIT). Two DIT molecules condense to form tetraiodothyronine (thyroxine, T_4). This is termed the coupling reaction and is thought to occur either when the two DIT molecules are attached to thyroglobulin (intramolecular coupling), or after DIT detaches from thyroglobulin (intermolecular coupling). Triiodothyronine (T_3) is formed when MIT condenses with DIT. Both T_3 and T_4 are biologically active. Reverse T_3 (RT_3) is formed when DIT condenses with MIT; this is inactive, and the synthesis of this may be increased in various disease states.

SECRETION

The thyroid cells ingest colloid by endocytosis and this produces the absorption lacunae seen in active glands. Within the cell, the globules of colloid fuse with lysosomes and thyroglobulin is broken down by proteases, liberating MIT, DIT, T_4 and T_3 into the cytoplasm of the cell. The thyroid hormones (T_3 and T_4) then diffuse out of the cell into the circulation. Any released free iodine is re-used by the cell and may provide more iodine than the iodine pump.

CONTROL OF THYROID HORMONE SECRETION

The thyroid is primarily controlled by the circulating level of TSH, which is dependent upon TRH from the hypothalamus. The hormones are under negative feedback control, T_4 and T_3 inhibiting the release of TSH and TRH, while TSH inhibits TRH release. TSH is a glycoprotein made up of two subunits (α and β) with 211 amino acids. The α subunit is common to LH, FSH, TSH and human chorionic gonadotrophin (hCG). The specificity of the molecule is conferred by the β subunit. The half-life of TSH is 60 min and it is metabolized mainly by the kidney, but also by the liver. Secretion is pulsatile, beginning at 21.00 h with a peak at midnight and then slowly declining through the day.

Effect of TSH on the thyroid

The TSH receptor is a typical serpentine receptor of the G-protein family and activates adenylyl cyclase to increase the production of intracellular cAMP when TSH is bound.

This causes an increase in the rate of iodide trapping and the synthesis of T_3, T_4, thyroglobulin and iodotyrosines. It causes the cells to change from squamous to cuboidal epithelium, and the weight of the gland increases with prolonged stimulation.

ACTION OF THYROID HORMONES

Thyroid hormones enter the cells and bind to intranuclear receptors. T_3 has the highest affinity for these receptors, and most of the T_4 is converted to T_3 at the tissue level. The hormone receptor complex then binds to DNA and alters the expression of various genes that ultimately affect cell function.

Most of the effects of thyroid hormones are widespread and secondary to the stimulation of increased oxygen consumption (calorigenic action). However, these hormones also have effects on growth and development, regulate lipid metabolism and elevate the rate of carbohydrate absorption from the gut. They have an effect on the oxygen haemoglobin dissociation curve, shifting it to the right by increasing red blood cell 2,3-DPG levels.

Calorigenic action

The thyroid hormones stimulate the oxygen consumption of all tissues except the brain, testes, uterus, lymphoreticular system and the anterior pituitary (the rate of TSH production is reduced). This effect on the metabolic rate is measurable after a few hours and persists for approximately a week. This calorigenic action causes an increase in protein and fat catabolism, an increase in body temperature and an increased need for vitamins and micronutrients. In the cardiovascular system, there is an increase in cardiac output and heart rate with a reduction in vascular resistance because of an increase in cardiac β-adrenergic receptors (this also results in increased cardiac excitability). Skeletal muscle is also affected and, in excess, the thyroid hormones cause a myopathy.

Thyroid hormones also affect carbohydrate and lipid metabolism, causing an increase in gut carbohydrate absorption, a reduction in the renal threshold for glucose and a reduction in serum cholesterol concentration as a result of an increase in hepatic LDL receptors. The hormones are also vital for normal growth and development, especially of neural tissue.

TRANSPORT OF THYROID HORMONES

Thyroid hormones are transported bound to several plasma proteins with varying affinities. These proteins include albumin, thyroxine-binding globulin (TBG) and thyroxine-binding prealbumin (TBPA). The hormones are in equilibrium between free and bound phases. Free circulating hormone forms the active phase, whereas the bound phase provides a reservoir of hormone. This allows a large pool of readily available hormone and promotes even distribution. Albumin has the largest capacity to bind T_4, but TBG has the highest affinity. Approximately 99.8% of T_4 and 99.8% of T_3 are bound.

METABOLISM

Thyroid hormones are metabolized by the liver, kidneys and other tissues. Approximately one-third of T_4 is converted to T_3, and half to inactive RT_3.

The hormones are conjugated to sulphate or glucuronide and are secreted into the intestinal lumen in the bile with some enterohepatic circulation.

PARATHYROID HORMONES AND CALCIUM HOMEOSTASIS

ANATOMY

Humans have four parathyroid glands, two on each side of the neck. The glands have a variable position in the neck and may even be found in the mediastinum. In common with all endocrine glands, they are richly vascularized with fenestrated capillaries. They derive their blood supply from the inferior thyroid arteries. There are two cell types in the parathyroid glands: chief cells have prominent endoplasmic reticulum, Golgi apparatus and numerous secretory vesicles; oxyphil cells are rich in mitochondria and oxyphilic granules. Chief cells are thought to be responsible for the synthesis and secretion of parathyroid hormone (PTH), while oxyphil cells are thought to be degenerated chief cells.

PARATHYROID HORMONE SYNTHESIS AND STORAGE

Parathyroid hormone is a linear polypeptide of molecular weight 9500 Da with 84 amino acids. It is synthesized initially as pre-proparathyroid hormone, which is subjected to post-translational modification to form PTH which is stored in secretory vesicles. The N terminal of PTH forms the active region of the molecule. It has a plasma half-life of 20 min and is metabolized by the Kupffer cells in the liver.

CONTROL OF PTH SECRETION

Negative feedback is mediated by the action of ionized calcium (Ca^{2+}) on the chief cells, the Ca^{2+} receptor being linked to a G-protein. Plasma magnesium ions (Mg^{2+}) directly inhibit the gland. High phosphate concentrations also stimulate PTH release, by lowering the Ca^{2+} concentration. 1,25-Dihydrocholecalciferol reduces preproPTH mRNA transcription.

ACTION OF PTH

Parathyroid hormone acts on the bones and the kidneys via a G-protein-linked receptor to cause an increase in intracellular cAMP. In bone, it acts on the osteocytes and osteoblasts by increasing their Ca^{2+} permeability. The osteoblasts then pump the Ca^{2+} into the extracellular fluid. 1,25-Dihydrocholecalciferol also stimulates this process. When PTH is produced in excess, bone resorption exceeds bone formation.

In the kidneys, PTH causes increased phosphate excretion in the urine by reducing the amount of phosphate reabsorbed in the proximal tubule. This allows for increased calcium reabsorption in the distal tubule. The net effect is to increase Ca^{2+} excretion because of the increased filtered load. PTH also stimulates 1,25-dihydrocholecalciferol production by the kidney.

CALCITONIN

The parafollicular cells (or clear [C] cells) of the thyroid gland produce calcitonin. It is a linear polypeptide of 34 amino acids with molecular weight 3500 Da.

Calcitonin secretion

Elevated Ca^{2+} concentrations are the stimulus to calcitonin release, but none is released until the Ca^{2+} level exceeds 2.4 mmol L^{-1}. It has a half-life of 10 min.

Action of calcitonin

Calcitonin acts via a G-protein-linked receptor in the bones and kidneys. It inhibits bone resorption and causes an increase in calcium excretion in the urine. Its exact physiological role is uncertain, as humans who have had a total thyroidectomy do not have calcium balance problems provided their parathyroid function is normal. Calcitonin may have a role in skeletal development and maturation, as large amounts are secreted in childhood.

VITAMIN D

In the skin, under the action of ultraviolet light, 7-cholecalciferol is converted into cholecalciferol (vitamin D_3). Vitamin D_3 is then transported in the circulation bound to vitamin D binding protein (DBP). Vitamin D_3 is also acquired from the diet.

In the liver, vitamin D_3 is converted to 25-hydroxycholecalciferol ($25OHD_3$). $25OHD_3$ is then converted to 1,25-dihydroxycholecalciferol ($1,25DOHD_3$) by the proximal tubules of the kidney.

Effects of vitamin D derivatives

$1,25DOHD_3$ is a steroid and acts on an intranuclear receptor to affect gene transcription. The result is to cause an increase in calcium absorption from the intestine and calcium reabsorption from the kidney. In bone, calcium and phosphate are mobilized by increasing the number of mature osteoclasts and stimulating osteoblasts.

Vitamin D regulation

The production of $1,25DOHD_3$ is regulated in a negative feedback fashion by Ca^{2+} concentrations. $25OHD_3$ is not closely regulated. PTH facilitates its production, whereas high concentrations of Ca^{2+} cause the kidneys to produce the inactive 23,25-dihydroxycholecalciferol.

CALCIUM HOMEOSTASIS

Calcium

In excess of 25 mol of calcium is present in the body and this represents almost 1.5% of body weight, with 99% of this present in the skeleton.

In the plasma, calcium is bound to plasma proteins, with the remainder free as the ionized form. The ionized phase of calcium is responsible for its physiological actions, such as nerve function, muscle contraction and blood coagulation. In the bones, calcium is present in two types, as a readily exchangeable reservoir (to allow regulation of plasma Ca^{2+}) and a much larger stable pool of bone. There is some exchange between the two.

Phosphorus

Phosphorus is present as phosphate and is not as strictly regulated as calcium. It forms part of the skeleton, but is also a part of proteins, ATP, cAMP and other nucleotides. Dietary absorption is related to intake, unlike calcium which is not absorbed when plasma concentrations are high.

PANCREATIC ENDOCRINE FUNCTION

The endocrinologically active parts of the pancreas are the islets of Langerhans. These ovoid clusters of cells, which comprise 1–2% of pancreatic mass, are scattered amongst the pancreas, but are more numerous in the head and tail. They have a large blood supply with fenestrated capillaries in keeping with their endocrine function. Blood from the pancreas drains into the hepatic portal vein.

Four cell types are found in human pancreatic islets (Table 28.4). The A, D and F cells are found in the periphery of the

Table 28.4 Cell types found in the islets of Langerhans

Cell type	Hormone secreted
A	Glucagon
B	Insulin
D	Somatostatin
F	Pancreatic polypeptide

islets, with the B cells in the centre. The B cells tend to be surrounded by A cells. There is a paracrine action between the cells, the hormones of each influencing the secretion of the others (see below).

INSULIN

Insulin consists of two polypeptide chains – A (21 amino acids) and B (30 amino acids) – has a half-life of 5 min and is metabolized by the kidney (80%) or when it is taken up by the tissue in which it is acting (see below).

Insulin is synthesized initially as preproinsulin. As preproinsulin enters the endoplasmic reticulum, a 23-amino-acid leader sequence is cleaved to form a molecule that is folded and disulphide bridges are formed between approximated cysteine moieties. At this stage, the molecule is still a single polypeptide chain and is called proinsulin. The C-peptide is then cleaved to form insulin, which consists of two polypeptide chains connected by disulphide bridges (Fig. 28.9). Insulin is stored in granules ready for release by endocytosis. Insulin and C-peptide are excreted in equimolar amounts.

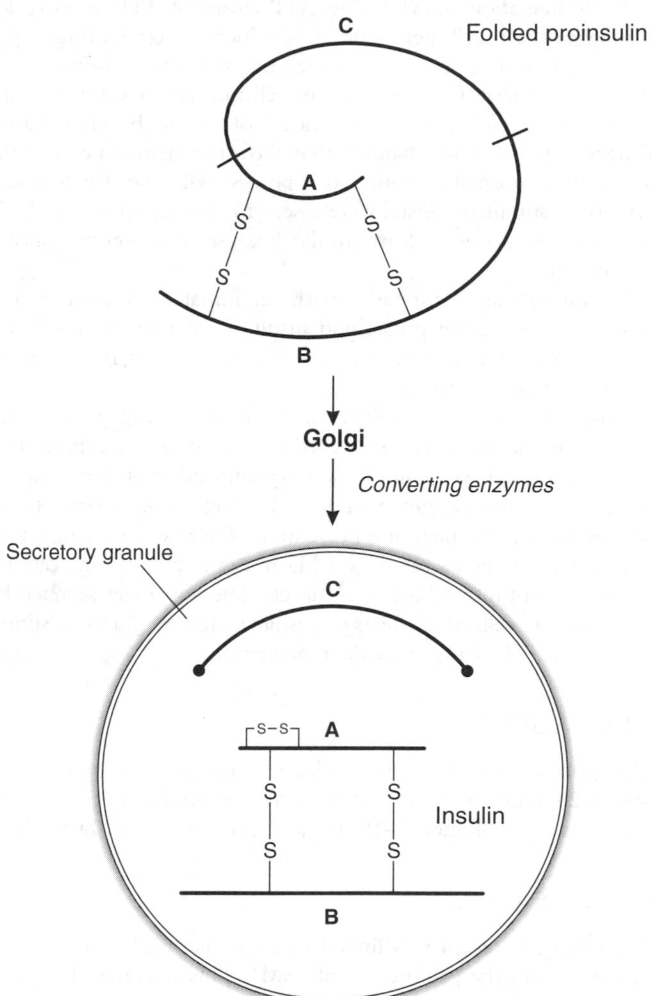

Fig. 28.9
Synthesis of insulin from proinsulin. (Adapted with permission from Ganong 1999.)

Effects of insulin

The actions of insulin are mediated by the insulin receptor, which is a tetramer made up of two α and two β subunits. All subunits come from a single mRNA chain. The α subunits form the extracellular domain and bind to insulin. The β subunits, which are intracellular and have tyrosine kinase activity, mediate the effects by phosphorylating and dephosphorylating various enzymes. When insulin binds, the receptors aggregate and the ligand–receptor complex is endocytosed and eventually destroyed by lysosomes.

The action of insulin depends on the tissue involved. Insulin is the major anabolic hormone; its effects may be classified into early, intermediate and late. The net result of these effects is to increase the storage of protein, fat and carbohydrate. Early (seconds) effects include accelerated entry of glucose, amino acids and potassium into cells. This action is used in the pharmacological treatment of hyperkalaemia. Intermediate effects include the inhibition of protein catabolism, stimulation of protein synthesis, the activation of glycogen synthase and glycolytic enzymes, and the inhibition of phosphorylase and gluconeogenic enzymes. Delayed effects include transcription of mRNA for lipogenic enzymes.

Glucose enters all cells by facilitated diffusion. Insulin increases the number of glucose transporter molecules on the cell membranes of muscle, adipose and other tissues. When inside the cell, glucose is phosphorylated rapidly to maintain its concentration gradient. Causing the induction of the enzyme hexokinase also increases the rate of glucose entry into hepatic cells. This enzyme is responsible for glucose phosphorylation.

In adipose tissue, there is an increase in FFA and glycerol synthesis, activation of lipoprotein lipase and the inhibition of hormone-sensitive lipase. In muscle, there is increased amino acid and ketone uptake, and protein and glycogen synthesis, together with reduced protein catabolism and release of ketogenic amino acids. In the liver, there is reduced ketogenesis and glucose output, with increased protein and lipid synthesis. The rate of glycogen synthesis is increased with a corresponding reduction in gluconeogenesis.

Control of insulin secretion

The normal basal rate of insulin secretion is approximately 1 U h^{-1} into the hepatic portal vein, which the pancreas can normally increase up to 10-fold. The major factor responsible for the release of insulin is glucose. Glucose enters the B cells by a non-insulin-dependent glucose transporter and is metabolized by glucokinase with the liberation of ATP. This ATP closes an ATP-sensitive K^+ channel in the B-cell membrane that reduces K^+ efflux, thus depolarizing the cell. This leads to opening of voltage-sensitive Ca^{2+} channels that allow Ca^{2+} to enter the cell and activate Ca^{2+}-dependent kinases, which trigger the release of insulin by endocytosis. Voltage-dependent K^+ channels that allow the membrane potential to return to normal terminate this process. Glucose, fructose and mannose stimulate insulin release. Mannoheptulose and 2-deoxyglucose do not release insulin because they prevent glucose metabolism.

Insulin release is biphasic, with an initial peak after 5 min (caused by release of preformed insulin) and then a slow initial increase, reaching a plateau at 20–40 min (caused by release of newly synthesized insulin).

Other factors may stimulate insulin release. Any process that increases intracellular ATP or cAMP causes release. Catecholamines have a dual effect on insulin release; α_2 stimulation prevents release, and β_2 stimulation augments releas. The net result of sympathetic nervous system stimulation is prevention of release. Parasympathetic stimulation augments release via M_4 muscarinic receptors, causing an elevation of intracellular Ca^{2+} levels. The hormones secreted by the other islet cells have effects on insulin secretion; glucagon stimulates release, whereas somatostatin prevents it.

GLUCAGON

Glucagon is secreted by the A cells. It is a linear polypeptide comprising 29 amino acids and has a molecular weight of 3500 Da. Its half-life is approximately 5–10 min and it is metabolized by the liver.

Effects of glucagon

The glucagon receptor is linked to a stimulating G-protein (G_s) that promotes the production of cAMP. This activates phosphorylase and causes the breakdown of glycogen and hence increases plasma glucose concentration. There is also a hepatic glucagon receptor linked to phospholipase C, which stimulates gluconeogenesis. Glucagon does not stimulate gluconeogenesis in muscle tissue. In large doses, it is a positive inotrope with limited arrhythmogenic effects on the heart (unlike catecholamines). This effect is used in the treatment of β-blocker overdose. It also stimulates the release of GH, insulin and pancreatic somatostatin.

Control of glucagon release

Release is stimulated by hypoglycaemia and prevented by hyperglycaemia. Interestingly, glucagon release is inhibited by γ-aminobutyric acid (GABA – this is released by the B cells when they release insulin). β-Adrenergic stimulation also causes release, and α-adrenergic stimulation prevents it. Other factors that stimulate release are a protein meal, cortisol, exercise, cholecystokinin (CCK) and gastrin. FFAs and ketones inhibit the process.

SOMATOSTATIN

This is a linear polypeptide secreted by the D cells. It occurs in both a 14- and 28-amino-acid form. Its main actions are to inhibit the release of insulin and glucagon.

Glucose and amino acids such as arginine and isoleucine stimulate its release.

PANCREATIC POLYPEPTIDE

This is a linear polypeptide with 36 amino acids and is secreted by the F cells. A protein meal, fasting, exercise and acute hypoglycaemia bring about its secretion. Somatostatin and glucose inhibit its release. Its exact physiological role is unclear, but it has been found to slow food absorption.

FURTHER READING

British National Formulary 2000 Number 40. British Medical Association, London

Ganong W F 1999 Medical review of physiology, 18th edn. Lange Medical Publications, Los Altos, CA

Guyton A C, Hall J E 2000 Textbook of medical physiology, 10th edn. W B Saunders, Philadelphia

Jameson J L 1996 Principles of hormone action. In: Weatherall D J, Ledingham J G G, Warrell D A (eds) Oxford textbook of medicine, 3rd edn. Oxford University Press, Oxford, ch 12, 1553–1573

Last R J 1994 Anatomy: regional and applied, 9th edn. Churchill Livingstone, Edinburgh

Laycock J, Wise P 1996 Essential endocrinology, 3rd edn. Oxford University Press, Oxford

29 Maternal and neonatal physiology

An understanding of the physiological changes induced by pregnancy is vital to the clinician involved in the care of pregnant women. The obstetric anaesthetist must understand maternal adaptation to pregnancy in order to manipulate physiological changes following general anaesthesia or regional analgesia and anaesthesia in such a way that the condition of the neonate at delivery is optimized.

The success of colleagues in other specialities now enables many more women with chronic disease processes to achieve pregnancy. The obstetric anaesthetist requires an understanding of the pathophysiological changes associated with the disease process and their interaction with the changes consequent upon pregnancy. The physiological changes of pregnancy are exaggerated in multiple pregnancy. The success of assisted conception implies that obstetric anaesthetists care for more women with twins, triplets and quadruplets.

There are few manufacturers' data on the effects of commonly used anaesthetic agents on pregnant women, fetuses and neonates. However, many unlicensed drugs are used in obstetric and paediatric anaesthesia, because no suitable alternatives exist. In such cases, the clinician must understand the altered pharmacology of such drugs.

Hormonal changes after ovulation initiate physiological preparation for pregnancy. Following conception, an increased blood volume occurs ahead of the metabolic demands of the developing fetoplacental unit. Safe parturition is effected by the complementary changes in coagulation and fibrinolysis. Maternal physiology returns to normal remarkably quickly after parturition. Similarly, the transition from fetal to infant physiology which begins dramatically at birth involves fundamental changes to the cardiac and respiratory systems.

PHYSIOLOGY OF PREGNANCY

PROGESTERONE

The hormone progesterone may be considered the most important physiological substance in pregnancy. It is secreted initially in increasing amounts during the second half of the menstrual cycle to prepare the woman for pregnancy. Following conception, the corpus luteum ensures adequate blood concentrations until placental secretion is adequate. The most important physiological role of progesterone is its ability to relax smooth muscle. All other physiological changes stem from this pivotal function (Fig. 29.1).

HAEMATOLOGICAL AND HAEMODYNAMIC CHANGES

The increase in blood volume from 60–65 to 80–85 ml kg^{-1} is caused mainly by expansion of plasma volume, which starts shortly after conception and implantation and is maximal at 30–32 weeks (Fig. 29.2). Red cell volume increases linearly but not as much as plasma volume. Haemoglobin concentration decreases from 14 to 12 g dl^{-1} (Table 29.1). Thus the haematocrit also decreases.

Although erythrocyte production is increased because of the stimulus of erythropoietin, red cell count is usually reduced to approximately $3.8 \times 10^{12}\ L^{-1}$. Mean cell volume increases and the cells become more spherical. There is no significant change in platelets or lymphocytes, although cell-mediated immunity is depressed. A neutrophilia increases the white cell count to $9 \times 10^{9}\ L^{-1}$ by the third trimester, peaking at $40 \times 10^{9}\ L^{-1}$ during labour. Haematological changes return to normal by the sixth day after delivery. The erythrocyte sedimentation rate (ESR) is increased. Blood viscosity decreases to assist the hyperdynamic circulation.

The development of the pulmonary artery catheter with the facility for measurement of cardiac output by thermodilution has led to central haemodynamic assessment of critically ill mothers. Interpretation of abnormal physiological variables is easier if based on a sound knowledge of the changes in normal pregnancy. Many of the early studies on cardiac output were performed before the full significance of aortocaval compression was appreciated. Modern technology has led to reassessment of the haemodynamic changes in pregnancy (Table 29.2).

Table 29.1 Haematological changes associated with pregnancy

Variable	Non-pregnant	Pregnant
Haemoglobin	14 g dl^{1}	12 g dl^{1}
Haematocrit	0.40–0.42	0.31–0.34
Red cell count	$4.2 \times 10^{12}\ L^{-1}$	$3.8 \times 10^{12}\ L^{-1}$
White cell count	$6.0 \times 10^{9}\ L^{-1}$	$9.0 \times 10^{9}\ L^{-1}$
Erythrocyte sedimentation rate	10	58–68

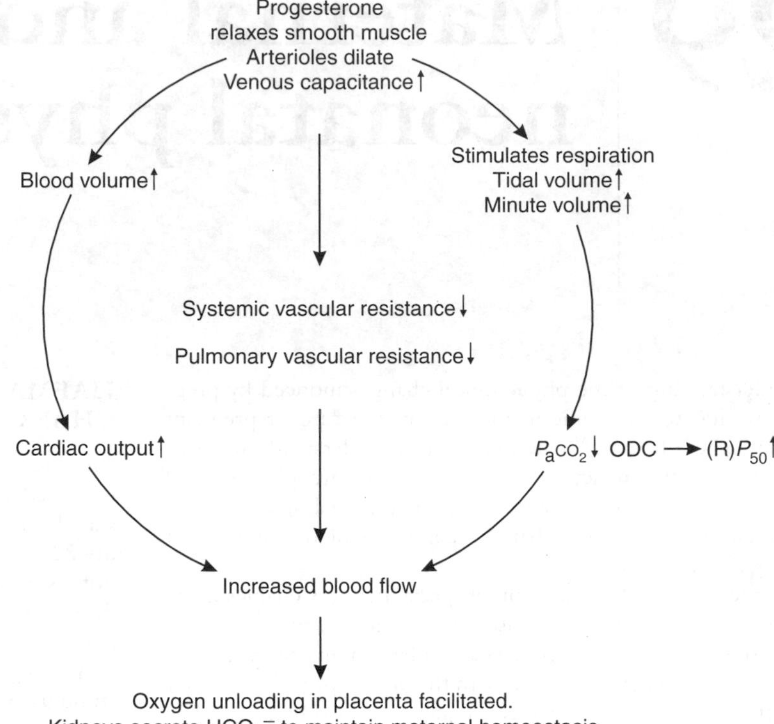

Fig. 29.1
Summary of the main actions of progesterone – it establishes the maternal physiological adaptation to pregnancy. P_aCO_2, arterial carbon dioxide tension; ODC, oxyhaemoglobin dissociation curve; P_{50}, partial pressure of oxygen when haemoglobin is 50% saturated at pH 7.4 and temperature 37°C; HCO_3^-, bicarbonate.

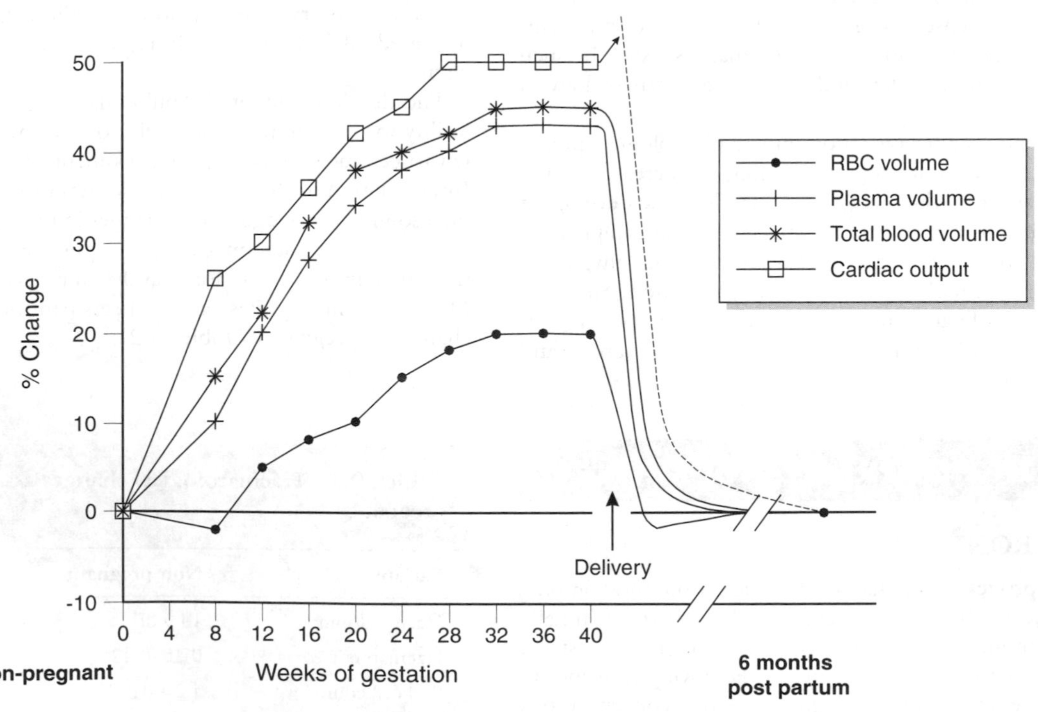

Fig. 29.2
Changes in blood, plasma and red cell volumes and cardiac output during pregnancy.

Table 29.2 Haemodynamic changes in pregnancy

Variable	Non-pregnant	Pregnant
Cardiac output ($L min^{-1}$)	4.3 ± 0.9	6.2 ± 1.0
Heart rate (beat min^{-1})	71 ± 10	83 ± 10
Systemic vascular resistance (dyne s cm^{-5})	1530 ± 520	1210 ± 266
Pulmonary vascular resistance (dyne s cm^{-5})	119 ± 47	78 ± 22
Colloid oncotic pressure (mmHg)	20.8 ± 1.0	18.0 ± 1.5
Central venous pressure (mmHg)	3.7 ± 2.6	3.6 ± 2.5
Pulmonary capillary wedge pressure (mmHg)	6.3 ± 2.1	7.5 ± 1.8

Data from Clark et al (1989).

The increase in blood volume is accompanied by an increase in cardiac output (Fig. 29.1) within the first 10–12 weeks by approximately 1.5 L min^{-1}. By the third trimester, cardiac output has increased by about 44% as a result of significant increases in heart rate (17%) and stroke volume (27%).

During labour, cardiac output may double, especially with the expulsive efforts of the second stage. There is a further increase in the immediate post-delivery period caused by autotransfusion at delivery. During this period, central venous pressure and pulmonary capillary wedge pressure (PCWP) increase and colloid osmotic pressure decreases as a result of movement of extravascular water into the circulating volume. This is the most dangerous time for the mother with intrinsic cardiac or renal disease. Women with pre-eclamptic toxaemia have widespread endothelial damage and multiorgan dysfunction and so are at risk of developing pulmonary oedema or acute respiratory distress syndrome (ARDS) at this time.

However, in normal pregnancy, despite the increased blood volume and hyperdynamic circulation, the PCWP and central venous pressure do not increase, because of the relaxant effect of progesterone on the smooth muscle of arterioles and veins. There are significant decreases in systemic (21%) and pulmonary vascular resistance (34%). These decreases permit the increased blood volume to be accommodated at normal vascular pressures. Although the stroke volume increases, the PCWP does not increase, because the left ventricle dilates.

The heart enlarges as a result of increases in both myocardial thickness and the volume of the chambers. It is raised by the elevated diaphragm and rotated forwards, the apex beat being moved upwards and laterally. On X-ray, the upper border of the heart is straightened and pulmonary vascularity is increased. There are also changes in the heart sounds; the first sound is frequently split and a third sound is common. A systolic ejection murmur is usual and an innocent diastolic murmur with the third heart sound may occur. Electrocardiogram (ECG) changes comprise left axis deviation, flattened or inverted T waves and occasionally ST depression. Cardiac arrhythmias may occur; these include atrial and ventricular extrasystoles. Supraventricular tachycardia is the commonest arrhythmia.

In essence, a large heart pumps a larger blood volume more quickly through an enlarged and expanding vascular bed which provides a low resistance to less viscous blood.

Despite the reductions in haemoglobin concentration and red cell mass, the physiological changes are geared to maximize oxygen transport to the placenta and eliminate carbon dioxide from the developing fetus.

Arterial and venous pressures

There is little change in systolic arterial pressure, but there is a marked decrease in diastolic pressure, which is lowest at mid-pregnancy. Pregnant women who lie supine may suffer from aortocaval compression. Arterial pressure decreases because the gravid uterus compresses the inferior vena cava to reduce venous return and therefore cardiac output. The aorta is also frequently compressed, so that femoral arterial pressure may be lower than brachial arterial pressure. Compensation for aortocaval compression occurs through sympathetic stimulation. However aortocaval compression becomes more significant in the presence of placental insufficiency, a compromised fetus, hypovolaemia or where the sympathetic response is attenuated by general or regional anaesthesia.

Venous pressure in the arms is not increased, but pressures in the femoral and other leg veins increase throughout pregnancy. This is a result of obstruction caused by the weight of the uterus on the iliac veins and inferior vena cava – hence the propensity for development of varicose veins.

Haematinics

Iron absorption increases from 5–10% to 40% by late pregnancy. Routine iron supplementation is not necessary in women with adequate nutrition and a singleton pregnancy.

Folate requirements increase. Folic acid is transported actively by the placenta even when there is folate deficiency. Fetal deformity, premature delivery and antepartum haemorrhage are associated with folate deficiency. Folate supplements are thought to prevent neural tube defects.

Vitamin B_{12} levels decrease in pregnancy because there is preferential transfer to the fetus. Vitamin B_{12} deficiency is associated with infertility and intrauterine death. Strict vegans require B_{12} supplementation during pregnancy.

Regional blood flow

There is an increased blood flow to various organs, especially the uterus and placenta, from 85 to 500 ml min^{-1} (Fig. 29.3). Uterine blood flow is reduced during aortocaval compression or maternal hypotension from other causes.

Renal blood flow is increased by about 400 ml min^{-1}. By 10–12 weeks, glomerular filtration rate (GFR) has increased by 50% and remains at that level until delivery. Twenty-four-hour creatinine clearance is increased; serum creatinine and urea concentrations decrease. Sodium balance is maintained because tubular reabsorption of water and electrolytes increases in proportion to the GFR and the effects of the mineralocorticoids. Glycosuria often occurs because of decreased tubular reabsorption and the increased load.

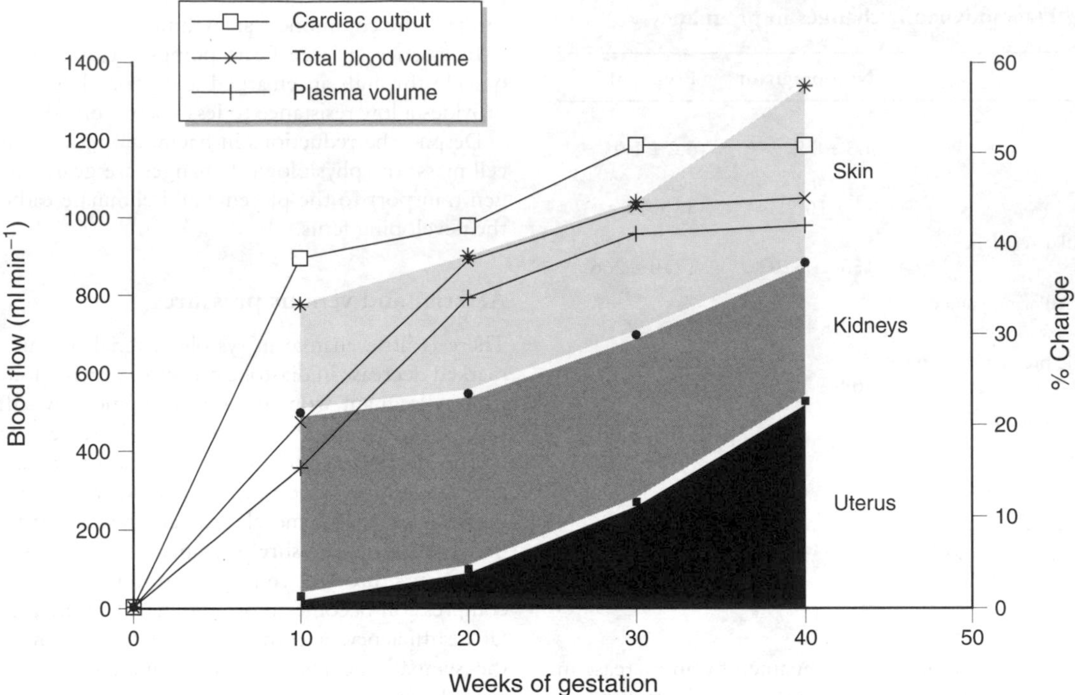

Fig. 29.3
Diagrammatic representation of changes in blood flow to various organs during pregnancy, together with percentage changes in cardiac output, and blood and plasma volumes.

Increased levels of aldosterone, cortisol and human placental lactogen contribute to the changes in renal function. The renal pelvis, calyces and ureters dilate as a result of the action of progesterone and intermittent obstruction from the uterus, especially on the right.

Liver blood flow is *not* increased. Serum concentrations of total proteins, especially albumin, are reduced in blood, further reducing plasma oncotic pressure. Serum alkaline phosphatase concentration is increased by a factor of 2–4, but the major source of this enzyme is the placenta (50%). The increase in liver alkaline phosphatase concentration may result from injuries to the canalicular membrane. Concentrations of aspartate aminotransferase (AST) and alanine aminotransferase (ALT) are altered only slightly in pregnancy; an increase in concentrations of these enzymes indicates liver dysfunction. Serum lipids and cholesterol concentrations are markedly increased. Plasma cholinesterase concentration decreases by 30%. This is probably only clinically significant in women who are heterozygous for an abnormal gene or who have had plasmapheresis for Rhesus isoimmunization.

Blood flow to the nasal mucosa is increased. Nasal intubation may be associated with epistaxis.

There is a great increase in blood flow to the skin, resulting in warm, clammy hands and feet. The purpose of this vasodilatation, together with that in the nasal mucosa, is to dissipate heat from the metabolically active fetoplacental unit.

RESPIRATORY CHANGES

Respiratory function undergoes several important modifications (Table 29.3), also as a result of the action of progesterone. The larger airways dilate and airway resistance decreases. The transverse and anteroposterior diameters of the thorax increase *early* in pregnancy. Chest wall compliance and total lung compliance decrease by about 30%. This enables the mechanical component of ventilation to facilitate the increase in tidal volume (from 10 to 12 weeks) and the minute volume (50%). Progesterone exerts a stimulant action on the respiratory centre and carotid body receptors.

Table 29.3 Changes in respiratory function in pregnancy

Variable	Non-pregnant	Term pregnancy
Tidal volume ↑	450 ml	650 ml
Respiratory rate	16 min^{-1}	16 min^{-1}
Vital capacity	3200 ml	3200 ml
Inspiratory reserve volume	2050 ml	2050 ml
Expiratory reserve volume ↓	700 ml	500 ml
Functional residual capacity ↓	1600 ml	1300 ml
Residual volume ↓	1000 ml	800 ml
P_aO_2 slight ↑	11.3 kPa	12.3 kPa
P_aCO_2 ↓	4.7–5.3 kPa	4 kPa
pH slightly ↑	7.40	7.44

P_aO_2, arterial oxygen tension; P_aCO_2, arterial carbon dioxide tension.

Forced expiratory volume in 1 s (FEV_1) and peak expiratory flow rate (PEFR) are unaffected.

Anatomical dead space is unchanged (until late pregnancy, when upper airway oedema may cause a reduction) but physiological dead space increases. The dead space/tidal volume (V_D/V_T) ratio is unchanged, as is the alveolar–arterial oxygen tension difference $P_{A-a}O_2$, although alveolar ventilation is increased by 20% at term.

Alveolar hyperventilation leads to a low arterial carbon dioxide tension (P_aCO_2) during the second and third trimesters. The significance of the low P_aCO_2 is apparent when gas exchange in the placenta is considered.

The functional residual capacity (FRC) is reduced by about 300 ml at term because of the enlarged uterus. The residual volume is also reduced by 20–30%. This substantial reduction, combined with the increase in tidal volume, results in large volumes of inspired air mixing with a smaller volume of air in the lungs. The composition of alveolar gas may be altered with unusual rapidity; inhalation induction of anaesthesia is rapid but alveolar and arterial hypoxia also develop more rapidly during apnoea or airway obstruction. In normal pregnancy, closing volume does not intrude into tidal volume.

Oxygen consumption ($\dot{V}O_2$) increases gradually from 200 to 250 ml min^{-1} at term (up to 500 ml min^{-1} in labour). Carbon dioxide production parallels oxygen consumption. Rapid desaturation occurs during apnoea at term. Desaturation occurs even more rapidly in women with multiple pregnancies and in morbidly obese pregnant women, illustrating the combined effect of increased oxygen consumption, decreased mechanical effectiveness of ventilation and an even lower FRC.

Arteriovenous oxygen difference is smaller in early pregnancy because the increase in cardiac output occurs before the increase in oxygen consumption. The average non-pregnant level is not achieved until the third trimester (i.e. oxygen-carrying capacity more than compensates for increased oxygen demand).

Blood gas tensions, acid–base balance and the oxyhaemoglobin dissociation curve

By the 12th week of pregnancy, P_aCO_2 may be as low as 4.1 kPa (P_aCO_2 gradually reduces during the premenstrual phase of the menstrual cycle). Progesterone also enhances the response of the respiratory centre to carbon dioxide; for every 0.13 kPa increase in P_aCO_2, the pregnant woman increases ventilation by about 6 L min^{-1} (2 L min^{-1} in non-pregnant subjects). The respiratory alkalosis is accompanied by a decrease in plasma bicarbonate concentration resulting from renal excretion (base excess decreases from 0 to −3.5 mmol L^{-1}). Arterial pH does not change significantly. Peripheral venous pH is higher because of the increase in peripheral blood flow. Progesterone also increases the concentration of carbonic anhydrase B in red cells, which tends to decrease P_aCO_2 independently of any change in ventilation.

The oxyhaemoglobin dissociation curve is shifted to the right because the increase in red cell 2,3-diphosphoglycerate (2,3-DPG) concentration outweighs the effects of a low PCO_2 and high pH, both of which normally shift the curve to the left. The P_{50} increases from about 3.5 to 4.0 kPa. Thus, oxygen delivery and carbon dioxide transport to and from the tissues (i.e. the fetoplacental unit) are enhanced. Changes in respiratory variables are shown in Table 29.3.

GASTROINTESTINAL CHANGES

These also stem from the effects of progesterone on smooth muscle.

A reduction in lower oesophageal sphincter pressure occurs before the enlarging uterus exerts its mechanical effects (an increase in intragastric pressure and a decrease in the gastro-oesophageal angle). These mechanical effects are greater when there is multiple pregnancy, hydramnios or morbid obesity. A history of heartburn denotes a lax gastro-oesophageal sphincter.

Placental gastrin increases gastric acidity. Together with the sphincter pressure changes, this makes regurgitation and inhalation of acid gastric contents more likely to occur during pregnancy.

Gastrointestinal motility decreases but gastric emptying is not delayed during pregnancy. However, it is delayed during labour but returns to normal by 18 h after delivery. Pain, anxiety and systemic opioids (including epidural and subarachnoid administration of opioids) aggravate gastric stasis. Small and large intestinal transit times are increased in pregnancy and may result in constipation.

The effects of labour on gastric emptying coupled with the mechanical changes cause the labouring woman to be at risk of regurgitation of gastric acid until approximately 18 h after delivery.

HAEMOSTATIC MECHANISMS IN PREGNANCY

As placental separation takes place following parturition, a blood flow of 500–800 ml min^{-1} must be arrested within a few seconds or serious blood loss may occur. Arrest of bleeding depends on the complex interaction of the three components of haemostasis:

Vasoconstriction. In the placental bed, this is dependent mainly on myometrial retraction. Prostacyclin is an unstable prostaglandin synthesized by blood vessels. It is a vasodilator and potent inhibitor of platelet aggregation, protecting the vessel wall from platelet deposition. Prostacyclin concentrations increase in pregnancy. It is synthesized in increasing quantities by the placenta and the uterus as pregnancy advances. Umbilical cord arteries also produce prostacyclin.

Formation of an adequate platelet plug at the site of injury. Platelets have a key role in the maintenance of vascular integrity and in blood coagulation. Platelet count and function (i.e. aggregation) remain unchanged in normal pregnancy. Platelets produce thromboxane A_2 (TXA_2), which causes vasoconstriction and platelet aggregation. There is a balance between production of prostacyclin by vessel walls and production of thromboxane by platelets. This dynamic equilibrium controls the tendency of the platelets to aggregate. Increased prostacyclin production in pregnancy helps to promote increased blood flow to the fetoplacental unit. The fetus is able to maintain a low arterial pressure in the umbilical arteries despite a high cardiac output.

In pre-eclampsia, the TXA_2/prostacyclin ratio is altered so that there is vasoconstriction and platelet aggregation. This leads to poor placental blood flow.

Activation of the clotting cascade. Blood becomes hypercoagulable and fibrinolytic activity is reduced. Although these changes prevent excessive blood loss at delivery, they predispose the pregnant woman to two apparently opposing hazards: haemorrhage and thrombosis.

Changes in clotting factors (Table 29.4)

In the intrinsic pathway, factor VIII concentration doubles; in the extrinsic pathway, factor VII concentration increases 10-fold. In the common pathway, factor X and fibrinogen concentrations increase (this alters the negative surface charge on red cells which form rouleaux, and increases the ESR). Concentrations of factors II and V increase in early pregnancy and then decrease steadily. Concentrations of antithrombin IIIa and factors XI and XIII decrease because of consumption at the placental site as a result of low-level coagulation with fibrin deposition (5–10% of total circulating fibrinogen). Bleeding time, prothrombin time and partial thromboplastin time remain within normal limits.

Plasma fibrinogen concentration increases from the 12th week to twice that in the non-pregnant state. A progressive inhibition of fibrinolysis occurs from 11 to 12 weeks. Plasminogen remains unchanged, plasminogen activator activity decreases and the concentrations of the inhibitors (antiplasmin and macroglobulin) increase, leading to delayed fibrinolysis, especially in late pregnancy. The hypercoagulable state of the blood and the reduced fibrinolytic activity represent a compensatory response to local utilization of fibrin and are advantageous for haemostasis at placental separation.

Table 29.4 Coagulation changes in late pregnancy
Fibrinogen increased from 2.5 (non-pregnant value) to 4.6–6.0 g L^{-1}
Factor II slightly increased
Factor V slightly increased
Factor VII increased 10-fold
Factor VIII increased – twice non-pregnant state
Factor IX increased
Factor X increased
Factor XI decreased 60–70%
Factor XII increased 30–40%
Factor XIII decreased 40–50%
Antithrombin IIIa decreased slightly
Plasminogen activator reduced
Plasminogen inhibitor increased
Fibrinogen-stabilizing factor falls gradually to 50% of non-pregnant value

THE EPIDURAL AND SUBARACHNOID SPACES

The volume of the vertebral canal is finite. An increase in volume of contents of one compartment reduces the compliance of the other compartments and increases the pressures throughout.

In pregnancy, the epidural veins are dilated by the action of progesterone. These valveless veins of Bateson form collaterals and become engorged as a result of aortocaval compression, during a uterine contraction or secondary to raised intrathoracic or intra-abdominal pressure, e.g. coughing, sneezing or expulsive efforts of parturition. The dose of local anaesthetic for epidural analgesia or epidural/subarachnoid anaesthesia is reduced by about one-third for the following reasons:

- Spread of local anaesthetic in either the subarachnoid or epidural space is more extensive as a result of the reduced volume.
- Progesterone-induced hyperventilation leads to a low P_aCO_2 and a reduced buffering capacity; thus, local anaesthetic drugs remain as free salts for longer periods.
- Pregnancy itself produces antinociceptive effects. The onset of nerve block is more rapid, and human peripheral nerves have been shown to be more sensitive to lidocaine during pregnancy. Increased plasma and cerebrospinal fluid (CSF) progesterone concentrations may contribute towards the reduced excitability of the nervous system.
- Increased pressure in the epidural space facilitates diffusion across the dura and produces higher concentrations of local anaesthetic in CSF.
- Venous congestion of the lateral foramina decreases loss of local anaesthetic along the dural sleeves.

In pregnancy, the epidural pressure is slightly positive and becomes negative a few hours after delivery. During contractions, the pressure may increase by 0.2–0.8 kPa and become very high (2.0–5.9 kPa) in the second stage of labour. Because the spread of local anaesthetics is exaggerated during contractions, top-ups should not be administered at that time.

The CSF pressure increases from about 2.2 to 3.8 kPa during contractions and 6.9 kPa in the second stage.

Even if precautions are taken to prevent it, intermittent aortocaval compression always occurs in association with maternal movement. Consequently, the epidural veins become intermittently and unpredictably engorged.

MATERNAL PHARMACOKINETICS

Changes in plasma volume, body water and fat, haematocrit, protein concentrations, protein binding, cardiac output and regional blood flow radically affect maternal handling of drugs. In addition to concerns regarding teratogenicity, doses of drugs for chronic disease such as epilepsy may need to be adjusted in pregnancy.

SUMMARY

There is a hyperdynamic circulation of an increased blood volume to the placenta. The metabolic changes caused by the respiratory system encourage haemoglobin to give up its oxygen and take up carbon dioxide. The kidneys rapidly filter the increased blood volume but maintain homeostasis.

Relaxed arterioles and venous capacitance vessels accommodate the increased blood volume. The increase in plasma volume with a reduction in serum albumin concentration reduces colloid osmotic pressure. Blood viscosity is reduced, which assists blood flow to all organs vital for the metabolic support of the pregnancy (e.g. liver) and preparation for nutrition of the newborn (e.g. breast).

The effect of the changes in blood volume and dilatation of epidural veins is also reflected in the altered physiology of the epidural and subarachnoid spaces, which changes the pharmacological profile of epidural and subarachnoid analgesia and anaesthesia.

THE PLACENTA

The placenta (Figs 29.4–29.6) is both a vital barrier and a vital link between maternal and fetal circulations. It also has hormonal and immunological functions.

The placenta consists of maternal and fetal tissue – the basal and chorionic plates, separated by the intervillous space. The structures, which enable the placenta to function, arise from these plates.

The basal plate comprises the following structures:

- The *decidua basalis*, forming the placental bed. Decidual septa arise from this layer. These septa do not reach the chorionic plate but greatly increase the surface area exposed to the intervillous space.
- *Decidua capsularis*, overlying the fetus.
- *Decidua parietalis* – a parietal layer which fuses with the amnion to form the amniochorionic membrane containing liquor.

The decidua basalis contains the final branch of the uterine vasculature – the spiral arteries. These end-arteries open into the intervillous space. The spiral arteries have no smooth muscle.

Chorionic villi are formed from the chorionic plate. The fertilized ovum, i.e. the blastocyst, is attached firmly to the endometrium via an outer layer of cells (the trophoblast) which proliferates into an inner layer (cytotrophoblast) and an outer layer (syncytiotrophoblast). Both layers arborize to form chorionic villi dipping into the intervillous space. Initially cuboidal, these cells become flatter with increased arborization. Microvilli enhance their surface area, facilitating transfer of gases and other substances.

The chorionic villi containing branches of the umbilical vein and artery are bathed by maternal blood from the spiral arteries (Figs 29.5 and 29.6). These either release spurts of blood into the intervillous space or wind round the chorionic villi. Thus the two circulations are separated by two layers of cells – the cytotrophoblast and the syncytiotrophoblast.

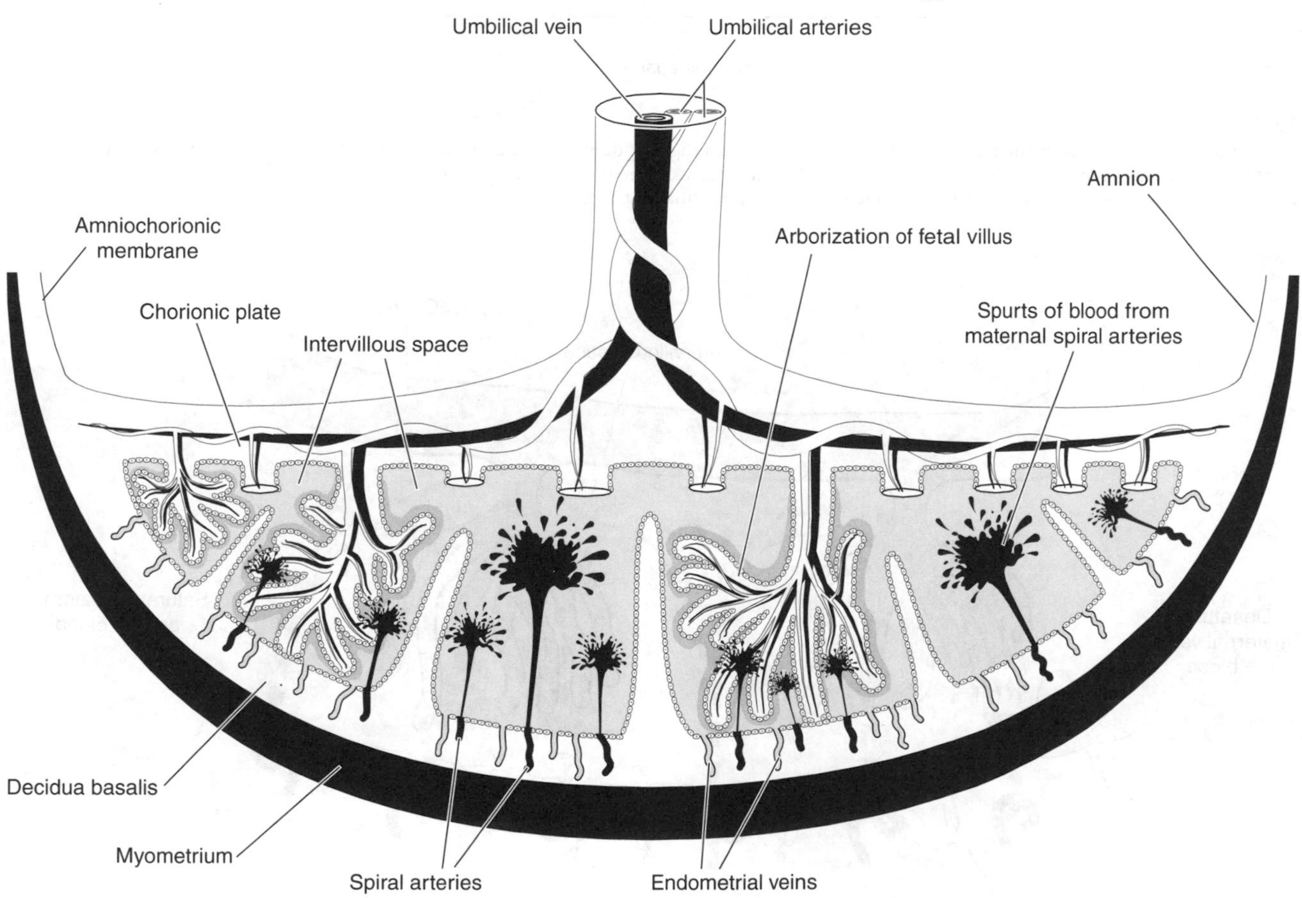

Fig. 29.4
The placenta.

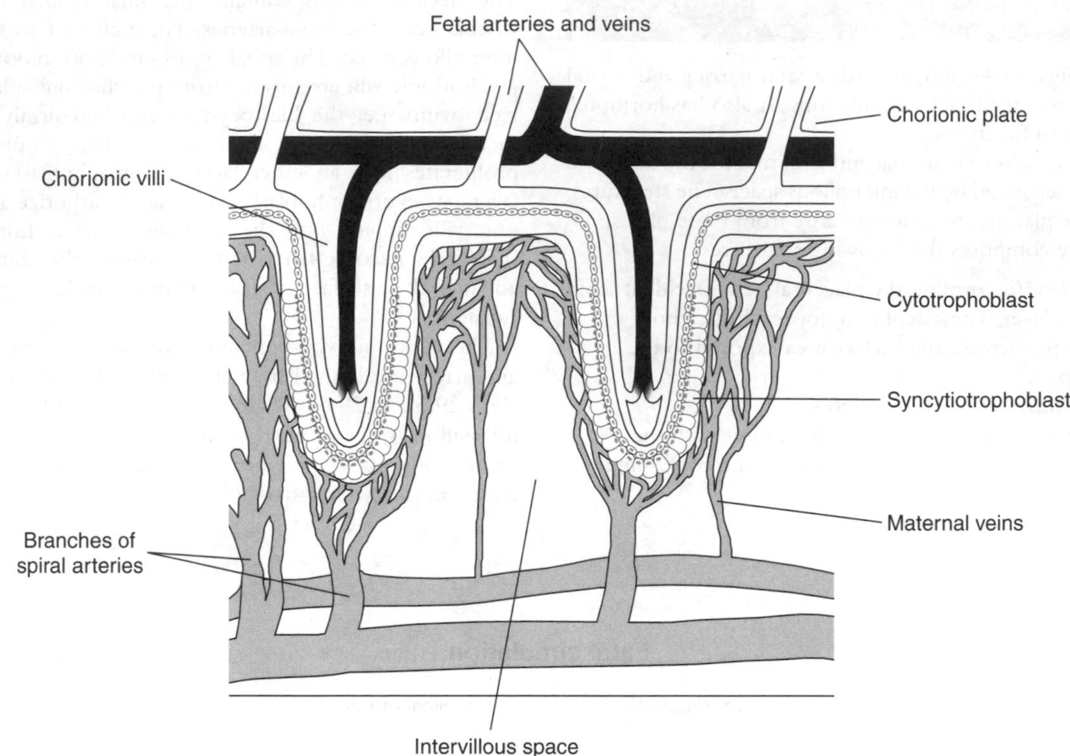

Fig. 29.5
Maternal and fetal blood vessels in the placenta. Chorionic villi are seen dipping down into the maternal circulation. Maternal vessels either envelop a chorionic villus or release spurts of blood directly into the intervillous space. The two circulations are separated by two layers of cells. These cells have microvilli and present a huge surface area for exchange of gases and essential nutrients.

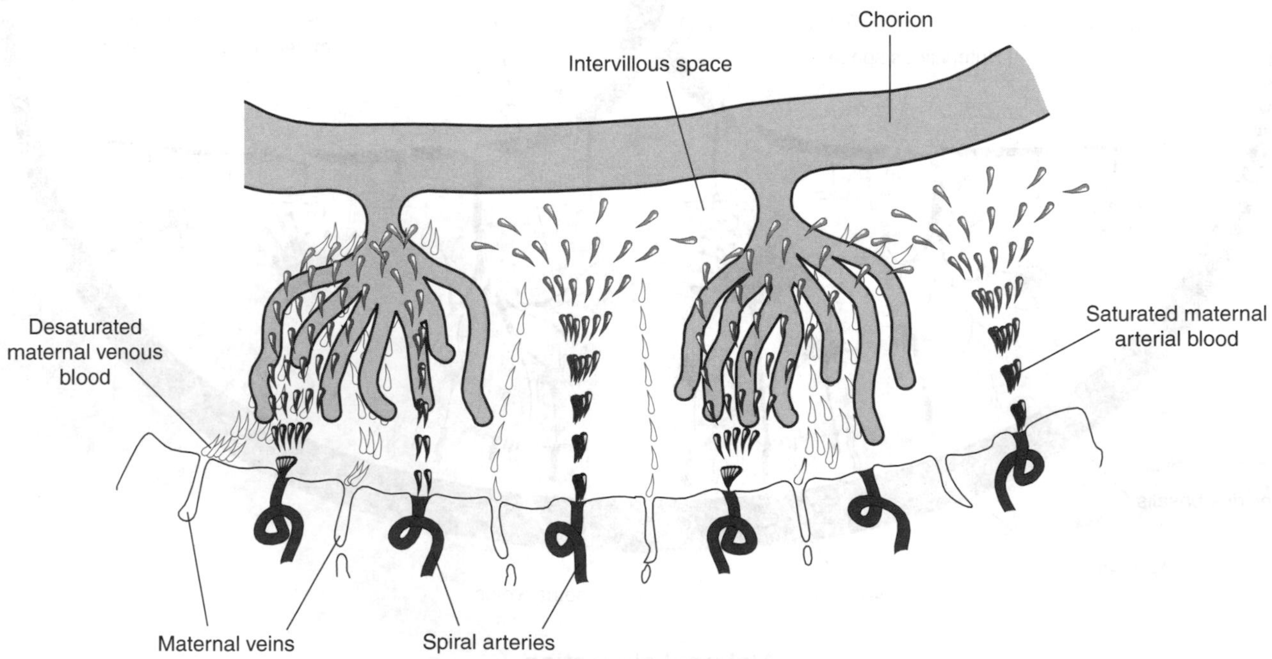

Fig. 29.6
Maternal blood bathes the fetal vessels in the chorionic villi. Some maternal blood circles the fetal villi before draining into the maternal veins; some enters the centre of a villus, and disperses laterally before draining; some is ejected from spiral arteries directly into the intervillous space.

With increasing gestation, the cytotrophoblast ceases to be a continuous layer and is represented by individual cells beneath the syncytiotrophoblast. In turn, syncytiotrophoblastic cells unite with fetal capillary endothelial cells to form a vasculosyncytial membrane.

PLACENTAL BLOOD FLOW

Fetal well-being depends on an adequate placental blood flow. At term, the uterine blood flow is approximately 500–700 ml min^{-1}, of which 70–90% is distributed to the placenta.

The smooth muscle in the spiral arteries disappears during placentation, thus providing a low resistance to the driving pressure of the maternal cardiac output, which forces blood into the intervillous space.

Placental blood flow depends on the balance between the perfusion pressure across the intervillous space and the resistance of the spiral arteries. Placental perfusion is therefore reduced by changes in cardiac output (e.g. haemorrhage) or uterine hypertonicity (e.g. overstimulation by Syntocinon). The spiral and uterine arteries possess α-receptors. Maternal sympathetic stimulation caused by hypotension or catecholamine release resulting from pain may markedly reduce placental perfusion.

Intervillous pressure is increased by intrauterine (i.e. amniotic fluid) pressure and by increased venous pressure (e.g. aortocaval compression).

$$\text{Placental blood flow} = \frac{\text{uterine arterial pressure} - (\text{intrauterine pressure} + \text{uterine venous pressure})}{\text{intrinsic resistance of spiral arteries} + \text{extrinsic resistance (myometrial tone)}}$$

The normal fetus may tolerate a 50% reduction in uteroplacental blood flow, because there is good circulatory reserve.

FUNCTIONS OF THE PLACENTA

Hormonal

Placental syncytiotrophoblasts secrete human chorionic gonadotrophin (hCG). hCG production commences in very early pregnancy, increases at a remarkable rate, peaks at 8–10 weeks, and declines until a few weeks before term when secretion starts to increase again. The rapid increase in early pregnancy is to stimulate the corpus luteum to secrete progesterone to maintain the viability of the pregnancy. No obvious biological function for hCG in late pregnancy has yet been defined.

Human placental lactogen (hPL) concentration increases from 0.3 μg L^{-1} at 10–14 weeks to 5.4 μg L^{-1} by 35–38 weeks. It increases lipolysis, inhibits gluconeogenesis and prevents glucose uptake by maternal tissues (i.e. an anti-insulin effect). hPL can be considered as a metabolic signal by which the fetus obtains nutrients.

Oestrogens. Four oestrogens are secreted: oestrone, oestradiol, oestriol and oestetrol. The role of oestrogens in pregnancy is not entirely clear, although their effect on the breast and the uterus are obvious. They also play a part in fetal development.

Progestogens. Progesterone is the most important hormone in this group and the physiological effects are necessary for the initiation and maintenance of maternal adaptation to pregnancy. Its role in late pregnancy has not been elucidated.

Other hormones. The placenta secretes alkaline phosphatase, cystine aminopeptidase and several other protein hormones. Their role in the physiology of pregnancy is not yet clear.

Immunological

The placenta modifies the immune systems of both mother and fetus so that the fetus is not rejected. The mechanism by which this occurs is poorly understood. In pregnancy there is a reduction in cell-mediated immunity. There is a reduction in the activity of T-cytotoxic cells and a reduction in numbers of T-helper cells. The trophoblast acts as an immunologically inert barrier between mother and fetus. However, there is an increase in numbers and activity of neutrophils. IgG is transferred to the fetus in utero and confers some passive immunity. It may produce fetal disease. Modification of the maternal immune system may be the cause of the rapid spread of some cancers during pregnancy and the rapidity with which some viral disorders become life-threatening, e.g. chickenpox with pneumonitis.

Transport of respiratory gases

This is the most important function of the placenta. Gas exchange between mother and fetus takes place in the intervillous space and is governed by the laws of diffusion, aided by the different oxygen affinities of maternal and fetal haemoglobins. Fetal haemoglobin (HbF) has a much higher affinity for oxygen than does adult haemoglobin (HbA). The high affinity of HbF is explained partly by diminished binding of 2,3-DPG in the central cavity which is formed by the gamma chains. Thus 2,3-DPG cannot facilitate release of oxygen in the placenta; HbF can carry more oxygen than can HbA.

The oxyhaemoglobin dissociation curve (ODC) of HbF is to the left of that for HbA. As the oxygen tension decreases on the normal oxygen cascade, HbA unloads 4.7 ml of oxygen from each 100 ml of blood, whereas HbF unloads only 3.0 ml of oxygen. However, between an oxygen tension of 2.0 kPa (fetal tissue) and 4.5 kPa (placenta), HbF loads 10.3 ml of oxygen to each 100 ml of blood, compared with 8.8 ml for HbA. The loading–unloading advantages of HbF are at *low* oxygen tensions.

The sequence of events in placental gas transfer is best considered in the following steps:

1. Fetal blood gives up carbon dioxide.
2. Fetal blood becomes more alkaline.
3. Fetal ODC shifts further to the left, increasing oxygen affinity.
4. Fetal carbon dioxide diffuses across to maternal blood.
5. Maternal pH decreases.
6. Maternal ODC shifts to the right (Bohr effect).
7. Oxygen release is facilitated.
8. Oxygen is taken up by left-shifted fetal ODC (double Bohr effect).
9. Within the placenta, HbF becomes more acidic with oxygenation.
10. HbF releases carbon dioxide (Haldane effect).
11. HbA becomes less acidic as it becomes increasingly deoxygenated.
12. HbA binds more carbon dioxide (double Haldane effect).
13. Carbon dioxide enters maternal cells.

14. HCO_3^- is formed and exchanged for chloride (reversed Hamburger phenomenon).
15. A fetomaternal diffusion gradient is maintained.
16. Maternal blood has carbonic anhydrase.
17. Therefore, maternal blood has higher carbon dioxide binding power.

In the intervillous space, the diffusion gradient for oxygen is approximately 4.0 kPa, and for carbon dioxide is approximately 1.3 kPa.

Placental exchange of oxygen is regulated mainly by a change in oxygen affinities of HbA and HbF caused principally by altered hydrogen ion and carbon dioxide concentrations on both sides of the placenta.

Without the double Bohr and double Haldane effects, the diffusion gradients or placental blood flow would have to be increased considerably to maintain the same efficiency of gas transfer.

PLACENTAL TRANSFER OF DRUGS

The barrier between maternal and fetal blood is a single layer of chorion united with fetal endothelium. The surface area of this is vastly increased by the presence of microvilli. Placental transfer of drugs occurs, therefore, by passive diffusion through cell membranes which are lipophilic. However, this membrane appears to be punctuated by channels which allow transfer of hydrophilic molecules at a rate that is around 100 000 times lower.

Hence drugs cross the placenta by simple diffusion of un-ionized lipophilic molecules. Fick's law of diffusion applies. The rate is directly proportional to the maternofetal concentration gradient and the area of the placenta available for transfer, and inversely proportional to placental thickness. Lipid solubility, degree of ionization and protein binding affect placental transfer, as do the dose and route of administration and absorption, distribution and metabolism in the mother.

Lipid solubility

The placental membrane is freely permeable to lipid-soluble substances which undergo flow-dependent transfer. As the rate of transfer depends on the concentration gradient of the drug across the membrane and blood flow on each side, maternal hypotension reduces placental blood flow and, consequently, transfer of lipid-soluble drugs.

Hydrophilic substances

The placental membrane carries an electrical charge; ionized molecules with the same charge are repelled, while those with the opposite charge are retained within the membrane. The rate of this permeability-dependent transfer is inversely proportional to molecular size. Size limitation for polar substances begins at molecular weights between 50 and 100 Da. Ions diffuse much more slowly. Factors affecting the degree of ionization alter the rate of transfer.

Maternal pH

This alters ionization of a partially ionized drug. The maternal–fetal pH gradient also affects transfer. The degree of ionization of acidic drugs is greater on the maternal side and lower on the fetal side. The converse applies for basic drugs.

Protein binding

A dynamic equilibrium exists between bound (unavailable) and unbound (available) drug. Protein binding is pH-dependent, e.g. acidosis reduces protein binding of local anaesthetics. Reduced albumin concentration increases the proportion of unbound drug. Many basic drugs are bound to α_1-glycoprotein, which is present in much lower concentrations in the fetus.

THE FETUS

The fetus has adapted to life in a hypoxic environment but adjusts quickly to extrauterine life.

Fetal circulation (Fig. 29.7)

Oxygenated blood in the umbilical vein divides into two branches passing though the ductus venosus and the portal sinus. The ductus venosus enters the inferior vena cava, bypassing the liver. The portal sinus supplies the left lobe of the liver. The blood in the right atrium divides into two streams. The main stream enters the left atrium via the foramen ovale and is carried ultimately to the head, brain and heart via the left ventricle and aorta.

A smaller stream, together with superior vena caval blood, enters the right ventricle. The right ventricle is dominant, ejecting 66% of the combined ventricular output. Blood in the right ventricle enters the pulmonary artery, but the high pulmonary vascular resistance ensures that blood is shunted to the aorta via the ductus arteriosus. Mixing of saturated and desaturated blood takes place, and this blood supplies the lower body of the fetus and enters the umbilical arteries. The low systemic vascular resistance of the placenta aids shunting away from the fetal lungs. The fetus has a high cardiac output (160 ml kg^{-1}) and operates a hierarchy of circulation:

1. non-negotiable – brain, heart, lung tissue
2. negotiable – liver, gut, spleen, kidney
3. expendable – bone, muscles, skin.

The non-negotiable blood flow is unreactive to α- and β-stimulation and very sensitive to changes in partial pressures of oxygen and carbon dioxide ($P\text{O}_2$, $P\text{CO}_2$) and pH; the negotiable and expendable circulations are sensitive to neurogenic and hormonal influences.

Fetal lung

Pulmonary circulation is essentially a high-pressure, low-flow circuit with little blood volume. The adult lung is essentially a low-pressure, high-flow circuit which also acts as a reservoir for the left ventricle. In the fetal lung, the vasomotor responses are greater and the large arteriolar muscle mass confers high resistance. There are very few autonomic nerve endings and the pulmonary blood flow is less sensitive to neurogenic and endocrine stimuli.

Surfactant

Although the respiratory function of the lungs is performed by the placenta before birth, blood supply to the fetal lung is much greater than that to the adult lung because alveolar cells are

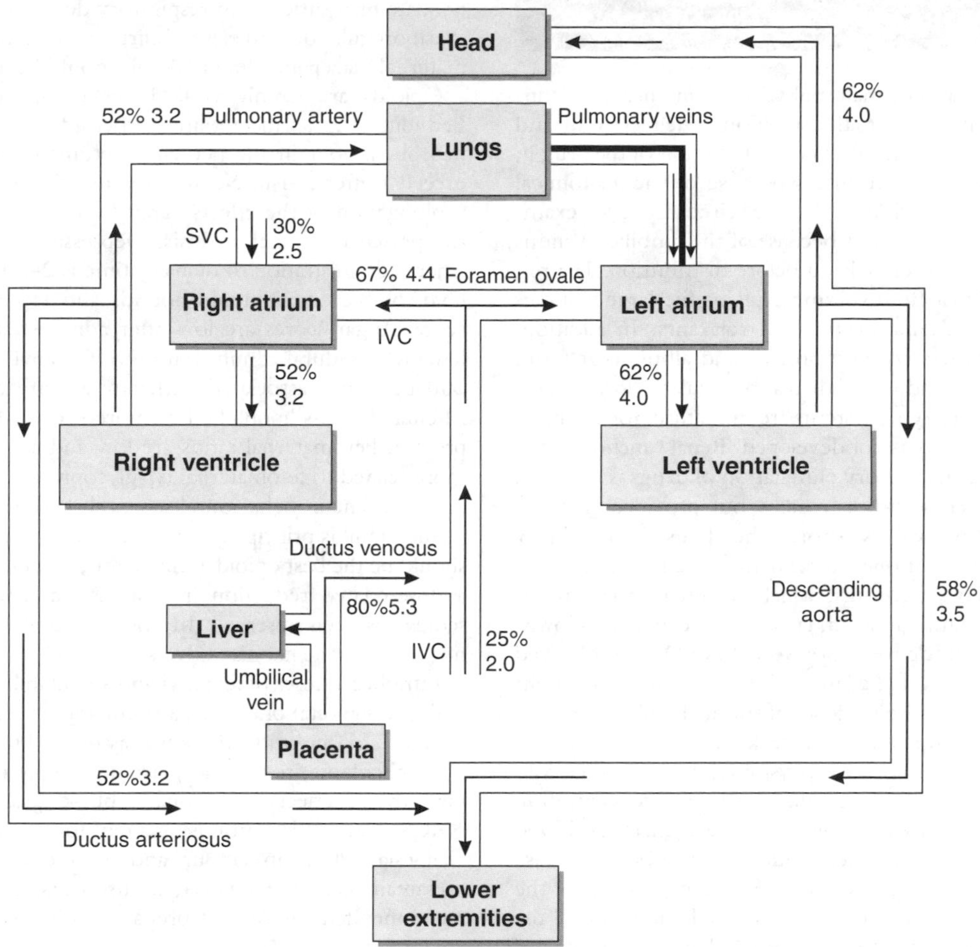

Fig. 29.7
Fetal circulation showing oxygen saturation (So_2, %) and oxygen tension (Po_2, kPa) in different parts of the circulation. SVC, superior vena cava; IVC, inferior vena cava.

metabolically very active. They manufacture surfactant, a complex glycoprotein which confers stability on alveoli. Surfactant is manufactured from 28 weeks' gestation.

Effects of drugs on the fetus

These effects depend on fetal distribution, metabolism and excretion; for example, polar substances cross the placenta slowly, but when they reach the fetus, they are excreted rapidly into the amniotic fluid. Lipophilic substances are transferred quickly, but it may take up to 40 min for equilibration to occur.

THE FIRST BREATH AND CHANGES IN CIRCULATION

The instant the umbilical cord is cut, the fetus becomes physiologically and legally an independent and separate individual. The events may be summarized as follows:

1. During delivery, the chest wall is squeezed.
2. Recoil of the chest wall assists expansion of the lungs against forces of surface tension; the FRC reaches 75% of its ultimate volume in a few minutes.
3. The first gasps may generate intrapleural pressures of –25 to –50 mmHg. Within a few breaths, the fetal P_aO_2 of 2–3.5 kPa becomes the neonatal P_aO_2 of 9–13 kPa.
4. As the lungs expand, pulmonary vascular resistance decreases, and pulmonary capillaries and post-alveolar vessels dilate. Arteriolar constriction decreases because of increasing alveolar Po_2; pulmonary blood flow increases.
5. Right atrial pressure decreases below left atrial pressure. There is functional closure of the foramen ovale.
6. Clamping the umbilical cord increases systemic vascular resistance, which helps to maintain left atrial pressure.
7. Closure of the foramen ovale results in blood from the venae cavae entering the pulmonary circulation.
8. The rapid increase in pulmonary blood flow is assisted by the developing low pulmonary vascular resistance.
9. Flow through the ductus arteriosus is gradually reduced; this, together with an increasing P_aO_2, leads to closure of the ductus.

In the first hour, there may be bidirectional shunting through the ductus but the right-to-left flow gradually decreases. There is a *transitional* circulation until the adult circulatory pattern is irreversibly developed.

EFFECTS OF DRUGS ON THE NEONATE

In many studies, the ratio of maternal vein to umbilical vein concentration is used; this indicates the situation at delivery only and gives little information on the effects or distribution of the drug in the neonate. The distribution differs because of the anatomical and physiological organization of the fetal circulation; for example, drugs accumulate in the liver because of the umbilical venous flow to the liver and are metabolized before distribution. The relatively high extracellular fluid volume explains the large volumes of distribution of local anaesthetics and relaxants. In addition, fetal plasma contains less α_1-glycoprotein and albumin at term, which affects protein binding of drugs, particularly local anaesthetics. Many hepatic enzyme systems are immature; for example, the hydroxylating pathway is not developed. Renal function in the neonate is immature, and urinary elimination of drugs is reduced.

Inhalation anaesthetics diffuse readily, but provided that the induction–delivery interval is short, the fetus is minimally affected. Neonatal elimination is dependent on ventilation.

Neuromuscular blocking drugs, which are quaternary ammonium compounds and fully ionized, cross the placenta very slowly. Fetomaternal ratios at delivery are very low. Only prolonged administration of a relaxant, e.g. in the intensive care unit, might lead to neonatal paralysis. Bolus doses of succinylcholine are safe.

Thiopental is highly lipid-soluble, weakly acidic, 75% protein-bound and less than 50% ionized at physiological pH. It therefore crosses the placenta rapidly, with umbilical vein concentration closely following the relatively rapid decrease in maternal blood concentration. Fetal plasma concentration continues to increase for around 40 min after single exposure. However, because of the relatively large fetal volume of distribution, fetal and neonatal tissue concentrations are lower than maternal. The maintenance of high maternal thiopental concentration by repeated boluses maintains a high diffusion gradient, producing prolonged placental transfer and neonatal sedation. Doses of thiopental greater than 8 mg kg^{-1} produce neonatal depression, whereas doses of less than 4 mg kg^{-1} produce no significant neonatal effects providing induction to delivery time is less than 5 min. Thiopental in such doses does not affect Apgar score or umbilical cord gas tensions, but may produce subtle changes in the neuroadaptive (NACS) score, such as reduction in muscular tone, decreased excitability and a predominant sleep state in the first day of life. A dose of thiopental of 4–7 mg kg^{-1} is commonly advocated for induction of general anaesthesia because it ensures unconsciousness. Widespread clinical use testifies to the safety of thiopental.

Propofol is highly protein-bound, neutral and lipophilic. Propofol has been used for both induction and maintenance of anaesthesia for caesarean section. There is conflicting evidence concerning the effects of propofol on the neonate. Clearly, if propofol is administered by infusion and uterine blood concentrations are maintained, a high diffusion gradient is maintained across the placenta and therefore persistently high transfer of propofol. Induction doses as low as 2–3 mg kg^{-1} and maintenance doses as low as 5 mg kg^{-1} h^{-1} have been shown to cause significant neonatal depression. Neonatal elimination of propofol is slower than that in adults. Unless thiopental is contraindicated, there seems little advantage in using propofol for caesarean section.

Diazepam is a sinister agent. It is a non-polar compound which is bound to albumin, but the fetomaternal ratio may reach 2. The neonate may suffer from respiratory depression, hypotonia, poor thermoregulation and raised bilirubin concentrations. Prolonged maternal diazepam administration should be avoided, if possible.

Opioids are mainly weak bases bound to α_1-glycoprotein. Pethidine and its metabolite norpethidine depress all aspects of neurobehaviour in the neonate. Fetomaternal ratios increase to exceed 1 after 2–4 h. Neonatal elimination is slower, resulting in prolongation of the effects. Transfer of pethidine is increased in the presence of fetal acidosis. Depressant effects are maximum where administration to delivery time is 2–3 h. Fentanyl is highly lipid-soluble and albumin-bound, and rapidly crosses the placenta. Apgar scores are low after administration of intravenous fentanyl. Epidural administration of fentanyl in doses of less than 200 µg is not associated with any adverse effect on the fetus. Alfentanil is less lipophilic but more protein-bound to α_1-glycoprotein. Fetomaternal ratios are low and at caesarean section are more related to fetomaternal α_1-glycoprotein levels. Theoretically, Apgar and neurobehavioural scores should be less affected.

Sufentanil is principally bound to α_1-glycoprotein. Therefore it should be the best opioid additive for epidural analgesia. However, a dose-related reduction in both Apgar and neurobehavioural scores has been observed. In doses of less than 30 µg, it appears not to affect the neonate adversely.

Intrathecal doses of fentanyl and sufentanil have been associated with sudden fetal bradycardia occurring within 30 min of administration. In one study, there was associated uterine hypertonicity.

Remifentanil crosses the placenta rapidly but appears to have few adverse effects on neonatal blood gas tensions, Apgar or NACS scores. It is a promising agent for use in patient-controlled analgesia (PCA) in labour and as a continuous infusion for caesarean section. However, its use outside clinical trials is not recommended. Its current preparation is unsuitable for spinal or epidural use.

ASSESSMENT OF THE NEONATE

Perinatal asphyxia is a relatively rare cause of permanent neurological damage. Neonates are commonly assessed clinically at birth and progress monitored if necessary. The Apgar score is not sensitive enough to detect neurobehavioural changes. The Brazelton neonatal assessment score is the basis of neonatal neurobehavioural assessment systems:

- *Early neonatal neurobehavioural scale (ENNS)*. This is based on the neonate's ability to adapt to the environment and depends on tests of habituation, reflexes, tone, placing and alertness, and is finalized by a general assessment of the neonate's behaviour. Although better than an Apgar score, it is very subjective.
- *Neurological and adaptive capacity score (NACS)*. This was introduced to assess the effects of medication on labour, perinatal asphyxia and birth trauma. It includes response and habituation to sound and light, consolability, active and passive tone, and primary reflexes, and is finalized by a general assessment.

Drugs produce generalized motor depression. Birth trauma or asphyxia may lead to unilateral or upper body hypotonia.

The long-term significance of transient neurobehavioural changes is difficult to assess. Capillary and umbilical blood gas tensions are being used increasingly as an assessment of peripartum asphyxia. Umbilical arterial pH is lower than venous pH and represents fetal blood. An umbilical venous pH below 7.0 is associated with a risk of hypoxic ischaemic encephalopathy (HIE) which becomes more common with a pH below 6.8.

LACTATION AND DRUGS IN OBSTETRIC ANAESTHESIA

Women are encouraged to breast feed. Oestrogen and progesterone stimulate mammary development during pregnancy. These hormones inhibit prolactin. This inhibition ceases at delivery. Suckling triggers lactation and stimulates the release of more prolactin and oxytocin, both of which promote production of milk.

Many women wish to suckle their infant immediately after delivery and are encouraged to do so. The anaesthetist should know, therefore, if the drugs used for obstetric anaesthesia and analgesia are secreted in the milk and, if so, whether they are likely to have an adverse effect either on the process of lactation itself or on the neonate.

The effects of a drug administered to the mother on a breast feeding neonate are determined by peak plasma concentration of the drug, its transfer into milk, composition of milk, volume ingested by the neonate, metabolism including first pass metabolism by the neonate, pharmacokinetics in the neonate and action in the neonate.

Many studies have relied on assessment of concentration of drug in milk with little consideration of resultant neonatal plasma concentration and the changing composition of breast milk.

Human breast milk consists of an isosmotic emulsion of fat in water, with lactose and protein in the aqueous phase. However, its composition varies with time. Colostrum (first milk) contains abundant protein and lactose but no fat. It has a high pH and specific gravity. Over the following 7–10 days, milk has less protein, less lactose and more fat. Colostrum is more likely to be contaminated by water-soluble drugs, whereas lipid-soluble drugs are secreted into mature milk. The volume of colostrum produced is around 10–120 ml, in contrast to ingestion of mature milk by the neonate of 130–180 ml kg^{-1} day^{-1} (600–1000 ml day^{-1}). Even in mature milk there is a significant diurnal variation in composition.

The maternal concentration of drug presented to the breast varies with dose, route of administration, volume of distribution, lipid solubility, ionization and protein binding.

The physicochemical properties of a drug which determine transfer into the milk are pK_a, the partition coefficient, degree of ionization and molecular weight. The pH of mature human milk is 7.09. Therefore, weak acids are less easily transferred than weak bases.

The total amount of drug contained in the milk depends on binding to milk protein, partition into milk lipid and the quantity which remains unbound in the aqueous phase, e.g. lipid-soluble drugs such as diazepam are concentrated in milk lipid. The dose of drug delivered to the neonate from the milk varies with the volume ingested. The higher gastric pH, different gastrointestinal flora and slow gastrointestinal transit of the neonate influence drug absorption.

The pharmacokinetics of drugs in the neonate may differ markedly from those in adults. Lipophilic and acidic drugs are bound to albumin and may displace unconjugated bilirubin. Metabolic pathways such as hydroxylation, conjugation and oxidation are immature. Immature renal function may delay excretion of drugs and active metabolites dependent on renal excretion.

Opioids. Morphine appears safe with conventional administration. PCA may increase maternal plasma concentration. It is transferred readily to breast milk but does not appear to cause neonatal depression, possibly because of first pass metabolism. Codeine and dihydrocodeine are metabolized to morphine and are not associated with neonatal depression. Pethidine is associated with neurobehavioural depression of the neonate. Short-acting opioids such as fentanyl and alfentanil are safe, even by continuous epidural infusion.

Non-steroidal anti-inflammatory drugs. The non-steroidal anti-inflammatory drugs ketorolac and diclofenac are safe. The neonate has immature biotransformation and excretory pathways. Aspirin should be avoided because high concentrations have been observed following a single oral dose. Neonates may be at risk of developing Reye's syndrome.

Paracetamol is minimally secreted into breast milk. However, it is cleared by the liver more slowly than in adults. It is considered safe.

Thiopental and propofol are detectable in milk and colostrum. However, the dose received by the neonate after a single induction dose is insignificant,

Diazepam and its metabolites are excreted in breast milk. As with placental transfer, there is the possibility of adverse effects on the neonate, especially with continuous administration.

Lidocaine and bupivicaine. The amounts excreted in breast milk are small or undetectable.

FURTHER READING

Philipp E, Selchell M, Ginsburg J 1991 Scientific foundations of obstetrics and gynaecology, 4th edn. Butterworth-Heinemann, London

Reynolds F (ed) 1993 Effects on the baby of maternal analgesia and anaesthesia. Saunders, London

Smith C A, Nelson N M (eds) 1976 The physiology of the newborn infant. CC Thomas, Springfield, IL

Van Zundert A, Ostheimer G W 1996 Pain relief and anesthesia in obstetrics. Churchill Livingstone, Edinburgh

30 Basic physics for the anaesthetist

THE APPLICATION OF PHYSICS IN ANAESTHESIA

Knowledge of simple physics is required in order to understand fully the function of many items of anaesthetic apparatus. This chapter is designed to emphasize the more elementary aspects of physical principles and it is hoped that the reader will be stimulated to read some of the excellent books which are designed for anaesthetists and examine this topic in greater detail (see 'Further reading'). Sophisticated measurement techniques may be required for more complex types of anaesthesia, in the intensive therapy unit and during anaesthesia for severely ill patients and an understanding of the principles involved in performing such measurements is required in the later stages of the anaesthetist's training.

This chapter does not describe all the physical principles which may be encountered in the early stages of anaesthetic training, but concentrates on the more common applications, including pressure and flow in gases and liquids, electricity and electrical safety. However, it is necessary first to consider some basic definitions.

BASIC DEFINITIONS

It is now customary in medical practice to employ the International System (SI) of units. Common exceptions to the use of the SI system include measurement of arterial pressure and, to a lesser extent, gas pressure. Arterial pressure is frequently measured using a mercury column and so 'mmHg' is retained. Pressures in gas cylinders are also referred to frequently in terms of the 'normal' atmospheric pressure of 760 mmHg; this is equal to 1.01 bar (or approximately 1 bar). Low pressures are expressed usually in the SI units of kPa whilst higher pressures are referred to in bar (100 kPa = 1 bar). The basic and derived units of the SI system are shown in Table 30.1.

The fundamental quantities in physics are mass, length and time.

Mass (m) is defined as the amount of matter in a body. The unit of mass is the kilogram (kg), for which the standard is a block of platinum held in a Physics Reference Laboratory.

Length (l) is defined as the distance between two points. The SI unit is the metre (m), which is defined as the distance occupied by a specified number of wavelengths of light.

Time (t) is measured in seconds. The reference standard for time is based on the frequency of resonation of the caesium atom.

From these basic definitions, several units of measurement may be derived:

Velocity is defined as the distance travelled per unit time:

$$\text{velocity } (v) = \frac{\text{distance}}{\text{time}} \text{ m s}^{-1}$$

Table 30.1 Physical quantities

Quantity	Definition	Symbol	SI unit
Length	Unit of distance	l	metre (m)
Mass	Amount of matter	m	kilogram (kg)
Density	Mass per unit volume (m/V)	ρ	kg m^{-3}
Time		t	second (s)
Velocity	Distance per unit time (l/t)	v	m s^{-1}
Acceleration	Rate of change of velocity (v/t)	a	m s^{-2}
Force	Gives acceleration to a mass (ma)	F	newton (N) (kg m s^{-2})
Weight	Force exerted by gravity on a mass (mg)	W	kg × 9.81 m s^{-2}
Pressure	Force per unit area (F/A)	P	N m^{-2}
Temperature	Tendency to gain or lose heat	T	kelvin (K) or degree Celsius (°C)
Work	Performed when a force moves an object (force × distance)	U	joule (J) (N m)
Energy	Capacity for doing work (force × distance)	U	joule (J) (N m)
Power	Rate of performing work (joules per second)	P	watt (W) (J s^{-1})

Acceleration is defined as the rate of change of velocity:

$$\text{acceleration } (a) = \frac{\text{velocity}}{\text{time}} \text{ m s}^{-2}$$

Force is that which is required to give a mass acceleration:

$$\text{force} = \text{mass} \times \text{acceleration}$$
$$= ma$$

The SI unit of force is the newton (N). One newton is the force required to give a mass of 1 kg an acceleration of 1 m s^{-2}:

$$1 \text{ N} = 1 \text{ kg m s}^{-2}$$

Weight is the force of the earth's attraction for a body. When a body falls freely under the influence of gravity, it accelerates at a rate of 9.81 m s^{-2}:

$$\text{weight} = \text{mass} \times g$$
$$= m \times g$$
$$= m \times 9.81 \text{ m s}^{-2}$$

Momentum is defined as mass multiplied by velocity:

$$\text{momentum} = m \times v$$

Work is undertaken when a force moves an object:

$$\text{work} = \text{force} \times \text{distance}$$
$$= F \times l$$
$$= U \text{ N m (or joules, J)}$$

Energy is the capacity for undertaking work. Thus it has the same units as those of work.

Power is the rate of doing work. The SI unit of power is the watt, which is equal to 1 J s^{-1}:

$$\text{power} = \text{work per unit time}$$
$$= \text{joules per second}$$
$$= \text{watt (W)}$$

Pressure is defined as force per unit area:

$$\text{pressure } (P) = \frac{\text{force}}{\text{area}}$$
$$= \text{N m}^{-2}$$
$$= \text{pascal (Pa)}$$

As 1 Pa is a rather small unit, it is more common in medical practice to use the kilopascal (kPa).

FLUIDS

Substances may exist in solid, liquid or gaseous form. These forms or phases differ from each other according to the random movement of their constituent atoms or molecules. In solids, molecules oscillate about a fixed point, whereas in liquids the molecules possess higher velocities and move more freely and thus do not bear a constant relationship in space to other molecules. The molecules of gases also move freely, but to an even greater extent.

Both gases and liquids are termed fluids. Liquids are incompressible and at constant temperature occupy a fixed volume, conforming to the shape of a container; gases have no fixed volume but expand to occupy the total space of a container.

Heating a liquid increases the kinetic energy of its molecules, permitting some to escape from the surface into the vapour phase. Random loss of molecules with higher kinetic energies from a liquid occurs in the process of vaporization. As these molecules possess higher kinetic states, this leads to a reduction in the energy state and cooling of the liquid.

Collision of randomly moving molecules in the gaseous phase with the walls of a container is responsible for the pressure exerted by a gas.

GAS PRESSURES

There are three important laws which determine the behaviour of gases and which are important to anaesthetists.

Boyle's law states that, at constant temperature, the volume (V) of a given mass of gas varies inversely with its absolute pressure (P):

$$PV = k_1$$

Charles' law states that, at constant pressure, the volume of a given mass of gas varies directly with its absolute temperature (T):

$$V = k_2T$$

The third gas law states that, at constant volume, the absolute pressure of a given mass of gas varies directly with its absolute temperature:

$$P = k_3T$$

Combining these three gas laws:

$$PV = kT$$

or

$$\frac{P_1V_1}{T_1} = \frac{P_2V_2}{T_2}$$

The behaviour of a mixture of gases in a container is described by *Dalton's law of partial pressures.* This states that, in a mixture of gases, the pressure exerted by each gas is the same as that which it would exert if it alone occupied the container.

Thus, in a cylinder of compressed air at a pressure of 100 bar, the pressure exerted by nitrogen is equal to 79 bar (as the fractional concentration of nitrogen is 0.79).

Avogadro's hypothesis

Avogadro's hypothesis states that equal volumes of gases at the same temperature and pressure contain equal numbers of molecules.

Avogadro's number is the number of molecules in 1 g molecular weight of a substance and is equal to 6.022×10^{23}.

Under conditions of standard temperature and pressure, 1 g molecular weight of any gas occupies a volume of 22.4 litres (L).

These data are useful in calculating, for example, the quantity of gas produced from liquid nitrous oxide. The molecular weight of nitrous oxide is 44. Thus, 44 g of N_2O occupy a volume of 22.4 L at standard temperature and pressure (STP). If a full cylinder of N_2O contains 3.0 kg of liquid, then vaporization of all the liquid would yield:

$$\frac{22.4 \times 3.0 \times 1000}{44} \text{ L}$$

$$= 1527 \text{ L at STP}$$

Critical temperature

The critical temperature of a substance is the temperature above which that substance cannot be liquefied by pressure, irrespective of its magnitude.

The critical temperature of oxygen is −118°C, that of nitrogen is −147°C, and that of air is −141°C. Thus, at room temperature, cylinders of these substances contain gases. In contrast, the critical temperature of carbon dioxide is 31°C and that of nitrous oxide is 36.4°C. The critical pressures are 73.8 and 72.5 bar, respectively; at higher pressures, cylinders of these substances contain a mixture of gas and liquid.

Clinical application of the gas laws

A ‘full’ cylinder of oxygen on an anaesthetic machine contains compressed gaseous oxygen at a pressure of 137 bar (2000 lb in^{-2}). If the cylinder of oxygen empties at constant temperature, the volume of gas contained is related linearly to its pressure (by Boyle’s law). In practice, linearity is not followed because temperature falls as a result of adiabatic expansion of the compressed gas; the term adiabatic implies a change in the state of a gas without exchange of heat energy with its surroundings.

In contrast, the pressure in a cylinder of nitrous oxide remains relatively constant as the cylinder empties to the point at which liquid has totally vaporized. Subsequently, there is a linear decline in pressure proportional to the volume of gas remaining within the cylinder.

Filling ratio

The degree of filling of a nitrous oxide cylinder is expressed as the mass of nitrous oxide in the cylinder divided by the mass of water that the cylinder could hold. Normally, a cylinder of nitrous oxide is filled to a ratio of 0.67. This should not be confused with the volume of liquid nitrous oxide in a cylinder. A ‘full’ cylinder of nitrous oxide at room temperature is filled to the point at which approximately 90% of the interior of the cylinder is occupied by liquid, the remaining 10% being occupied by gaseous nitrous oxide. Incomplete filling of a cylinder is necessary because thermally induced expansion of the liquid in a totally full cylinder may cause an explosion.

Entonox

Entonox is the trade name for a compressed gas mixture containing 50% oxygen and 50% nitrous oxide. The mixture is compressed into cylinders containing gas at a pressure of 137 bar (2000 lb in^{-2}). The nitrous oxide does not liquefy because the two gases in this mixture ‘dissolve’ in each other at high pressure. In other words, the presence of oxygen reduces the critical temperature of nitrous oxide. The critical temperature of the mixture is −7°C. Cooling of a cylinder of Entonox to a temperature below −7°C results in separation of liquid nitrous oxide. Use of such a cylinder results in oxygen-rich gas being released initially, followed by a hypoxic nitrous oxide-rich gas. Consequently, it is recommended that when an Entonox cylinder may have been exposed to low temperatures, it should be stored horizontally for a period of not less than 24 h at a temperature of 5°C or above. In addition, the cylinder should be inverted several times before use.

Pressure notation in anaesthesia

Although the use of SI units of measurement is generally accepted in medicine, a variety of ways of expressing pressure is still used, reflecting custom and practice. Arterial pressure is still referred to universally in terms of mmHg because a column of mercury is one of the most common means of measurement of pressure and is used also to calibrate electronic devices.

Similarly, measurement of central venous pressure is referred to customarily in cmH_2O.

Atmospheric pressure (P_B) exerts a pressure sufficient to support a column of mercury of height 760 mm (Fig. 30.1).

1 atmospheric pressure = 760 mmHg
= 1.01325 bar
= 760 torr
= 1 atmosphere absolute (ata)
= 14.7 lb in^{-2}
= 101.325 kPa
= 10.33 m H_2O

In considering pressure, it is necessary to indicate whether or not atmospheric pressure is taken into account. Thus, a diver working 10 m below the surface of the sea may be described as compressed to a depth of 1 atmosphere or working at a pressure of 2 atmospheres absolute (2 ata).

In order to avoid confusion when discussing compressed cylinders of gases, the term gauge pressure is used. This refers to the difference between the pressure of the contents of the cylinder and the ambient pressure. Thus, a full cylinder of oxygen has a gauge pressure of 137 bar, but the contents are at a pressure of 138 bar absolute.

PRESSURE RELIEF VALVES

The Heidbrink valve is a common component of many anaesthesia breathing systems. In the Magill breathing system, the anaesthetist may vary the force in the spring(s), thereby controlling the pressure within the breathing system (Fig. 30.2). At equilibrium, the force exerted by the spring is equal to the force exerted by gas within the system:

$$\text{Force } (F) = \text{gas pressure } (P) \times \text{disc area } (A)$$

Modern anaesthesia systems contain a variety of pressure relief valves, in each of which the force is fixed so as to provide a gas escape mechanism when pressure reaches a preset level. Thus, an anaesthetic machine may contain a pressure relief valve operating at 35 kPa, situated on the back bar of the machine between the vaporizers and the breathing system. Modern ventilators may contain a pressure relief valve set at 7 kPa. A much lower pressure is set in relief valves which form part of anaesthetic scavenging systems and these may operate at pressures of 0.2–0.3 kPa.

PRESSURE-REDUCING VALVES (PRESSURE REGULATORS)

Pressure regulators have two important functions in anaesthetic machines:

- They reduce high pressures of compressed gases to manageable levels (acting as pressure-reducing valves).

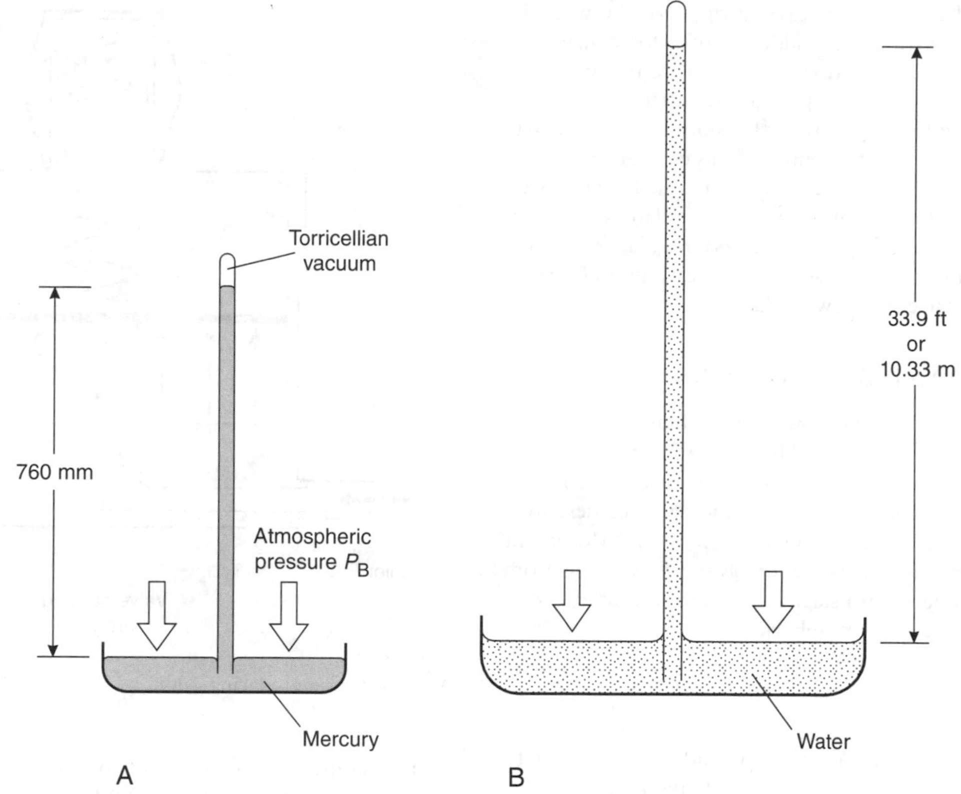

Fig. 30.1
The simple barometer described by Torricelli. **A**. Filled with mercury. **B**. Filled with water.

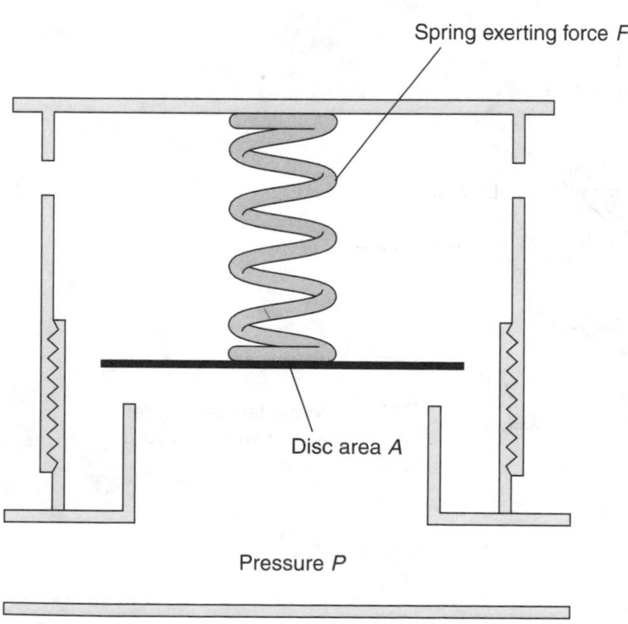

Fig. 30.2
A pressure relief valve.

- They minimize fluctuations in the pressure within an anaesthetic machine, which would necessitate frequent manipulations of flowmeter controls.

Modern anaesthetic machines are designed to operate with an inlet gas supply at a pressure of 3–4 bar (usually 4 bar in the UK). Hospital pipeline supplies also operate at a pressure of 4 bar and therefore pressure regulators are not required between a hospital pipeline supply and an anaesthetic machine. In contrast, the contents of cylinders of all medical gases (i.e. oxygen, nitrous oxide and carbon dioxide) are at much higher pressures. Thus, cylinders of these gases require a pressure-reducing valve between the cylinder and the flowmeter.

The principle on which the simplest type of pressure-reducing valve operates is shown in Figure 30.3. High-pressure gas enters through the valve and forces the flexible diaphragm upwards, tending to close the valve and prevent further ingress of gas from the high-pressure source.

If there is no tension in the spring, the relationship between the reduced pressure (p) and the high pressure (P) is very approximately equal to the ratio of the areas of the valve seating (a) and the diaphragm (A):

$$\frac{p}{P} = \frac{a}{A}$$

By tensing the spring, a force F is produced which offsets the closing effect of the valve. Thus, p may be increased by increasing the force in the spring.

Without the spring, the simple pressure regulator has the disadvantage that reduced pressure decreases proportionally with the decrease in cylinder pressure. The addition of a force from the spring considerably reduces but does not eliminate this problem, and in order to overcome it newer pressure regulators contain an extra closing spring. During high flows, the input to the valve may not be able to keep pace with the output. This can cause the regulated pressure to fall. A two-stage regulator can be employed in order to overcome this. Simple one-stage regulators are often designed for use with a specific gas. A universal regulator in which the body is used for all gases but has different seatings and springs fitted for each particular gas is now available.

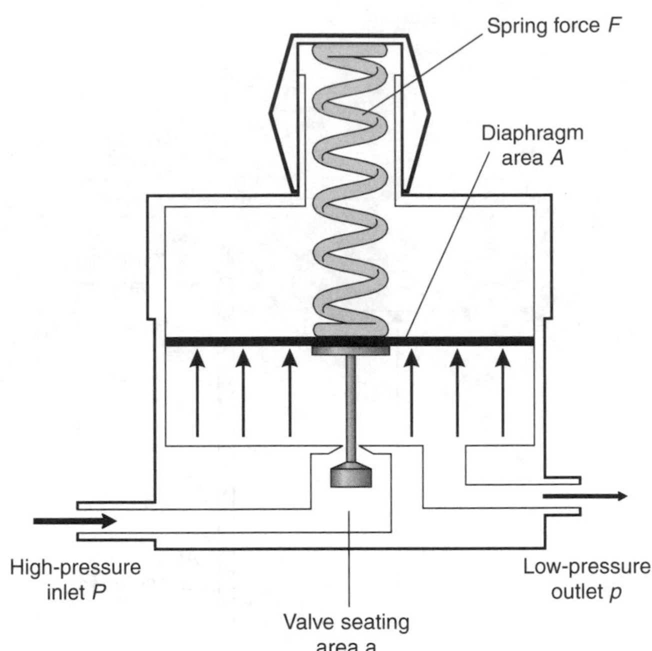

Fig. 30.3
A simple pressure-reducing valve.

PRESSURE DEMAND REGULATORS

These are regulators in which gas flow occurs when an inspiratory effort is applied to the outlet port. The Entonox valve is a two-stage regulator and its mode of action is demonstrated in Figure 30.4. The first stage is identical to the reducing valve described above. The second-stage valve contains a diaphragm. Movement of this diaphragm tilts a rod, which controls the flow of gas from the first-stage valve. The second stage is adjusted so that gas flows only when pressure is below atmospheric.

FLOW OF FLUIDS

Viscosity is defined as that property of a fluid that causes it to resist flow. The coefficient of viscosity (η) is defined as:

$$\eta = \frac{\text{force}}{\text{area}} \times \text{velocity gradient}$$

In this context, velocity gradient is equal to the difference between velocities of different fluid molecules divided by the distance between molecules (Fig. 30.5B). The units of the coefficient of viscosity are Pascal seconds (Pa s).

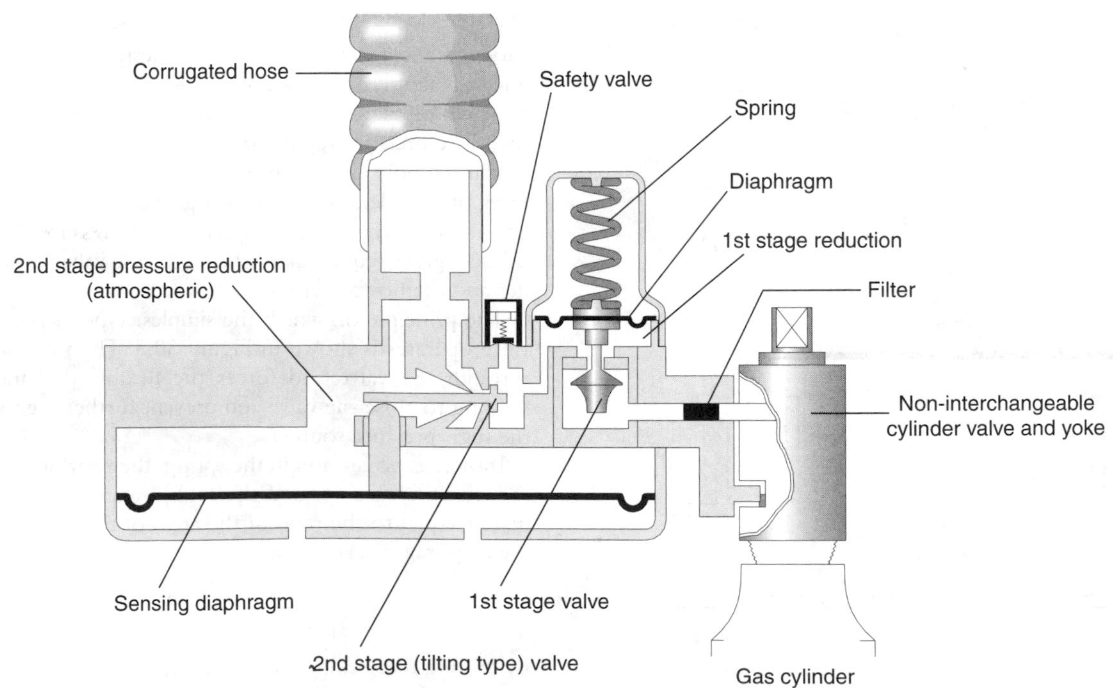

Fig. 30.4
The Entonox two-stage pressure demand regulator.

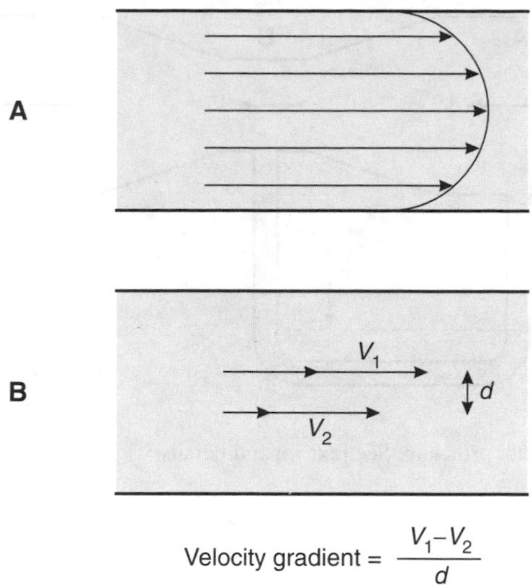

Fig. 30.5
A. Diagrammatic illustration of laminar flow. **B.** Velocity gradient.

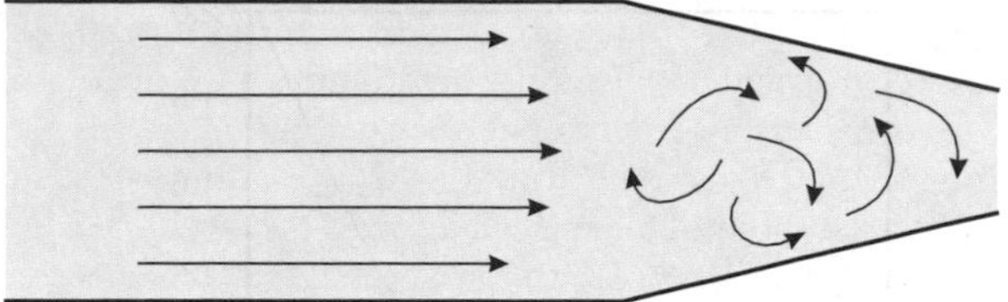

Fig. 30.6
Diagrammatic illustration of turbulent flow.

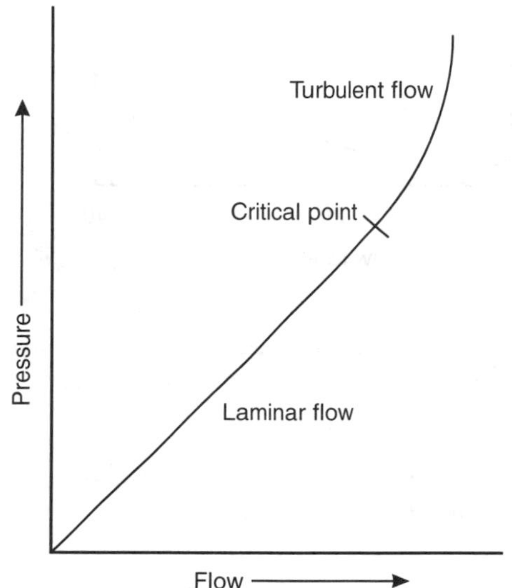

Fig. 30.7
The relationship between pressure and flow in a fluid is linear up to the critical point, above which flow becomes turbulent.

Fluids that obey this formula are referred to as Newtonian fluids and η is a constant for each fluid. However, some biological fluids are non-Newtonian. A prime example is blood; viscosity changes with the rate of flow of blood (as a result of change in distribution of cells) and, in stored blood, with time (blood thickens on storage).

Viscosity of liquids diminishes with increase in temperature, whereas viscosity of a gas increases with increase in temperature.

Laminar flow

Laminar flow through a tube is illustrated in Figure 30.5A. In this situation, there is a smooth, orderly flow of fluid such that molecules travel with the greatest velocity in the axial stream, whilst the velocity of those in contact with the wall of the tube may be virtually zero. The linear velocity of axial flow may be twice the average linear velocity of flow.

In a tube, the factors determining flow are given by the Hagen–Poiseuille formula:

$$\dot{Q} = \frac{\pi \Delta P r^4}{8\eta l}$$

where $\dot{Q}$ is the flow, ΔP is the pressure gradient along the tube, r is the radius of the tube, η is the viscosity of fluid, and l is the length of the tube.

The Hagen–Poiseuille formula applies only to Newtonian fluids. In non-Newtonian fluids such as blood, increase in velocity of flow may alter viscosity because of variation in the dispersion of cells within plasma.

Turbulent flow

In turbulent flow, fluid no longer moves in orderly planes but swirls and eddies around in a haphazard manner as illustrated in Figure 30.6. Although viscosity affects laminar flow, it should be noted that this does not apply to turbulent flow, which is affected by changes in density.

It may be seen from Figure 30.7 that the relationship between pressure and flow is linear within certain limits. However, as velocity increases, a point is reached (the critical point or critical velocity) at which the characteristics of flow change from laminar to turbulent. The critical point is dependent upon several factors, which were investigated by the physicist Reynolds. The factors are related by the formula used for calculation of Reynolds' number:

$$\text{Reynolds' number} = \frac{v\rho r}{\eta}$$

where v is the linear velocity, r is the radius of the tube, ρ is the density, and η is the viscosity.

Studies with cylindrical tubes have shown that if Reynolds' number exceeds 2000, flow is likely to be turbulent, whereas a Reynolds' number of less than 2000 is usually associated with laminar flow.

Flow of fluids through orifices

In an orifice, the diameter of the fluid pathway exceeds the length. The flow rate of a fluid through an orifice is dependent upon:

- the square root of the pressure difference across the orifice
- the square of the diameter of the orifice

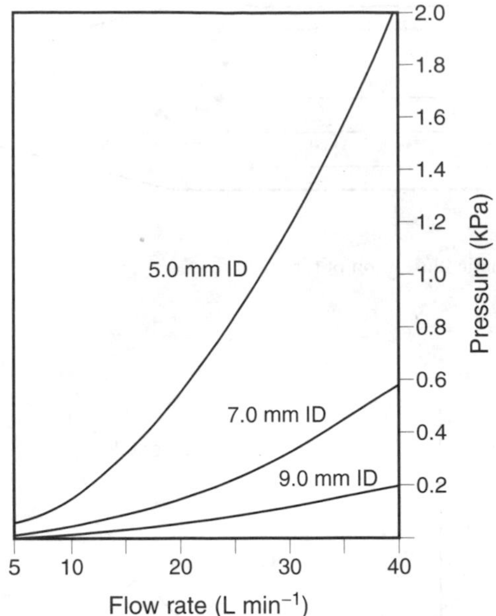

Fig. 30.8
Resistance to gas flow through tracheal tubes of different internal diameter (ID).

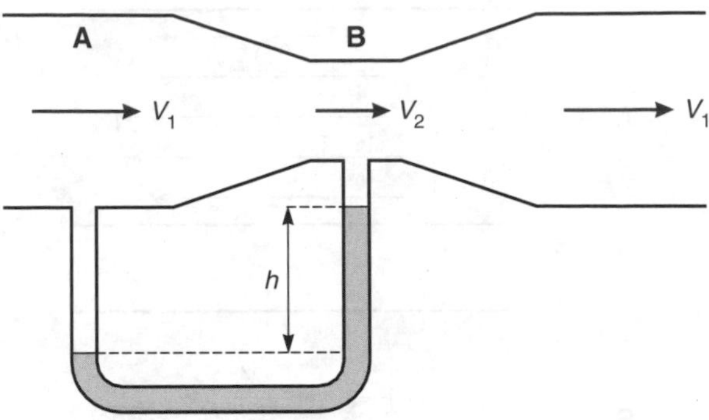

Fig. 30.9
The Bernoulli principle. See text for full details.

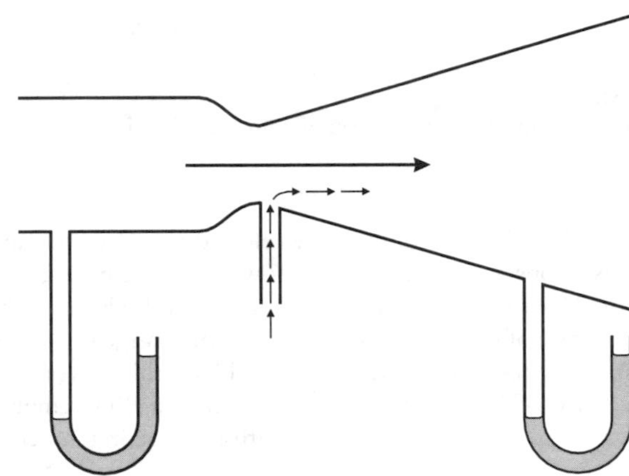

Fig. 30.10
Fluid entrainment by a Venturi injector.

- the density of the fluid, as flow through an orifice inevitably involves some degree of turbulence.

Applications in anaesthetic practice

- In upper respiratory tract obstruction of any severity, flow is inevitably turbulent; thus for the same respiratory effort, a lower tidal volume is achieved than when flow is laminar. The extent of turbulent flow may be reduced by reducing gas density; clinically it is common practice to administer oxygen-enriched helium rather than oxygen alone (the density of oxygen is 1.3 and that of helium is 0.16).
- In anaesthetic breathing systems, a sudden change in diameter of tubing or irregularity of the wall may be responsible for a change from laminar to turbulent flow. Thus, tracheal and other breathing tubes should possess smooth internal surfaces, gradual bends and no constrictions, and should be of as large a diameter and as short a length as possible.
- Resistance to breathing is much greater when a tracheal tube of small diameter is used (Fig. 30.8).

THE INJECTOR

The injector is frequently termed a Venturi, although the principles governing such an apparatus were formulated by Bernoulli in 1778, some 60 years earlier than Venturi. The principle is illustrated in Figure 30.9. As fluid passes through a constriction, there is an increase in velocity of the fluid; beyond the constriction, velocity decreases to the initial value. At point A, the energy in the fluid is both potential and kinetic, but at point B the amount of kinetic energy is much greater because of the increased velocity. As the total energy state must remain constant, potential energy is reduced at point B and this is reflected by a reduction in pressure. Venturi's contribution to the injector lay in the design of the tube distal to the site of the constriction. For optimum performance, it is necessary for fluid flow to remain laminar in such a tube. In the Venturi tube, the pressure is least at the site of maximum constriction and, by gradual opening of the tube beyond the constriction, a subatmospheric pressure may be induced distal to the constriction (Fig. 30.10).

The injector principle may be seen in anaesthetic practice in the following situations:

- *Oxygen therapy.* Several types of Venturi oxygen masks are available which provide oxygen-enriched air. With an appropriate flow of oxygen (usually exceeding 4 L min^{-1}), there is a large degree of entrainment of air. This results in a total gas flow that exceeds the patient's peak inspiratory flow rate, thus ensuring that the inspired oxygen concentration remains constant, and it prevents an increase in apparatus dead space which always accompanies the use of low-flow oxygen devices (see p. 534).
- *Nebulizers.* These are used to entrain water from a reservoir. If the water inlet is suitably positioned, the entrained water may be broken up into a fine mist by the high gas velocity.

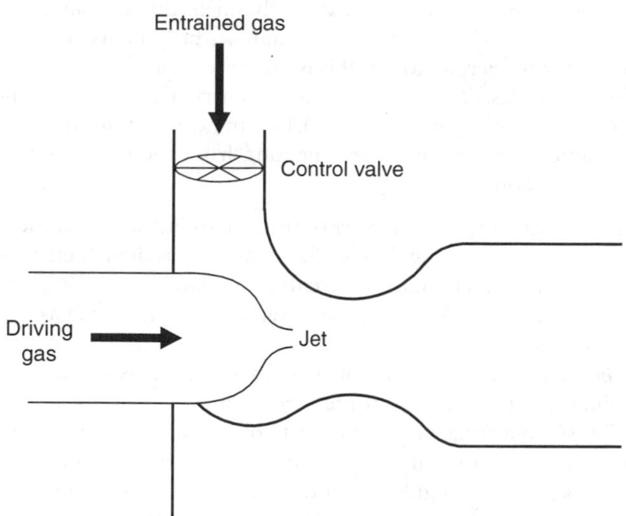

Fig. 30.11
A simple injector.

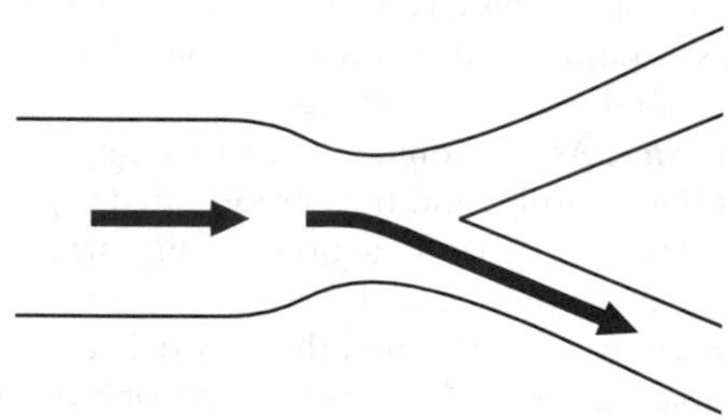

Fig. 30.12
The Coanda effect.

- *Portable suction apparatus.*
- *Oxygen tents.*
- *As a driving gas in a ventilator* (Fig. 30.11).

The Coanda effect

The Coanda effect describes a phenomenon whereby gas flow through a tube with two Venturis tends to cling either to one side of the tube or to the other. The principle has been used in anaesthetic ventilators (termed fluidic ventilators), as the application of a small pressure distal to the restriction may enable gas flow to be switched from one side to another (Fig. 30.12).

HEAT AND TEMPERATURE

Temperature is a measure of the tendency of an object to gain or lose heat. Heat is the energy which can be transferred from a body at a hotter temperature to one at a colder temperature.

THERMOMETRY

In the SI system, the unit of temperature is the kelvin (K). The zero reference point on this scale is absolute zero (0 K or −273.15°C) and the upper point is the triple point of water (the temperature at which water exists simultaneously in solid, liquid and gaseous states); this corresponds to 273.16 K or 0.01°C. The Celsius scale is also widely used. The intervals on this scale are identical to those on the kelvin scale (K) and the relationship between the two scales is as follows:

$$\text{temperature (K)} = \text{temperature (°C)} + 273.15$$

Temperature is measured in clinical practice by one of the following techniques:

- *Liquid expansion thermometer.* Mercury and alcohol are the more commonly used liquids.
- *Thermistor.* This is a semiconductor, which exhibits a reduction in electrical resistance with increase in temperature.
- *Thermocouple.* This relies on the Seebeck effect. When two metal conductors are joined together to form a circuit, a potential difference is produced which is proportional to the difference in temperatures of the two junctions. In order to measure temperature, one junction has to be kept at a constant temperature.
- *Chemical thermometers.* These thermometers are described in more detail in Chapter 31.

HEAT CAPACITY

The heat capacity of a body is the amount of heat required to raise the temperature of the body by 1°C; in the SI nomenclature, heat capacity is measured in units of joules per kelvin (J K^{-1}).

Specific heat capacity

The specific heat capacity of a substance is the energy required to raise the temperature of 1 kg of a substance by 1 K. Thus:

$$\text{heat capacity} = \text{mass} \times \text{specific heat capacity}$$

The specific heat capacity of different substances is of interest because anaesthetists are frequently concerned with maintenance of body temperature in unconscious patients.

Heat is lost from patients by the processes of:

- conduction
- convection
- radiation
- evaporation.

The specific heat capacity of gases is up to 1000 times smaller than that of liquids. Consequently, humidification of inspired gases is a more important method of conserving heat than warming dry gases; in addition, the use of humidified gases minimizes the very large energy loss produced by evaporation of fluid from the respiratory tract.

The skin acts as an almost perfect radiator; radiant losses in susceptible patients may be reduced by the use of reflective aluminium foil ('space blanket').

VAPORIZATION AND VAPORIZERS

In a liquid, molecules are in a state of continuous motion because of mutual attraction by Van der Waal's forces. Some molecules may develop velocities sufficient to escape from these forces, and if they are close to the surface of a liquid these molecules may escape to enter the vapour phase. Increasing the temperature of a liquid increases its kinetic energy and a greater number of molecules escape. As the faster moving molecules escape into the vapour phase, the net velocity of the remaining molecules reduces; thus the energy state and therefore temperature of the liquid phase are reduced. The amount of heat required to convert a unit mass of liquid into a vapour without a change in temperature of the liquid is termed the heat of vaporization.

In a closed vessel containing liquid and gas, a state of equilibrium is reached when the number of molecules escaping from the liquid is equal to the number of molecules re-entering the liquid phase. The vapour concentration is then said to be saturated at the specified temperature. Saturated vapour pressure of liquids is independent of the ambient pressure, but increases with increasing temperature.

The boiling point of a liquid is the temperature at which its saturated vapour pressure becomes equal to the ambient pressure. Thus, on the graph in Figure 30.13, the boiling point of each liquid at 1 atmosphere is the temperature at which its saturated vapour pressure is 101.3 kPa.

VAPORIZERS

Vaporizers may be classified into two types:

- drawover vaporizers
- plenum vaporizers.

In the former type, gas is pulled through the vaporizer when the patient inspires, creating a subatmospheric pressure. In the latter type, gas is forced through the vaporizer by the pressure of the fresh gas supply. Consequently, the resistance to gas flow through a drawover vaporizer must be extremely small; the resistance of a plenum vaporizer may be high enough to prevent its use as a drawover vaporizer, although this is not necessarily so.

The principles of both devices are similar. If we consider the simplest form of vaporizer (Fig. 30.14), the concentration (C) of anaesthetic in the gas mixture emerging from the outlet port is dependent upon:

- *The saturated vapour pressure* of the anaesthetic liquid in the vaporizer. Thus, a highly volatile agent such as diethyl ether is present in a much higher concentration than a less volatile agent (i.e. with a lower saturated vapour pressure) such as halothane.
- *The temperature* of the liquid anaesthetic agent, as this determines its saturated vapour pressure.
- *The splitting ratio*, i.e. the flow rate of gas through the vaporizing chamber (F_V) in comparison with that through the bypass ($F - F_V$). Regulation of the splitting ratio is the usual mechanism whereby the anaesthetist controls the output concentration from a vaporizer.
- *The surface area* of the anaesthetic agent in the vaporizer. If the surface area is relatively small during use, the flow of gas through the vaporizing chamber may be too rapid to achieve complete saturation with anaesthetic molecules of the gas above the liquid.
- *Duration of use*. As the liquid in the vaporizing chamber evaporates, its temperature, and thus its saturated vapour pressure, decreases. This leads to a reduction in concentration of anaesthetic in the mixture leaving the exit port.
- *The flow characteristics* through the vaporizing chamber. In the simple vaporizer illustrated, gas passing through the vaporizing chamber may fail to mix completely with vapour as a result of streaming because of poor design. This lack of mixing is flow-dependent.

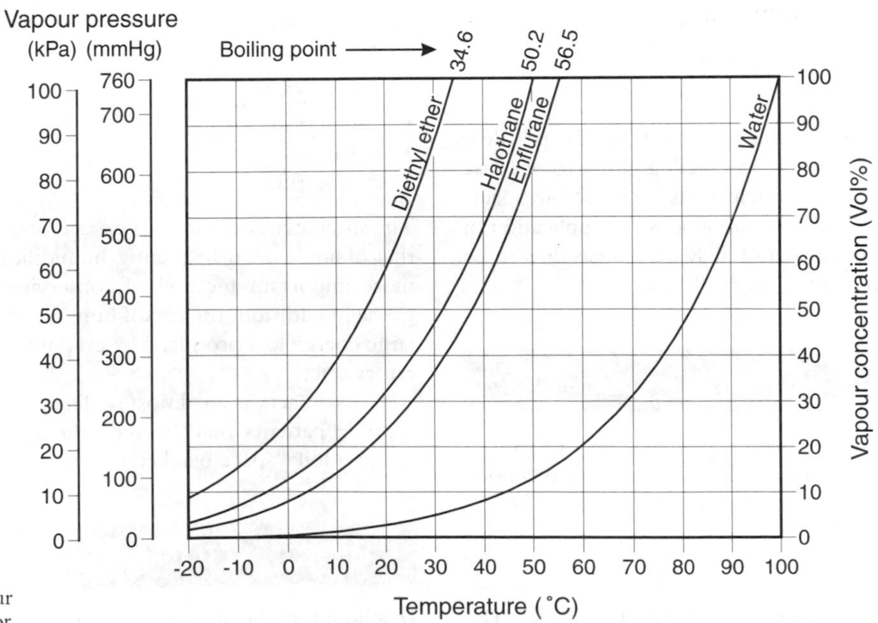

Fig. 30.13
Relationship between vapour pressure and temperature for different anaesthetic agents.

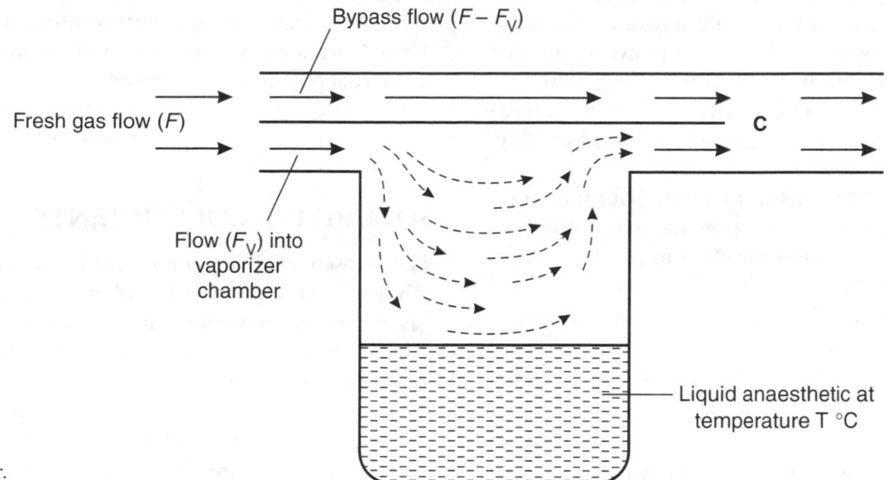

Fig. 30.14
A simple type of vaporizer.

Modern anaesthetic vaporizers overcome many of the problems described above. Maintenance of full saturation may be achieved by making available a large surface area for vaporization. In the TEC series of vaporizers, this is achieved by the use of wicks which draw up liquid anaesthetic and provide a very large surface area. Efficient vaporization and prevention of streaming of gas through the vaporizing chamber are achieved by ensuring that gas travels through a concentric helix, which is bounded by the fabric wicks. Another method of ensuring full saturation is to bubble gas through liquid anaesthetic via a sintered disc. This method is used in the Halox vaporizer and in the Copper Kettle vaporizer. In both these types of vaporizer, the final concentration is determined by mixing a known flow of fresh gas with a measured flow of fully saturated vapour.

Temperature compensation

Temperature-compensated vaporizers possess a mechanism which produces an increase in flow through the vaporizing chamber (i.e. an increased splitting ratio) as the temperature of liquid anaesthetic decreases. In the TEC vaporizers, a bimetallic strip controls (by bending) a valve which alters flow through the exit port of the vaporizing chamber. In the EMO and Ohio vaporizers, a bellows mechanism is used to regulate the valve (by shortening with decreased temperature), whilst in the Drager Vapor 19 vaporizers, a metal rod acts in a similar fashion.

In the Copper Kettle and Halox vaporizers, the temperature in the vaporizer is measured and the flow rate adjusted according to a calibration chart. In addition, reduction in temperature is minimized in the Copper Kettle vaporizer by the method of construction; this comprises a large mass of copper, which provides a large heat capacity, and efficient conduction of heat from the anaesthetic machine to which the vaporizer is attached.

Back pressure (pumping effect)

Some gas-driven mechanical ventilators (e.g. Manley) produce a considerable increase in pressure in the outlet port and back bar of the anaesthetic machine. This pressure is highest during the inspiratory phase of ventilation. If the simple vaporizer shown in Figure 30.14 is attached to the back bar, the increased pressure during inspiration compresses the gas in the vaporizer; some gas in the region of the outlet port of the vaporizer is forced back into the vaporizing chamber, where more vapour is added to it. Subsequently, there is a temporary surge in anaesthetic concentration when the pressure decreases at the end of the inspiratory cycle.

This effect is minimal with efficient vaporizers (i.e. those which saturate gas fully in the vaporization chamber) because gas in the outlet port is already saturated with vapour. However, when pressure reduces at the end of inspiration, some saturated gas passes retrogradely out of the inspiratory port and mixes with the bypass gas. Thus, a temporary increase in total vapour concentration may still occur in the gas supplied to the patient. Methods of overcoming this problem include:

- incorporation of a one-way valve in the outlet port
- construction of a bypass chamber and vaporizing chamber which are of equal volumes so that the gas in each is compressed or expanded equally
- construction of a long inlet tube to the vaporizing chamber so that retrograde flow from the vaporizing chamber does not reach the bypass channel (as in the Mark 3 TEC vaporizers).

HUMIDITY AND HUMIDIFICATION

Absolute humidity is the mass of water vapour present in a given volume of gas. Relative humidity is the ratio of mass of water vapour in a given volume of gas to the mass required to saturate that volume of gas at the same temperature.

Relative humidity (RH) may be expressed as:

$$\text{RH} = \frac{\text{actual vapour pressure}}{\text{saturated vapour pressure}}$$

In normal practice, relative humidity may be measured using:

- *The hair hygrometer.* This operates on the principle that a hair elongates if humidity increases; the hair length controls a pointer. This simple device may be mounted on a wall. It is reasonably accurate only in the range 15–85% relative humidity.

- *The wet and dry bulb hygrometer.* The dry bulb measures the actual temperature, whereas the wet bulb measures a lower temperature as a result of the cooling effect of evaporation of water. The rate of vaporization is related to the humidity of the ambient gas and the difference between the two temperatures is a measure of ambient humidity; the relative humidity is obtained from a set of tables.
- *Regnault's hygrometer.* This consists of a thin silver tube containing ether and a thermometer to show the temperature of the ether. Air is pumped through the ether to produce evaporation, thereby cooling the silver tube. When gas in contact with the tube is saturated with water vapour, it condenses as a mist on the bright silver. The temperature at which this takes place is known as the *dew point*, from which relative humidity is obtained from tables.

HUMIDIFICATION IN THE RESPIRATORY TRACT

Air drawn into the respiratory tract becomes fully saturated in the trachea at a temperature of 37°C. Under these conditions, the SVP of water is 6.3 kPa (47 mmHg); this represents a fractional concentration of 6.2%. The concentration of water is 44 mg L^{-1}. At 21°C, saturated water vapour contains 2.4% water vapour or 18 mg L^{-1}. Thus, there is a considerable capacity for patients to lose both water and heat when the lungs are ventilated with dry gases.

There are three means of humidifying inspired gas:

- heated humidifier (water vaporizer)
- nebulizer
- condenser humidifier (also known as heat and moisture exchanging humidifier).

The hot water bath humidifier is a simple device for heating water to 45–60°C. These devices have several potential problems, including infection if the water temperature decreases below 45°C, scalding the patient if the temperature exceeds 60°C (these high temperatures may be employed to prevent growth of bacteria), and condensation of water in the inspiratory anaesthetic tubing. These devices are approximately 80% efficient.

Some nebulizers are based upon a Venturi system; a gas supply entrains water, which is broken up into a large number of droplets. The ultrasonic nebulizer operates by dropping water onto a surface, which is vibrated at a frequency of 2 MHz. This breaks up the water particles into extremely small droplets. The main problem with these nebulizers is the possibility that supersaturation of inspired gas may occur and the patient may be overloaded with water.

The condenser humidifier (or artificial nose) may consist of a simple wire mesh, which is inserted between the tracheal tube and the anaesthetic breathing system. More recently, humidifiers constructed of rolled corrugated paper have been introduced. These devices are approximately 70% efficient.

SOLUTION OF GASES

Henry's law states that, at a given temperature, the amount of a gas which dissolves in a liquid is directly proportional to the partial pressure of the gas in equilibrium with the liquid. If a liquid is heated and its temperature rises, the partial pressure of its vapour increases. As the total ambient pressure remains constant, the partial pressure of any dissolved gas must decrease.

It is customary to confine the term 'tension' to the partial pressure of a gas exerted by gas molecules in solution.

SOLUBILITY COEFFICIENTS

The Bunsen solubility coefficient is the volume of gas which dissolves in unit volume of liquid at a given temperature when the gas in equilibrium with the liquid is at a pressure of 1 atmosphere.

The Ostwald solubility coefficient is the volume of gas which dissolves in unit volume of liquid at a given temperature. Thus, the Ostwald solubility coefficient is independent of pressure.

The partition coefficient is the ratio of the amount of substance in one phase compared with a second phase, each phase being of equal volume and in equilibrium. As with the Ostwald coefficient, it is necessary to define the temperature but not the pressure. The partition coefficient may be applied to two liquids, but the Ostwald coefficient applies to partition between gas and liquid.

DIFFUSION AND OSMOSIS

If two different gases or liquids are separated in a container by an impermeable partition which is then removed, gradual mixing of the two different substances occurs as a result of the kinetic activity of each molecule. This is illustrated in Figure 30.15. The principle governing this process is described by Fick's law of diffusion, which states that the rate of diffusion of a substance across unit area is proportional to the concentration gradient. Graham's law (which applies to gases only) states that the rate of diffusion of a gas is inversely proportional to the square root of its molecular weight.

In the example shown in Figure 30.15B, the interface between fluids X and Y after removal of the partition would be the surface

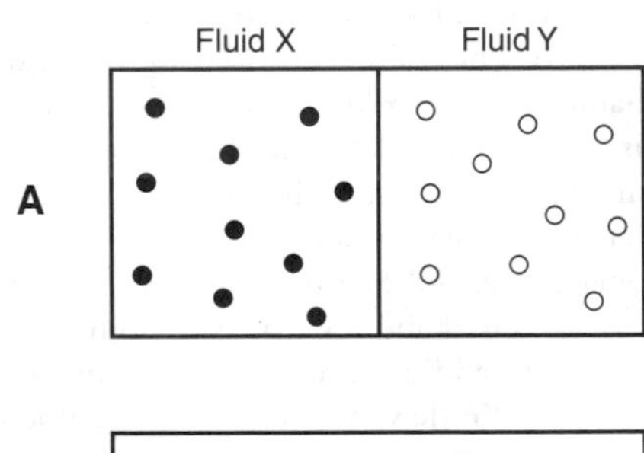

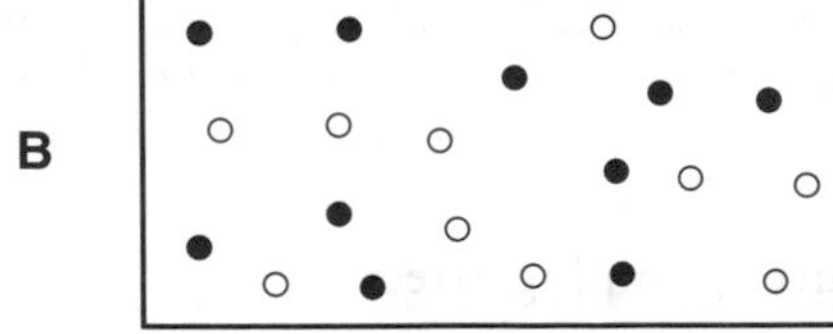

Fig. 30.15
Illustration of diffusion in fluids. **A.** Fluid X and Y separated by partition. **B.** Mixing of fluids after removal of partition.

of the fluid. In biology, however, there is normally a membrane separating gases or separating gas and liquids.

The rate of diffusion of gases may be affected by the nature of the membrane. In the lungs, the alveolar membrane is moist and may be regarded as a water film. Thus, diffusion of gases through the alveolar membrane is dependent not only on the properties of diffusion described above but also on the solubility of gas in the water film. As carbon dioxide is highly soluble compared with oxygen, it diffuses more rapidly across the alveolar membrane, despite the larger partial pressure gradient for oxygen.

OSMOSIS

In the examples given above, the membranes are permeable to all substances. However, in biology, membranes are frequently semipermeable, i.e. they allow the passage of some substances but are impermeable to others. This is illustrated in Figure 30.16. In Figure 30.16A, initially equal volumes of water and glucose solution are separated by a semipermeable membrane. Water molecules pass freely through the membrane to dilute the glucose solution (Fig. 30.16B). By application of a hydrostatic pressure (Fig. 30.16C), the process of transfer of water molecules can be prevented; this pressure (*P*) is equal to the osmotic pressure exerted by the glucose solution.

Substances in dilute solution behave in accordance with the gas laws. Thus, 1 g molecular weight of a dissolved substance occupying 22.4 L of solvent exerts an osmotic pressure of 1 bar at 273 K. Dalton's law also applies; the total osmotic pressure of a mixture of solutes is equal to the sum of osmotic pressures exerted independently by each substance.

The osmotic pressure of a solution depends on the number of dissolved particles per litre. Thus, a molar solution of a substance which ionizes into two particles exerts twice the osmotic pressure exerted by a molar solution of a non-ionizing substance.

The term osmolarity refers to the osmotic pressure produced by all substances in a fluid. Thus, it is the sum of the individual molarities of each particle.

The term osmolality refers to the number of osmoles per kilogram of water or other solvent (whilst osmolarity refers to osmoles per litre of solution). Thus, osmolarity may vary slightly from osmolality as a result of changes in density due to the effect of temperature on volume, although in biological terms the difference is extremely small.

In the circulation, water and the majority of ions are freely permeable across the endothelial membrane, but plasma proteins do not traverse into the interstitial fluid. The term oncotic pressure is used to describe the osmotic pressure exerted by the plasma proteins alone. Plasma oncotic pressure is relatively small (approximately 1 mosmol L^{-1} equivalent to 25 mm Hg) in relation to total osmotic pressure exerted by plasma (approximately 300 mosmol L^{-1} equivalent to 6.5 bar).

ELECTRICAL SAFETY

The anaesthetist is in daily contact with a large amount of equipment which is powered by mains supply electricity; this includes monitoring equipment, some ventilators, suction apparatus, defibrillators and diathermy equipment.

Whilst a total understanding of this equipment and its mode of action may depend upon a detailed knowledge of electronics, the equipment can usually be used safely as a type of 'black box' – i.e. the inside of the box may be a mystery, but the anaesthetist must be familiar with the operating controls and the ways in which the apparatus may malfunction or, if a recording instrument, give rise to artefacts.

It is not possible in this brief chapter to provide a synopsis of the basic principles of electricity and electronics, but it is essential to stress some elements, which have a bearing on the safety of both the patient and the anaesthetist in the operating theatre.

In the UK, the mains electricity is supplied at a voltage of 240 V with a frequency of 50 Hz, and in the USA at a voltage of 110 V and a frequency of 60 Hz. These voltages are potentially dangerous, although the danger is related predominantly to the current which flows through the patient:

$$\text{current } (I) = \frac{\text{voltage } (V)}{\text{resistance } (R)} \quad \text{(Ohm's law)}$$

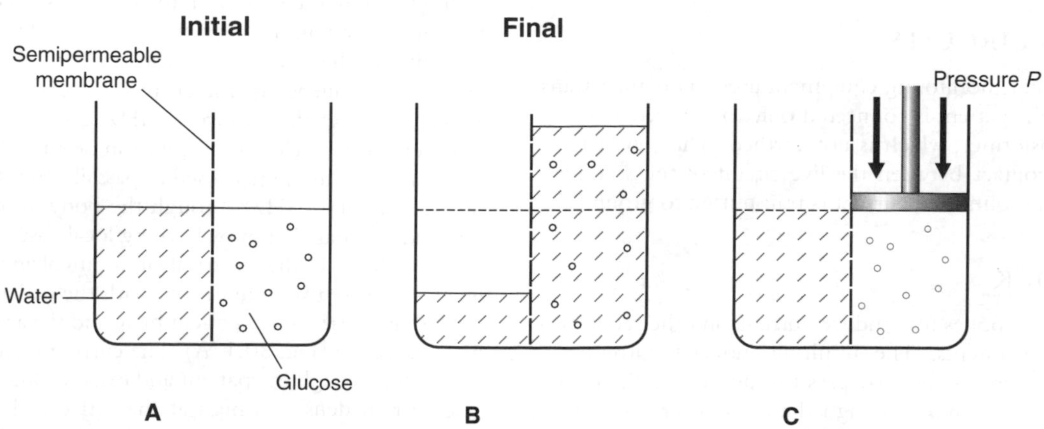

Fig. 30.16
Diagram to illustrate osmotic pressure. **A.** Water and glucose placed into two compartments separated by a semipermeable membrane. **B.** At equilibrium, water has passed into the glucose compartment to balance the pressure. **C.** The magnitude of osmotic pressure of the glucose is denoted by a hydraulic pressure *P* applied to the glucose to prevent any movement of water into the glucose compartment.

When dealing with alternating current, it is necessary to use the term impedance in place of resistance, as impedance takes into account the presence of capacitors and resistors. Direct current cannot pass through capacitors; the resistance of a capacitor is inversely proportional to the frequency of an alternating current.

If an increasing electrical current at 50 Hz passes through the body, there is initially a tingling sensation at a current of 1 mA. Increase in the current produces increasing pain and muscle spasm until, at 80–100 mA, arrhythmias and ventricular fibrillation may occur.

The damage to tissue by alternating current is related also to the current density; a current passing through a small area is more dangerous than the same current passing through a much larger area. Other factors relating to the likelihood of ventricular fibrillation are the duration of passage of the current and its frequency. Radio frequencies (such as those used in diathermy) have no potential for fibrillating the heart.

It is clear from Ohm's law that the size of the current is dependent upon the size of the impedance to current flow. A common way of reducing the risk of a large current injuring the anaesthetist in the operating theatre is to wear antistatic shoes and to stand on the antistatic floor. This provides a high impedance (see below).

There are three classes of electrical insulation which are designed to minimize the risk of a patient or anaesthetist forming part of an electrical circuit between the live conductor of a piece of equipment and ground:

- *Class I equipment* (fully earthed). The main supply lead has three cores (live, neutral and earth). The earth is connected to all exposed conductive parts, and in the event of a fault developing which short-circuits current to the casing of the equipment, current flows from the case to earth and blows a fuse.
- *Class II equipment* (double-insulated). This has no protective earth. The power cable has only live and neutral conductors and these are 'double-insulated'. The casing is normally made of non-conductive material.
- *Class III equipment* (low voltage). This relies on a power supply at a very low voltage produced from a secondary transformer situated some distance away from the device. Potentials do not exceed 24 V (AC) or 50 V (DC). Electric heating blankets, for example, are rendered safer in this way.

ISOLATION CIRCUITS

All modern patient-monitoring equipment uses an isolation transformer so that the patient is connected only to the secondary circuit of the transformer, which is not earthed. Thus, even if the patient makes contact between the live circuit of the secondary transformer and ground, no current is transmitted to ground.

MICROSHOCK

Mains electricity supplies may induce currents in other circuits or on cases of instruments. The resulting induced currents are termed leakage currents and may pass through either the patient or anaesthetist to ground. Although the currents are very small, they may present problems to patients with an intracardiac pacemaker or a saline-filled intracardiac monitoring catheter.

The International Electrotechnical Commission has produced recommendations (adopted by the British Standards Institute) defining the levels of permitted leakage currents and patient currents from different types of electromedical equipment. Whenever new equipment is bought for a hospital, it should be subjected to tests, which will verify that the leakage currents and other electrical safety characteristics are within the allowed specifications. Regular servicing of equipment should be carried out to ensure that these safe characteristics are maintained.

THE DEFIBRILLATOR

Capacitance is the ability to store electric charge. Electric charge is the measure of the amount of electricity and its SI unit is the coulomb (C).

The coulomb is the quantity of electric charge that passes some point when a current of 1 ampere (A) flows for a period of 1 s:

$$\text{coulombs (C)} = \text{amperes (A)} \times \text{seconds (s)}$$

The defibrillator is an instrument in which electric charge is stored in a capacitor and then released in a controlled fashion. Direct current (DC) rather than alternating current (AC) energy is used. DC energy is more effective, causes less myocardial damage and is less arrhythmogenic than AC energy. Defibrillators are set according to the amount of energy stored and this depends on both the stored charge and the potential:

$$\text{available energy (J)} \propto \text{stored charge (C)} \times \text{potential (V)}$$

To defibrillate a heart, two electrodes are placed on the patient's chest; one is placed just to one side of the sternum and the other over the apex of the heart. When it is discharged, the energy stored in the capacitor is released as a current pulse through the patient's chest and heart. This current pulse gives a synchronous contraction of the myocardium after which a refractory period and normal or near-normal beats may follow. The voltage may be up to 5000 V with a stored energy of up to 400 J. In practice, an inductor is included in the output circuit to ensure that the electric pulse has an optimum shape and duration. The inductor absorbs some of the energy which is discharged by the capacitor.

DIATHERMY

The effect of passing electric current through the body varies from slight physical sensation, through muscle contraction to ventricular fibrillation. The severity of these effects depends on the amount and the frequency of the current. These effects become less as the frequency of the current increases, being small above 1 kHz and negligible above 1 MHz. However, the heating and burning effects of electric current can occur at all frequencies.

A diathermy machine is used to pass electric current of high frequency (about 1 MHz) through the body in order to cause cutting and/or coagulation by burning local tissue where the current density is high. In the electrical circuit involving diathermy equipment, there are two connections with the patient. In the unipolar diathermy, these are the patient plate and the active electrode used by the surgeon (Fig. 30.17A). The current travels from the active electrode, through the patient and exits through the patient plate. The current density is high at the active end where burning or cutting occurs, but it is low at the plate end where no injury occurs. If for any reason (e.g. a faulty plate) the current flows from the patient through a small area of contact between the patient and earth, then a burn can occur at the point of contact.

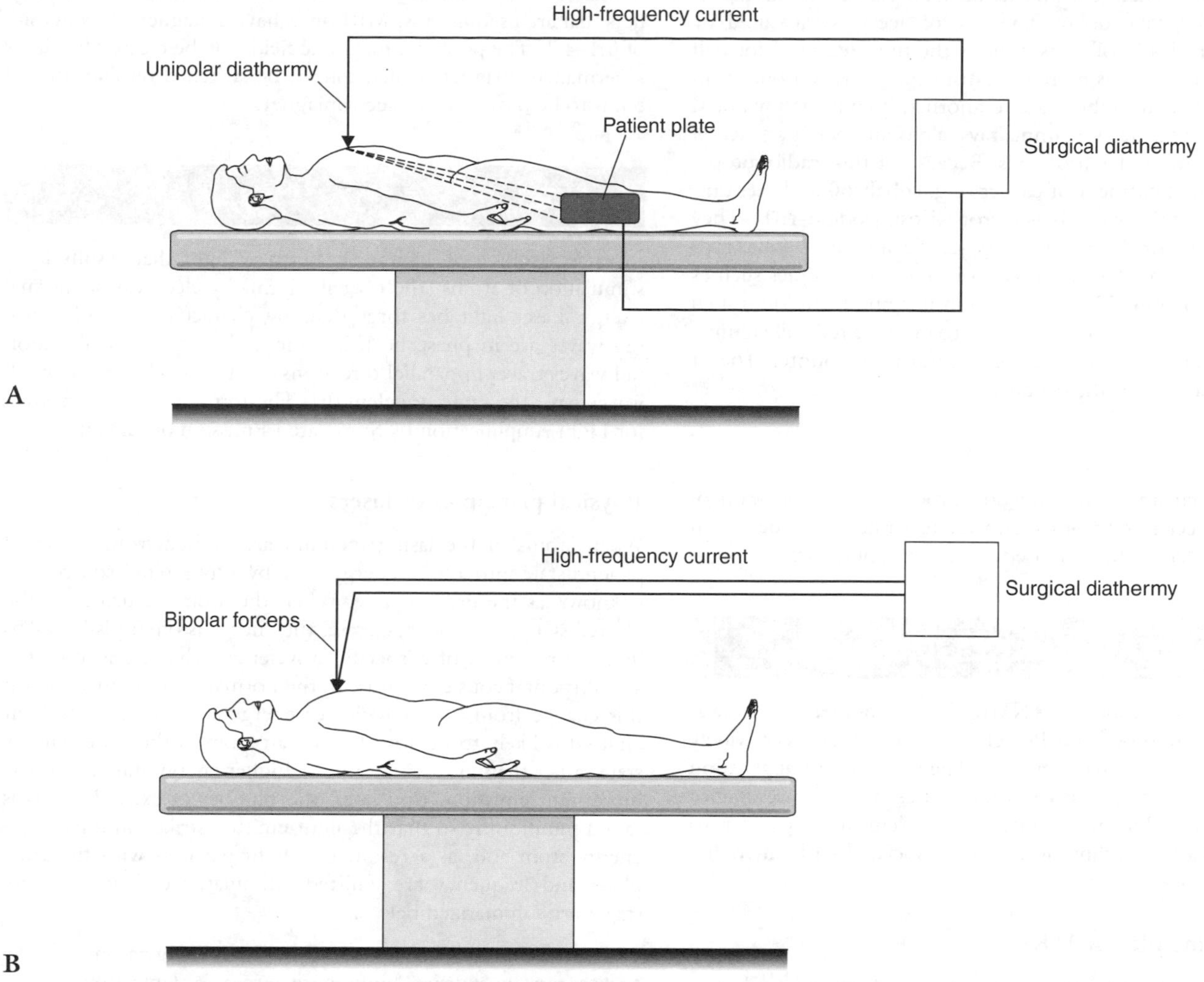

Fig. 30.17
Principle of the surgical diathermy system. **A.** Unipolar diathermy. **B.** Bipolar diathermy.

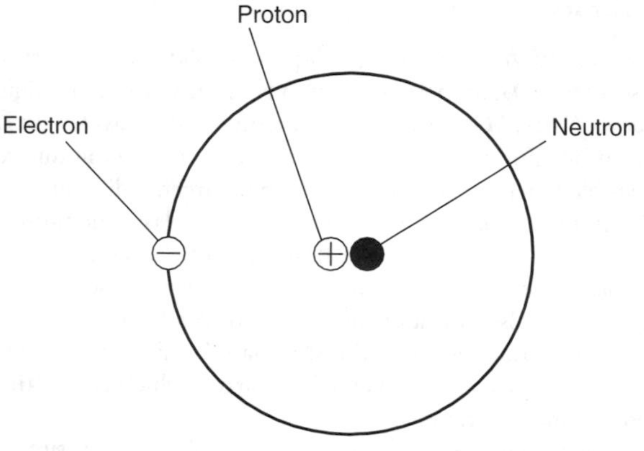

Fig. 30.18
Basic structure of an atom.

In the bipolar diathermy, there is no patient plate, but the current travels down one side of the diathermy forceps and out through the other side (Fig. 30.17B). This type of diathermy uses low power and, because the current does not travel through the patient, it is advisable to use this in patients with a cardiac pacemaker.

ISOTOPES AND RADIATION

An atom consists of electrons which are negatively charged and these orbit around a nucleus which contains protons (positive charge) and neutrons (no charge) (Fig. 30.18). Isotopes are variations of similar atoms but with different numbers of neutrons. Isotopes with unstable nuclei are known as radioisotopes and are radioactive.

The process of change from one unstable isotope to another is known as radioactive decay. The rate of decay is measured by the half-life. Half-life of an isotope is the time required for half of the radioactive atoms present to disintegrate. When one atom changes from one unstable state to another, it emits gamma rays, or alpha or beta particles. Gamma rays, alpha and beta particles all cause damage to or death of cells. Because of this, radioisotopes are used for the treatment of cancer (e.g. cobalt-60 and caesium-137) and for conditions such as thyrotoxicosis (iodine-131). They can also be used for diagnostic purposes. Technetium-99m, krypton-81m and xenon-133 are used in imaging techniques such as scanning. Chromium-51 is used in non-imaging techniques such as labelling of red blood cells in order to measure red cell volume.

Radiation can be detected using a scintillation counter. The SI unit for radioactivity is the becquerel.

X-rays

X-rays are electromagnetic radiation produced when a beam of electrons is accelerated from a cathode to strike an anode (often made of tungsten). They are used for imaging purposes.

MAGNETIC RESONANCE IMAGING

Nuclear magnetic resonance (NMR) is a phenomenon that was first described by Bloch and Purcell in 1945 and has been widely used in chemistry and biochemistry. The more recent application of NMR to imaging came to be known as magnetic resonance imaging (MRI). The word nuclear was removed in order to emphasize that this technique was not associated with any radiation risk.

Physical principles of MRI

Due to the presence of protons, all atomic nuclei possess a charge. In addition, the nuclei of some atoms spin. The combination of the spinning and the charge results in a local magnetic field. When some nuclei are placed in a powerful static magnetic field, they tend to align themselves longitudinally with the field. Approximately one-half of the nuclei are aligned parallel to the field and the other half antiparallel to it. However, there is an excess of nuclei which are parallel to the field and it is this population of nuclei which are of interest in the principles of MRI. When such a population of nuclei is intermittently subjected to a second magnetic field which is oscillating at the resonant frequency of the nucleus and at right angles to the static field, they tend to precess (i.e. they rotate about an axis different from the one about which they are spinning). The precession of the nuclei produces a rotating magnetic field and this is measured from the magnitude of the electrical signal induced in a set of coils within the MRI unit. The atoms then revert to their normal alignment. As they do so, images are made at different phases of relaxation known as T1, T2 and other sequences. These sequences are recorded. From the timings of these sequences, referred to as different weightings, the recorded images are compared with each other. The detected signals are then used to form an image of the body.

Hydrogen ion is commonly used for the imaging because it is abundant in the body and it has a strong response to an external magnetic field. Phosphorus may also be used.

The SI unit for magnetic flux density is the tesla (T) and magnets that are used in most MRI units have a magnetic flux density of 0.1–4 T. The powerful magnetic field may be created by either a permanent magnet (which cannot be switched on and off and tends to be heavy) or an electromagnet.

LASERS

Laser is a source of an intense beam of light that results from stimulation of atoms (the laser medium) by electrical or thermal energy. Laser light has three defining characteristics: coherence (all waves are in phase both in time and in space), collimation (all waves travel in parallel directions) and monochromaticity (all waves have the same wavelength). The term laser is an acronym for Light Amplification by Stimulated Emission of Radiation.

Physical principles of lasers

When atoms of the lasing medium are excited from a normal ground state into a high-energy state by a 'pumping' source, this is known as the excited state. When the atoms return from the excited state to the normal state, the energy is often dissipated as light or radiation of a specific wavelength characteristic of the atom (spontaneous emission). In the normal circumstances, when this change from higher to lower energy state occurs, the light emitted is likely to be absorbed by an atom in the lower energy state rather than meet an atom in a higher energy state and cause more light emission. In a laser, the number of excited atoms is raised significantly so that the light emitted strikes another high-energy atom and, as a result, two light particles with the same phase and frequency are emitted (stimulated emission). These stages are summarized below:

- *Excitation*: stable atom + energy → high energy atom
- *Spontaneous emission*: high-energy atom → stable atom + a photon of light
- *Stimulated emission*: photon of light + high energy atom → stable atom + 2 photons of light

The light emitted is reflected back and forth many times between mirrored surfaces giving rise to further stimulation. This amplification will continue as long as there are more atoms in the excited state than in the normal state.

A laser system has four components: (Fig. 30.19).

- *The laser medium* may be gas, liquid or solid. Common surgical lasers are CO_2, argon gas and neodymium-yttrium-aluminium-garnet (Nd-YAG) crystal. This determines the wavelength of the radiation emitted. The Nd-YAG and CO_2 lasers emit infrared invisible radiation and argon gives blue-green radiation.
- *The pumping source* supplies energy to the laser medium and this can be either an intense flash of light or electric discharge.
- *An optical cavity* is the container in which the laser medium is encased. It also contains mirrors used to reflect light in order to increase the energy of the stimulated emission. One of the mirrors is a partially transmitting mirror, which allows the laser beam to escape.
- *The light guide* directs the laser light to the surgical site. This may be in the form of a hollow tube or a flexible fibreoptic guide.

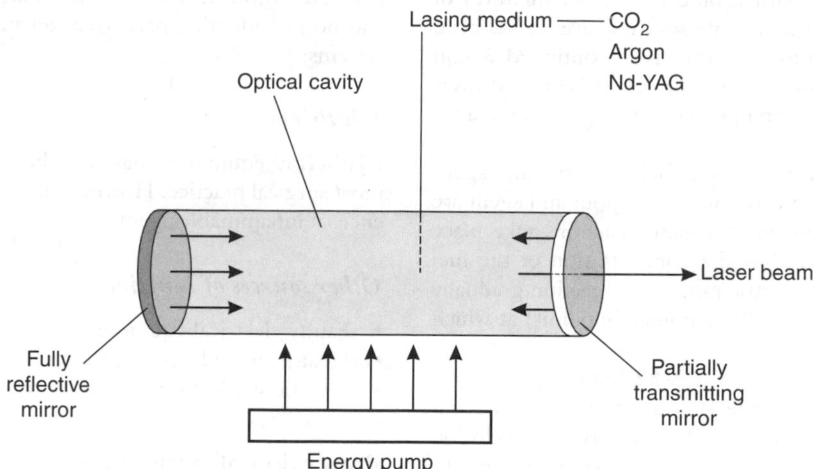

Fig. 30.19
Principle of a laser system.

The longer the wavelength of the laser light, the more strongly it is absorbed, and the power of the light is converted to heat in shallower tissues, e.g. CO_2. The shorter the wavelength, the more scattered is the light, and the light energy is converted to heat in deeper tissues, e.g. Nd-YAG.

Lasers are categorized according to the degree of hazard they afford into four classes: class 1 is the least dangerous and class 4 the most dangerous. Surgical lasers which are specifically designed to damage tissue are class 4.

OPTICAL FIBRES

Optical fibres are used in the design of endoscopes and bronchoscopes in order to be able to see around corners. Optical fibres use the principle that when light passes from one medium to another, it is refracted (i.e. bent). If the direction of the light is altered, the light may be totally reflected instead and this allows transmission of the light along the optical fibres (Fig. 30.20). As a result, if light passes into one end of a fibre of glass or other transparent material, it may pass along the fibre by being continually reflected from the glass/air boundary. Endoscopes and bronchoscopes contain bundles of the flexible transparent fibres.

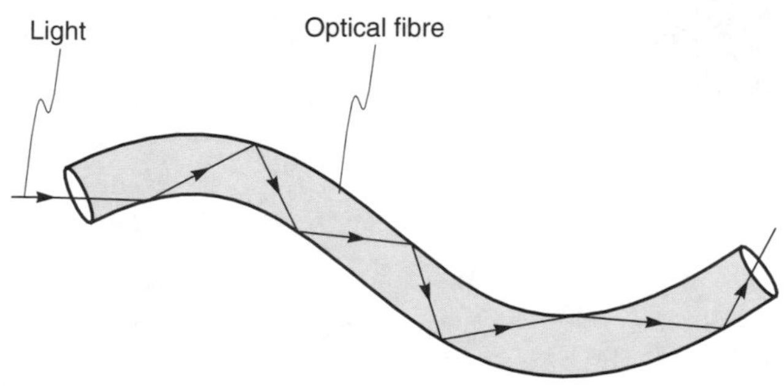

Fig. 30.20
Principle of the optical fibre.

FIRES AND EXPLOSIONS

Although the use of inflammable anaesthetic agents has declined greatly over the last two to three decades, ether is still used in some countries. In addition, other inflammable agents may be utilized in the operating theatre, e.g. alcohol for skin sterilization. Thus the anaesthetist should have some understanding of the problems and risks of fire occurring in the operating theatre.

Fires are produced when fuels undergo combustion. A conflagration differs from a fire in having a more rapid and more violent rate of combustion. A fire becomes an explosion if the combustion is sufficiently rapid to cause pressure waves that, in turn, cause sound waves. If these pressure waves possess sufficient energy to ignite adjacent fuels, the combustion is extremely violent and termed a detonation.

Fires require three ingredients:

- fuel
- oxygen or other substance capable of supporting combustion
- source of ignition, i.e. a source of heat sufficient to raise the fuel temperature to its ignition temperature. This quantity of heat is termed the activation energy.

FUELS

The modern volatile anaesthetic agents are non-flammable and non-explosive at room temperature in either air or oxygen.

Oils and greases are petroleum-based and form excellent fuels. In the presence of high pressures of oxygen, nitrous oxide or compressed air, these fuels may ignite spontaneously, an event termed dieseling (an analogy with the diesel engine). Thus oil or grease must not be used in compressed air, nitrous oxide or oxygen supplies.

Surgical spirit burns readily in air and the risk is increased in the presence of oxygen or nitrous oxide. Other non-anaesthetic inflammable substances include methane in the gut (which may be ignited by diathermy when the gut is opened), paper dressings and plastics found in the operating theatre suite.

Ether burns in air slowly with a blue flame, but mixtures of nitrous oxide, oxygen and ether are always explosive. It has been suggested that if administration of ether is discontinued 5 min before exposure to a source of ignition, the patient's expired gas is unlikely to burn provided that an open circuit has been used after discontinuation of ether.

The stoichiometric concentration of a fuel and oxidizing agent is the concentration at which all combustible vapour and agent are completely utilized. Thus the most violent reactions take place in stoichiometric mixtures, and as the concentration of the fuel moves away from the stoichiometric range, the reaction gradually declines until a point is reached (the flammability limit) at which ignition does not occur.

The inflammability range for ether is 2–82% in oxygen, 2–36% in air, and 1.5–24% in nitrous oxide. The stoichiometric concentration of ether in oxygen is 14% and there is a risk of explosion with ether concentrations of approximately 12–40% in oxygen. In air, the stoichiometric concentration of ether is 3.4% and explosions do not occur.

SUPPORT OF COMBUSTION

It should always be remembered that as the concentration of oxygen increases, so does the likelihood of ignition of a fuel and the conversion of the reaction from fire to explosion.

Nitrous oxide supports combustion. During laparoscopy, there is a risk of perforation of the bowel and escape of methane or hydrogen into the peritoneal cavity. Consequently, the use of nitrous oxide to produce a pneumoperitoneum for this procedure is not recommended; carbon dioxide is to be preferred, as it does not support combustion (and, in addition, has a much greater solubility in blood than nitrous oxide, thereby diminishing the risk of gas embolism).

SOURCES OF IGNITION

The two main sources of ignition in the operating theatre are static electricity and diathermy.

Static electricity

Electrostatic charges are produced on non-conductive material, such as rubber mattresses, plastic pillow cases and sheets, woollen blankets, nylon, terylene, hosiery garments, rubber tops of stools and non-conducting parts of anaesthetic machines and breathing systems.

Diathermy

Diathermy equipment has now become an essential element of most surgical practice. However, it should not be used in the presence of inflammable agents.

Other sources of ignition

- Faulty electrical equipment.
- Heat from endoscopes, thermocautery, lasers, etc.
- Electric sparks from motor switches, X-ray machines, etc.

Prevention of static charges

Where possible, antistatic conducting material should be used in place of non-conductors. The resistance of antistatic material should be between 50 kΩ cm^{-1} and 10 MΩ cm^{-1}.

All material should be allowed to leak static charges through the floor of the operating theatre. However, if the conductivity of the floor is too high, there is a risk of electrocution if an individual forms a contact between mains voltage and ground. Consequently, the floor of the operating theatre is designed to have a resistance of 25–50 kΩ when measured between two electrodes placed 1 m apart. This allows the gradual discharge of static electricity to earth. Personnel should wear conducting shoes, each with a resistance of between 0.1 and 1 MΩ.

Moisture encourages the leakage of static charges along surfaces to the floor. The risk of sparks from accumulated static electricity charges is reduced if the relative humidity of the atmosphere is kept above 50%.

FURTHER READING

Davis P D, Parbrook G D, Kenny G N C 1998 Basic physics and measurement in anaesthesia, 4th edn. Heinemann, London

Mushin W W, Jones P L 1987 Physics for the anaesthetist, 4th edn. Blackwell Scientific Publications, Oxford

Scurr C, Feldman S, Soni N 1991 Scientific foundation of anaesthesia, the basis of intensive care, 4th edn. Butterworth-Heinemann, London

31 Clinical measurement

Modern anaesthetic practice depends on reliable measurement of the physiological and pharmacological state of the patient and the physical functioning of supportive anaesthetic equipment. The anaesthetist is responsible for the correct use of sophisticated instruments for clinical measurement which extend clinical observations beyond the human senses and enhance patient care. This requires vigilance and awareness of the limitations of measurement and the many causes of error. Failure to appreciate the host of factors that may influence clinical measurements, inappropriate practical application and the uncritical acceptance of the recordings of monitoring equipment, even in the face of contradictory evidence, are common and indefensible errors. Unreliable measurements that are taken at face value and used to change patient management compromise the safety and effectiveness of care.

Clinical measurement is limited by four major constraints:

- *Feasibility of measurement.* The sensitivity and inherent variability of a clinical measurement depend on complex interactions and technical difficulties at the biological interface between the patient and the instrument.
- *Reliability* of measurements is determined by the properties of the measurement system. This is influenced by the calibration and correct use of the instrument in a demanding clinical environment. Simple examples include the correct placement of ECG electrodes, or the appropriate size of cuff for non-invasive measurement of arterial pressure. Delicate equipment, e.g. a blood gas analyser, requires regular maintenance and calibration.
- *Interpretation* depends on the critical faculties of the anaesthetist who interprets the significance of measurements in the context of complex physiological systems. Arterial pressure may be within the normal range despite severe hypovolaemia or derangement of cardiovascular function within the limits of physiological compensation. Global measurements of end-tidal CO_2 or pulse oximetry are influenced by many factors in a highly complex system; more information is required to deduce the cause of a change in the measurement.
- *Value* of clinical measurements in patient care is defined by the role of a measurement in improving the processes of patient care. This includes the ease, convenience, continuity and usefulness of a clinical measurement, and evidence of improvement in patient safety and clinical outcome.

This chapter describes the feasibility and reliability of clinical measurements relevant to anaesthetic practice. The correct interpretation of measurements and appropriate actions in the context of the condition of the patient, and the value of an instrument to the process of anaesthesia and outcomes for the patient are important but separate issues.

PROCESS OF CLINICAL MEASUREMENT

STAGES OF CLINICAL MEASUREMENT

There are four stages of clinical measurement:

- detection of the biological signal, by a sensing device which responds to a characteristic signal in the form of electrical, mechanical, electromagnetic, chemical or thermal energy
- transduction in which the output from the sensor is converted into another form, usually to a continuous electrical signal
- amplification and signal processing to extract and magnify the relevant features of the signal and reduce unwanted noise
- display and storage – the output from the instrument is presented to the operator. Storage for future use may be achieved using mechanical markers, printed copy or computer memory.

Mechanical instruments use the signal energy to drive a display, with minimal intermediate processing. The height of a fluid-column manometer provides a visible index of pressure. The expansion of mercury within the confines of a thin glass column is a measure of temperature. Mechanical springs and gearing translate the rotation of a vane into the recording of expired volume on a dial. However, the overwhelming trend is for non-electrical signals to be converted by a transducer to an electrical signal suitable for electronic processing by digital computers.

THE MICROPROCESSOR REVOLUTION

The development of digital microprocessors over the last 25 years has revolutionized anaesthetic practice. Beautifully engineered mechanical instruments, e.g. the von Recklinghausen oscillotonometer, are now obsolete in developed countries.

Advantages of digital signal processing include:

- continuous real-time detection, processing and recording of measurements
- increased range of measurements possible
- miniaturization of complicated and powerful instruments
- sophisticated artefact rejection and noise reduction algorithms

- complex on-line mathematical and statistical signal processing in upgradeable software, e.g. Fourier analysis of the EEG
- automated control of the apparatus and the timing and process of measurement, and integration of alarms
- storage in memory, permitting trend analysis, future display and further analysis
- user-friendly audiovisual display of recordings, integrating many simultaneous clinical measurements, and able to be customized by the user
- less maintenance than analogue instruments.

There are a few important disadvantages:

- dependence on electrically powered equipment
- degradation of clinical skills and alternative manual measurements through disuse
- impoverished understanding of the principles of complex measuring equipment and the requirements for correct use
- illusion of the unquestionable accuracy of measurements produced by expensive computer-controlled equipment and presented on an impressive display or typed copy.

ESSENTIAL REQUIREMENTS FOR CLINICAL MEASUREMENT

All clinical measurement systems detect a biological signal and reproduce the input signal in the form of a display or record that is presented to the operator. The degree to which a discrete measurement is a true reflection of the underlying signal is defined by the accuracy and precision.

Accuracy is the difference between the measurements and the real biological signal, or in practice, a different and superior 'gold standard' measurement. Calibration against predetermined signals is used to test and optimally adjust measuring instruments. For absolute measurements, e.g. arterial pressure, one point must be a fixed reference or 'zero'.

Precision describes the reproducibility of repeated measurements of the same biological signal. This dispersion is usually described by summary statistics, standard deviation for normally distributed measurements, or the range for non-normal distributions. A single recording is unreliable when the measurement is imprecise. This is especially true of tests which require patient cooperation, practised skill or effort, e.g. peak expiratory flow rate. Repeated measurements demonstrate the variability in response.

The importance of repeated measurements

Differences in clinical measurements arise from three causes:

- change in the clinical condition of the patient
- variability inherent in the biological signal or measuring instrument
- confounding errors – the recorded measurement does not reflect the signal.

The anaesthetist must be satisfied with the accuracy and precision of any clinical measurement used in patient management. Repeated measurements that are consistent ensure that the measurement is representative, i.e. precise, but do not ensure accuracy. For example, repeated recordings of invasive arterial pressure may be extremely consistent but completely erroneous if the transducer is not calibrated against the correct zero point. Defences against the uncritical acceptance of inaccurate measurements include meticulous care in calibrating instruments and the recording of clinical measurements, and reflection on clinical measurements that do not fit the clinical state of the patient or other related measurements. A discrepant result should be rechecked, using a different measurement technique if possible, before it is used to change patient management. This is especially true of complex, operator-dependent techniques such as measurement of cardiac output.

MEASUREMENT OF CONTINUOUS SIGNALS OVER TIME

Continuous signals, which include the majority of modern clinical measurements such as biological electrical signals and the electrical output of signal transducers, introduce the complication of the response of the measuring instrument to a changing signal over time. The reliability with which a continuous signal is reproduced is defined by the relationship between input and output of the measurement system over the clinical range of signal magnitude and frequency. The input–output function of an accurate clinical measurement system would demonstrate good zero and gain stability, minimal amplitude non-linearity and hysteresis, and an adequate frequency response. This cannot be taken for granted, particularly with older equipment or with variations in environmental temperature or humidity.

Zero stability

The ability of a measurement to maintain a zero reading on the display or record when the input signal is zero defines the zero stability. The importance of zero instability depends on the magnitude relative to the signal; for example, a zero drift of a few millimetres of mercury is much less important for the recording of arterial pressure than it is for intracranial pressure.

Gain stability

The majority of biological signals are amplified before reproduction. This 'gain' may be fixed or controlled by the user. When set, this should remain constant over the period of recording.

Amplitude linearity

The degree of amplification of the signal should be constant over the whole range of signal amplitudes. Manufacturers usually specify the degree of linearity of electronic components over a certain amplitude range. The amplitude linearity of a complete clinical system may be confirmed easily in an electronics laboratory by comparing the output to known, standardized test signals.

Hysteresis

Certain instruments such as thermistors and humidity sensors may display hysteresis. This is a special case of non-linearity, in which the output differs depending on whether the input signal is increasing or decreasing.

Frequency response

Many biological signals vary in a complicated and rapidly changing pattern. Accurate reproduction of a complex waveform requires that all of the component frequencies that make up the waveform are processed in an identical manner. This requires more than equal amplification irrespective of frequency, i.e. no amplitude distortion. It also implies that the relative positions of the various frequency components of the waveform are not shifted, i.e. no phase distortion. In practice, accurate reproduction up to the 10th harmonic of the fundamental frequency is sufficient for clinical purposes, e.g. 30 Hz for an arterial pressure waveform associated with heart rates up to 180 beats min^{-1} (3 Hz).

Signal-to-noise ratio

Biological signals are obscured to a variable degree by unwanted or extraneous signals which have similar physical characteristics and are described as noise, e.g. heart sounds become difficult to detect in the presence of continuous, noisy breath sounds. The efficiency of isolation of the signal from unwanted biological signals and electronic noise sources in the equipment is defined by the signal-to-noise ratio. The variability of the amplitudes of signal and noise is enormous and the signal-to-noise ratio is described using a logarithmic scale of decibels. Microvolt EEG measurements are particularly susceptible to noise from many sources. Biological noise includes contaminating ECG and EMG potentials, particularly from the scalp muscles, and interference from electrochemical activity at the skin–electrode interface. Electrostatic and electromagnetic linkage between the recording wires and nearby sources of mains electricity generates noise that is predominantly 50 Hz frequency and harmonics. Radiofrequency noise from diathermy or transmitters may also be picked up at this stage. Physical disturbance of the recording wires causes tiny changes in capacitative potentials and may add low-frequency noise, called microphony. Thermal noise is added during amplification, particularly at the input stage when the signal is in the microvolt range. Good amplifier design, electronic filtering of unwanted frequencies and modern techniques of digital signal processing can extract small signals from considerable background noise, but this inevitably introduces some distortion of the signal. Prevention of contamination of the signal by minimizing sources of noise before the signal is amplified is always preferable. The operator is responsible for correctly using measuring instruments to optimize the signal and for applying knowledge of the physical principles of the measurement to minimize contamination by noise.

ANALOGUE AND DIGITAL PROCESSING

Following signal detection and appropriate transduction, the continuously variable analogue signal is amplified, processed and displayed for the attention of the clinician.

Mechanical measuring instruments

Measuring instruments based on mechanical principles lack the flexibility and automated control of computerized devices, but use ingenious methods for processing and displaying analogue measurements. For example, mechanical spirometers use precision-engineered gears to translate the movement of a piston or vane into the rotation of a calibrated dial.

Analogue computers

Analogue computers use hardware comprising electronic circuits and operational amplifiers. Signals are represented by continuously variable electric potentials. Solid state hardware components can perform a wide variety of mathematical functions on a rapidly changing input waveform. Continuous integration and differentiation are formidable mathematical tasks for a digital computer, which can be solved simply and cheaply using analogue circuits. Integration of the flow signal from a pneumotachograph produces a volume waveform.

Microcomputers and digital signal processing

Digital signal processing offers a powerful alternative to mechanical processing and analogue computation. A fundamental step in this process is the conversion of a continuous analogue electrical signal into a discrete digital form. This analogue-to-digital conversion is achieved by measuring or 'sampling' the continuous input signal at regular intervals, to produce a series of discrete measurements over time which are in a suitable format for digital computation. The overwhelming advantage of digital processing is that the manipulation of the digitized signal is performed by a flexible and unlimited series of software calculations which range from mathematical functions to the analysis of statistical properties and trends.

Analogue to digital conversion

The core processing units of digital computers assume one of two stable states, i.e. a binary, rather than decimal, code. This imposes a limit on the resolving power of the digital processor. A binary number of eight digits (called 8 bits) may represent a range of integer decimal numbers, from binary 00000000 = decimal 0 to binary 11111111 = decimal 255. In short, an 8-bit converter can resolve an analogue signal with an accuracy of one part in 255, i.e. with an amplitude resolution of 0.4% of full scale. A 12-bit converter is more accurate, with a resolving power of one part in 4095 or 0.02% of full scale. The cost of this improvement in resolution is more expensive hardware to digitize, process and store considerably more digital information.

Amplitude resolution is not the only determinant of the accuracy of analogue-to-digital conversion. Resolution over time, determined by the sampling frequency, is also important. A relatively low sampling frequency may provide a representative sample of values for a slowly changing waveform; it may inadequately represent high-frequency components and introduce aliasing error. The Nyquist theorem suggests that the minimum sampling frequency to maintain the integrity of the waveform is at least twice the highest frequency component with significant amplitude in the input signal waveform; for example, a sampling frequency of 100 Hz would adequately capture the fastest rate of change in a physiological pressure signal.

The immensely powerful and complicated hardware and software programming instructions responsible for performing the tasks of digitizing, processing, storing and displaying the input signal are hidden from view in the commercial 'black box'.

DATA DISPLAY

Useful instruments communicate measurements in an appropriate and user-friendly manner.

Analogue displays

A continuously variable signal, such as pressure or temperature, is represented by an analogue display in terms of the amplitude of a physical quantity on a calibrated scale, dial, electrical meter or printed record. The glass thermometer incorporates a wedge-shaped lens which magnifies the appearance of the mercury column against the calibrated background scale. The height of a water column manometer is a linear, visual scale of pressure. Simple mechanical displays are accurate and easily understood, but are inconvenient to read and most suitable for intermittent discrete measurements.

Mechanical spirometers and flowmeters record flow on a dial driven by gears. Electrical moving coil meters use a coil of wire suspended in a magnetic field which rotates in proportion to the applied current and moves a pointer on a calibrated dial. Alternatively, the amplified and filtered electrical signal could drive a chart recorder which produces a continuous printed record of the amplitude of measurements against time. Limitations common to these mechanical devices include fragile moving parts and inertia, which impairs the frequency response to rapidly changing signals.

The cathode ray oscilloscope continues to be an effective screen-based display for continuous electrical signals. A heated cathode generates a stream of electrons which are focused and accelerated onto phosphorescent coating which lines the flat surface of the tube to generate a bright spot. The position of the electron beam in both *x*- and *y*-axes is controlled by electrostatic plates. The continuously varying input signal is applied to the *y*-plates so that deflection in the vertical *y*-axis is proportional to the amplitude of the signal. The absence of mechanical parts results in a high-frequency response. An electronic time-base circuit can deliver a sawtooth voltage to the *x*-plates which drives the electron beam across the *x*-axis at a constant rate and returns the beam to the left-hand side at the start of each sweep. This produces a dynamic image of signal amplitude against time. Alternatively, a second input signal may be applied to the *x*-plates to produce an *x*–*y* graphical plot, e.g. pressure–volume loop. Cathode ray oscilloscopes are widely used in electronic engineering and signal processing, but have been replaced in clinical practice by microprocessor-controlled displays.

Microprocessor-controlled displays

Digital signal processing has revolutionized clinical measurement. However, digital information in the form of a list of numbers is extremely difficult to interpret quickly and easily. Digital records are appropriate for discrete measurements such as drug concentrations or blood gas tensions, but a digital time series of a continuously varying signal, such as pressure in the form of a list of numbers, would be incomprehensible. The human brain is accustomed to continuous analogue sensory input and modern microprocessor-controlled measuring instruments convert the discrete digital record back into the continuous analogue waveforms for display on a monitor in a manner familiar to anaesthetists.

This paradox illustrates the real power of digital signal processing to manipulate and present information in a relevant and user-friendly manner. Continuous waveforms, e.g. invasive pressure, may be displayed alongside discrete numerical measurements of amplitude or frequency and a graphical display of trends over time. These can be recreated or processed in other ways from the original digital signal, which is stored in a digital computer record without degradation of the quality of the signal.

BIOLOGICAL ELECTRICAL SIGNALS

The detection and recording of biological electrical potentials are important clinical measurements which incorporate many of the important principles of clinical measurement.

Depolarization of the cell membrane of excitable cells is fundamental to the action of these cells and generates a transient potential difference between the active cell and surrounding tissues. The summation of synchronous extracellular potentials from a large number of excitable cells generates a widespread electric field which can be detected by electrodes on the body surface.

The electrocardiogram is a well established measure of myocardial electrical activity. The synchronous depolarization and prolonged action potentials in cardiac muscle summate to generate a potential field of high amplitude. Body surface ECG recordings are approximately 1 mV in amplitude, with a frequency content in the range 0.05–100 Hz.

The electroencephalogram is a smaller and more complex signal, with an amplitude of 50–200 μV and a frequency content that is classified conventionally into four categories:

- delta waves: 0–4 Hz
- theta waves: 4–8 Hz
- alpha waves: 8–13 Hz
- beta waves: 13 Hz and above.

The spiking, transient depolarization, then repolarization, of action potentials in neurones in the brain is sufficiently asynchronous and transient to be unrecordable from the scalp or surface of the brain. It is believed that the electroencephalogram is generated by the summation of synchronous postsynaptic potentials on the dendrites of sheets of large and symmetrically arranged pyramidal cells in cortical layers III and IV. Recording of these microvolt signals with acceptable levels of artefact and interference is difficult.

Evoked potentials are small, specific changes in the EEG in response to a series of auditory, visual or somatosensory stimuli. These tiny evoked potentials are overwhelmed by the larger background EEG. They are, however, time-locked to the stimulus and can be extracted from the asynchronous background EEG by the digital signal processing technique of signal-averaging of several hundred responses.

DETECTION OF BIOLOGICAL ELECTRICAL SIGNALS: ELECTRODES

Modern electrodes are constructed of silver, coated electrolytically with silver chloride. Low, stable impedances minimize mains interference. Symmetrical electrode impedance and insignificant polarization control drift. However, care is still required to achieve optimum results. The silver chloride layer is very thin, prone to deterioration and only suitable for single use. Movement artefacts which alter the electrode potential and impedance are greatly reduced if the electrode surface is separated from the skin by a foam pad impregnated with electrolyte gel. It is no longer necessary to abrade the skin to achieve ultra-low impedance, but de-greasing with alcohol before applying the electrode helps to reduce skin impedance and ensures satisfactory adhesion.

Needle electrodes deliver poor electrical performance, are sensitive to movement and increase the risk of diathermy burns.

AMPLIFIERS FOR BIOLOGICAL SIGNALS

The amplitude of tiny bioelectrical signals must be increased by amplification, and unwanted noise and interference minimized. Calibration voltages may be incorporated for correct adjustment of the gain of the amplifier.

Input impedance and common mode rejection

Amplifiers for biological signals require high common mode rejection and high input impedance. The input and electrode impedances act as a potential divider; high electrode impedance and low amplifier input impedance attenuates the electrical signal across the amplifier. The input impedance of modern amplifiers exceeds 5 MΩ to avoid problems, and careful attention must be paid to minimizing electrode impedance, particularly for EEG recordings.

Differential amplification is a powerful method of reducing unwanted noise. The potential difference between two input signals is amplified, but electrical signals common to both are attenuated. This feature is termed 'common mode rejection' and very effectively reduces mains interference in all biological signals and electrocardiographic contamination of much smaller electroencephalographic signals. The common mode rejection ratio (CMRR) for a typical differential amplifier exceeds 10 000:1. In other words, a signal applied equally to both input terminals would need to be 10 000 times larger than a signal applied between them for the same change in output.

Frequency response

The bandwidth of the amplifier must cover the range of frequencies that are important in the signal. In practice, amplifiers require a flat frequency response for ECG from 0.14 to 50 Hz, for EEG from 0.5 to 100 Hz, and for EMG from 20 Hz to at least 2 kHz.

Low-frequency interference, largely caused by slow fluctuating potentials generated in the electrodes, produces baseline instability and drift. This is removed by incorporating a network of resistors and capacitors which function as a simple high-pass filter allowing biological signals to pass, but attenuating slow drift. This introduces a compromise in amplifier design between signal trace fidelity and stability of recording. For example, amplifiers designed for diagnostic electrocardiography have long time constants with optimal reproduction of the waveform at the expense of baseline instability, especially to movement. In comparison, continuity of recording is more important when the electrocardiogram is used for monitoring during anaesthesia; high-pass filtering produces a short time constant and good baseline stability at the expense of waveform reproduction. Low-frequency elements of the ECG, such as the T wave, may become differentiated by phase shift in the high-pass filter and appear distorted or biphasic.

Other filters can attenuate particular frequencies. Highly selective band reject filters attenuate 50 Hz interference from the signal. Low-pass filters are used to eliminate higher frequency artefacts from an EEG signal. The purpose of filtering is to reduce unwanted noise relative to the signal; when the frequency range of signal and noise overlap, some degree of signal degradation is inevitable.

Noise and interference

Electrical noise arising from the patient, the patient–electrode interface or the surroundings may seriously interfere with accurate recording of biological potentials.

Noise originating from the patient

Millivolt ECG potentials on the body surface are hundreds of times larger than microvolt EEG signals on the scalp. EMG signals may be even larger, and muscular activity, especially shivering, causes severe interference. Two features of electronic amplifier design substantially improve the EEG signal-to-noise ratio. ECG potentials are essentially the same across the scalp and are ignored by amplifiers with a high common mode rejection. EMG activity has a higher frequency content than the EEG signal, and may be minimized by a low-pass filter which attenuates the higher frequency response of the amplifier to a level which does not interfere with the characteristics of the EEG.

Noise originating from the patient–electrode interface

Recording electrodes do not behave as passive conductors. All skin–metal electrode systems employ a metal surface in contact with an electrolyte solution. Polarization describes the interaction between metal and electrolyte which generates a small electrical gradient. Electrodes comprising metal plated with one of its own salts, e.g. silver:silver chloride, avoid this problem because current in each direction does not significantly change the electrolyte composition. Mechanical movement of recording electrodes may also cause significant potential gradients – alteration in the physical dimensions of the electrode changes the cell potential and skin–electrode impedance. Differences in potential between two electrodes connected to a differential amplifier are amplified and asymmetry of electrode impedance seriously impairs the common mode rejection ratio of the recording amplifier.

Noise originating outside the patient

Electrical interference. Mains frequency interference with the recording of biological potentials may be troublesome, particularly in electromagnetically noisy clinical environments. Patients function physically as large unscreened conductors and interact with nearby electrical sources through the processes of capacitative coupling and electromagnetic induction.

Capacitance permits alternating current to pass across an air gap. A live mains conductor and nearby patient behave as the two plates of a capacitor. The very small mains frequency current that flows through the patient is of no clinical significance, but confounds the detection and amplification of biological potentials, creating unwanted interference in the recording. Capacitatively coupled interference is minimized by reducing the capacitance and the alternating potential difference. This is achieved by moving the patient away from the source of interference and by screening mains powered equipment with a conductive surround which is maintained at earth potential by a low resistance earth connection and by surrounding leads with a braided copper screen – stray capacitances couple with the screen instead of the lead.

Alternating currents in a conductor generate a magnetic flux. This induces voltages in any nearby conductors which lie in the changing magnetic flux, including the patient or signal leads to the amplifier, which function as inefficient secondary transformers. This source of interference is minimized by keeping patients as far as possible from powerful sources of electromagnetic flux, especially mains transformers. Electromagnetic inductance may be minimized by ensuring that all patient leads are the same length, closely bound or twisted together until very close to the electrodes. This ensures that the induced signals are identical in all leads and therefore susceptible to common mode rejection.

The importance of low electrode impedance. Low electrode impedance may exaggerate the effects of surrounding electrical interference. Capacitative and inductive coupling produce very small currents in the recording leads. If the electrode impedance is low, the potential at the amplifier input must remain close to the potential at the skin surface, so that minimal interference results. If electrode impedance is high, the small induced currents may create significant potential difference across that impedance, leading to severe 50 Hz interference.

Radiofrequency interference from diathermy is a severe problem for the recording of biological potentials. ECG amplifiers may be provided with some protection by filtering the signal before it enters the isolated input circuit, filtering the power supply to block mains-borne radiofrequencies and enclosing the electronic components in a double screen: the outer earthed and the inner at amplifier potential.

MECHANICAL SIGNALS: MEASUREMENT OF ARTERIAL PRESSURE

Several physical principles and a wide range of instruments are used to measure pressure. Liquid column manometers display pressure according to the height of a column of fluid relative to a predefined zero-point, and the density of the fluid. Mechanical pressure gauges are used widely, particularly in high-pressure gas supplies; pressure-dependent mechanical movement is amplified by a gearing mechanism which drives a pointer across a scale.

For most physiological pressure measurements, diaphragm gauges are used – a flexible diaphragm moves according to the applied pressure. Mechanical display of diaphragm movement is limited by poor sensitivity to small pressures, inertia to changing pressure and a narrow range of linear response. In modern diaphragm gauges used for sensing dynamic pressures, movement of the diaphragm is sensed by a device which converts the mechanical energy imparted to the diaphragm into electrical energy.

ELECTROMECHANICAL TRANSDUCERS

The first step in transduction is movement of the diaphragm caused by the relationship to applied pressure. This depends on the stiffness of the diaphragm and substantially determines the operating characteristics of the transducer. Linearity of amplitude and frequency response are improved by using small stiff diaphragms, but require a more sensitive mechanism for sensing diaphragm movement.

Wire strain gauges are based on the principle that stretching or compression of a wire changes the electrical resistance. Changes in capacitance or inductance have also been coupled to movement of a diaphragm. Silicon strain gauges utilize the changes in resistance in a thin slice of silicon crystal that occur when it is compressed or expanded. They are very sensitive and suitable for incorporation into a small stiff diaphragm with excellent frequency response, but non-linearity and temperature dependence are difficult technical problems.

Optical transduction senses movement of the diaphragm by reflecting light from the silvered back of the convex diaphragm onto a photocell. Applied pressure causes the silvered surface to become more convex. This causes the reflected light beam to diverge, reducing the intensity of reflected light sensed by the photoelectric cell. This design is used in a fibreoptic cardiac catheter for intravascular pressure measurement. These miniature pressure transducers are expensive but have a high-frequency response and fibreoptic light sources eliminate the risk of microshock.

DIRECT MEASUREMENT OF INTRAVASCULAR PRESSURE

Liquid manometers remain a simple, cheap and useful method of measuring central venous pressure. However, electromechanical transducers are commonly used for the invasive measurement of intravascular pressures; cost and complexity are compensated by convenience, accuracy, continuity of measurement and an electrical output which can be processed, stored and displayed according to the requirements.

Fourier showed that all complex waveforms may be described as a mixture of simple sine waves of varying amplitude, frequency and phase. These consist of a fundamental wave, in this case at the pulse frequency, and a series of harmonics. The lower harmonics tend to have the greatest amplitude and a reasonable approximation to the arterial pressure waveform may be obtained by accurate reproduction of the fundamental and first 10 harmonics. In other words, to reproduce an arterial waveform at 120 beats min^{-1} accurately would require transduction with a linear frequency response up to a frequency of at least $120 \times 10/60 = 20$ Hz. Accurate reproduction of a waveform requires that both the amplitude and phase difference of each harmonic are faithfully reproduced. This requires a transduction system with a natural frequency higher than the significant frequency components of the system, and the correct amount of damping.

The commonest method for the direct measurement of intravascular pressure uses a pressure transducer connected to the lumen of the vessel by a fluid-filled catheter. The fluid and diaphragm of the transducer constitute a mechanical system which oscillates in simple harmonic motion at the natural resonant frequency. This determines the frequency response of the measurement system (Fig. 31.1). The resonant frequency of a catheter–transducer

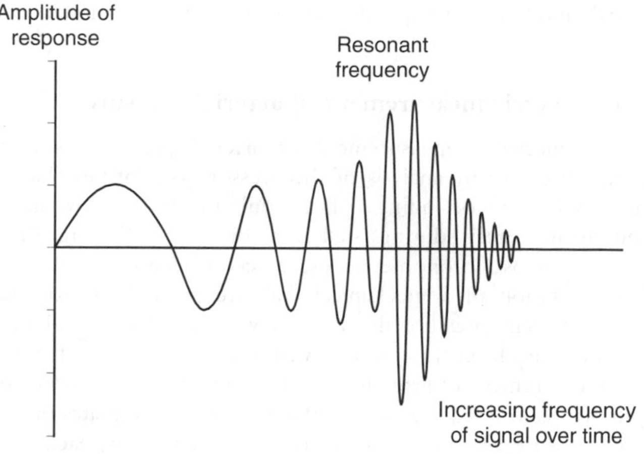

Fig. 31.1
Simulation of the output of a catheter-transducer system with increasing frequency of a constant amplitude input signal. The linearity of response is lost as the frequency approaches the resonant frequency of the system.

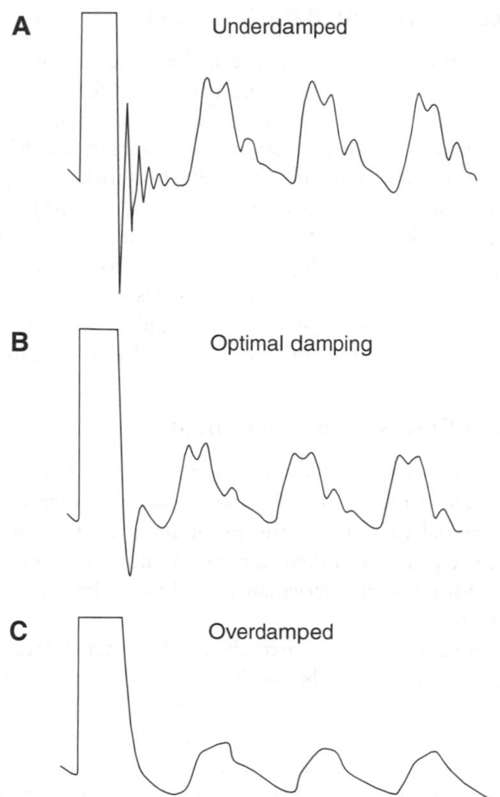

Fig. 31.2
Damping of arterial pressure waves and the response to a square wave signal from the fast flush device.

measuring system is highest, and the frictional resistance to fluid flow which dampens the frequency response is lowest, when the velocity of movement of fluid in the catheter is minimized. This is achieved with a stiff, low-volume displacement diaphragm and a short, wide, rigid catheter.

Transduced vascular pressures should always be displayed; inspection of the arterial waveform provides a qualitative assessment of the adequacy of the frequency response and damping. Modern instruments calculate mean arterial pressure automatically by integrating the area under the pressure waveform. This measurement is affected less by non-linear characteristics of the catheter–transducer system and is more accurate and precise than the peak systolic and trough diastolic pressure. It is also more relevant to the physiology of organ perfusion.

DETERMINATION OF THE RESONANT FREQUENCY AND DAMPING

The resonant frequency and the effects of damping may be estimated by applying a step change in pressure to the catheter–transducer system and recording the response (Fig. 31.2). The underdamped system responds rapidly but overshoots and oscillates close to the natural resonant frequency of the system; frequency components of the pressure wave close to the resonant frequency are exaggerated. In contrast, the overdamped system responds slowly and records a correct amplitude of response, but the speed of response is slow and the recorded signal decreases slowly to reach the baseline with no overshoot. High-frequency oscillations are damped, underestimating the true pressure changes. These extremes are undesirable.

Optimal damping

Optimal damping maximizes the frequency response of the system, minimizes resonance and represents the best compromise between speed of response and accuracy of transduction. A small overshoot represents approximately 7% of the step change in pressure, with the pressure then following the arterial waveform (Fig. 31.2).

Damping is relatively unimportant when the frequencies being recorded are less than two-thirds of the natural frequency of the catheter–transducer system. Modern transducer systems using small compliance transducers connected to a short, stiff catheter, with a minimum of constrictions or connections, approximate to this ideal. Air bubbles in the system, clotting or kinking in the vascular catheter and arterial spasm lower the natural resonant frequency and increase the damping.

In clinical practice, the resonant frequency of the whole system is uncomfortably close to the frequency content of the signal, and accurate measurements require optimal damping. However, damping is difficult to measure and control, and is poor compensation for an inadequate frequency response in the pressure recording system. Adjustment of damping is difficult to achieve and mechanical methods which include inserting constrictions or a compliant tube into the system to increase damping, or using a commercial damping device (Accudynamic), further reduce the resonant frequency. Electronic damping of the electrical output from the transducer cannot correct for non-linear amplification and attenuation of frequencies in the pressure wave before transduction.

INDIRECT METHODS FOR MEASURING ARTERIAL PRESSURE (see Ch. 38)

Indirect methods of measuring arterial pressure do not depend on contact between arterial blood and the system for signal recognition and transduction. The majority depend on signals generated by the occlusion of a major artery using a cuff; the Riva–Rocci method. Clinical methods of signal detection include palpation to estimate the systolic pressure at the return of a palpable distal pulse, and auscultation of the Korotkoff sounds for systolic and diastolic pressures. Measuring devices depend on the detection of movement of the arterial wall using changes in pressure or sound below audible frequencies and detection of blood flow using the Doppler shift of an ultrasound signal or plethysmography.

Accuracy of pressure measurements

The accuracy of pressure measurements, particularly using indirect methods, needs to be considered. Invasive direct measurement of arterial pressure is the usual standard for comparison. However, the catheter–transducer system must be carefully set up and tested for optimal performance, and this is hard to achieve in clinical practice.

Arterial pressure varies throughout the arterial tree and the measured pressure depends on the site of measurement. As the pulse wave travels from the ventricle to peripheral arteries, changes in vessel diameter and elasticity affect the pressure waveform which becomes narrower with increased amplitude. Differences in arterial pressure between limbs are common, particularly in patients with arterial disease.

Indirect methods using an occluding cuff make intermittent measurements, with the systolic and diastolic readings reflecting the conditions in the artery at two instants at which the endpoints are detected. In contrast, direct pressure measurements are the average of a number of cycles more precisely reflecting mean pressures. Indirect measurements may be compromised by taking a small number of infrequent samples from a variable signal.

Oscillometric measurement of arterial pressure

The oscillometric measurement of arterial pressure estimates arterial pressure by analysis of the pressure oscillations that are produced in an occluding cuff by pulsatile blood flow in the underlying artery during deflation of the cuff (Fig. 31.3). Mechanical oscillotonometers use a second sensing cuff which drives rotation of a mechanical dial. Automated oscillometers sense transient pressure fluctuations with an electromechanical pressure transducer. In common with other instruments for indirect measurement of arterial pressure, accurate estimation of the systolic pressure requires slow cuff deflation and estimates of diastolic pressure are unreliable. During slow deflation, each pulse wave produces a pressure transient in the cuff which may be distinguished from the slowly decreasing ambient pressure in the cuff. Above systolic pressure, the transients are small, but suddenly increase in magnitude when the cuff pressure reaches the systolic point. As the cuff pressure decreases further, the amplitude reaches a peak and then starts to diminish. The mean arterial pressure correlates closely with the lowest cuff pressure at which the maximum amplitude is maintained. As the cuff pressure reaches diastolic pressure, the transients abruptly diminish in amplitude.

Commercial instruments incorporate mechanisms for improving the reliability of the measurement. For example, at each successive plateau pressure during the controlled deflation, successive pressure fluctuations are compared and accepted only if they are similar. All automatic oscillometric instruments require a regular cardiac cycle with no great differences between successive pulses. Accurate and consistent readings may be impossible to record in patients with an irregular rhythm, particularly atrial fibrillation.

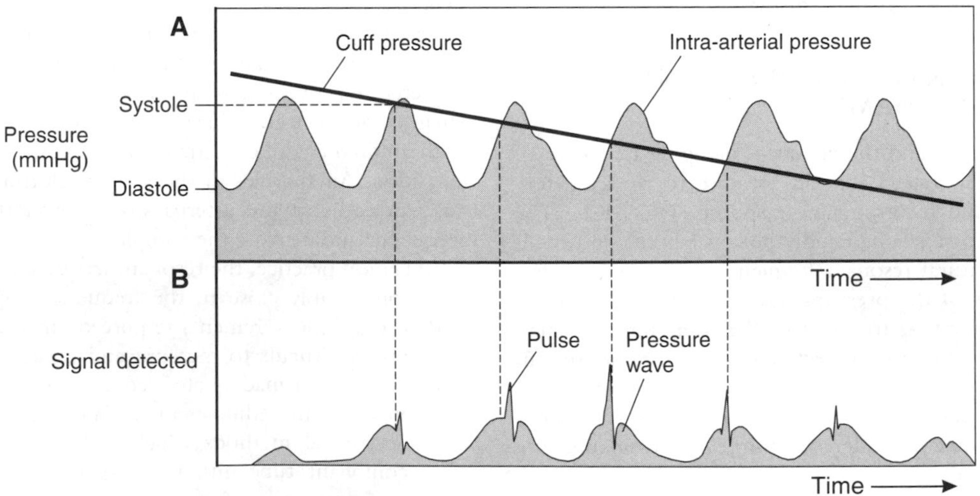

Fig. 31.3
Diagram showing: **A** relationship between cuff pressure and intra-arterial pressure as cuff pressure decreases during oscillometry; **B** the signal created by the relative pressure changes in **A**. The sharp spikes of pressure in **B** are created by the walls of the artery opening and closing. These spikes are detected by a transducer first when the cuff pressure is just below systolic arterial pressure; their amplitude reaches a peak at mean arterial pressure and they cease when the cuff pressure is below diastolic pressure.

Clinical studies comparing automatic oscillometric instruments with direct arterial pressure have demonstrated good correlation for systolic pressure with a tendency to overestimate at low pressures and underestimate at high pressures. Mean and diastolic pressures were less reliable. The 95% confidence interval for all three indices exceeded 15 mmHg.

MEASUREMENT OF BLOOD FLOW: CARDIAC OUTPUT

Three different approaches to the measurement of cardiac output that are based on different and contrasting principles are discussed:

- indicator dilution, and other techniques based on the Fick principle
- Doppler ultrasonography
- thoracic electrical bioimpedance.

More detail concerning these and other techniques of measuring blood flow are described in the reference texts.

The Fick principle

The Fick principle defines flow by the ratio of the uptake or clearance of a tracer within an organ to measurements of the arteriovenous difference in concentration. It may be used to measure cardiac output, notably when applied to oxygen uptake or indicator dilution, and also regional blood flow, e.g. cerebral blood flow using the uptake of nitrous oxide, and renal blood flow from the excretion of compounds cleared totally by the kidney, such as para-aminohippuric acid.

In subjects with minimal cardiac shunt and reasonable pulmonary function, pulmonary blood flow can be calculated from the oxygen consumption and the difference in oxygen content between arterial and mixed venous blood, as follows:

$$\text{Pulmonary blood flow} = \frac{\text{oxygen consumption}}{\text{arteriovenous oxygen content difference}}$$

Oxygen consumption from a reservoir is measured using an accurate spirometer, and oxygen content of blood requires a cooximeter. The patient should be at steady state when the measurements are made, with constant inspired oxygen concentration and blood samples obtained slowly whilst the oxygen consumption is being determined. True mixed venous blood samples must be obtained from a pulmonary artery catheter, in which case alternative indicator dilution techniques described below are less demanding. The effects of ventilation and beat-to-beat variation in cardiac output are averaged over the long period of measurement of oxygen consumption. Errors in measurement of oxygen consumption limit the accuracy of this technique (± 10%).

INDICATOR DILUTION

An indicator is injected as a bolus into the right heart and the concentration reaching the systemic side of the circulation is plotted against time (Fig. 31.4). The average concentration is calculated from the area under the concentration–time curve divided by the duration of the curve. The cardiac output during the period of this measurement is the ratio of the dose of indicator to the average concentration.

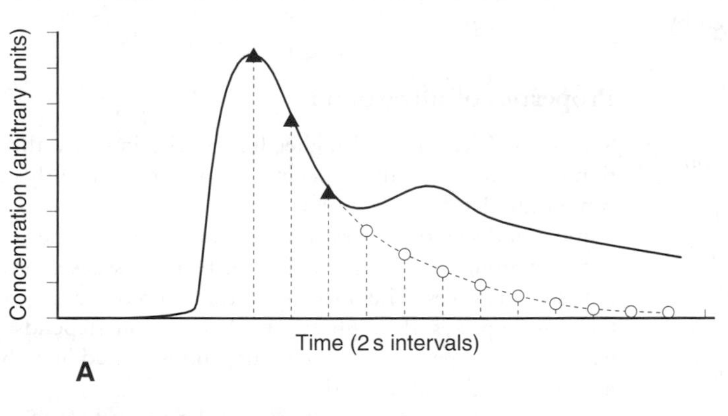

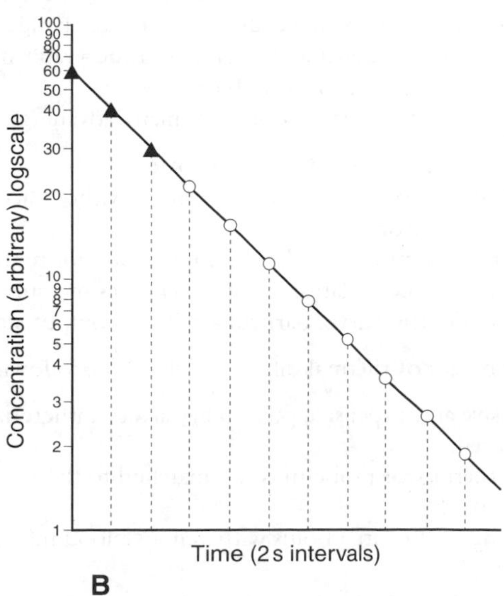

Fig. 31.4
A Single injection indicator dilution curve showing distortion of downslope produced by recirculation. **B** Re-plot on semi-logarithmic paper.

▲ = points taken from the downslope in **A** to establish the slope of the re-plot in **B**; ○ = points taken from **B** to plot tail of curve in **A**.

Reproduced from Fig. 16.13, page 216, in Principles of Measurement and Monitoring in Anaesthesia and Intensive Care, by Sykes MK, Vickers MD and Hull CJ, third edition, published 1991. Permission from Blackwell Scientific Publication.

The general formula is:

$$\text{Cardiac output (L min}^{-1}) = \frac{\text{indicator dose (units)} \times 60}{\text{average concentration (units L}^{-1}) \times \text{time (s)}}$$

Recirculation of the indicator before the downslope is complete is a problem (Fig. 31.4). This may be circumvented by extrapolation of the early exponential downslope to define the tail of the curve which would have been recorded if recirculation had not occurred. The area under the curve is calculated by integration.

Chemical indicator dilution

Indocyanine green is the commonest chemical indicator. It is non-toxic and has a relatively short half-life so that repeated measurements may be made. It also has a peak spectral absorption at 800 nm, which is the wavelength at which absorption of oxygenated haemoglobin is identical to that of reduced haemoglobin. The measurement is therefore not affected by arterial saturation.

Chemical indicator dilution techniques have been overtaken by the use of pulmonary flotation catheters and heat energy as the signal indicator.

Thermal indicator dilution

This technique is used commonly in the intensive care patient where a pulmonary artery catheter is required frequently for monitoring of cardiac output and left-sided pressures. The principle of the method is similar to other indicator dilution methods, but the injection and sampling are performed on the right side of the heart. A bolus of 10 ml of saline at room temperature is injected into the right atrium and the temperature change is recorded by a thermistor in the pulmonary artery. The recorded temperatures generate an exponential dilution curve with no recirculation. The 'heat dose' is the product of the difference in temperature between the injectate and blood multiplied by the density, specific heat and volume of the injectate. The average change in heat content is the area under the temperature–time graph multiplied by the density and specific heat of blood.

Thermal dilution techniques offer many advantages:

- The indicator is cheap and non-toxic.
- Repeated measurements may be made without accumulation of the indicator.
- Arterial puncture and blood sampling are not required.
- Absence of recirculation greatly facilitates measurement of the area under the curve, particularly in low output states.

Disadvantages of thermal dilution include the following:

- Invasive and expensive pulmonary artery catheterization is required.
- The thermistor probe must be matched to the cardiac output processor.
- Mixing of the large bolus with venous blood may be incomplete.
- Pulmonary artery flow varies more with respiration than does systemic flow.
- Corrections are required, e.g. for changes in injectate temperature during injection through the catheter.

The measurement of cardiac output using both dye and thermal dilution is now automated with computer-controlled sampling, calculation of indicator dilution curves, rejection algorithms for artefacts or curves which are not exponential, and on-line calculation of cardiac output.

Instruments with rapidly responding thermistors and a heating element incorporated in the pulmonary flotation catheter can measure the stoke volume of a single right ventricular contraction, and derive a continuous estimate of cardiac output.

DOPPLER ULTRASONOGRAPHY

Ultrasound techniques can detect the shape, size and movement of tissue interfaces, especially soft tissues and blood, including the echocardiographic measurement of blood flow and the structure and function of the heart. Sound waves are transmitted by the oscillation of particles in the direction of wave transmission and are defined by the amplitude of oscillation (the difference between ambient and peak pressures) and the wavelength (distance between successive peaks) or frequency (inversely proportional to wavelength, the number of cycles per second). These characteristics are measured by a pressure transducer placed in the path of an oncoming wave. The human ear can detect frequencies within the range of 20–20 000 Hz. Diagnostic ultrasound uses frequencies in the range of 1–10 MHz. Short-term diagnostic use of ultrasound appears to be free from hazard.

Generation and detection of ultrasound

Generation and sensing of ultrasound are performed by transducers which are manufactured from ceramic materials containing lead zirconate and lead titanate which display the piezoelectric effect. These substances are cheap, easily shaped and very efficiently transform mechanical to electrical energy and vice versa. Pressure on the surface of these materials generates a related and measurable electric charge. Conversely, applying a high-frequency alternating potential difference across the transducer changes the thickness and generates ultrasound of the same frequency as the applied voltage.

Properties of ultrasound

Shorter wavelengths and higher frequencies improve the resolution of distance, but tissue penetration is simultaneously reduced. Amplitude determines the intensity of the ultrasound beam, the number and size of echoes recorded and therefore the sensitivity of the instrument. Ultrasound is absorbed by tissues and reflected at tissue interfaces. The intensity of the beam decreases exponentially as it passes through tissue. Attenuation depends on the nature and temperature of the tissue, and is related linearly to the frequency of the ultrasound.

The reflection of the ultrasound beam from the junction between two tissues or from tissue–fluid or tissue–air interfaces forms the basis of the majority of diagnostic techniques. Reflections at most soft tissue interfaces are therefore weak, but bone-fat and tissue-air interfaces reflect the majority of incident energy. Structures lying behind a bone or air interface cannot be studied using ultrasound.

Ultrasound scanning techniques have been developed which are suited to different applications and which have extremely sophisticated two-dimensional, real-time, brightness-and colour-modulated displays under microprocessor control.

Detection of motion by the Doppler effect: cardiac output

The frequency of ultrasound waves reflected from a stationary object is the same as that of the transmitted waves. However, if the reflector is moving towards the transmitter, it encounters more oscillations in a given time than a stationary reflector, so that the frequency of the waves impinging on the reflector is apparently increased. This physical phenomenon is termed the Doppler effect. The apparent increase in frequency is directly proportional to the velocity of the reflecting object relative to the source and two constants, the frequency of the transmitted ultrasound and the velocity of ultrasound in the medium. This difference in frequency lies within the range of hearing and provides a vivid audible description of pulsatile blood flow. A Doppler signal proportional to blood flow may be obtained from the ascending aorta via the suprasternal notch or the aortic root from a trans-oesophageal probe which provides a non-invasive index of cardiac output.

The blood flow velocity curve is integrated to calculate the average velocity over each cardiac cycle. The stroke volume is calculated by multiplying the average velocity per cycle by an echocardiographic estimation of the cross-sectional area of the aorta. Multiplication of the stroke volume by heart rate yields cardiac output.

There are three major problems with Doppler measurements of cardiac output:

- Aortic diameter must be measured accurately. This may be done reasonably accurately by echocardiography, but errors also arise because the aorta is not completely circular, it expands by up to 12% during systole, and the sites of measurement of diameter and velocity may differ.
- The shape of the velocity profile is not uniform, with central streaming in the large diameter aorta. Low and unrepresentative velocities may be recorded if the ultrasound beam is not aligned exactly along the central core of the aorta.
- The Doppler shift depends on the direction of the ultrasound beam relative to the axis. Provided that the angle is less than 20°, the error in cardiac output is only about 6%.

Unacceptable variation in measurements, operator dependence and poor correlation with thermal dilution for absolute measurements of cardiac output have limited the application of Doppler ultrasonography in clinical practice. However, it is less invasive with fewer serious complications, records a continuous measurement and provides a useful indication of trends in cardiac output.

THORACIC ELECTRICAL BIOIMPEDANCE

Tissue impedance depends on blood volume. Measurement of thoracic impedance provides an index of stroke volume. Two circumferential electrodes are placed around the neck and two around the upper abdomen. A small (< 1 mA) constant, high-frequency (>1 kHz) alternating current is passed between the outer electrodes and the resulting potential difference is detected by the inner pair. This potential is rectified, smoothed and filtered to record voltage fluctuations which reflect changes in impedance due to respiration and cardiac activity. The cardiac activity is extracted by signal-averaging relative to the ECG R wave. This represents changes in thoracic blood volume and clearly resembles the pulse waveform.

Modern instruments show a modest agreement with invasive measurements of cardiac output, although trends and rapid changes in cardiac output are reliably demonstrated. This method is inaccurate when there are intracardiac shunts or arrhythmias, and underestimates cardiac output in a vasodilated circulation.

MEASUREMENT OF GAS FLOW AND VOLUME

The relationships between volume, flow and velocity are central to understanding gas flow and volume. Flow rate is defined as the volume passing a fixed point in unit time, i.e. volume per second. Integration of a continuous flow signal is the volume that has flowed over a defined period. Velocity is the distance moved by gas molecules in unit time. These are related directly and depend upon the cross-sectional area of flow:

$$\text{Velocity} = \text{flow rate}/\text{area}$$

The concept of velocity is important in flow measurement because several instruments measure the velocity of flow and not the flow rate. The velocities of all molecules in a gas or liquid are not the same. Axial streaming is characteristic of laminar flow (Fig. 31.5).

Methods of measuring gas volume and flow are considered in three groups:

- volume measurements
- steady gas flow rates
- unsteady gas flow rates.

VOLUME MEASUREMENTS

Measurements of gas volume depend on collecting the gases in a calibrated spirometer or passing the gases through some type of gas meter.

Spirometers

Wet spirometers consist of a rigid cylinder suspended over an underwater seal and counterbalanced. Gas entering the bell causes

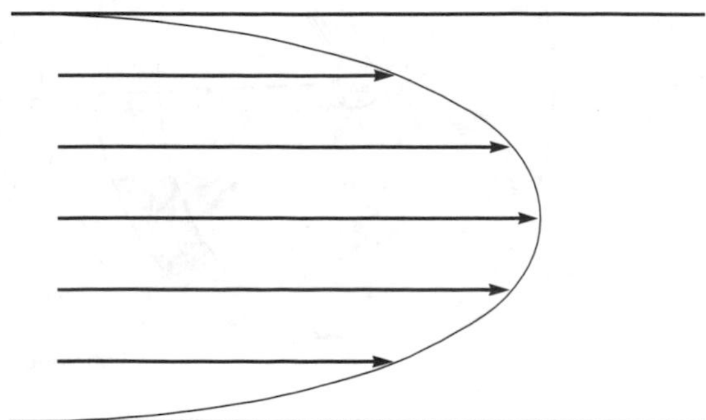

Fig. 31.5
Velocity profile during laminar flow. Velocity is zero at the walls of the containing tube and maximal in the axial stream.

it to rise. This linear displacement is proportional to the volume of gas. Wet spirometers are accurate at steady state and have been used to calibrate other volume-measuring devices. However, they are bulky and inconvenient to use, and the frequency response is damped by friction between the moving parts, causing the instrument to under-read with rapidly changing rates of flow.

Dry spirometers are more convenient for clinical work. Gas displaces a rolling diaphragm or bellows and the expansion is recorded and related to gas volume. The 'Vitalograph' is a specialized type of bellows spirometer used for lung function testing. The patient makes a maximal forced exhalation into the spirometer through a wide-bore tube. The expansion of the wedge-shaped bellows is recorded by a stylus on a pressure-sensitive chart. The stylus moves across the *x*-axis (time) at a constant rate. The resultant plot represents the volume–time plot of the patient's expiration (Fig. 31.6). The FVC is the maximal volume expired. Understanding of technique and active cooperation of the patient are essential for accurate and precise recordings. The patient must make an airtight seal with the mouthpiece and the nose is occluded with a nose clip. Expiration should be as forcible and rapid as possible. Several attempts are recorded. The highest value recorded is documented (as the technique is dependent on voluntary effort which usually improves with practice).

Gas meters

Dry gas meters are widely used in the gas industry and are used also in medicine, e.g. in some mechanical ventilators, to measure large volumes of gas. Displacement of bellows controls valves which alternately direct gas flow to fill and empty the bellows, and also drives the pointer on a calibrated recording dial. Irregularities within each cycle disappear when the meter has returned to the same position in the cycle; hence, accuracy of measurements improves with increasing multiples of meter volume.

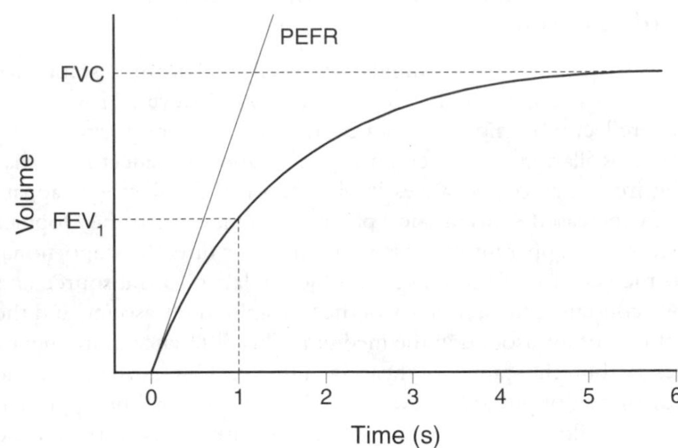

Fig. 31.6
Forced vital capacity (FVC), forced expiratory volume in 1 second (FEV_1), and peak expiratory flow rate can all be derived from the volume-time plot (Sykes et al 1991).

The Dräger volumeter

The volume of gas that flows through the Dräger volumeter is related to the rotation of two light, interlocking, dumbbell-shaped rotors. It is a simple meter and accurate when dry, but is affected by moisture.

The Wright respirometer

This device contains a light mica vane which rotates within a small cylinder (Fig. 31.7). Inflowing air is directed on to the vane by tangential slits. Rotation of the vane drives a gear chain and

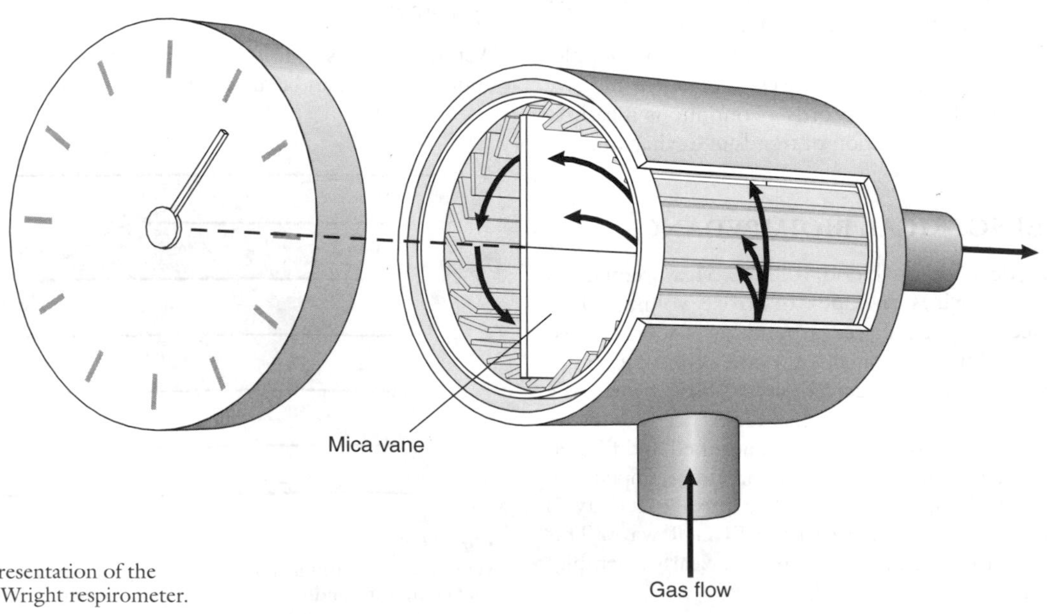

Fig. 31.7
Diagrammatic representation of the mechanism of the Wright respirometer.

pointer on a dial. This mechanism is described as inferential because it does not measure either the volume or the flow of all of the gas flowing through the device. It is calibrated for normal tidal volumes and breathing rates by a sine wave pump. However, the meter seriously over-reads at high tidal volumes and under-reads at low tidal volumes because of the inertia of the moving parts.

Integration of the flow signal

The flow signal from a rapidly responding flowmeter may be integrated electronically over time to calculate volume. However, the process of integration exaggerates the effect of baseline drift; a small and insignificant change in the baseline of the flow signal may produce substantial and increasing error in the volume signal over time. This effect is minimized by limiting the duration of integration, e.g. to a single tidal volume, by resetting the integrator to zero at the end of each inspiration.

Indirect methods of measuring tidal volume

Methods which depend on measuring inspired or expired gases require a leak-free connection. This is feasible with tracheal intubation. A physiological mouthpiece and connection to the measuring apparatus may change the pattern of breathing and is suitable only for short-term use. Several indirect methods have been developed which enable tidal volume to be derived from measurements of chest wall movement.

Pneumography

Pneumographs sense changes in chest and abdominal circumference. Non-elastic tapes are placed around the chest and abdomen and the ends are connected to a displacement sensor. The output may be calibrated to provide a tidal volume signal. However, these devices are sensitive to position and require frequent calibration.

Respiratory inductance plethysmography

Respiratory inductance plethysmograph uses a wire coil sewn into an elasticated strap. Expansion of the chest or abdomen increases the space between the coils and so alters the inductance generated by a high-frequency alternating (AC) current. The change in inductance depends on the cross-sectional area enclosed by the coil which is closely related to change in volume. Inductance plethysmography has been used in various physiological studies and to monitor postoperative respiratory depression and apnoea.

MEASUREMENT OF GAS FLOW RATE

Volume–time methods

Flow rate may be calculated from spirometric measurements of volume of gas per unit time. These methods are accurate when corrected for temperature and pressure and are used widely to calibrate other flowmeters, but are slow, cumbersome and have limited clinical application.

Most clinical methods are based on the relationship between pressure decrease and flow across a resistance – either a fixed pressure decrease across a variable orifice or a variable pressure change across a fixed orifice

Variable orifice (constant pressure change) flowmeters

The orifice through which gas flows enlarges with the flow rate so that the pressure difference across the orifice remains constant.

Rotameter

This is the physical principle of the Rotameter which consists of a vertical glass tube inside which rotates a light metal alloy bobbin (Fig. 31.8). The flow of gas is controlled by the fine-adjustment flow control valve at the bottom of the rotameter, and when this is opened the pressure of the gas forces the bobbin up the tube. The inside of the tube is shaped like an inverted cone, so that the cross-sectional area of the annular space exactly opposes the downward pressure resulting from the weight of the bobbin. The pressure decrease remains constant throughout the range of flows for which the tube is calibrated and the bobbin rotates freely in the steady stream of gas. Each Rotameter must be calibrated for a specific gas. Laminar flow predominates at low flow rates and depends on the viscosity of gas. Turbulent flow increases at higher flow rates and the density of the gas becomes an important factor. Both density and viscosity of a gas vary with temperature and pressure, and each Rotameter must be calibrated for one specific gas in appropriate conditions.

The peak flowmeter

This useful clinical instrument is capable of measuring flow rates up to 1000 L min^{-1}. Air flow causes a vane to rotate or a piston to move against the constant force of a light spring. This opens orifices which permit air to escape. The position adopted by the vane or piston depends primarily on the flow rate and on the area of the orifice which must be exposed to the air flow to maintain a constant pressure. The light moving vane or piston rapidly attains a maximum position in response to the peak expiratory flow. It is held in this position by a ratchet. The reading is obtained from a mechanical pointer which is attached to the vane or piston.

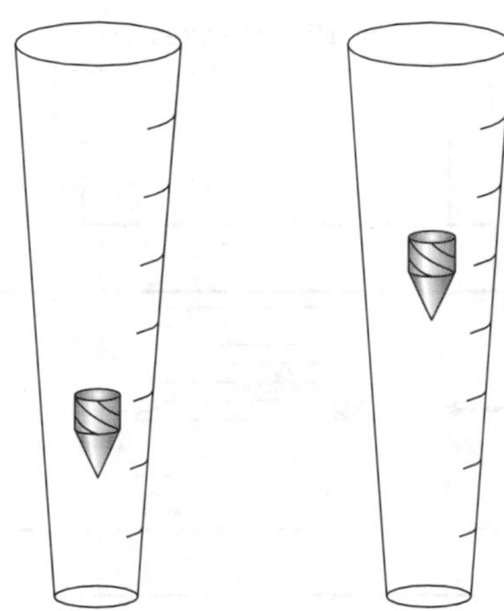

Fig. 31.8
Physical principle of the Rotameter flowmeter. The weight of the bobbin is exactly opposed by the pressure drop across the cross-sectional area of the annular space around the bobbin.

Accurate results demand good technique. These devices must be held horizontally to minimize the effects of gravity on the position of the moving parts. The patient must be encouraged to exhale as rapidly as possible. Consistency of repeated recordings suggests maximal effort and the peak expiratory flow rate is the maximum reading recorded.

Variable pressure change (fixed orifice) flowmeters

The resistance is maintained constant so that changes of flow are accompanied by changes in pressure across the resistance element.

Bourdon gauge flowmeter

A Bourdon gauge is used to sense the pressure change across an orifice and is calibrated to the gas flow rate. These rugged meters are not affected by changes in position and are useful for metering the flow from gas cylinders at high ambient pressure. Back-pressure causes over-reading of the actual flow rate.

Pneumotachograph

The pneumotachograph measures flow rate by sensing the pressure change across a small but laminar resistance. Careful design ensures that the differential manometer senses the true lateral pressure exerted by the gas on each side of the resistance element (Fig. 31.9). The differential manometer needs to be very sensitive to record the tiny changes in pressure across the resistance and transduce them to a continuous electrical output. This signal may be integrated to give volume and the manometer must have good zero and gain stability.

Pneumotachographs are sensitive instruments with a rapid response to changing gas flow and are used widely for clinical measurement of gas flows in respiratory and anaesthetic practice. The principles are easy to understand and they are used widely in the clinical measurement of respired gases. However, practical application requires frequent calibration and correction or compensation for differences in temperature, humidity, gas composition and pressure changes during mechanical ventilation.

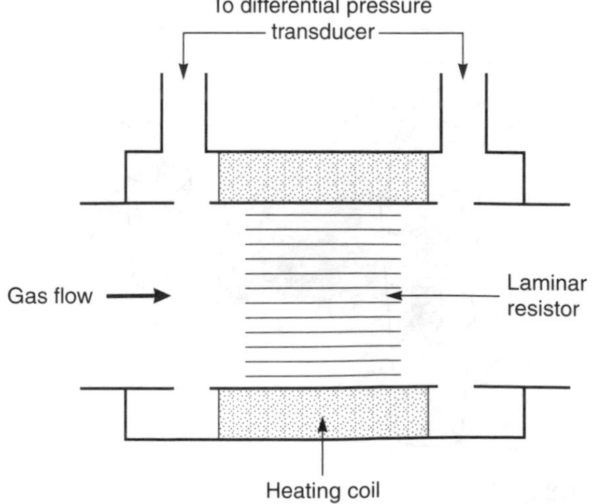

Fig. 31.9
The Fleisch pneumotachograph.

Other devices for measuring gas flow

Measurements other than pressure change across an orifice have been used to measure flow.

Hot wire flowmeters

These employ the rate of cooling of a heated wire which depends on the gas flow rate and is measured by sensing the change in temperature. It also depends on the thermal conductivity of the gas, which is affected by changes in the gas composition and the presence of water vapour.

Ultrasonic flowmeters

These flowmeters use the vortex-shedding technique. Gas is passed through a tube containing a rod 1–2 mm in diameter, mounted at right angles to the direction of gas flow. Vortices form downstream of the rod, the number of vortices formed being directly related to the flow rate. The vortices are detected using ultrasound and integrated to give a volume signal. Measurement is not affected greatly by temperature, humidity or changes in gas composition. A critical flow rate is required for the formation of vortices and the flowmeter is most accurate when the tidal volume is large.

GAS AND VAPOUR ANALYSIS

Three main applications of gas and vapour analysis are used in anaesthetic practice:

- to establish identity and concentrations of gases and vapours delivered to the patient
- to detect atmospheric pollution
- to assess metabolic or cardiorespiratory function either by analysis of the respired gases (O_2, CO_2 and N_2) or by the use of inert tracer gases such as helium, carbon monoxide or argon.

CHEMICAL METHODS

Chemical methods are important historically for measurement of oxygen and carbon dioxide concentrations. They involve the removal of fractional volumes from the gas phase by chemical reactions to non-gaseous compounds, the fractional concentration being determined by the reduction in volume that occurs:

$$\text{Fractional concentration} = \frac{\text{reduction in gas volume}}{\text{original volume}}$$

Several types of apparatus have been described, e.g. the Haldane. Carbon dioxide is absorbed in a strongly alkaline potassium hydroxide solution. Subsequently, oxygen is absorbed in alkaline pyrogallol or sodium anthraquinone.

PHYSICAL METHODS

In contrast with chemical methods, instruments based on the physical properties of a gas or vapour are convenient, responsive and more suitable for continuous operation.

Speed of response of the system is determined by two components:

- *Transit time* required for the sample to flow along the sampling catheter usually accounts for the greater part of the total delay. It is minimized by using a narrow and short sampling catheter with a rapid sampling flow rate.
- *Response time* required for the instrument to react to the change in gas concentration. It consists of the time required to wash out the analysis cell and delays imposed by the sensing mechanism.

Zero drift and variations in gain are common problems and most gas analysers have to be calibrated frequently, ideally against gas mixtures of known composition.

NON-SPECIFIC METHODS

Non-specific methods use a property of the gas which is common to all gases, but which is possessed by each gas to a differing degree.

Thermal conductivity

A gas with a high thermal conductivity conducts heat more readily than one with a low conductivity. In the katharometer, gas is passed over a heated wire and the degree of cooling of the wire depends on the temperature of the gas, the rate of gas flow and the thermal conductivity of the gas. The reduction in temperature of the wire reduces its resistance and produces an electrical signal related to the gas concentration. In clinical practice, katharometers are usually used for the measurement of CO_2 and He, and as detectors in gas chromatography systems.

Refractive index: interference refractometers

The speed of light slows through transparent materials to a degree determined by the refractive index of that substance. The delay caused by the passage of light through the gas depends on the number of gas molecules present; hence the refractive index also depends on the pressure and temperature of the gas. This extremely small delay is measured using the phase lag by the principle of interference. When light waves from a common source are passed through two linear slits in an opaque sheet and focused onto a screen, an interference pattern is produced. Bright areas where light from the two sources in phase is reinforced alternating with dark bands where the light paths differ in length by half a wavelength, i.e. they are out of phase and attenuating each other. When a gas is introduced into one light path, it delays transmission of the light waves with a reduction in wavelength and an alteration in the position of the dark bands. If the refractive index of the gas is known, the change in position may be related to the number of gas molecules in the light path and hence to the partial pressure of the gas. Interference refractometers are calibrated using known concentrations of gas or vapour. The response is essentially linear and after calibration remains stable.

This method of analysis is used to calibrate flowmeters and vaporizers accurately. Portable devices are useful for monitoring pollution by anaesthetic gases and vapours.

SPECIFIC METHODS

Specific methods identify and measure a gas using some unique property and are particularly suitable for complex mixtures of gases.

Magnetic susceptibility

Most gases are repelled by a magnetic field and are termed diamagnetic. Two unpaired electrons spinning in the same direction in the outer electron shell of the oxygen atom make the molecules strongly paramagnetic, i.e. attracted into a magnetic field.

The first paramagnetic analyser consisted of a cell containing the pole pieces of a permanent magnet. Two small spheres filled with a weakly diamagnetic gas such as nitrogen were connected by a short bridge and suspended by a taut wire in the strongest part of a non-homogeneous magnetic field. Molecules of a paramagnetic gas such as oxygen were attracted to the centre of the magnetic field and displaced the glass spheres with a force related to the concentration of oxygen molecules. This rotational force was detected by a reflected light spot or by the current required by an opposing induction coil to maintain the sensing element in the zero position. Accuracy was high but the mechanism was delicate and the response time slow.

Alternative designs of oxygen analyser are based on the paramagnetic property of oxygen. A fast differential paramagnetic oxygen sensor has been designed on the pneumatic bridge principle. The sample and reference gas are drawn by a common pump through two tubes surrounded by an electromagnet alternating at 110 Hz. Pressure differences between the two tubes are related to the paramagnetic properties of the sample and reference gases. The phasic changes in pressure are extremely small and measured with a miniature microphone. The output of the device is linear, very stable and has a fast response time of less than 150 ms.

Absorption of radiation

All gases absorb electromagnetic radiation in either the infrared or ultraviolet regions of the spectrum. The wavelengths are specific for each gas and depend on the molecular configuration.

Infrared gas analysers

Infrared radiation (1–15 μm) is absorbed by all gases with two or more dissimilar atoms in the molecule. The infrared spectrophotometer uses infrared light dispersed through a prism or diffraction grating into a spectrum of different wavelengths, which is absorbed to different degrees by the gas to be analysed, in a concentration-dependent manner, and the resulting absorption spectrum is specific to the gas. Modern infrared analysers use special photocells to detect and transduce the infrared radiation to a continuous electrical output.

There are several sources of error with infrared analysis:

- The absorption wavebands of different gases are coincident. For instance, the peak absorption bands for carbon dioxide, nitrous oxide and carbon monoxide are at 4.3, 4.5 and 4.7 μm, respectively, and the absorption spectra inevitably overlap. Error is minimized by narrowing the band of infrared light.

- The phenomenon of 'collision broadening' describes the apparent widening of the absorption spectrum of CO_2 by the physical presence of certain other gases, notably N_2 and N_2O. Correction factors have been described , but the error may be minimized by calibrating the instrument with similar background gas mixtures as the gas to be analysed.
- Absorption is related to the number of molecules in the absorbent gas in the cuvette, i.e. partial pressure. The reading is affected by changes in atmospheric pressure, pressurization of a breathing system or variation in the resistance of the sampling flow line.

Modern CO_2 analysers for clinical use are very stable but require regular calibration of the zero point and scale. Accuracy at normal breathing frequencies also requires a satisfactory response time, typically a 90 or 95% rise time less than 150 ms. Slow response is usually caused by blockage of the sampling line with condensation or sputum, or failure of the suction pump.

Mass spectrometry

Mass spectrometers are capable of separating the components of complex gas mixtures according to their mass and charge by deflecting the charged ions in a magnetic field. Molecules of sample gas are drawn into an evacuated ionization chamber where they are bombarded by a transverse beam of electrons. The positively charged ions then diffuse out of a slit in the chamber wall and are accelerated by a plate to which a negative voltage is applied. A magnetic field from plates or parallel cylindrical rods deflects the ions according to their mass:charge ratio. The ions impinge on a detector in proportion to the partial pressure of the sample gas. Streams of ions of different masses are detected by varying the accelerating and focusing voltages. A mass spectrum is produced by relating the detector output on the *y*-axis (calibrated to concentration of gas) to the accelerating voltage on the *x*-axis (calibrated to molecular weight).

Mass spectrometers are bulky and expensive, but have a very short response time (approx. 100 ms for a 95% response) and require very small sample flow rates (approx. 20 ml min^{-1}). All mass spectrometers operate under conditions of a very high vacuum which takes time to achieve and must be maintained.

Some molecules may lose two electrons and become doubly charged – they behave like ions with half the mass. Some fragmentation of molecules also occurs in the ionization process, resulting in the production of a mass spectrum rather than a single peak for each molecule. These secondary peaks may be used to advantage, e.g. in the identification and quantification of CO_2 and N_2O, both of which share a parent peak at 44 Da, but produce secondary peaks at 12 and 30 Da, respectively.

Gas–liquid chromatography

Gas–liquid chromatographs achieve separation of the components of a mixture using the principle of partition chromatography. The molecules of a solute partition between two solvents in a way that reflects the balance of attractive and repulsive forces between solute and solvent. One solvent is absorbed onto an inert material such as firebrick granules or a diatomaceous earth. This 'stationary phase' is packed into a narrow, stainless steel or glass tube (up to 2 m long) to form the chromatographic column. The second solvent is a moving stream of gas which flows through the column. The mixture to be analysed is injected as a bolus into this stream of carrier gas and its constituents then partition between the two solvents as the mixture is carried down the column. Components which have a high volatility or low solubility in the stationary phase are eluted before the less volatile or more soluble compounds and are the first to appear at the outlet of the column. Increasing temperature also pushes the partition in favour of the gaseous phase. This speeds the elution of the compound from the column. Careful control of temperature is used to separate two substances which have a similar solubility in the liquid phase, but different volatility.

The various components of the mixture thus emerge at varying intervals after injection and pass to a non-specific detector unit which yields an electronic signal proportional to the quantity of each substance present. Commonly used detectors include katharometers, flame ionization and electron capture detectors. Identification of the source of a deflection produced by a non-specific detector remains a problem in normal practice. Identification of known mixtures may be determined by the retention time for each constituent in the chromatograph column. The combination of a gas chromatograph and mass spectrometer is a particularly powerful analytical tool – the mass spectrometer identifies the molecular fragments present in any component eluted from a chromatograph column.

In addition to gas analysis, the gas–liquid chromatograph may be used to analyse blood samples containing volatile or local anaesthetic agents, anticonvulsants and intravenous anaesthetic drugs.

BLOOD GAS ANALYSIS

THE GLASS pH ELECTRODE

A potential difference is generated across hydrogen ion-sensitive glass depending on the gradient of hydrogen ions. The hydrogen ion concentration within the pH electrode is fixed by a buffer solution, so that the potential across the glass is dependent on the hydrogen ion concentration in the sample (Fig. 31.10).

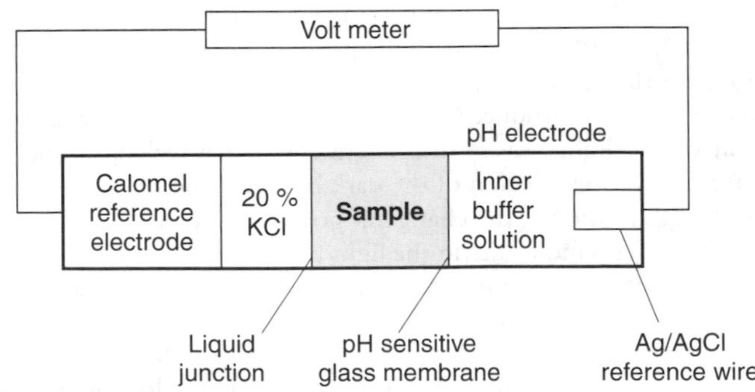

Fig. 31.10
Component parts of the pH electrode. Reproduced from the Radiometer Reference Manual. Permission from Radiometer A/S, Åkandevej 21, DK-2700 Brønshøj, Denmark.

Measurement of this potential gradient is complicated by the difficulty of making stable electrical contact with the sample and buffer solutions. Two silver:silver chloride electrodes generate an electrode potential, but this is constant at a fixed temperature and provides a stable electrical connection with the buffer solution in the pH electrode, and with a potassium chloride solution in the reference electrode separated from the test sample by a semi-permeable membrane. The potential difference between the electrodes is determined by the pH of the test solution and the temperature, and is calibrated using two phosphate buffers of known and fixed pH. Careful daily calibration is required to maintain accuracy and the electrodes must be regularly cleaned of protein deposits. Reliable measurement of blood pH also depends on the quality of the blood sample, which must be free from air bubbles, heparinized and analysed promptly.

Dissociation of acids and bases is temperature-dependent and the electrodes and blood sampling channel are maintained at 37°C. The measured pH is then corrected to indicate the pH at the temperature of the patient.

THE CO_2 ELECTRODE

The main methods of measuring carbon dioxide tension in liquids are based on pH measurement: carbon dioxide equilibrates in solution with hydrogen and bicarbonate ions. A glass pH electrode is in contact with a thin layer of bicarbonate buffer. The buffer is trapped in a nylon mesh spacer and separated by a thin Teflon or silicone membrane which is permeable to CO_2 but not to blood cells, plasma or charged ions.

The whole unit is maintained at 37°C. Carbon dioxide diffuses from the blood into the buffer, and so changes the hydrogen ion concentration. The electrode is calibrated by equilibrating the buffer with two known CO_2 concentrations to establish the relationship between pH and $P\text{CO}_2$.

OXYGENATION

Oxygenation may be assessed by measuring the tension, saturation or content of oxygen, the relationship between these three measurements being determined by the shape and position of the oxygen dissociation curve. There are many causes of variations in both the shape and position of the curve and it is usually necessary to measure the oxygen tension or saturation directly. Tension measurements are required for most respiratory problems, although saturation or content may be required for calculation of the percentage shunt.

Oxygen tension is usually measured using an oxygen electrode.

Content is measured by vacuum extraction and chemical absorption, by driving the O_2 into solution and measuring the increase in $P\text{O}_2$ or by galvanic cell analyser.

Saturation is determined by photometric techniques, involving the transmission or reflection of light at certain wavelengths.

Oxygen tension

Oxygen electrode: the polarographic method

The oxygen electrode (Clark) consists of a platinum wire, nominally 2 nm in diameter, embedded in a rough surfaced glass rod. This is immersed in a phosphate buffer which is stabilized with KCl and contained in an outer jacket which incorporates an oxygen-permeable polyethylene or polypropylene membrane (Fig. 31.11). A polarizing voltage of between 600 and 800 mV is applied to the platinum wire and as oxygen diffuses through the membrane electro-oxidoreduction occurs at the cathode:

$$O_2 + 4e^- \rightarrow 2O_2^-$$

$$2O_2^- + 2H_2O \rightarrow 4OH^-$$

Corresponding oxidation occurs at the Ag:AgCl anode:

$$4Ag \rightarrow 4Ag^+ + 4e^-$$

$$4Ag^+ + 4Cl^- \rightarrow 4AgCl$$

Thus a half cell is set up and a tiny current is generated dependent on the oxygen tension at the platinum cathode. The change in current is measured as a change in voltage using the same potentiometric circuit as the pH and $P\text{CO}_2$ measurement systems. The oxygen electrode may be used with gas mixtures or blood. Two-point calibration includes zero with an oxygen-free reference gas or an electronic zero with no electrode output, and the second point with 12% O_2. Temperature control is important and the electrode is maintained at 37°C. Accuracy is compromised by protein deposits or perforation of the delicate plastic membrane which must be regularly inspected. Oxygen continues to be consumed in blood samples which should be taken anaerobically, heparinized and analysed promptly.

Galvanic or fuel cell

Galvanic cells convert energy from an oxidation–reduction chemical process into electrical energy. The potential generated is dependent on the oxygen concentration.

A gold mesh cathode catalyses the reduction of oxygen by reaction with water to hydroxyl ions, while lead is oxidized at the

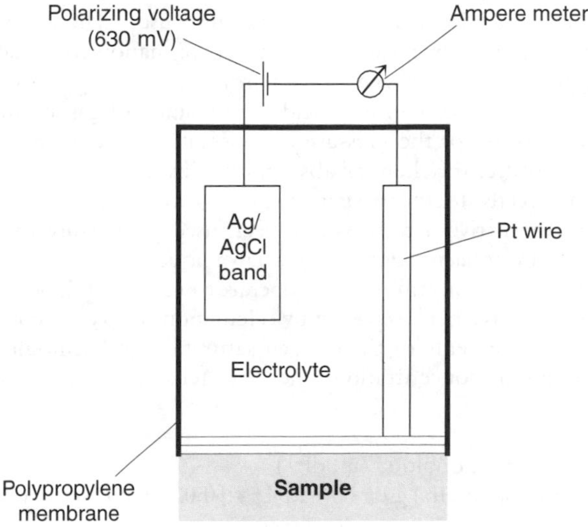

Fig. 31.11
The oxygen electrode. Reproduced from the Radiometer Reference Manual. Permission from Radiometer A/S, Åkandevej 21, DK-2700 Brønshøj, Denmark.

anode. Unlike the oxygen electrode, no battery is required. The reaction in the fuel cell generates a potential gradient. The chemical reaction uses up the components of the cell, so that its life depends on the concentration of oxygen to which it is exposed and on the duration of exposure: in practice, 6–12 months. Fuel cells are widely used in reliable and portable oxygen analysers which incorporate a digital readout and audible alarms. These are cheap and require little maintenance. Inaccurate responses to calibration with oxygen and air suggest that the fuel cell is exhausted and should be replaced.

Transcutaneous electrodes

Transcutaneous electrodes are non-invasive and used extensively for monitoring neonatal blood gas tensions. The electrodes are based on principles similar to those used in blood gas analysers but also incorporate a heating element. The electrode is attached to the skin to form an airtight seal using a contact liquid and the area is heated to 43°C. At this temperature, the blood flow to the skin increases and the capillary oxygen diffuses through the skin allowing measurement of the diffused gases by the attached electrode. The values obtained from the transcutaneous electrode are lower than those from a simultaneous arterial specimen. Many factors affect the transcutaneous measurement of oxygen tension, including the skin site and thickness. Most importantly, the electrode depends on local capillary blood flow and reads low with hypotension and microcirculatory perfusion failure. Problems occur with surgical diathermy; the heating current circuit provides a return path for the cutting current which may cause the transcutaneous electrode to overheat.

Other methods of measuring oxygen tension in blood include mass spectrometry and optodes, which employ the quenching of fluorescence from illuminated dye.

Oxygen content

The total amount of oxygen in blood may be measured directly, but this is technically demanding and rarely used. The van Slyke technique uses a chemical and volumetric or manometric analysis of oxygen content. Oxygen is driven from a small sample by denaturing the haemoglobin with acid. The volume of gas at atmospheric pressure, or the pressure at constant volume, is recorded before and after the chemical absorption of oxygen. The change is related directly to the oxygen content of the fixed volume of blood. Alternative detectors have been used to measure oxygen displaced from haemoglobin, e.g. a galvanic cell.

These time-consuming and operator-dependent laboratory techniques have been replaced by calculation of oxygen content from measurements of the oxygen saturation of haemoglobin, haemoglobin concentration and the tension of oxygen in blood:

$$\text{Oxygen content of blood (ml dl}^{-1}\text{)} = [S\text{O}_2\ (\%) \times \text{Hb (g dl}^{-1}\text{)} \times 1.34] + [0.0225 \times P\text{O}_2\ \text{(kPa)}]$$

Accurate estimates require that the oxygen saturation of haemoglobin is measured directly, and not calculated from oxygen tension and an arbitrary but unmeasured oxygen dissociation curve.

Oximetry: measurement of oxygen saturation

In vitro oximetry

Oximetry relies on the differing absorption of light at different wavelengths by the various states of haemoglobin. The absorption of radiation passing through a sample is measured. The degree of absorption of light, defined by the ratio of incident to emergent light intensities on a logarithmic scale, is proportional to the concentration of the molecules absorbing light (Beer's law) and the thickness of the absorbing layer (Lambert's law).

Oxyhaemoglobin and deoxyhaemoglobin differ at both the red and infrared portions of the spectrum (Fig. 31.12). The differential absorption of two wavelengths of red and infrared light permits the calculation of the ratio of the concentration of oxygenated and reduced haemoglobins. Additional wavelengths are added in co-oximeters for the calculation of the proportions of other species of haemoglobin, such as carboxyhaemoglobin and methaemoglobin, and the absolute absorbance is used to estimate total haemoglobin concentration from the sum of the various haemoglobins. This is important in measurements of oxyhaemoglobin for use in the calculation of oxygen content.

Commercial co-oximeters draw a small blood sample which is haemolysed before entering a cuvette. Light is filtered to produce monochromatic beams, shone through the cuvette and detected by a photocell. The absorption by the sample is the difference in the intensity of both incident and transmitted light and both must be measured. Spectrophotometers apply a double-beam technique which improves the accuracy and precision. Light from the monochromator is split into two beams, which pass through the test sample or a reference sample. Photocells generate two signals corresponding to the sample and the reference light intensities. Electronic processing compares the two signals and generates an output proportional to the difference. This greatly improves the signal-to-noise ratio because any variation which affects both the sample and reference beams equally is ignored and the difference remains constant.

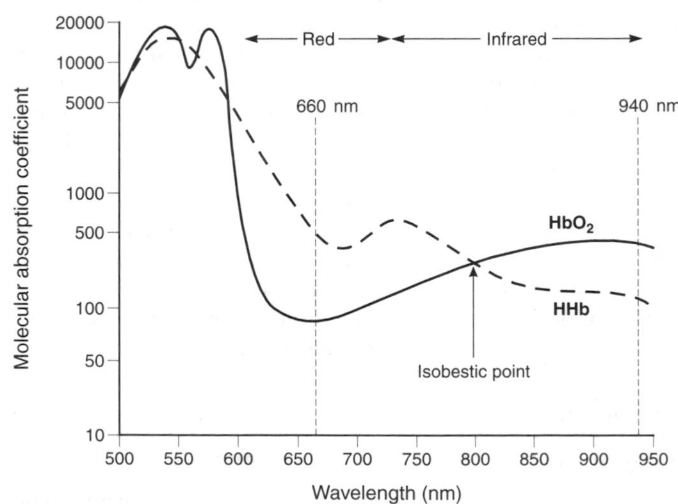

Fig. 31.12
Absorption spectra of reduced (HHb) and oxygenated (HbO_2) haemoglobin.

The saturation of mixed venous blood may be measured using an oximeter incorporated into a pulmonary artery catheter. Fibreoptic cables transmit incident light of at least two wavelengths, and reflected light from red blood cells back to a detector.

The same spectrophotometric principles used by co-oximeters in vitro on haemolysed blood samples have been applied to patients in vivo.

Pulse oximetry

Light transmitted through tissues is absorbed not only by arterial blood, but also by other tissue pigments and venous blood. However, the variation in light absorption with each pulse beat results almost entirely from pulsatile arterial blood flow. Two light-emitting diodes – red (660 nm) and infrared (940 nm) – shine light through a finger or earlobe and a photocell detects the transmitted light. The output of the sensor is processed to display a pulse waveform and the arterial oxygen saturation.

To identify the absorption at each wavelength, the LEDs are switched on and off at 30 Hz to detect the cyclical changes in the signal due to pulsatile arterial blood flow. The electrical output from the photodetector consists of a steady (DC) signal which depends on the strength of the light source, absorption by the tissues and by the arterial, venous and capillary blood. On this is superimposed a pulsatile (AC) signal resulting from absorbance associated with the greater volume of blood in the light path with each pulse wave (Fig. 31.13). These raw signals require complex processing. The AC level is scaled relative to the DC component so that it is no longer a function of the incident light intensity. The ratio of the amplitude of the red and infrared pulsatile signals is related to arterial saturation using an algorithm which is non-linear and derived from empirical measurements.

Several important sources of error are common in the measurement of pulse oximetry:

- The AC signal sensed by the pulse oximeter is less than 5% of the DC signal when the pulse volume is normal. Inadequate signals are caused by vasoconstriction or poor perfusion from whatever cause. Modern instruments display a continuous waveform and include algorithms which warn of inadequate pulsation or probe misplacement.
- Errors in measurement are underestimated. Calibration points in the range 80–100% are derived from volunteer studies and values below this are extrapolated and unreliable. Accuracy within the working range is ± 3%, and the variability between different instruments is significantly higher.
- The response time is slow and includes two separate components: instrument delay and circulatory delay. Instrument delay is caused by averaging times of 10–15 s which are designed to improve reliability. Circulatory delay depends on the distribution of blood from the lungs to the tissues. Response time at the fingertip may exceed 1 min in normal subjects, and is exaggerated by low cardiac output or vasoconstriction.
- Having only two transmitted wavelengths does not permit pulse oximeters to differentiate oxyhaemoglobin from other species of haemoglobin, especially carboxyhaemoglobin and methaemoglobin. Dyes, including methylene blue and bilirubin, may also cause interference.

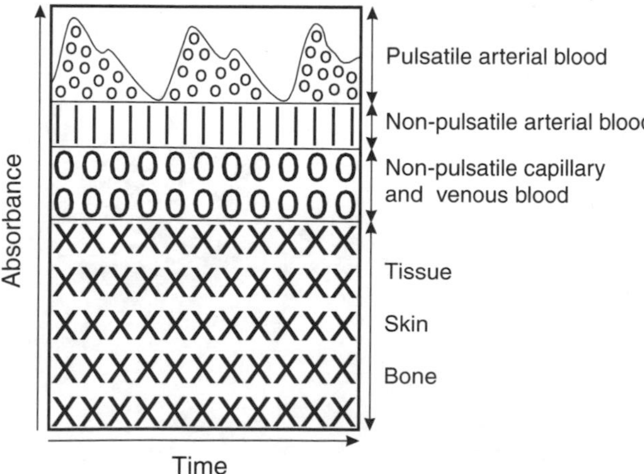

Fig. 31.13
Schematic representation of the contribution of pulsatile anterial blood, non-plusatile blood and tissues to the absorbance of light.

THERMOMETRY

Several temperature-dependent phenomena have been incorporated in commercial thermometers.

DIRECT READING NON-ELECTRICAL THERMOMETERS

Liquid expansion thermometers

Liquid expansion thermometers are simple, reliable instruments. A glass bulb is filled with a liquid (generally alcohol or mercury) and connected to an evacuated, closed capillary tube. The temperature is recorded by the position of the meniscus in the capillary tube against a calibrated scale. If the cross-sectional area of the capillary tube is constant, movement of the meniscus with changing temperature is linear.

Several simple and elegant design features improve usability. A large bulb and very narrow capillary increase the sensitivity. Visibility of the narrow capillary is improved by shaping the thermometer so that the glass forms a lens and by incorporating a strip of white glass behind the capillary. A constriction in the capillary tube permits the mercury to expand but hinders its return to the bulb so that the reading is preserved until the mercury is shaken down. However, glass thermometers are fragile. A large thermal capacity results in a slow response. The instrument is hand-held, awkward to read and reset, and cannot be used for remote measurement or recording.

Dial thermometers

Dial thermometers exploit the increase in pressure caused by the temperature-dependent expansion of a liquid or gas in an enclosed cavity. This is sensed by a Bourdon pressure gauge and recorded on a dial. Although cheap and robust, they are relatively inaccurate, slow to respond and are only suitable for large temperature changes in heated equipment, e.g. autoclaves.

Bimetallic strip thermometers

If strips of two metals with different coefficients of expansion are fastened together throughout their length, the combined strip will bend when heated. Sensitivity is improved by using a long strip which is usually bent in a spiral or coil, with one end fixed and the other connected to a recording pointer. This technique is used for temperature compensation in some anaesthetic vaporizers, and in cheap mechanical thermometers for measuring air temperature.

CHEMICAL THERMOMETERS

Thermometers based on temperature-dependent changes in chemical mixtures have been marketed. Reversible chemical thermometers contain several cells filled with liquid crystals, each of slightly different composition. At a critical temperature, the optical properties change because of realignment of the molecules, causing reflection instead of absorption of the incident light. An alternative technique consists of rows of cells filled with chemical mixtures which melt at specific temperatures releasing a dye; this single-use, disposable design prevents cross-infection but is relatively expensive.

REMOTE READING INSTRUMENTS

Temperature-dependent electrical properties may be incorporated into thermometers suitable for automation.

Resistance-wire thermometers

Resistance-wire thermometers are based on the principle that the resistance of certain metal wires increases as their temperature increases. Platinum resistance thermometers have a large temperature coefficient of resistance and are very sensitive to small changes in temperature, but are fragile and slow to respond. Single-use probes which incorporate a tiny copper element have been marketed with an acceptable clinical accuracy and response time.

Thermistor thermometers

Thermistors are semiconductors made from the fused oxides of heavy metals such as cobalt, manganese and nickel. They demonstrate marked and non-linear variation in resistance with temperature, which is usually compensated by electronic processing. Disadvantages include inconsistent variation between individual thermistors, change in resistance over time, and hysteresis during rapid heating and cooling. However, the large temperature coefficient permits the detection of small temperature changes and the tiny 'pin-head' size results in a rapid response. They are used widely in invasive temperature monitoring, e.g. in pulmonary artery catheters.

Thermocouple thermometers

If two dissimilar metals are joined to create an electrical circuit and the junctions are at different temperatures, a current flows from one metal to the other. The potential difference that is generated is a function of the temperature difference between the two junctions. All junctions made from the same metals have identical properties. The reference junction must be kept at a constant temperature, or incorporate temperature compensation into the measurement. Common combinations of metals include copper–-constantan or platinum–rhodium. The output is small (about 40 mV per °C temperature difference between the junctions), but this is sufficient to be sensed by a galvanometer.

FURTHER READING

Cruikshank S 1998 Mathematics and statistics in anaesthesia. Oxford Medical Publications, Oxford

Parbrook G D, Davis P D, Kenny G 1995 Basic physics and measurement in anaesthesia, 4th edn. Butterworth-Heinemann, Oxford

Scurr C, Feldman S A, Soni N 1991 Scientific foundations of anaesthesia, 4th edn. Butterworth-Heinemann, Oxford

Sykes M K 1992 Clinical measurement and clinical practice. Anaesthesia 47: 425–432

Sykes M K, Vickers M D, Hull C J 1991 Principles of clinical measurement, 3rd edn. Blackwell Scientific Publications, Oxford

32 Anaesthetic apparatus

Anaesthetists must have a sound understanding and firm knowledge of the functioning of all anaesthetic equipment in common use. Although primary malfunction of equipment has not featured highly in surveys of anaesthetic-related morbidity and mortality, failure to understand the use of equipment features in these reports as a cause of morbidity and mortality. This is true especially of ventilators, where lack of knowledge regarding the function of equipment may result in a patient being subjected to the dangers of hypoxaemia and/or hypercapnia.

It is essential that anaesthetists check that all equipment is functioning correctly before they proceed to anaesthetize patients (see Ch. 36). In some respects, the routine of testing anaesthetic equipment resembles the airline pilot's checklist, which is an essential preliminary to aircraft flight.

The purpose of this chapter is to describe briefly apparatus which is used in delivery of gases, from the sources of supply to the patient's lungs. Clearly, it is not possible to describe in detail equivalent models produced by all manufacturers. Consequently, this chapter concentrates only on principles and some equipment which is used commonly.

It is convenient to describe anaesthetic apparatus sequentially from the supply of gases to point of delivery to the patient. This sequence is shown in Table 32.1.

Table 32.1 Classification of anaesthetic equipment described in this chapter

Supply of gases
- From outside the operating theatre
- From cylinders within the operating theatre, together with the connections involved

The anaesthetic machine
- Unions
- Cylinders
- Reducing valves
- Flowmeters
- Vaporizers

Safety features of the anaesthetic machine

Anaesthetic breathing systems

Ventilators

Apparatus used in scavenging waste anaesthetic gases

Apparatus used in interfacing the patient to the anaesthetic breathing system
- Laryngoscopes
- Tracheal tubes

Accessory apparatus for the airway
- Anaesthetic masks and airways
- Forceps
- Laryngeal sprays
- Bougies
- Mouth gags
- Stilettes
- Catheter mounts

Suction apparatus

GAS SUPPLIES

BULK SUPPLY OF ANAESTHETIC GASES

In the majority of modern hospitals, piped medical gases and vacuum (PMGV) systems have been installed. These obviate the necessity for holding large numbers of cylinders in the operating theatre suite. Normally, only a few cylinders are kept in reserve, attached usually to the anaesthetic machine.

The advantages of the PMGV system are reductions in cost, in the necessity to transport cylinders and in accidents caused by cylinders becoming exhausted. However, there have been several well-publicized incidents in which anaesthetic morbidity or mortality has resulted from incorrect connections in piped medical gas supplies.

The PMGV services comprise five sections:

- bulk store
- distribution pipelines in the hospital
- terminal outlets, situated usually on the walls or ceilings of the operating theatre suite and other sites
- flexible hoses connecting the terminal outlets to the anaesthetic machine
- connections between flexible hoses and anaesthetic machines.

Responsibility for the first three items lies with the engineering and pharmacy departments. Within the operating theatre, it is partly the anaesthetist's responsibility to check the correct functioning of the last two items.

BULK STORE

Oxygen

In small hospitals, oxygen may be supplied to the PMGV from a bank of several oxygen cylinders attached to a manifold.

Oxygen cylinder manifolds consist of two groups of large cylinders (size J). The two groups alternate in supplying oxygen to the pipelines. In both groups, all cylinder valves are open so that they empty simultaneously. All cylinders have non-return valves. The supply automatically changes from one group to the other when the first group of cylinders is nearly empty. The changeover also activates an electrical signalling system which alerts staff to change the empty cylinders.

However, in larger hospitals, pipeline oxygen originates from a liquid oxygen store. Liquid oxygen is stored at a temperature of approximately −165°C at 10.5 bar in a giant Thermos flask – a vacuum insulated evaporator (VIE). Some heat passes from the environment through the insulating layer between the two shells of the flask, increasing the tendency to evaporation and pressure increase within the chamber. Pressure is maintained constant by transfer of gaseous oxygen into the pipeline system (via a warming device). However, if the pressure increases above 17 bar (1700 kPa), a safety valve opens and oxygen runs to waste. When the supply of oxygen resulting from the slow evaporation from the surface in the VIE is inadequate, the pressure decreases and a valve opens to allow liquid oxygen to pass into an evaporator, from which gas passes into the pipeline system.

Liquid oxygen plants are housed some distance away from hospital buildings because of the risk of fire. Even when a hospital possesses a liquid oxygen plant, it is still necessary to hold reserve banks of oxygen cylinders in case of supply failure.

Oxygen concentrators

Recently, oxygen concentrators have been used to supply hospitals and it is likely that the use of these devices will increase in future. The oxygen concentrator depends upon the ability of an artificial zeolight to entrap molecules of nitrogen. These devices cannot produce pure oxygen, but the concentration usually exceeds 90%; the remainder comprises nitrogen, argon and other inert gases. Small oxygen concentrators are provided for domiciliary use.

Nitrous oxide

Nitrous oxide and Entonox may be supplied from banks of cylinders connected to manifolds similar to those used for oxygen.

Medical compressed air

Compressed air is supplied from a bank of cylinders into the PMGV system. Air of medical quality is required, as industrial compressed air may contain fine particles of oil (see Ch. 13).

Piped medical vacuum

Piped medical vacuum is provided by large vacuum pumps which discharge via a filter and silencer to a suitable point, usually at roof level, where gases are vented to atmosphere. Although concern has been expressed regarding the possibility of volatile anaesthetic agents dissolving in the lubricating oil of vacuum pumps and causing malfunction, this fear has not been substantiated.

TERMINAL OUTLETS

There has been standardization of terminal outlets in the UK since 1978, but there is no universal standard.

Six types of terminal outlet are found commonly in the operating theatre. The terminals are colour-coded and also have non-interchangeable connections specific to each gas:

- Vacuum (coloured yellow) – a vacuum of at least 53 kPa (400 mmHg) should be maintained at the outlet, which should be able to take a free flow of air of at least 40 L min^{-1}.
- Compressed air (coloured white/black) at 4 bar – this is used for anaesthetic breathing systems and ventilators.
- Air (coloured white/black) at 7 bar – this is to be used only for powering compressed air tools and is confined usually to the orthopaedic operating theatre.
- Nitrous oxide (coloured blue) at 4 bar.
- Oxygen (coloured white) at 4 bar.
- Scavenging – there is a variety of scavenging outlets from the operating theatre. The passive systems are designed to accept a standard 30 mm connection.

Whenever a new pipeline system has been installed or servicing of an existing pipeline system has been undertaken, a designated member of the pharmacy staff should test the gas obtained from the sockets, using an oxygen analyser. Malfunction of an oxygen/air mixing device may result in entry of compressed air into the oxygen pipeline, rendering an anaesthetic mixture hypoxic. Because of this and other potential mishaps, it has been advocated that oxygen analysers be used routinely during anaesthesia.

GAS SUPPLIES

Gas supplies to the anaesthetic machine should be checked at the beginning of each session to ensure that the gas which issues from the pipeline or cylinder is the same as that which passes through the appropriate flowmeter. This ensures that pipelines are not connected incorrectly. Both the machine in the operating theatre and that in the anaesthetic room should be checked. Checking of anaesthetic machine and medical gas supplies is discussed fully in Chapter 36.

CYLINDERS

Modern cylinders are constructed from molybdenum steel. They are checked at intervals by the manufacturer to ensure that they can withstand hydraulic pressures considerably in excess of those to which they are subjected in normal use. One cylinder in every 100 is cut into strips to test the metal for tensile strength, flattening impact and bend tests. Medical gas cylinders are tested hydraulically every 5 years and the tests recorded by a mark stamped on the neck of the cylinder.

The cylinders are provided in a variety of sizes, and colour-coded according to the gas supplied. The cylinders comprise a body and a shoulder containing threads into which are fitted a pin index valve block, a bull-nosed valve or a handwheel valve.

The pin index system was devised to prevent interchangeability of cylinders of different gases. Pin index valves are provided for the smaller cylinders of oxygen and nitrous oxide (and also carbon dioxide) which may be attached to anaesthetic machines. The pegs on the inlet connection slot into corresponding holes on the cylinder valve.

Full cylinders are supplied usually with a plastic dust cover in order to prevent contamination by dirt. This cover should not be removed until immediately before the cylinder is fitted to the anaesthetic machine. When fitting the cylinder to a machine, the yoke is positioned and tightened with the handle of the yoke spindle. After fitting, the cylinder should be opened to make sure that it is full and that there are no leaks at the gland nut or the pin index valve junction, caused, for example, by absence of or damage to the washer. The washer used is normally a Bodok seal which has a metal periphery designed to keep the seal in good condition for a long period.

Cylinder valves should be opened slowly to prevent sudden surges of pressure and should be closed with no more force than is necessary, otherwise the valve seating may be damaged.

The sealing material between the valve and the neck of the cylinder may be constructed from a fusable material which melts in the event of fire and allows the contents of the cylinder to escape around the threads of the joint.

The colour codes used for medical gas cylinders are shown in Table 32.2 and the cylinder sizes and capacities are shown in Table 32.3.

THE ANAESTHETIC MACHINE

The anaesthetic machine comprises:

- a means of supplying gases either from attached cylinders or from piped medical supplies via appropriate unions on the machine
- methods of measuring flow rate of gases
- apparatus for vaporizing volatile anaesthetic agents
- breathing systems and a ventilator for delivery of gases and vapours from the machine to the patient
- apparatus for scavenging anaesthetic gases in order to minimize environmental pollution.

SUPPLY OF GASES

In the UK, gases are supplied at a pipeline pressure of 4 bar (400 kPa, 60 lb in^{-2}) and this pressure is transferred directly to the bank of flowmeters and back bar of the anaesthetic machine. The flexible colour-coded hoses connect the pipeline outlets to the anaesthetic machine. The anaesthetic machine end of the hoses should be permanently fixed using a nut and liner union where the thread is gas-specific and non-interchangeable. The non-interchangeable screw thread (NIST) is the British Standard.

Table 32.2 Medical gas cylinders in the UK

	Colour		Pressure at 15°C	
	Body	**Shoulder**	**lb in^{-2}**	**bar**
Oxygen	Black	White	1987	137
Nitrous oxide	Blue	Blue	638	44
CO_2	Grey	Grey	725	50
Helium	Brown	Brown	1987	137
Air	Grey	White/black quarters	1987	137
O_2 / helium	Black	White/brown quarters	1987	137
O_2 / CO_2	Black	White/grey quarters	1987	137
N_2O/O_2 (Entonox)	Blue	White/blue quarters	1987	137

Table 32.3 Medical gas cylinder sizes and capacities

Cylinder size	A	B	C	D	E	F	G	J
Height (in)	**10**	**10**	**14**	**18**	**31**	**34**	**49**	**57**
Capacities (L)								
Oxygen			170	340	680	1360	3400	6800
Nitrous oxide			450	900	1800	3600	9000	
CO_2			450	900	1800			
Helium				300		1200		
Air							3200	6400
O_2 / helium					600	1200		
O_2 / CO_2						1360	3400	
Entonox							3200	6400

375

The gas issuing from other medical gas cylinders is at a much higher pressure, necessitating the interposition of a pressure regulator between the cylinder and the bank of flowmeters. In some older anaesthetic machines (and in some other countries), the pressure in the pipelines of the anaesthetic machine may be 3 bar (300 kPa, 45 lb in^{-2}).

PRESSURE REGULATORS

Pressure regulators are used on anaesthetic machines for three purposes:

- to reduce the high pressure of gas in a cylinder to a safe working level
- to prevent damage to equipment on the anaesthetic machine, e.g. flow control valves
- as the contents of the cylinder are used, the pressure within the cylinder decreases and the regulating mechanism maintains a constant outlet pressure, obviating the necessity to make continuous adjustments to the flowmeter controls.

The principles underlying the operation of flowmeters are described in detail in Chapter 30.

Flow restrictors

Pressure regulators are omitted usually when anaesthetic machines are supplied directly from a pipeline at a pressure of 4 bar. Changes in pipeline pressure would cause changes in flow rate, necessitating adjustment of the flow control valves. This is prevented by the use of a flow restrictor upstream of the flowmeter (flow restrictors are simply constrictions in the low-pressure circuit).

A different type of flow restrictor may be fitted also to the downstream end of the vaporizers to prevent back-pressure effects (see Ch. 30). The absence of such a flow restrictor may be detected if a ventilator such as the Manley is used, as this leads to fluctuations in the positions of the flowmeter bobbins during the respiratory cycle.

Pressure relief valves on regulators

Pressure relief valves are often fitted on the downstream side of regulators to allow escape of gas if the regulators were to fail (thereby causing a high output pressure). Relief valves are set usually at approximately 7 bar for regulators designed to give an output pressure of 4 bar.

FLOWMETERS

The principles of flowmeters are described in detail in Chapter 30.

Problems with flowmeters

- *Non-vertical tube.* This causes a change in shape of the annulus and therefore variation in flow. If the bobbin touches the side of the tube, resulting friction causes an even more inaccurate reading.
- *Static electricity.* This may cause inaccuracy (by as much as 35%) and sticking of the bobbin, especially at low flows. This may be reduced by coating the inside of the tube with a transparent film of gold or tin.
- *Dirt* on the bobbin may cause sticking or alteration in size of the annulus and therefore inaccuracies.
- *Back-pressure.* Changes in accuracy may be produced by back-pressure. For example, the Manley ventilator may exert a back-pressure and depress the bobbin; there may be as much as 10% more gas flow than that indicated on the flowmeter. Similar problems may be produced by the insertion of any equipment which restricts flow downstream, e.g. Selectatec head, vaporizer.
- *Leakage.* This results usually from defects in the top sealing washer of a flowmeter.

It is unfortunate that in the UK the standard position of the oxygen flowmeters is on the left followed by either nitrous oxide or air (if all three gases are supplied). On several recorded occasions, patients have suffered damage from hypoxia because of leakage from a broken flowmeter tube in this type of arrangement, as oxygen, being at the upstream end, passes out to the atmosphere through any leak. This problem is reduced if the oxygen flowmeter is placed downstream (i.e. on the right-hand side of the bank of flowmeters) as is standard practice in the USA. In the UK, this problem is now avoided by designing the outlet from the oxygen flowmeter to enter the back bar downstream from the outlets of other flowmeters (Fig. 32.1). Most modern anaesthetic machines do not have a flowmeter for carbon dioxide.

The emergency oxygen flush is a non-locking button which, when pressed, delivers pure oxygen from the anaesthetic outlet. On modern anaesthetic machines, the emergency oxygen flush lever is situated downstream from the flowmeters and vaporizers. A flow of about 35–45 L min^{-1} at pipeline pressure is delivered. This may lead to dilution of the anaesthetic mixture with excess oxygen if the emergency oxygen tap is opened partially by mistake and may result in awareness. There is also a risk of barotrauma

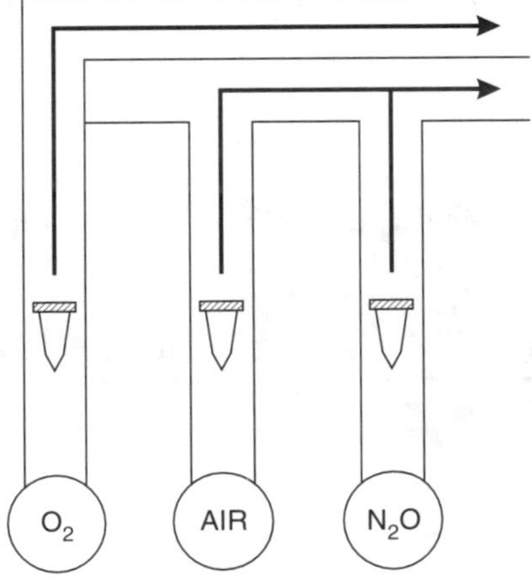

Fig. 32.1
Oxygen is the last gas to be added to the gas mixture being delivered to the back bar.

should the high pressure be accidentally delivered directly to the patient's lungs.

Quantiflex

The Quantiflex mixer flowmeter (Fig. 32.2) eliminates the possibility of reducing the oxygen supply inadvertently. One dial is set to the desired percentage of oxygen and the total flow rate is adjusted independently. The oxygen passes through a flowmeter to provide evidence of correct functioning of the linked valves. Both gases arrive via linked pressure-reducing regulators. The Quantiflex is useful in particular for varying the volume of fresh gas flow (FGF) from moment to moment whilst keeping the proportions constant. In addition, the oxygen flowmeter is situated downstream of the nitrous oxide flowmeter.

Linked flowmeters

The majority of modern anaesthetic machines such as that shown in Figure 32.3 possess a mechanical linkage between the N_2O and O_2 flowmeters. This causes the N_2O flow to decrease if the oxygen flowmeter is adjusted to give less than 25–30% O_2 (Fig. 32.4).

VAPORIZERS

The principles of vaporizers are described in detail in Chapter 30.

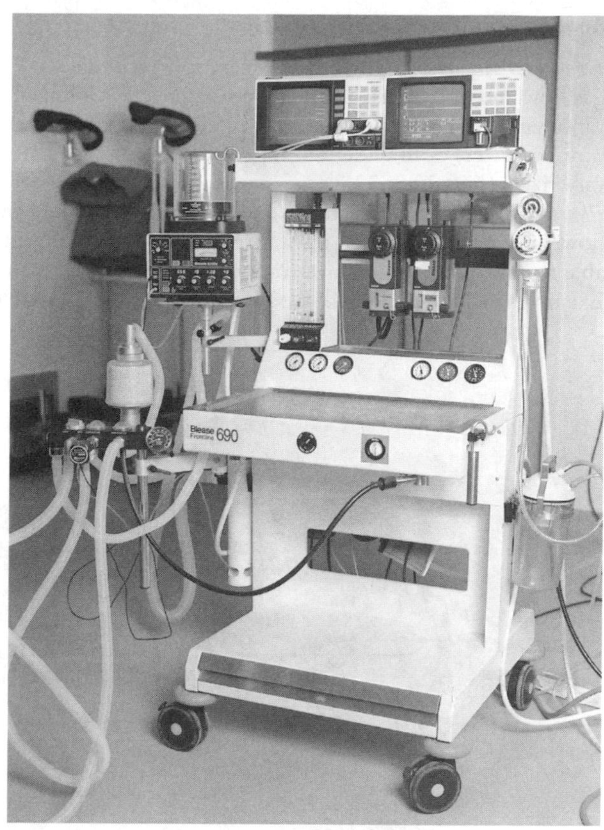

Fig. 32.3
A Blease Frontline anaesthetic machine.

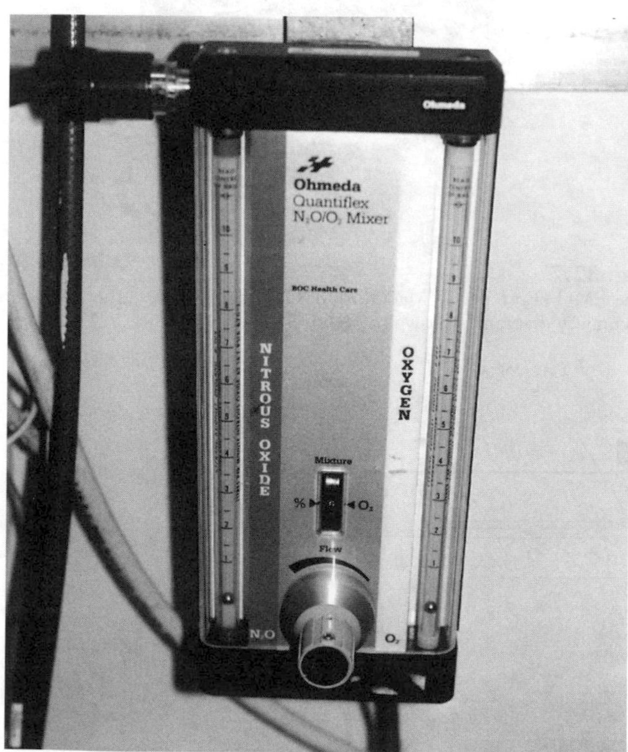

Fig. 32.2
A Quantiflex flowmeter. The required oxygen percentage is selected using the dial, and total flow of the oxygen/nitrous oxide mixture is adjusted using the black knob.

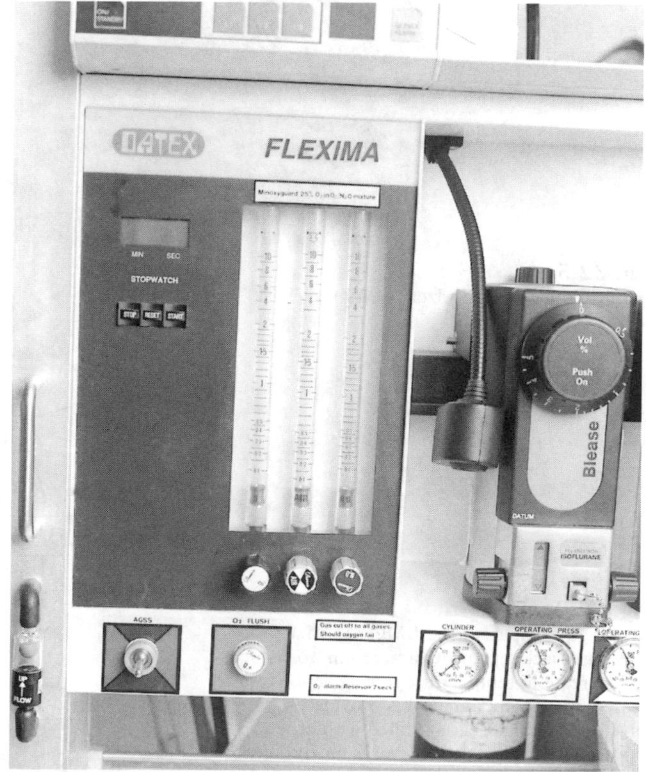

Fig. 32.4
Flowmeters with mechanical linkage between nitrous oxide and oxygen.

Modern vaporizers may be classified as:

- *Drawover vaporizers.* These have a very low resistance to gas flow and may be used in a circle system (e.g. Goldman vaporizer), for emergency use in the field (e.g. Oxford miniature vaporizer) or in underdeveloped countries (e.g. EMO vaporizer) (Figs 32.5–32.8).
- *Plenum vaporizers.* These are intended for unidirectional gas flow, have a relatively high resistance to flow and are unsuitable for use either as drawover vaporizers or in a circle system. Examples include the 'TEC' type in which there is a variable

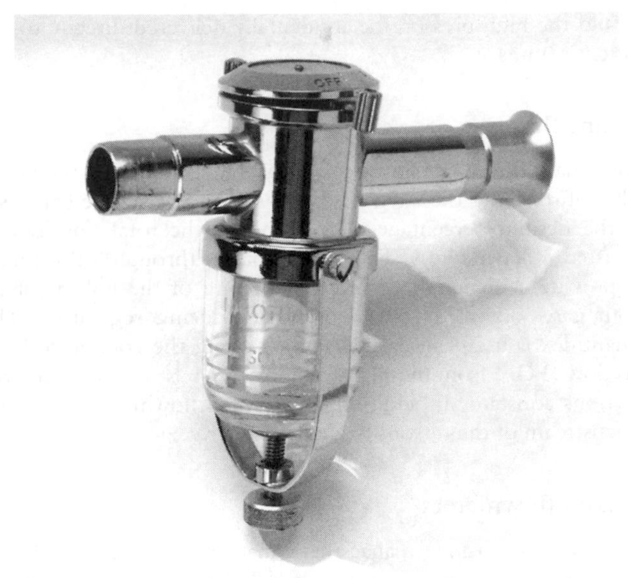

Fig. 32.6
The Goldman drawover vaporizer.

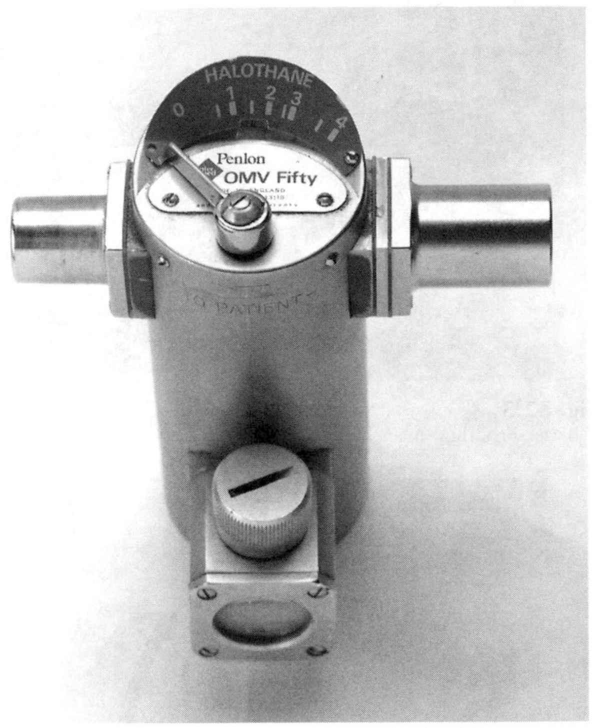

Fig. 32.5
Oxford miniature vaporizer (OMV).

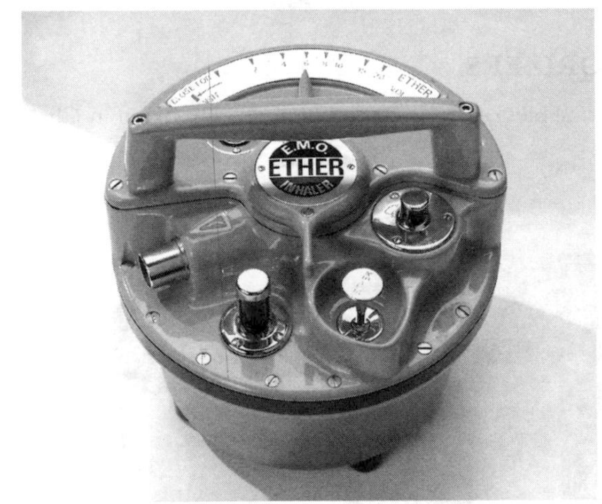

Fig. 32.7
The EMO (Epstein and Macintosh of Oxford) drawover ether vaporizer. A cutaway diagram is shown in Figure 32.8.

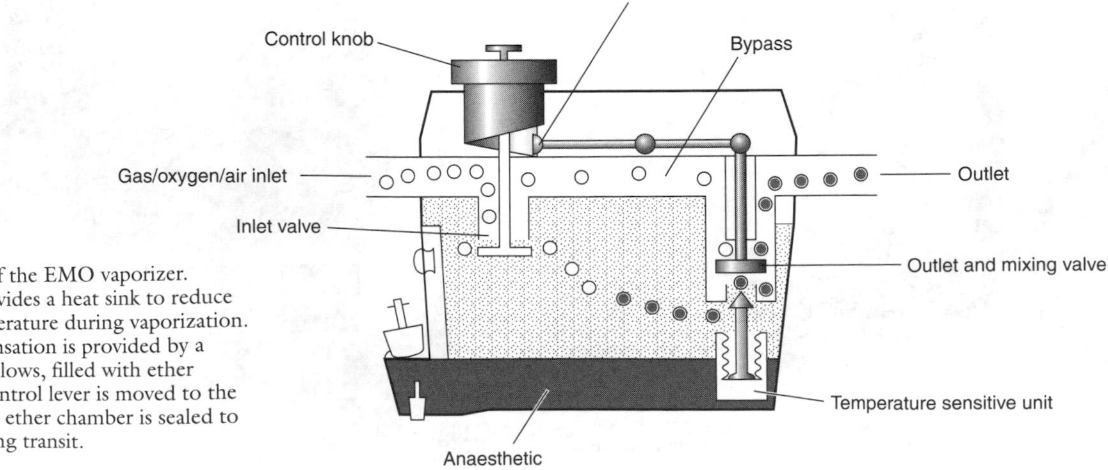

Fig. 32.8
Working principles of the EMO vaporizer. The water jacket provides a heat sink to reduce the decrease in temperature during vaporization. Temperature compensation is provided by a valve operated by bellows, filled with ether vapour. When the control lever is moved to the 'closed' position, the ether chamber is sealed to prevent spillage during transit.

bypass flow, and the Kettle type in which measured flows are used. Commonly used types of equipment are shown in Figures 32.9–32.11.

Methods of temperature regulation include a bimetallic strip (TEC), bellows (EMO and Blease Universal vaporizer) and manual compensation (Drager Vapor and Copper Kettle).

There has been more than one model of the 'TEC' type of vaporizer. The TEC Mark 2 vaporizer is now obsolete. The TEC Mark 3 had characteristics which were an improvement on the Mark 2. These included improved vaporization as a result of increased area of the wicks, reduced pumping effect by having a long tube through which the vaporized gas leaves the vaporizing chamber, improved accuracy at low gas flows and a bimetallic strip which is situated in the bypass channel and not the vaporizing chamber. In the Mark 4 the improvements were as follows: no spillage into the bypass channel if the vaporizer is accidentally inverted and the inability to turn two vaporizers on at the same time when they are on the back bar of the anaesthetic machine. The TEC Mark 5 vaporizer (Fig. 32.10) has improved surface area for vaporization in the chamber, improved key-filling action and an easier mechanism for switching on the rotary valve and lock with one hand.

Desflurane presents a particular challenge as it possesses a boiling point of 23.5°C and above this temperature the liquid changes to as. In order to combat this problem, a new vaporizer, the TEC 6, was developed (Fig. 32.11). It is heated electrically to 35°C with a pressure of 1550 mmHg. The vaporizer has electronic monitors of vaporizer function and alarms. The FGF does not enter the vaporization chamber. Instead, desflurane vapour enters into the path of the FGF. A percentage control dial regulates the flow of desflurane vapour into the FGF. The dial calibration is from 1 to 18%. The vaporizer has a back-up 9 volt battery should there be a mains failure. The

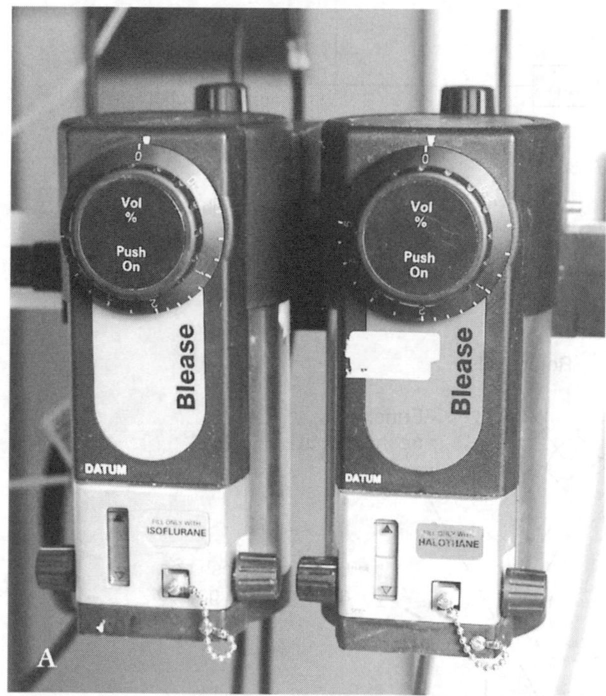

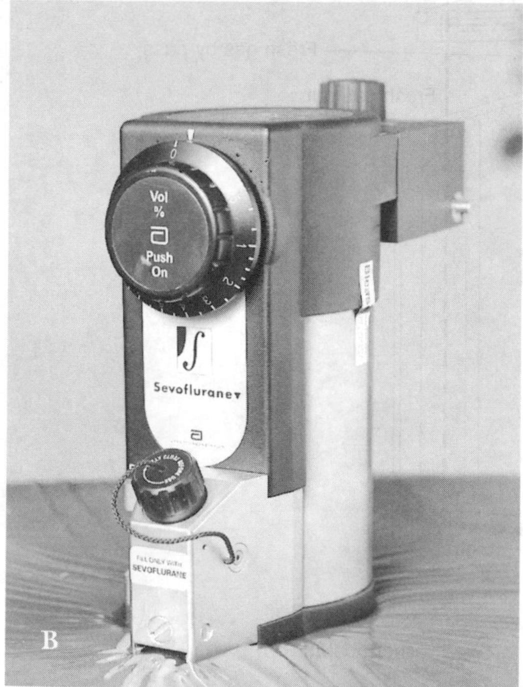

Fig. 32.9
Modern vaporizers. **A.** Blease isoflurane and halothane vaporizers. **B.** Blease sevoflurane vaporizer.

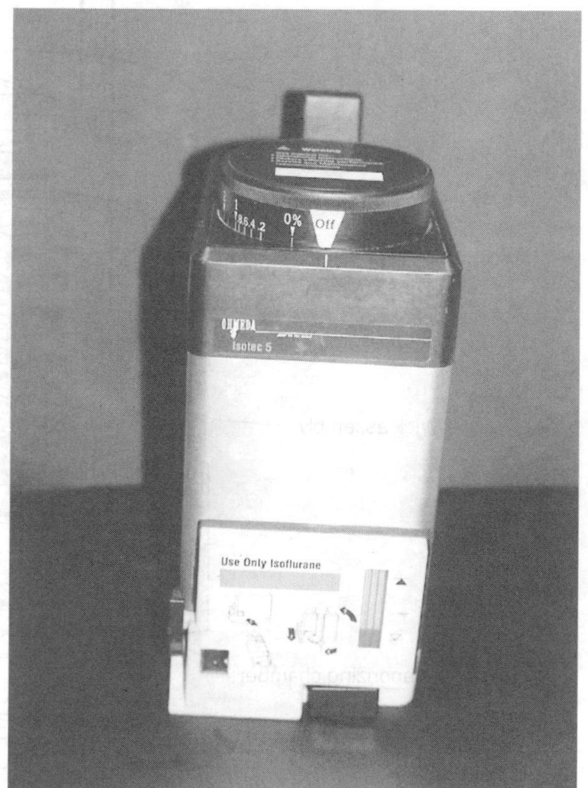

Fig. 32.10
A. A Mark 5 TEC vaporizer.

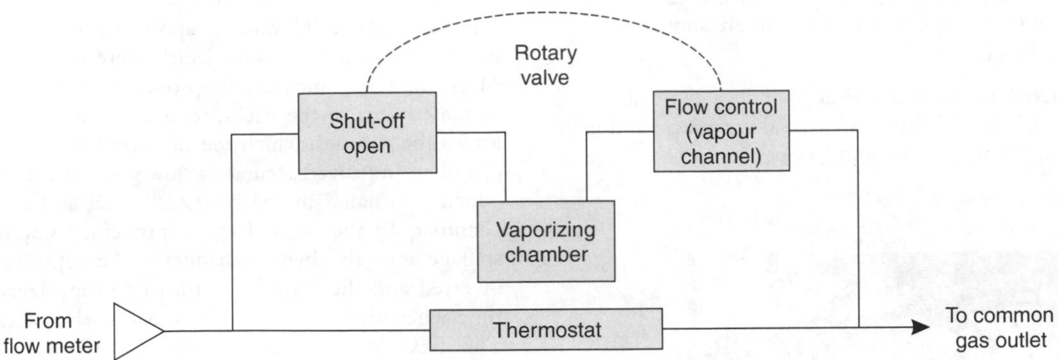

Fig. 32.10
B. Schematic diagram of the Mark 5 TEC vaporizer.

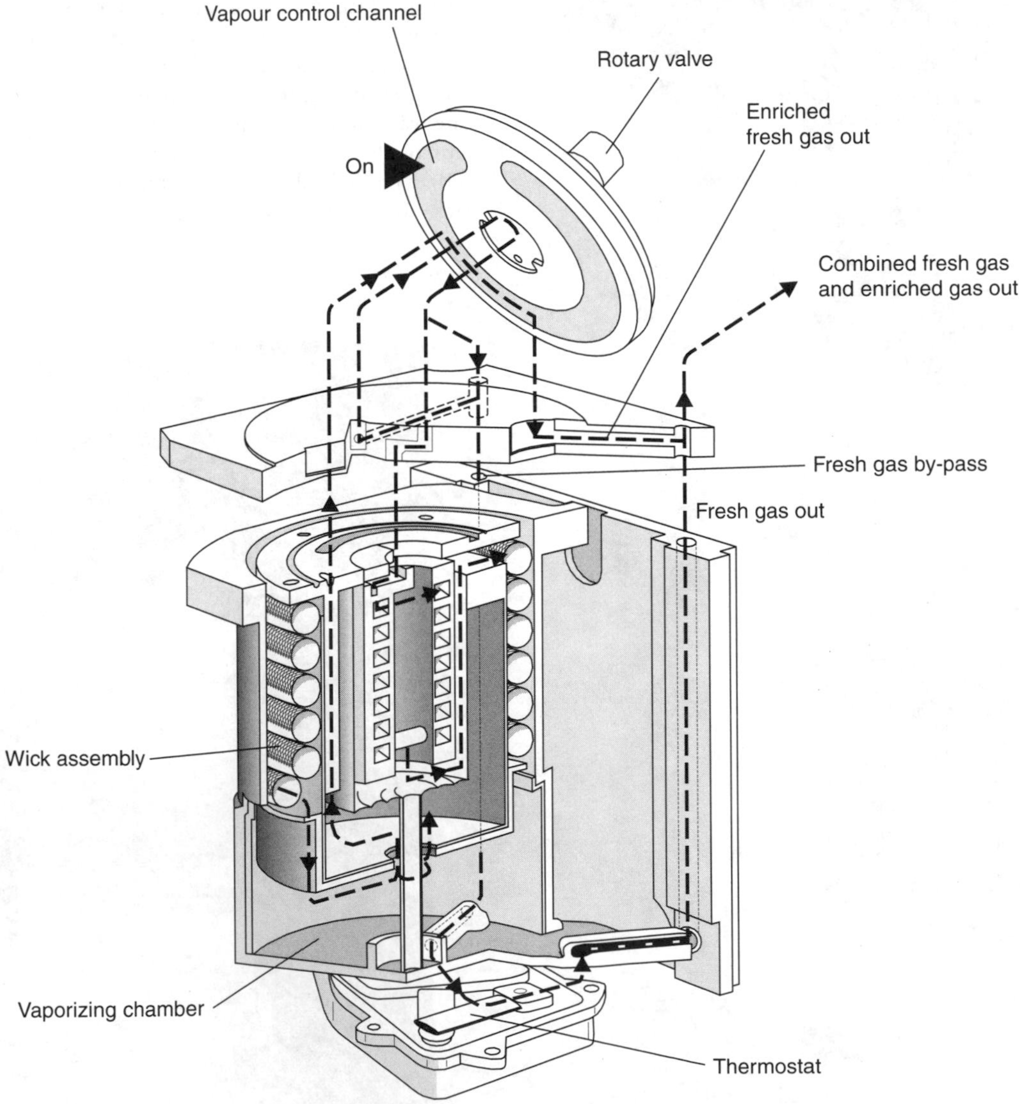

Fig. 32.10
C. Diagram of the Mark 5 TEC vaporizer.

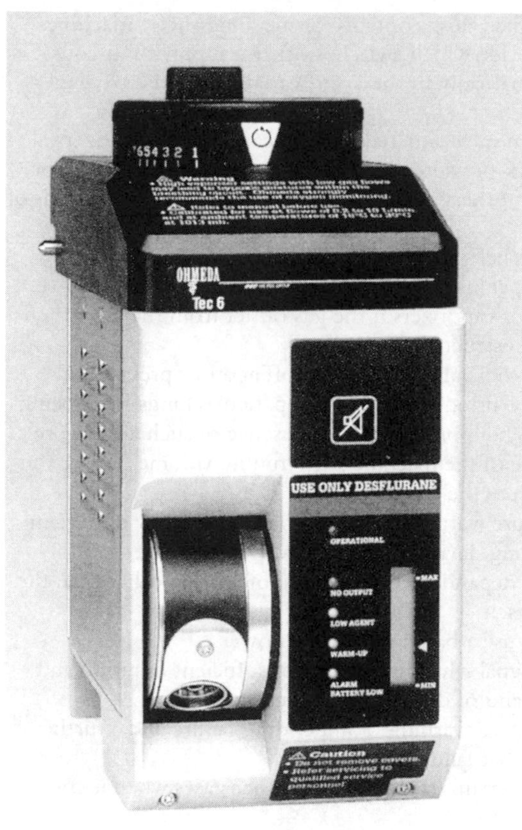

Fig. 32.11
The TEC 6 desflurane vaporizer.

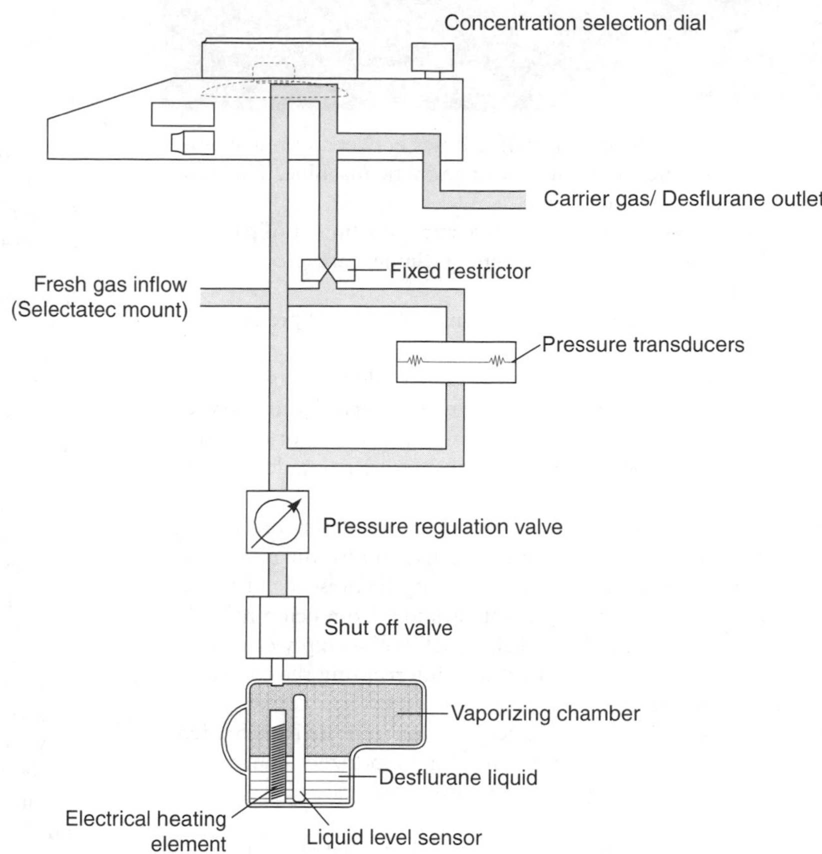

Fig. 32.12
The TEC 6 desflurane vaporizer. Liquid in the vaporizing chamber is heated and mixed with fresh gas; the pressure-regulating valve balances both fresh gas pressure and anaesthetic vapour pressure.

functioning of the vaporizer is shown diagrammatically in Figure 32.12.

Anaesthetic-specific connections are available to link the supply bottle (container of liquid anaesthetic agent) to the appropriate vaporizer (Fig. 32.13). These connections reduce the extent of spillage (and thus atmospheric pollution) and also the likelihood of filling the vaporizer with an inappropriate liquid. In addition to being designed specifically for each liquid, the connections themselves may be colour-coded (e.g. purple for isoflurane, yellow for sevoflurane, orange for enflurane, red for halothane).

Halothane contains a non-volatile stabilizing agent (0.01% thymol) to prevent breakdown of the halothane by heat and ultraviolet light. Thymol is less volatile than halothane and its concentration in the vaporizer increases as halothane is vaporized. If the vaporizer is used and refilled regularly, the concentration of thymol may become sufficiently high to impair vaporization of halothane. In addition, very high concentrations may result in a significant degree of thymol vaporization, which may be harmful to the patient. Consequently, it is recommended that halothane vaporizers be drained once every 2 weeks. Enflurane and isoflurane vaporizers require to be emptied at much less frequent intervals.

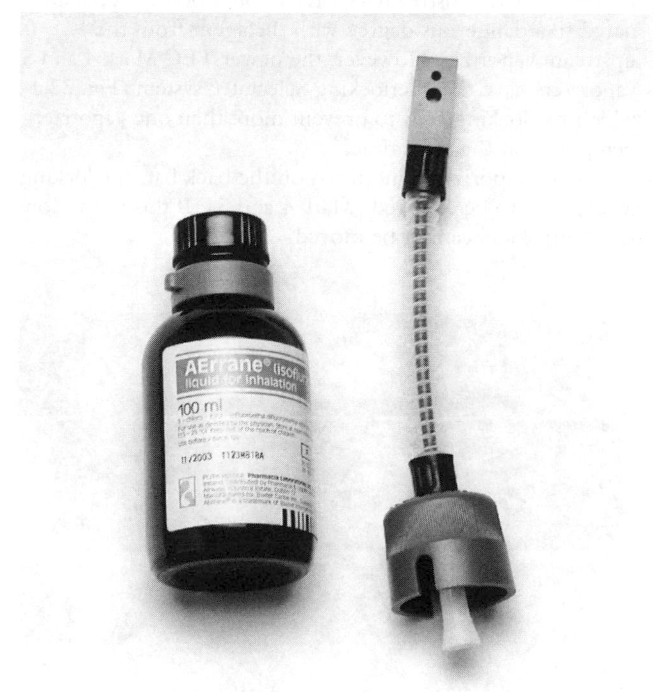

Fig. 32.13
An agent-specific connector for filling a vaporizer.

SAFETY FEATURES OF THE MODERN ANAESTHETIC MACHINES

- Specificity of probes on flexible hoses between terminal outlets and connections with the anaesthetic machine. The flexible hoses are colour-coded.
- Pin index system to prevent incorrect attachment of gas cylinders to anaesthetic machine. Cylinders are also colour-coded.
- Pressure relief valves on the downstream side of pressure regulators.
- Flow restrictors on the upstream side of flowmeters.
- Arrangement of the bank of flowmeters such that the oxygen flowmeter is on the right (i.e. downstream side) or oxygen is the last gas to be added to the gas mixture being delivered to the back bar (Fig. 32.1).
- Non-return valves. Sometimes a single regulator and contents meter is used both for cylinders in use and for the reserve cylinder. When one cylinder runs out, the presence of a non-return valve prevents the empty cylinder from being refilled by the reserve cylinder and also enables the empty cylinder to be removed and replaced without interrupting the supply of gas to the patient.
- An oxygen bypass valve (emergency oxygen) delivers oxygen directly to a point downstream of the vaporizers. When operated, the oxygen bypass should give a flow rate of at least 35 L min^{-1}.
- Mounting of vaporizers on the back bar. There is concern about contamination of vaporizers if two vaporizers are turned on at the same time. Temperature-compensated vaporizers contain wicks and these can absorb a considerable amount of anaesthetic agent. If two vaporizers are mounted in series, the downstream vaporizer could become contaminated to a dangerous degree with the agent from the upstream vaporizer. However, the newer TEC Mark 4 and 5 vaporizers have the interlocking Selectatec system (Fig. 32.14) which has locking rods to prevent more than one vaporizer being used at the same time.

  When a vaporizer is mounted on the back bar, the locking lever needs to be engaged (Mark 4 and 5). If this is not done, the control dial cannot be moved.

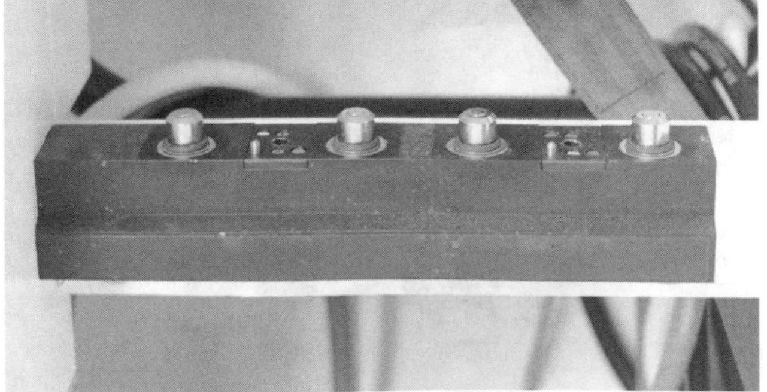

Fig. 32.14
A Selectatec block on the back bar of an anaesthetic machine. This permits the vaporizer to be changed rapidly without interrupting the flow of carrier gas to the patient.

- Pressure-linked flow controls. Some anaesthetic machines possess a device which switches off the supply of nitrous oxide automatically in the event of failure of the oxygen supply.
- A non-return valve situated downstream of the vaporizers prevents back-pressure (e.g. when using a Manley ventilator) which might otherwise cause output of high concentrations of vapour.
- A pressure relief valve may be situated downstream of the vaporizer, opening at 34 kPa to prevent damage to the flowmeters or vaporizers if the gas outlet from the anaesthetic machine is obstructed.
- A pressure relief valve set to blow off at a low pressure of 5 kPa may be fitted to prevent the patient's lungs from being damaged by high pressure. The presence of such a valve prevents the use of the machine with minute volume divider ventilators, such as the Manley.
- Oxygen failure warning devices. There is a variety of oxygen failure warning devices. The ideal warning device:
  - — does not depend on the pressure of any gas other than the oxygen itself
  - — does not use a battery or mains power
  - — gives a signal which is audible, of sufficient duration and volume, and of distinctive character
  - — should give a warning of impending failure and a further warning that failure has occurred
  - — should interrupt the flow of all other gases when it comes into operation.

  The breathing system should open to the atmosphere, the inspired oxygen concentration should be at least equal to that of air, and accumulation of carbon dioxide should not occur. In addition, it should be impossible to resume anaesthesia until the oxygen supply has been restored.
- The reservoir bag in an anaesthetic breathing system is highly distensible and seldom reaches pressures exceeding 5 kPa.

BREATHING SYSTEMS

The delivery system which conducts anaesthetic gases from the machine to the patient is termed colloquially a 'circuit' but is described more accurately as a breathing system. Terms such as 'open circuits', 'semi-open circuits' or 'semi-closed circuits' should be avoided. The 'closed circuit' or circle system is the only true circuit, as anaesthetic gases are recycled.

Adjustable pressure-limiting valve

Most breathing systems incorporate an adjustable pressure-limiting valve (APL valve, spill valve, 'pop-off' valve, expiratory valve) which is designed to vent gas when there is a positive pressure within the system. During spontaneous ventilation, the valve opens when the patient generates a positive pressure within the system during expiration; during positive pressure ventilation, the valve is adjusted to produce a controlled leak during the inspiratory phase.

Several valves of this type are available. They comprise a lightweight disc (Fig. 32.15) which rests on a 'knife edge' seating to minimize the area of contact and reduce the risk of adhesion

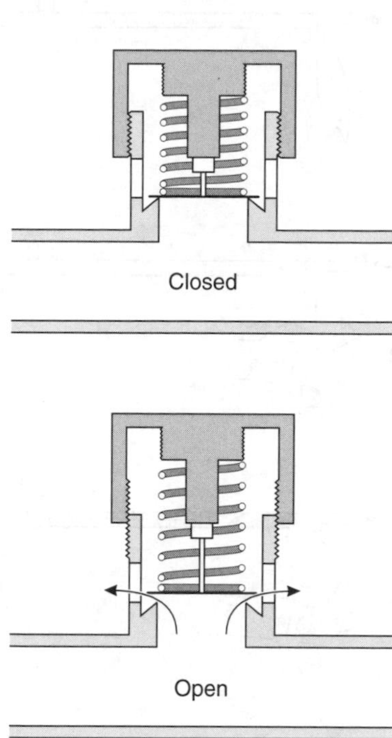

Fig. 32.15
Diagram of a spill valve. See text for details.

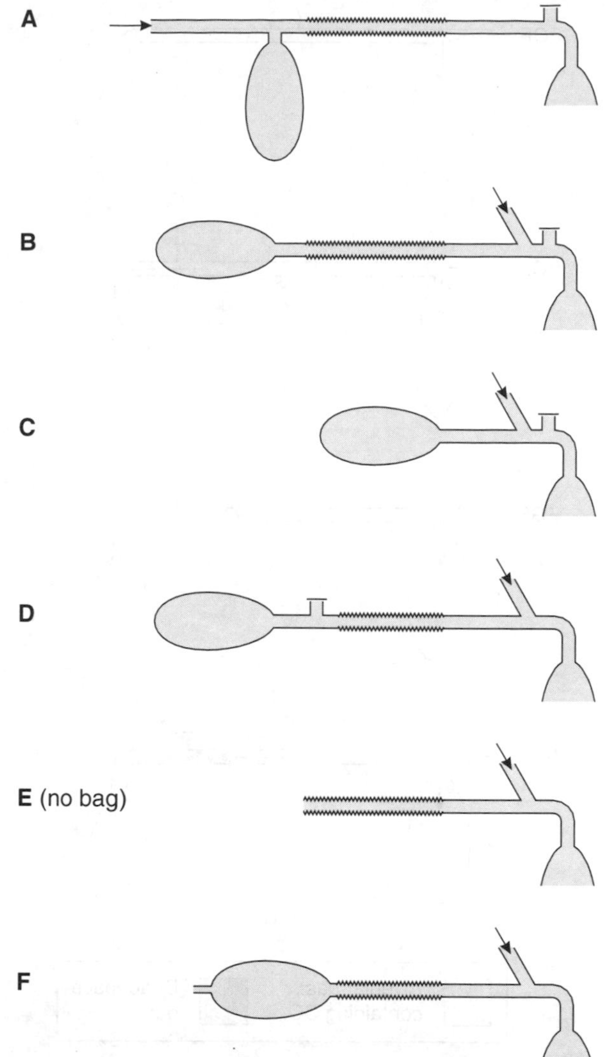

Fig. 32.16
Mapleson classification of anaesthetic breathing systems. The arrow indicates entry of fresh gas to the system.

resulting from surface tension of condensed water. The disc has a stem which acts as a guide to position it correctly. A light spring is incorporated in the valve so that the pressure required to open it may be adjusted. During spontaneous breathing, the tension of the spring is low so that the resistance to expiration is minimized. During controlled ventilation, the valve top is screwed down to increase the tension in the spring so that gas leaves the system at a higher pressure than during spontaneous ventilation.

CLASSIFICATION OF BREATHING SYSTEMS

In 1954, Mapleson classified anaesthetic breathing systems into five types (Fig. 32.16); the Mapleson E system was modified subsequently by Rees, but is classified as the Mapleson F system. The systems differ considerably in their 'efficiency ', which is measured in terms of the fresh gas flow (FGF) rate required to prevent rebreathing of alveolar gas during ventilation.

Mapleson A systems

The most commonly used version is the Magill attachment. The corrugated hose should be of adequate length (usually approximately 110 cm). It is the most efficient system during spontaneous ventilation, but one of the least efficient when ventilation is controlled.

During spontaneous ventilation (Fig. 32.17), there are three phases in the ventilatory cycle: inspiratory, expiratory and the expiratory pause. Gas is inhaled from the system during inspiration (Fig. 32.17B). During the initial part of expiration, the reservoir bag is not full and thus the pressure in the system does not increase; exhaled gas (the initial portion of which is dead space gas) passes along the corrugated tubing towards the bag (Fig. 32.17C), which is filled also by fresh gas from the anaesthetic machine. During the latter part of expiration, the bag becomes full, the pressure in the system increases and the spill valve opens, venting all subsequent exhaled gas to atmosphere. During the expiratory pause, continued flow of fresh gas from the machine pushes exhaled gas distally along the corrugated tube to be vented through the spill valve (Fig. 32.17D). Provided that the FGF rate is sufficiently high to vent all *alveolar* gas before the next inspiration, no rebreathing takes place from the corrugated tube. If the system is functioning correctly and no leaks are present, a FGF rate equal to the patient's alveolar minute ventilation is sufficient to prevent rebreathing. In practice, a higher FGF is selected in order to compensate for leaks; the rate selected is usually equal to

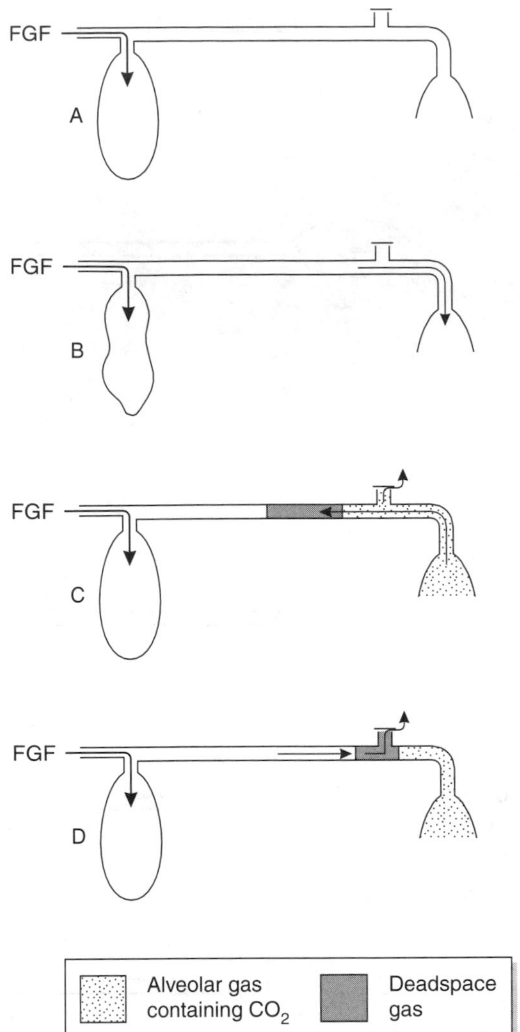

Fig. 32.17
Mode of action of Magill attachment during spontaneous ventilation. See text for details. FGF, fresh gas flow.

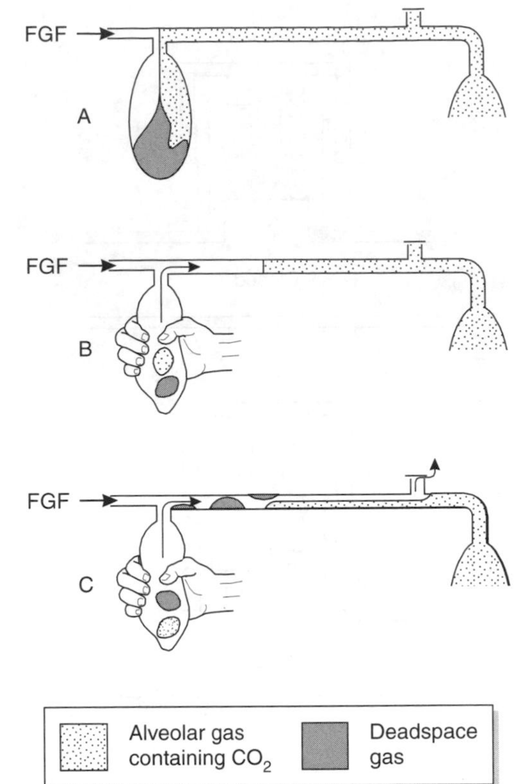

Fig. 32.18
Mode of action of Magill attachment during controlled ventilation. See text for details. FGF, fresh gas flow.

the patient's total minute volume (approximately 6 L min^{-1} for a 70 kg adult).

The system increases dead space to the extent of the volume of the anaesthetic face mask and angle piece to the spill valve. The volume of this dead space may amount to 100 ml or more for an adult face mask. Paediatric face masks reduce the extent of dead space, but it remains too high to allow use of the system in infants or small children (< 4 years old).

The characteristics of the Mapleson A system are different during controlled ventilation (Fig. 32.18). At the end of inspiration (produced by the anaesthetist squeezing the reservoir bag), the bag is usually less than half full (see below). During expiration, dead space and alveolar gas pass along the corrugated tube and are likely to reach the reservoir bag, which therefore contains some carbon dioxide (Fig. 32.18A). During inspiration, the valve does not open initially because its opening pressure has been increased by the anaesthetist in order to generate a sufficient pressure within the system to inflate the lungs. Thus, alveolar gas re-enters the patient's lungs and is followed by a mixture of fresh, dead space and alveolar gases (Fig. 32.18B). When the valve does open, it is this mixture which is vented (Fig. 32.18C). Consequently, FGF rate must be very high (at least three times alveolar minute volume) to prevent rebreathing. The volume of gas squeezed from the reservoir bag must be sufficient both to inflate the lungs and to vent gas from the system.

The major disadvantage of the Magill attachment during surgery is that the spill valve is attached close to the mask. This makes the system heavy, particularly when a scavenging system is used, and it is inconvenient if the valve is in this position during surgery of the head or neck. The Lack system (Fig. 32.19B) is a modification of the Mapleson A system with a coaxial arrangement of tubing. This permits positioning of the spill valve at the proximal end of the system. The inner tube must be of sufficiently wide bore to allow the patient to exhale with minimal resistance. The Lack system is not quite as efficient as the Magill attachment.

Mapleson B and C systems

These systems cause mixing of alveolar and fresh gas during spontaneous or controlled ventilation. Very high FGF rates are required to prevent rebreathing. There is no clinical role for the Mapleson B system. The Mapleson C system is used in some hospitals to ventilate the lungs with oxygen during transport, but a self-inflating bag with a non-rebreathing valve is preferable.

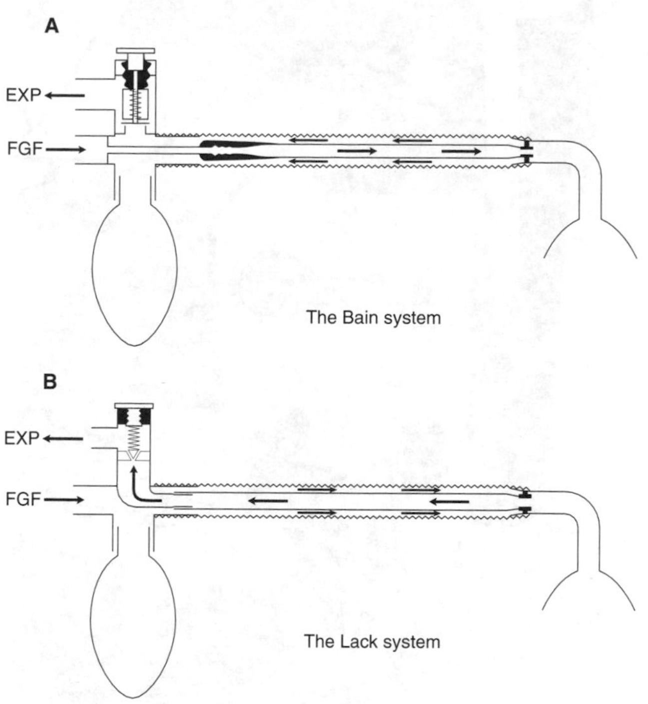

Fig. 32.19
Coaxial anaesthetic breathing systems. **A.** Bain system (Mapleson D). **B.** Lack system (Mapleson A). FGF: fresh gas flow.

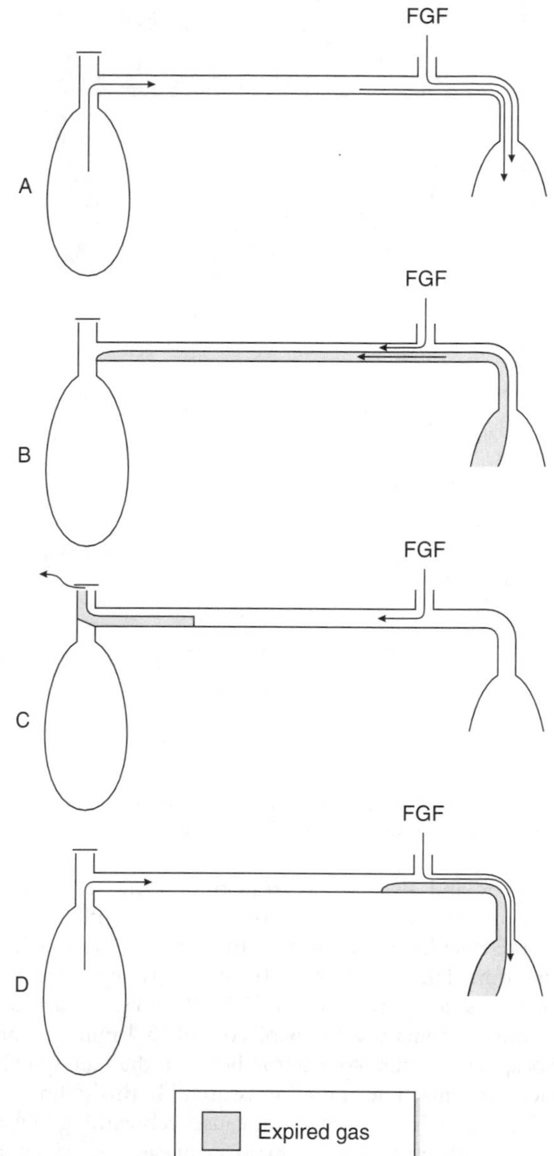

Fig. 32.20
Mode of action of Mapleson D breathing system during spontaneous ventilation. See text for details. FGF, fresh gas flow.

Mapleson D system

The Mapleson D arrangement is inefficient during spontaneous breathing (Fig. 32.20). During expiration, exhaled gas and fresh gas mix in the corrugated tube and travel towards the reservoir bag (Fig. 32.20B). When the reservoir bag is full, the pressure in the system increases, the spill valve opens and a mixture of fresh and exhaled gas is vented; this includes the dead space gas, which reaches the reservoir bag first (Fig. 32.20C). Although fresh gas pushes alveolar gas towards the valve during the expiratory pause, a mixture of alveolar and fresh gases is inhaled from the corrugated tube unless FGF rate is at least twice as great as the patient's minute volume (i.e. at least 12 L min^{-1} in the adult); in some patients, a FGF rate of 250 ml kg^{-1} min^{-1} is required to prevent rebreathing.

However, the Mapleson D system is more efficient than the Mapleson A during controlled ventilation (Fig. 32.21), especially if an expiratory pause is incorporated into the ventilatory cycle. During expiration, the corrugated tubing and reservoir bag fill with a mixture of fresh and alveolar gas (Fig. 32.21A). Fresh gas fills the distal part of the corrugated tube during the expiratory pause (Fig. 32.21B). When the reservoir bag is squeezed, this fresh gas enters the lungs, and when the spill valve opens a mixture of fresh and alveolar gas is vented. The degree of rebreathing may thus be controlled by adjustment of the FGF rate, but this should always exceed the patient's minute volume.

The Bain coaxial system (Fig. 32.19A) is the most commonly used version of the Mapleson D system. FGF is supplied through a narrow inner tube. This tube may become disconnected, resulting in hypoxaemia and hypercapnia. Before use, the system should be tested by occluding the distal end of the inner tube transiently with a finger or the plunger of a 2 ml syringe; there should be a reduction in the flowmeter bobbin reading during occlusion and an audible release of pressure when occlusion is discontinued. Movement of the reservoir bag during anaesthesia does not necessarily indicate that fresh gas is being delivered to the patient.

The Bain system may be used to ventilate the patient's lungs with some types of automatic ventilator (e.g. Penlon Nuffield 200; Fig. 32.22). A 1 m length of corrugated tubing is interposed between the patient valve of the ventilator and the reservoir bag mount (Fig. 32.23); the spill valve *must* be closed completely. An appropriate tidal volume and ventilatory rate are selected on the ventilator and anaesthetic gases are supplied to the Bain system. During inspiration, the gas from the ventilator pushes a mixture

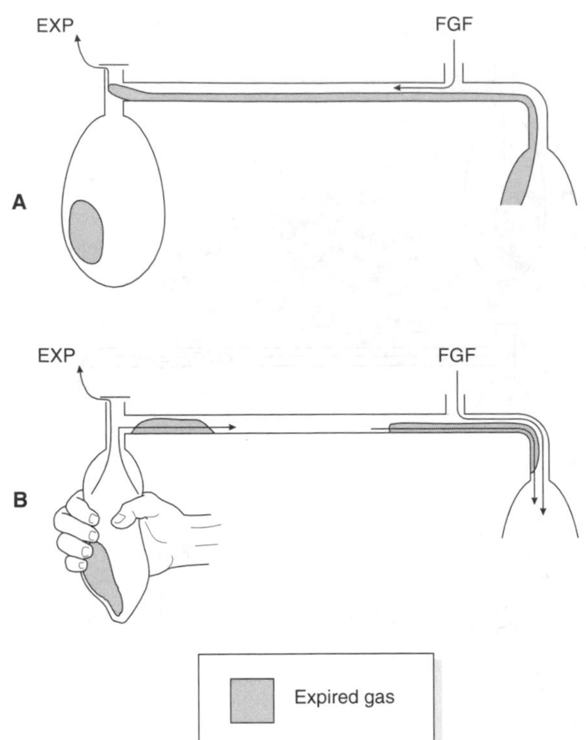

Fig. 32.21
Mode of action of Mapleson D breathing system during controlled ventilation. See text for details. FGF, fresh gas flow.

of anaesthetic and alveolar gas from the corrugated outer tube into the patient's lungs; during expiration, the ventilator gas and some of the alveolar gas are vented through the exhaust valve of the ventilator. The degree of rebreathing is regulated by the anaesthetic gas flow rate; a flow of 70–80 ml kg^{-1} min^{-1} should result in normocapnia and a flow of 100 ml kg^{-1} min^{-1} in moderate hypocapnia. A secure connection between the Bain system and the anaesthetic machine must be assured. If this connection is loose, a leak of fresh gas occurs; this causes rebreathing of ventilator gas and results in awareness, hypoxaemia and hypercapnia.

Mapleson E and F systems

The Mapleson E system, or Ayre's T-piece, has virtually no resistance to expiration and was used extensively in paediatric anaesthesia before the advantages of continuous positive airways pressure (CPAP) were recognized. It functions in a manner similar to the Mapleson D system in that the corrugated tube fills with a mixture of exhaled and fresh gas during expiration and with fresh gas during the expiratory pause. Rebreathing is prevented if the FGF rate is 2.5–3 times the patient's minute volume. If the volume of the corrugated tube is less than the patient's tidal volume, some air may be inhaled at the end of inspiration; consequently, a FGF rate of at least 4 L min^{-1} is recommended with a paediatric Mapleson E system.

During spontaneous ventilation, there is no indication of the presence, or the adequacy, of ventilation. It is possible to attach a visual indicator, such as a piece of tissue paper or a feather, at the end of the corrugated tube, but this is not very satisfactory.

Intermittent positive pressure ventilation (IPPV) may be applied by occluding the end of the corrugated tube with a finger.

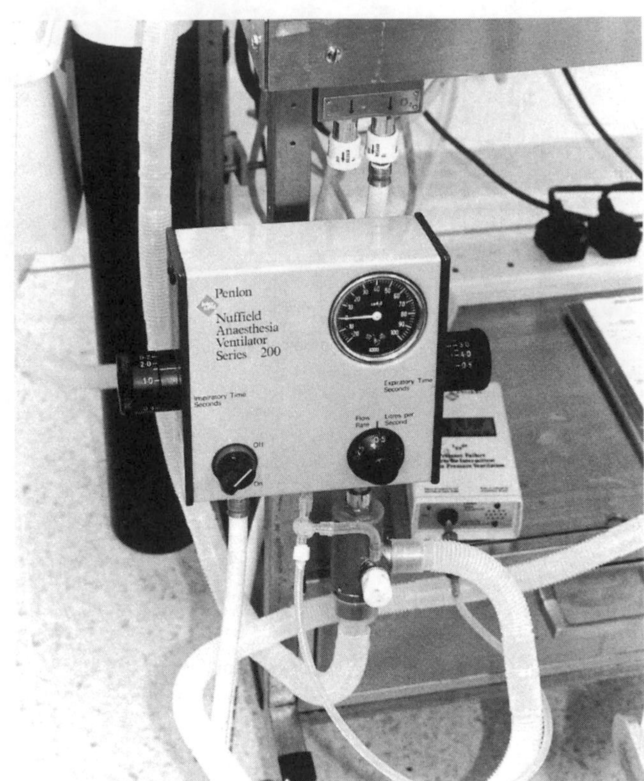

Fig. 32.22
The Penlon Nuffield 200 ventilator.

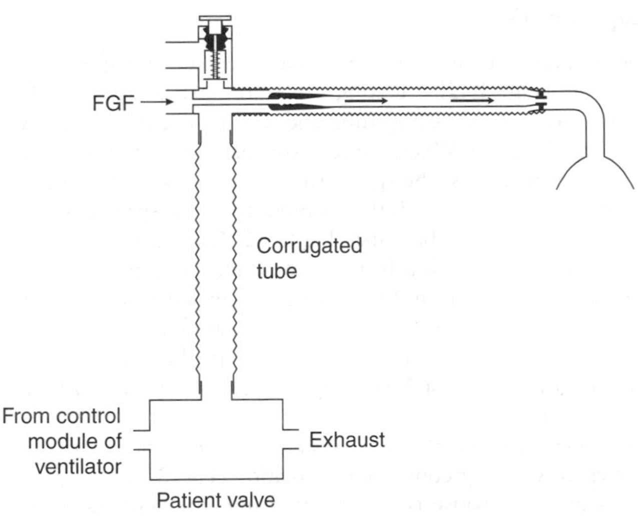

Fig. 32.23
The Bain system for controlled ventilation by a mechanical ventilator (e.g. Penlon Nuffield 200). A 1 m length of corrugated tubing with a capacity of at least 500 ml is required to prevent gas from the ventilator reaching the patient's lungs. P_aCO_2 is controlled by varying the fresh gas flow rate (FGF).

However, there is no way of assessing the pressure in the system and there is a possibility of exposing the patient's lungs to excessive volumes and pressures.

The Mapleson F system, or Rees' modification of the Ayre's T-piece, includes an open-ended bag attached to the end of the corrugated tube. This confers several advantages:

- It provides visual evidence of breathing during spontaneous ventilation.
- By occluding the open end of the bag temporarily, it is possible to confirm that fresh gas is entering the system.
- It provides a degree of CPAP during spontaneous ventilation and positive end-expiratory pressure (PEEP) during IPPV.
- It provides a convenient method of assisting or controlling ventilation. The open end of the reservoir bag is occluded between the fourth and fifth fingers and the bag is squeezed between the thumb and index finger; the fourth and fifth fingers are relaxed during expiration to allow gas to escape from the bag. It is possible with experience to assess (approximately) the inflation pressure and to detect changes in lung and chest wall compliance.

However, one main disadvantage of the Mapleson F system is that efficient scavenging is unsatisfactory and is non-standard.

Mapleson ADE system

This system provides the advantages of the Mapleson A, D, and E systems. It can be used efficiently for spontaneous and controlled ventilation in both children and adults.

It consists of two parallel lengths of 15 mm bore tubing; one delivers fresh gas and the other carries exhaled gas. One end of the tubing connects to the patient via a Y-connection and the other end contains the Humphrey block (Fig. 32.24). The Humphrey block (Fig 32.25) consists of an APL valve, a lever to select spontaneous or controlled ventilation, a reservoir bag, a port to connect a ventilator and a safety pressure relief valve which opens at a pressure above 6 kPa.

When the lever is in the A mode (up), the reservoir bag is connected to the breathing system as it would be in the Mapleson A system. The breathing hose connecting the bag to the patient is the inspiratory limb. The expired gases travel along the other tubing back to the APL valve, which is connected to the scavenging system.

With the lever in the D/E mode (down), the reservoir bag and the APL valve are isolated from the breathing system. What was the inspiratory limb in the A mode now delivers gas to the patient. The hose returning gas to the Humphrey block now functions as a reservoir to the T-piece. This hose would open to atmosphere via a port adjacent to the bag mount, but in practice this port is connected to a ventilator such as the Nuffield Penlon.

In adults, an appropriate FGF is 50–60 ml kg^{-1} min^{-1} in spontaneously breathing patients and 70 ml kg^{-1} min^{-1} in ventilated patients.

Drawover systems

Occasionally, it is necessary to administer anaesthesia at the scene of a major accident. If inhalation anaesthesia is required, it is necessary to use simple, portable equipment. The Triservice apparatus has been designed by the British armed forces for use in battle conditions (Fig. 32.26). It comprises a self-inflating bag, a non-rebreathing valve (e.g. Ambu E, Rubens) which vents all

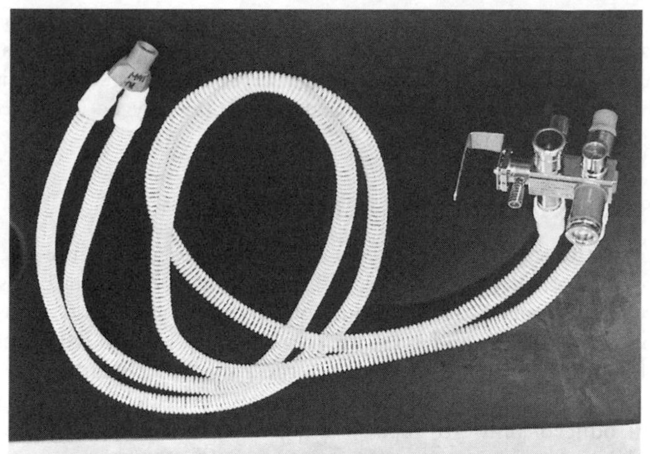

Fig. 32.24
The ADE system.

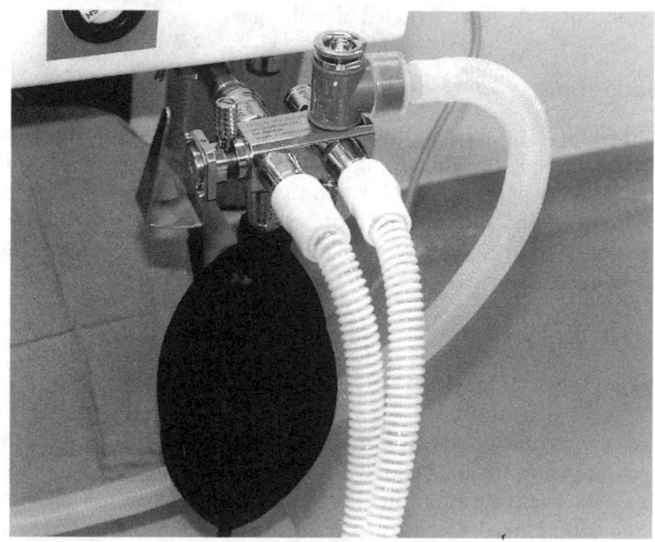

Fig. 32.25
The Humphrey block. This consists of an APL valve, a lever to select spontaneous or controlled ventilation, a reservoir bag, a port to connect to the ventilator and a safety pressure relief valve.

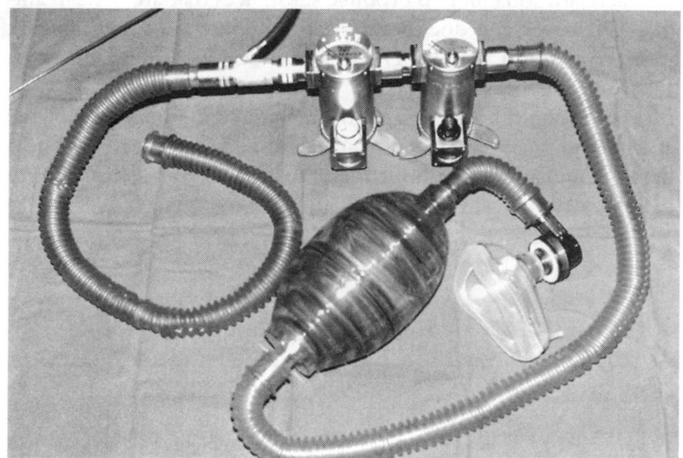

Fig. 32.26
The Triservice apparatus (courtesy of Dr S. Kidd).

expired gases to atmosphere, one or two Oxford miniature vaporizers (which have a low internal resistance), an oxygen supply and a length of corrugated tubing which serves as an oxygen reservoir. Either spontaneous or controlled ventilation may be employed using this apparatus.

REBREATHING SYSTEMS

Anaesthetic breathing systems in which some gas is rebreathed by the patient were designed originally to economize in the use of cyclopropane. In addition, they reduce the risk of atmospheric pollution and increase the humidity of inspired gases, thereby reducing heat loss from the patient. Rebreathing systems may be used as 'closed ' systems, in which fresh gas is introduced only to replace oxygen and anaesthetic agents absorbed by the patient. More commonly, the system is used with a small leak through a spill valve, and the fresh gas supply exceeds basal oxygen requirements. Because rebreathing occurs, these systems must incorporate a means of absorbing carbon dioxide from exhaled alveolar gas.

Soda lime

Soda lime is the substance used most commonly for absorption of carbon dioxide in rebreathing systems. The composition of soda lime is shown in Table 32.4. The major constituent is calcium hydroxide, but sodium and potassium hydroxides may also be present. Absorption of carbon dioxide occurs by the following chemical reactions:

$$CO_2 + 2NaOH \rightarrow Na_2CO_3 + H_2O + \text{heat}$$

$$Na_2CO_3 + Ca(OH)_2 \rightarrow 2NaOH + CaCO_3$$

Water is required for efficient absorption. There is some water in soda lime and more is added from the patient's expired gas and from the chemical reaction. The reaction generates heat and the temperature in the centre of a soda lime canister may exceed 60°C. Trichloroethylene degenerates at high temperatures, forming toxic substances including the neurotoxin dichloroacetylene; consequently, trichloroethylene must never be used in rebreathing systems which contain soda lime. Sevoflurane has been shown to interact with soda lime to produce substances that are toxic in animals. However, this does not appear to impose any significant risk in humans (see Ch. 13). There is new evidence suggesting that the presence of strong alkalis such as sodium and potassium hydroxide could be the trigger of the interaction between volatile agents and soda lime. New carbon dioxide absorbers are now being manufactured without these hydroxides in order to reduce this interaction.

Table 32.4 Composition of soda lime

$Ca(OH)_2$	94%
NaOH	5%
KOH	<1% or nil
Silica	0.2%
Moisture content	14–19%

The size of soda lime granules is important. If granules are too large, the surface area for absorption is insufficient; if they are too small, the narrow space between granules results in a high resistance to breathing. Granule size is measured by a mesh number. Soda lime consists of granules in the range of 4–8 mesh. (A 4-mesh strainer has four openings per inch and an 8-mesh strainer has eight openings). Silica is added to soda lime to reduce the tendency of the granules to disintegrate into powder. In addition, soda lime contains an indicator which changes colour as the active constituents become exhausted. The rate at which soda lime becomes exhausted depends on the capacity of the canister, the FGF rate and the rate of carbon dioxide production. In a completely closed system, a standard 450 g canister becomes inefficient after approximately 2 h.

Baralyme

Baralyme is another commonly used carbon dioxide absorber. It is a mixture of approximately 20% barium hydroxide and 80% calcium hydroxide. It may also contain some potassium hydroxide, an indicator and moisture. Barium hydroxide contains eight molecules of water of crystallization, which help to fuse the mixture so that it retains the granular structure under various conditions of heat and moisture. The granules of Baralyme are similar to those of soda lime.

'To-and-fro ' (Waters') system

This breathing system comprises a Mapleson C breathing system with a canister of soda lime interposed between the spill valve and the reservoir bag (Fig. 32.27). The soda lime granules nearest the patient become exhausted first, increasing the dead space of the system; in addition, the canister is positioned horizontally and gas may be channelled above the soda lime unless the canister is packed tightly. The system is cumbersome and there is a risk that patients may inhale soda lime dust from the canister.

Circle system

This system has replaced the 'to-and-fro ' system in most centres. The soda lime canister is mounted on the anaesthetic machine, and inspiratory and expiratory corrugated tubing conducts gas to

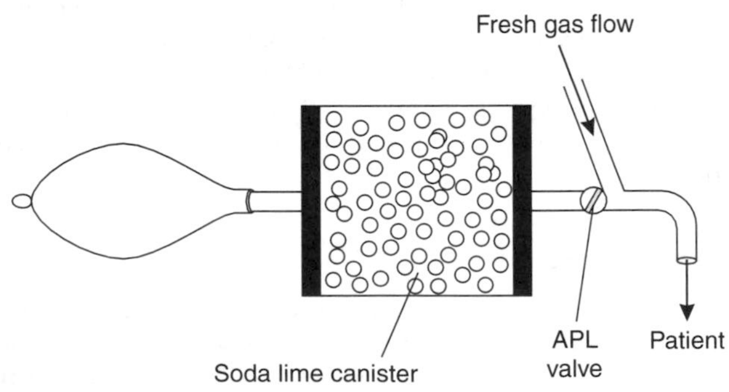

Fig. 32.27
Waters' anaesthetic breathing system, incorporating a canister of soda lime.

and from the patient (Fig. 32.28). The system incorporates a reservoir bag and spill valve and two low-resistance one-way valves to ensure unidirectional movement of gas (Fig 32.29). These valves are normally mounted in glass domes so that they may be observed to be functioning correctly. The spill valve may be mounted close to the patient or beside the absorber; during surgery to the head or neck, it is more convenient to use a valve near the absorber. Fresh gas enters the system between the absorber and the inspiratory tubing.

The soda lime canister is mounted vertically and thus channelling of gas through unfilled areas is not possible. The canister cannot contribute to dead space; consequently, a large canister may be used and the soda lime needs to be changed less often.

The major disadvantage of the circle system arises from its volume. If the system is filled with air initially, low flow rates of anaesthetic gases are diluted substantially and adequate concentrations cannot be achieved. Even if the system is primed with a mixture of anaesthetic gases, the initial rapid uptake by the patient results in a marked decrease in concentrations of anaesthetic agents in the system, resulting in light anaesthesia. Consequently, it is necessary usually to provide a total FGF rate of 3–4 L min^{-1} to the system initially. This flow rate may be reduced subsequently, but it must be remembered that dilution of fresh gas continues at low flow rates and that rapid changes in depth of anaesthesia cannot be achieved.

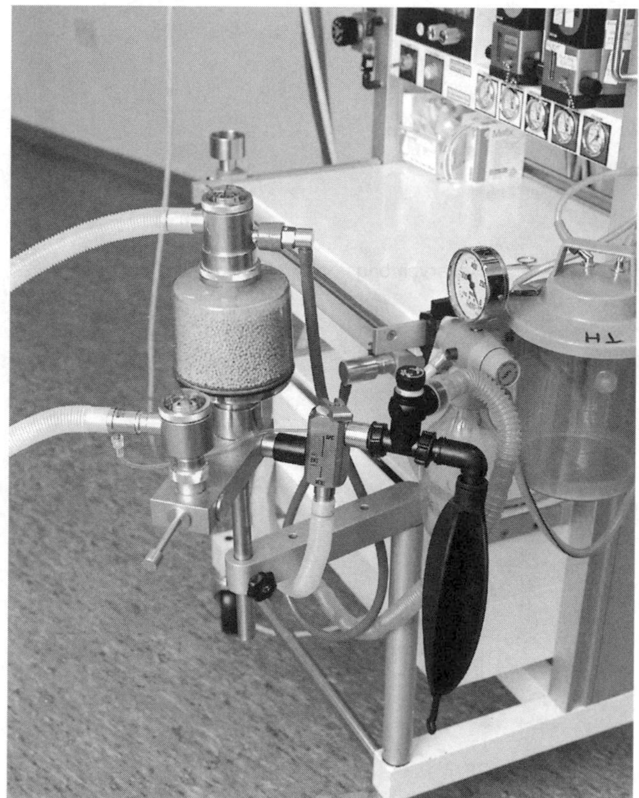

Fig. 32.28
The circle breathing system mounted on an anaesthetic machine.

Volatile anaesthetic agents may be delivered to a circle system in two ways:

- *Vaporizer outside the circle (VOC)* (Fig. 32.30A). If a standard vaporizer (e.g. TEC series) is used, it must be placed on the back bar of the anaesthetic machine because of its high internal resistance. If low FGF rates (< 1 L min^{-1}) are used, the change in concentration of volatile anaesthetic agent achieved in the circle system is very small because of dilution, even if the vaporizer is set to deliver a high concentration (Fig. 32.30A). It may be necessary to change FGF rate rather than the vaporizer setting in order to achieve a rapid change in depth of anaesthesia. The concentration of volatile agent in the system depends on the patient's expired concentration (which is recycled), the rate of uptake by the patient (which decreases with time and is slower with agents of low blood/gas solubility coefficient), the concentration of agent supplied and the FGF rate.
- *Vaporizer inside the circle (VIC)* (Fig. 32.30B). Drawover vaporizers with a low internal resistance (e.g. Goldman) may be placed within the circle system. During each inspiration, vapour is added to the inspired gas mixture. In contrast to a VOC system, the inspired concentration is higher at low FGF rates because the expired concentration is diluted to a lesser extent (Fig. 32.31B) and the vaporizer *adds* to the concentration present in the expired gas. Very high concentrations of volatile agent may be inspired if minute volume is large; this risk is greatest if IPPV is employed.

If FGF rate is low, the use of the circle system by the inexperienced anaesthetist may result either in inadequate anaesthesia or in severe cardiovascular and respiratory depression. In addition, a hypoxic gas mixture may be delivered if low flow rates of a nitrous oxide/oxygen mixture are supplied, because after 10–15 min oxygen is taken up in larger volumes than nitrous oxide. These difficulties may be overcome by monitoring the inspired concentration of oxygen, carbon dioxide and volatile anaesthetic agent continuously (see Ch. 20). The trainee anaesthetist *must* be aware that:

- It is inadvisable to use a VIC system unless inspired concentrations of anaesthetic agents are monitored continuously.
- IPPV must *never* be used with a VIC system unless inspired concentrations of anaesthetic agents are monitored continuously, because of the risk of generating very high concentrations of volatile agent.
- Nitrous oxide must *not* be used in any circle system if the total FGF rate is less than 1000 ml min^{-1}, unless inspired oxygen concentration is measured continuously.
- It is strongly advisable to monitor inspired concentration of oxygen and inhalation anaesthetic agent and expired concentration of carbon dioxide when using the circle system.
- One-way valves may stick. These should be checked both at the pre-anaesthetic check of the machine and during anaesthesia.
- Because the circle system has many connections, the anaesthetist should be vigilant about checking for any leak or disconnection.

The advantages and disadvantages of the circle system are summarized in Table 32.5.

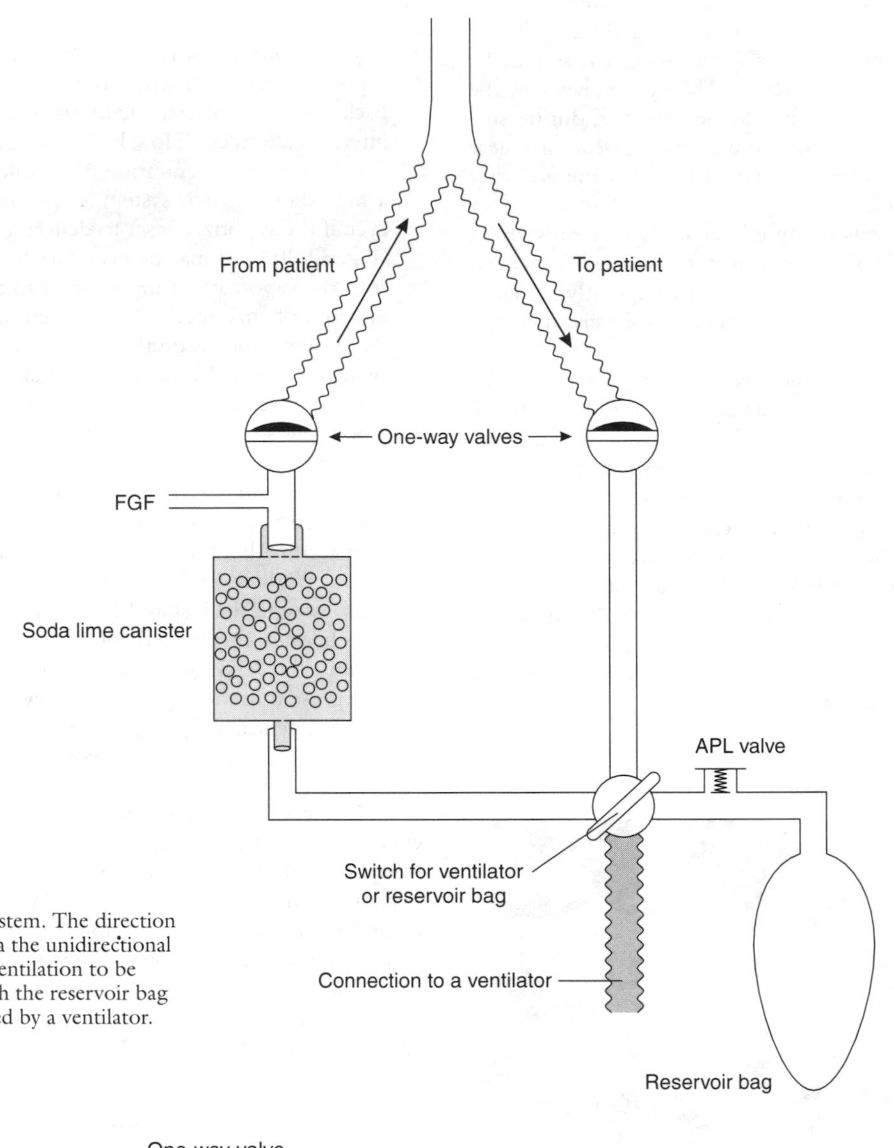

Fig. 32.29
Mechanism of the circle system. The direction of gas flow is controlled via the unidirectional valves. A lever allows the ventilation to be either spontaneous through the reservoir bag and APL valve or controlled by a ventilator.

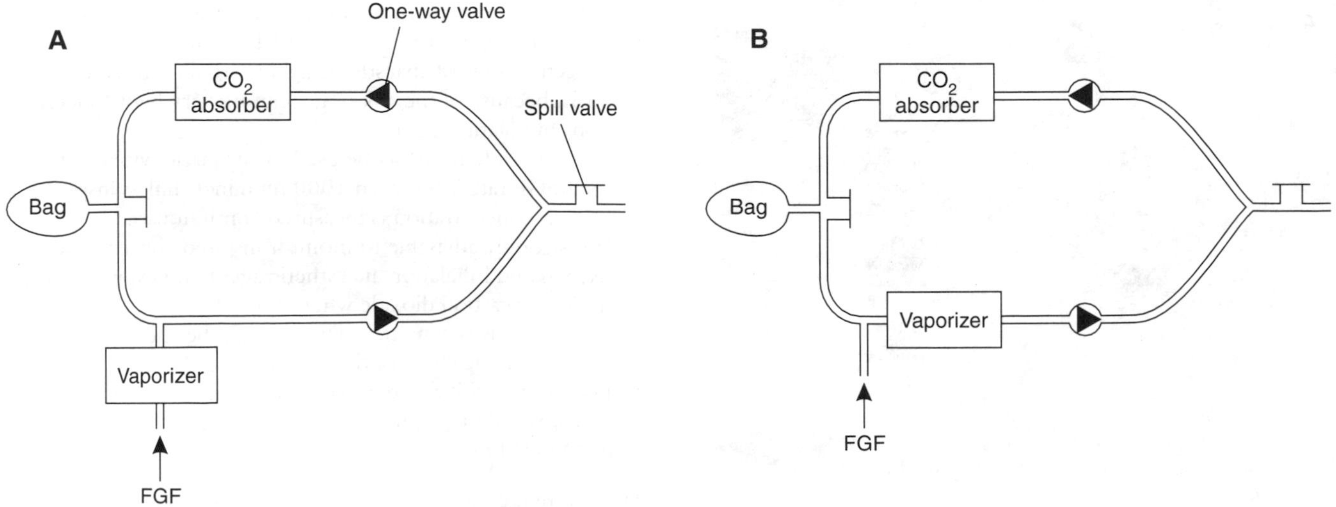

Fig. 32.30
Diagrammatic representation of circle system. **A.** Vaporizer outside the circle (VOC). **B.** Vaporizer inside the circle (VIC).

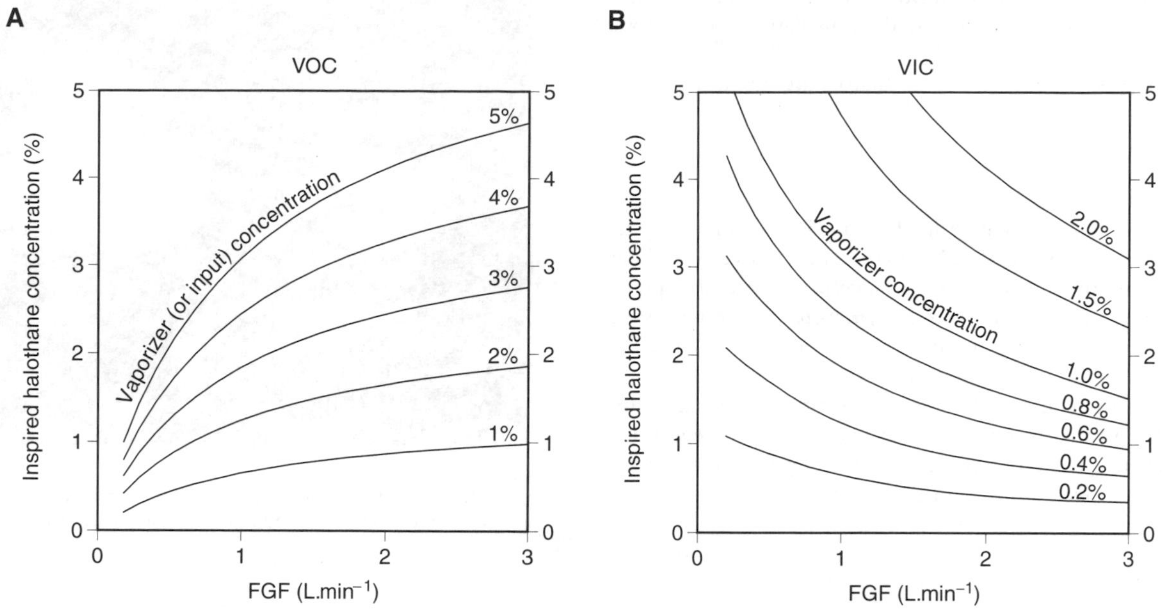

Fig. 32.31
Variation of inspired concentration of halothane with fresh gas flow rate. Total minute ventilation is 5 L min^{-1}. **A.** Vaporizer outside the circle (VOC); note that dilution of the fresh gas results in much lower concentrations in the circle system than the concentration set on the vaporizer unless fresh gas flow rate approaches 3 L min^{-1}. **B.** Vaporizer inside the circle (VIC); at low flow rates, lack of dilution of expired halothane concentrations, with additional halothane vaporized during each inspiration, results in inspired concentrations much higher than those set on the vaporizer. Even at a fresh gas flow rate of 3 L min^{-1}, inspired concentration is approximately 50% higher than the vaporizer setting.

Table 32.5 Disadvantages and advantages of the circle system

Disadvantages	Advantages
Cumbersome equipment	Inspired gases are humidified and warmed
Risk of delivering hypoxic mixture	Economical
Increased resistance to breathing	Minimal pollution
Slow change in the depth of anaesthesia	
Risk of awareness	
Risk of a rise in end-tidal CO_2	
Risk of unidirectional valves sticking	
Not ideal for paediatric patients breathing spontaneously	
Some inhalation agents may interact with soda lime	

VENTILATORS

Mechanical ventilation of the lung may be achieved by several mechanisms, including the generation of a negative pressure around the whole of the patient's body except the head and neck (cabinet ventilator or 'iron lung '), a negative pressure over the thorax and abdomen (cuirass ventilators) or a positive pressure over the thorax and abdomen (inflatable cuirass ventilators). However, during anaesthesia, and in the majority of patients who require mechanical ventilation in the intensive care unit, ventilation is achieved by the application of positive pressure to the lungs through a tracheal tube. Only this mode of ventilation is described here.

An enormous selection of ventilators exists and it is possible in this section to discuss only the principles involved in their use. Before using any ventilator, it is *essential* that the trainee understands its functions fully; failure to do so may result in the delivery of a hypoxic gas mixture, rebreathing of carbon dioxide and/or delivery of a mixture that contains no anaesthetic gases. If an unfamiliar ventilator is encountered, it may be helpful to use a 'dummy lung ' (a small reservoir bag on the patient connection) and to discuss the capabilities and limitations of the machine with a senior colleague. In addition, the manufacturer's 'user handbook' may be consulted or details may be obtained from a specialist book.

Continuous clinical monitoring is essential when any ventilator is used, even those which incorporate sophisticated monitoring and warning devices. In addition to standard clinical monitoring systems attached to the patient (see Ch. 20), the minimum acceptable monitoring of ventilator function includes measurement of expired tidal volume, airway pressure and inspired oxygen concentration; in addition, a ventilator disconnection alarm should be incorporated in the system. Continuous monitoring of end-tidal carbon dioxide, pulse oximetry and inspired anaesthetic gas concentrations is essential.

The incorporation of a humidifier in the inspiratory limb, or of a condenser humidifier at the connection with the tracheal tube, is essential in long-term ventilation in the ICU. Bacterial filters (Fig. 32.32) are now recommended in all patients undergoing anaesthesia.

The principles of operation of ventilators are described best by considering each phase of the ventilatory cycle.

Inspiration

The pattern of volume change in the lung is determined by the characteristics of the ventilator. Ventilators may deliver a predetermined flow rate of gas (*constant flow generators*) or exert a predetermined pressure (*constant pressure generators*), although some machines produce a pattern which does not conform to either category. Most flow generators produce a constant flow of gas during inspiration, although a few generate a sinusoidal flow pattern if the ventilator bellows is driven via a crank, e.g. Cape-Waine ventilator. The characteristics of constant flow and constant pressure generators are shown in Figure 32.33.

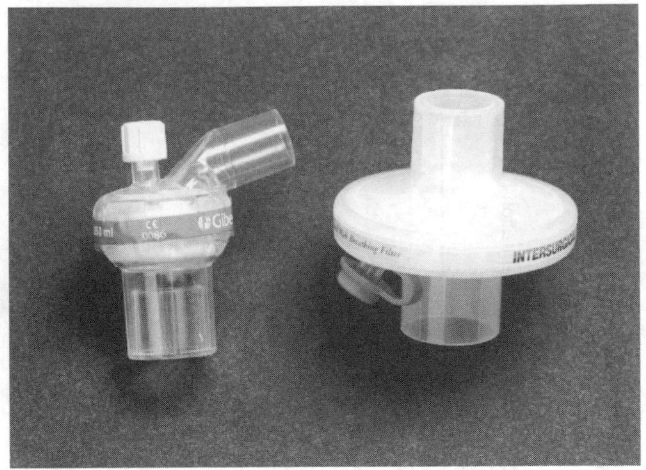

Fig 32.32
Bacterial filters and humidifiers which are used in breathing systems: *left* – a paediatric filter incorporated into an angle piece; *right* – an adult filter.

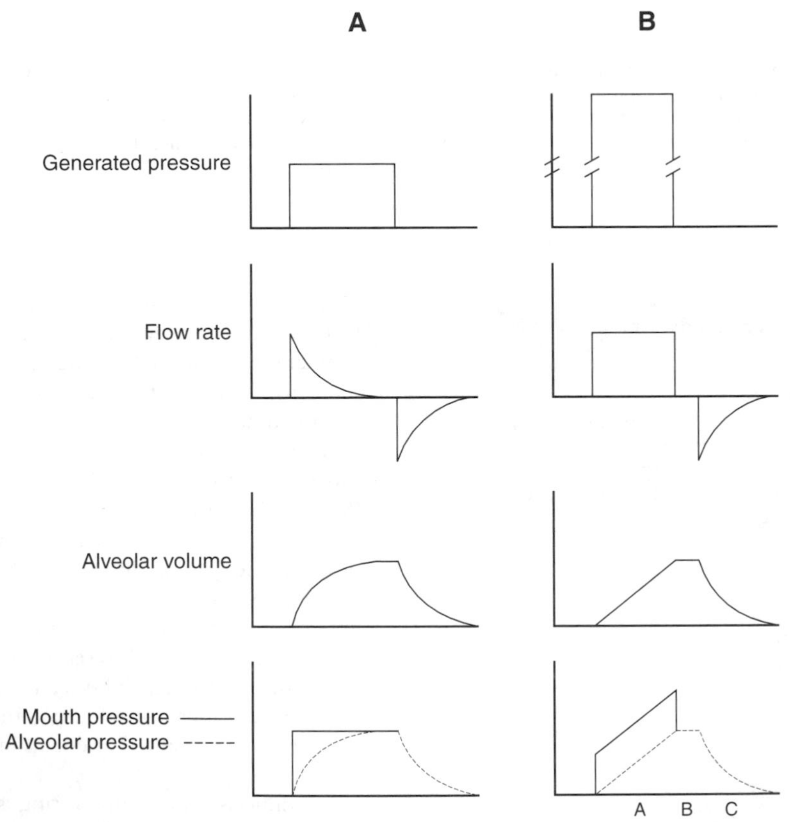

Fig. 32.33
Graphs of generated pressure, mouth (or tracheal tube) and alveolar pressures, flow rate and alveolar volume changes during inspiration and subsequent expiration produced by a constant pressure generator **A** and a constant flow generator **B**. A constant pressure generator exerts a low pressure (e.g. 1.5 kPa, 15 cmH_2O). At the start of inspiration, the pressure in the alveoli is zero. Gas flows rapidly into the alveoli at a rate determined by airways resistance, resulting in rapid increases in alveolar volume and pressure. The mouth–alveolar pressure gradient decreases and flow rate, and consequently the rate of increase of alveolar volume and pressure, decrease also. When the alveolar pressure equals the ventilator pressure, flow ceases. A constant flow generator generates a very high internal pressure (e.g. 400 kPa) but has a high internal resistance to limit flow rate. The pressure gradient between machine and alveoli remains virtually constant throughout inspiration and thus flow rate is constant. The increases in alveolar volume and (assuming constant compliance) pressure are linear. Because flow rate is constant, the pressure gradient between mouth and alveoli is constant throughout inspiration (A). Mouth pressure decreases to equal alveolar pressure during the inspiratory pause when flow ceases (B). Gas flow out of the lung during expiration (C) is passive.

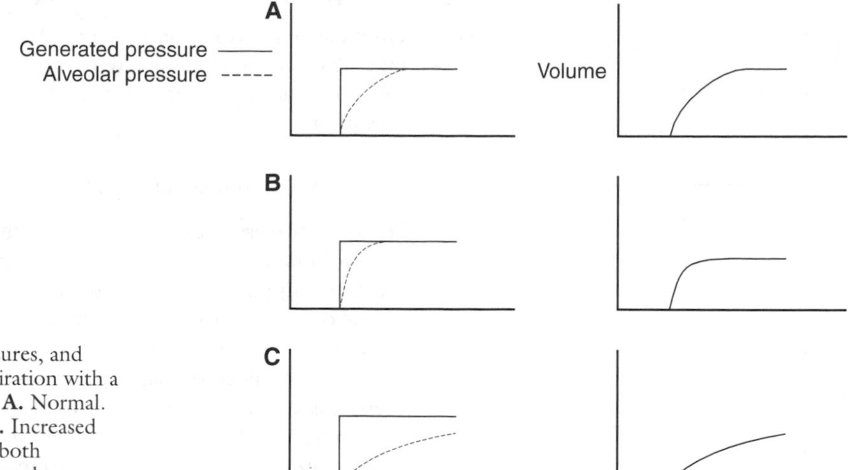

Fig. 32.34
Generated and alveolar pressures, and alveolar volume, during inspiration with a constant pressure generator. **A.** Normal. **B.** Decreased compliance. **C.** Increased airway resistance. Note that both abnormalities reduce alveolar volume.

Constant pressure generator

The East-Radcliffe ventilator is the only true constant pressure generator. This machine contains bellows with a capacity that greatly exceeds the normal tidal volume. The inspiratory pressure is generated by weights on top of the bellows. The bellows cease to empty when the pressure generated by the weights equals the pressure in the patient's alveoli. To some extent, the machine may compensate for leaks, as the bellows are large and continue to empty until a predetermined pressure has been achieved in the lungs. However, that pressure may be achieved after delivery to the lungs of different volumes of gas if the lung/chest wall compliance changes (Fig. 32.34). For example, if the patient is tipped head-down, compliance decreases and a smaller tidal volume is delivered [compliance = Δ(volume)/ Δ(pressure)]. If airways resistance increases, the flow rate of gas is decreased and the pressure in the lungs may not reach bellows pressure before the end of the inspiratory cycle; consequently, tidal volume decreases. Tidal volume is decreased also if a large leak develops.

Constant flow generator

Changes in resistance or compliance make little difference to the volume delivered (unless the ventilator is pressure-cycled; see below), although airway and alveolar pressures may change (Fig. 32.35). For example, decreased compliance results in delivery of a normal tidal volume; however, the rate of increase of alveolar pressure is greater than normal (i.e. the slope is greater) and airway pressure is correspondingly higher to maintain a gradient between the tracheal tube and the alveoli. If airway resistance increases, the pressure at the tracheal tube (and the gradient between tracheal tube and alveolar pressures) is higher than normal throughout inspiration, but alveolar pressure and the slopes of both pressure curves are normal. Constant flow generators do not compensate for leaks; the tidal volume delivered to the lungs decreases.

Some ventilators, e.g. Blease Brompton, generate a pressure rather higher than that required to inflate the lungs but not high enough to maintain constant flow throughout inspiration. The flow, volume and pressure changes within the lung are shown in Figure 32.36.

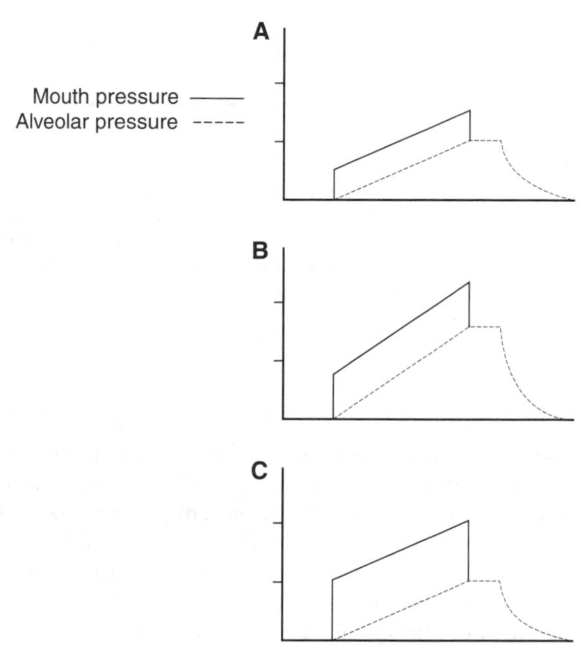

Fig. 32.35
Mouth and alveolar pressures during inspiration with a constant flow generator. **A.** Normal. **B.** Decreased compliance. **C.** Increased airway resistance. Alveolar volume remains constant because flow rate is constant. Decreased compliance results in an increased rate of increase of alveolar pressure; mouth pressure also increases more steeply, but the gradient between mouth and alveolar pressures remains normal. Increased airway resistance increases the mouth–alveolar pressure gradient.

Change from inspiration to expiration

This is termed 'cycling ' and may be achieved in one of three ways:

Volume-cycling. The ventilator cycles into expiration whenever a predetermined tidal volume has been delivered. The duration of inspiration is determined by the inspiratory flow rate.

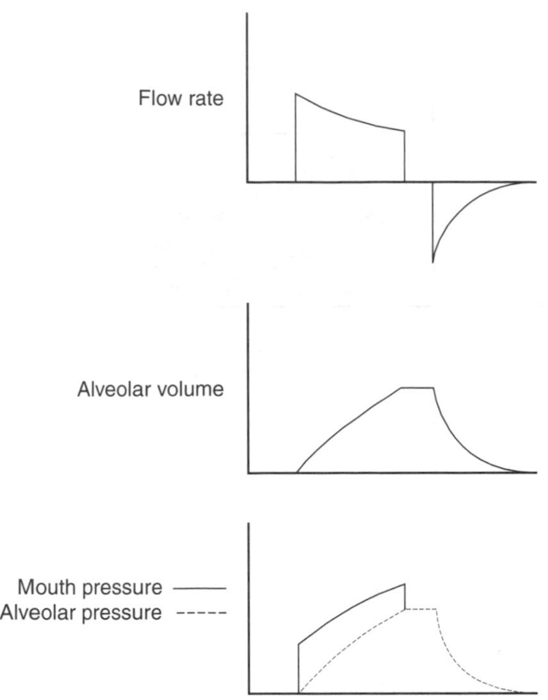

Fig. 32.36
Pressure, flow and alveolar volume characteristics during inspiration with a ventilator with a moderately high internal pressure (e.g. Blease Brompton). At higher bellows pressures, and in a patient with normal compliance and airway resistance, the characteristics approximate to those of a constant flow generator (Fig. 32.35). At low bellows pressures, if compliance decreases or if airway resistance increases, the pattern is similar to that of a constant pressure generator.

Pressure-cycling. The ventilator cycles into expiration when a present *airway* pressure is achieved. This allows compensation for small leaks but, in common with a constant pressure generator, a pressure-cycled ventilator delivers a different tidal volume if compliance or resistance changes. In addition, inspiratory time varies with changes in compliance and resistance.

Time-cycling. This is the method used most commonly by modern ventilators. The duration of inspiration is predetermined. With a constant flow generator, it may be desirable to preset a tidal volume; when this has been delivered, there is a short inspiratory pause (which improves gas distribution within the lung) before the inspiratory cycle ends. The use of this 'volume-preset' mechanism must be differentiated from volume-cycling. When a constant pressure generator is time-cycled, the tidal volume delivered depends on the compliance and resistance of the lungs and on the pressure within the bellows.

Expiration

Usually, the patient is allowed to exhale to atmospheric pressure; flow rate decreases exponentially. Subatmospheric pressure should not be used during expiration as it induces small airways closure and air trapping. PEEP may be applied in some circumstances (see Ch. 60).

Change from expiration to inspiration

On most ventilators, this is achieved by time-cycling. However, it may be desirable occasionally to use pressure-cycling in response to a subatmospheric pressure generated by the patient's inspiratory effort.

Delivery of anaesthetic gas

Some ventilators deliver a minute volume determined by a preset tidal volume and rate. When used in anaesthesia, these machines must be supplied with a flow rate of anaesthetic gases which equals or exceeds the minute volume delivered, otherwise air, or gas used to drive the ventilator, is entrained and delivered to the patient. A number of ventilators which are driven by the anaesthetic gas supply may deliver only that gas and divide it into predetermined tidal volumes (***minute volume dividers***).

Ventilators may be used to compress bellows in a separate system which contains anaesthetic gases ('bag-in-a-bottle'); it is possible to provide IPPV in a circle system in this way. The bag-in-a-bottle ventilator (Fig. 32.37) consists of a chamber with a tidal volume range of 0–1500 ml (adult mode) or 0–400 ml (paediatric mode) and ascending bellows which accommodate FGF. The control unit has controls, displays and alarms and these may include tidal volume, respiratory rate, I/E ratio, airway pressure and an on/off/standby switch. Compressed air is used as the driving gas. On entering the chamber, the compressed air forces the bellows down, delivering the FGF within the bellows to the patient. The driving gas in the chamber and the FGF in the bellows remain separate.

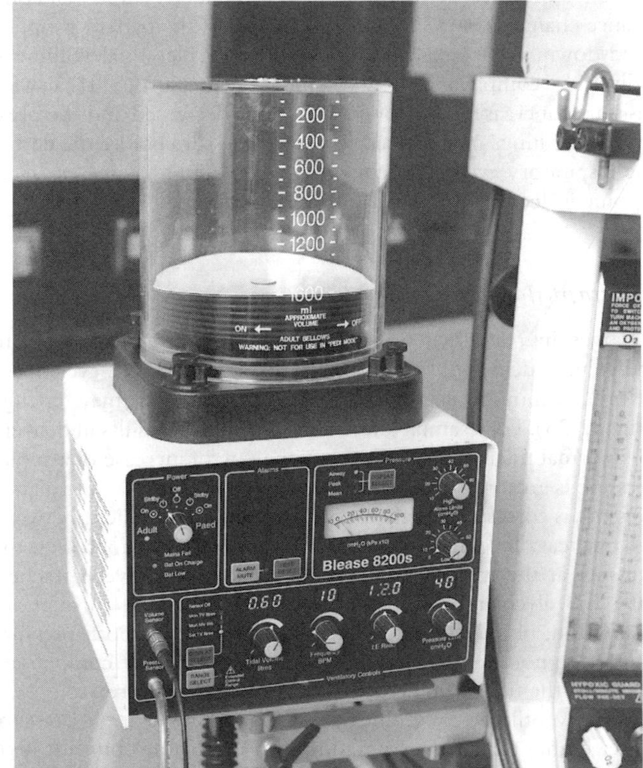

Fig. 32.37
Blease bag-in-a-bottle ventilator.

Table 32.6 Classification of some common ventilators used during anaesthesia

Ventilator	Driven by	Cycling to expiration	Cycling to inspiration	Pressure/flow generator	Minute volume divider	Volume preset
Manley MP2, MN2, NO3	Anaesthetic gases	Time	Time	Pressure	Yes	Yes
Manley Pulmovent	Anaesthetic gases	Volume	Time	Flow	Yes	Yes
Blease Brompton	Anaesthetic gases	Volume or time	Time	Mixed	Yes	Yes
Manley Servovent	Compressed air or oxygen	Volume	Time	Flow	No	Yes
Oxford	Compressed air or oxygen	Time	Time	Flow	No	Yes
Nuffield 200	Compressed air or oxygen	Time	Time	Flow	No	No
Servo 900	Anaesthetic gases	Time (electrically operated valves)	Time (electrically operated valves)	Flow (usually)	No	Yes
Bag-in-bottle	Compressed air or oxygen	Time	Time	Flow	No	Yes

The Penlon Nuffield 200 ventilator is an intermittent blower (Fig. 32.22). It is a very versatile ventilator which may be used in different age groups and using different breathing systems. The control unit consists of an airway pressure gauge (cmH_2O), inspiratory and expiratory time dials (seconds), inspiratory flow rates ($L\ s^{-1}$) and an on/off switch. Below the control unit, there is a connection for the driving gas (oxygen or air) and the valve block. A small tubing connects the valve block to an airway pressure monitor and to a ventilator alarm. The valve block consists of a port for tubing to connect to the breathing system reservoir bag mount (Bain system) or the ventilator port (ADE system), an exhaust port which can be connected to the scavenging system and a pressure relief valve which opens at 60 cmH_2O. With this standard valve, the ventilator is a time-cycled flow generator. The valve block can be changed to a paediatric Newton valve and this then converts the ventilator to a time-cycled pressure generator.

The characteristics of several common ventilators are summarized in Table 32.6.

HIGH-FREQUENCY VENTILATION

High-frequency ventilation (HFV) may be defined as ventilation at a respiratory rate of greater than four times the resting respiratory rate of the subject. The different modes of HFV are shown in Table 32.7.

Table 32.7 Types of high frequency ventilation

Type of ventilation	Rate of ventilation (cycles min^{-1})
High-frequency positive pressure ventilation (HFPPV)	60–100
High-frequency jet ventilation (HFJV)	100–400
High-frequency oscillation ventilation (HFOV)	400–2400

Of the three types of HFV, high-frequency jet ventilation (HFJV) is the most commonly used. The tidal volume used in HFJV is small compared with conventional ventilation. This is delivered at high pressure (up to 5 bar) through a cannula or catheter placed in the trachea. Inspiratory flow rates of up to 100 L min^{-1} may be required. The inspiratory time is adjustable from 20 to 50% of the cycle. The mechanism by which HFV is able to maintain gas exchange is not clear. Typical values for adult ventilation are:

- ventilation rate – 100–150 cycles min^{-1}
- driving pressure 100–200 kPa
- inspiratory cycle of 20–40%.

HFJV is used during some operations on the larynx, trachea or lung and in a small number of patients in the ICU. Gases should be humidified when using HFJV. Gas exchange may be unpredictable and the technique should not be used by the trainee without supervision. Figure 32.38 illustrates a type of ventilator used for HFJV.

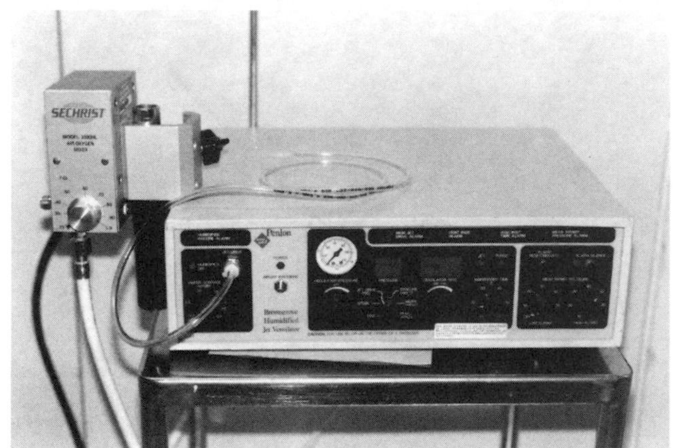

Fig. 32.38
Penlon Bromsgrove jet ventilator.

VENTURI INJECTOR DEVICE

The Venturi injector consists of a high-pressure oxygen source (at about 400 kPa from either the anaesthetic machine or direct from a pipeline), an on/off trigger and connection tubing that can withstand high pressure (Fig. 32.39). This is connected to the side of a rigid bronchoscope, to a transtracheal catheter or to a cannula through the cricothyroid membrane. A 14G cannula or a specially designed cannula (Fig. 32.40) inserted through the cricothyroid membrane may be used to ventilate using the Venturi injector device. The injector is controlled manually. A Venturi effect is created which entrains atmospheric air and allows intermittent insufflation of the lungs with oxygen-enriched air at airway pressures of 2.5–3.0 kPa. It is used in operations on the larynx, trachea or lung. Possible complications include barotrauma, gastric distension and awareness if inadequate intravenous anaesthetic drugs are administered. When Venturi injector devices are employed, it is essential to ensure that gas is able to leave the lungs though the upper airway during expiration.

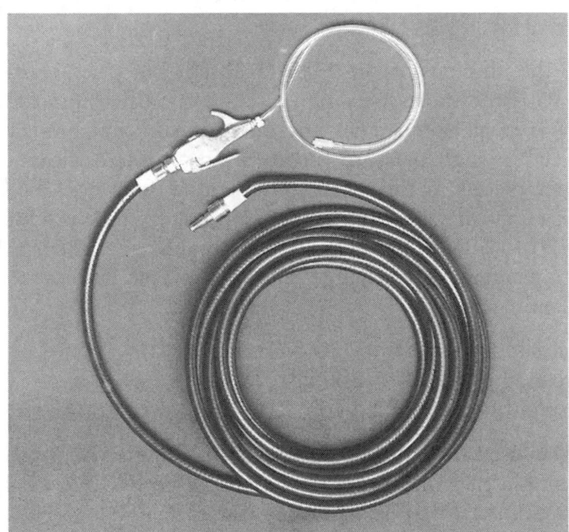

Fig. 32.39
Manually controlled Venturi injector.

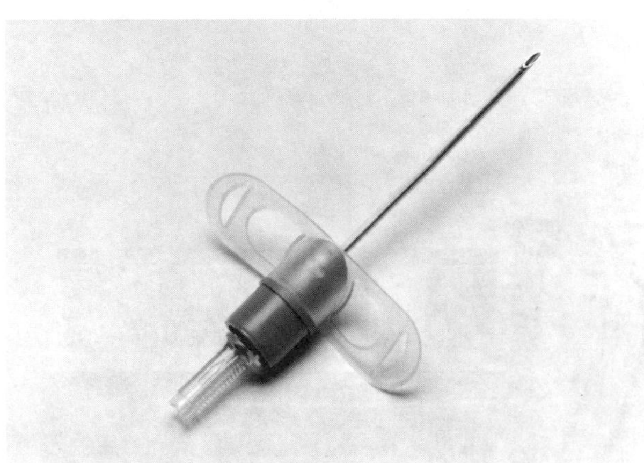

Fig. 32.40
A cricothyroid cannula to use with a Venturi injector device.

SCAVENGING

The possible adverse effects of pollution on staff in the operating theatre environment are discussed in Chapter 33. The principal sources of pollution by anaesthetic gases and vapours include:

- discharge of anaesthetic gases from ventilators
- expired gas vented from the spill valve of anaesthetic breathing systems
- leaks from equipment, e.g. from an ill-fitting face mask
- gas exhaled by the patient after anaesthesia. This may occur in the operating theatre, corridors and recovery room
- spillage during filling of vaporizers.

Although most attention has centred on removing gas from the expiratory ports of breathing systems and ventilators, other methods of reducing pollution should also be considered:

Reduced use of anaesthetic gases and vapours. The use of the circle system reduces the potential for atmospheric pollution. The use of inhalation anaesthetics may be obviated totally by using total intravenous anaesthesia or local anaesthetic techniques.

Air conditioning. Air conditioning units which produce a rapid change of air in the operating theatre reduce pollution substantially. However, some systems recycle air, and older operating theatres, dental surgeries and obstetric delivery suites may not be equipped with air conditioning.

Care in filling vaporizers. Great care should be taken not to spill volatile anaesthetic agent when a vaporizer is filled. The use of agent-specific connections (see Fig. 32.13) reduces the risk of spillage. In some countries, vaporizers may be filled only in a portable fume cupboard.

SCAVENGING APPARATUS

Anaesthetic gases vented from the breathing system are removed by a collecting system. A variety of purpose-built scavenging spill valves is available; an example is shown in Figure 32.41. Waste gases from ventilators are collected by attaching the scavenging system to the expiratory port of the ventilator. Connectors on

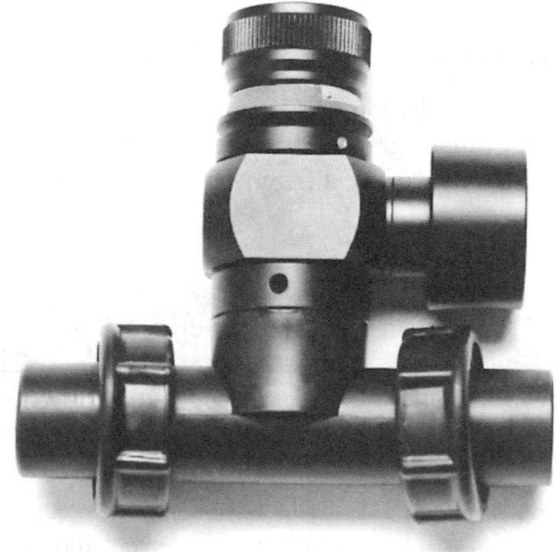

Fig. 32.41
An APL valve with scavenging attachment.

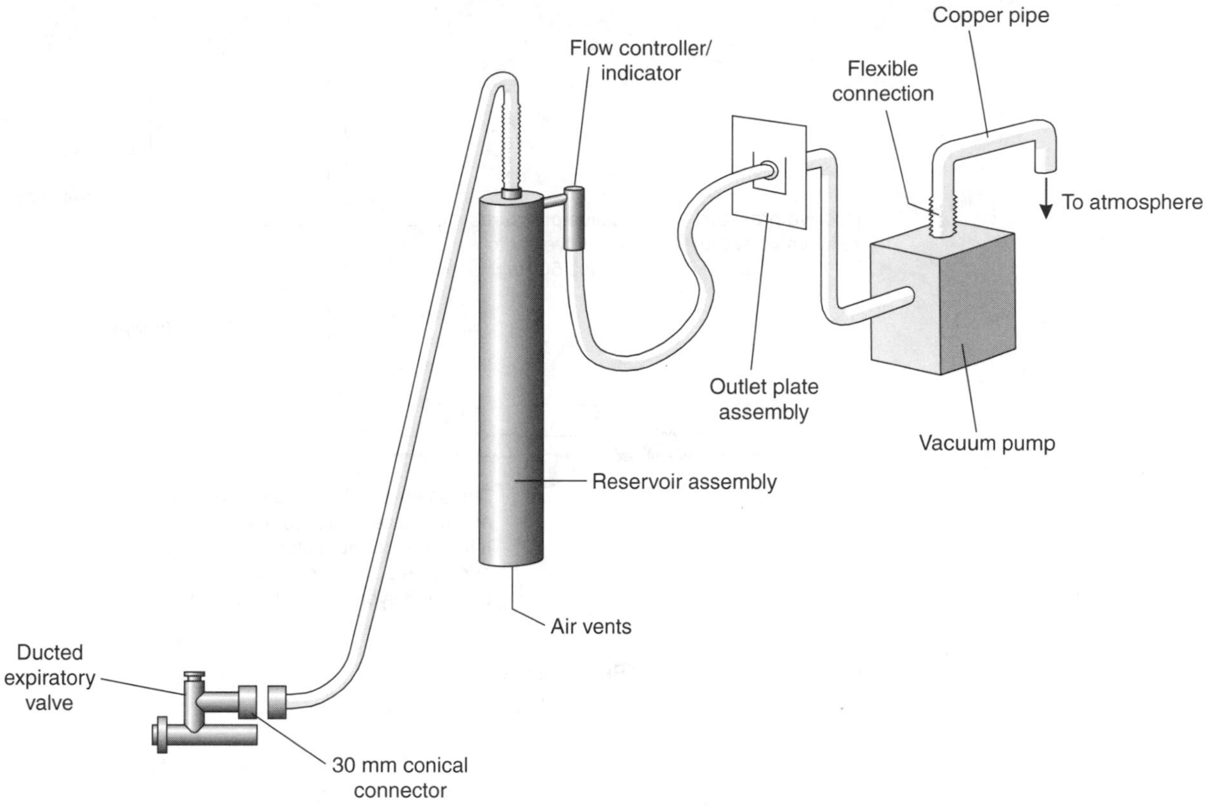

Fig. 32.42
An active scavenging system.

scavenging systems have a diameter of 30 mm to ensure that inappropriate connections with anaesthetic apparatus cannot be made.

Disposal systems may be active, semi-active or passive.

Active systems

These employ apparatus to generate a negative pressure within the scavenging system to propel waste gases to the outside atmosphere. The system may be powered by a vacuum pump (Fig. 32.42) or a Venturi system (Fig. 32.43). The exhaust should be capable of accommodating 75 L min^{-1} continuous flow with a peak of 130 L min^{-1}. Usually, a reservoir system is used to permit high peak flow rates to be accommodated. In addition, there must be a pressure-limiting device within the system to prevent the application of negative pressure to the patient's lungs.

Semi-active systems

The waste gases may be conducted to the extraction side of the air-conditioning system, which generates a small negative pressure within the scavenging tubing. These systems have variable performance and efficiency.

Passive systems

These systems vent the expired gas to the outside atmosphere (Fig. 32.44). Gas movement is generated by the patient. Consequently, the total length of tubing must not be excessive or resistance to expiration is high. The pressure within the system may be altered by wind conditions at the external terminal; on occasions, these may generate a negative pressure, but may also generate high positive pressures. Each scavenging location should have a separate external terminal to prevent gases being vented into adjacent locations. Relief valves must be incorporated to prevent negative or high positive pressures within the system.

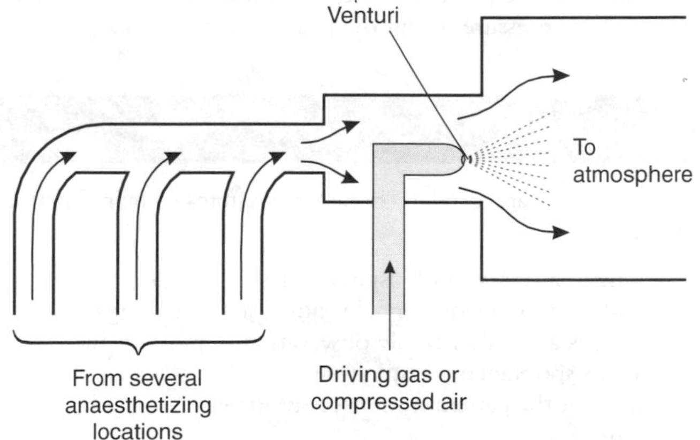

Fig. 32.43
A Venturi system for active scavenging of anaesthetic gases.

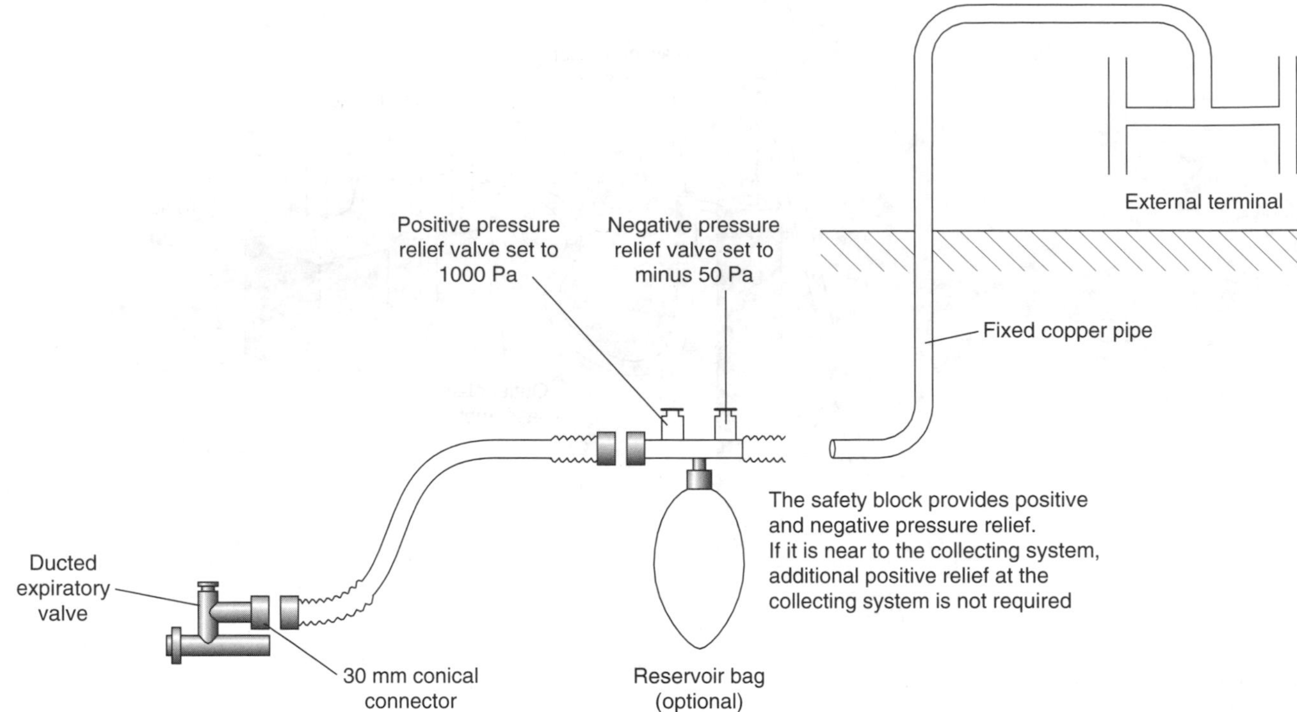

Fig. 32.44
A passive scavenging system.

Irrespective of the type of disposal system, tubing used for scavenging must not be allowed to lie on the floor of the operating theatre, as compression (e.g. by feet or by items of equipment) results in increased resistance to expiration and may generate dangerously high pressure within the patient's lungs.

RESERVOIR BAGS

Reservoir bags are used in breathing systems. Their functions include:

- serving as a reservoir of inspired gases
- providing a means of manual ventilation of the lungs
- serving as a visual or tactile observation to monitor the patient's spontaneous respiration
- protecting the patient from excessive pressure in the breathing system.

The reservoir bag may accommodate an increase in pressure in the breathing system to a maximum of approximately 50 cmH_2O (5 kPa).

The standard adult size is 2 L and the paediatric size is 0.5 L (Fig. 32.45). However, the size of reservoir bags may vary from 0.5 to 6 L. The larger reservoir bags are used in ventilators.

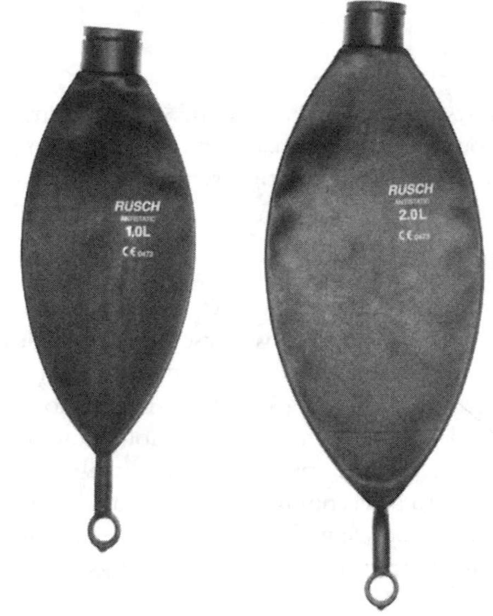

Fig. 32.45
Reservoir bags.

LARYNGOSCOPES

A laryngoscope consists of a blade which elevates the lower jaw and tongue, a light source near the tip of the blade to illuminate the larynx, and a handle to apply leverage to the blade. There are many forms of blade and handle.

Curved blade

The most commonly used adult laryngoscope blade is the Macintosh curved blade, which is manufactured in several sizes (Figs 32.46 and 32.47).

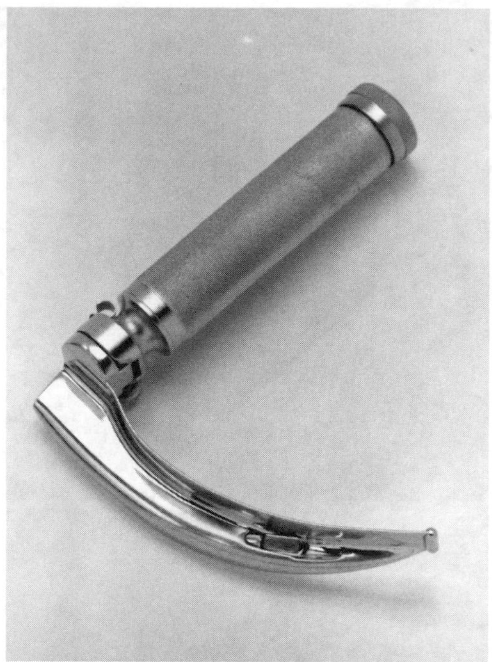

Fig. 32.46
A laryngoscope with the Macintosh adult blade.

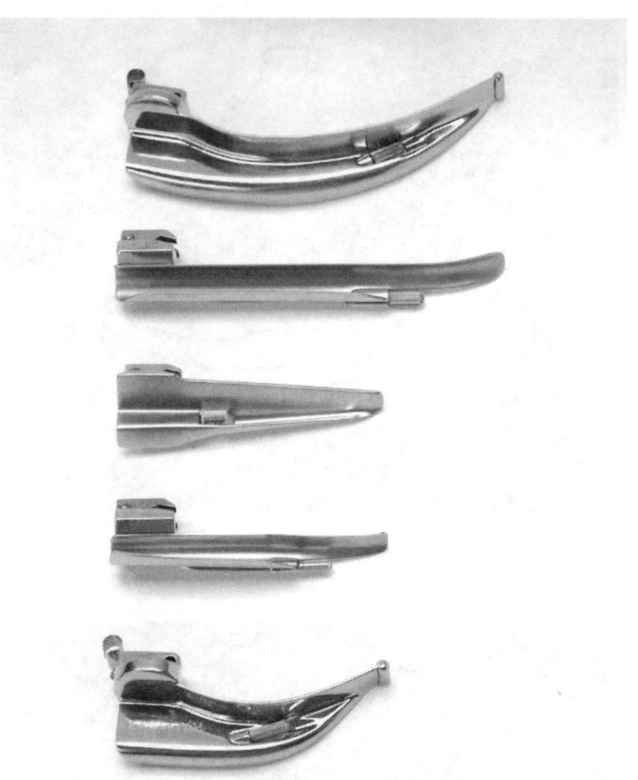

Fig. 32.47
A selection of laryngoscope blades. From the top downwards: Macintosh adult blade, Miller adult blade, Soper infant blade, Wisconsin infant blade and Macintosh infant blade.

The tip of the laryngoscope blade is advanced carefully over the surface of the tongue until it reaches the vallecula (see Fig. 37.3). The tip of the blade is rotated upwards and the laryngoscope lifted along the axis of the handle to lift the larynx; the incisor teeth must not be used as a fulcrum to lever the tip of the blade upwards. When the arytenoids and posterior part of the cords are seen, gentle pressure on the larynx using the right thumb, or provided by an assistant, may help to improve the view.

Straight blade

Straight-bladed laryngoscopes are useful adjuncts in safe airway management. However, they are not always as easy to use as curved blades. The technique of laryngoscopy is slightly different when a straight-bladed laryngoscope is used (see Fig. 37.3). Instead of placing the tip of the blade in the vallecula, it is advanced over the posterior border of the epiglottis, which is then lifted directly by the blade to provide a view of the larynx. This technique is useful particularly in babies, in whom the epiglottis is rather floppy and may obscure the view of the larynx if a curved blade is used. However, bruising of the epiglottis is more likely with a straight blade. The straight-bladed laryngoscopes available include the Miller, Magill, Soper, Wisconsin and Henderson laryngoscopes. The last of these is still undergoing evaluation.

Light source

Most laryngoscopes are powered by batteries contained within the handle; these must be replaced regularly to prevent failure during laryngoscopy. On many laryngoscopes, the light source is a bulb which screws into a socket on the blade; a tight connection should be ensured before laryngoscopy is attempted. It is usual for the electrical circuit between the batteries and the bulb to be closed by a switch which operates automatically when the blade is opened. However, the electrical contacts of the switch may become corroded, causing a reduction in power or total failure. Because of these potential problems, it is important that the function of the laryngoscope is checked carefully before use. It is also wise to have a spare functioning laryngoscope and a variety of blades available. Some designs place the bulb in the handle and the light is transmitted to the blade by means of fibreoptics.

Laryngoscope handle

The standard handle may result in difficult laryngoscopy in obese patients, and in women with large breasts. Short handles are available for the use in these situations (Fig. 32.48). The short handle has almost replaced the use of the Polio blade (Fig. 32.49) in obstetric practice.

The McCoy laryngoscope (Fig. 32.50A) is based on the standard Macintosh blade but has a hinged tip. This is operated by a lever mechanism attached to the handle. When the lever is pressed (Fig. 32.50B), the tip of the blade bends forward and this improves the view of the larynx.

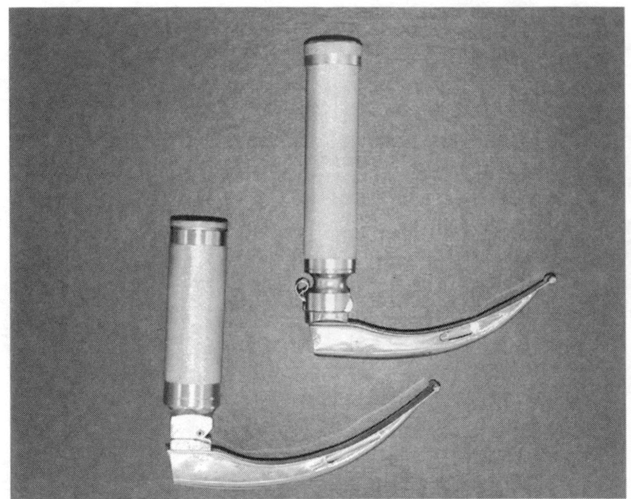

Fig. 32.48
Short and standard laryngoscope handles.

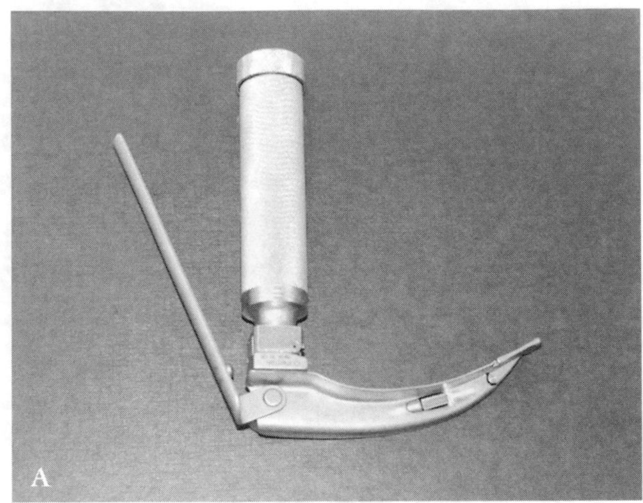

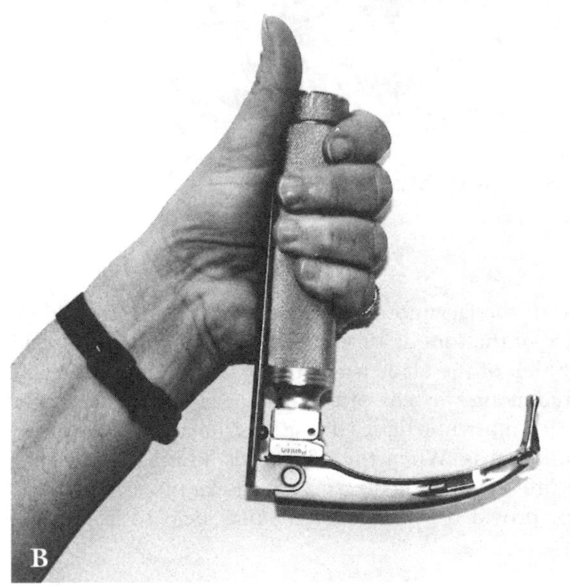

Fig. 32.50
A. The McCoy laryngoscope. **B.** The McCoy laryngoscope, demonstrating the hinged blade tip.

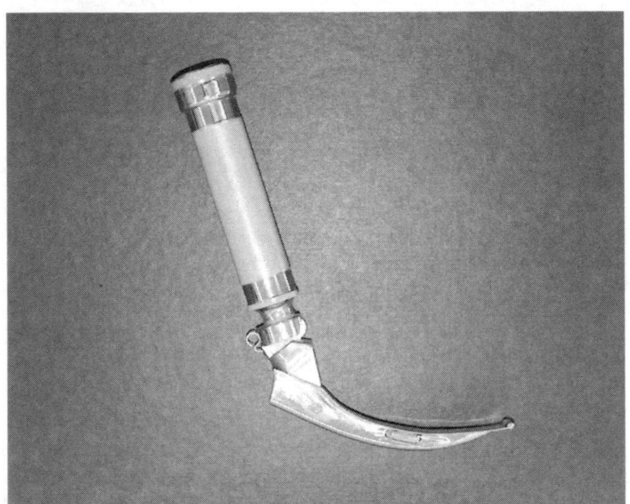

Fig. 32.49
The Polio blade

FIBREOPTIC LARYNGO/BRONCHOSCOPE

The fibreoptic scope (Fig. 32.51) is an endoscope which is used to view the upper and lower airway through either the nose or the mouth. The principle of the fibreoptic system is that light from a powerful external light source is transmitted through a flexible instrument and an image of the area is returned to an eyepiece or camera. The fibres which transmit the light have a diameter of approximately 20 μm and are made up of a central glass core coated with a thin layer of glass material with a lower refractive index. The light passing down the fibre is repeatedly reflected down the inner glass.

The fibreoptic scope consists of a light source, a universal cord and light guide connector, a control unit, an eyepiece and an insertion tube. The light source (Fig 32.52) is usually powered by mains electrical supply and contains either a xenon or a halogen lamp. The universal cord and light guide connector contain the light guide fibre bundle and transmit light from a light source to the fibreoptic bundle in the insertion tube.

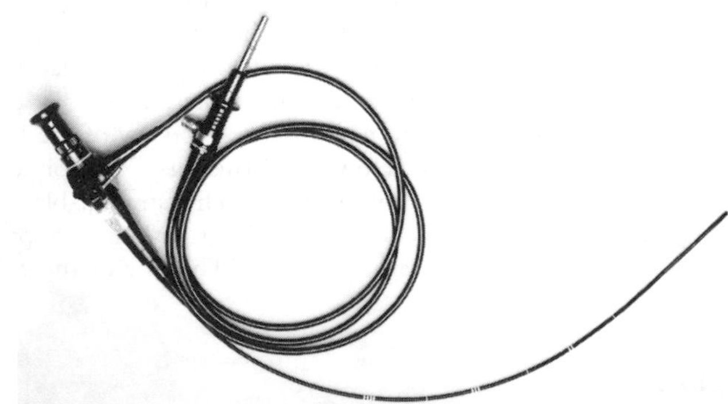

Fig. 32.51
The fibreoptic intubating laryngoscope which consists of the universal cord and light guide connector, the control unit and the insertion cord.

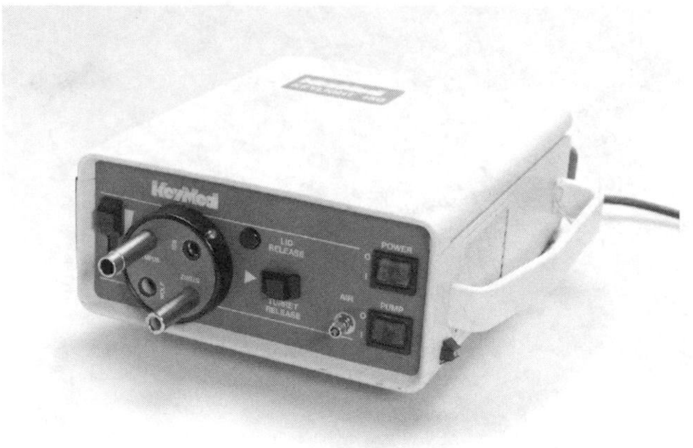

Fig. 32.52
The light source for the fibreoptic intubating laryngoscope.

The control unit consists of an angulation control lever, suction port and a biopsy port. The angulation lever controls the deflection of the tip of the scope. The suction port is for connecting to a suction pump but it can also be used for insufflation of oxygen. The biopsy channel can be used for taking biopsy specimens but it can also be used to attach a syringe to instil local anaesthetic into the airway.

The eyepiece consists of the viewing lens and the dioptre adjustment ring. A camera can be attached to the eyepiece either to take photographs or to transmit the pictures to a television monitor.

The insertion tube contains two optical fibre bundles: the light guide and the image guide. The fibres transmitting light (light guide) are arranged in a random fashion but those returning the image (image guide) are precisely located relative to each other. The insertion tube also contains the suction channel and the biopsy channel. At the distal end of each optical fibre, there is a lens. The size of the insertion tube varies from 1.8 to 6.4 mm to fit inside tracheal tubes of internal diameter 3.0–7.0 mm.

TRACHEAL TUBES

Most tracheal tubes are constructed of red rubber, silicone rubber or plastic. Red rubber tubes are re-usable, although they may start to show signs of deterioration after 2–3 years. Today, disposable plastic tubes are the preferred choice (Fig 32.53) as they eliminate the need to collect, clean, sterilize and check tubes after use. Plastic tubes are presented in a sterile pack and should be cut to an appropriate length before use. The plastic disposable tubes have a cuff and a pilot balloon with a self-sealing valve. The cuff can be inflated with air, nitrous oxide or saline. The internal diameter of the tube is marked on the side of the tube in mm and the length of the tube is marked along the length of the tube in cm. The tube also has a radio-opaque line running along its length. This enables the position of the tube to be determined on a chest X-ray.

Some tracheal tubes contain latex and must not be used in patients who have a history of latex allergy. Silicone rubber is increasingly being used in the manufacture of tracheal tubes. These are more expensive than the plastic tubes but they may be sterilized and re-used. They are softer than red rubber or plastic endotracheal tubes and they are non-irritant.

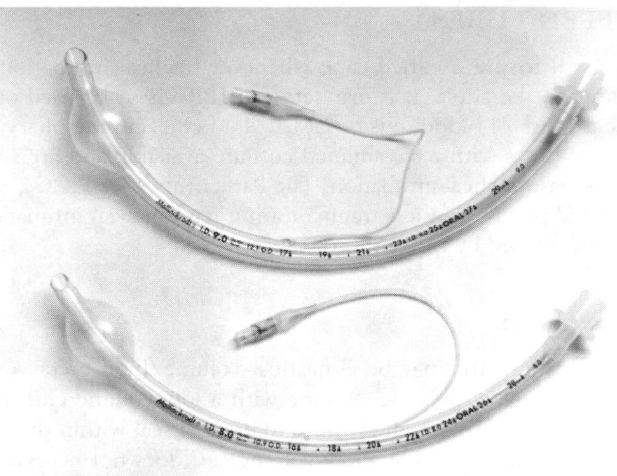

Fig. 32.53
Size 8 and 9 plastic disposable endotracheal tubes.

TUBE SIZE

In adults, there is little to be gained in the way of reduced resistance to breathing by selecting a tube larger than 8.0 mm internal diameter. However, it is common to use a tube of 9.0–9.5 mm internal diameter for male and 8.0–8.5 mm for female adults. Tubes of wide diameter may exert pressure on the laryngeal cords after insertion. Appropriate sizes of tracheal tubes for children are shown in Appendix IX.

PLAIN TUBES

Uncuffed tubes are used in children (Fig. 32.54). A cuff is unnecessary to secure an airtight fit if the correct diameter of tube is selected, because the narrowest part of the airway is in the trachea at the level of the cricoid cartilage. However, the larynx is the narrowest part of the airway in the adult and a leak occurs if an uncuffed tube is used; in addition, there is a risk of aspiration of fluid from the pharynx into the trachea. Nasotracheal intubation is less traumatic if an uncuffed tube is used. The incidence of sore throat is not influenced by the presence of a cuff on the tracheal tube.

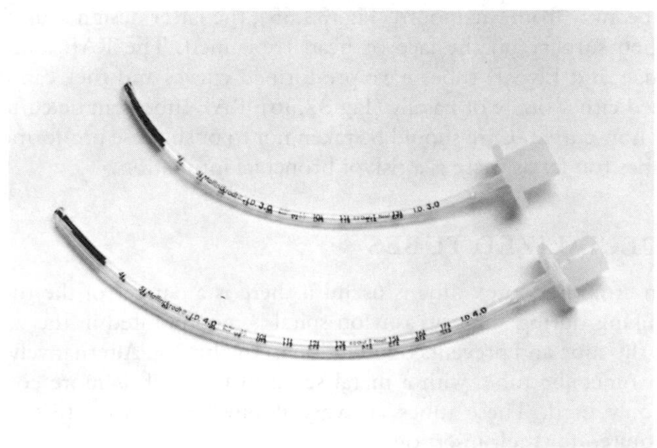

Fig. 32.54
Paediatric uncuffed plastic endotracheal tubes.

CUFFED TUBES

It is usual to use a cuffed tube whenever tracheal intubation is required in the adult. It is mandatory if IPPV is to be used or if there is a risk of blood, pus or gastric fluid entering the pharynx. Tracheal tubes with a streamlined cuff are available and are suitable for nasotracheal intubation. The Parker tube (see Fig. 32.59) is claimed to result in less trauma during nasotracheal intubation than that caused by conventional tubes.

Cuff volume

Tracheal tube cuffs may be either low-volume/high-pressure or high-volume/low-pressure. A tube with a low-volume cuff may require inflation to a high pressure to effect a seal within the trachea. The pressure within a low-volume cuff does not necessarily relate to the pressure exerted by the cuff on the tracheal mucosa. However, a high pressure may be exerted on the mucosa if the cuff is overinflated. This may occur inadvertently during anaesthesia because nitrous oxide diffuses through some types of plastic. Some anaesthetists inflate the cuff with an oxygen/nitrous oxide mixture to obviate this problem. Alternatively, the cuff volume may be readjusted after 10–15 min of anaesthesia.

High-volume, low-pressure ('floppy') cuffs cover a larger area of tracheal wall and may effect a seal with less pressure exerted on the mucosa. However, they may cause more trauma during insertion and may become puckered in a relatively small trachea.

Herniation of an overinflated cuff may occlude the distal end of the tracheal tube and cause partial or total airway obstruction.

SHAPE OF TUBE

In most centres, a curved tracheal tube is used. These should be cut to the correct length as there is a risk of accidental intubation of a bronchus (usually the right main bronchus) if the tip is inserted too far. The Oxford tube is L-shaped and the angle of the tube lies in the pharynx; the distal end is of a fixed length. It is claimed that the use of an Oxford tube reduces the risk of bronchial intubation. There may be less risk of an Oxford tube kinking if the head is flexed during surgery. However, an introducer is required to pass an Oxford tube through the larynx.

Some plastic tracheal tubes are pre-formed in shapes which either fit the pharyngeal contour or carry the proximal end of the tube away from the mouth (Fig. 32.55); the latter design is useful when surgery on the face or head is planned. The RAE (Ring, Adair and Elwyn) tubes have pre-formed curves and they can be used either orally or nasally (Fig 32.56). RAE tubes can be cuffed or non-cuffed. Care should be taken not to push these pre-formed tubes too far as there is a risk of bronchial intubation.

SPECIALIZED TUBES

An armoured latex tube is useful if there is a danger of the tube kinking during surgery; a nylon spiral is incorporated in the wall of the tube and prevents obliteration of the lumen. Alternatively, a flexometallic tube, with a metal spiral in the wall, is more commonly used. These tubes are very floppy and a wire stilette is required for their insertion.

The flexometallic tubes are available in either uncuffed paediatric sizes or cuffed adult sizes (Fig. 32.57). These tracheal tubes are long

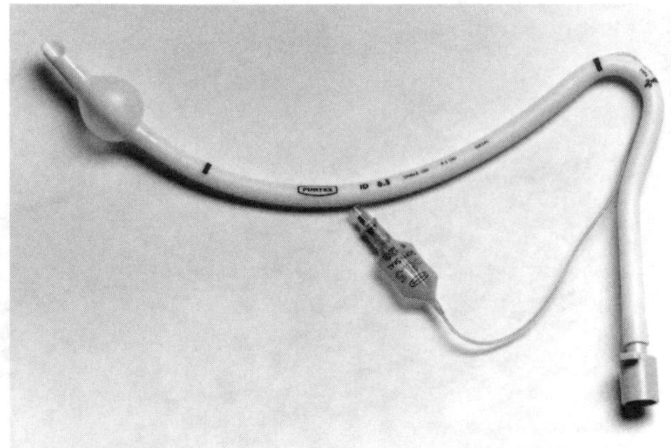

Fig. 32.55
Pre-formed north-facing nasotracheal tube.

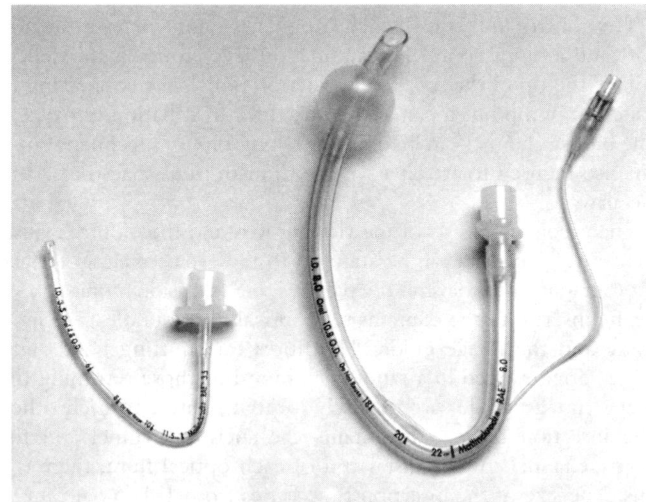

Fig. 32.56
Pre-formed RAE disposable plastic tracheal tubes. The cuffed adult tube and the uncuffed paediatric tube.

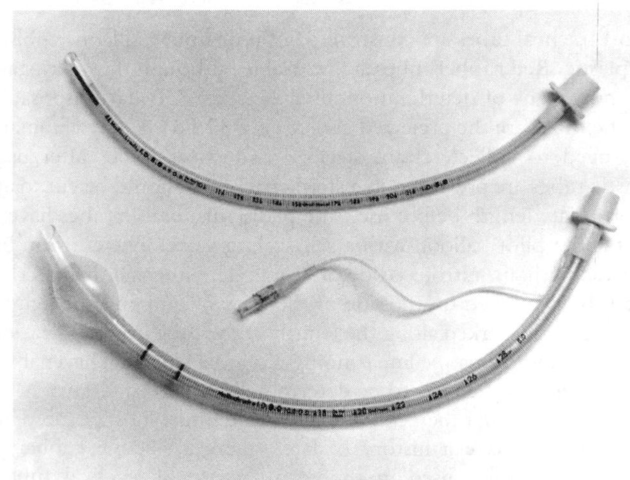

Fig. 32.57
The reinforced tracheal tube – the adult cuffed and paediatric uncuffed tubes.

and cannot be shortened because they have a fixed tracheal tube connector. Therefore, when inserting them into the trachea, care should be taken to avoid bronchial intubation. The adult cuffed tubes have two black rings and the paediatric uncuffed tubes have a black line at the distal end. These give guidance as to where the vocal cords should be, in order to avoid bronchial intubation.

A flexible metal tube (Fig. 32.58) may be used during procedures that require the use of lasers in the airway; plastic tubes may ignite if struck by the laser beam. Some designs have two cuffs. This ensures a tracheal seal should the upper cuff be damaged by laser. An air-filled cuff may ignite if it is hit by a laser beam. Therefore it is recommended that the cuffs are filled with saline instead of air.

The Parker tube (Fig 32.59) has a curved bevel on the inner curvature of the tube. The bevel therefore lies on the anterior aspect of the tube during insertion. The manufacturer claims that it is less likely than the conventional tube to cause trauma to the larynx or trachea, particularly during insertion over a bougie or fibreoptic laryngoscope.

The Combitube (Fig. 32.60) is a double-lumen airway which is designed to be inserted blindly in difficult and emergency situations. When inserted, it allows establishment of an effective airway whether it is placed into the oesophagus or the trachea. It combines the function of an oesophageal obturator and conventional tracheal tube and it protects the airway against aspiration of gastric contents. The tube has two cuffs, a proximal larger pharyngeal cuff (85–100 ml) and the smaller distal cuff (10–15 ml). The distal cuff may be placed in either the oesophagus or the trachea. Ninety-four to 98% of blind insertions usually result in oesophageal placement. In this situation, the breathing system is attached to the longer blue connecting tube and the Combitube acts as a pharyngeal airway (Fig. 32.61A). If the tube enters the trachea, ventilation of the lungs should be carried out using the shorter connecting tube and it acts as an ordinary endotracheal tube (Fig. 32.61B).

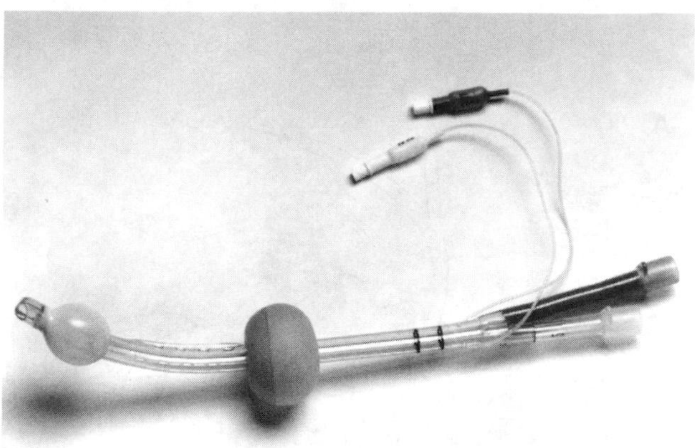

Fig 32.60
The Combitube, showing the larger proximal pharyngeal cuff and smaller distal cuff.

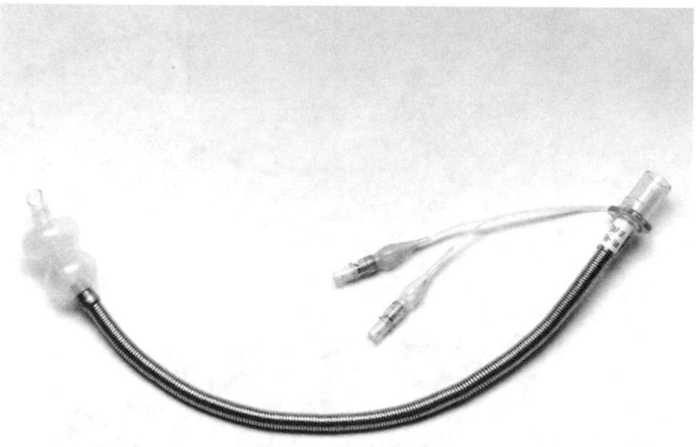

Fig. 32.58
Flexible metal tube suitable for use during laser surgery to the airway.

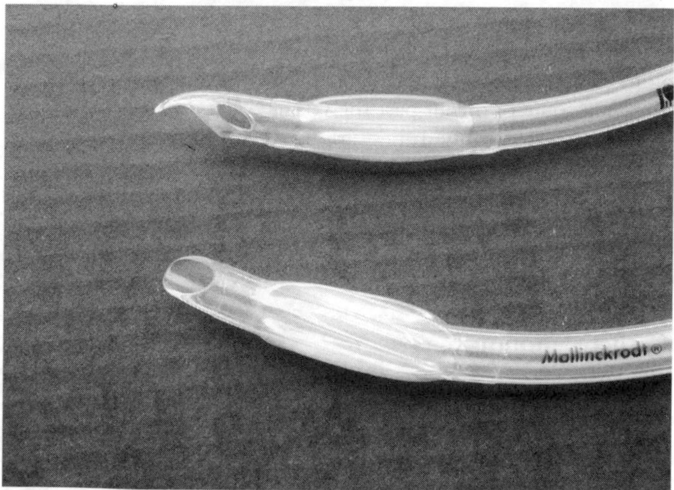

Fig. 32.59
The distal ends of a Parker (upper) and a conventional bevelled tracheal tube.

Double-lumen endobronchial tubes are used during thoracic surgery when there is a need for one lung to be deflated. They allow selective deflation of one lung whilst maintaining ventilation of the other lung. The older Robertshaw double-lumen tubes are made of red rubber and are therefore re-usable. The disposable Bronchocath double-lumen tubes (Fig. 32.62), which are made of plastic, are used more commonly now.

Laryngectomy tubes (Fig. 32.63) are designed to be inserted through a tracheostomy into the trachea to maintain the airway during surgery for laryngectomy. Because of its shape, the connection to the breathing system is some distance away from the surgical field and this gives the surgeon a relatively clear field in which to operate.

A microlaryngeal tube is a small tube (usually 5 mm internal diameter) with an adult-sized cuff which is used during surgery on the larynx. It allows better surgical access to the larynx.

TRACHEOSTOMY TUBES

There are many types of tracheostomy tube. They may be cuffed or non-cuffed. The proximal end of a tracheostomy tube has a standard 15 mm connector and there are two wings with slots to which the securing tape is attached (Fig. 32.64). Tracheostomy tubes have a replaceable inner cannula which facilitates insertion and is removed once the tracheostomy tube is in place.

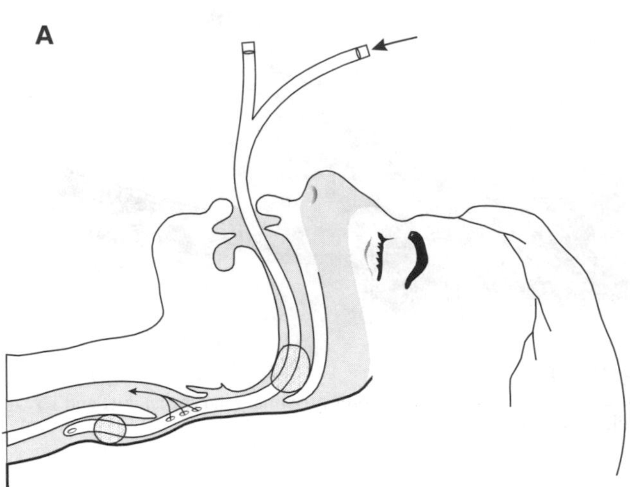

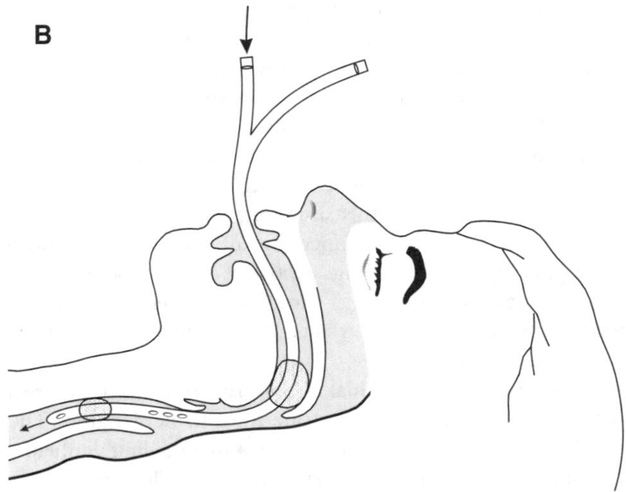

Fig. 32.61
The two possible positions of the Combitube. **A.** Combitube inserted in the oesophagus. **B.** Combitube inserted in the trachea.

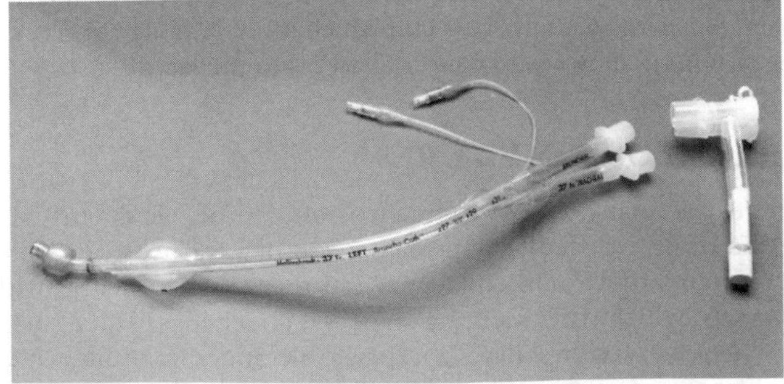

Fig. 32.62
Bronchocath double-lumen endobronchial tube with catheter mount.

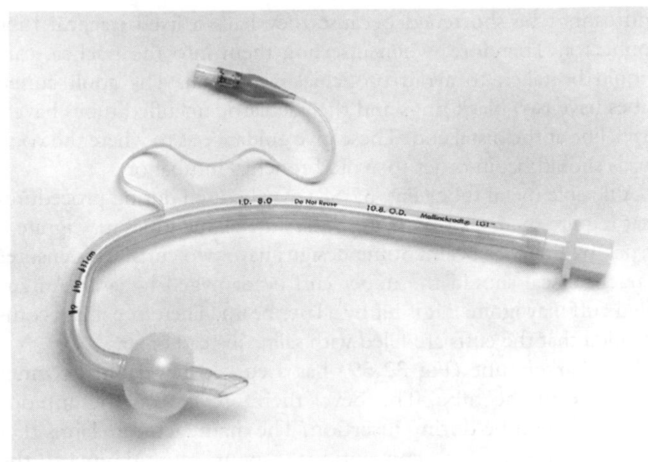

Fig. 32.63
Laryngectomy tube.

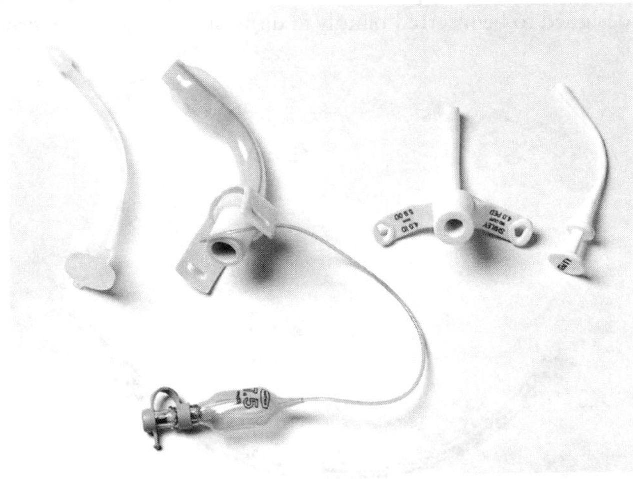

Fig. 32.64
Tracheostomy tubes. Adult cuffed (size 7) and paediatric Shiley uncuffed tube with the replaceable inner cannulae.

The fenestrated tracheostomy tube has a hole (fenestration) along its greater curvature. This allows the patient to speak by directing some of the air past the vocal cords.

Silver tracheostomy tubes are used in many patients who require long-term intubation. They have an inner tube which may be removed for cleaning. Some designs have a one-way flap valve to allow the patient to speak. Silver is non-irritant and bactericidal.

CONNECTIONS

Catheter mount

This is a flexible link between the breathing system and a tracheal tube, laryngeal mask airway, face mask or tracheostomy tube (Fig. 32.65). It may be made of rubber or plastic and some have a gas sampling port. The proximal end, which attaches to the breathing system, has a standard 22 mm connection and the distal end is a 15 mm connector. The length of catheter mounts varies from 45 to 170 mm.

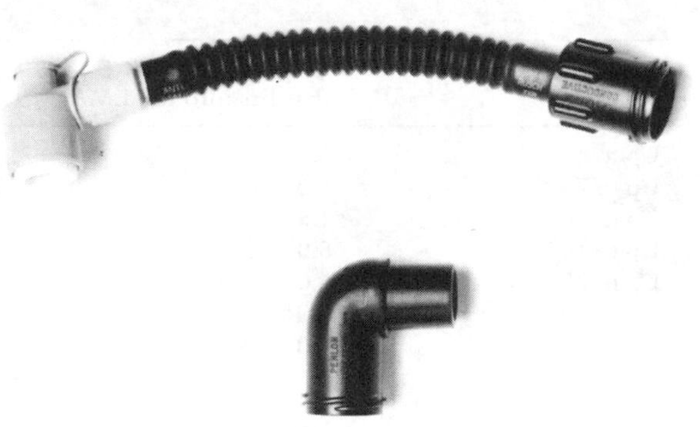

Fig. 32.65
Catheter mount to connect the endotracheal tube to the breathing system (top). An angle piece to connect a face mask or tracheal tube to the breathing system (bottom).

Tracheal tube connectors

Disposable 15 mm diameter connectors are provided with plastic disposable tubes; the diameter of the distal end is of an appropriate size to fit the internal diameter of the tube. Several other connections (Fig. 32.66) may be used with plastic or rubber tracheal tubes. The Nosworthy connector is less bulky than the 15 mm disposable connector and is used often in paediatric practice. The Magill connector is useful, particularly during surgery of the head or neck.

Angle pieces

These are connectors which fit between the breathing system and the tracheal tube or mask (Fig. 32.65). They incorporate a 90° bend and have either 15 or 22 mm connectors at each end. Some angle pieces have a condenser humidifier, bacterial filter and a port for gas sampling incorporated into them (Fig. 32.32).

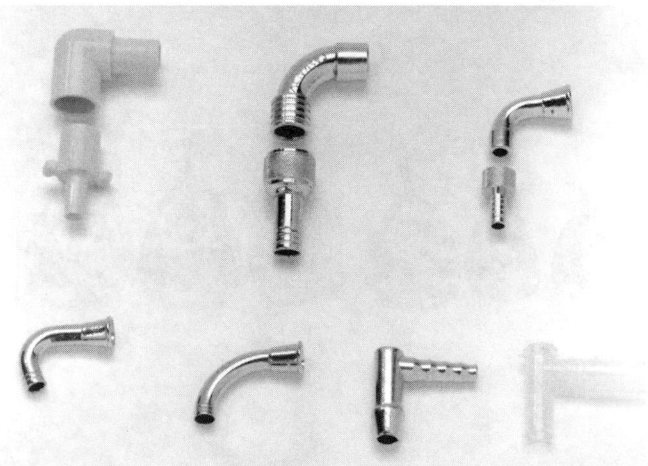

Fig. 32.66
A variety of tracheal tube connectors. From top left in clockwise rotation: Portex with 15 mm tracheal tube connector, Nosworthy, Knight's paediatric connector, Cobbs, Rowbotham, Magill oral, Magill nasal.

THE LARYNGEAL MASK AIRWAY (LMA)

This device consists of a shortened conventional silicone tube with an elliptical cuff, inflated through a pilot tube, attached to the distal end (Fig. 32.67). The cuff, which resembles a miniature face mask, has been designed to form a (relatively) airtight seal around the posterior perimeter of the larynx (Fig. 32.68). A variety of sizes of cuff are available, ranging from size 1 which is used in the neonate to size 5 which is used in large adults. The mask is inserted and the cuff inflated until no air leak is detected. It is important to ensure that the maximum inflation volume is not exceeded (Table 32.8). The device is very effective in maintaining a patent airway in the spontaneously breathing patient. Positive

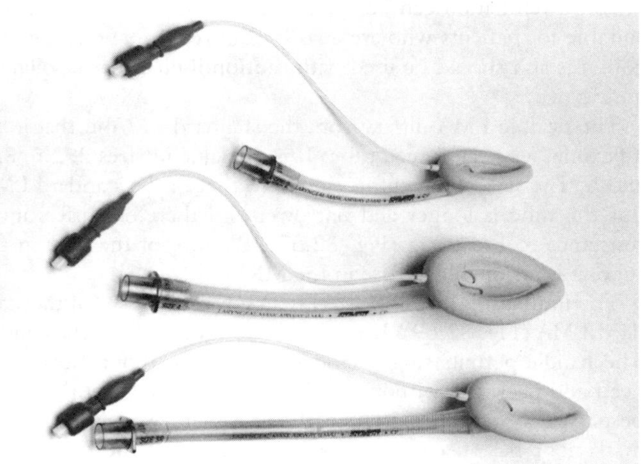

Fig. 32.67
Laryngeal masks. A paediatric size 2 mask, an adult size 4 mask, and a size 3 reinforced LMA.

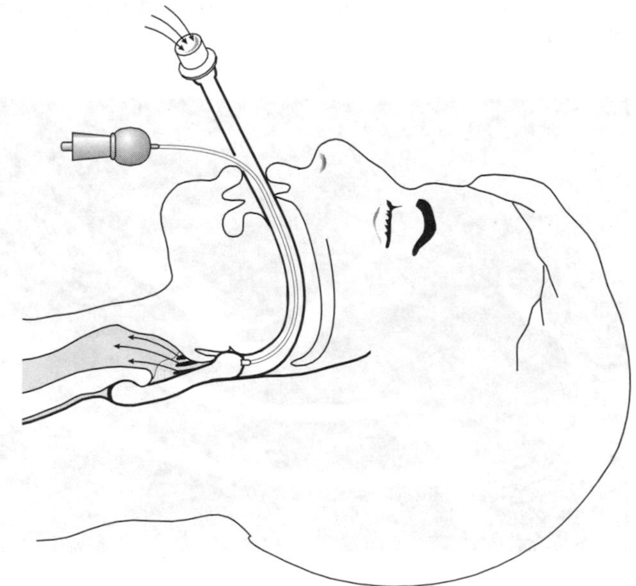

Fig. 32.68
A laryngeal mask in situ.

Table 32.8 Characteristics of laryngeal mask airways (LMAs)

Size of LMA	Length of LMA	Size of patient	Volume of cuff (ml)	Largest size of ETT that fits into the LMA
1	8	Neonates and infants up to 6.5 kg	Up to 4	3.5
1.5	10	Infants 5–10 kg	Up to 7	4.0
2	11	Infants and children 10–20 kg	Up to 10	4.5
2.5	12.5	Children 20–30 kg	Up to 14	5.0
3	16	Children and small adults 30–50 kg	Up to 20	6.0
4	16	Normal adults 50–70 kg	Up to 30	6.0
5	18	Large adults > 70 kg	Up to 40	7.0

pressure ventilation can be applied if necessary. The mask is not suitable for patients who are at risk from regurgitation of gastric contents and should be used with caution if pharyngeal soiling is anticipated.

The flexible LMA differs from the standard LMA in that it has a flexible, wire reinforced tube. It is available in sizes 2, 2.5, 3, 4 and 5. The size of the cuff is similar to that of the standard LMA but the tube is longer and narrower and therefore offers more resistance to breathing (Fig. 32.67). Because of the wire in the tube, it is unsuitable for use in the MRI unit.

The intubating LMA (ILMA) is an advanced form of the standard LMA (Fig. 32.69). It has a shorter tube and a metal handle. The handle permits single-handed insertion without moving the head and neck and without placing fingers in the mouth. It may be passed through an interdental gap as narrow as 20 mm. The mask floor has an elevating bar which replaces the two bars in the standard LMA. The caudal end of the bar is not fixed to the mask floor and this allows a tracheal tube to be passed in order to intubate the trachea. The ILMA is available in sizes 3, 4 and 5. The recommended cuff volumes are similar to the corresponding sizes of the standard LMA. The rigid curved airway has a standard 15 mm connector at the proximal end. The tube is wide enough to allow passage of a cuffed 8 mm tracheal tube. The ILMA is a re-usable device which may be cleaned and sterilized up to 40 times.

OTHER APPARATUS

FACE MASKS

These are designed to fit the face perfectly so that no leak of gas occurs, but without applying excessive pressure to the skin (Fig. 32.70). An appropriate size of face mask must be selected to ensure a proper fit, but the smallest size possible should be used to minimize dead space. Masks made of transparent material are available. These allow the detection of vomitus or secretions.

A harness system (e.g. Clausen harness) is used by some anaesthetists to hold the mask on the face during surgery. However, airway obstruction may occur at any time and the excursion of the reservoir bag must be observed constantly. In most countries, the LMA is now used during maintenance of anaesthesia in almost all situations in which a face mask was formerly used.

INTUBATING FORCEPS

The most commonly used intubating forceps is that designed by Magill (Fig. 32.71). The instrument is employed to manipulate a nasotracheal or nasogastric tube through the oropharynx and into the correct position. A laryngoscope is used to obtain a view of the oropharynx.

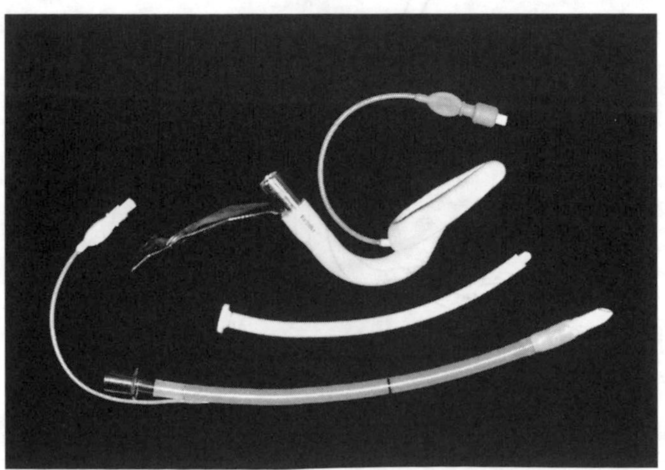

Fig. 32.69
An intubating laryngeal mask with the silicone endotracheal tube and the introducer.

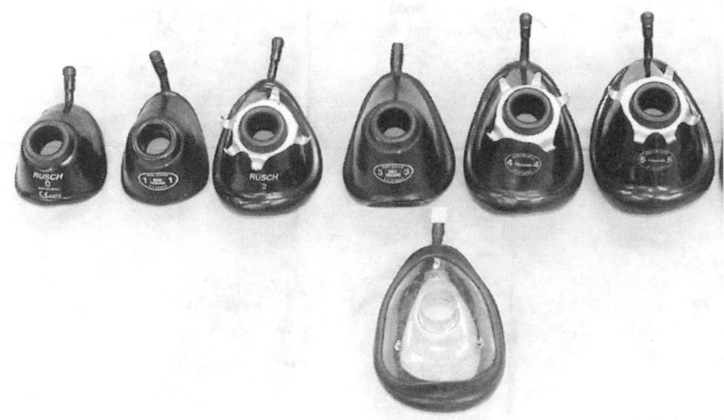

Fig. 32.70
Face masks.

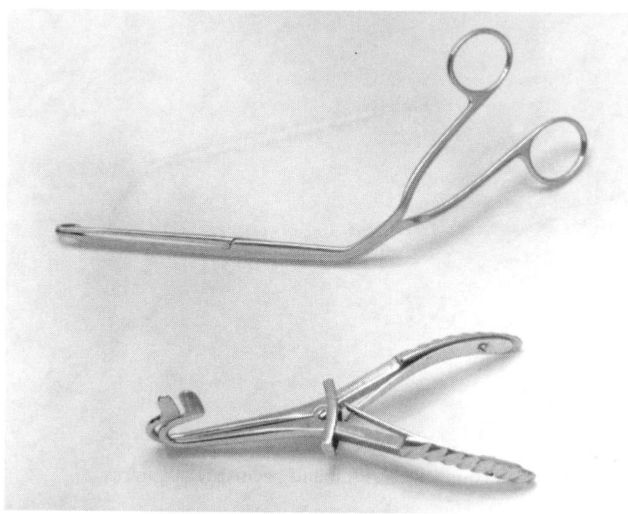

Fig. 32.71
Magill intubating forceps (above). The Ferguson mouth gag (below).

LARYNGEAL SPRAY

This is used to deposit a fine mist of local anaesthetic solution (usually lidocaine 4 or 10%) on the mucosa of the larynx and upper trachea (Fig. 32.72). These sprays are particularly useful in applying local anaesthetic to the upper airway during awake fibre-optic intubation.

MOUTH GAG

A mouth gag (Fig. 32.71) may be used during dental anaesthesia and is required occasionally to open the mouth in patients with trismus, or if masseter spasm is present. It is positioned between the molar teeth and must be used with great care to avoid dental trauma.

GUM ELASTIC BOUGIE

If the larynx cannot be seen adequately during laryngoscopy, or if the tracheal tube cannot be manoeuvred into the laryngeal inlet, a gum elastic bougie may be used as an aid to tracheal intubation. The lubricated bougie is inserted into the trachea to act as a guide for the tracheal tube. The tube should be rotated so that the bevel does not become lodged against the aryepiglottic fold.

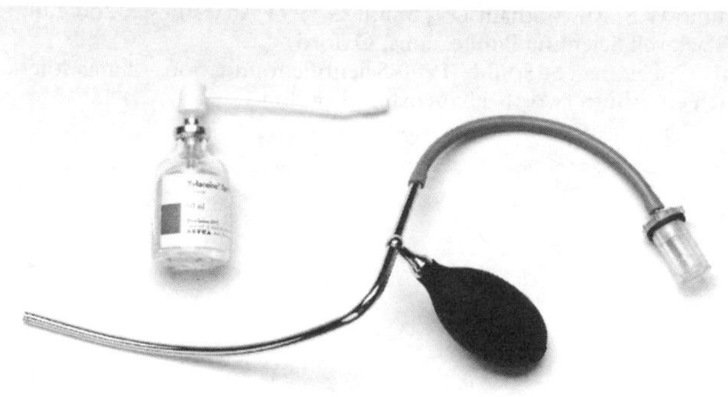

Fig. 32.72
Laryngeal sprays. Forrester spray and the 10% lidocaine pre-filled laryngeal spray.

STILETTES

A malleable metal stilette may be used to adjust the degree of curvature of a tracheal tube as an aid to its insertion. The stilette must not protrude from the distal end of the tube.

AIRWAYS

An *oropharyngeal* airway (Guedel airway, Fig. 32.73) may be required to prevent obstruction caused by the tongue or collapse of the pharynx in the patient without a tracheal tube. A *nasopharyngeal* airway (Fig. 32.73) is better tolerated during light anaesthesia and may also be used if it is difficult to insert an oropharyngeal airway, e.g. trismus. However, the use of nasopharyngeal airways may be associated with significant bleeding from the nose.

The cuffed oropharyngeal airway (COPA, Fig. 32.74) is essentially a Guedel airway with an extended pharyngeal section in which an inflatable cuff is embedded. Inflation of the cuff is designed to produce an airtight seal in the oropharynx and lift the tongue. It may be attached to the anaesthetic breathing system. It

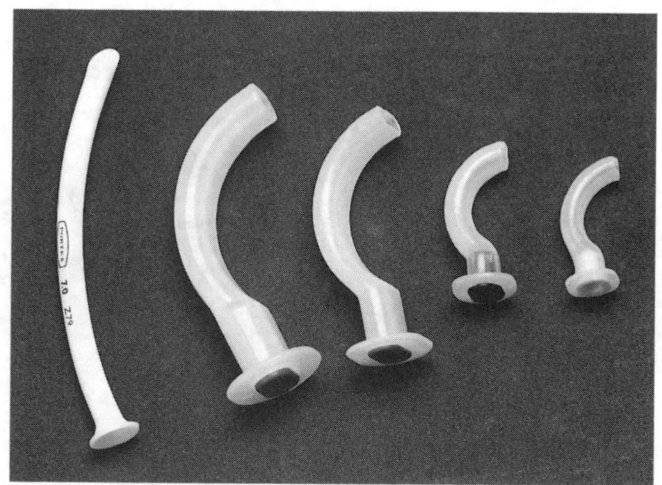

Fig. 32.73
Guedel airways and a nasopharyngeal airway.

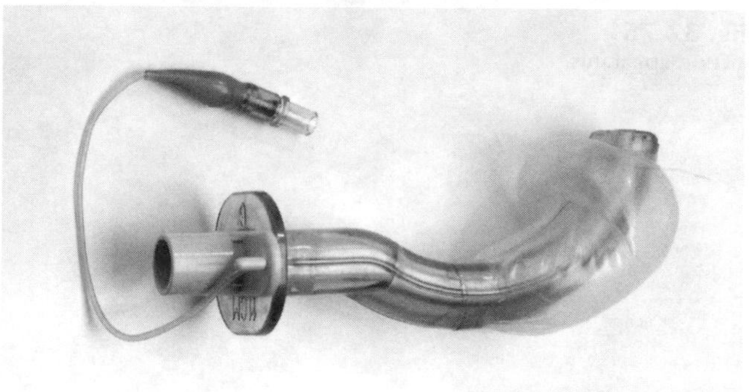

Fig. 32.74
The cuffed oropharyngeal airway (COPA).

is designed to avoid tracheal intubation and is easier to place than the LMA. The advantages and disadvantages of this device are similar to those of the LMA, although it possibly does not form as good a sealed airway as the LMA.

SUCTION APPARATUS

Suction apparatus is vital during anaesthesia and resuscitation to clear the airway of any mucus, blood or debris. It is also used during surgery to clear the operating field of either blood or fluid.

Suction apparatus consists of a source of vacuum, a suction unit and suction tubing. The source of vacuum can be either piped vacuum or electrically or manually operated units. Piped vacuum is the most commonly used source in many operating theatres.

The suction unit consists of a reservoir jar, bacterial filter, vacuum control regulator and a vacuum gauge (Fig. 32.75). The reservoir jar is graduated so that the volume of aspirate may be estimated. It contains a cut-off valve. The cut-off valve has a float that rises as the fluid level increases and shuts off the valve when the reservoir jar is full. This prevents liquid from the suction jar entering the suction system. There is a bacterial filter between the cut-off valve and the suction control unit to prevent air that has been contaminated during passage through the apparatus infecting the atmosphere when it is blown out. The filter also traps any particulate or nebulized matter. Filters should be changed at regular intervals.

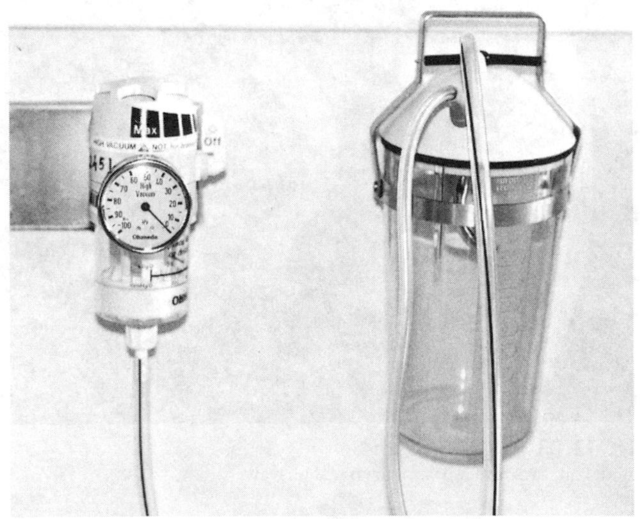

Fig. 32.75
Suction apparatus.

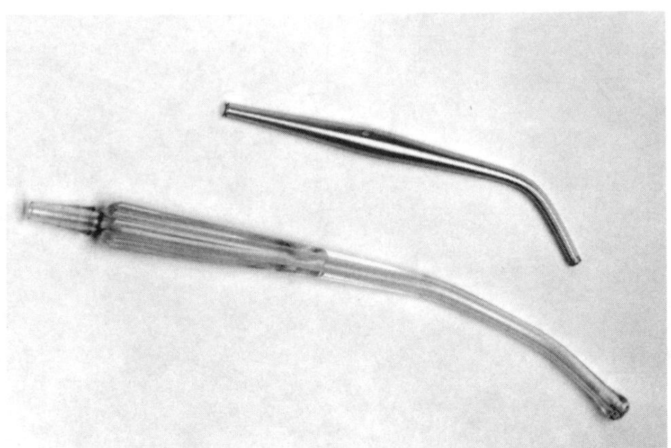

Fig. 32.76
Yankauer suction connectors. Adult and paediatric apparatus.

The vacuum regulator adjusts the degree of vacuum. The vacuum is indicated on the pressure gauge. This is normally marked in mmHg or kPa. The needle on the gauge goes in an anticlockwise direction as the vacuum increases. Suction units can achieve flows of greater than 25 L min^{-1} and a vacuum of greater than 67 kPa. However, flows and vacuum as high as these are seldom necessary and can cause harm if used inappropriately, particularly in children.

The suction reservoir jar is connected to the patient via a suction tubing and either a Yankauer handpiece (Fig. 32.76) or suction catheters.

FURTHER READING

Al-Shaikh B and Stacey S 1999 Essentials of anaesthetic equipment, 1st edn. Churchill Livingstone, London

Association of Anaesthetists of Great Britain and Ireland 1997 Checklist for anaesthetic apparatus 2. AAGBI, London

Davey A, Moyle J T B, Ward C S 1992 Anaesthetic equipment, 3rd edn. W B Saunders, London

Dorsch J A, Dorsch S E 1999 Understanding anaesthetic equipment, 4th edn. Williams and Wilkins, London

Nimmo W S, Rowbotham D J, Smith G 1994 Anaesthesia, 2nd edn. Blackwell Scientific Publications, Oxford

Scurr C, Feldman S, Soni N 1990 Scientific foundations of anaesthesia, 4th edn. Butterworth-Heinemann, London

33 The operating theatre environment

Until the middle of the 19th century, surgery was carried out in any convenient room, frequently one which was used for other purposes. Although the introduction of antisepsis resulted in the washing of instruments and operating table, the operating room itself was ignored as a source of infection. Operating rooms were designed with tiers of wooden benches around the operating table for spectators; thus the term operating *theatre* was introduced. During the early part of the 20th century, large windows were incorporated, as artificial light was relatively ineffective, and high ceilings were introduced to improve ventilation. Additional facilities became necessary for preparing and anaesthetizing the patient, for sterilization of instruments and for the surgeon and other theatre staff to change clothes and scrub up. In addition, the design of operating theatres changed, and smaller theatres were introduced to facilitate frequent cleaning.

A modern operating theatre incorporates the following design features:

- environmental controls of varying degrees of complexity, to reduce the risk of airborne infection
- services for surgical and anaesthetic equipment
- an operating table on which the patient may be placed in the position required for surgery
- artificial lighting appropriate for the requirements of both surgeon and anaesthetist
- measures to ensure the safety of patient and staff.

In addition, provision should be made immediately adjacent to the operating theatre for anaesthetizing the patient, preparing instruments, cleaning dirty instruments and for the surgeon to scrub up. There should also be separate areas for reception and recovery of patients. It is now common practice for each hospital to have a suite of theatres, rather than operating theatres close to each of the surgical wards. The use of theatre suites permits more flexible and efficient use of staff and resources.

THE OPERATING THEATRE SUITE

The number of operating theatres required is difficult to calculate, but approximates in most British cities to one for every 40 000 of the population served. Ideally, the operating theatre suite should be close to the surgical wards, and adjacent to, and on the same floor as, the accident and emergency department, intensive care unit, X-ray department, day-case ward and sterile supplies unit. It is logical for the anaesthetic department to be immediately adjacent to, or an integral part of, the operating theatre suite, although this seldom occurs in practice.

Table 33.1 Zones of cleanliness in the operating theatre suite

Outer zone – hospital areas up to and including the reception area

Clean zone – the circulation area used by staff after they have changed, and the route taken by patients from the transfer bay to the anaesthetic room

Aseptic zone – scrub-up and gowning area, anaesthetic room, theatre preparation room, operation room, exit bay

Disposal zone – disposal area for waste products and soiled or used equipment and supplies

The main purpose of the operating theatre environment is to minimize the risk of transmission of infection to the patient from the air, the building or the staff. The operating theatre suite contains four zones of increasing degree of cleanliness (Table 33.1).

TRANSFER OF PATIENT

There is some evidence that anxiety in the surgical patient peaks as transfer from the ward to the operating theatre begins, and it is important that facilities for transfer minimize stress. A nurse from the ward usually accompanies the patient, but it is customary for the ward nurse to leave adult patients before anaesthesia has been induced. In paediatric practice, it is now the normal routine that a ward nurse and parent remain with the child during induction of anaesthesia.

On arrival at the reception area, the patient's identity and surgical procedure are checked. In a theatre suite, it may be necessary for patients to wait for some time in the reception area to prevent delays in the operating schedules. Consequently, adequate space should be provided for several beds, and there should be screens for patients who wish privacy. The staff in the reception area should include nurses. The décor should be cheerful, and the lighting subdued.

Transport should involve the minimum number of changes of trolley. A trolley is used commonly to transfer the patient to the operating theatre suite, but changes of trolley may be required to enter the clean area and also for transfer to the operating table after anaesthesia has been induced.

Alternatively, the patient's own bed may be taken to the operating theatre suite. If the patient is infirm or in severe pain, the bed may be taken to the anaesthetic room, and transfer delayed until after induction of anaesthesia, but this is appropriate only if the bed has the facility to be tipped head-down if necessary. In some hospitals, a single transfer is effected by transporting the patient to the theatre suite in bed, where the patient is moved on to the operating theatre table-top, which is mounted on a wheeled frame. After induction of anaesthesia, the table-top is wheeled into the theatre and the top attached to a fixed base, which allows it to be positioned for surgery.

There is no universal method of transferring patients from one trolley to another. This may be achieved by the use of canvas and poles, rollers or other 'sliding' devices, or lifting the patient bodily. There is increasing awareness of the risk of injury to operating theatre personnel as a result of lifting patients, and thus an increasing tendency to install transfer systems which do not require great physical effort.

All trolleys in the operating theatre suite should be equipped with oxygen, and this should be administered routinely to patients during transfer from theatre to the recovery room at the end of the procedure if general anaesthesia has been used or if there is any other clinical indication.

ANAESTHETIC ROOM

In several countries, the anaesthetic room has developed from a small annexe to the theatre to an integral part of the operating theatre suite. However, this is not universal, and in many parts of the world anaesthesia is induced in the operating theatre after the patient has been transferred onto the operating table. The main advantages of the anaesthetic room are:

- The patient's anxiety may be reduced by avoiding the sights and sounds of the operating theatre. This is of special importance in children.
- The equipment which may be necessary during induction of anaesthesia may be stored in a readily accessible form.
- Time is saved by inducing anaesthesia while surgery is being completed on another patient. This is useful particularly if preparation is prolonged, e.g. performance of local anaesthetic blocks or establishment of invasive cardiovascular monitoring, but is safe only if at least two anaesthetists are present.

However, there are several disadvantages:

- Anaesthetic and monitoring equipment must be duplicated, or moved to the operating theatre with the patient; this usually necessitates temporary disconnection from electrical or gas supplies.
- Hazards are involved in transferring an unconscious patient from a trolley to the operating table.
- Construction and maintenance of anaesthetic rooms are expensive.

Even in countries where anaesthetic rooms are used, it is customary to induce anaesthesia in the high-risk patient on the operating table, as the delay between onset of unconsciousness and the start of surgery must be kept to a minimum, e.g. for emergency caesarean section or severe haemorrhage.

The design of the anaesthetic room should allow easy access all round the patient's trolley, and should provide space for anaesthetic and monitoring equipment, and storage cupboards and shelves. The minimum floor area recommended by the Department of Health in the UK is 17 m^2, but this is inadequate. A floor area of 21m^2 is more appropriate. Piped gases and suction and electrical sockets are required near the head of the trolley. An anaesthetic machine, mechanical ventilator and monitoring system are also necessary. Cupboards must be available to store equipment and drugs, and worktops must be of sufficient size to allow syringes, needles, cannulae and drugs to be prepared. There should be a clock with a second hand.

OPERATING ROOM

The operating room is designed around its centrally situated operating table with overhead lighting and ventilation systems. The ideal shape for the operating room is circular, but this is inefficient and most operating rooms are square or nearly square. In 1980, the Royal College of Surgeons of England suggested that the floor should be 625 ft^2 (approximately 58 m^2) in area, and no smaller than 484 ft^2 (approximately 45 m^2). Theatres for specialized surgery may require a larger area to accommodate bulky equipment.

Outlets for piped gases and electrical sockets must be positioned close to the head of the operating table; they are provided most conveniently by a boom or stalactite system. Electrical cables should not lie across the floor. The operating room should be of sufficient size to allow all types of surgery without moving the position of the head of the table; this location should be reached easily and without complex manoeuvres as the patient enters the theatre from the anaesthetic room.

Temperature, humidity and ventilation

The temperature in the operating theatre and anaesthetic room should be sufficiently high to minimize the risk of inducing hypothermia in the patient, but must be comfortable for theatre staff. The patient may develop hypothermia at an ambient temperature of less than 21°C. Temperatures of 22–24°C are usually acceptable in the operating room, with a relative humidity of 50–60%; a higher environmental temperature is required during surgery in the neonate or infant. Slightly lower temperature and humidity are acceptable in other parts of the theatre suite. Controls for temperature and humidity should be located within the operating theatre so that adjustments can be made by theatre staff.

Heating and humidity are controlled usually by an air-conditioning and ventilation system, which provides an ambient pressure inside the operating room slightly higher than atmospheric. In general, air is introduced directly over the operating table, and leaves at the periphery through ducts positioned near floor level. In the area of the table, 400 air changes per hour are required to minimize the risk of airborne transmission of infection. More effective systems of ventilation, involving radial exponential air flow away from the operating table, or laminar flow, are used in some centres for some types of surgery, e.g. total hip replacement, in which infection is especially undesirable. High-flow systems may accelerate cooling of the patient.

Light

Daylight is not necessary in the operating theatre, although it is more pleasant for staff if there are windows in the theatre suite, e.g. in corridors and common rooms. A high level of illumination is required over the operating table, and ceiling-mounted lamps are standard; it is preferable if they can be positioned directly by the surgeon.

The intensity and colour temperature of general lighting are very important to the anaesthetist, as appreciation of skin colour is affected by the spectrum of the source of illumination. The spectrum provided by lighting tubes should be similar to that of daylight, with an emission temperature of 4000–5000 K. The colour of the décor should be neutral and uniform. The intensity of general illumination should be up to 325 lm m^{-2} in the operating theatre, and it should be diffuse to avoid glare. In the anaesthetic room and recovery area, a light intensity of approximately 220 lm m^{-2} is acceptable, but a spotlight should be available if increased illumination is required for specific procedures.

SAFETY IN THE OPERATING THEATRE

Electrocution and gas explosions are the two main hazards to staff and patients in the operating theatre. In addition, there may be a risk to staff from pollution of the atmosphere with anaesthetic gases and vapours, and of contracting infection, particularly human immunodeficiency virus (HIV) or hepatitis, from infected patients.

Electrical safety

Although some mention is made of electrical hazards in the operating theatre in Chapter 30, a detailed description is beyond the scope of this book, and the reader is referred to the article by Hull (1978). The electrical supply to the operating theatre and all electrical equipment connected to the patient incorporate design features which minimize the risk of electrical currents being transmitted through the patient to earth.

Explosions

The use of explosive anaesthetic gases and vapours has diminished greatly in recent years. However, diethyl ether is still used occasionally in some countries. Ether burns in air, but forms an explosive mixture with oxygen. An explosion may be initiated by a spark of very low energy (< 1 μJ) or by contact with a temperature of 300°C or higher. The risk of explosion is highest within and close to the anaesthetic breathing system because of the presence of a high oxygen concentration. Beyond a distance of 10 cm from the breathing system, the oxygen concentration diminishes and the risk is reduced.

The construction of anaesthetic apparatus is designed to minimize explosion hazards from generation of sparks caused by cumulation of static electricity. All rubber is conductive, so that electrical charges leak to earth, and non-conductive substances are treated with antistatic material. In most existing theatres, the operating theatre floor has a high but finite resistance, so that static charges leak to earth but electrocution risks are minimized. Theatre footwear is also designed to earth static charges. Sparks may be generated by clothing made of synthetic materials such as nylon. The risk of accumulation of static electricity on walls and equipment is reduced if the environment humidity exceeds 70%. Diathermy must not be used if explosive anaesthetics are employed. However, the use of these agents has virtually ceased in the UK and most other developed countries, and many of the precautions, particularly the use of expensive antistatic flooring, are becoming unnecessary. In addition, modern monitoring apparatus is unsuitable for use with flammable or explosive anaesthetics. Most new operating theatres are built without antistatic precautions, but this must be indicated clearly by labels so that explosive agents are not used.

Fire is still a hazard if alcohol-based solutions are used by the surgeon to sterilize the skin; the usual ignition source is a spark from the diathermy probe.

Atmospheric pollution

There has been considerable controversy regarding the risk to theatre staff from atmospheric pollution by anaesthetic gases and vapours. Earlier investigations suggested that theatre staff are more likely than other hospital personnel to suffer from hepatic and renal disease, to have non-specific neurological symptoms and for their children to have an increased risk of congenital abnormality. However, none of these problems has been substantiated.

There was more convincing evidence from the early studies that female staff who worked in the operating theatre during the early months of pregnancy suffered an increased incidence of spontaneous abortion, and there is experimental evidence to suggest that constant exposure of rats to a concentration of more than 1000 ppm of nitrous oxide produces adverse results on their reproduction. However, the most recent, comprehensive and only randomized prospective investigation of operating theatre staff failed to demonstrate any increased health risk.

Trace concentrations of anaesthetic gases have been implicated in another area of concern – impairment of professional performance. Motor and intellectual performance were shown in an early laboratory study in volunteers to deteriorate in the presence of concentrations of nitrous oxide of 500 ppm, with or without halothane 15 ppm. However, subsequent studies failed to confirm these findings, and the consensus of several studies is that concentrations of 8–12% nitrous oxide are required before significant impairment of performance occurs. Such concentrations might be inhaled if the anaesthetist is close to an unscavenged expiratory valve, or during inhalation induction of anaesthesia, but exceed those present in other areas of an adequately ventilated operating theatre.

Nevertheless, it is sensible to minimize atmospheric pollution in the operating theatre, and hospital regulations in both western Europe and North America require the installation of anaesthetic gas-scavenging systems in all areas where anaesthesia is administered. In the USA, the National Institute of Occupational Safety and Hygiene (a federal regulatory body) dictates that environmental concentrations of anaesthetic gases should not exceed a value of 25 ppm of nitrous oxide and 2 ppm of volatile agent. In the UK, the Health and Safety Executive introduced maximum limits of exposure to anaesthetic agents in January 1996; these are shown in Table 33.2, and may necessitate major alterations in anaesthetic techniques. Scavenging systems are described in Chapter 32.

Anaesthetic gases are not the only source of environmental pollution in the operating theatre; volatile skin-cleaning fluids and

Table 33.2 Maximum levels of exposure to anaesthetic agents in the operating theatre suite over an 8 h time-weighted average reference period, as laid down in the UK by the Health and Safety Executive

Agent	Maximum concentration (ppm)
Nitrous oxide	100
Halothane	10
Enflurane	50
Isoflurane	50

aerosol sprays, e.g. iodine or plastic skin dressing, should be used sensibly, and inhalation of vapours should be avoided. Ethyl chloride is used by some anaesthetists to produce local anaesthesia of the skin before venepuncture or to test cutaneous sensation after a regional block has been performed; ethyl chloride is both explosive and an atmospheric pollutant, and should not be used for these purposes.

Infection

The most serious types of acquired infection in operating theatre staff are HIV and hepatitis, which may be contracted by contact with blood or body fluids from an infected patient. Several health care workers have been infected in this way, either by a needlestick injury or through cuts and abrasions. The risk of percutaneous transmission of HIV is believed to be extremely low; the incidence of seroconversion after occupational exposure to HIV is 0.39%. However, the risk is 5–30% after an occupational inoculation injury.

Two thousand cases of hepatitis B are reported each year in the UK, although the true incidence is probably very much higher. Hepatitis B surface antigen persists for at least 6 months in 5–10% of infected individuals. The virus is highly infectious, and minute amounts of blood may transmit the disease. The Association of Anaesthetists of Great Britain and Ireland (AAGBI) recommends that all anaesthetists should receive active immunization against hepatitis B. A single dose of hepatitis B immunoglobulin combined with active immunization is required immediately if an unprotected individual is inoculated with infected material.

Hepatitis C and D viruses are also blood-borne. Up to 50% of people infected with the hepatitis C virus develop chronic liver disease. Occupational transmission of this virus has been reported.

The incidence of acquired immunodeficiency syndrome (AIDS) continues to increase and is not confined to homosexuals and drug abusers. For every patient with fully developed AIDS, there are estimated to be five with a less severe form of the disease, and up to 50 asymptomatic carriers. At present, it is unclear what proportion of these develop AIDS, but it may approach 100%. Thus, anaesthetists are likely to be exposed to an increasing number of patients who may transmit HIV. At present, compulsory screening of hospital patients for HIV is regarded as unacceptable. Consequently, precautions must be taken in patients who are believed to be at high risk of being HIV-positive; these include homosexual or bisexual men, haemophiliacs and sexual partners of high-risk patients. In some locations, it has been recommended that precautions should be taken with all patients.

Human T-cell leukaemia virus (HTLV-1) is also of potential importance.

The following precautions are recommended to reduce the risks of transmission of HIV; these are also applicable when patients infected with other blood-borne viruses are anaesthetized.

- Gloves must be worn during induction of anaesthesia, performance of venepuncutre or insertion of any intravascular cannula, and during insertion or removal of airways and tracheal tubes. A plastic apron, mask and eye protection should be worn if substantial spillage of blood is anticipated, e.g. during insertion of an arterial cannula. Gloves should normally be discarded on taking the patient into the operating theatre and a fresh pair donned when any of these procedures is carried out during or at the end of anaesthesia. Equipment, notes and other articles must not be handled with contaminated gloves.
- Needles which have been in contact with the patient must not be resheathed or handed from one person to another.
- All needles and other sharp objects should be disposed of in an appropriate tough disposal bin; cardboard bins are unsatisfactory.
- Cuts or abrasions on the anaesthetist's hands should be covered with a waterproof dressing. An anaesthetist with considerable skin lesions, such as eczema, chapping or several scratches, is particularly at risk of being infected.
- If a needlestick injury or contamination of a cut or abrasion occurs, bleeding should be encouraged and the skin washed thoroughly with soap and water.
- Advice should be obtained immediately from the hospital's occupational health department if there is reason to believe that contamination has occurred.
- Disposable equipment should be used where possible. Non-disposable equipment should be decontaminated with 2% glutaraldehyde, washed with soap and water and left in glutaraldehyde for a further 3 h. Contaminated floors and surfaces should be washed with 1% hypochlorite solution. Gloves must be worn.

It has been recommended that a bacterial filter should be placed between the tracheal tube or airway and the anaesthetic breathing system in all patients to prevent cross-infection from a patient with undiagnosed infection.

RECOVERY ROOM

A recovery room or ward is an essential requirement in the operating theatre. All patients require close surveillance in the immediate postoperative period and for up to 24 h after major surgery.

The recovery room should be an integral part of the operating theatre suite and should be located within the clean area. Department of Health guidelines suggest that there should be 1.5 places in the recovery area for each operating theatre, although a greater number may be required if surgery with a high turnover, e.g. gynaecology or day-case surgery, is common. Each place requires a minimum floor area of approximately 10 m^2, and there must be sufficient space to move a patient without disturbing the remainder.

It is appropriate for most patients to lie on a trolley in the recovery room, but beds should be available for those who are likely to stay for more than 30–45 min, e.g. patients who have undergone major surgery, or ASA grade III or IV patients who may require prolonged observation even after minor surgery. Each place should have piped oxygen and suction outlets on the wall, with an oxygen flowmeter and suction apparatus attached to a wall rail. Lighting should conform to the same standards as apply to the operating theatre, and additional spotlights should be provided. It is not common practice in the UK to monitor the electrocardiogram in all patients in the recovery ward, but oxygen saturation and blood pressure should be monitored routinely. Most large recovery areas have two or three places which are fully equipped with piped nitrous oxide, a mechanical ventilator and complete cardiovascular monitoring facilities.

An anaesthetic machine, defibrillator and equipment, and drugs for resuscitation must be available in the recovery room. Oxygen is usually administered by disposable face mask, but each place should have a self-inflating resuscitation bag and anaesthetic mask.

Drug cupboards and storage space for equipment should be provided and, in a large recovery area, special telephones are required. Nursing staff spend most of their time with the patient, but require a nursing station at which notes may be written and theatres and wards contacted by telephone. At least one nurse is required for each three bed spaces. At present there is no specific training course in the UK for recovery room nurses. Student nurses receive only 1 week of training in this area.

In many hospitals, it is possible to provide supervision of patients in the recovery ward for up to 24 h after major surgery. This is highly desirable in the absence of a separate high-dependency unit, as intensive care facilities are often overwhelmed in large hospitals.

Clinical aspects of recovery room care are discussed in Chapter 41.

HIGH-DEPENDENCY UNIT

A high-dependency unit is an area for patients who require more invasive observation, treatment and nursing care than can be provided on a general ward. It would not normally accept patients requiring mechanical ventilation, but could manage those who require invasive monitoring. A survey conducted by the AAGBI (1991) indicated that many intensive care units admitted patients who could have been managed appropriately in a high-dependency unit. An unknown number of patients return from the recovery area to a general ward requiring monitoring or an intensity of nursing or medical care which cannot be provided safely in that location.

The facilities required to provide high-dependency care vary. Essential features are a high nurse-to-patient ratio, provision of piped oxygen and suction at every bed, and appropriate monitoring equipment. Protocols must be in place for admission and discharge criteria, and medical staffing must be clearly defined. In large hospitals, several units may be desirable, each dedicated to the care of specific groups of patients; in smaller hospitals, a single, multi-user unit may be more appropriate.

OTHER ACCOMMODATION

Storage space is required for large items of equipment. In most modern operating theatre suites, instruments are sterilized in a separate department, which should be situated in close proximity. Access to blood gas analysis and measurement of serum electrolyte concentrations are essential, especially if major surgery is to be undertaken, and large operating theatre suites usually contain a small laboratory.

Staff accommodation includes changing rooms and rest rooms. There should be facilities for beverages and snacks. Offices are provided for the theatre supervisor and senior operating department assistants, and there should be a tutorial or seminar room for staff training. Some theatre suites incorporate an office for the anaesthetic department.

OTHER ANAESTHETIZING LOCATIONS

The anaesthetist is often required to work in areas outside the operating theatre suite. Many hospitals have peripheral theatres for some types of surgery, e.g. a self-contained day-case unit. In addition, patients may require anaesthesia in the accident and emergency unit, the radiology and radiotherapy departments or, in some instances (e.g. paediatric oncology), the side room of a ward. In these circumstances, where conditions are frequently not ideal, it is essential that the same precautions are taken as in the operating theatre suite to ensure that the identity of the patient is checked, that equipment is functioning correctly, that skilled help for the anaesthetist is available and that recovery facilities and staff are satisfactory. It is wise to avoid sending junior and inexperienced anaesthetists to these remote locations without direct senior supervision.

ANCILLARY STAFF

Skilled and dedicated help should be available to the anaesthetist at all times. In the majority of hospitals in the UK, this is provided by operating department practitioners (ODPs), who undergo a 2-year training programme in recognized institutions and are required to sit examinations. In some hospitals, anaesthetic nurses assist the anaesthetist. It is important to differentiate between anaesthetic nurses and the nurse anaesthetists who are trained to deliver anaesthesia in some countries (e.g. CRNAs in the USA). The anaesthetic nurse performs essentially the same functions as the ODP. These include:

- Preparation and preliminary checking of equipment. It should be stressed that this does not absolve the anaesthetist from the responsibility of checking the equipment fully before an operating list is started.
- Alleviation of anxiety by reassurance and constant communication with the patient while awaiting anaesthesia.
- Checking the correct identity of the patient. However, it is the joint responsibility of the surgeon and anaesthetist to ensure that the appropriate procedure is undertaken on the correct patient, and this is one of the many reasons why the anaesthetist must see every patient preoperatively.
- Preparation of intravenous infusions, cardiovascular monitoring transducers, etc.
- Assistance during anaesthesia, particularly during induction, when special manoeuvres such as cricoid pressure may be required, and after transfer to the operating theatre to assist in re-establishment of monitoring.
- Assistance in positioning the patient for local or regional blocks.

- Assistance in obtaining drugs or equipment if complications arise during anaesthesia.
- Assistance in the immediate postoperative period before the patient is transferred to the recovery room.

The ODP or anaesthetic nurse should *never* be left alone with an anaesthetized patient unless a dire emergency requires the anaesthetist's presence elsewhere.

THE MEDICOLEGAL ENVIRONMENT

The increasing volume of litigation instituted by patients in respect of alleged or actual injury arising from treatment is causing great concern within the medical profession. Insurance premiums for medical practice have escalated rapidly. Anaesthesia represents a high insurance risk, because anaesthetists manipulate the physiology of the cardiovascular and respiratory systems to administer potentially lethal drugs for reasons which are not primarily therapeutic; consequently, when a serious accident occurs, it may result in death or permanent neurological damage. In addition, even minor morbidity caused by anaesthesia or the anaesthetist may be regarded by the patient as unacceptable when it does not appear to be related to the primary illness.

MORTALITY ASSOCIATED WITH ANAESTHESIA

The overwhelming majority of anaesthetics are uneventful. However, both surgery and anaesthesia carry a finite risk. Mortality is usually related to the extent of surgery and the preoperative condition of the patient (see Ch. 34). However, avoidable deaths occur. In 1982, Lunn & Mushin estimated that the risk of death attributable to anaesthesia alone was approximately 1 in 10 000. In a subsequent study of more than half a million operations (Confidential Enquiry into Perioperative Deaths; CEPOD), the overall death rate after anaesthesia and surgery was 0.7% (Buck et al 1987). Anaesthesia alone was responsible for death in approximately 1 in 1 800 000 operations, but *contributed* to 14% of all deaths; in almost one-fifth of these deaths, avoidable errors occurred. Factors which contributed to death in these instances are listed in Table 33.3.

Table 33.3 Factors involved in deaths attributable in part to anaesthesia, in decreasing order of frequency (CEPOD report)

Failure to apply knowledge
Lack of care
Failure of organization
Lack of experience
Lack of knowledge
Drug effect
Failure of equipment
Fatigue

MORBIDITY ASSOCIATED WITH ANAESTHESIA

The incidence of major morbidity (causing permanent disability) related to anaesthesia is difficult to assess. Its causes are often similar to those associated with mortality. Table 33.4 lists the causes of death or cerebral damage reported to the Medical Defence Union between 1970 and 1982; Table 33.5 shows the detailed causes of the incidents resulting from errors in technique. Permanent disability may result also from spinal cord damage.

Table 33.5 Causes of anaesthetic-related death or cerebral damage reported to the Medical Defence Union and thought to be the result of errors in technique

Cause	% of total
Errors associated with tracheal intubation	31
Misuse of apparatus	23
Inhalation of gastric contents	14
Errors associated with induced hypotension	8
Hypoxia	4
Obstructed airway	4
Accidental pneumothorax/haemopericardium	4
Errors associated with extradural analgesia	3
Use of nitrous oxide instead of oxygen	2
Use of carbon dioxide instead of oxygen	2
Errors associated with Bier's block	2
Underventilation	1
Use of halothane with epinephrine	1
Mismatched blood transfusion	<1
Vasovagal attack	<1

Table 33.4 Causes of anaesthetic-related death or cerebral damage reported to the Medical Defence Union between 1970 and 1982

Mainly misadventure	%	Mainly error	%
Coexisting disease	14	Faulty technique	43
Unknown	6	Failure of postoperative care	9
Drug sensitivity	5	Drug overdosage	5
Hypotension/blood loss	4	Inadequate preoperative assessment	3
Halothane-associated hepatic failure	3	Drug error	1
Hyperpyrexia	2	Anaesthetist's failure	1
Embolism	2		

Other, albeit less serious, incidents may result in distress or physical injury to patients. Table 33.6 lists untoward events, other than death and cerebral damage, reported to the Medical Defence Union.

CRITICAL INCIDENTS

These are incidents that could or do lead to death, permanent disability or prolongation of hospital stay. Most critical incidents in anaesthesia are detected before damage occurs; their incidence is 400–500 times greater than that of death or serious injury attributable to anaesthesia. It has been estimated that a critical incident occurs on average once in every 80 anaesthetics. Analysis of the causes of critical incidents is valuable in indicating the potential causes of anaesthetic-related mortality and major morbidity. Human error is responsible for approximately 70% of critical incidents in anaesthesia; the commonest errors are shown in Table 33.7. Factors associated with critical incidents are shown in Table 33.8.

Table 33.6 Untoward anaesthetic-related events (other than death or cerebral damage) reported to the Medical Defence Union between 1970 and 1982

Event	% of total
Damage to teeth	52
Peripheral nerve damage	9
Extradural foreign bodies (needles, catheter tips)	7
Superficial thrombophlebitis and minor injuries (e.g. abrasions)	7
Awareness	7
Spinal cord damage	4
Pneumothoraces	3
Extravasation of injected drugs	2
Lacerations, falls from table	2
Impaired renal function (mismatched blood)	1
Burns	1
Other	5

Table 33.7 Types of human error contributing to critical incidents during anaesthesia

Type of error	% of total
Wrong drug administered	24
Misuse of anaesthetic machine	22
Problem with airway management	16
Problem with breathing system	11
Fluid therapy mismanagement	5
Intravenous infusion disconnection	6
Failure of monitoring	4
Others	12

Table 33.8 Associated factors producing critical incidents during anaesthesia, in decreasing order of frequency

Failure to check
First experience of procedure
Inadequate experience
Inattention/carelessness
Haste
Unfamiliarity
Visual restriction
Fatigue

MINIMIZING THE RISK

The most effective means of reducing the risk of an anaesthetic accident is to ensure that every aspect of anaesthetic management is conducted competently (Table 33.9). Preoperative assessment (see Ch. 34) is essential. In the anaesthetic room, the anaesthetist must check the identity of the patient before proceeding. The information contained in Tables 33.4–33.8 indicates areas of particular concern regarding intraoperative management. All anaesthetic equipment must be checked before use. The anaesthetist must understand the principles of all the equipment used, especially mechanical ventilators. Drug doses must be calculated carefully and syringes labelled. After induction of anaesthesia, the correct placement of the tracheal tube must be confirmed on every occasion.

Studies of critical incidents indicate that the time of highest risk is during maintenance of anaesthesia. For this reason, appropriate clinical and instrumental monitoring (see Ch. 38) must be used throughout anaesthesia. After operation, the anaesthetist is responsible for the patient until consciousness has returned and until the

Table 33.9 Summary of important factors which should minimize the risk of accidents during anaesthesia and the risk of litigation against the anaesthetist

- Careful preoperative assessment should be undertaken to identify risk factors such as concurrent disease, chronic medication history of allergy or other untoward reactions to anaesthesia, and potential difficulties in tracheal intubation
- Anaesthetic equipment must be maintained according to the manufacturers' recommendations, and checked thoroughly before every operating theatre session, or when the equipment is changed during an operating session
- The anaesthetic technique should be recognized as appropriate for the individual patient and for the proposed type of surgery
- The anaesthetist must be present at all times during anaesthesia
- Appropriate monitoring, in accordance with national recommendations, should be used at all times during anaesthesia and in the immediate recovery period. Alarms should be set at appropriate levels and must not be disabled
- At the end of anaesthesia, the anaesthetist should transfer the care of the patient only to an appropriately qualified recovery room nurse
- All anaesthetists should be taught how to manage uncommon emergencies, such as failed intubation, anaphylaxis or malignant hyperthermia. It is advisable to have protocols available in every anaesthetizing location to act as an *aide-memoire* for uncommon emergencies, and anaesthetists and operating room staff should rehearse emergency management on a regular basis
- The anaesthetist should keep careful records

cardiovascular and respiratory systems are stable. He or she may be required to defend a decision to delegate the care of the patient to a nurse in the recovery room.

The following factors should also be considered:

Awareness. Patients may recall intraoperative events, and may experience pain and discomfort, if the doses or concentrations of anaesthetic drugs are insufficient (see p. 517). In high-risk groups, it may be advisable to warn the patient of the possibility of awareness.

Anaesthetic record. A legible and comprehensive record must be made of every anaesthetic. The record should include details of preoperative findings, the doses and timing of all drugs administered during anaesthesia, frequent and regular recordings of cardiovascular and respiratory measurements, and notes regarding any untoward intraoperative event. This is an important document because it provides information which may assist other anaesthetists in the future and because a comprehensive record is *essential* in the event of medicolegal proceedings.

Communication. If a mishap occurs, failure on the part of the anaesthetist to communicate with the patient or relatives may arouse feelings of anger and suspicion. While no admission (or accusations) of liability should be made, an explanation should be offered. An interview with a patient or relatives in these circumstances requires skill and tact; the trainee should discuss the event with a consultant, and, if possible, the consultant should be present at the interview.

Each anaesthetic department should ensure that the channels of communication between trainees and consultants are clear, especially with regard to emergency procedures.

Audit. Standards of anaesthetic practice may be improved by identifying areas in which patient care has been suboptimal. Although case reports published in anaesthetic journals form a useful source of information, local meetings to discuss morbidity and mortality related to anaesthesia and surgery, together with critical incident analysis, should be convened regularly.

FURTHER READING

Association of Anaesthetists of Great Britain and Ireland 1991 The high dependency unit: acute care in the future. AAGBI, London

Association of Anaesthetists of Great Britain and Ireland 1992 HIV and other blood borne viruses: guidance for anaesthetists. AAGBI, London

Aitkenhead A R 1994 The pattern of litigation against anaesthetists. British Journal of Anaesthesia 73: 10

Buck N, Devlin H B, Lunn J N 1987 The report of a confidential enquiry into perioperative deaths. Nuffield Provincial Hospitals Trust, London

Drain C B, Christoph S S 1987 The recovery room, 2nd edn. WB Saunders, Philadelphia

Johnston I D A, Hunter A R (eds) 1984 The design and utilization of operating theatres. Edward Arnold, London

Hull C J 1978 Electrical hazards in the operating theatre. British Journal of Anaesthesia 50: 647

Lunn J N, Mushin W W 1982 Mortality associated with anaesthesia. Nuffield Provincial Hospitals Trust, London

Runciman W B, Sellen A, Webb R K, Williamson J A, Currie M, Morgan C A, Russell W J 1993. Errors, incidents and accidents in anaesthetic practice. Anaesthesia and Intensive Care 21: 506

Spence A A 1987 Environmental pollution by inhalation of anaesthetics. British Journal of Anaesthesia 59: 96

Taylor T H, Major E (eds) 1994 Hazards and complications of anaesthesia, 2nd edn. Churchill Livingstone, Edinburgh

34 Preoperative assessment and premedication

All patients scheduled to undergo surgery should be assessed in advance with a view to planning optimal preparation and perioperative management. This is one mechanism by which the standard and quality of care provided by an individual anaesthetist or an anaesthetic department may be measured. Failure to undertake this activity places the patient at increased risk of perioperative morbidity or mortality.

The overall aims of preoperative assessment should include the following.

- Confirm that the surgery proposed is realistic when comparing the likely benefit to the patient with the possible risks involved.
- Anticipate potential problems and ensure that adequate facilities and appropriately trained staff are available to provide satisfactory perioperative care.
- Ensure that the patient is prepared correctly for the operation, improving where feasible any existing factors which may increase the risk of an adverse outcome.
- Provide appropriate information to the patient and obtain consent for the planned anaesthetic technique.
- Prescribe premedication and/or other specific prophylactic measures if required.

It is implicit that the anaesthetist requires sufficient knowledge and experience to predict the potential progress of an individual patient during the perioperative period. Appropriate skills must be achieved and maintained by respecting an ongoing commitment to education both individually and within the profession overall. Within individual hospitals there are organizational issues which must be addressed in order that preoperative assessment and preparation of patients may be accomplished successfully.

THE PROCESS OF PREOPERATIVE ASSESSMENT

WHO, WHEN AND WHERE?

The decision regarding the need for an operation is normally made by an experienced surgeon on the basis of the patient's presenting pathology. The patient subsequently undergoes a more extensive assessment of general health closer to the time of admission for surgery. This is undertaken usually by the least experienced member of the surgical team, and in some circumstances is delegated (in part) to an experienced nurse practitioner. Identification of potential problems by these individuals relies upon their application of general medical knowledge and common sense, often assisted by the use of screening protocols developed specifically by the anaesthetic department. When a patient is recognized to be at special risk, referral to an appropriate anaesthetist should be made. This need not be the anaesthetist ultimately responsible for the patient's care if surgery is not urgent, provided that decisions made regarding preoperative preparation are communicated and recorded clearly in the medical notes. If surgery is more imminent then it becomes relevant to involve the anaesthetist who will be responsible for the patient's perioperative care.

The need to improve efficiency of hospital bed occupancy has led to the increasing use of pre-admission clerking appointments, arranged to allow completion of the majority of the necessary administrative details. This is an ideal opportunity for anaesthetic assessment to take place, but in reality it is often not feasible to guarantee the availability of an experienced anaesthetist for these sessions. One direct consequence of this change is that patients are subsequently admitted onto the ward close to the time of surgery, allowing significantly less time for the anaesthetist to organize perioperative management. In order to optimize preparation for surgery within this system, many hospitals now use preoperative questionnaires which are completed by the patient in advance of clerking and are designed specifically to identify key features in the medical history which need further clarification. In addition, guidelines may be provided by the anaesthetic department for the surgical team or nurse practitioner to ensure that appropriate investigations are undertaken and suitable action taken if problems are identified.

Regardless of the timing and the individual personnel involved in clerking patients before surgery, the fundamental process of taking a detailed history and performing a systematic clinical examination remains the foundation on which preoperative assessment relies. This allows the anaesthetist to concentrate on areas of particular relevance to perioperative care.

HISTORY

Direct questions should be asked about the following items of specific relevance to anaesthesia.

Presenting condition and concurrent medical history

The indication for surgery determines its urgency and thus influences aspects of anaesthetic management. There are many surgical conditions which have systemic effects and these must be sought and quantified, e.g. bowel cancer may be associated with malnourishment, anaemia, and electrolyte imbalance. The presence of coexisting medical disease must also be identified, together with an assessment of the extent of any associated limitations to normal activity. The most relevant tend to be related to cardiovascular and respiratory diseases because of their potential effect on perioperative management. Specific questioning should ascertain the degree of exertional dyspnoea, paroxysmal nocturnal dyspnoea, orthopnoea, angina of effort, etc. Limitations to exercise because of other factors should be identified, e.g. intermittent claudication, arthritis, etc., so that effort-related symptoms such as dyspnoea and angina may be interpreted correctly.

Anaesthetic history

Details of the administration and outcome of previous anaesthetic exposure should be documented, especially if problems were encountered. Some sequelae such as sore throat, headache, or postoperative nausea may not seem of great significance to the anaesthetist but may form the basis of considerable preoperative anxiety for the patient. Previous anaesthetic records should be examined if available, as more serious problems such as difficulty with tracheal intubation should have been documented. Because of the risk of postoperative hepatotoxicity, the Committee on Safety of Medicines recommends that repeated exposure to halothane should be avoided within a 3-month period unless specifically indicated.

Family history

There are several hereditary conditions which influence planned anaesthetic management, such as malignant hyperthermia, cholinesterase abnormalities, porphyria, some haemoglobinopathies and dystrophia myotonica. Some of these disorders may not limit the patient's normal activities, but their presence is usually confirmed by asking about details of anaesthetic problems encountered by immediate family members and any subsequent investigations required; the family history is particularly important in patients who have not undergone surgery and anaesthesia previously.

Drug history

A complete history of concurrent medication must be documented carefully. Many drugs interact with agents or techniques used during anaesthesia, but problems may occur if drugs are withdrawn suddenly during the perioperative period (Table 34.1). Knowledge of pharmacology is essential to permit the anaesthetist to adjust the doses of anaesthetic agents appropriately and to avoid possibly dangerous interactions. In addition, the anaesthetist must maintain up-to-date knowledge of pharmacological advances as new drugs continue to emerge on the market. Any potential interactions observed with new drugs must always be reported to the Committee on Safety of Medicines.

Table 34.1 Drugs with potential anaesthetic interaction during anaesthesia

Drug group	Comments
Cardiovascular	
Angiotensin-converting enzyme inhibitors Captopril Enalapril Lisinopril	Hypotensive effects may be potentiated by anaesthetic agents. Sudden withdrawal tends not to produce haemodynamic effects, perhaps because of relatively long duration of action
Angiotensin II receptor antagonists Losartan Valsartan	May be associated with severe hypotension at induction or during maintenance of anaesthesia; consideration should be given to stopping treatment 24 h preoperatively
Antihypertensives Clonidine Guanethidine Methyldopa Reserpine	Hypotension with all anaesthetic agents, requiring extreme care with dosage and administration. *Clonidine* (or *dexmedetomidine*) allows reduction in dosage of anaesthetic agents and opioids. Acute withdrawal of long-term treatment may result in a hypertensive crisis. *Guanethidine* potentiates effect of sympathomimetics. *Reserpine* depletes norepinephrine stores, so attenuating the action of pressor agents acting via norepinephrine release.
Beta-blockers	Negative inotropic effects additive with anaesthetic agents to cause exaggerated hypotension. Mask compensatory tachycardia. Caution with concomitant use of any cardiovascular depressant drugs. Acute withdrawal may result in angina, ventricular extrasystoles, or even precipitate myocardial infarction
Ca^{2+} channel blockers	
Verapamil	Depresses AV conduction and excitability. Interacts with volatile anaesthetic agents leading to bradyarrhythmias and decreased cardiac output.
Diltiazem Nifedipine	Negative inotropic effect and vasodilatation interact with volatile anaesthetic agents to cause hypotension. May augment action of competitive muscle relaxants. Acute withdrawal may exacerbate angina
Others	
Digoxin	Arryhthmias enhanced by calcium. Toxicity is enhanced by hypokalaemia, which must be corrected preoperatively. Succinylcholine enhances toxicity, and should therefore be used with caution. Beware of bradyarrhythmias

Table 34.1 (Cont)

Drug group	Comments
Diuretics	Can cause hypokalaemia which may potentiate the effect of competitive muscle relaxants
Magnesium	Potentiates action of muscle relaxants, the dosage of which may need to be reduced
Quinidine	Intravenous administration can produce neuromuscular blockade, notable particularly following succinylcholine
Central nervous system	
Anticonvulsants	Cause liver enzyme induction. May increase requirements for sedative or anaesthetic agents. Recommended to avoid enflurane. Caution with propofol. Sudden withdrawal may produce rebound convulsive activity
Benzodiazepines	Additive effect with many CNS-depressant drugs. Caution with dosage of intravenous anaesthetic agents and opioids. Additive effect with competitive muscle relaxants, causing potentiation of their action. Action of succinylcholine may be antagonized
Monoamine oxidase inhibitors (MAOIs)	React with opioids causing coma or CNS excitement. Severe hypertensive response to pressor agents. Treatment of regional anaesthetic-induced hypotension may be difficult, especially as indirect sympathomimetics (e.g. ephedrine) are contraindicated due to unpredictable and exaggerated release of norepinephrine. Adverse effects do not always occur, but recommended to withdraw drugs 2–3 weeks before surgery and use alternative medication
Tricyclic antidepressants	Inhibit the metabolism of catecholamines, increasing the likelihood of arrhythmias. Imipramine potentiates the cardiovascular effects of epinephrine. Delay gastric emptying
Phenothiazines *Butyrophenones*	Interact with other hypotensive agents, necessitating care with administration of all agents with potential cardiovascular effect
Others	
Lithium	Potentiates non-depolarizing muscle relaxants. Consider changing to alternative treatment 48–72 h prior to anaesthesia
L-Dopa	Risks of tachycardia and arrhythmias with halothane. Actions antagonized by droperidol. Augments hyperglycaemia in diabetes. Some suggest discontinuing on day of surgery, but this must be balanced against possible detrimental effects as a result
Antibiotics	
Aminoglycosides	Potentiation of neuromuscular block. Caution with the use of muscle relaxants. Effect may be partially antagonized with Ca^{2+}
Sulphonamides	Potentiation of thiopental
Non-steroidal anti-inflammatory drugs	Interfere with platelet function to varying degrees by inhibition of platelet cyclooxygenase. Possible effect on coagulation mechanism makes use of regional anaesthesia controversial
Steroids	Potential adrenocorticoid suppression. Additional steroid cover may be required for the perioperative period
Anticoagulants	Problems with minor trauma resulting from cannulation, laryngoscopy and intubation (especially nasotracheal), intramuscular injections, and the use of local anaesthetic blocks. Full anticoagulation is an absolute contraindication to the use of regional anaesthetic techniques. Surgical haemorrhage more likely. Preoperative management of anticoagulant therapy is discussed elsewhere
Anticholinesterases	
Ecothiopate eye drops *Organophosphorus insecticides*	Rarely encountered nowadays. Inhibition of plasma cholinesterase. Caution should be exercised with the use of succinylcholine
Oral contraceptive pill	Increased risk of thromboembolic complications with oestrogen-containing formulations. Recommended that OCP is stopped 4 weeks before elective surgery or that some form of prophylactic therapy is provided
Antimitotic agents	Inhibition of plasma cholinesterase. Caution should be exercised with the use of succinylcholine

In general terms, administration of most drugs should be continued up to and including the morning of the operation, although some adjustment in dose may be required (e.g. antihypertensives, insulin). Consideration must also be given to possible perioperative events which influence subsequent drug administration (e.g. postoperative ileus), and appropriate plans made to use an alternative route or an alternative product with similar action. It is advised that some drugs should be discontinued several weeks before surgery (e.g. the oral contraceptive pill, long-acting monoamine oxidase inhibitors), because of the potential severity of perioperative complications with which they are associated.

There are occasions when patients with an illicit drug habit present for surgery. The patterns of abuse geographically are prone to frequent change, as are the specific drugs taken.

Abuse of opioids and cocaine is not uncommon and there is significant information available about potential perioperative problems related to acute or chronic toxicity; however, the same is not true for the increasing number of 'designer drugs' available.

History of allergy

A history of allergy to specific substances must be sought, whether it is a drug, foods or adhesives, and the exact nature of the symptoms and signs should be elicited in order to distinguish true allergy from some other predictable adverse reaction. Latex allergy is becoming an increasing problem and requires specific equipment to be used perioperatively. Atopic individuals do not have an increased risk of anaphylaxis, but may demonstrate increased cardiovascular or respiratory reactivity to any vasoactive mediators (e.g. histamine) released following administration of some drugs.

A small number of patients describe an allergic reaction to previous anaesthetic exposure. A careful history and examination of the relevant medical notes should clarify the details of the problem, together with the documentation of any postoperative investigations.

Smoking

Long-term deleterious effects of smoking include vascular disease of the peripheral, coronary and cerebral circulations, carcinoma of the lung and chronic bronchitis. It has been suggested that there are good theoretical reasons for advising all patients to cease cigarette smoking for at least 12 h prior to surgery, although there is little evidence to suggest that this influences patients' behaviour in this period.

There are several potential mechanisms by which cigarette smoking can contribute to an adverse perioperative outcome. The cardiovascular effects of smoking are caused by the action of nicotine on the sympathetic nervous system, producing tachycardia and hypertension. Furthermore, smoking causes an increase in coronary vascular resistance; cessation of smoking improves the symptoms of angina. Cigarette smoke contains carbon monoxide, which converts haemoglobin to carboxyhaemoglobin. In heavy smokers, this may result in a reduction in available oxygen by as much as 25%. The half-life of carboxyhaemoglobin is short and therefore abstinence for 12 h leads to an increase in arterial oxygen content. Finally, the effect of smoking on the respiratory tract leads to a sixfold increase in postoperative respiratory morbidity. It has been suggested that abstinence for 6 weeks results in reduced bronchoconstriction and mucus secretion in the tracheobronchial tree.

Alcohol

Patients may present with acute intoxication from alcohol or sequelae of chronic consumption. The latter are mainly non-specific features of secondary organ damage such as cardiomyopathy, pancreatitis and gastritis. Establishing the diagnosis may be far from straightforward, and needs to be complemented by a decision about whether to allow continued alcohol consumption during the hospital admission or risk the development of a withdrawal syndrome.

PHYSICAL EXAMINATION

A full physical examination should be performed on every patient admitted for surgery and the findings documented in the medical notes. It might be argued that this is unnecessary in young healthy patients undergoing short or minor procedures. However, the exercise is a simple and safe method for confirming good health or otherwise, and provides important information in case unexpected morbidity arises postoperatively, e.g. foot drop as a result of incorrect positioning on the operating theatre table, prolonged sensory anaesthesia following local anaesthetic techniques, etc. The information obtained from clinical examination should complement the patient's history and allows the anaesthetist to focus further on features of relevance (Table 34.2).

In addition, the anaesthetist must predict any potential difficulty in maintaining the patient's airway during general anaesthesia. The teeth should be inspected closely for the presence of caries, caps, loose teeth and particularly protruding upper incisors. The extent of mouth opening is assessed together with the degree of flexion of the cervical spine and extension of the atlanto-occipital joint. The thyromental distance should also be documented. Specific features associated with difficulty in performing tracheal intubation are described elsewhere (p. 512).

SPECIAL INVESTIGATIONS

In general, the results of many investigations may be predicted if a detailed history and examination have been performed. Routine laboratory tests in patients who are apparently healthy on the basis of the history and clinical examination are invariably of little use and a waste of resources. Before ordering extensive investigations, the following questions should be considered:

- Will this investigation yield information not revealed by clinical assessment?
- Will the results of the investigation alter the management of the patient?

Table 34.2 Features of the clinical examination relevant to the anaesthetist

System	Features of interest
General	Nutritional state, fluid balance Condition of the skin and mucous membranes (anaemia, perfusion, jaundice) Temperature
Cardiovascular	Peripheral pulse (rate, rhythm, volume) Jugular venous pressure and pulsation Arterial pressure Heart sounds Carotid bruits Dependent oedema
Respiratory	Central vs. peripheral cyanosis Observation of dyspnoea Auscultation of lung fields
Airway	Mouth opening Neck movements Thyromental distance Dentition
Nervous	Any dysfunction of the special senses, other cranial nerves, or peripheral motor and sensory nerves

In order to reduce the volume of routine preoperative investigations, the following suggestions are made. It should be noted that these are guidelines only and should be modified according to the assessment obtained from the history and clinical examination (Table 34.3).

Urine analysis

This should be performed in every patient. It is inexpensive and may occasionally reveal undiagnosed diabetes mellitus or the presence of urinary tract infection. Positive results should be confirmed by further evidence of pathology.

Full blood count

This provides information about the haemoglobin concentration, white blood cell count and platelet count, together with details of red cell morphology. Haemoglobin concentration tends to be of greatest interest to the anaesthetist. Patients whose ethnic origin or family history suggests that a haemoglobinopathy may be present should have haemoglobin concentration measured and haemoglobin electrophoresis undertaken if it has not been performed previously or if the result is not available. If such patients are scheduled for emergency surgery, a Sickledex test should be performed; if this is positive, haemoglobin electrophoresis should be undertaken as soon as possible but should not delay emergency surgery.

Blood chemistry

The measurements available include the serum concentrations of urea, creatinine and electrolytes, blood glucose concentration and liver function tests. There are specific conditions in which knowledge of preoperative values is important (e.g. diuretic therapy, chronic alcohol abuse). Beyond these situations, the value of preoperative screening is less clear, and detection of an unexpected abnormality seldom alters anaesthetic management. Blood sugar measurement is required in patients receiving corticosteroid drugs and in those who have diabetes mellitus or vascular disease; a fasting sample is usually required.

Chest X-ray

This investigation should be reserved for an older population (e.g. over 60 years of age) and patients with a clear indication. It probably has little value as a preoperative baseline because postoperative abnormalities are treated predominantly on the basis of their clinical relevance.

Other X-rays

Cervical spine X-rays should be considered in any patient in whom there is a possibility of vertebral instability, e.g. in the presence of rheumatoid arthritis. Thoracic inlet X-rays are required in patients with thyroid enlargement.

ECG

A 12-lead electrocardiogram can demonstrate many acute or long-standing pathological conditions affecting the heart, particularly changes in rhythm or the occurrence of myocardial ischaemia or infarction. It has some value as a preoperative baseline in patients with known or potential cardiovascular disease, although in the resting state the trace may appear normal despite the presence of clinically significant coronary artery disease. More extensive investigations are available in many departments to supplement the 12-lead ECG and these are discussed elsewhere (Chs 35 and 59).

Pulmonary function tests

Peak expiratory flow rate, forced vital capacity (FVC) and forced expiratory volume in 1 s (FEV_1) should be measured in all patients with significant dyspnoea on mild or moderate

Table 34.3 Guidelines for preoperative investigations

Urinalysis	All patients
Full blood count	Males over 50 years of age All female adults Before surgery which is likely to result in significant blood loss When indicated clinically, e.g. history of blood loss, previous anaemia or haemopoietic disease, cardiovascular disease, malnutrition, etc.
Urea, creatinine and electrolytes	All patients over 65 years, or with a positive urinalysis result Any patient with cardiopulmonary disease, or taking cardiovascular active medication, diuretics or corticosteroids Patients with renal or liver disease, diabetes or abnormal nutritional status Patients with a history of diarrhoea, vomiting or metabolic disorder Patients receiving intravenous fluid therapy for greater than 24 h
Blood glucose	Fasting sample in patients with diabetes mellitus, vascular disease or taking corticosteroids
Liver function tests	Any history of liver disease, alcoholism, previous hepatitis or an abnormal nutritional state
Coagulation screen	Any history of a coagulation disorder, drug abuse, significant chronic alcohol abuse, acute or chronic liver disease or anticoagulant medication
ECG	Male smokers older than 45 years; all others older than 50 years Any history (actual or suspected) of heart disease or hypertension Any patient taking medication active on the cardiovascular system or a diuretic Patients with chronic or acute-on-chronic pulmonary disease.
Chest X-ray	History suggesting a possible abnormality, e.g. cardiovascular disease, pulmonary disease with localizing signs, possible lung tumour (1° or 2°), thyroid enlargement (combined with a thoracic inlet view) Previous abnormal chest X-ray

exertion. This acts as a valuable preoperative baseline reference in assessing the effects of postoperative complications, although the results may not be predictive of such problems. Arterial blood gas analysis is required in all patients with dyspnoea at rest and in patients scheduled for elective thoracotomy; the information is a useful supplement to spirometry values. In patients with progressive disease, these investigations serve as a useful reference for future admissions.

Coagulation studies

Coagulation tests (PTTK and INR; see p. 26) are required in patients who give a history of bleeding disorders, in patients receiving anticoagulant therapy and in those with liver disease. Assessment of platelet function is worth considering in patients with potential inherited or acquired disturbances, especially if a regional anaesthetic technique is being proposed; however, this involves measurement of the bleeding time or thromboelastography.

PREDICTION OF PERIOPERATIVE MORBIDITY OR MORTALITY

After the patient's history, examination and relevant investigations have been collated the anaesthetist must answer two questions.

- Is the patient in optimum physical condition for anaesthesia and surgery?
- Are the anticipated benefits of surgery greater than the combined risks of undergoing anaesthesia and surgery, taking into account any concurrent disease?

In principle, if there is any medical condition which may be improved (e.g. pulmonary disease, hypertension, cardiac failure, chronic bronchitis, renal disease), surgery should be postponed and appropriate therapy instituted. The reasoning behind such a decision must be recorded clearly in the patient's medical notes, with the anticipated time required to achieve reasonable improvement. At this stage, the patient should be reassessed and the decision about when or whether to proceed with surgery reviewed.

There is continued interest in quantifying factors preoperatively which correlate with the occurrence of postoperative morbidity and mortality. Some accuracy is possible for populations of patients, but precision does not extend to accurate prediction of risk for an individual patient. Frequently, the decision to proceed may be made only by discussion between surgeon and anaesthetist.

Scoring systems for determining the likelihood of adverse outcome may be divided into two main groups:

- general scoring systems designed to predict non-specific undesirable events
- systems which focus on prediction of specific morbidity or technical difficulty, e.g. adverse cardiac events, difficulty with tracheal intubation.

PREDICTION OF NON-SPECIFIC ADVERSE OUTCOME

Over a broad range of operations and age, the overall mortality rate from surgery is of the order of 0.6%. This is many times greater than the incidence of deaths in which anaesthesia has made a significant contribution or has been the sole cause (approximately 1 in 10 000). In many large studies of mortality, e.g. NCEPOD reports, common factors which have emerged as contributing to anaesthetic mortality include inadequate assessment of patients in the preoperative period, inadequate supervision and monitoring in the intraoperative period and inadequate postoperative supervision and management. However, it remains difficult to evaluate formally whether it is the patient's characteristics, the surgical features or the anaesthetic technique that is the most influential in terms of final outcome. This is primarily a result of the high standards of practice which exist, the relative infrequency with which significant perioperative morbidity or mortality occurs, and the multifactorial background for many adverse events.

Any prospective studies intended to evaluate predictive factors of perioperative risk rely upon the incorporation of large numbers of patients and scrupulous design. Those that have been published tend to agree on several factors identified from physiological, demographic and laboratory data which can combine to indicate the likelihood of adverse outcome (Table 34.4).

ASA grading

The ASA grading system (Table 34.5) was introduced in the 1960s as a simple description of the physical state of a patient, along with an indication of whether surgery is elective or emergency. Despite its apparent simplicity, it remains one of the few prospective descriptions of the patient that correlates with the risks of anaesthesia and surgery. However, it does not embrace all aspects of anaesthetic risk, as there is no allowance for inclusion of many criteria such as age or difficulty in intubation. In addition, it does not take into account the severity of either the presenting disease or the surgery proposed, nor does it identify factors which can be improved preoperatively in order to influence outcome. Nevertheless, it is extremely useful and should be applied to all patients who present for anaesthesia.

PREDICTION OF SPECIFIC ADVERSE EVENTS

The difficult airway

There are specific medical or surgical conditions which are associated with potential airway problems during anaesthesia, such as obesity, the later stages of pregnancy, a large neck, mediastinal tumours and some faciomaxillary deformities. Apart from these, it requires an experienced anaesthetist to collate various physical features which can predict likely difficulty. Several classifications or scoring systems have been designed for this purpose, although none is entirely reliable; they are discussed elsewhere (p. 511).

Adverse cardiac events

Over 20 years ago, Goldman and colleagues published a retrospective analysis of preoperative risk factors which were associated with an adverse cardiac event following non-cardiac surgery (Table 34.6). This topic has been re-evaluated extensively in the intervening years, with many studies agreeing broadly with Goldman's conclusions. However, conflicting opinions exist regarding identification of the most accurate predictors, prob-

Table 34.4 Typical features which may increase the likelihood of significant perioperative complications or mortality

Preoperative feature		
Demographic/surgical	**Physiological**	**Laboratory**
Age > 70 years	Dyspnoea at rest or on minimal exertion	Plasma urea > 20 mmol L^{-1}
Major thoracic, abdominal or cardiovascular surgery	MI < 6 months previously	Serum albumin < 30 gL^{-1}
Perforated viscus (excluding appendix), pancreatitis or intraperitoneal abscess	Cardiac symptoms requiring medical treatment	Haemoglobin < 10 g dL^{-1}
Intestinal obstruction	Confusional state	
Palliative surgery	Clinical jaundice	
Smoking	Significant weight loss (> 10%) in 1 month	
Cytotoxic or corticosteroid treatment	Productive cough with sputum, especially if persistent	
Controlled diabetes	Haemorrhage or anaemia requiring transfusion	

MI, myocardial infarction.

Table 34.5 ASA classification of physical status and the associated mortality rates (for elective and emergency cases)

ASA rating	Description of patient	Mortality rate (%)
Class I	A normally healthy individual	0.1
Class II	A patient with mild systemic disease	0.2
Class III	A patient with severe systemic disease that is not incapacitating	1.8
Class IV	A patient with incapacitating systemic disease that is a constant threat to life	7.8
Class V	A moribund patient who is not expected to survive 24 h with or without operation	9.4
Class E	Added as a suffix for emergency operation	

ably as a result of the diversity of methods used in these studies, together with the significant and continued advances made in the understanding and management of cardiovascular pathophysiology.

Respiratory complications

Patients at risk of developing postoperative pulmonary complications include smokers, those with pre-existing lung disease, the obese and those undergoing thoracic or abdominal surgery. Unfortunately, predicting the likelihood and severity of such adverse events remains difficult. Sophisticated tests of pulmonary function (e.g. functional residual capacity, closing capacity, pulmonary diffusing capacity, etc.) are no more valuable in assessment of lung disease than simple spirometric tests, particularly vital capacity, FVC and FEV_1. Blood gas analysis should be performed preoperatively if there is concern about postoperative lung function; the presence of a preoperative arterial oxygen tension of less than 9 kPa, together with the presence of dyspnoea at rest, is the most sensitive method of predicting the need for mechanical ventilation in the postoperative period.

PREOPERATIVE PREPARATION

Having taken a full clinical history, performed a physical examination and reviewed the relevant investigations, the anaesthetist should decide if further measures are required to prepare the patient satisfactorily before proceeding to anaesthesia and surgery. This is the time to address any factors which place the patient at increased risk of adverse outcome and which could be improved to the patient's benefit before surgery. It is also appropriate to consider factors such as preoperative fasting; providing information to the patient and obtaining consent to proceed; ensuring blood products are available during the perioperative period if this is

Table 34.6 Goldman's index of cardiac risk in non-cardiac procedures (modified)

Risk factor	Points
Third heart sound or jugular venous distension	11
MI in preceding 6 months	10
Rhythm other than sinus or premature atrial contractions	7
More than five ventricular ectopic beats per min	7
Abdominal, thoracic or aortic operation	3
Age > 70 years	5
Important aortic stenosis	3
Emergency operation	4
Poor condition as defined by any one of:	3
P_aO_2 < 8 kPa	
P_aCO_2 > 6.5 kPa	
K^+ < 3.0 mmol L^{-1}	
HCO_3' < 20 mmol L^{-1}	
Urea > 7.5 mmol L^{-1}	
Creatinine > 270 μmol L^{-1}	
SGOT abnormal	
Chronic liver disease	
Total	53

0–5 points: major cardiac complications 0.3–3%
6–12 points: major cardiac complications 1–10%
13–25 points: major cardiac complications 3–30%
26–53 points: major cardiac complications 19–75%.

thought necessary; and organizing appropriate staff and equipment within the operating theatre suite.

POSTPONING SURGERY FOR CLINICAL REASONS

There are several common reasons for postponing surgery, some of which are mentioned below. One key issue relates to communication; the reason(s) for the decision to postpone surgery must be clear to the patient, the surgical team and any other staff who have been contacted to review the patient (e.g. cardiologists, physiotherapists). This helps to ensure that the time course for any improvement remains realistic and apparent to everyone involved, and that it can be balanced against the possible detriment of delaying surgery.

Acute upper respiratory tract infection

Although many patients may admit to the presence of a cold, clarification of such an admission should be made. In general, the presence of nasal secretions, pyrexia or the unexpected presence of physical signs on clinical examination of the chest suggest that non-urgent surgery should be postponed for a few weeks until the patient has recovered.

Coexisting medical disease and drug therapy

If the patient has coexisting medical disease which may affect outcome adversely if not under optimum control, there is a strong argument to postpone non-urgent surgery until further specialized advice has been sought.

Emergency surgery for which the patient has not been resuscitated adequately

Postponement may be necessary for only 1–2 h to permit restoration of circulating blood volume. This important principle may be breached if haemorrhage is extensive and continuous.

Recent ingestion of food

In general, anaesthesia for elective surgery should not be undertaken within 6 h of ingestion of food, although clear fluids may be taken up to 2 h before surgery (see below).

Failure to obtain consent

Consent for surgery should be obtained from all adult patients unless the patient is incapable of providing consent and the treatment proposed is clearly in his or her best interests (see below). If there is any doubt regarding the validity of the consent then surgery should be postponed where feasible until appropriate advice has been obtained.

PREOPERATIVE FASTING

The time of last oral intake of solid and fluid must be established. One of the commonest causes of anaesthetic-related mortality and morbidity is aspiration of gastric contents.

Many anaesthetic departments are currently re-evaluating their standing orders on the issue of preoperative fasting for clear fluids in light of clinical studies which have demonstrated the speed of gastric emptying in healthy adults. Several important points need to be emphasized on this topic.

- There are many factors which can increase the likelihood of significant gastric content regardless of the period of starvation (e.g. pain, anxiety, some drugs and premedication, paralytic ileus, later stages of pregnancy, etc.).
- The normal daily secretion of gastric fluid can approach 2000 ml in adults; consequently the stomach is never truly 'empty'.
- Clinical studies which encourage changes in practice should be scrutinized carefully to ensure that the results are not extrapolated beyond the sample of the population upon which they were based.

PROVIDING INFORMATION TO THE PATIENT AND OBTAINING CONSENT

Consent for anaesthesia is a vital part of preoperative preparation. It must be obtained by an individual with sufficient knowledge of the procedure and the risks involved. In order for consent to be valid, it must encompass three elements.

- The patient must have the capacity to consent to the treatment offered.
- The patient must have sufficient information to enable him/her to make a balanced decision to consent.
- The consent must be voluntary.

Capacity to consent refers to the patient's ability to comprehend the information provided, come to a decision on what is involved, and communicate that decision. There is no fixed age limit below which a minor cannot consent to treatment, although caution should be exercised when dealing with patients less than 16 years old; if in doubt, consent should also be sought from a person with parental responsibility. Capacity may also be invalidated by a patient's confusion, pain, shock or fatigue, and administration of some drugs such as opioid analgesics or benzodiazepine premedication. Appropriate advice should be sought if there is any concern.

Patients are confronted by a barrage of information on arrival in hospital, in addition to having to comply with an often alien environment with its own routines and practices. It is common for surgical consent forms to include consent to anaesthesia, despite the fact that the surgical team rarely has the knowledge to inform the patient fully on this subject. During the preoperative visit, the anaesthetist must ensure that the patient has been given an adequate amount of information about the proposed anaesthetic technique, and in particular its nature and consequences. The amount of information provided should be determined by an assessment of the needs of the patient to receive detailed information and the likelihood of adverse events:

- All patients should be told of common complications associated with the proposed anaesthetic technique (e.g. succinylcholine pains, postdural puncture headache).
- All patients should be told what they may experience in the perioperative period, including temporary numbness and weakness in the postoperative period if a local or regional technique is to be used.
- If a technique of a sensitive nature (e.g. insertion of an analgesic suppository) is to be used during anaesthesia, the patient should be informed.
- Patients should be informed of any increased risk related to their preoperative condition (e.g. damage to loose or crowned teeth, or cardiac complications in the presence of severe coronary artery disease).
- All patients should be given the opportunity to ask questions, and specific questions relating to anaesthesia must be answered honestly; if the questions relate to surgery, then the anaesthetist should ensure that a surgeon speaks to the patient before anaesthesia is induced.
- A summary of the matters discussed, the risks explained and the techniques agreed should be documented on the anaesthetic record.

BLOOD TRANSFUSION REQUESTS

Blood products are an expensive commodity and blood transfusion carries small but finite risks of incompatibility reactions and transmission of infection. In addition, there is the potential for supplies to be short, and the need for transfusion should be considered very carefully. The object of transfusion is to ensure that adequate oxygen delivery to the tissues can be maintained throughout the perioperative period. The amount of blood ordered from the blood transfusion service depends upon both the patient's preoperative haemoglobin concentration and the anticipated extent of surgery. Consideration should also be given to the use of anaesthetic techniques which reduce intraoperative blood loss, the use of cell salvage techniques perioperatively if available, preoperative red cell donation immediately before surgery, or acute normovolaemic haemodilution.

PREOPERATIVE ORGANIZATION OF THE OPERATING THEATRE AND THE POSTOPERATIVE PERIOD

The process of preoperative assessment provides the anaesthetist with a wealth of information about the patient and the proposed surgery. This allows the anaesthetist to plan various aspects of perioperative management. Some aspects must be conveyed to staff in the operating theatre suite in advance. Examples include the planned use of invasive monitoring, issues related to patient positioning, and any special needs the patient might have, such as an interpreter. If senior anaesthetic assistance is needed, this should be arranged in advance, and organization of appropriate postoperative care should also be initiated.

PREMEDICATION AND OTHER PROPHYLACTIC MEASURES

Premedication refers to the administration of drugs in the period 1–2 h before induction of anaesthesia. It is no longer a routine part of preoperative preparation, but the need for premedication must be considered after all of the relevant factors have been identified. The objectives of premedication are to:

- allay anxiety and fear
- reduce secretions
- enhance the hypnotic effect of general anaesthetic agents
- reduce postoperative nausea and vomiting
- produce amnesia
- reduce the volume and increase the pH of gastric contents
- attenuate vagal reflexes.
- attenuate sympathoadrenal responses.

Relief from anxiety

Surgical patients have a high incidence of anxiety and there is a significant inverse relationship between anxiety and smoothness of induction of anaesthesia. Relief from anxiety is accomplished most effectively by non-pharmacological means, which may be termed psychotherapy. This is effected at the preoperative visit by establishment of rapport, explanation of events which occur in the perioperative period and reassurance regarding the patient's anxieties and fears. There is good evidence that this approach has a significant calming effect.

In some patients, reassurance and explanation may be insufficient to allay anxiety. In these patients, it is appropriate to offer anxiolytic medication; the benzodiazepine drugs are the most effective for this purpose.

Reduction in secretions

Ether stimulated the production of secretions from pharyngeal and bronchial glands and premedication with an anticholinergic agent was common. This problem occurs rarely with modern anaesthetic agents, and anticholinergic premedication is no longer used as a routine. However, premedication with an anticholinergic drug is advisable for patients in whom an awake fibreoptic intubation is planned (when excessive salivation can create extra difficulty), or before using ketamine.

Sedation

Sedation is not synonymous with anxiolysis. Some drugs, e.g. the barbiturates and to a lesser extent the opioids, provide sedative but have no anxiolytic properties. In general, it is unnecessary to use a sedative preoperatively. An exception to this may be in paediatric practice. It is unwise to administer any sedative medication if the patient is in a critical condition, particularly if the airway and/or respiratory function are at risk of compromise.

Postoperative antiemesis

Nausea and vomiting are extremely common after anaesthesia. Opioid drugs administered during and after operation are often responsible. Occasionally, antiemetics may be given with the premedication, but they are more effective if administered intravenously during anaesthesia.

Amnesia

Under some circumstances, it may be desirable for patients, especially children, to be amnesic throughout the perioperative period in case unpleasant memories cause difficulties if subsequent operations are required. Some anaesthetists believe that amnesia should not be induced in children, lest they associate natural sleep with awakening to find a surgical incision. Although claims have been made for retrograde amnesia, it is unlikely that this can be achieved by pharmacological means. However, anterograde amnesia (loss of memory of events after administration of a drug) is produced commonly by the benzodiazepines; in this respect, lorazepam is two to five times more potent than diazepam. It is inappropriate to prescribe an amnesic drug with the object of reducing the risks of awareness during general anaesthesia.

Reduction in gastric volume and elevation of gastric pH

In patients who are at risk of vomiting or regurgitation (e.g. emergency patients with a full stomach or elective patients with hiatus hernia), it may be desirable to promote gastric emptying and elevate the pH of residual gastric contents. Gastric emptying may be enhanced by the administration of metoclopramide, which also possesses some antiemetic properties, whilst elevation of the pH of gastric contents may be produced by administration of sodium citrate. This topic is described in greater detail in Chapter 51.

Reduction in vagal reflexes

Premedication with an anticholinergic drug may be considered in specific situations in which vagal bradycardia may occur:

- Traction of the eye muscles, particularly the rectus medialis, during squint surgery may result in bradycardia and/or arrhythmias (the oculocardiac reflex). Premedication with atropine protects against this, but it is not as effective as the intravenous administration of atropine at induction of anaesthesia or in anticipation of traction of the muscles.
- Repeated administration of succinylcholine often results in bradycardia, which sometimes proceeds to asystole. Administration of atropine should always precede the administration of a second dose of succinylcholine.
- Induction of anaesthesia with halothane, particularly in children, may be associated with bradycardia.
- Surgical stimulation during a balanced anaesthetic technique may be associated with bradycardia.
- The administration of propofol to patients with a slow heart rate may result in dangerous degrees of bradycardia.

Limitation of sympathoadrenal responses

Induction of anaesthesia and tracheal intubation may be associated with marked sympathoadrenal activity, manifest by tachycardia, hypertension and elevation of plasma catecholamine concentrations. These responses are undesirable in the healthy individual and may be harmful in patients with hypertension or ischaemic heart disease. β-Blocker drugs or clonidine may be given as premedication in order to attenuate these responses.

DRUGS USED FOR PREMEDICATION

Some of the objectives listed above may be achieved by administration of drugs at induction or during maintenance of anaesthesia. The ability to achieve all objectives by administration of a variety of drugs either preoperatively or at induction is responsible for the wide variation in prescribing habits amongst anaesthetists.

Benzodiazepines

The benzodiazepines possess several properties which are useful for premedication, including anxiolysis, sedation and amnesia. The extent of each of these effects differs among individual drugs. Diazepam was the first drug of this group to be used commonly, although temazepam (10–30 mg) is now often preferred because of its shorter duration of action. Lorazepam (1–5 mg) produces a greater degree of amnesia than the other drugs in this group. Benzodiazepines produce anxiolysis in doses that do not produce excessive sedation, and this is advantageous if respiratory function is compromised; however, great caution should be exercised in these patients because depression of ventilation may be precipitated even by small doses. Some benzodiazepines may be administered by intramuscular injection, but evidence suggests that oral administration gives better results. There is a very wide variation in response to benzodiazepines and effects may be unpredictable. Although physostigmine was used in the past to reverse excessive sedation produced by benzodiazepines, a specific antagonist (flumazenil) is now available.

Opioid analgesics

It is necessary to prescribe opioid analgesic drugs for premedication only when patients are in pain preoperatively. This is uncommon except in some patients who require surgery as an emergency. Nevertheless, opioid drugs were used commonly for premedication in the past. The opioids cause sedation, but are not good anxiolytic agents. Although they produce euphoria in the presence of pain, they tend to cause dysphoria in its absence. They contribute to a smoother intraoperative course, and premedication with an opioid with a long half-life may provide some analgesia in the early postoperative period. Tachypnoea, which occurs during spontaneous breathing of volatile agents, is reduced and a lower concentration of anaesthetic agent is required for maintenance of anaesthesia. However, it is more logical to administer an opioid intravenously at or after induction of anaesthesia rather than intramuscularly for premedication.

There are several important side-effects of the opioids:

- Depression of ventilation and delayed resumption of spontaneous ventilation at the end of anaesthesia in which a muscle relaxant has been used.
- Nausea and vomiting, produced by stimulation of the chemoreceptor trigger zone in the medulla, are extremely common. Opioids should always be used in combination with an antiemetic agent.
- Morphine causes spasm of the sphincter of Oddi and this may result in right upper quadrant pain in patients presenting for surgery on the biliary tract.

Butyrophenones

Of the two butyrophenones, haloperidol and droperidol, only the latter enjoys popularity in anaesthetic practice. This drug possesses neuroleptic effects (which may be manifest as withdrawal and seclusion), α-blocking actions and antiemetic effects. Occasionally, droperidol may produce dose-dependent dysphoric reactions and extrapyramidal side-effects. Butyrophenones possess a very long duration of action and may delay recovery from anaesthesia, particularly in elderly patients. The commonest use for droperidol in anaesthetic practice is as an antiemetic agent, administered either with premedication in a dose of 2.5 mg or intravenously during anaesthesia in a dose of 1.25 mg or less.

Phenothiazines

These have been regarded as useful agents for premedication because they produce the following effects:

- central antiemetic action
- sedation
- anxiolysis
- H_2-receptor antagonism
- α-adrenergic antagonism
- anticholinergic properties
- potentiation of opioid analgesia.

Disadvantages include extrapyramidal side-effects, synergism with opioids which may delay postoperative recovery, and potentiation of the hypotensive effects of anaesthetic agents. Postoperatively (particularly in children given trimeprazine) the patient may exhibit pallor with mild tachycardia and hypotension, mimicking the signs of hypovolaemia.

Anticholinergic agents

The three anticholinergic agents used commonly in anaesthesia are atropine, hyoscine and glycopyrronium. Atropine and hyoscine are tertiary amines that cross the blood–brain barrier; glycopyrronium is a quarternary amine which does not cross the blood–brain barrier and which is not absorbed from the gastrointestinal tract. Although atropine is absorbed from the gastrointestinal tract, this occurs in an unpredictable manner and is dependent upon gastric content, pH and motility.

These three drugs differ in respect of their dose–response effects at various cholinergic receptors. In standard clinical doses, hyoscine 0.4 mg produces a greater antisialagogue effect than atropine 0.6 mg and has little action on cardiac vagal receptors. Hyoscine possesses sedative and amnesic actions and, in contrast to atropine, does not cause stimulation of higher centres. Hyoscine should be avoided in the elderly (over 60 years of age) as it can produce dysphoria and restlessness. Glycopyrronium has no central effects, a much longer duration of action and, in a standard clinical dose of 0.4 mg, causes less change in heart rate than atropine 0.6 mg.

Anticholinergic drugs are used clinically to produce the following effects:

- *Antisialagogue effects.* Glycopyrronium and hyoscine are more potent than atropine in this respect. These drugs block secretions when irritant anaesthetic gases are used and reduce excessive secretions and bradycardia associated with succinylcholine when it is given either repeatedly or as an infusion.
- *Sedative and amnesic effects.* In combination with morphine, hyoscine produces powerful sedative and amnesic effects.
- *Prevention of reflex bradycardia.* Anticholinergics are given for both prophylaxis and treatment of bradycardia. Atropine is used commonly as premedication in ophthalmic surgery to block the oculocardiac reflex in patients undergoing squint surgery and is used also in small children to reduce the bradycardia which may occur in association with halothane anaesthesia.

Side-effects of anticholinergic drugs include the following:

- *CNS toxicity.* The central anticholinergic syndrome is produced by stimulation of the CNS (usually by atropine). Symptoms include restlessness, agitation and somnolence and, in extreme cases, convulsions and coma. With hyoscine there is more commonly prolonged somnolence. Physostigmine 1–2 mg i.v. has been recommended to reverse the central anticholinergic syndrome and should be given in combination with glycopyrronium to prevent profound muscarinic effects produced by physostigmine.
- *Reduction in lower oesophageal sphincter tone.* Theoretically, a reduction in tone may lead to an increased risk of gastro-oesophageal reflux, although in clinical practice there is no suggestion that the use of anticholinergics for premedication is associated with an increased incidence of regurgitation and aspiration.
- *Tachycardia*, which should be avoided in patients with cardiac disease (e.g. obstructive cardiomyopathy, valvular stenosis or ischaemic heart disease) or when a hypotensive anaesthetic technique is planned.
- *Mydriasis and cycloplegia*, which lead to visual impairment. This may be troublesome, but is not a serious side-effect. Theoretically, mydriasis may be associated with reduced drainage of aqueous humour from the anterior chamber of the eye, thereby increasing intraocular pressure in patients with glaucoma. However, this effect is not important in practice

Table 34.7 Prophylactic measures against specific complications

Complication	Methods of prophylaxis
Deep vein thrombosis	Early postoperative mobilization Leg exercises (active/passive) Pneumatic compression of limbs Electrical stimulation of calf muscles Graduated stockings Low-dose subcutaneous heparin Warfarin anticoagulation Dextran-70 (Regional anaesthetic techniques, especially for orthopaedic lower-limb procedures)
Aspiration of gastric contents	Nil by mouth Antacids: sodium citrate H_2-antagonists Omeprazole Metoclopramide
Infection	
Surgical procedure	Directed by local or national practice with advice of microbiologists
Infective endocarditis	Follow guidelines of the Endocarditis Working Party
Adrenocortical suppression – suggested for patients who have received exogenous systemic steroids during the 2 months preceding surgery	Hydrocortisone 50 mg 4-hourly or 80 mg 6-hourly, or continue usual steroids if this is in excess of the current requirements (i.e. > 300 mg hydrocortisone equivalent, which is the maximum daily production in response to stress)

and atropine may be prescribed safely to patients with glaucoma provided that appropriate therapy is maintained.

- *Pyrexia*. By suppressing secretion of sweat, anticholinergics predispose to an increase in body temperature. These drugs should therefore be avoided in the presence of pyrexia, particularly in children.
- *Excessive drying*. Although anticholinergics are given for the specific purpose of producing antisialagogue effects, this may be most unpleasant for the patient.
- *Increased physiological dead space*. Atropine and hyoscine increase physiological dead space by 20–25%, but this is compensated for by an increase in ventilation.

β-Blockers

The use of β-blockers (e.g. atenolol) during the perioperative period limits the haemodynamic response to nociceptive stimuli, such as tracheal intubation and surgical stimulation, and inhibits the neuroendocrine stress response. Recent studies suggest that the use of β-blockers in patients at risk of coronary artery disease may be associated with improved outcome. However, their use incurs a limitation on appropriate increases in cardiac output during the perioperative period, and their administration to patients with impairment of left ventricular function should be considered very cautiously.

Clonidine and dexmedetomidine

These are α_2-agonists which potentiate anaesthetics by decreasing central noradrenergic activity. Dexmedetomidine is more specific for the α_2-receptor and probably has greater potential as a premedicant. Administration results in decreased intraoperative requirements for inhaled anaesthetic agents or propofol, although recovery times may be prolonged. These agents may also have a role in attenuating sympathoadrenal responses at induction of anaesthesia.

OTHER PROPHYLACTIC MEASURES

Thought should be given to the value of giving prophylactic treatment for the specific situations summarized in Table 34.7.

FURTHER READING

Fee J P H, McCaughey W 1994 Preperative preparation, premedication and concurrent drug therapy. In: Nimmo W S, Rowbotham D J, Smith G (eds) Anaesthesia. Blackwell Scientific Publications, London, p 677-703

Mason R A 1994 Anaesthesia databook, 2nd edn. A clinical practice compendium. Churchill Livingstone, Edinburgh

Strunin L 1993 How long should patients fast before surgery? Time for new guidelines. British Journal of Anaesthesia 70: 1–3

35 Intercurrent disease and anaesthesia

An increasing proportion of patients presenting for surgery suffer from unrelated disease, and many are receiving drug treatment. The patient with multiple co-morbidities and a complex drug regimen is now commonplace. These factors may interact with anaesthesia and surgery in several ways:

- The course of the disease may be modified by anaesthesia or surgery.
- The disease may influence the effects of anaesthesia.
- Drug treatment may influence the effects of anaesthesia.
- Both disease and drug treatment may influence choice of anaesthetic technique.
- Drug treatment may modify the normal compensatory physiological responses, e.g. cardiovascular agents such as β-blockers.

The aims of anaesthetic management in such patients are:

- to assess the extent of the medical problem
- to optimize the patient's condition as much as possible in the time available before surgery (this may vary widely between emergency and elective surgery)
- to conduct anaesthesia using drugs and techniques which have the least detrimental effect on the medical condition
- to use monitoring of a level appropriate to the clinical circumstances, taking into account chronic disability, acute physiology, the surgical technique and any drugs which the patient is receiving
- to extend these principles into the postoperative period.

The ability to achieve these aims varies widely depending on the urgency of surgery, and thus the time available. All patients who present for surgery require a full clinical history and examination. A past medical history, including previous anaesthesia, drug and allergy history and examination of previous anaesthetic records (if available) may be particularly important. In addition, special investigations may be necessary depending on the age and fitness of the patient and the nature of the surgery (see Ch. 34). The patient should be 'risk assessed' for a number of aspects of care (Table 35.1).

Table 35.1 Risk assessment: what does the patient need?

Senior involvement
Specialist opinion/investigation
Invasive monitoring
Basic resuscitation
Pre-optimization
HDU/ICU care

CARDIOVASCULAR DISEASE

GENERAL PRINCIPLES

Anaesthesia for patients with cardiovascular disease involves the application of several basic principles:

- Myocardial and tissue oxygenation should be optimized by maintenance of adequate oxygenation.
- Cardiac output must be maintained at a level commensurate with adequate tissue perfusion.
- Systemic arterial pressure must be adequate to maintain major organ perfusion (particularly for cerebral, coronary, renal and hepatic blood flow).
- The balance of myocardial oxygen supply and demand must be preserved, thus minimizing the risk of perioperative ischaemia and infarction (Table 35.2). Maintenance of oxygen-carrying capacity by blood transfusion, and optimization of circulating blood volume and intracardiac filling are essential.

Table 35.2 Factors affecting myocardial oxygen supply and consumption

Supply
Coronary perfusion pressure (diastolic pressure – LVEDP)
Arterial oxygen tension
Haemoglobin concentration
Coronary vascular resistance
Intraluminal obstruction
External compression
Heart rate
LVEDP
Autoregulation – dependent on myocardial oxygen consumption
Consumption
Heart rate
Contractility
Wall tension
LVEDP
Arterial pressure
Contractility
External work
Cardiac output
Arterial pressure

LVEDP, left ventricular end-diastolic pressure.

This approach demands a knowledge of the physiological mechanisms governing cardiac output, myocardial oxygen availability and consumption, and the adjustments that occur in disease states. An understanding of the effects of intravenous (i.v.) and volatile anaesthetic agents and muscle relaxants allows a choice to be made of appropriate drugs and techniques. Reversible risk factors (e.g. cardiac failure, myocardial ischaemia or hypertension) must be detected and treated preoperatively.

PREOPERATIVE ASSESSMENT

History

Symptoms of cardiovascular disease include dyspnoea, chest pain, palpitations, ankle swelling and intermittent claudication. Severity of symptoms assessed by a history of exercise tolerance is the most useful estimate of severity of cardiovascular disease.

Past medical history and previous medical records can usually reveal the nature and severity of disease. Several factors relating to history, clinical examination and proposed surgery are associated with an increased risk of perioperative cardiac complications, such as myocardial infarction (see Table 34.6). For example, the date of a previous myocardial infarction must be noted and elective surgery should not be performed within 6 months of that date. Unstable angina may also be associated with an increased risk of perioperative infarction, and should be investigated fully and treated before elective surgery. This may necessitate coronary arteriography. Previous thromboembolic disease necessitates prophylactic measures, e.g. low-dose s.c. heparin or intermittent calf compression.

Concurrent drug treatment

β-Adrenergic blockers

In most instances, β-blockade should be maintained throughout the perioperative period, although the dose of β-blocker should be reduced if undue bradycardia (heart rate less than 55 beats min^{-1}) is present. Sudden preoperative cessation may be associated with rebound angina, myocardial infarction, arrhythmia or hypertension perioperatively. Intravenous atropine or glycopyrrolate may be given before induction or, if undue bradycardia occurs, intraoperatively. β-Blockers may contribute to and mask the signs of hypoglycaemia. Most patients are now treated with long-acting cardioselective agents taken once daily, such as atenolol or bisoprolol.

Calcium channel blockers

These drugs (Table 35.3) block the slow influx of calcium ions which contribute to depolarization. *Verapamil*, which acts predominantly on the atrioventricular (AV) node, is used in the management of supraventricular tachyarrhythmias, angina, hypertension and hypertrophic obstructive cardiomyopathy. As it increases AV block, concurrent use with digoxin or β-blockers should be avoided, as should halothane and enflurane anaesthesia. *Nifedipine*, which acts predominantly on vascular smooth muscle, is used in the management of angina, hypertension and in Raynaud's phenomenon. *Amlodipine* has a similar profile of effects to that of *nifedipine*, but its once-daily formulation leads to less overshoot hypotension. *Diltiazem* lies between verapamil and nifedipine in terms of its effect. There is some evidence that the risk of myocardial ischaemia is increased as a result of coronary steal when isoflurane is used in patients receiving nifedipine. *Nimodipine* is predominantly a cerebral vasodilator and is used to prevent vasospasm associated with subarachnoid haemorrhage.

Table 35.3 Calcium channel blockers

Mostly vasodilator: nifedipine, nicardipine, amlodipine
Vasodilator, negative chronotrope: diltiazem
Negative inotrope and chronotrope, vasodilator: verapamil

Angiotensin-converting enzyme (ACE) inhibitors

These drugs produce vasodilatation by inhibiting conversion of angiotensin I to angiotensin II, a potent vasoconstrictor and stimulant of aldosterone secretion. Their main uses are in the treatment of cardiac failure, in which reduction of afterload improves left ventricular function and cardiac output, and in hypertension. They may predispose to renal failure, particularly in the presence of renovascular disease or if hypotension occurs, and can cause hyperkalaemia.

Angiotensin II receptor antagonists

These drugs, e.g. losartan and valsartan, are specific angiotensin II receptor antagonists with similar effects to ACE inhibitors. Hypotension may occur particularly in the presence of hypovolaemia, and hyperkalaemia occasionally occurs.

Digoxin

The dose should be assessed on the basis of age, weight and renal function, and reduced in the elderly, in patients with impaired renal function or if the plasma digoxin concentration exceeds the therapeutic range. Serum potassium concentration should always be measured and is commonly abnormal when there is concurrent diuretic therapy. Symptoms of digoxin toxicity, e.g. nausea and vomiting, should be sought. Heart rate and rhythm require assessment. In excessive dosage, especially with concurrent hypokalaemia, ventricular arrhythmias or heart block may occur.

The presence of vasodilator or heart rate-limiting drugs of whatever type, whether alone or in combination, has an adverse effect on the patient's ability to tolerate the effects of anaesthetic agents or acute hypovolaemia. In some situations, it may be appropriate to stop drugs, e.g. ACE inhibitors, preoperatively.

Diuretics

Serum potassium concentration should always be measured, and hypokalaemia corrected.

Anticoagulants

Where long-term therapy is indicated, perioperative control must be monitored closely. Warfarin should be stopped 48 h preoperatively, and the prothrombin time monitored daily; it should not be greater than 1.5 times control at the time of surgery. If prolonged, administration of vitamin K is indicated, while for emergency surgery, or if undue bleeding occurs, fresh frozen plasma should be given. After minor surgery, warfarin may be restarted on the first postoperative day; after major surgery, an infusion of unfractionated heparin may be used to maintain anticoagulation (with control by thrombin time estimations) until warfarin therapy is restarted. This allows rapid reversal of anticoagulation with protamine 1 mg for every 100 units of heparin if bleeding occurs. This is preferable to low molecular weight heparin in this situation as it may be monitored more easily and reversal titrated more accurately. Protamine should be administered slowly to avoid hypotension and, if given in excessive dosage, is itself an anticoagulant.

Antiplatelet drugs (aspirin/clopidogrel: spinals/epidurals)

In practical terms, if regional blockade is indicated, antiplatelet agents are not an absolute contraindication provided that the block is performed by an experienced operator. In these circumstances, the risk of haematoma is small, particularly with intrathecal blockade. Postoperative care should include a high clinical awareness of the risk of epidural haematoma to allow prompt identification and effective management (see Ch. 43).

Examination

Preoperative cardiovascular examination should include measurement of heart rate and rhythm, arterial pressure, assessment of peripheral perfusion and detection of signs of cardiac failure. The presence of a third heart sound or an elevated jugular venous pressure have been shown to have prognostic significance for perioperative cardiac morbidity. Hypertension and cardiac murmurs are not infrequently a chance finding, and require further assessment before surgery. The murmur most commonly encountered as an incidental preoperative finding is an aortic systolic murmur. This may represent aortic sclerosis or stenosis. It is particularly important to define whether significant stenosis exists. A normal-character pulse, normal pulse pressure and normal second heart sound suggest that aortic stenosis is less likely. Echocardiography should be performed if aortic stenosis is possible.

Investigations

In addition to routine haematological and biochemical investigations, an electrocardiogram (ECG) is important as a baseline before surgery for the diagnosis of arrhythmias, to provide confirmatory evidence of ischaemic heart disease and to assess the severity of cardiac disease, e.g. hypertension, cor pulmonale and valvular heart disease. However, a normal ECG is common in ischaemic heart disease, and exercise testing may disclose ischaemia in these patients. Holter 24 h ECG monitoring is useful in revealing transient ST-segment changes or arrhythmias.

Chest X-ray provides information on heart and chamber sizes, the state of the pulmonary vasculature and evidence of pulmonary oedema and infection.

Echocardiography is used to diagnose valve lesions, to detect intracardiac thrombus and pericardial effusion, and to assess global or segmental cardiac function. Cardiac Doppler examination allows assessment of pressure gradients across valves. Transoesophageal echocardiography may be particularly useful.

Cardiac catheterization and coronary angiography are rarely indicated before routine non-cardiac surgery.

Preoperative treatment

Cardiac failure, arrhythmias, hypertension and angina should be controlled before surgery. The conventional treatment of cardiac failure with diuretics has been augmented by the use of ACE inhibitors such as enalapril. This has been shown to improve symptoms and reduce mortality in patients with left ventricular dysfunction (New York Heart Association, grades III and IV). Anaemia should be treated – if necessary with blood transfusion – at least 48 h before surgery; supplementary diuretic cover may be necessary during transfusion. Haemoglobin concentration should be greater than $10 g dl^{-1}$ before surgery.

Premedication

In ischaemic heart disease and hypertension, premedication should be adequate to allay anxiety. A benzodiazepine such as temazepam is usually satisfactory. In patients with low or fixed cardiac output states (e.g. mitral or aortic stenosis, constrictive pericarditis) or congestive cardiac failure, premedication should be light, and in poor-risk patients it may be preferable to omit premedication altogether. The patient's usual cardiac medications should normally be continued and be included in the premedication.

Anaesthesia

In practical terms, this involves maintenance of a normal heart rate, and an arterial pressure adequate to maintain coronary perfusion and oxygenation without increasing cardiac work and thus myocardial oxygen requirements. Excessive myocardial depression should be avoided.

The high-risk periods during anaesthesia are:

- *Induction.* Most induction agents are cardiovascular depressants, and in patients with low or fixed cardiac output, hypertension or hypovolaemia, hypotension may occur. Of the agents currently available, etomidate has the least depressant effect on the cardiovascular system; propofol or thiopental may cause significant hypotension as a result of direct myocardial depression and reduction of systemic vascular resistance. Of the numerous neuromuscular blocking drugs, atracurium, rocuronium and vecuronium produce fewest (and negligible) cardiovascular effects.
- *Intubation.* Tracheal intubation is commonly associated with hypertension and tachycardia. The administration of a short-acting opioid such as alfentanil or fentanyl before induction allows reduction in induction dose and may limit the hypertensive response to intubation.
- *Postoperative period.* Rebound hypertension occurs commonly in association with pain and peripheral vasoconstriction. Good analgesia is necessary, as is careful attention to optimization of intravascular volume.

Careful monitoring is essential and must always include heart rate, arterial pressure and ECG. It should be instituted before induction, and maintained throughout the immediate postoperative period (if necessary in the high-dependency unit [HDU] or intensive care unit [ICU]). The common ECG configuration used for anaesthetic monitoring is standard limb lead II. Whilst this is useful for differentiating arrhythmias, myocardial ischaemia occurs most commonly in the left ventricle and is detected more sensitively with a CM5 configuration (see Fig. 38.2). The use of pulse oximetry is mandatory to detect any period of desaturation, while end-tidal carbon dioxide monitoring allows ventilation to be set to maintain normocapnia and gives early warning of acute haemodynamic disturbances. In high-risk patients undergoing major surgery, intra-arterial cannulation and central venous pressure (CVP) measurements are indicated. The use of oesophageal Doppler cardiac output monitoring as a guide to fluid and vasoactive drug administration has been suggested. Placement of a pulmonary artery flotation catheter (PAFC) is indicated in patients with severe ischaemic heart disease, left ventricular failure or shock, and in those scheduled for more major vascular or cardiac surgery. The PAFC allows measurement of pulmonary artery pressure, pulmonary artery occlusion pressure (PAOP; wedge pressure) and cardiac output, and sampling of pulmonary artery blood for mixed venous oxyhaemoglobin saturation ($S_{\bar{v}}O_2$). The PAOP reflects left ventricular end-diastolic pressure (LVEDP), a major determinant of myocardial oxygen supply and demand, while cardiac output is a major determinant of tissue oxygen delivery. Fibreoptic pulmonary artery catheters allow continuous monitoring of S_vO_2, which closely reflects cardiac output in low-flow states and may be of most practical use in theatre. Use of a PAFC may greatly aid preoperative optimization of cardiac function in patients with severe cardiac dysfunction.

HYPERTENSION

Untreated hypertension is associated with increased perioperative morbidity and mortality, and increased risk of cerebrovascular accident and myocardial infarction. Even mild hypertension has an important effect on long-term mortality. Because arterial pressure increases with age, an acceptable maximum pressure is difficult to define, but elective surgery should rarely be undertaken when the resting diastolic pressure exceeds 110 mmHg. Control of hypertension is usually achieved using a thiazide diuretic, with the possible addition of a β-blocker and/or a vasodilator, such as a calcium channel blocker, e.g. amlodipine. β-Blockers are often contraindicated in the presence of obstructive airways disease, left ventricular dysfunction, peripheral vascular disease and bradyarrhythmias, and in these situations a peripheral vasodilator calcium channel blocker would be preferred. ACE inhibitors may be used if left ventricular dysfunction or failure is present. The combination of ACE inhibitor and β-blocker is becoming more commonly used, particularly in patients with left ventricular dysfunction.

If hypertension is an unexpected preoperative finding, surgery should be delayed, if possible, until investigations are performed and treatment started. Endocrine and renal causes should be excluded. Complications of hypertension (e.g. myocardial ischaemia, cardiac failure and renal impairment) should be sought, and unstable angina and cardiac failure controlled before surgery. Appropriate investigations might include chest X-ray, ECG, echocardiography and renal ultrasound. Antihypertensive therapy should be continued throughout the perioperative period, although the dose of β-blocker may need to be reduced depending upon resting heart rate.

Anaesthesia

Premedication should be generous. Anaesthetic management should be directed towards avoidance of both hypotension and hypertension. Close monitoring of arterial pressure and ECG is required from before induction through anaesthesia and into the postoperative period. Blood loss should also be monitored carefully, and deficits replaced promptly. Hypertensive patients are particularly vulnerable to the development of hypotension following induction of anaesthesia or following establishment of subarachnoid or epidural blockade. Etomidate has fewest cardiovascular effects, but thiopental is acceptable if administered carefully. Propofol may produce excessive hypotension. Ketamine is contraindicated in anaesthetic dosages. Pancuronium should be avoided in severe hypertension; atracurium, rocuronium and vecuronium are suitable relaxants. Tracheal intubation may cause hypertension, tachycardia and arrhythmias. Administration of a rapidly acting opioid (fentanyl 3–5 μg kg^{-1} or alfentanil 20 μg kg^{-1}) before induction attenuates this response and also reduces the requirements for the induction agent.

For maintenance of anaesthesia, a balanced anaesthetic technique using N_2O and opioids with careful use of volatile or i.v. agents is appropriate. Volatile agents possess marked cardiovascular depressant effects and require careful administration. However, they are suitable for minor procedures with a spontaneous breathing technique. The effects of anaesthetic agents on the circulation are discussed in Chapters 13 and 14.

Intraoperatively, nodal arrhythmias may occur commonly, especially with halothane, and may produce a decrease in cardiac output. Depending on heart rate, i.v. atropine or glycopyrrolate (or a decrease of the inspired halothane concentration) may be effective in treating arrhythmias. The reduced left ventricular compliance and more rigid vascular tree found in hypertensive patients make them more vulnerable to small changes in blood volume. Furthermore, β-blockers prevent the physiological heart rate response to intraoperative blood loss, while vasodilators prevent vasoconstriction. Thus, careful monitoring of blood and fluid loss (and of CVP) is important, and prompt replacement of fluid deficits is necessary to avoid undue hypotension. Local anaesthetic preparations containing catecholamine vasoconstrictors should be avoided.

Postoperative hypertension occurs frequently, partly as a result of inadequate analgesia and partly because of peripheral vasoconstriction which occurs during prolonged surgery with associated heat loss and bleeding. Plasma epinephrine concentrations may be increased markedly. Hypertension increases myocardial work and oxygen demand, and may cause subendocardial ischaemia or infarction in patients with left ventricular hypertrophy or enlargement. Good analgesia is essential, and continuous epidural analgesia is safe in treated hypertensive patients if monitored closely.

Hypertension should be treated promptly; metoprolol in 1 mg i.v. boluses up to 5 mg over 10 min or labetalol titrated in 10–20 mg i.v. bolus doses, followed if necessary by an infusion, is usually effective. The ultra-short-acting agent esmolol is a useful alternative if there is concern about the cardiodepressant effects. In the presence of peripheral vasoconstriction, a vasodilator (e.g. glyceryl trinitrate 1–5 mg h^{-1} or hydralazine by 5–10 mg bolus) is usually effective. Nifedipine may be administered using the sublingual route until there is reliable restoration of gastrointestinal function.

If the patient has been managed preoperatively with oral β-blockers, a long-acting agent, e.g. atenolol or bisoprolol, should be given before surgery, and oral treatment recommenced on the day after surgery. In some instances, nasogastric administration or i.v. infusion may be necessary. Labetalol is an appropriate agent for infusion.

All hypotensive therapy requires careful arterial pressure monitoring, with a low threshold for intra-arterial measurement.

ISCHAEMIC HEART DISEASE

Five per cent of patients over 35 years of age have asymptomatic ischaemic heart disease. In patients who have had a previous myocardial infarction, anaesthesia and surgery within 3 months of infarction until recently carried a 40% risk of perioperative re-infarction. This rate decreases to 15% at 3–6 months and 5% thereafter. Research findings suggest that, with intensive perioperative monitoring, much lower rates of reinfarction can be achieved (at less than 3 months and at 3–6 months). Mortality from postoperative infarction is 40–60%. Elective surgery should generally be postponed until 6 months after infarction unless it is urgent.

Unstable angina is particularly associated with an increased risk of perioperative myocardial infarction. Low-dose aspirin (enteric-coated 300 mg or soluble 150 mg once daily) and systemic heparinization decrease the incidence of acute myocardial infarction in this situation. Angina should also be controlled with β-blockade and i.v. nitrate infusion before surgery. There is no evidence that the incidence of postoperative infarction is reduced by using local or regional anaesthetic techniques. Consideration should be given to coronary arteriography with a view to angioplasty or stenting.

Factors which precipitate further infarction are those which increase myocardial work, and thus oxygen requirement, or which decrease coronary blood flow (Table 35.2).

Anaesthesia

Preoperatively, left ventricular failure should be treated with diuretics, ACE inhibitors and nitrates. Anaemia should be corrected. Premedication should be adequate to allay anxiety. Oxygen therapy may be considered appropriate with premedication in some patients. The demands of anaesthetic management are similar to those which apply in the hypertensive patient: close monitoring, avoidance of tachycardia and bradycardia, maintenance of normotension or slight hypotension and careful choice of anaesthetic agent. β-Blockade should be maintained, and this necessitates care in fluid replacement and concurrent drug administration.

Enflurane dilates the peripheral circulation in addition to depressing myocardial contractility. Overall, it causes a decrease in arterial pressure comparable with that resulting from administration of halothane.

Isoflurane causes less reduction in cardiac output than does enflurane or halothane. It is a potent vasodilator and has been implicated as a cause of coronary steal in patients with myocardial ischaemia. Although there is some dispute about the importance of this effect at high doses, it is likely that low concentrations of isoflurane (< 0.5%) do not cause coronary steal. Sevoflurane has similar effects to those of isoflurane but causes less vasodilatation and increase in heart rate and possibly less effect on the coronary circulation.

Halothane depresses contractility and myocardial oxygen consumption, but coronary blood flow is depressed to a proportionately lesser extent; thus, halothane is tolerated well in low concentrations. However, high concentrations of halothane may produce excessive myocardial depression with a profound decrease in cardiac output, increased LVEDP and myocardial ischaemia. These effects may be potentiated by β-blockade.

Interactions between calcium channel blockers and volatile anaesthetic agents may cause serious hypotension (Table 35.3).

Normocapnia should be maintained, because hypercapnia may provoke arrhythmias, while hypocapnia causes peripheral and coronary vasoconstriction and shifts the oxyhaemoglobin dissociation curve to the left. Postoperative monitoring, management of analgesia and control of arterial pressure must be meticulous, and HDU or ICU admission may be appropriate.

CARDIAC FAILURE

Anaesthesia and surgery in patients with cardiac failure carry an increased risk of morbidity and mortality. The cause of heart failure should be elucidated, and treatment instituted before surgery.

Left heart failure causes pulmonary congestion and oedema, and decreases pulmonary compliance; respiratory work is increased and hypoxaemia occurs. Signs indicating left ventricular failure include tachycardia, gallop rhythm, mitral regurgitation, cyanosis, tachypnoea, crepitations and wheeze. Causes include ischaemic heart disease, hypertension, rheumatic heart disease and congestive cardiomyopathy. It may be precipitated by arrhythmias, e.g. atrial fibrillation, or by drugs, e.g. β-blockers.

Treatment involves delivery of a high inspired oxygen concentration (with continuous positive airways pressure [CPAP] or mechanical ventilation in severe cases), intravenous opioid, nitrate (by infusion if failure is severe) and loop diuretic. The aim of treatment is to optimize both the left ventricular filling pressure and cardiac output. If left ventricular failure is precipitated by arrhythmias, these should be treated, avoiding negatively inotropic drugs.

Right ventricular failure generally results from pulmonary hypertension. This is usually secondary either to left heart failure or to chronic lung disease (cor pulmonale). ECG evidence of right atrial enlargement and ventricular hypertrophy raises the suspicion of pulmonary hypertension. Hypoxaemia in such patients causes an exaggerated increase in pulmonary vascular resistance, provoking right ventricular failure. Acute right heart failure occurs commonly when patients with chronic obstructive pulmonary disease (COPD) suffer an acute infective exacerbation with hypoxaemia. Preoperative treatment of infection is important, and intraoperative and postoperative maintenance of the airway and avoidance of hypoxaemia are imperative.

The clinical features of biventricular failure may also be associated with salt and water overload and hypoalbuminaemia, e.g. in renal or hepatic disease.

Low subarachnoid or epidural block may be useful in some patients with cardiac failure, as the sympathetic block produces venodilatation and reduction in preload; however, a high block should be avoided.

SHOCK

Surgery should not usually be undertaken until adequate resuscitation of the patient has been achieved. In cases of severe haemorrhage, only initial resuscitation may be possible before surgery, and resuscitation must be continued during operation until bleeding is controlled, e.g. penetrating trauma. Such patients require adequate oxygenation and ventilation, guided by regular blood gas measurements. The degree of base deficit is helpful in assessing severity and response to treatment.

Monitoring required during resuscitation and anaesthesia includes direct arterial pressure, heart rate, CVP and urine output. Core–peripheral temperature gradient is generally recommended as a useful measure of peripheral perfusion in shock. However, it is of less value in septic shock where vasoregulation is lost, and it is of limited value as a measure of either volume status in hypovolaemic shock or cardiac output in cardiogenic shock. Pulmonary artery catheterization for measurement of PAOP, cardiac output and oxygen transport variables is essential to direct appropriate fluid and vasoactive drug therapy in cardiogenic or septic shock which proves not to be readily reversible with volume resuscitation.

Anaesthesia in shock

Adequate venous access with large-gauge cannulae (at least two; 14G or pulmonary artery catheter introducer) should be ensured before induction of anaesthesia. Monitoring should be commenced pre-induction. Anaesthetize in theatre. Early ICU involvement is recommended. Minimal doses of induction agent should be used. Etomidate is associated with least cardiovascular disturbance, but other agents, e.g. thiopental, may be used with care in very low dosage. A balanced technique, is usually appropriate. In theatre, maintenance of oxygen saturation and an adequate mean arterial pressure are prime objectives. It may not be practicable to begin full haemodynamic monitoring preoperatively, but this should be achieved as soon as possible, and continued into the ICU postoperatively. Where hypotension is difficult to reverse, epinephrine by small bolus injection (10 μg aliquots: 1 ml of 1 in 100 000 solution) or by infusion is appropriate first-line therapy. The management of shock is discussed in Chapters 51 and 60.

ARRHYTHMIAS (see also Chs 7 and 40)

Arrhythmias which are present preoperatively should be treated before surgery (which should be postponed if necessary). The most commonly occurring arrhythmia is probably atrial fibrillation, which is usually caused by ischaemic heart disease, mitral valve disease, hypertensive heart disease or thyrotoxicosis. The ventricular rate should be controlled with digoxin. If the ventricular rate is normal, digoxin should usually be started preoperatively to prevent an increase in ventricular rate during surgery.

Intraoperative arrhythmias

Approximately 12% of patients undergoing anaesthesia develop arrhythmias, but this frequency increases to 30% in patients with cardiovascular disease. Treatment may not be required, depending on the nature of the arrhythmia and its effect on cardiac output. Single supraventricular or ventricular ectopic beats and slow supraventricular rhythms do not require treatment unless cardiac output is compromised.

Factors affecting intraoperative arrhythmias include the following:

Spontaneous ventilation. Raised arterial carbon dioxide tension ($P_{a}CO_2$) may cause ventricular extrasystoles.

Hypoxaemia. Initially this causes tachycardia, then bradycardia.

Anaesthetic agents. Halogenated hydrocarbons, e.g. halothane, are associated with an increased incidence of ventricular arrhythmias, especially if $P_{a}CO_2$ is raised.

Catecholamines. Local anaesthetic preparations containing epinephrine may provoke ventricular arrhythmias, especially in patients anaesthetized with halothane in the presence of a raised $P_{a}CO_2$. A maximum of 100 μg of epinephrine (10 ml of 1:100 000 solution) may be injected over any 10 min period (maximum 300 μg in 1 h). Enflurane is less likely to be associated with epinephrine-induced arrhythmias, and isoflurane and sevoflurane do not sensitize the myocardium to catecholamines.

Hypokalaemia may be associated with ventricular arrhythmias, especially in the presence of digoxin. Hyperkalaemia delays ventricular conduction, with eventual cardiac arrest.

Reflex arrhythmias tend to occur during light anaesthesia as a result of sympathetic or parasympathetic stimulation. They include tachyarrhythmias, e.g. in response to laryngoscopy and intubation (diminished by β-blockers), ventricular arrhythmias following dental extraction (partially blocked by local anaesthetic infiltration) and bradyarrhythmias, e.g. the oculocardiac reflex, or in response to peritoneal traction (prevented or treated by atropine or glycopyrrolate). Reflex arrhythmias in general are prevented by deepening anaesthesia. The treatment of intraoperative arrhythmias depends on the nature of the arrhythmia and the haemodynamic decompensation caused. Supraventricular (SVT) and ventricular tachycardias (VT) differ in their clinical significance and treatment, and should be distinguished (Table 35.4).

Treatment of SVT under GA consists of:

- carotid sinus massage
- adenosine 3–12 mg i.v.–contraindicated in asthma
- direct current (DC) cardioversion (25–50 J) if haemodynamic decompensation is present; synchronized DC shock is also indicated for atrial flutter
- if no decompensation, verapamil 5 mg, titrated i.v.
- in sepsis-related or refractory SVT, volume loading plus amiodarone 300 mg i.v. by infusion over 20 min, then 900 mg over 24 h

Table 35.4 Diagnostic features of ventricular tachycardia

Clinical
Cannon waves in JVP
Variable first heart sound
Often recent MI or IHD
ECG
Rate usually 120–250 beat min^{-1}, usually regular
Broad complexes usual in VT
Independent atrial activity: P waves dissociated from QRS
Fusion beats
Capture beats

JVP, jugular venous pulse; VT, ventricular tachycardia; MI, myocardial infarction; IHD, ischaemic heart disease; ECG, electrocardiogram.

- in thyrotoxicosis or phaeochromocytoma, β-blocker (in the latter case, not before α-blockade).

Intravenous verapamil should not be given to patients already receiving β-blockers as it may cause refractory asystole. The role of adenosine intraoperatively is, as yet, undefined. It is used as treatment for SVT and in diagnosis of regular broad complex tachycardia.

Synchronized DC cardioversion should be used if VT is associated with decompensation. Compensated VT usually responds to i.v. lidocaine 50–100 mg followed by an infusion, but if unsuccessful, bretylium or amiodarone may be tried. Other measures include correction of hypercapnia, hypoxaemia or hypokalaemia, i.v. magnesium and reduction of the volatile concentration.

HEART BLOCK

The extent of the conduction deficit should be determined preoperatively from a 12-lead ECG or 24 h tape if no clear evidence is seen on ECG. If the patient has syncopal attacks or is in cardiac failure, long-term pacing is indicated.

If the patient with heart block presents for surgery without a pacemaker in situ, preoperative insertion of a temporary pacing line is usually indicated in:

- complete heart block
- second-degree heart block, of Mobitz type 2 variety
- first-degree heart block with bifascicular block (right bundle branch block with left anterior or posterior hemiblock)
- sick sinus syndrome (see below).

The availability of external pacing as a 'safety net' may probably limit the number of temporary transvenous lines inserted.

A decision on whether long-term pacing is indicated or not may be made by a cardiologist after the immediate postoperative period. During anaesthesia, ECG should be monitored continuously, a standby pacemaker should be available and care should be taken to avoid undue blood loss or vasodilatation as heart rate is unable to increase in compensation.

Diathermy should be avoided if possible because it may interfere with pacemaker function. Where unavoidable, the diathermy plate should be sited as far away as possible from the pacemaker generator, or bipolar diathermy should be used. Temporary generators and demand permanent generators are most often affected. Demand pacemakers should be converted to fixed-rate before surgery if the use of diathermy is essential. During transurethral prostatectomy, the 'cutting' current may affect the pacemaker, while the 'coagulation' current has no effect; with some pacemakers, the reverse may occur. Diathermy should be used in short bursts only and pacemaker threshold should be checked postoperatively. If first-degree heart block only is present, not necessitating temporary pacing, drugs which slow AV conduction should be avoided, e.g. β-blockers, digoxin, verapamil, halothane.

SICK SINUS SYNDROME

This term covers several conduction defects which affect the sinoatrial node, ranging from sinus bradycardia to sinus arrest. Sinoatrial block may be associated with runs of SVT (so-called tachycardia–bradycardia syndrome). Long-term pacing is indicated if the patient has syncopal episodes. Sinus bradycardia usually responds to atropine, while in complete sinoatrial block atropine accelerates nodal escape rhythm. In the tachycardia–bradycardia group, temporary pacing is indicated to cover anaesthesia and surgery, because treatment of tachycardia with, for example, β-blocker, calcium channel blocker or digoxin may provoke severe bradycardia.

VALVULAR HEART DISEASE

In both aortic and mitral stenosis, there is a low, fixed cardiac output, which leaves no reserve to compensate for changes in heart rate or vascular resistance.

Aortic stenosis

Isolated aortic stenosis is associated most commonly with calcification, often on a congenital bicuspid valve. In rheumatic heart disease, aortic stenosis occurs rarely in the absence of mitral disease and is usually combined with regurgitation. The diagnosis is suggested by the findings of an ejection systolic murmur, low pulse pressure, and clinical and ECG evidence of left ventricular hypertrophy. Aortic systolic murmurs in elderly patients are frequently ascribed to aortic sclerosis, and an assessment of the degree of stenosis rests on examination. A slow-rising low-volume pulse with reduced pulse pressure, reduced intensity of the second heart sound and the presence of a click are suggestive of stenosis, and evidence of left ventricular hypertrophy on ECG usually indicates severe stenosis. Echocardiography with Doppler flow monitoring aids diagnosis and assessment. On chest X-ray, heart size is normal until late in the disease, while symptoms of angina, effort syncope and left ventricular failure indicate advanced disease.

Perioperative mortality is increased in patients with aortic stenosis; arrhythmias are common and are associated with precipitous decreases in cardiac output. The myocardial oxygen balance is upset by the decreases in coronary perfusion pressure and subendocardial blood flow, and the increase in ventricular afterload. Successful management demands precise maintenance of heart rate, arterial pressure and myocardial contractility. Bradycardia causes a decrease in cardiac output because stroke volume is fixed; tachycardia decreases the time available for coronary filling, and therefore both should be avoided.

Vasodilatation causes severe hypotension because cardiac output cannot increase significantly; coronary perfusion pressure is reduced if hypotension occurs.

All anaesthetic induction agents must be used with extreme caution. Etomidate is the agent of choice. The relaxant of choice is atracurium or vecuronium. Volatile agents which depress ventricular contractility (halothane, enflurane) may also seriously decrease cardiac output; in addition, halothane predisposes to arrhythmias. Isoflurane produces vasodilatation and causes decreases in diastolic pressure and coronary perfusion pressure. A balanced general technique is the best anaesthetic option. Replacement of blood must be prompt. Intensive monitoring is important and should include measurement of intra-arterial pressure and, in severe disease, PAOP measurement.

Mitral stenosis

This is usually a manifestation of rheumatic heart disease. Characteristic features include atrial fibrillation, arterial embolism, pulmonary oedema, pulmonary hypertension and right heart failure. Acute pulmonary oedema may follow the onset of atrial fibrillation.

Patients with mitral stenosis who present for surgery are frequently receiving digoxin, diuretics and anticoagulants. Preoperative control of atrial fibrillation, treatment of pulmonary oedema and management of anticoagulant therapy (see Ch. 23) are necessary. During anaesthesia, control of heart rate is important. Tachycardia reduces diastolic ventricular filling and thus cardiac output, while bradycardia also results in a decreased cardiac output because stroke output is limited. As with aortic stenosis, drugs which produce vasodilatation may cause severe hypotension.

As a result of pre-existing pulmonary hypertension, patients are particularly vulnerable to hypoxaemia, including transient episodes. Both hypoxaemia and acidosis are potent pulmonary vasoconstrictors and may produce right ventricular failure. Thus, opioid analgesics should be prescribed cautiously, and airway obstruction avoided.

Aortic regurgitation

Acute aortic regurgitation, e.g. resulting from infective endocarditis, causes rapid left ventricular failure and may require emergency valve replacement, even in the presence of unresolved infection.

Chronic aortic regurgitation is asymptomatic for many years. Left ventricular dilatation occurs, with eventual left ventricular failure.

Patients with mild or moderate aortic regurgitation without left ventricular failure or massive ventricular dilatation tolerate anaesthesia well. A slightly increased heart rate of approximately 100 beats min^{-1} is desirable because this reduces left ventricular dilatation. Bradycardia causes ventricular distension and should be avoided. Vasodilator therapy increases net forward flow by decreasing afterload and is useful in severe aortic regurgitation; isoflurane anaesthesia may be beneficial. Careful monitoring is required, preferably with PAOP measurement, if severe hypotension is to be avoided.

Mitral regurgitation

Acute mitral regurgitation commonly results from infective endocarditis, or myocardial infarction with papillary muscle dysfunction or ruptured chordae tendineae. Acute pulmonary oedema results, and urgent valve replacement is required. Left ventricular failure with ventricular dilatation may cause functional mitral regurgitation.

Chronic mitral regurgitation is commonly associated with mitral stenosis. In pure mitral regurgitation, left atrial dilatation occurs with a minimal increase in pressure. The degree of regurgitation may be reduced by reducing the size of the left ventricle and the impedance to left ventricular ejection. Thus, inotropic agents and vasodilators may be useful. A slight increase in heart rate is desirable unless there is concomitant stenosis.

Infective endocarditis

This is caused predominantly by the *viridans* group of streptococci, occasionally by Gram-negative organisms or enterococci and also by staphylococci, especially after cardiac surgery or in drug addicts. *Coxiella burnetii* also accounts for a few cases. Patients with rheumatic or congenital heart disease, including asymptomatic lesions, e.g. bicuspid aortic valve, are at risk. Infection is caused by transient bacteraemia, most frequently after dental extraction or genitourinary investigation or surgery.

Antibiotic cover should be given for all surgical procedures in at-risk patients. Appropriate regimens are detailed in the *British National Formulary* or comparable recent sources of advice. Flucloxacillin or an alternative antistaphylococcal agent should be included in regimens for cardiac surgery.

ROLE OF LOCAL AND REGIONAL ANAESTHESIA

In appropriate patients with cardiovascular disease, local infiltration, peripheral nerve blocks or plexus blocks provide satisfactory anaesthesia with low risk of side-effects, allow a reduction in requirement for general anaesthetic and improve postoperative analgesia. This can reduce cardiovascular depression and risk. Local anaesthetic preparations which contain epinephrine may produce tachycardia and should be used with caution in patients with severe cardiovascular disease.

Patients undergoing lower abdominal, pelvic or lower limb surgery may be managed satisfactorily with low subarachnoid or epidural anaesthesia. With higher blocks, sympathetic block produces vasodilatation, reducing preload and afterload. While controlled vasodilatation may have beneficial effects in ischaemic heart disease, hypertension and cardiac failure, patients anaesthetized with subarachnoid or epidural block must be managed very carefully in respect of posture, and fluid preloading and replacement to avoid undue hypotension. This may pose a particular problem in patients with untreated hypertension, low cardiac output states, constrictive pericarditis, severe valvular disease or a fixed heart rate resulting from heart block or β-blocker therapy. However, patients with congestive cardiac failure may benefit from the preload reduction caused by sympathetic block, and patients with peripheral vascular disease may benefit from peripheral vasodilatation.

In general, anaesthetists with limited experience in regional anaesthesia should avoid subarachnoid and epidural blocks in patients with severe cardiac disease.

RESPIRATORY DISEASE

Successful anaesthetic management of the patient with respiratory disease is dependent on accurate assessment of the nature and extent of functional impairment, and an appreciation of the effects of surgery and anaesthesia on pulmonary function.

ASSESSMENT

History

Of the six cardinal symptoms of respiratory disease (cough, sputum, haemoptysis, dyspnoea, wheeze and chest pain), dyspnoea provides the best indication of functional impairment. Specific questioning is required to elicit the extent to which activity is limited by dyspnoea. Dyspnoea at rest or on minor exertion clearly indicates severe disease. A cough productive of purulent sputum indicates active infection. Chronic copious sputum production may indicate bronchiectasis. A history of heavy smoking or occupational exposure to dust may suggest pulmonary pathology.

A detailed drug history is important. Long-term steroid therapy within 3 months of the date of surgery necessitates augmented cover for the perioperative period and may cause hypokalaemia and hyperglycaemia. Bronchodilators should be continued during the perioperative period. Patients with cor pulmonale may be receiving digoxin and diuretics.

Examination

A full physical examination is required, with emphasis on detecting signs of airway obstruction, increased work of breathing, active infection which can be treated preoperatively, and evidence of right heart failure. The presence of obesity, cyanosis or dyspnoea is noted. In addition, a simple forced expiratory manoeuvre may reveal prolonged expiration, and a simple test of exercise tolerance may be useful.

Investigations

Chest X-ray

The preoperative chest X-ray is a poor indicator of functional impairment but is important for several reasons:

- as a baseline for assessing postoperative radiographs
- to discover any localized disease of lungs and pleura not detected on clinical examination, e.g. neoplasm, collapse, consolidation, effusion
- to reveal underlying generalized lung disease in patients presenting with acute pulmonary symptoms, e.g. pulmonary fibrosis, emphysema.

ECG

This may indicate right atrial or ventricular hypertrophy (P pulmonale in II; dominant R wave in III, V_{1-3}) while associated ischaemic heart disease is common.

Haematology

Polycythaemia occurs secondary to chronic hypoxaemia, while anaemia aggravates tissue hypoxia. Leucocytosis may indicate active infection.

Sputum culture

Sputum culture is essential in patients with chronic lung disease or suspected acute infection.

Pulmonary function tests (see Appendix VIII)

Peak expiratory flow rate, forced expiratory volume in 1 s (FEV_1) and forced vital capacity (FVC) may be measured easily at the bedside. The FEV_1:FVC ratio is decreased in obstructive lung disease and normal in restrictive disease. In the presence of obstructive disease, the test should be repeated 5–10 min after administration of a bronchodilator aerosol to provide an indication of reversibility. An FVC < 1–1.5 L is indicative of limited ability to take large sigh breaths, expand lung bases and clear secretions by coughing.

Fuller investigation involves measurement of functional residual capacity (FRC), residual volume and total lung capacity, but these are rarely of value in determining clinical management.

Blood gas measurement

This is indicated in patients with chronic respiratory disease undergoing significant surgery and also if there is suspected acute hypoxaemia. It is also advisable when pulmonary function tests are markedly abnormal, e.g. in obstructive disease where the FEV_1 is less than 1.5 L. A raised P_aCO_2 is a prognostic indication that pulmonary complications are likely to develop postoperatively. With a P_aCO_2 of 6.7 kPa (50 mmHg) or greater, elective postoperative ventilation may be required after all but minor surgery. The combination of a low preoperative arterial oxygen tension (P_aO_2) and dyspnoea at rest is also associated with a high likelihood of the need for elective ventilation after abdominal surgery.

EFFECTS OF ANAESTHESIA AND SURGERY

Fitness for anaesthesia and surgery in patients with respiratory disease depends on the type and magnitude of surgery. The effects of anaesthesia alone on respiratory function are generally minor and short-lived, but may tip the balance towards respiratory failure in patients with severe disease. These effects include mucosal irritation by anaesthetic agents, ciliary paralysis, introduction of infection by aspiration or tracheal intubation and respiratory depression by relaxants, opioid analgesics or volatile anaesthetic agents. In addition, anaesthesia is associated with a decrease in FRC, especially in the elderly and in obese patients, which leads to basal airways closure and shunting of blood through underventilated areas of lung, an effect which is magnified by inhibition of the hypoxic pulmonary vasoconstrictor reflex.

Following recovery from anaesthesia, residual concentrations of anaesthetic agents inhibit the hyperventilatory responses to both hypercapnia and hypoxaemia, so that without close monitoring, e.g. with pulse oximetry, serious hypoxaemia and hypercapnia may occur.

Following thoracic and upper abdominal surgery, the decrease in FRC is more profound and persists for 5–10 days after surgery, with a parallel increase in alveolar–arterial oxygen tension difference ($P_{A-a}O_2$; see Fig. 41.3). Complications including atelectasis and pneumonia occur in approximately 20% of these patients. Clearly, patients with pre-existing respiratory disease are at much greater risk following upper abdominal surgery than after limb, head and neck or lower abdominal surgery.

Laparoscopic surgery

The use of laparoscopic techniques for cholecystectomy, fundoplication and other abdominal procedures has markedly reduced postoperative pulmonary morbidity, with the result that patients with severe pulmonary disease can usually undergo these procedures without the need for postoperative ventilatory support. The reasons for reduced morbidity include the relative lack of postoperative pain and the preservation of lung volumes postoperatively. These techniques should be encouraged in patients with chronic pulmonary disease. Nevertheless, cardiopulmonary function may be considerably compromised intraoperatively, and judicious use of invasive monitoring has been recommended in patients with severe cardiorespiratory disease.

CHRONIC OBSTRUCTIVE PULMONARY DISEASE

Chronic bronchitis is characterized by the presence of productive cough for at least 3 months in two successive years. Airways obstruction is caused by bronchoconstriction, bronchial oedema and hypersecretion of mucus. In the postoperative period, pulmonary atelectasis and pneumonia result if sputum is not cleared. COPD may be classified into two groups – the bronchitis group (blue bloaters) and the emphysematous group (pink puffers) – although in practice most patients have mixed pathologies. The former group is characterized by hypoxaemia, hypercapnia and right ventricular failure, while patients in the latter group are usually markedly dyspnoeic.

Preoperative management

This should include the following:

Detection and treatment of active infection. Amoxycillin, co-amoxiclav or ceftriaxone are usually appropriate, the common infecting organisms being *Streptococcus pneumoniae* and *Haemophilus influenzae*. Sputum for culture and sensitivities should be obtained to allow an appropriate choice of antibiotic. Chest physiotherapy and humidification of inspired gases aid expectoration.

Treatment of airways obstruction. Some patients respond to bronchodilator therapy with a β_2-agonist (e.g. salbutamol), anticholinergic agent (e.g. ipratropium bromide) or phosphodiesterase inhibitor (e.g. aminophylline). Existing bronchodilator therapy should be continued perioperatively, while in patients receiving no bronchodilator, a trial of oral aminophylline (Phyllocontin) 225 mg b.d. and salbutamol 200 µg or ipratropium 40 µg (two puffs) by inhalation may decrease airways obstruction. Steroids may occasionally improve airways obstruction.

Chest X-ray examination should be carried out to exclude spontaneous pneumothorax or emphysematous bullae.

Assessment of the patient's ventilatory response to carbon dioxide can be made by serial blood gas estimation with different levels of fractional inspired concentration of oxygen (F_IO_2). Patients dependent on a hypoxic stimulus can thus be recognized preoperatively.

Treatment of cardiac failure. Biventricular failure resulting from concurrent ischaemic heart disease and cor pulmonale frequently complicates chronic pulmonary disease. Diuretics are indicated, while nitrates or digoxin may have a role.

Weight reduction should be encouraged before elective surgery in obese patients with respiratory disease.

Smoking. Ideally, smoking should be stopped for at least 6 weeks before elective surgery.

Premedication

Opioids should be avoided if severe disease exists. Atropine is useful if copious secretions are present. Temazepam is satisfactory to allay anxiety.

Regional anaesthesia

Regional anaesthesia for operations on the head, neck or limbs offers freedom from respiratory side-effects, while avoiding the complications of general anaesthesia. For brachial plexus blockade, the axillary route is preferred in these patients to avoid the possible complications of pneumothorax associated with the supraclavicular route and phrenic nerve blockade with the interscalene approach. Low subarachnoid or epidural anaesthesia for lower abdominal and pelvic surgery have a similar advantage. However, if the block is sufficiently high to affect the intercostal muscles, peak expiratory flow rate is reduced and the ability to expectorate is impaired. Overall, the morbidity resulting from general anaesthesia for such operations is low, and it is only perhaps in the respiratory cripple that any significant advantage accrues from the use of a regional technique. In these patients, sedation should be kept to a minimum.

In upper abdominal and thoracic surgery, where changes in respiratory function are more profound and prolonged, there is no evidence that epidural anaesthesia is associated with lower morbidity than general anaesthesia. The advantages accruing from avoidance of volatile anaesthetics, muscle relaxants and opioids are balanced by the effect of epidural blockade on expiratory muscles, decreasing vital capacity. However, the use of epidural analgesia postoperatively allows pain-free coughing and clearing of secretions. Furthermore, it may reduce postoperative hypoxaemia by diminishing the decrease in FRC, and its use may result in fewer pulmonary complications.

General anaesthesia

Two approaches may be taken in the presence of severe COPD.

Elective spontaneous ventilation

This involves using minimal sedation, avoiding opioid analgesics and maintaining spontaneous ventilation, usually with a face mask or laryngeal mask airway. Tolerance to tracheal intubation is improved by spraying the larynx with local anaesthetic solution. Analgesia is best provided by a local or regional technique.

Elective mechanical ventilation

A deliberate decision is made to undertake intermittent positive-pressure ventilation (IPPV) during anaesthesia and for a variable period after operation, at least until elimination of muscle relaxants and anaesthetic agents has occurred. This also permits optimal provision of analgesia without fear of opioid-induced depression of ventilation. This technique is usually preferred if the preoperative P_aCO_2 is greater than 6.7 kPa (50 mmHg) or if major thoracic or abdominal surgery is planned. After surgery, salt and water retention occurs and, in combination with over-enthusiastic fluid administration, and perhaps a decrease in cardiac output, may result in an increase in lung water, which in turn may cause small airways closure and hypoxaemia.

There is an increased risk of pneumothorax, especially if high inflation pressures are used.

Postoperative care

Postoperative care of the patient with severe COPD should be conducted in a HDU or ICU.

Elective postoperative controlled ventilation allows adequate oxygenation, analgesia without respiratory depression, clearance of secretions by physiotherapy, tracheal suction and, if necessary, fibreoptic bronchoscopy. Cardiac output and peripheral perfusion should be optimized before restoration of spontaneous ventilation. Unless there is pre-existing pulmonary infection, a period of 24 h of elective controlled ventilation is usually adequate. Institution of analgesia by regional (e.g. paravertebral or epidural) blockade often allows earlier return to spontaneous ventilation when the respiratory-depressant effects of anaesthetics and relaxants have terminated.

Oxygen

With spontaneous ventilation, controlled oxygen is required using a 24 or 28% Ventimask with frequent checks on arterial blood gases to ensure an adequate P_aO_2 (> 8 kPa) without excessive carbon dioxide retention (P_aCO_2 < 7.5–8 kPa). Using a pulse oximeter, the F_IO_2 can be titrated to achieve an S_pO_2 of around 90%. Hypoxaemia may seriously aggravate existing pulmonary hypertension and precipitate right ventricular failure.

Analgesia

Simple, non-opioid analgesics and/or local and regional techniques should be used if possible. Non-steroidal anti-inflammatory drugs (NSAIDs) such as diclofenac and piroxicam are useful in reducing the opioid requirements following major surgery, and may be adequate on their own after minor surgery. Fifty per cent nitrous oxide in oxygen (Entonox) is useful for physiotherapy and painful procedures. Opioid analgesics are best administered, where necessary, in small i.v. doses, e.g. morphine 2 mg, under direct supervision, or using patient-controlled analgesia. Physiotherapy, bronchodilators and antibiotics should be continued postoperatively. Doxapram by infusion (2 mg kg^{-1} over a period of 30 min to 4 h) may decrease marginally the extent of postoperative alveolar collapse and infection, although the evidence for this is controversial.

A technique of percutaneous cricothyroid puncture and insertion of a small-diameter tube into the trachea (minitracheotomy) permits aspiration of secretions while preserving the ability of the patient to cough and speak.

The application of CPAP via a close-fitting face mask in the spontaneously breathing patient increases FRC and reduces the incidence of atelectasis in postoperative patients with pulmonary disease. It may reduce the need for mechanical ventilation, although it is not tolerated by all patients. Intermittent positive pressure breathing using face mask or mouth piece also expands the lungs and aids clearance of secretions.

RESTRICTIVE LUNG DISEASE

This category includes a wide range of conditions which affect the lung and chest wall. Lung diseases include sarcoidosis and fibrosing alveolitis, while lesions of chest wall include kyphoscoliosis and ankylosing spondylitis. Pulmonary function tests reveal a decrease in both FEV_1 and FVC, with a normal $FEV_{1.0}$/FVC ratio and a decreased FRC and total lung capacity (TLC). Small airways closure occurs during tidal ventilation, with resultant shunting and hypoxaemia. Lung or chest wall compliance is decreased; thus, the work of breathing is increased and the ability to cough and clear secretions is impaired. There is an increased risk of postoperative pulmonary infection.

Anaesthesia causes little additional decrease in lung volumes and is tolerated well, provided that hypoxaemia is avoided. Postoperatively, however, inadequate basal ventilation and retention of secretions may occur, partly as a result of pain, opioid analgesics and the residual effects of anaesthetic agents. High concentrations of oxygen may be used without risk of respiratory depression. A short period of mechanical ventilation may be necessary in patients with severe disease to allow adequate analgesia and clearing of secretions. High epidural anaesthesia should be avoided in these patients as it causes a further reduction in vital capacity.

BRONCHIECTASIS

The patient should be admitted several days before surgery and regular postural drainage carried out. Appropriate antibiotics, based on sputum culture, should be prescribed. Disease localized in one lung should be isolated using a double-lumen tube.

BRONCHIAL CARCINOMA

Patients with bronchial carcinoma frequently suffer from coexisting chronic bronchitis. In addition, there may be infection and collapse of the lung distal to the tumour. Patients with bronchial carcinoma may have myasthenic syndrome (see p. 452), while oat-cell tumours may secrete a number of hormones, among the commonest being adrenocorticotrophic hormone (ACTH), producing Cushing's syndrome, and antidiuretic hormone (ADH), producing dilutional hyponatraemia (syndrome of inappropriate ADH secretion).

TUBERCULOSIS

Tuberculosis should be considered in patients with persistent pulmonary infection, especially if associated with haemoptysis or weight loss. If active disease is present, all anaesthetic equipment should be sterilized after use to avoid cross-infection of other patients.

BRONCHIAL ASTHMA

This common disease, which affects all age groups, is characterized by recurrent generalized reversible airways obstruction, caused by bronchial smooth-muscle spasm, mucus plugs and bronchial oedema. Asthma may be classified into two types: *extrinsic*, where an external allergen is demonstrable, and *intrinsic*. Intrinsic asthma tends to occur in adults, is more chronic and continuous and often requires long-term steroid therapy.

Preoperative management

The current state of the patient's disease is assessed by:

- *History* – frequency and severity of attacks, factors provoking attacks, drug history
- *Examination* – presence or absence of wheeze, prolonged expiratory phase, overdistension, evidence of infection

- *Pulmonary function tests* – peak expiratory flow rate or FEV_1/FVC before and after inhalation of bronchodilator. Blood gas analysis may be required in severe disease.

Elective surgery should not be undertaken until asthma is well-controlled. This involves the use of one or more of a number of drugs: inhaled β_2-adrenoceptor agonists, e.g. salbutamol; steroids, systemic or inhaled; oral phosphodiesterase inhibitors, e.g. aminophylline. In patients already on theophyllines, the plasma concentration should be checked. Pulmonary infection requires treatment where appropriate. A suitable bronchodilator regimen in the preoperative period comprises salbutamol 200 μg (two puffs) 4- to 6-hourly by inhaler, possibly in combination with oral aminophylline (Phyllocontin) 225 mg b.d. Patients with intrinsic asthma sometimes respond well to ipratropium bromide, an anticholinergic agent, 40 μg (two puffs) by inhaler. A dose of bronchodilator should be given with the premedication 1 h before induction of anaesthesia.

Patients with severe asthma who are receiving topical or systemic steroid therapy, or not responding to conventional bronchodilator therapy, require systemic steroid therapy to cover the anaesthetic and postoperative periods. Prednisolone 40–100 mg daily may be given preoperatively, with hydrocortisone 100 mg four times daily for the first postoperative day. An equivalent dose of oral prednisolone (Table 35.5) should be substituted when oral intake is resumed, and the dose gradually reduced as the severity of asthma permits.

Premedication should consist of a sedative agent, e.g. diazepam.

Anaesthesia

All volatile anaesthetic agents are bronchodilators, and are therefore well tolerated. Bronchoconstriction may be triggered by tracheal intubation or by surgical stimulation during light anaesthesia. The larynx and trachea should be sprayed with local anaesthetic and adequate depth of anaesthesia maintained. The use of the laryngeal mask airway can reduce stimulation of adverse airway reflexes. Drugs which are associated with histamine release (atracurium and morphine) are best avoided; vecuronium and fentanyl are preferable. β-Blocking drugs should also be avoided. With controlled ventilation, a prolonged expiratory phase is required if there is evidence of severe airways obstruction; the inspiratory time should be adequate to avoid unduly high inflation pressures. Pneumothorax is a possible complication and requires early detection and prompt drainage. Humidification is necessary if ventilation is prolonged.

Table 35.5 Equivalent doses of glucocorticoids

Glucocorticoid	Dose
Betamethasone	3mg
Cortisone acetate	100mg
Dexamethasone	3mg
Hydrocortisone	80mg
Methylprednisolone	16mg
Prednisolone	20mg
Prednisone	20mg
Triamcinolone	16mg

If bronchospasm occurs, it may result from easily remedied causes such as light anaesthesia or tracheal tube irritation, and these should be corrected. If bronchospasm persists, aminophylline 250–500 mg or salbutamol 125–250 μg should be administered by slow i.v. injection under ECG monitoring. The dose should be halved if the patient is receiving oral theophylline. Thereafter, an infusion of aminophylline, up to 0.5–0.8 mg kg^{-1} h^{-1}, or salbutamol, possibly in combination with nebulized salbutamol by positive-pressure ventilation (solution of 50–100 μg ml^{-1} of water), should be maintained until improvement occurs. Hydrocortisone 200 mg i.v. should be given simultaneously, although it has no immediate effect. Intravenous ketamine has also been used with success when other agents have failed to relieve acute bronchospasm.

Postoperative management consists of close respiratory monitoring, treatment of bronchospasm and provision of adequate analgesia, humidified oxygen and physiotherapy. Salbutamol is best administered by nebulization (2.5 mg in 2.5 ml saline 4- to 6-hourly) and aminophylline by i.v. infusion (0.5–0.8 mg kg^{-1} h^{-1}). The dose should be reduced if the patient is receiving oral theophylline. There is no loss of carbon dioxide responsiveness in asthmatic patients, and high inspired oxygen concentrations are tolerated well.

GASTROINTESTINAL DISEASE

DYSPHAGIA

Patients with dysphagia resulting from oesophageal stricture, tumour or achalasia may be severely malnourished and fluid-depleted. Fluid and electrolyte depletion should be corrected preoperatively, and anaesthetic drug doses should be reduced appropriately to avoid hypotension at induction of anaesthesia. There may be a considerable quantity of food debris in the oesophagus, and the standard approach with preoxygenation and a rapid-sequence induction of anaesthesia, with cricoid pressure, should be taken to avoid regurgitation and aspiration.

HIATUS HERNIA

There is a risk of regurgitation and inhalation of gastric contents, especially in the obese patient and in the lithotomy position. In addition to the usual measures to avoid aspiration, administration of a histamine H_2-receptor antagonist, e.g. ranitidine (150 mg on the night before surgery, followed by 150 mg with premedication), together with 0.3 mol L^{-1} sodium citrate 30 ml 5 min before induction may decrease the risk of pneumonitis if aspiration occurs.

INTESTINAL OBSTRUCTION

The principal anaesthetic problems in these patients are extreme fluid and electrolyte depletion with consequent risk of cardiovascular collapse on induction of anaesthesia, and increased risk of vomiting and inhalation of gastric contents. A large nasogastric tube should be used to empty the stomach as effectively as possible before induction. A rapid-sequence induction with cricoid pressure is mandatory, but the dose of induction agent requires fine judgement.

Patients who have severe vomiting and diarrhoea also pose problems in relation to fluid and electrolyte depletion. All such patients undergoing surgery require appropriate fluid and electrolyte replacement preoperatively; the volume and composition depend on blood urea and electrolyte measurements and CVP monitoring.

Subarachnoid and epidural anaesthesia should be avoided if significant fluid depletion is suspected.

LIVER DISEASE

Anaesthesia and surgery may affect liver function adversely even in previously normal patients. Pre-existing liver dysfunction may have effects on the conduct of anaesthesia, e.g. on the metabolism of anaesthetic drugs.

Preoperative assessment should be directed towards detection of jaundice, ascites, oedema and signs of hepatic failure (encephalopathy with flapping tremor). Routine preoperative investigations should include a coagulation screen, measurement of haemoglobin concentration, white cell and platelet counts, and concentrations of serum bilirubin, alkaline phosphatase, transaminases, urea, electrolytes, proteins (including albumin) and blood sugar. Blood should also be taken to screen for viral hepatitis. Appropriate measures must be taken to protect theatre staff from possible contamination.

Particular problems relevant to the anaesthetist include the following:

Acid–base and fluid balance. Many patients are overloaded with fluid. Hypoalbuminaemia results in oedema and ascites, and predisposes to pulmonary oedema. Secondary hyperaldosteronism produces sodium retention (even though plasma sodium concentration may be low) and hypokalaemia. Diuretic therapy, often including spironolactone, may also affect serum potassium concentration. In hepatic failure, a combined respiratory and metabolic alkalosis may occur, which shifts the oxygen dissociation curve to the left, impairing tissue oxygenation.

Hepatorenal syndrome. This may be defined as acute renal failure developing in patients with pre-existing chronic liver failure. Jaundiced patients are at risk of developing postoperative renal failure. This may be precipitated by hypovolaemia. Prevention involves adequate preoperative hydration, with i.v. infusion for at least 12 h before surgery, and close monitoring of urine output, intra- and postoperatively. Intravenous 20% mannitol 100 ml is recommended immediately preoperatively and is indicated postoperatively if the hourly urine output decreases below 50 ml. Close cardiovascular monitoring is essential.

Bleeding problems. Production of clotting factors II, VII, IX and X is reduced as a result of decreased vitamin K absorption. Production of factor V and fibrinogen is also reduced. Thrombocytopenia occurs if portal hypertension is present. Vitamin K should be administered preoperatively and fresh frozen plasma given to provide clotting factors during surgery, with regular checks made on coagulation. Infusion of platelet concentrate is indicated to cover surgery in cases of severe thrombocytopenia (platelet count $< 50 \times 10^9$ L^{-1}) or if there is overt bleeding in a thrombocytopenic patient.

Drug metabolism. Impairment of liver function slows elimination of drugs, including anaesthetic induction agents, opioid analgesics, benzodiazepines, succinylcholine, local anaesthetic agents and many others. Since the duration of action of many of these drugs is determined initially by redistribution, prolongation of action may not become apparent until a subsequent dose has been given.

In addition, many drugs have toxic effects on the liver. Rarely, halothane is associated with postoperative hepatitis, usually when administered more than once within a period of a few weeks. The mechanism appears to be induction of reductive enzymes in the liver, which, in the presence of hypoxia, causes an increase in hepatotoxic reductive metabolites. Halothane should not be used within 3 months of a previous halothane anaesthetic or if there is a history of unexplained jaundice or abnormal liver function tests after any previous halothane anaesthetic. Enflurane and isoflurane have also been implicated in postoperative hepatic dysfunction.

Hepatic failure. In such patients, all sedative drugs should be administered with extreme care, as they aggravate encephalopathy. All opioids and benzodiazepines are eliminated by the liver. Benzodiazepines are probably the best sedatives to use in small doses, with midazolam being first choice. Patients with hepatic failure require management in an ICU, including invasive haemodynamic monitoring with an arterial cannula and a pulmonary artery catheter. The classic picture in the fluid-replete individual is of high cardiac output, warm peripheries and hypotension which often requires vasopressor therapy, e.g. norepinephrine. Careful metabolic, fluid and electrolyte monitoring is essential. Hypoglycaemia, which occurs as a result of depleted liver glycogen stores, should be avoided by the administration of glucose infusion, and sodium intake should be restricted. Amino acids, fat emulsions and fructose should be avoided. Patients are very vulnerable to infective complications, and close bacteriological surveillance should be maintained. Mechanical ventilation is often required, and this diminishes the risks of sedative administration. In hepatic coma, mechanical ventilation is mandatory and intracranial pressure monitoring should be considered even in the presence of coagulopathy. *N*-acetylcysteine may be of value, even when given late in paracetamol-induced hepatic failure, and there is preliminary evidence for its efficacy in other forms of fulminant hepatic failure.

Conduct of anaesthesia

If liver function is severely impaired, no premedication should be given. Otherwise, a light benzodiazepine premedication is suitable.

The liver is particularly vulnerable to hypovolaemia, hypotension and hypoxia. During anaesthesia, cardiac output should be kept as stable as possible. Blood loss should be replaced promptly, and overall fluid balance maintained with CVP monitoring. Drugs which depress cardiac output or arterial pressure, including volatile anaesthetic agents and β-blockers, should be used with caution to avoid decreasing hepatic blood flow unduly.

The muscle relaxants of choice are those with cardiovascular stability and a short duration of action; atracurium may be preferable because its elimination is independent of liver and renal function. Opioid analgesic drugs should be administered with caution unless ventilatory support is planned postoperatively. Pethidine may be preferable to morphine and is best titrated initially against pain in small i.v. doses, e.g. 20 mg, in the immediate postoperative period. NSAIDs should be avoided.

Controlled ventilation to a normal P_aCO_2 is important, as hypocapnia is associated with decreased hepatic blood flow. Hypoxaemia should be avoided throughout, and oxygen saturation should be monitored (with blood gas analysis if necessary) into the postoperative period. In the adequately volume-expanded patient hypotension can be reversed by infusion of norepinephrine. However, in the unstable patient, expert help should be sought and monitoring should include the measurement of cardiac output and PAOP with a PAFC.

RENAL DISEASE

Renal dysfunction has several important implications for anaesthesia, and therefore full assessment is required before even minor surgical procedures are contemplated.

Measurement of blood urea and electrolyte concentrations should be undertaken before all major surgery and in all elderly or potentially unhealthy patients; a raised blood urea concentration demonstrated preoperatively may be the first indication of renal disease. Severity of renal dysfunction may be assessed further by measurement of serum creatinine concentration and creatinine clearance, urinary:plasma osmolality ratio and urinary urea and electrolyte excretion (Table 35.6).

PRE-ANAESTHETIC ASSESSMENT

Pre-anaesthetic assessment of the patient should be directed to several specific problems which require correction before embarking on anaesthesia.

Fluid balance

In acute renal failure, fluid overload may develop suddenly and is uncompensated. In chronic renal failure, overload may be controlled with diuretic therapy or dialysis. Pulmonary oedema and hypertension may result from overload and must be treated before induction of anaesthesia. This may require dialysis or haemofiltration.

In patients with nephrotic syndrome, hypoalbuminaemia results in oedema and ascites. Circulating blood volume in these patients is often decreased, and care should be taken at induction of anaesthesia to avoid hypotension.

Electrolyte disturbances

Sodium retention occurs in renal failure, and through increased secretion of ADH is associated with water retention, oedema and hypertension.

Hyponatraemia is also common in renal disease. It is the result either of sodium losses through the kidney or gastrointestinal tract, or of water overload causing dilutional hyponatraemia. The renal tubules may have a reduced ability to conserve sodium (e.g. in pyelonephritis, analgesic nephropathy or recovering acute renal failure), or sodium may be lost through diuretic therapy, vomiting or diarrhoea. Dilutional hyponatraemia is caused by either inappropriate fluid administration (glucose 5%) or inappropriate ADH secretion, or both. Following transurethral prostatectomy, hyponatraemia may result from absorption of glycine irrigation fluid. Diagnosis of the cause of hyponatraemia involves measurement of urinary and plasma osmolality and urinary sodium concentration.

Hyperkalaemia occurs typically in renal failure, frequently in association with metabolic acidosis. It causes delayed myocardial conduction and, if untreated, leads to cardiac arrest in asystole or ventricular fibrillation.

Hyperkalaemia should be treated promptly when the serum potassium concentration exceeds 6 mmol L^{-1} or when ECG changes are evident:

1. Calcium chloride 10% up to 10–20 ml i.v. to antagonize the cardiac effects of hyperkalaemia, under ECG guidance.
2. Glucose 50%, 50 ml with 12 units of soluble insulin followed by an infusion of 20% glucose with insulin as required, depending on BM-test blood sugar estimation.
3. Sodium bicarbonate to correct the metabolic acidosis partly.
4. Haemodialysis or haemofiltration. The former is more effective in lowering serum potassium concentration rapidly, but haemofiltration may be more easily set up as an emergency in a general ICU.
5. An ion exchange resin (e.g. calcium polystyrene sulphonate 15 g t.i.d. orally or 30 g retention enema) provides longer-term control in chronic renal failure. Succinylcholine should be avoided in hyperkalaemic patients in view of its effect of releasing potassium from muscle cells. An increase of up to 0.6 mmol L^{-1} may be expected in normal dosage. Rocuronium may be a suitable alternative.

Hypokalaemia occurs commonly in patients receiving diuretic therapy. These patients require preoperative measurement of serum potassium concentration, and replacement if necessary. Hypokalaemia is associated with ventricular irritability, notably in patients taking digoxin.

Retention of phosphate and vitamin D depletion (1,25-dihydroxycholecalciferol) in chronic renal failure lead to hyperparathyroidism. The development of a parathyroid adenoma leads to hypercalcaemia (tertiary parathyroidism).

Table 35.6 Urinary measurements in prerenal and renal failure

Variable	Prerenal	Renal
Specific gravity	High > 1.020	1.010–1.012
Sodium	Low < 20 mmol L^{-1}	High > 40 mmol L^{-1}
U:P urea ratio	High > 20	Low < 10
U:P creatinine ratio	High > 40	Low < 10
U:P osmolality ratio	High > 2.1	Low < 1.2

U, urine; P, plasma

Cardiovascular effects

Hypertension may occur for several reasons. A raised plasma renin concentration secondary to decreased perfusion of the juxtaglomerular apparatus results in hypertension through increased secretion of angiotensin and aldosterone.

Fluid retention also causes hypertension by increasing the circulating blood volume. Conversely, hypertension from other causes results in renal impairment. The precise cause of hypertension in these patients should be sought and the hypertension treated. Anaesthesia for hypertensive patients is discussed on page 432.

Both pulmonary and peripheral oedema may occur from a combination of fluid overload, hypertensive cardiac disease and hypoproteinaemia. Cardiac failure should be treated preoperatively. Uraemia may cause pericarditis and a haemorrhagic pericardial effusion, which may embarrass cardiac output and require aspiration. Good control of blood urea with haemodialysis or haemofiltration will often prevent this complication and is essential for its resolution.

Neurological effects

Uraemia causes drowsiness and eventually coma. Electrolyte disturbances and rapid fluid shifts, e.g. during dialysis, may also affect conscious level by causing cerebral oedema. Sedative drugs, including morphine, should be used with care in these patients, as renally excreted metabolites accumulate. In addition, a combined motor and sensory peripheral neuropathy may occur in uraemic patients.

Haematology

Patients with chronic renal failure suffer from normochromic anaemia, which results from marrow depression, partly as a result of erythropoietin deficiency. They also have an increased incidence of gastrointestinal bleeding, and so an iron-deficiency component may be present. These patients are usually well compensated, with an increased cardiac output; excessive preoperative blood transfusion should be avoided.

Other factors

Patients with chronic renal failure are frequently undernourished. They tend to be vulnerable to infection. Patients who have received a renal transplant and are immunosuppressed are particularly vulnerable to opportunistic pathogens, e.g. *Pneumocystis carinii*. Patients undergoing chronic haemodialysis are occasionally carriers of hepatitis B antigen, and, if so, appropriate precautions should be taken by theatre staff.

Drug treatment

Many patients with renal disease are receiving diuretics, antihypertensive therapy including β-blockers and digoxin. The doses of drugs excreted renally (e.g. digoxin and aminoglycoside antibiotics) should be reduced; monitoring of plasma concentrations is essential in determining appropriate dosage.

The widespread use of NSAIDs both as analgesics and for arthritis has considerable implications for renal function. They inhibit vasodilator prostaglandin production in the kidney and thus reduce glomerular blood flow and sodium excretion, which may be critical in septic or shocked patients, or those undergoing surgery associated with major blood loss. Their use should be restricted in such high-risk patients.

ACE inhibitors dilate the post-glomerular arterioles in the kidney and thus reduce glomerular filtration pressure. They may therefore precipitate renal failure in hypotensive patients. Patients receiving these agents should be monitored carefully and fluid should be replaced adequately to avoid hypotension. It may be prudent to omit the immediate pre-anaesthetic dose in the high-risk patient. ACE inhibitors may also cause hyperkalaemia, particularly in patients with renal dysfunction.

ANAESTHESIA

A light premedication with benzodiazepine or opioid analgesic is satisfactory. Minor procedures, e.g. to establish vascular access for dialysis, are carried out most satisfactorily under regional anaesthesia: brachial plexus block for upper limb and combined femoral and sciatic block for lower limb.

Patients who suffer from acute renal failure, and those receiving long-term dialysis for chronic renal failure, may require dialysis before surgery to correct fluid overload, acid–base disturbances and hyperkalaemia. Ideally, there should be some delay before surgery to allow correction of anticoagulation.

The i.v. cannula for induction and fluid infusion should be sited in the contralateral limb from the arteriovenous shunt or fistula (in patients undergoing dialysis) and care should be taken to protect the fistula during the operation. Careful monitoring of arterial pressure and ECG is required, and CVP measurement is indicated in patients who are clinically overloaded with fluid. Intravenous fluid administration should be cautious, and in some instances titrated against CVP measurements. Excessive sodium administration should be avoided, and potassium-containing solutions completely avoided in renal failure. If the patient is anaemic preoperatively, intraoperative blood loss should be replaced promptly.

Drugs excreted primarily via the kidneys should be used with caution in renal failure. In anaesthetic practice, the principal drugs involved are the muscle relaxants. Atracurium (elimination of which is independent of kidney and liver function, and which has minimal cardiovascular effects) is the relaxant of choice. All other relaxants depend to some extent on renal elimination and should be avoided. In addition, many drugs, including morphine, are conjugated in the liver before excretion in the urine. Depending on the activity of the conjugated metabolite, these drugs may have adverse effects following repeated doses. Morphine-6-glucuronide, an active metabolite of morphine, accumulates in renal failure and may result in prolongation of clinical effects after administration of morphine.

Enflurane is partly metabolized to fluoride ion, which affects the concentrating ability of the kidney through an effect on the distal tubule, and should be used with caution in patients with severe renal impairment. Isoflurane, which undergoes minimal metabolism in the body, is currently the volatile agent of choice in renal disease, although desflurane, which is metabolized even less, is also suitable.

POSTOPERATIVE RENAL FAILURE

In the absence of severe sepsis or pre-existing renal dysfunction, this is now relatively uncommon. In patients undergoing major surgery which involves large blood loss, in surgery following trauma and in most septic patients, avoidance of renal failure involves close monitoring of the cardiovascular state, including CVP and urinary output, avoidance of hypoxaemia and hypotension, and adequate fluid and blood replacement. In many instances, e.g. in patients with pre-existing renal dysfunction, shock, sepsis or liver disease, a pulmonary artery catheter is required to optimize cardiac output and oxygen delivery, and to guide vasoactive drug therapy. Low-dose (2–5 μg kg^{-1} min^{-1}) dopamine is frequently recommended to prevent renal failure in such situations, but its efficacy is unproven and its use may confuse the situation by inducing diuresis through stimulation of dopaminergic receptors in the renal tubules. The only proven therapy in the prevention and early treatment of acute renal failure is adequate fluid resuscitation titrated against CVP or PAOP, and maintenance of an adequate cardiac output and mean arterial pressure (> 80 mmHg).

Other measures, such as use of an osmotic diuretic (mannitol 100 ml of 20% solution over 15 min) or loop diuretic (furosemide by bolus or infusion), are of doubtful value. Mannitol continues to be recommended in jaundiced patients at risk of developing the hepatorenal syndrome, and in patients with rhabdomyolysis. In some cases of oliguric acute renal failure, where resuscitation has failed to achieve diuresis, furosamide i.v. does appear to 'kick-start' a urine output which is then maintained.

Postoperative oliguria may also be the result of postrenal causes. Patients with prostatic enlargement are particularly liable to develop acute urinary retention. Examination to exclude a full bladder and catheterization should always be carried out in the anuric postoperative patient. Abdominal ultrasound may be useful in more complicated cases.

CONNECTIVE TISSUE DISORDERS

RHEUMATOID ARTHRITIS

Rheumatoid arthritis is a multisystem disease, with a number of implications for anaesthesia which must be considered at the time of preoperative assessment.

Airway problems. The arthritic process may involve the temporomandibular joints, rendering laryngoscopy and intubation difficult. The cervical spine may be fixed or subluxed, and thus unstable, especially when the patient is anaesthetized and paralysed. Cricoarytenoid involvement should be suspected if hoarseness or stridor is present.

Respiratory function. Costochondral involvement causes a restrictive defect with reduced vital capacity. Pulmonary involvement with interstitial fibrosis produces ventilation/perfusion ($\dot{V}/\dot{Q}$) abnormalities, a diffusion defect and thus hypoxaemia.

Cardiovascular system. Endocardial and myocardial involvement may occur. Coronary arteritis, conduction defects and peripheral arteritis are other uncommon features. Immobility caused by arthritis may mask symptoms of cardiorespiratory disease.

Anaemia. A chronic anaemia, hypo- or normochromic, but refractory to iron, occurs. Preoperative transfusion to a haemoglobin concentration of approximately 10g dl^{-1} is advisable before major surgery. Treatment with salicylates or other NSAIDs may cause gastrointestinal blood loss.

Renal failure, or nephrotic syndrome, may occur as a result of amyloidosis or drug treatment.

Steroid therapy. Many patients are receiving long-term steroid therapy and require augmented steroid cover for the perioperative period (see p. 447). They are more vulnerable to postoperative infection.

Routine preoperative investigation should include full blood count, urea and electrolytes, chest X-ray, cervical spine X-ray and ECG. Other investigations, e.g. pulmonary function tests, may be required in some instances.

Conduct of anaesthesia

Particular care should be taken with venepuncture and placing of i.v. infusions because of atrophy of skin and subcutaneous tissues and fragility of veins. Careful positioning of the patient on the operating table is required because these patients may have multiple joint involvement. Padding may be required to prevent pressure sores.

The anaesthetist should be prepared for difficult intubation; spinal, epidural or regional techniques are useful for many limb or lower abdominal operations because they obviate the need for tracheal intubation. Where intubation is essential, an awake fibreoptic-assisted intubation may be the technique of choice.

OTHER CONNECTIVE TISSUE DISEASES

Connective tissue diseases can present in many ways. Their manifestations include vasculitis, glomerulonephritis, pulmonary fibrosis, arthropathies and myocarditis or pericarditis. The diffuse nature of the vasculitis may also result in neurological involvement. Steroid and immunosuppressive therapy are other potential problems.

Scleroderma

Scleroderma (systemic sclerosis) is characterized by many of the above features, including restricted mouth opening, lower oesophageal involvement with increased risk of regurgitation, pulmonary involvement, renal failure, steroid therapy and peripheral vascular disease.

Systemic lupus erythematosus

Anaemia, renal and respiratory involvement may be severe. Cardiac involvement may include mitral valve disease. Steroid therapy is usual.

Ankylosing spondylitis

The rigid spine makes intubation difficult, and spinal and epidural anaesthesia may be technically impossible. Costovertebral joint involvement restricts chest expansion.

Marfan's syndrome

This is a disorder of connective tissue of autosomal dominant inheritance, which is characterized by long, thin extremities, high arched palate, lens subluxation and aortic and mitral regurgitation. Regurgitation may be severe, and the valve lesions may be complicated by infective endocarditis. Antibiotic cover is necessary for dental and other surgical procedures.

NUTRITIONAL PROBLEMS

OBESITY

Obesity poses several problems to the anaesthetist and surgeon.

Cardiovascular function. Obesity is associated with increased blood volume, increased cardiac work, hypertension and cardiomegaly. Atherosclerosis and coronary artery disease are common. Diabetes mellitus may coexist.

Respiratory function. Vital capacity and FRC are decreased. Closing volume is increased. As a result, increased shunting occurs through underventilated, dependent lung regions, with consequent hypoxaemia. These changes, brought about by abdominal splinting of the diaphragm, are accentuated in the supine, Trendelenburg and lithotomy positions. Total thoracic compliance is decreased, the work of breathing increased, and increased oxygen consumption and carbon dioxide production cause hyperventilation.

Other factors. There may be difficulty in achieving venous access, and blood pressure measurement may be inaccurate unless the appropriate size of cuff is used. Assessment of volume state is generally more difficult. Surgery is technically more difficult, with heavy blood loss and increased incidences of wound infection and wound dehiscence. Hiatus hernia with risk of regurgitation is more common, and maintenance of the airway and tracheal intubation may be more difficult.

Obese patients require careful preoperative respiratory and cardiovascular assessment (see Ch. 34). The inspired oxygen fraction should be increased to 0.4. Fluid balance should be monitored carefully. Elective postoperative ventilation should be considered, especially after abdominal surgery. Pulmonary, thromboembolic and wound complications are more common, and appropriate prophylactic measures and/or early recognition and treatment are important.

PICKWICKIAN SYNDROME

Pickwickian syndrome is characterized by a combination of obesity, episodic somnolence and hypoventilation with cyanosis, polycythaemia, pulmonary hypertension and right ventricular failure. Avoidance of hypoxaemia is important, and elective postoperative ventilation may be necessary, especially after abdominal surgery.

MALNUTRITION

As a result of persistent anorexia, dysphagia or vomiting, malnourished patients may have severe depletion of fluid and electrolytes. Anaemia and hypoproteinaemia are common. The anaemia may result from iron, vitamin B_{12} or folate deficiency, and if megaloblastic in nature, it may be associated with thrombocytopenia.

Preoperative correction of fluid and electrolyte deficits is required, with CVP monitoring in severe cases. Infusion of albumin may be advisable in some instances to raise the colloid osmotic pressure. A multivitamin preparation should be administered in view of probable thiamine deficiency. Induction agents should be administered carefully to avoid hypotension, while smaller doses of relaxants are required.

ENDOCRINE DISEASE

PITUITARY DISEASE

The clinical features of pituitary disease depend on the local effects of the lesion and its effects on the secretion of pituitary hormones. Local effects include headache and visual field disturbances. The effects on hormone secretion depend on the cells involved in the pathological process.

Acromegaly

Acromegaly is caused by increased secretion of growth hormone from eosinophil cell tumours of the anterior pituitary gland. If this occurs before fusion of the epiphyses, gigantism results. Problems for the anaesthetist include the following:

- Upper airway obstruction may result from an enlarged mandible, tongue and epiglottis, thickened pharyngeal mucosa and laryngeal narrowing. Maintenance of a clear airway and tracheal intubation may be difficult, and postoperative care of the airway must be meticulous.
- Cardiac enlargement, hypertension and congestive cardiac failure occur commonly and require preoperative treatment.
- Growth hormone increases blood sugar concentration. Hyperglycaemia should be controlled perioperatively.
- Thyroid and adrenal function may be impaired because of decreased release of thyroid-stimulating hormone (TSH) and ACTH. Thyroxine and steroid replacement may be required.

Treatment involves hypophysectomy, which requires steroid cover preoperatively, and steroid, thyroxine and possibly ADH replacement thereafter.

Cushing's disease

Cushing's disease results from basophil adenomas, which secrete ACTH (see below).

Hypopituitarism (Simmonds' disease)

Causes include chromophobe adenoma, tumours of surrounding tissues (e.g. craniopharyngioma), skull fractures, infarction following postpartum haemorrhage and infection. Clinical features include loss of axillary and pubic hair, amenorrhoea, features of hypothyroidism and adrenal insufficiency, including hypotension, but with a striking pallor, in contrast to the pigmentation of Addison's disease (see p. 447).

The fluid and electrolyte disturbances are not as marked as in primary adrenal failure as a result of intact aldosterone production, but may be unmasked by surgery, trauma or infection. Anaesthesia in these patients requires steroid cover (p. 447), cautious administration of induction agent and volatile anaesthetic agents, and careful cardiovascular monitoring.

Diabetes insipidus

This is caused by disease or damage affecting the hypothalamic–posterior pituitary axis. Common causes are pituitary tumours, craniopharyngiomas, basal skull fracture and infection, or it may occur as a sequel to pituitary surgery. In 10% of cases, diabetes insipidus is renal in origin.

Dehydration with hypernatraemia follows excretion of large volumes of dilute urine. Patients require fluid replacement and treatment with vasopressin (DDAVP; desmopressin 2–4 μg i.m. daily or 1 μg i.v. in the acute situation).

THYROID DISEASE

Goitre

Thyroid swelling may result from iodine deficiency (simple goitre), autoimmune (Hashimoto's) thyroiditis, adenoma, carcinoma or thyrotoxicosis. Nodules of the thyroid gland may be 'hot' (secreting thyroxine) or 'cold'.

The goitre may occasionally cause respiratory obstruction. Retrosternal goitre may in addition cause superior vena caval obstruction. The presence of a goitre should alert the anaesthetist to the possibility of tracheal compression or displacement. A preoperative X-ray of neck and thoracic inlet may be useful, and a selection of small-diameter, armoured tracheal tubes should be available. Preoperative assessment of thyroid function is essential.

Thyrotoxicosis

This is characterized by excitability, tremor, tachycardia and arrhythmias (commonly atrial fibrillation), weight loss, heat intolerance and exophthalmos. Diagnosis is confirmed by measurement of total serum thyroxine, tri-iodothyronine (T_3) and TSH concentrations.

Elective surgery should not be carried out in hyperthyroid patients; they should first be rendered euthyroid with carbimazole or radioactive iodine. However, urgent surgery and elective subtotal thyroidectomy may be carried out safely in hyperthyroid patients using β-adrenergic blockade alone or in combination with potassium iodide to control thyrotoxic symptoms and signs. Emergency surgery carries a significant risk of thyrotoxic crisis. Control is best achieved in these circumstances by i.v. potassium iodide and a broad-spectrum β-blocker (e.g. propranolol). If patients are unable to absorb oral medication, i.v. infusion is indicated (for propranolol, the daily i.v. dose is approximately one-tenth of the oral dose).

The doses of sedative drugs for premedication, and of anaesthetic agents, should be increased to compensate for faster distribution and elimination. Larger doses of sedative drugs than normal are required to avoid anxiety when procedures are carried out under regional anaesthesia.

Preparation for thyroidectomy

Previous conventional management involved at least 6–8 weeks' administration of carbimazole to render the patient euthyroid, followed by potassium iodide 60 mg t.i.d. for 10 days to decrease the vascularity of the gland.

Many anaesthetists now use β-blockers to prepare the hyperthyroid patient for thyroidectomy. Propranolol 160–480 mg daily for 2 weeks preoperatively and a further 7–10 days postoperatively provides adequate control in most patients. However, control with β-blockers depends on maintaining an adequate plasma concentration of the drug. Since β-blockers, in common with other drugs, are cleared more rapidly than normal in thyrotoxic patients, propranolol should be prescribed more frequently (e.g. four times daily). Alternatively, a long-acting β-blocker, e.g. atenolol once daily (including the morning of surgery), provides satisfactory control and avoids the problem of impaired drug absorption immediately after operation. A combination of β-blocker and potassium iodide 60 mg t.i.d. provides reliable control in even the most severely thyrotoxic patient.

Hypothyroidism

This may result from primary thyroid failure, Hashimoto's thyroiditis, as a consequence of thyroid surgery, or secondary to pituitary failure. The diagnosis is suggested by tiredness, cold intolerance, loss of appetite, dry skin and hair loss. It may be confirmed by the finding of a low serum thyroxine concentration, associated, in primary thyroid failure, with a raised serum TSH concentration.

Basal metabolic rate is decreased. Cardiac output is decreased, with little myocardial reserve, and hypothermia may be present. Treatment is with thyroxine, which should be started in a small dose of 25–50 μg daily. Rapid correction of hypothyroidism may be achieved using i.v. T_3, but this is inadvisable in elderly patients and those with ischaemic heart disease, which is common in hypothyroidism, as the sudden increase in myocardial oxygen demand may provoke infarction. ECG monitoring is advisable during treatment. Elective surgery should be avoided in myxoedematous patients, but if emergency surgery is necessary, close cardiovascular, ECG and blood gas monitoring is essential. Drug distribution and metabolism are slowed, and thus all anaesthetic agents must be administered in reduced doses.

DISEASE OF THE ADRENAL CORTEX

Clinical symptoms are associated with increased or decreased secretion of cortisol or aldosterone.

Hypersecretion of cortisol (Cushing's syndrome)

Most instances are caused by pituitary adenomas which secrete ACTH and thus cause bilateral adrenocortical hyperplasia (Cushing's disease). In 20–30% of patients, an adrenocortical adenoma or carcinoma is present. Rarely, an oat-cell carcinoma of bronchus, secreting ACTH, is the cause. ACTH and corticosteroid therapy present similar pictures. Clinical features include obesity, hypertension, proximal myopathy and diabetes mellitus. Biochemically, there is a metabolic alkalosis with hypokalaemia. Depending on the cause, treatment may involve hypophysectomy or adrenalectomy.

Anaesthetic management of these patients involves preoperative treatment of hypertension and congestive cardiac failure, and correction of hypokalaemia. Intraoperative management is directed towards careful monitoring of arterial pressure and maintenance of cardiovascular stability, with careful choice and administration of anaesthetic agents and muscle relaxants. Etomidate and atracurium or vecuronium would be an appropriate choice of induction agent and relaxant. Postoperative steroid cover is required for hypophysectomy and adrenalectomy (see below).

Fludrocortisone 0.1–0.3 mg daily is required after bilateral adrenalectomy.

Primary hypersecretion of aldosterone (Conn's syndrome)

Conn's syndrome is caused by an adenoma of the zona glomerulosa of the adrenal cortex and presents with hypertension, hypernatraemia, hypokalaemia and oliguria. Anaesthetic management involves preoperative treatment of hypertension, the administration of spironolactone and potassium replacement; meticulous intra- and postoperative monitoring of arterial pressure is essential.

Adrenocortical hypofunction

Primary adrenocortical insufficiency (Addison's disease) may be caused by an autoimmune process, tuberculosis, amyloid, metastatic carcinoma, or bilateral adrenalectomy. Haemorrhage into the glands during meningococcal septicaemia may cause acute adrenal failure in association with septic shock. Secondary failure results from hypopituitarism or prolonged corticosteroid therapy. In secondary failure resulting from pituitary insufficiency, aldosterone secretion is maintained, and fluid and electrolyte disturbances are less marked.

Clinical features include weakness, weight loss, hyperpigmentation, hypotension, vomiting, diarrhoea and volume depletion. Hypoglycaemia, hyponatraemia, hyperkalaemia and metabolic acidosis are characteristic biochemical findings. The stress of infection, trauma or surgery provokes profound hypotension. Diagnosis is made by measurement of plasma cortisol concentrations and the response to ACTH stimulation.

All surgical procedures in these patients must be covered by increased steroid administration (see below). Patients with acute adrenal insufficiency require urgent fluid and sodium replacement with arterial pressure and CVP monitoring, glucose infusion to combat hypoglycaemia and hydrocortisone 100 mg 6-hourly i.v. Antibiotics are advisable to cover the possibility that infection has provoked the crisis. In cases of primary adrenal failure, mineralocorticoid replacement with fludrocortisone is required. If emergency surgery is required in acute adrenal failure, all precautions necessary for anaesthetizing the shocked patient should be taken (p. 619).

Congenital adrenal hyperplasia (adrenogenital syndrome)

This is associated with overproduction of androgens as a result of deficiency of the hydroxylase enzyme required for production of cortisol. Hydrocortisone treatment overcomes adrenal insufficiency and, by suppressing ACTH production, decreases androgen accumulation. Augmented steroid cover is required for surgery in these patients.

STEROID THERAPY

Replacement therapy in cases of primary adrenocortical failure and hypopituitarism is given as oral hydrocortisone 20 mg in the morning and 10 mg in the evening. Fludrocortisone 0.05–0.1 mg daily is given additionally to replace aldosterone in primary adrenocortical failure. Equivalent doses of other steroid preparations are shown in Table 35.5. Prednisolone and prednisone have less mineralocorticoid effect, while betamethasone and dexamethasone have none. Requirements increase following infection, trauma or surgery.

Corticosteroids are also prescribed for a wide range of medical conditions, including asthma and collagen diseases. Prolonged therapy suppresses adrenocortical function.

Steroid cover for anaesthesia and surgery

Indications for augmented perioperative steroid cover include the following:

- patients with pituitary–adrenal insufficiency, on steroid replacement therapy
- patients undergoing pituitary or adrenal surgery
- patients receiving systemic steroid therapy for more than 2 weeks before surgery
- patients receiving systemic steroid therapy for more than 1 month in the year before surgery.

Topical fluorinated steroid preparations applied widely to the skin and high-dose inhaled steroids may be absorbed sufficiently to produce adrenal suppression. Preoperative assessment should involve appropriate fluid and electrolyte correction. Evidence of infection should be sought in patients receiving long-term steroid therapy.

Corticosteroid cover for operation should be given as follows:

- minor diagnostic procedures – single dose of hydrocortisone 100 mg i.m. 1 h preoperatively
- intermediate operations (e.g. inguinal herniorrhaphy) – hydrocortisone 100 mg i.m. with premedication; 100 mg 6-hourly for 24 h
- major surgery – hydrocortisone 100 mg 6-hourly for 72 h starting with premedication.

The requirements may need to be increased if infection is present, or be continued beyond 3 days if infection or the effects of major trauma persist. Oral steroid preparations may be preferred for premedication and then resumed after 24 h.

If steroids are prescribed for asthma or other medical conditions, the perioperative dosage may require modification according to the activity of the disease.

DISEASE OF THE ADRENAL MEDULLA

Phaeochromocytoma

This is discussed on p. 675.

DIABETES MELLITUS

Fifty per cent of all diabetic patients present for surgery during their lifetime, most commonly for ophthalmic or vascular disease or for drainage of an abscess. Perioperative morbidity and mortality are greater in diabetic than in non-diabetic patients. This may result partly from controllable factors such as regulation of perioperative blood glucose concentration, but unavoidable complications of diabetes, such as ischaemic heart disease, autonomic neuropathy and infection, may affect anaesthetic management.

The problems of managing diabetics who undergo surgery are associated with its attendant period of starvation and the metabolic effects of surgery. The aim is to minimize the metabolic disturbance by ensuring an adequate intake of glucose, calories and insulin, thus controlling hyperglycaemia and reducing proteolysis, lipolysis and production of lactate and ketones. Adequate control of blood glucose concentration must be established preoperatively and maintained until oral feeding is resumed after operation. Hypoglycaemia, which may not be detectable readily in the anaesthetized patient, must be avoided. Modern techniques for frequent monitoring of blood glucose (Dextrostix, Ames: BM-Test-Glycemie, Boehringer-Mannheim, preferably used in conjunction with a reflectance colorimeter) have simplified management considerably.

Precise management depends upon the nature of the diabetes and its treatment (insulin-dependent or non-insulin-dependent), the magnitude of the surgery contemplated (including the estimated time to resumption of oral intake) and the time available for control of the diabetes.

PREOPERATIVE ASSESSMENT

Preoperative assessment is aimed at evaluating blood glucose control, the treatment regimen used and the presence of complications.

Control of blood glucose

This is assessed by inspection of the patient's urine-testing or BM-testing records, by random blood glucose measurements, by a 24 h blood glucose profile in patients receiving insulin, and by measurement of glycosylated haemoglobin (Hb A_{1c}). Whenever possible, blood glucose concentration should be maintained between 6 and 10 mmol L^{-1}, and insulin dosages should be adjusted to achieve this, with the introduction of twice-daily short- and intermediate-acting insulins if necessary. The serum potassium concentration may decrease on commencing insulin treatment and serum urea and electrolyte concentrations should be checked.

Treatment regimens

Oral hypoglycaemic agents are of two types. The sulphonylureas stimulate release of insulin from the pancreatic islets. Chlorpropamide has a very prolonged duration of action and may cause hypoglycaemia unless it is withdrawn 48 h before surgery. A change to a shorter-acting agent such as glipizide or gliclazide is preferable.

Biguanides, which increase peripheral uptake of glucose and decrease gluconeogenesis, are used in obese maturity-onset diabetics either alone or in combination with sulphonylureas. These agents may cause lactic acidosis, usually, but not exclusively, in patients with even mild renal or hepatic impairment. Guidelines for the administration of i.v. contrast media include the instructions to withhold metformin for 24 h before and 48 h after the investigation. Lactic acidosis carries a very high mortality; consequently, metformin, the only biguanide now available, should be discontinued at least 24 h before surgery.

The last dose of oral hypoglycaemic agent should be administered 24 h before surgery and no further treatment is required until the morning of surgery if blood glucose control is satisfactory.

Insulin

Some of the insulin preparations in common use are listed in Table 35.7. The best control is achieved by twice-daily injections of short- and intermediate-acting insulin. Increasingly, younger diabetics are managed with a background once-daily ultra-long-acting preparation coupled with a pen injector delivering small doses of short-acting insulin. The type of preparation must be noted, and if a change is made in the type of insulin (bovine, porcine, human) the dose must be adjusted, because increased sensitivity to the latter two may lead to hypoglycaemia. Insulin with the human sequence of amino acids is produced biosynthetically (chain recombinant DNA technology using bacteria, CRB) or semisyn-

Table 35.7 Newer insulin preparations

Proprietary name	Type and source	Onset (h)	Peak action (h)	Duration of action (h)	Dosage
Humulin S	Short-acting, soluble, CRB	0.5	1–3	5–7	t.i.d. alone or b.d. + intermediate preparation
Human Velosulin	Short-acting, soluble, EMP	0.5	1–3	8	
Actrapid MC	Short-acting, soluble, porcine	0.5	2–5	8	
Humulin I	Intermediate, isophane, CRB	1.0	2–8	18–20	b.d. + short-acting preparation
Insulatard	Intermediate, isophane, porcine	1.5	4–12	24	b.d. + short-acting preparation
Semitard	Insulin zinc suspension amorphous semilente, porcine	1.5	5–10	16	b.d. + short-acting preparation
Humulin M2	Mixed 20% soluble, 80% isophane, CRB	0.5	1–8	14–16	b.d.
Mixtard 30/70	Mixed 30% soluble, 70% isophane, porcine	0.5	4–8	24	b.d.
Monotard MC	Long-acting, insulin zinc suspension, 30% amorphous, 70% crystalline, lente, porcine	2.5	7–15	22	daily or b.d.
Humulin Zn	Long-acting, insulin zinc suspension, crystalline CRB	3.0	6–14	20–24	daily or b.d.

CRB, chain recombinant DNA technology using bacteria; EMP, enzyme modification of porcine material.

thetically (by enzyme modification of porcine material, EMP) from purified porcine insulin. The biosynthetic preparations are less expensive than purified porcine preparations and may become the principal commercial preparations. Insulin with the human sequence is associated with a less severe degree of antigenicity and is thus the preparation of choice for newly diagnosed diabetics and for patients requiring short-term therapy (e.g. in the perioperative period).

In well-controlled diabetics, it is not necessary to change to a short-acting insulin regimen on the day before surgery, provided that the dose of the intermediate- or long-acting insulin is not excessive (40 units of long-acting or 24-unit evening dose of intermediate insulin); all too often a change of regimen results in poorer control.

The poorly controlled diabetic

Whether the patient is normally insulin-dependent or not, elective surgery should be delayed until improved control is achieved by administration of short-acting insulin three times daily. If surgery is urgent, a glucose, insulin and potassium regimen (Table 35.8) should be instituted to achieve rapid blood glucose control.

Complications of diabetes mellitus

Cardiovascular disorders (coronary artery, cerebrovascular and peripheral vascular) are common in diabetics, and there is an increased risk of perioperative myocardial infarction. Careful preoperative assessment of cardiovascular function, appropriate choice of anaesthetic technique and precise perioperative monitoring are essential.

Renal disease. Microvascular damage produces glomerulosclerosis with proteinuria, oedema and eventually chronic renal failure. Anaesthetic implications of renal disease are discussed on page 442.

Table 35.8 Perioperative management of the mature-onset diabetic

Preoperative	
Check random glucose, urea and electrolyte concentrations:	
Poor control:	Start insulin (t.i.d. soluble) and delay surgery
	Urgent surgery: glucose insulin infusion (Table 35.9)
Good control:	Chlorpropamide – change to a shorter acting agent
	All agents terminated 24 h preoperatively
Day of surgery	
Check fasting blood glucose (BM stix, Dextrostix)	
No oral hypoglycaemic agent	
Minor surgery:	If blood glucose < 10 mmol L^{-1}, no specific therapy
Major surgery:	Treat as insulin-dependent diabetic (Table 35.9)
Postoperative	
Check blood glucose (BM stix, Dextrostix)	
Minor surgery:	Restart oral hypoglycaemic agent with first meal
Major surgery:	Treat as insulin-dependent diabetic (Table 35.9)
	When oral diet is resumed, t.i.d. soluble insulin 8–12 units before each meal; restart oral therapy when daily requirement is less than 20 units

Ocular problems. Cataracts, exudative or proliferative retinopathy, vitreous haemorrhage and retinal detachment may occur. In the long term, good blood glucose control has been shown to reduce the frequency of such complications.

Infection. Diabetics are prone to infection and an increased risk of septicaemia and abscess formation. Infection is associated with increased insulin requirements, which return to normal on its eradication, e.g. after surgical drainage of an abscess.

Neuropathy. Chronic sensory peripheral neuropathies are common; mononeuropathies and acute motor neuropathies (amyotrophy) are associated with poor control of blood glucose. Loss of sensation together with peripheral vascular disease can lead to ulceration after trivial trauma; consequently, care in positioning patients in the operating theatre is important. Local anaesthetic nerve or plexus blocks should be avoided in patients with an acute neuropathy, as neurological deficits may be attributed to the local anaesthetic solution.

Autonomic neuropathy may cause postoperative urinary retention or vasomotor instability, e.g. postural hypotension or hypotension during anaesthesia. IPPV or subarachnoid or epidural block may be associated with severe hypotension; adequate preoperative volume resuscitation, precise cardiovascular monitoring and careful anaesthetic management are essential.

Concurrent drug therapy

Thiazide diuretics, diazoxide, adrenergic agents (e.g. salbutamol) and corticosteroids tend to increase the blood glucose concentration. Hypotensive drugs, e.g. β-adrenergic blockers, tend to potentiate hypoglycaemia and may mask its clinical signs. Blood glucose concentrations should be monitored if any of these drugs is administered, and insulin dosage altered accordingly.

Some drugs, including phenylbutazone, displace sulphonylureas from protein-binding sites and potentiate their hypoglycaemic effect.

PERIOPERATIVE DIABETIC MANAGEMENT

A combination of glucose and insulin is the most satisfactory method of overcoming the deleterious metabolic consequences of starvation and surgical stress in the diabetic patient.

Although satisfactory control of blood glucose may be achieved using a no-glucose/no-insulin regimen, the raised blood urea concentration which often occurs in the postoperative period is indicative of increased protein breakdown, accompanying lipolysis and ketosis. Minor procedures may be carried out at the start of an operating list by delaying the morning dose of insulin until a late breakfast is taken after recovery from anaesthesia. A low-dose insulin infusion on its own (0.5 unit h^{-1} by syringe pump) is effective for minor surgery, but is not adequate for major surgery.

Subarachnoid and epidural anaesthesia have some advantages in the diabetic patient; avoidance of general anaesthesia allows hypoglycaemia to be recognized, while early resumption of oral diet eases postoperative management.

Tables 35.8 and 35.9 (both of which are based on Alberti's recommendations) describe schemes for the precise management of patients receiving oral hypoglycaemic agents or insulin therapy who require minor or major surgery. Minor surgery includes endoscopic procedures and body-surface surgery.

The combination of i.v. glucose solution with insulin added to the bag is a safety precaution; one cannot be infused inadvertently without the other, and thus hyperglycaemia, and more particularly hypoglycaemia, are avoided. Glucose 10% is used to provide adequate carbohydrate and energy without excessive volume. The glucose/insulin solution should be administered through an i.v. cannula separate from that used for other i.v. fluids; it is preferable to use an infusion pump to regulate the rate of infusion.

This scheme provides 250 g of glucose (1000 kcal) and an average of 50 units of insulin over 24 h. If the patient has high insulin demands normally or is obese, additional insulin may be required (e.g. 5 units per bag more than the amount stated in Table 35.9). Patients who normally receive oral hypoglycaemic agents may be more sensitive and require less insulin.

Blood transfusion may increase insulin requirements as the elevated citrate concentration stimulates gluconeogenesis. Ringer's lactate (Hartmann's) solution elevates blood glucose concentration for the same reason and should be avoided.

It is now common practice to control blood glucose concentration using a separate insulin infusion delivered by a syringe pump, with regulation of the insulin infusion rate determined by 2-hourly blood glucose measurements (Table 35.10).

Emergency surgery and diabetic ketoacidosis

Diabetic ketoacidosis results from inadequate insulin dosage or increased insulin requirements, often precipitated by infection, trauma or surgical stress. Diabetics who require emergency surgery often have a grossly elevated blood glucose concentration and occasionally overt ketoacidosis. Such patients require rehydration, correction of sodium depletion, correction of subsequent potassium depletion and i.v. soluble (Humulin S) insulin by infusion at an initial rate of 4–8 unit h^{-1}.

Initial fluid replacement should consist of isotonic (0.9%) saline: 1 L in the first 30 min, 1 L in the next hour and a further 1 L over the next 2 h.

Progress is monitored by regular measurements of blood glucose, sodium and potassium concentrations, and arterial pH and blood gas tensions. Correction of acidosis with bicarbonate is rarely, if ever, required. Cellular potassium depletion is present from the outset, but hyperkalaemia or normokalaemia may be found initially because potassium shifts out of the cells in the presence of acidosis. Potassium replacement is required as the plasma concentration begins to decrease with the correction of the acidosis. Magnesium 5–10 mmol is also required. An infusion of glucose 5% should be given when the blood glucose concentration decreases to approximately 15 mmol L^{-1}. When volume resuscitation is under way, and some reversal of acidosis and hyperglycaemia has been achieved, surgery may be carried out while management of the diabetes is continued intra- and postoperatively.

Table 35.9 Perioperative management of the insulin-dependent diabetic

Preoperative
Blood glucose profile; urea and electrolytes; urine ketones
Adjust insulin therapy; most patients b.d. soluble + isophane

Poor control: change to t.i.d. soluble insulin and delay surgery

Urgent surgery: glucose/insulin infusion (see below)

Day of surgery
Check fasting blood glucose; repeat 2-hourly
No subcutaneous insulin

Start infusion of 10% glucose (500 ml) with soluble (Humulin S) insulin 10 units and KCl 10 mmol at 0800 h to run 4–6 hourly

Adjust insulin in bag as follows depending on blood glucose:
- < 4 mmol L^{-1}: no insulin
- 4–6 mmol L^{-1}: insulin 5 units per 500 ml glucose 10%
- 6–10 mmol L^{-1}: infusion as above
- 10–20 mmol L^{-1}: insulin 15 units per 500 ml glucose 10%
- > 20 mmol L^{-1}: insulin 20 units per 500 ml glucose 10%

Adjust potassium dosage depending on plasma K^+concentration
- < 3 mmol L^{-1}: add KCl 20 mmol L
- > 5 mmol L^{-1}: omit KCl

Postoperative
Check blood glucose 2–6 hourly; check urea and electrolytes daily

Continue 4–6-hourly infusion until oral diet re-established

If delayed, change to decreased volume of 20–50% glucose with independent insulin infusion by syringe pump

When oral diet resumed, t.i.d. soluble insulin s.c.; daily dosage as preoperative

When requirements stable, restart normal regimen

Table 35.10 Sliding scale for infusion of insulin

Glucose concentration (mmol L^{-1})	Infusion rate of insulin (unit h^{-1})
<4.0	–
4.1–7	1
7.1–9	1.5
9.1–11	2
11.1–17	3
17.1–28	4
>28	6

Insulin administered via separate cannula from syringe pump. Infusion comprises 50 units of human Actrapid insulin in 49.5 ml normal saline.
Glucose 4%/saline 0.18% solution is given via a separate cannula at a rate of 1.5 ml kg^{-1} h^{-1}
Blood glucose concentration is measured at 1-hourly intervals (initially) using BM stix and rate of insulin infusion adjusted according to sliding scale. When stability has been achieved blood glucose concentration may be measured at 4-hourly intervals.

NEUROLOGICAL DISEASE

There are several points of significance:

Respiratory impairment. Motor neuropathy from various causes, e.g. motor neurone disease, acute polyneuritis (Guillain–Barré syndrome), disorders of the neuromuscular junction and high spinal cord lesions may produce respiratory inadequacy. These patients are sensitive to anaesthetic agents, opioids and relaxants, and if intraoperative IPPV is undertaken, a period of elective postoperative ventilation may be necessary until full recovery from the effects of anaesthesia has occurred. If possible, procedures should be carried out under local or regional block. If bulbar muscles are involved, protection of the airway from regurgitation and aspiration may require prolonged tracheal intubation or tracheostomy. Surgery should be postponed if a chest infection is present preoperatively.

Altered innervation of muscle, and potassium shifts. An altered ratio of intracellular to extracellular potassium tends to produce a sensitivity to non-depolarizing, and resistance to depolarizing, relaxants. If there is widespread denervation of muscle with lower motor neurone damage, e.g. in Guillain–Barré syndrome, disorganization of the motor end-plate occurs, resulting in hypersensitivity to acetylcholine and succinylcholine, with increased permeability of muscle cells to potassium. A similar potassium efflux occurs in the presence of direct muscle damage, widespread burns involving muscle, upper motor neurone lesions, spinal cord lesions with paraplegia, and tetanus. In upper motor neurone and spinal cord lesions, the reason for this shift is less clear. Patients undergoing mechanical ventilation in the ICU who are suffering from sepsis and multiple organ failure may develop a critical illness polyneuropathy, with a similar hyperkalaemic response to succinylcholine.

The resulting increase in serum potassium concentration after succinylcholine may be 3 mmol L^{-1} (in comparison with 0.5 mmol L^{-1} in the normal patient) and may occur from 24 h after acute muscle denervation or damage until 6–12 months later. In such patients, succinylcholine is clearly contraindicated.

Autonomic disturbances may occur as part of a polyneuropathy, e.g. diabetes mellitus, Guillain–Barré syndrome and porphyria. Sympathetic stimulation, e.g. during light anaesthesia, tracheal intubation or following administration of pancuronium or catecholamines, may produce severe hypertension and arrhythmias. More commonly, blood loss, head-up posture or IPPV may be associated with severe hypotension.

Conscious level. Patients with pre-existing marked reduction in conscious level for whatever reason require tracheal intubation and ventilation of the lungs for airway protection and control of CO_2 and O_2 levels (see p. 726).

Increased intracranial pressure. Elective surgery should be postponed if raised intracranial pressure is suspected, until investigation by CT scan and treatment have been undertaken. Anaesthetic agents which cause an increase in cerebral blood flow must be avoided. Hypercapnia must also be avoided, and controlled ventilation to a P_aCO_2 of approximately 4 kPa (30 mmHg) is indicated. This is discussed fully in Chapter 57.

Medicolegal. Perioperative alteration in neurological deficit may be attributed to anaesthesia. This may render subarachnoid or epidural anaesthesia inadvisable in some patients.

EPILEPSY

Epilepsy may be associated with birth injury, hypoglycaemia, hypocalcaemia, drug overdose or withdrawal, fever, head injury, cerebrovascular disease and cerebral tumour, the most likely cause depending on the age of onset. In most patients with epilepsy, no identifiable cause can be found. Epilepsy developing after the age of 20 years usually indicates organic brain disease.

Anaesthesia

Patients should be maintained on anticonvulsant therapy throughout the perioperative period. Some anaesthetic agents, e.g. enflurane and methohexital, have cerebral excitatory effects and should be avoided. Sevoflurane and isoflurane do not cause cerebral excitation. Convulsions and abnormalities of muscle posture have been reported after operation in patients who have received propofol, and it is currently recommended that this drug should not be used in known epileptics. Thiopental is a potent anticonvulsant and is the i.v. induction agent of choice, while isoflurane is currently the volatile agent of choice. Local anaesthetic agents may cause convulsions at lower than normal concentrations and the safe maximum dose should be reduced. The anticonvulsants phenobarbital and phenytoin induce hepatic enzymes and accelerate elimination of drugs metabolized by the liver.

In cases of late-onset epilepsy, where increased intracranial pressure may be present as a result of tumour, controlled ventilation is advisable to avoid any further increase in intracranial pressure.

Status epilepticus

Management is aimed at cessation of the fits while maintaining tissue oxygenation. Initial treatment should be Diazemuls, titrated intravenously in a dose of up to 10–20 mg or until fitting ceases. An alternative is lorazepam 2–4 mg i.v. slowly. A loading dose of phenytoin 10–15 mg kg^{-1} should be administered i.v. under ECG monitoring over 30–60 min. High-flow oxygen should be administered, and the airway maintained throughout. If the convulsions persist or conscious level diminishes to the extent of compromising the airway and ventilation, the patient should be anaesthetized, the trachea intubated and mechanical ventilation commenced. While propofol has been associated with convulsive episodes when used for standard general anaesthesia, it is also highly effective in the treatment of status epilepticus, and indeed may be the anaesthetic agent of choice in this condition. Propofol can be used in seizures refractory to benzodiazepines and phenytoin both as the anaesthetic induction agent and as maintenance by infusion.

The conventional anaesthetic induction agent employed is thiopental. The infusion of thiopental may be discontinued when control of the fits has been achieved.

With status epilepticus, patients undergoing mechanical ventilation should not be paralysed, but if they are, a cerebral function monitor/electroencephalogram monitor must be used so that continued fitting is noted and treated.

MULTIPLE SCLEROSIS

Deterioration of symptoms tends to occur after surgery, but no specific anaesthetic technique has been implicated. It is usually advisable to avoid epidural and subarachnoid anaesthesia, but only for medicolegal reasons, as there is no evidence that these techniques affect the disease adversely; they may be used if indicated strongly, provided that a full explanation has been given to the patient, e.g. in obstetrics.

If a large motor deficit of recent onset is present, there may be increased potassium release from muscle following administration of succinylcholine, which should be avoided.

PERIPHERAL NEUROPATHIES

These may exhibit axonal 'dying back' degeneration or segmental demyelination. They are classified by anatomical distribution, the commonest being a symmetrical peripheral polyneuropathy.

Motor, sensory and autonomic fibres are involved. Causes include:

- metabolic (diabetes, porphyria)
- nutritional deficiency
- toxic (heavy metals, drugs)
- collagen disease
- carcinoma
- infective
- inflammatory.

Problems for the anaesthetist include the effects of autonomic neuropathy, and respiratory and bulbar involvement.

Acute inflammatory polyneuropathy (Guillain–Barré syndrome)

This polyneuropathy appears some days after a pyrexial illness. Progression is very variable, ranging from near total paralysis in 24 h to progression over several weeks. Respiratory and bulbar muscles may be affected, and if so, tracheal intubation followed by tracheostomy and IPPV are required. Several techniques can be employed for induction of anaesthesia and intubation. We recommend either the combination of an i.v. induction agent with rocuronium or the combination of propofol and alfentanil. The patient's general state, particularly the presence of cardiovascular instability, will dictate which agents should be used. Autonomic neuropathy may result in hypotension after commencing IPPV. This may be minimized by adequate fluid preloading and gradual increases in minute volume. Succinylcholine should be avoided. There is evidence that either high-dose immunoglobulin therapy or plasmapheresis beneficially modifies the course of the disease, although mortality is not affected.

MOTOR NEURONE DISEASE (PROGRESSIVE MUSCULAR ATROPHY, AMYOTROPHIC LATERAL SCLEROSIS, PROGRESSIVE BULBAR PALSY)

Motor neurone disease is characterized by slow onset and progressive deterioration in motor function. Several patterns of motor loss occur with both upper and lower motor neurone loss. Problems for the anaesthetist include sensitivity to all anaesthetic agents and muscle relaxants, respiratory inadequacy and laryngeal incompetence. Local anaesthetic techniques may be useful.

HEREDITARY ATAXIAS

Friedreich's ataxia is the most common. Spinocerebellar, corticospinal and posterior columns are involved, and the course of the disease is slowly progressive. Problems for the anaesthetist include scoliosis, respiratory failure and cardiomyopathy with cardiac failure and arrhythmias.

SPINAL CORD LESIONS WITH PARAPLEGIA

Release of potassium from muscle cells by succinylcholine precludes its use within 6–12 months of cord injury. Assessment of ventilatory function is important, as impaired cough and poor inspiration may indicate a need for postoperative ventilation.

HUNTINGTON'S CHOREA

It has been reported that thiopental may cause prolonged apnoea, and decreased serum cholinesterase activity may prolong the action of succinylcholine.

MYASTHENIA GRAVIS

This disease usually occurs in young adults and is characterized by episodes of increased muscle fatigability, caused by decreased numbers of acetylcholine receptors at the neuromuscular junction. Treatment comprises an anticholinesterase (pyridostigmine 60 mg q.i.d. or neostigmine 15 mg q.i.d.) with a vagolytic agent (atropine or propantheline) to block the muscarinic side-effects. Steroid therapy is useful in some cases and thymectomy may benefit many patients considerably, especially young women with myasthenia of recent onset.

The principal problems concern adequacy of ventilation, ability to cough and clear secretions, and the increased secretions resulting from anticholinesterase therapy. If there is evidence of respiratory infection, surgery should be postponed. Serum potassium concentration should be normal, as hypokalaemia potentiates myasthenia. Local and regional anaesthesia, including low subarachnoid or epidural block, may be suitable alternatives to general anaesthesia, although the maximum dose of local anaesthetic agents should be reduced because of their neuromuscular blocking action. The minimum possible dose of induction agent should be used and relaxants should be avoided if possible. For major procedures requiring relaxation, the anticholinesterase may be omitted for 4 h preoperatively, and a small dose of relaxant may be given if necessary. Atracurium is the relaxant of choice because of its short duration of action, and should be administered in a reduced dose (10–20% of normal). Succinylcholine has a variable effect in myasthenia and is best avoided.

Postoperatively, the patient's lungs should be ventilated electively after major surgery (usually for a few hours, but in some cases for up to 48 h). Frequent chest physiotherapy and tracheal suction are required. Steroid cover is given if appropriate. If extreme muscle weakness occurs, i.v. atropine 0.6–1.2 mg and neostigmine 1–2 mg may be given. Care must be taken to titrate the doses of anticholinesterase carefully, or a cholinergic crisis may occur, characterized by a depolarizing neuromuscular block, with sweating, salivation and pupillary constriction. An infusion of neostigmine is required if resumption of oral intake is delayed after surgery; 0.5 mg i.v. is equal to 15 mg neostigmine or 60 mg pyridostigmine orally. Edrophonium may be used to test the end-plate response to acetylcholine.

A myasthenic state may also be associated with carcinoma, thyrotoxicosis, Cushing's syndrome, hypokalaemia and hypocalcaemia. In these patients, non-depolarizing relaxants should be avoided or used in reduced dosage.

FAMILIAL PERIODIC PARALYSIS

This is also associated with prolonged paralysis after administration of non-depolarizing muscle relaxants.

Table 35.11 Safety of drugs commonly used in clinical anaesthesia for patients with acute porphyrias

Drug group						
Intravenous induction agents	Propofol	PS	Ketamine	C	Barbiturates	U
	Midazolam	PS			Etomidate	PU
Inhalation agents	Nitrous oxide	S	Halothane	C	Enflurane	PU
	Cyclopropane	S	Isoflurane	ND		
	Diethyl ether	S				
Muscle relaxants	Curare	S	Atracurium	ND	Alcuronium	PU
	Succinylcholine	S	Pancuronium	C		
	Vecuronium	PS				
Neuromuscular blockade reversal	Atropine	S	Glycopyrronium	ND		
	Neostigmine	S				
Local anaesthetics	Procaine	S	Lidocaine	C	Mepivacaine	PU
	Tetracaine	PS	Prilocaine	C		
			Bupivacaine	C		
Analgesics	Morphine	S	Alfentanil	ND	Pentazocine	U
	Pethidine	S	Sufentanil	ND	Tilidine	U
	Fentanyl	S				
	Buprenorphine	S				
	Naloxone	PS				
	Paracetamol	S				
Anxiolytics	Temazepam	S	Diazepam	C	All other benzodiazepines	U
	Lorazepam	PS	Oxazepam	C		
	Droperidol	S				
	Phenothiazines	S				
Antiarrhythmics	Procainamide	S	Lidocaine	C	Verapamil	U
	β-blockers	S	Mexiletine	ND	Nifedipine	U
			Bretylium	ND	Diltiazem	U
			Disopyramide	C		
Other cardiovascular drugs	Epinephrine	S	β-Agonists	ND	Hydralazine	U
	Phentolamine	S	α-Agonists	ND	Phenoxybenzamine	U
			Sodium nitroprusside	ND		
Bronchodilators	Corticosteroids	PS	Hexaprenaline	ND	Aminophylline	U
	Salbutamol	S				
Gastric – for caesarean section	Metoclopramide	PS	Ranitidine	C	Cimetidine	PU
	Domperidone	S				

PS, possibly safe; S, safe; C, contentious; ND, no data; U, unsafe; PU, probably unsafe

PROGRESSIVE MUSCULAR DYSTROPHY

Several types of muscular dystrophy exist, of varying patterns of heredity and described according to their anatomical distribution. Muscular weakness occurs and must be distinguished from myasthenia and lower motor neurone disease. The anaesthetic complications comprise sensitivity to relaxants, opioids and other sedative and anaesthetic drugs, and liability to respiratory infection. Myocardial involvement may occur.

DYSTROPHIA MYOTONICA

This is a disease of autosomal dominant inheritance characterized by muscle weakness and muscle contraction persisting after the termination of voluntary effort. Other features may include frontal baldness, cataract, sternomastoid wasting, gonadal atrophy and thyroid adenoma. Problems which affect anaesthetic management include the following.

Respiratory muscle weakness. Respiratory function should be fully assessed before operation. Respiratory depressant drugs, e.g. thiopental or opioids, should be used with care; there is sensitivity also to non-depolarizing relaxants. Elective IPPV may be required after surgery. Postoperative care of the airway must be meticulous because of muscle weakness. Chest infections are common.

Cardiovascular effects. There may be a cardiomyopathy and conduction defects. Arrhythmias are common, particularly during anaesthesia, and may result in cardiac failure. Careful monitoring is essential.

Muscle spasm. This may be provoked by administration of depolarizing muscle relaxants or anticholinesterases; succinylcholine and neostigmine should thus be avoided. The spasm is not abolished by non-depolarizing relaxants.

MISCELLANEOUS DISORDERS

CARCINOID SYNDROME

This is discussed on page 674.

MYELOMA

This neoplastic condition affects plasma cells and has several features of significance to the anaesthetist:

- Widespread skeletal destruction occurs and careful handling of the patient on the operating table is essential. Pathological fractures are common.
- Bone pain may be severe and often requires large doses of analgesics. Thus, tolerance to opioids may occur.
- Hypercalcaemia occurs as a result of bony destruction and may precipitate renal failure.
- Chronic renal failure may also result from myeloma directly.
- Anaemia is almost invariable, and preoperative blood transfusion is often necessary.
- Patients are liable to infection, including chest infection, especially during chemotherapy with neutropenia.
- During cytotoxic therapy, thrombocytopenia is common.
- Increased plasma immunoglobulin concentrations may raise blood viscosity, predisposing to arterial and venous thrombosis. Drug binding may be affected.
- Neurological manifestations include spinal cord and nerve root compression.

PORPHYRIA

The porphyrias are an inherited group of disorders of porphyrin metabolism characterized by increased activity of D-aminolaevulinic acid synthetase with excessive production of porphyrins or their precursors. In the UK, *acute intermittent porphyria* is the most common type. It is characterized by acute attacks which may arise spontaneously or be precipitated by infection, starvation, pregnancy or administration of some drugs. Inheritance is Mendelian dominant and thus a family history of porphyria requires further investigation. Clinical features include the following:

- Gastrointestinal – abdominal pain and tenderness, vomiting, constipation and occasionally diarrhoea.
- Neurological – a motor and sensory peripheral neuropathy is common. It may involve bulbar and respiratory muscles. Epileptic fits and psychological disturbance may occur.
- Cardiovascular – hypertension and tachycardia often occur during the attacks. Hypotension has also been reported.
- Fever and leucocytosis occur in 25–30% of patients. Drugs which provoke the attack include alcohol, barbiturates, chlordiazepoxide, steroid hormones, chlorpropamide, pentazocine, phenytoin and sulphonamides.

Anaesthesia in such patients is directed to avoiding drugs which may provoke attacks. Induction with propofol, followed by muscle relaxation with succinylcholine or vecuronium, ventilation with nitrous oxide, and oxygen and analgesic supplementation with morphine or fentanyl is satisfactory (Table 35.11). If fits occur, diazepam is a suitable anticonvulsant, while chlorpromazine, promethazine or promazine are suitable sedatives.

FURTHER READING

Benumof J L (ed) 1998 Anesthesia and uncommon diseases, 4th edn. W B Saunders, Philadelphia
Miller R D 2000 Anesthesia, 5th edn. Churchill Livingstone, London
Stoelting R K, Dierdorf S R 1993 Anaesthesia and co-existing disease, 3rd edn. Churchill Livingstone, London
Vickers M D, Power Z (eds) 1999 Medicine for anaesthetists, 4th edn. Blackwell Science, Oxford.

36 Preoperative checking of equipment and environment

Anaesthesia is a complex activity during which the anaesthetist assumes responsibility for a patient's well-being and safety whilst using potent drugs and complex apparatus. It is never certain that anaesthesia will proceed uneventfully: idiosyncratic drug reactions or anaphylaxis are rare and unpredictable; however, there are other factors that contribute to anaesthetic risk which may be reduced by thorough preparation and anticipation. Drug- and procedure-related risk may be reduced (but not completely eliminated) by adequate preoperative preparation (e.g. adequate history-taking, examination and preparation of the patient, and appropriate planning of the anaesthetic for each patient), and these aspects are discussed in Chapter 34.

When considering preoperative checks, anaesthetists tend to concentrate on the equipment (anaesthetic and monitoring apparatus) which they intend to use, but in addition to these specific equipment checks there are other, less obvious, checks which should be considered and which contribute to overall safety levels; such checks are important for patient and personal safety.

RISK MANAGEMENT

Risk management and assessment seek to minimize the risks involved in any process or activity by estimating the probability, likelihood and severity of any possible adverse occurrence and taking the appropriate steps to prevent it. Risks may be reduced (but can never be entirely eliminated) by correct training and education of staff, by ensuring that the correct equipment is available, functional and serviceable, and by ensuring that an environment exists which is conducive to good working practice.

Knowledge of the local environment, including the physical layout of the operating theatre suite, contributes to general safety and may be considered as part of general risk management.

THE THEATRE ENVIRONMENT

Whilst carrying out the relatively informal (but nonetheless important) preoperative environmental check, attention should be paid to the actual layout of the operating theatre. Operating theatres are generally safe environments, although they do have their own peculiar hazards, and their layout is a compromise for all the users. This introduces several hazards into the operating theatre environment which should be considered as part of the preoperative check.

Hazards

Trailing electrical wires, gas supply hoses, ventilator tubing, intravenous tubing and monitoring cables are commonly seen in operating theatres. These represent a hazard to everyone, particularly in an emergency. Staff may trip and suffer injury, and it is easy to disconnect the electrical supply to vital equipment. If the power to a modern anaesthetic machine is disconnected, monitoring, ventilators and gas supplies fail simultaneously. Attention has been paid in many industrial processes to the ergonomic design of equipment, but the positioning and design of much anaesthetic equipment and monitoring are often haphazard. The position of anaesthetic and other apparatus should be altered as necessary, and as far as is practicable, in order to minimize these hazards. The result of the preoperative check should be to position equipment appropriately, so that information may be obtained rapidly and assimilated with ease.

The equipment in operating theatres is designed to take into account potential hazards (some examples of which are shown in Table 36.1), and is constructed and tested to minimize the possibility of accidents, e.g. splashing water onto electric cables and contacts; anaesthetic gases and vapours are potentially harmful, and occupational exposure to these substances is controlled under the COSHH (control of substances hazardous to health) regulations, so adequate scavenging of the theatre atmosphere is needed.

There is a conflict between the temperature requirements of patients and staff. Temperatures and humidity levels which are comfortable for staff are not appropriate for anaesthetized patients, who are unable to control their temperature and are therefore at risk of intraoperative hypothermia. The very young and the very old may be particularly at risk. It is therefore wise to check the theatre temperature before starting an operating session.

Now that flammable anaesthetic agents are no longer used, the risk of fire or explosion in operating theatres has declined, but has not completely disappeared. Flammable substances are still present

Table 36.1 Potential hazards in the operating theatre
Electricity
Liquids
Gases and vapours
Temperature
Humidity
Fire
Cables and tubes

in an operating theatre (e.g. spirit for skin preparation), together with sources of ignition (e.g. diathermy) and oxygen. Although a serious fire is unlikely, all personnel should be aware of the location of the fire alarms, fire-fighting equipment, fire exits and local fire procedures. Much of this information (fire procedures, health and safety issues) should be dealt with during induction courses, but it is important not to become complacent and to attend regular refresher courses. Anaesthetic staff should be aware of the location of the shut-off valves for piped medical gases, in case of fire.

OTHER ENVIRONMENTS

Operating theatres may be familiar to anaesthetists, but when they are required to anaesthetize in unfamiliar places – e.g. X-ray suites, endoscopy and MRI rooms – problems may arise. These locations are not designed for the needs of anaesthesia and anaesthetized patients, and it then becomes important to ensure that adequate equipment (and back-up) is available and that the local environmental hazards are assessed before commencing anaesthesia. These locations are often cramped because of the presence of other fixed apparatus, which may be hazardous to patients and anaesthetists in terms of physical access, monitoring, etc. Darkness and radiation add to the hazards.

Particularly hazardous in these areas is the possibility that anaesthetic gases may be supplied from machine-mounted cylinders rather than from pipelines. Most anaesthetists in the UK now have little experience of working with anaesthetic apparatus which is not supplied with gases from a central supply point. In situations where gas supply is exclusively from cylinders, it is essential that both the primary and reserve cylinders are checked before commencing anaesthesia, to ensure that an adequate gas supply is present. Normally, it is not necessary to test the oxygen failure warning alarm when working from a piped gas supply, but when using a cylinder supply it is essential that this alarm is tested before anaesthesia commences.

EQUIPMENT CHECKS

Good anaesthetic practice reduces risk. Good practice is not just that which happens in the operating theatre; it encompasses a whole spectrum of education, training, organization and equipment, creating a working environment which is to the benefit of everyone involved, including both staff and patients.

Equipment should be up to date, maintained regularly and the instruction manuals should be available and accessible. Monitoring should be in accordance with existing guidelines, appropriate alarm limits must be set and alarms must not be disabled. An equipment check must be completed before commencing an anaesthetic session, because apart from human error, a major cause of anaesthetic misadventure involves the use of a machine which has not been checked adequately by an anaesthetist. An adequate check of anaesthetic apparatus, using a checklist and associated procedures, should be seen as an integral part of good practice and training in anaesthesia. Although anaesthetists rely greatly on memory for essential facts when carrying out many anaesthetic procedures, a written checklist should be used to minimize the possibility of missing out an important part of machine checks. The list published by the Association of Anaesthetists of Great Britain and Ireland (AAGBI) is recommended (Table 36.2).

Table 36.2 Checklist for anaesthetic apparatus. (Reproduced with permission from AAGBI 1997)

The following checks should be made prior to each operating session:

- Check that the anaesthetic machine is connected to the electricity supply (if appropriate) and switched on
- Check that an oxygen analyser is present on the anaesthetic machine
  — place the oxygen sensor where it can monitor the gases leaving the common gas outlet
- Identify and take note of the gases which are supplied by pipeline, confirming with a 'tug test' that each pipeline is correctly and securely inserted into the appropriate gas supply terminal
  — check that there is a reserve supply of oxygen; check that adequate supplies of other gases are available; check that all pipeline pressure gauges indicate 400 kPa
- Check the operation of all flowmeters
- Check the vaporizer(s)
  — adequate filling; correct seating and locking on the back bar; check for leaks with vaporizer on and off
- Check the breathing system to be employed
  — visual check for correct assembly; check for leaks; pressure-limiting valves; one-way valves (circle system)
- Check that the ventilator is configured appropriately for its intended use
  — tubing, valves, controls, disconnection alarm
  — ensure that an alternative means of ventilating the patient's lungs is available
- Check the scavenging system
  — switched on, correctly attached and functioning
- Check that all ancillary equipment which may be needed is present and working
  — intubation equipment, suction, tipping trolley
- Ensure that the appropriate monitoring equipment is present, switched on and calibrated ready for use
  — check and set alarm limits, as appropriate

Equipment checks fall into two groups: those carried out immediately before use by the anaesthetist who is to use the equipment, and those which may have been carried out by another individual prior to this. Operating theatre staff usually carry out checks when setting up an operating theatre for use, or after apparatus has been serviced or repaired, but the final responsibility for ensuring that apparatus is safe for its intended use rests with the anaesthetist. The recommended procedures do not replace sophisticated complex engineering tests as might be required after major servicing. They should be performed particularly carefully after a machine has been serviced, as control settings may have been altered.

The final pre-use check is the sole responsibility of the anaesthetist who is to use the machine. It cannot be delegated to any other person. It is relatively easy to ensure that the equipment is in proper working order and safe to use. The series of checks described can be performed in a few minutes and should be undertaken before the commencement of every operating session.

It is strongly recommended that a record of the checks performed should be kept and this is best done by the use of a specific logbook attached to the anaesthetic machine, in which should be recorded the date and time that the equipment was checked, the name of the individual carrying out the check, and any faults encountered (however minor). All faults should be recorded and drawn to the attention of the appropriate person. Serious faults should result in a machine being withdrawn from service. There is no justification for proceeding with an anaesthetic with seriously deficient apparatus. More minor faults should be recorded, reported and attended to as soon as possible. If a problem occurs and there is no record of an adequate preoperative check having been performed, it is very difficult to defend an accusation of negligence.

CHECKING THE ANAESTHETIC MACHINE

At its most basic, the essential function of an anaesthetic machine is to enable the anaesthetist to administer to a patient oxygen under pressure without leaks. If all else fails, this enables the anaesthetist to preserve life.

Anaesthetic apparatus should be checked in a logical sequence as recommended in the checklist in Table 36.2. The checking procedure is based on the premise that an oxygen analyser is present on the machine. Without such a device, it is not safe to proceed, particularly when low-flow anaesthesia using a circle system is planned. An oxygen analyser ensures the purity of the initial gas supply to the anaesthetic machine, and then acts as a safeguard against the administration of a hypoxic gas mixture to the patient.

The check procedure is written in very general terms and is applicable, with only minor modifications, to any anaesthetic machine in clinical use. The microprocessor-based anaesthetic machines now entering service have 'checking routines' built into their software, but this does not relieve the user of the responsibility to ensure that the 'self-check' routine is performed correctly. It could be argued that a machine which is checking itself should be observed closely during this period in case of errors in the routine. The intention of the check is to ensure that the machine is safe to use and can deliver gases under pressure without leaks.

Training

In most industries in which complex equipment is used, full training is provided for users, but in the past anaesthetists have appeared reluctant to undertake such training, apparently preferring to believe that they intuitively understood their apparatus. With increasing complexity and more stringent concepts of user liability, this is no longer acceptable. This may be regarded as part of risk management for anaesthesia. Anyone using a piece of anaesthetic equipment for the first time should ensure full familiarity with it. Those new to the speciality require detailed instruction and training in the use of the equipment, but even experienced anaesthetists may need help when faced with newer equipment. This is particularly true of the advanced electronically based anaesthetic machines now available.

The familiarization process may entail study of the instruction manual, particularly when faced with new equipment. Similarly, should any equipment be assembled in a configuration which is unfamiliar, it should be checked thoroughly before use.

ANAESTHETIC MACHINE

The anaesthetic machine and associated ancillary equipment should be connected to the mains electrical supply (as appropriate) and switched on. Microprocessor-based machines may now commence their self-check routines, and should be observed throughout. A visual check of the apparatus confirms that all essential equipment is present and correctly assembled. In particular, an oxygen analyser must be present and should be placed where it monitors the gases leaving the common gas outlet. The analyser should be switched on, checked and calibrated according to the manufacturer's instructions. Should the oxygen analyser not be functioning correctly, it is not safe to proceed further or to use this anaesthetic machine.

MEDICAL GAS SUPPLIES

Pipelines

It is essential to know which gases are being supplied by pipeline from a central supply, and to confirm that the connections between the anaesthetic machine and the pipelines are secure and correct. The anaesthetist should visually check the connections and then perform a 'tug test' on each pipeline connection to confirm that the connections are correctly and securely made. The Schrader sockets and probes are manufactured to ensure that misconnection is almost impossible, but nonetheless crossed pipeline connections have occurred in the past. Anaesthetic machines are also moved between operating theatres and pipelines and then reconnected, again with the potential for misconnection. After checking that the connections are correct at both ends of the flexible supply hoses, the anaesthetist should check that the pipeline pressure displayed on the anaesthetic machine should indicate 400 kPa.

Cylinders

Machine-mounted cylinders provide reserve gas supplies, although on occasion they may be the sole gas supply. The anaesthetist should ensure that cylinders are installed in the correct position. The pin-index system is designed to prevent incorrect installation, (Ch. 32) but no system is foolproof, and vigilance is always needed. Leaks caused by faulty connections or missing Bodok seals should be evident, because of the high pressures involved. Cylinders should be seated securely and turned off after checking their contents.

An adequate reserve supply of oxygen should be available from a spare cylinder, and the pressure in the cylinder should be checked. A check should be made that adequate supplies of other gases are available and connected as appropriate. There is a debate about the need for a reserve of nitrous oxide, and this is a matter for individual decision.

Carbon dioxide is not required in modern practice, and therefore carbon dioxide cylinders should not normally be present on the anaesthetic machine. Many anaesthetic machines no longer have a mounting point for carbon dioxide, but blanking plugs should be fitted to all unused cylinder yokes to prevent backflow and leakage in the extremely unlikely event of a failure within the machine piping.

Oxygen failure alarm

When the primary oxygen supply is by pipeline, it is no longer considered necessary to check the oxygen failure warning device as part of the daily routine. Unscheduled oxygen pipeline failure is extremely rare. There are occasional anecdotal accounts of oxygen pipeline failure, but in the UK no such incidents were brought to the notice of the Medical Devices Agency in the 10-year period from 1987 to 1997 (C. Bray, personal communication). Routinely checking the oxygen failure alarm requires the pipelines to be disconnected and reconnected with a potential for damage and misconnection. The virtual absence of unplanned failure renders this process unnecessary. However, in the absence of a pipeline supply of oxygen, a test of the oxygen failure alarm is essential.

Although the oxygen failure alarm is not tested routinely during the daily (or sessional) machine check, all anaesthetists must be aware of the presence and warning tone of such an alarm.

Flowmeters

The operation of all flowmeters should be checked. Flowmeter tubes should be inspected visually to ensure that they are seated correctly and devoid of cracks, and should be operated through their full range. Flowmeter tubes are calibrated for particular gases, and inspection should confirm that the correct tubes are in position. This is especially important after servicing, as it has been known for flowmeter tubes to be refitted in the incorrect position, with consequent inaccuracy.

At this stage, the purity of the oxygen supply may be verified by closing all but the oxygen flowmeter (on which a flow of 2–3 L min^{-1} is set) and checking that the oxygen analyser display approaches 100%. Close the flowmeter, and then operate the emergency oxygen bypass control. There should be no significant decrease in the pipeline supply pressure during this manoeuvre, and again the oxygen analyser display should approach 100%. When the emergency oxygen bypass control is released, it must cease to operate. Older machines (many of which are still in service) have a locking device which locks the emergency oxygen in the 'on' position. Failure to ensure its release carries a potential for causing severe barotrauma to a patient's lungs. Machines with such a locking device are potentially hazardous and should be used with caution. Having checked the gas supply, the remainder of the machine should now be checked to ensure that there are no leaks.

Vaporizers

Vaporizers and their mountings are a not uncommon source of leaks within an anaesthetic machine. Such leaks lead primarily to inadequate vapour delivery to the patient, with consequent awareness, or if there is no possibility of entrainment of air into the anaesthetic circuit, total failure of gas supply to the patient. Careful checking and care in the use of vaporizers prevent this. The commonest cause of leaks associated with vaporizers is a missing or defective 'O'-ring on the mounting port. The presence and integrity of these 'O'-rings must therefore be verified before any vaporizer is installed on an anaesthetic machine. Failure to ensure proper mounting of a vaporizer is also a source of leaks. When a vaporizer is fitted to a machine, ensure that it is correctly seated, with the back bar locking mechanism fully engaged. If more than one vaporizer is fitted, each should be turned on (and off again) in turn and checked for leaks by occluding the common gas outlet, when there should be no audible gas leaks or leak of liquid from the vaporizer.

There are several types of vaporizers in use, some of which are fitted with interlock devices which ensure that only one vaporizer can be operated at a time, to avoid the inadvertent delivery of mixed anaesthetic agents. However, the interlock systems are not uniform in design and may themselves contribute to misconnection and consequent patient awareness when additional vaporizers are fitted. There is also a large number of older vaporizers in use which are not fitted with an interlock device. Whilst such situations persist, careful checking of vaporizers and their fitments is essential.

It is occasionally necessary to change an anaesthetic vaporizer during the course of an operating list; should this become necessary, it is essential that the new vaporizer is fitted carefully, and the system rechecked for leaks. Failure to do so is a common cause of critical incidents.

BREATHING SYSTEMS

It is beyond the scope of this chapter to describe every system which is available for use, but it is essential to be familiar with the construction and workings of the system. The general principle is the same for all. They should be inspected visually for correct configuration and assembly. All connections within the system itself, and between the system and the anaesthetic machine, should be checked carefully. It is important to note that all connections are completed by a 'push and twist' action in order to make a firm connection, the slight twisting action being very important to the security of the connection. A pressure leak test should be performed on the breathing system, and it is particularly important to perform an occlusion test on the inner tube of the Bain-type coaxial system, as a fault here would result in failure of gas delivery to the patient.

Even if it is not proposed to use a mechanical ventilator during the course of the anaesthetic, the ventilator tubing should be checked at this stage, and must be assembled correctly and secured.

Ventilators

The advice for checking of ventilators is the same for all types. In particular, all should be checked for their ability to generate an adequate inspiratory pressure. The anaesthetist must ensure that the ventilator is configured correctly and the controls set appropriately; the ventilator tubing has already been checked, but a further quick check at this stage is performed easily. It is essential that the pressure relief valve functions correctly, at the desired pressure, in order to prevent barotrauma. There must be a pressure disconnection alarm within the system and its presence must be sought and correct function ascertained before commencing anaesthesia. It is important to ensure that the pressure and timings are set correctly for each patient. The high-pressure alarm is also adjustable and its settings should be checked before use.

Whenever anaesthesia is undertaken, there must always be available, reasonably close to hand, an alternative means to ventilate the patient's lungs in the event that the ventilator or anaesthetic apparatus malfunctions. All anaesthetists should therefore know where to find a self-inflating (e.g. AMBU) bag within the operating theatre.

Scavenging

The final item on the anaesthetic apparatus is the scavenging system, which should be checked for adequate function. The scavenging tubing must be attached correctly to the appropriate expiratory ports of breathing systems and ventilators.

MONITORING

In the UK, recommendations on minimum standards for monitoring during anaesthesia have been published by the AAGBI and are widely accepted. These standards should be regarded as the minimum for every anaesthetic, and part of the safety check before commencing anaesthesia is to ensure that all necessary monitoring equipment is available and fully functional. Oxygen analysers should be switched on and calibrated according to the manufacturer's instructions. The alarm settings on all monitoring equipment should be reviewed and the upper and lower limits set appropriately. The manufacturer's default settings may be considered inappropriate and it is essential that the anaesthetist selects appropriate alarm levels. As an example, the default value for the lower oxygen concentration alarm on most monitors is set at 18%; most anaesthetists would regard this as an inadequate F_IO_2 and the limit should be adjusted to a more acceptable level.

The importance of this step when undertaking pre-use checks cannot be overemphasized. Failure to set alarm variables correctly has been identified by the medical defence organizations in the UK as a major risk factor for adverse outcomes of anaesthesia. Incorrect settings of alarms, failure to use alarms settings or ignoring alarms arguably amount to dangerous practice.

ANCILLARY EQUIPMENT

The preoperative equipment check is completed by ensuring that all ancillary equipment which may be needed (e.g. laryngoscopes, intubation aids [forceps, bougies, etc.]) are available and close at hand in the anaesthetic room. Appropriate face masks, airways, tracheal tubes and connectors must be available. Tracheal tubes should be ready for use, with cuffs checked, cut to the correct length and with all connections secured.

Consideration should be given to the need for blood warmers, warm air blowers and warming blankets if needed. The anaesthetist takes responsibility for maintenance of the patient's body temperature and must ensure that adequate equipment is available.

Suction apparatus should be functional and all connections should be secure. It should be tested before commencing anaesthesia, to ensure that an adequate negative pressure is developed rapidly. The patient trolley, bed or operating table must be capable of rapid head-down tilt. As with all other equipment, the anaesthetist must be familiar with the operating mechanism before commencing anaesthesia.

EMERGENCIES

Safe practice requires that everyone has the information required to conduct anaesthesia safely, or easy access to that information. Some eventualities are unpredictable, but there are many action plans available to guide individuals during emergency situations, and such protocols, guidelines and action plans should be displayed prominently in the theatre suite. It may be that the individual anaesthetist does not check, on every occasion, that these protocols are available, but departmental standards, directed towards the maintenance of good practice, should ensure that these conditions are met. Everyone must know where the defibrillator is situated in the theatre suite. Similarly, all should know the location of a fibreoptic laryngoscope. Rare emergencies such as malignant hyperthermia call for prompt action and the availability of large quantities of ice and dantrolene. It is therefore important that all anaesthetists know, particularly when working in a hospital or operating theatre for the first time, where dantrolene is to be found and where ice may be obtained. Good departmental practice should ensure that everyone knows the location and availability of these substances.

Most of this chapter is common sense. However, it bears repetition in some detail because the continuing saga of anaesthetic misadventure and mishap indicates that not all equipment checks are as adequate or as frequent as they should be. Good clinical practice requires thorough preparation, which begins with ensuring not only that the environment is safe to work in, but also that all equipment is in good working order and that the individual anaesthetist knows how to use this equipment. Adherence to the principles outlined in this chapter should ensure safe anaesthetic practice.

FURTHER READING

Association of Anaesthetists of Great Britain and Ireland (AAGBI) 1997 Checklist for anaesthetic apparatus 2. AAGBI, London

Association of Anaesthetists of Great Britain and Ireland (AAGBI) 2000 Recommendations for standards of monitoring during anaesthesia and recovery 3. AAGBI, London

Cartwright D P, Freeman M F 1999 Vaporisers. Anaesthesia 54: 519–520

Moyle J T B, Davey A 1992 Ward's anaesthetic equipment, 4th edn. W B Saunders, London

37 The practical conduct of anaesthesia

Planning the conduct of anaesthesia starts normally after details concerning the surgical procedure and the medical condition of the patient have been ascertained at the preoperative visit. Preoperative assessment and selection of appropriate premedication are discussed in Chapter 34.

PREPARATION FOR ANAESTHESIA

Before starting the anaesthetic, consideration should be given to the induction and maintenance of anaesthesia, the position of the patient on the operating table, the equipment necessary for monitoring, the use of intravenous (i.v.) fluids or blood for infusion and the postoperative care and recovery facilities that will be required.

The anaesthetic machine to be used must be tested for leaks, misconnections and proper function. A checklist, e.g. that published by the Association of Anaesthetists of Great Britain and Ireland (AAGBI), is recommended. This is discussed in Chapter 36. The breathing system to be used should be new for each patient, or a filter of appropriate size should be placed between the patient and the system and a new filter used for each patient according to the recommendations of the Blood Borne Advisory Group of the AAGBI, 1996.

The availability and function of all anaesthetic equipment should be checked before starting (see Table 37.1). After the patient's arrival in the anaesthetic room, the anaesthetist should be satisfied that the correct operation is being performed upon the correct patient and that consent has been given. The patient must be on a tilting bed or trolley and the anaesthetist should have a competent assistant.

Table 37.1 Equipment required for tracheal intubation
Correct size of laryngoscope and spare (in case of light failure)
Tracheal tube of correct size + an alternative smaller size
Tracheal tube connector
Wire stilette
Gum elastic bougies
Magill forceps
Cuff-inflating syringe
Artery forceps
Securing tape or bandage
Catheter mount(s)
Local anaesthetic spray – 4% lidocaine
Cocaine spray/gel for nasal intubation
Tracheal tube lubricant
Throat packs
Anaesthetic breathing system and face masks–tested with O_2 to ensure no leaks present

INDUCTION OF ANAESTHESIA

Anaesthesia is induced using one of the following techniques.

INHALATION INDUCTION

The most common indications for induction of anaesthesia by an inhalation technique are listed in Table 37.2.

The proposed procedure should be explained to the patient before starting. A 'no-mask' technique using a cupped hand around the fresh gas delivery tube may be preferred for young children. When an Ayre's T-piece is used for inhalation induction in young children, it is recommended that a filter is not used as its presence provides excessive resistance to gas flow, diverting fresh gas flow to the efferent limb and slowing induction. The mask or hand is introduced *gradually* to the face from the side, as the sight of a black mask descending onto the face may be disturbing. While talking to the patient and encouraging him/her to breathe normally, the anaesthetist adjusts the mixture of the fresh gas flow and observes the patient's reactions. Initially, nitrous oxide 70% in oxygen is used and anaesthesia is deepened by the gradual introduction of increments of a volatile agent, e.g. halothane 1–3%. However, sevoflurane may be used starting at an inspired

Table 37.2 Indications for inhalation induction
Young children
Upper airway obstruction, e.g. epiglottitis
Lower airway obstruction with foreign body
Bronchopleural fistula or empyema
No accessible veins

concentration of 8% which achieves more rapid induction than its use incrementally. Maintenance concentrations of halothane (1–2%), enflurane (1.5–2.5%), isoflurane (1–2%) or sevoflurane (2-3%) are used when anaesthesia has been established.

A single-breath technique of inhalation induction has been advocated for patients who are able to cooperate. One vital capacity breath from a prefilled 4 L reservoir bag containing a high concentration of volatile agent (e.g. halothane 5%) in oxygen (or nitrous oxide 50% in oxygen) results in smooth induction of anaesthesia within 20–30 s.

Observation of the colour of the patient's skin and pattern of ventilation, palpation of the peripheral pulse, ECG and S_pO_2 monitoring and measurement of arterial pressure are important accompaniments to the technique of inhalation induction.

If spontaneous ventilation is to be maintained throughout the procedure, the mask is applied more firmly as consciousness is lost and the airway is supported manually. Insertion of an oropharyngeal airway, a laryngeal mask airway or a tracheal tube may be considered when anaesthesia has been established.

Complications and difficulties

- slow induction of anaesthesia
- problems particularly during stage 2 (see below)
- airway obstruction, bronchospasm
- laryngeal spasm, hiccups
- environmental pollution.

INTRAVENOUS INDUCTION

Induction of anaesthesia with an i.v. agent is suitable for most routine purposes and avoids many of the complications associated with the inhalation technique. It is the most appropriate method of rapid induction for the patient undergoing emergency surgery, in whom there is a risk of regurgitation of gastric contents during induction. All drugs which may be required at induction should be prepared and a cannula inserted into a suitable vein before starting. The anaesthetist should wear rubber gloves for this and other procedures during induction of anaesthesia and during airway manipulations such as insertion of an airway or tracheal tube.

If an existing i.v. cannula is to be used, its function must be checked. Cannulae with a side injection port ('Venflon' type) are useful; large cannulae (e.g. 16G, 14G) are necessary for transfusion of fluids or blood. A vein in the forearm or on the back of the hand is preferable; veins in the antecubital fossa are best avoided because of the risks of intra-arterial injection and elbow flexion. After selection of a suitable vein, skin preparation is performed using iodine or alcohol. Subcutaneous local anaesthetic should be used for large cannulae. Alternatively, local anaesthetic cream (EMLA or tetracaine) may have been applied preoperatively. Intravenous entry is confirmed with blood aspiration and the device is secured firmly with tape. 'Opsite' dressings may be used when long-term use is anticipated.

Monitoring should be commenced before induction of anaesthesia, including S_pO_2, ECG and arterial pressure measurement. Preoxygenation may be started, using a close-fitting face mask, and 100% oxygen delivered, for example, by a Magill breathing system for 5 min. Alternatively, three to four large (vital capacity) breaths may be used. Preoxygenation before routine elective induction of anaesthesia avoids transient hypoxaemia before establishment of effective lung ventilation.

Table 37.3 Intravenous induction agents

Agent	Induction dose (mg kg^{-1})
Thiopental	3–5
Methohexital	1–1.5
Etomidate	0.3
Propofol	1.5–2.5
Ketamine	2

Doses of the common i.v. agents are shown in Table 37.3. The induction dose varies with the patient's weight, age, state of nutrition, circulatory status, premedication and any concurrent medication. A small test dose is commonly administered and its effects are observed. Slow injection is recommended in the aged and in those with a slow circulation time (e.g. shock, hypovolaemia, cardiovascular disease) while the effects of the drug on the cardiovascular and respiratory systems are monitored.

A rapid-sequence induction technique is indicated for patients undergoing emergency surgery and for those in whom vomiting or regurgitation is a potential problem. After i.v. induction, a rapid transition to stage 3 anaesthesia (see below) is achieved; this is maintained by the introduction of an inhalation agent or by repeated bolus injections or a continuous infusion of an i.v. anaesthetic agent. Emergency anaesthesia is discussed fully in Chapter 51.

Complications and difficulties

Regurgitation and vomiting. If regurgitation occurs, the patient should be placed immediately into the Trendelenburg position and material aspirated with suction apparatus. Should inhalation of gastric contents occur, treatment is with 100% oxygen, bronchodilators, tracheal suction and toilet. Steroids and antibiotics should be considered. Continued IPPV may be required if the resultant pneumonitis is severe.

Intra-arterial injection of thiopental. This rare complication should be avoided by the appropriate choice of venous site, use of a 'plastic' cannula and checking its function before injection. Pain and blanching in the hand and fingers occurs as a result of crystal formation in the capillaries. The needle should be left in the artery and 5 ml 0.5% procaine and 40 mg papaverine injected. Further treatment includes stellate ganglion block, brachial plexus block or sympathetic block with i.v. guanethidine.

Perivenous injection. This causes blanching and pain and may result in a small degree of tissue necrosis. Methohexital and propofol produce less tissue damage than thiopental. Hyaluronidase may be used to speed dispersal of the drug.

Cardiovascular depression. This is likely to occur particularly in the elderly, the hypovolaemic or the untreated hypertensive patient. Reducing the dose and speed of injection is recommended in these patients. Infusion of i.v. fluid (e.g. 500 ml colloid or 1000 ml crystalloid solution) is usually successful in restoring arterial pressure.

Respiratory depression. Slow injection of an induction agent may reduce the extent of respiratory depression. Respiratory adequacy must be assessed carefully and the anaesthetist should be ready to assist ventilation of the lungs if necessary.

Histamine release. Thiopental or methohexital may cause release of histamine with subsequent formation of typical wheals. Severe reactions may occur to individual agents, and appropriate drugs and fluids should be available in the anaesthetic room for treatment. Guidelines for emergency management of acute major anaphylaxis are available (AAGBI) and may be displayed in the anaesthetic room. This is discussed further in Chapter 40.

Porphyria. An acute porphyric episode may be precipitated by barbiturates in susceptible individuals.

Other complications. Pain on injection (especially with methohexital, etomidate or propofol), hiccup or muscular movements may occur. The use of lidocaine mixed with propofol reduces the incidence of pain on injection.

POSITION OF PATIENT FOR SURGERY

After induction of anaesthesia, the patient is placed on the operating table in a position appropriate for the proposed surgery. When positioning the patient, the anaesthetist should take into account surgical access, patient safety, anaesthetic technique, monitoring and position of i.v. lines, etc.

Some commonly used positions are shown in Figure 37.1. Each may have adverse effects in terms of skeletal, neurological, ventilatory and circulatory effects.

The lithotomy position may result in nerve damage on the medial or lateral side of the leg from pressure exerted by the stirrups, which must be well padded. Care must be taken to elevate both legs simultaneously so that pelvic asymmetry and resultant backache are avoided. The sacrum should be supported on the operating table and not allowed to slip off the end.

The lateral position may result in asymmetrical lung ventilation (see Ch. 58). Care is required with arm position and i.v. infusions. The pelvis and shoulders must be supported to prevent the patient from rolling either backwards (with a risk of falling from the table) or forwards into the recovery position.

The prone position may cause abdominal compression which may result in ventilatory and circulatory embarrassment. To prevent this, support must be provided beneath the shoulders and iliac crests. Excessive extension of the shoulders should be avoided. The face, and particularly the eyes, must be protected from trauma. The tracheal tube must be secured firmly in place as it is almost impossible to reinsert it with the patient in this position.

The Trendelenburg position may produce upward pressure on the diaphragm because of the weight of the abdominal contents. Damage to the brachial plexus may occur as a result of pressure from shoulder supports, especially if the arms are abducted.

The sitting position requires careful support of the head. In addition, venous pooling and resultant cardiovascular instability may occur.

The supine position carries the risk of the supine hypotensive syndrome during pregnancy (see Ch. 52) or in patients with a large abdominal mass.

Positioning during anaesthesia is discussed extensively by Martin & Warner (1997).

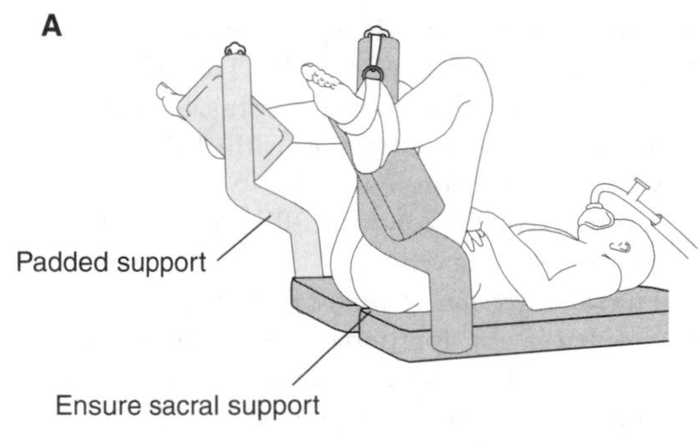

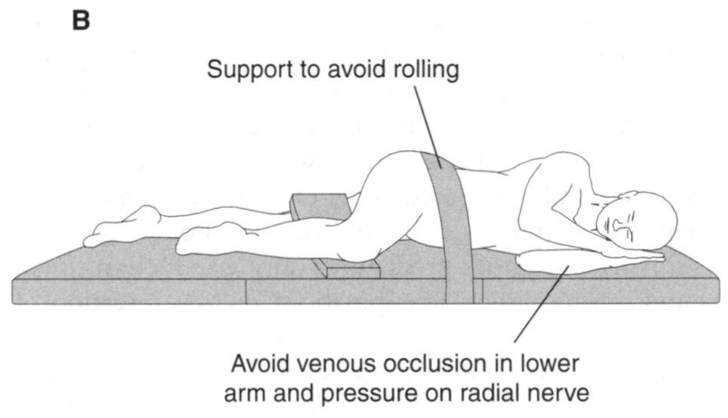

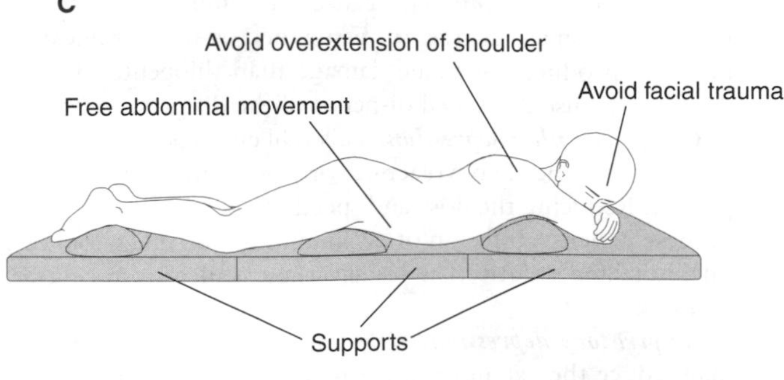

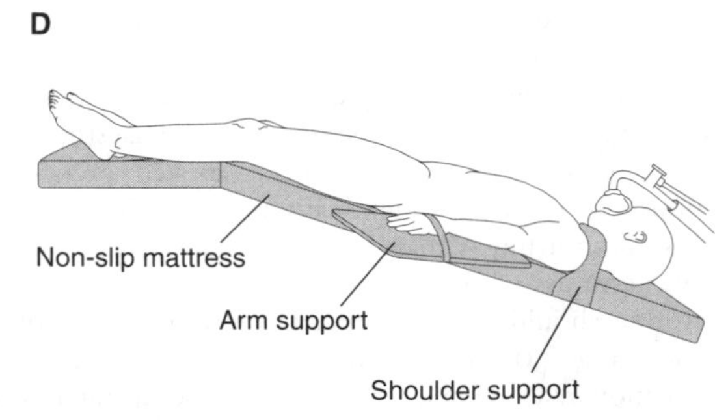

Fig. 37.1
Positions on the operating table. **A.** Lithotomy position. **B.** Lateral position. **C.** Prone position. **D.** Trendelenburg position.

MAINTENANCE OF ANAESTHESIA

Anaesthesia may be continued using inhalation agents, i.v. anaesthetic agents or i.v. opioids either alone or in combination. Tracheal intubation with or without muscle relaxants may be used. Regional anaesthesia may be used to supplement any of these techniques to achieve the components of the familiar anaesthetic triad of sleep, muscular relaxation and analgesia.

INHALATION ANAESTHESIA WITH SPONTANEOUS VENTILATION

This is an appropriate form of maintenance for superficial operations, minor procedures which produce little reflex or painful stimulation and operations for which profound muscle relaxation is not required.

Conduct

After induction of anaesthesia, inhalation and/or volatile agents may be used in the spontaneously breathing patient. Depending on the nature of surgery, the provision of analgesia in premedication (if used), and the patient's response (assessed by observation of ventilation, circulation and heart rate and rhythm), isoflurane 1–2% inspired concentration may be used in a mixture with nitrous oxide 70% in oxygen; enflurane 1.5–2.5%, halothane 1–2% or sevoflurane 2–3% are alternatives.

Minimum alveolar concentration (MAC)

MAC is the minimum alveolar concentration of an inhaled anaesthetic agent which prevents reflex movement in response to surgical incision in 50% of subjects. MAC values of commonly used inhalation agents are shown in Appendix II (p. 766). MAC varies little with metabolic factors but is reduced by opioid premedication and in the presence of hypothermia. MAC is higher in neonates and is reduced in the elderly (see Ch. 13).

The effects of inhalation anaesthetics are additive; thus 1 MAC-equivalent could be achieved by producing an alveolar concentration of 70% nitrous oxide (0.67 MAC) and 0.4% isoflurane (0.33 MAC).

The rate at which MAC is attained may be increased by raising the inspired concentration and by avoidance of airway obstruction. Increasing ventilation at a constant inspired concentration produces more rapid equilibration between inspired and alveolar concentrations. The time taken for equilibration increases with the blood/gas solubility coefficient of the agent; those with a high blood/gas solubility coefficient do not reach equilibrium for several hours (see Ch. 13). It follows, therefore, that the inspired concentration must be considerably higher than MAC to produce an adequate alveolar concentration when such agents are used.

Control of depth of anaesthesia by varying the inspired concentration of volatile agent requires constant assessment of the patient's reaction to anaesthesia and surgery to produce adequate anaesthesia, while avoiding overdosage and excessively 'deep' anaesthesia. This rapid control is one of the main advantages of inhalation anaesthesia. The signs of inadequate depth of anaesthesia include tachypnoea, tachycardia, hypertension and sweating.

Signs of anaesthesia (Fig. 37.2)

Guedel's classic signs of anaesthesia are those seen in patients premedicated with morphine and atropine and breathing ether in air. The clinical signs associated with anaesthesia produced by other inhalation agents follow a similar course, but the divisions between the stages and planes are less precise.

Stage 1: the stage of analgesia. This is the stage attained when using nitrous oxide 50% in oxygen, as employed in the technique of relative analgesia (see Ch. 54).

Stage 2: stage of excitement. This is seen with inhalation induction, but is passed rapidly during i.v. induction. Respiration is erratic, breath-holding may occur, laryngeal and pharyngeal reflexes are active and stimulation of pharynx or larynx, e.g. by insertion of a Guedel or laryngeal mask airway, can produce laryngeal spasm. The eyelash reflex (used as a sign of unconsciousness with i.v. induction) is abolished in stage 2, but the eyelid reflex (resistance to elevation of eyelid) remains present.

Stage 3: surgical anaesthesia. This deepens through four planes (in practice, three – light, medium, deep) with increasing concentration of anaesthetic drug. Respiration assumes a rhythmic pattern and the thoracic component diminishes with depth of anaesthesia. Respiratory reflexes become suppressed but the carinal reflex is abolished only at plane IV (therefore, a tracheal tube which is too long may produce carinal stimulation at an otherwise adequate depth). The pupils are central and gradually enlarge with depth of anaesthesia. Lacrimation is active in light planes but absent in planes III and IV – a useful sign in a patient not premedicated with an anticholinergic.

Stage 4: stage of impending respiratory and circulatory failure. Brainstem reflexes are depressed by the high anaesthetic concentration. Pupils are enlarged and unreactive. The patient should not be permitted to reach this stage. Withdrawal of the anaesthetic agents and administration of 100% oxygen lightens anaesthesia.

Observation of other reflexes provides a guide to depth of anaesthesia. Swallowing occurs in the light plane of stage 3. The gag reflex is abolished in upper stage 3. Stretching of the anal sphincter produces reflex laryngospasm even at plane III of stage 3.

Complications and difficulties

Airway obstruction. This is relieved by appropriate positioning and equipment (see below).

Laryngeal spasm. This may occur as a result of stimulation above light–medium stage 3. Treatment is to stop the stimulation and gently deepen anaesthesia. If spasm is severe, 100% oxygen is applied with the face mask held tightly, while the airway is maintained by hand and pressure is applied to the reservoir bag. Attempts to ventilate the patient's lungs usually result only in gastric inflation. However, as the larynx partially opens, 100% oxygen flows through under pressure. Further gentle deepening of anaesthesia may then take place. In severe laryngeal spasm, i.v. succinylcholine may be required, and after the lungs have been inflated with oxygen it is advisable to intubate the trachea.

Bronchospasm. This may occur if volatile anaesthetic agents are introduced rapidly, particularly in smokers with excessive bronchial secretions. Humidification and warming of gases may minimize the problem. Bronchospasm may accompany laryngospasm. Administration of bronchodilators may be required. These respiratory reflexes are induced more readily in the presence of, or shortly after, a respiratory tract infection.

Malignant hyperthermia. Volatile agents, succinylcholine or amide-type local anaesthetic agents may trigger this syndrome in susceptible individuals (see Ch. 40).

Raised intracranial pressure (ICP). All volatile agents may produce an increase in ICP and this is accentuated by retention of CO_2 which accompanies the use of volatile agents in the spontaneously breathing patient. A spontaneous ventilation technique is therefore contraindicated in patients with an intracranial space-occupying lesion or cerebral oedema.

Atmospheric pollution. The use of the appropriate scavenging apparatus helps to reduce levels of theatre pollution by volatile and gaseous agents (see Ch. 32).

Delivery of inhalation agents – airway maintenance

Maintenance of the airway is one of the most important of the anaesthetist's tasks. Inhalation agents may be delivered via a face mask, a laryngeal mask airway (LMA) or a tracheal tube. Insufflation techniques, although once popular, are now rarely used.

Use of the face mask

Inhalation anaesthesia usually involves the use of a face mask which is applied after loss of consciousness at anaesthetic induction. The face mask has many variants of type and size, and selection of the correct fit is important to provide a gas-tight seal.

For children, a mask with excessive dead space should be avoided. Nasal masks are required during dental anaesthesia. The patient's head position during mask anaesthesia is important; the mandible is held 'into' the mask by the anaesthetist, with his or her fingers holding the mandible itself rather than pressing into the soft tissues, which may result in airway obstruction (especially in children). The mandible is held forward, helping to prevent posterior movement of the tongue and obstruction of the airway.

The importance of observation of the airway during mask anaesthesia cannot be overemphasized. Soft tissue indrawing in the suprasternal and supraclavicular areas is evidence of obstruction of the upper airway. Noisy ventilation or inspiratory stridor provides further evidence that airway obstruction requires correction. Maintenance of the airway may be assisted further by the use of an oropharyngeal (Guedel) airway. An appropriate stage of anaesthesia must be reached before insertion of the airway, as stimulation of the pharynx at stage 2 or at light stage 3 produces coughing, laryngospasm or breath-holding. The use of local anaesthetic spray or jelly to coat the airway may permit its insertion at an earlier stage. A nasopharyngeal airway may be tolerated better.

The face mask is used in current practice only before tracheal intubation or insertion of the laryngeal mask or during short non-invasive procedures, e.g. dental anaesthesia and orthopaedic manipulations. To ensure patency of the airway, other airway adjuncts such as an oropharyngeal or a nasopharyngeal airway may be used.

STAGE	RESPIRATION	PUPILS	EYE REFLEXES	URT & RESPIRATORY REFLEXES
1 Analgesia	Regular Small volume			
2 Excitement	Irregular	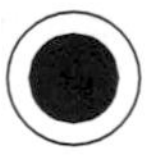	Eyelash absent	
3 Anaesthesia Plane I	Regular Large volume		Eyelid absent Conjunctival depressed	Pharyngeal & vomiting depressed
Plane II	Regular Large volume		Corneal depressed	
Plane III	Regular Becoming diaphragmatic Small volume			Laryngeal depressed
Plane IV	Irregular Diaphragmatic Small volume	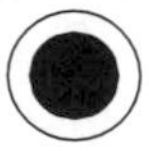		Carinal depressed
4 Overdose	Apnoea			

Fig. 37.2
Stages of anaesthesia (modified from Guedel).

Use of the laryngeal mask airway (LMA)

Indications

- To provide a clear airway without the need for the anaesthetist's hands to support a mask.
- To avoid the use of tracheal intubation during spontaneous ventilation.
- In a case of difficult intubation, to facilitate subsequent insertion of a tracheal tube either via the intubating LMA or after use of a gum elastic bougie (see Ch. 32).

Contraindications

- A patient with a 'full stomach' or with any condition leading to delayed gastric emptying.
- A patient in whom regurgitation of gastric contents into the oesophagus is likely (e.g. hiatus hernia).
- Where surgical access (e.g. to the pharynx) is impeded by the cuff of the LMA.

Conduct of LMA insertion. An appropriate depth of anaesthesia is required for successful insertion of the LMA. Fewer difficulties are encountered after i.v. induction of anaesthesia with propofol than with thiopental because of the greater tendency of the former to suppress pharyngeal reflexes. The patient's head is extended, the mouth is opened and, if necessary, the mandible can be held down by an assistant. The LMA cuff is evacuated and the LMA is inserted into the pharynx in a direction along the axis of the hard palate so that the cuff encounters the posterior pharyngeal wall and is swept distally into the laryngopharynx. This may be assisted by use of the gloved fingers in the 'classic' technique. The cuff then lies posterior to the larynx. Air is then injected into the cuff and the breathing system is attached via a catheter mount to the 22 mm proximal connector. The LMA is secured in place with tape or a bandage after confirmation of correct placement by observation of movement of the reservoir bag or the chest after a gentle manual inflation of the lungs.

TRACHEAL INTUBATION

Indications

- Provision of a clear airway, e.g. anticipated difficulty in using mask anaesthesia in the edentulous patient.
- An 'unusual' position, e.g. prone or sitting. A reinforced non-kinking tube may be necessary.
- Operations on the head and neck, e.g. ENT, dental. A nasotracheal tube may be required.
- Protection of the respiratory tract, e.g. from blood during upper respiratory tract or oral surgery and from inhalation of gastric contents in emergency surgery or patients with oesophageal obstruction. The use of a cuffed tube for adults is mandatory in these circumstances.
- During anaesthesia using IPPV and muscle relaxants.
- To facilitate suction of the respiratory tract.
- During thoracic operations.

Contraindications. There are few contraindications. In emergency situations, hypoxaemia must be relieved if at all possible before insertion of a tracheal tube.

Preparation

Before starting, the anaesthetist must check the availability and function of the necessary equipment. He or she should have a 'dedicated' and experienced assistant. Laryngoscopes of the correct size are chosen and the function of bulb and batteries checked, the patency of the tracheal tube is checked and the integrity of the cuff ensured. Various aids to intubation must also be present (see Table 37.1).

Choice of equipment

Laryngoscopes

Laryngoscopes are manufactured in many shapes and sizes. There are two basic types of blade – straight or curved. Straight-blade laryngoscopes (e.g. Magill) are favoured for children, in whom the epiglottis is floppy, and are designed to pass posterior to the epiglottis and to lift it anteriorly, exposing the larynx. The curved blade (e.g. Macintosh) is designed so that the tip lies anterior to the epiglottis in the vallecula, pressing on the hyoepiglottic ligament and moving it anteriorly to expose the larynx and vocal cords (Fig. 37.3). The McCoy blade is a relatively recent introduction where the distal tip of the blade is movable to facilitate a view of the glottis in some patients.

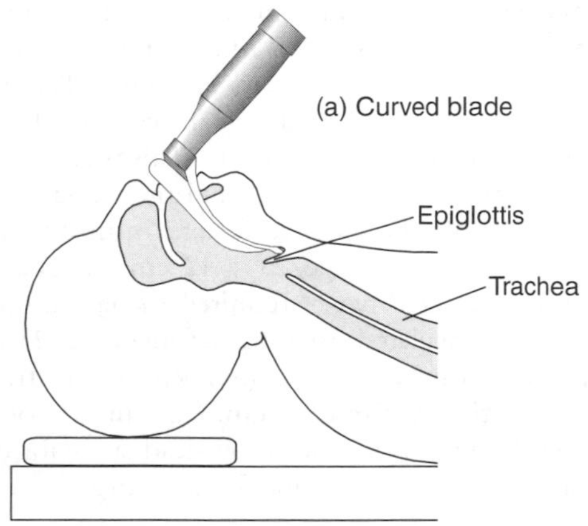

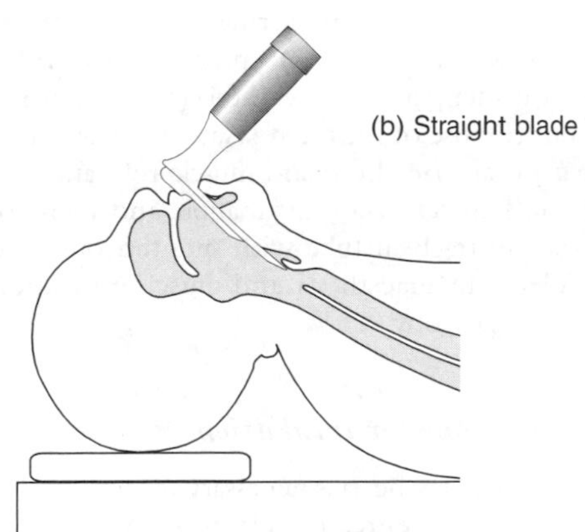

Fig. 37.3
Use of the laryngoscope.

Tracheal tubes

Modern tracheal tubes are disposable and made from PVC which is 'implant tested' for its inert effect upon the tissues. In some circumstances, e.g. head and neck or throat surgery, the tracheal tube may be subject to direct or indirect pressure and standard tubes may kink or become compressed. It may be appropriate to use a tube which is reinforced with a nylon or steel spiral in such cases. Tracheal tubes are introduced usually through the mouth, although it may be preferable to pass the tube through the nose, particularly for oral surgery. The supplied length of disposable tubes exceeds that required normally for oral intubation and the tube should be cut to the appropriate length before use. During thoracic surgery, it may be necessary to ventilate the lungs independently and a bronchial or double-lumen tube is required (see Ch. 58).

In order to seal the airway, most tracheal tubes are manufactured with an inflatable cuff at the distal end. The cuff may be of low or high volume; low-volume cuffs produce a seal over a smaller area of tracheal mucosa and tend to exert a high pressure on the mucosal cells, reducing the capillary blood supply and rendering the cells potentially ischaemic. High-volume cuffs cover a wide area of mucosa; the pressure exerted varies during the respiratory cycle, but on average is lower than that produced by a low-volume cuff. A medium-volume, low-profile cuffed tube represents a compromise and has some practical advantages.

Tracheal tubes of different sizes are required. The size quoted is the internal diameter (ID). Adult males normally require a tube of 9–9.5 mm ID and females 8–8.5 mm. For oral intubation, the tube should normally be 20–23 cm in length. The appropriate internal diameter of tube for paediatric use can be calculated from the following formula: (age/4) + 4 mm. This is an approximation and a tube 0.5 mm smaller and 0.5 mm larger should also be prepared. The length of tube required for oral intubation in children is approximately equal to (age/2) + 12 cm. A tube of slightly smaller internal diameter may be required for nasal intubation and its length may be calculated from the formula (age/2) + 15 cm.

An appropriate connector is required between the tracheal tube and the anaesthetic breathing system, e.g. curved connector for nasal tube, lightweight plastic with low dead space for children or a connector with a suction port for thoracic surgery.

Anaesthesia for tracheal intubation

Tracheal intubation may be performed under local anaesthesia (using topical spray, transtracheal spray and superior laryngeal nerve block) or under general anaesthesia (either i.v. or inhalation, with or without the use of muscle relaxation). The usual approach is to provide general anaesthesia and muscle relaxation, to perform laryngoscopy and direct vision intubation and then to maintain anaesthesia via the tracheal tube with spontaneous or controlled ventilation. Adequate anaesthesia and muscle relaxation must be provided for laryngoscopy.

Inhalation technique for intubation

Adequate depth of anaesthesia is necessary to depress the laryngeal reflexes and provide a degree of relaxation of the laryngeal and pharyngeal muscles. Halothane in concentrations up to 4% or sevoflurane 8% provides rapid attainment of the necessary depth, which can be judged from the pattern of respiration with predominance of diaphragmatic breathing (a useful sign in children is the 'dissociation' of the thoracic and abdominal excursion). The mask is removed and laryngoscopy and intubation performed. The anaesthetic circuit is then connected to the tracheal tube and anaesthesia maintained at a depth appropriate for surgery.

Relaxant anaesthesia for intubation

After i.v. or inhalation induction of anaesthesia, the short-acting depolarizing muscle relaxant succinylcholine may be used to provide relaxation for tracheal intubation. After loss of consciousness, the patient breathes 100% oxygen or 50% nitrous oxide in oxygen and succinylcholine is administered in a dose of 1–1.5 mg kg^{-1}. Assisted ventilation is maintained via the face mask until muscle relaxation occurs (except in emergency patients and those likely to regurgitate) and laryngoscopy and intubation are performed. Inhalation anaesthesia may be continued with manual ventilation until the effects of the relaxant have ceased, whereupon spontaneous ventilation is resumed. Alternatively, non-depolarizing neuromuscular blockade is produced and ventilation controlled.

Conduct of laryngoscopy

The position of the patient's head and neck is important. The neck should be flexed and the head extended with the support of a pillow; thus the oral, pharyngeal and tracheal axes are brought into alignment (Fig. 37.4). The laryngoscope is designed for left hand use and is introduced into the right side of the mouth while the right hand opens the mouth, parting the lips to avoid interposing them between laryngoscope and teeth. The teeth may be protected from blade trauma with the fingers or the use of a plastic 'guard'. The laryngoscope blade deflects the tongue to the left and the length of the blade is passed over the contour of the tongue. The laryngoscope is lifted upwards and forwards, avoiding a levering movement which can damage the upper teeth. Using a straight blade, the tip is passed posterior to the epiglottis, which is lifted anteriorly, and the vocal cords are seen. With a curved blade, the tip is inserted into the vallecula and pressure on the hyoepiglottic ligament moves the epiglottis to expose the vocal cords. External pressure on the thyroid cartilage by an assistant may aid laryngeal vision at this stage. Alternatively, using the McCoy adaptation of the Macintosh blade, the distal lever may be used to elevate the epiglottis to assist in viewing the larynx.

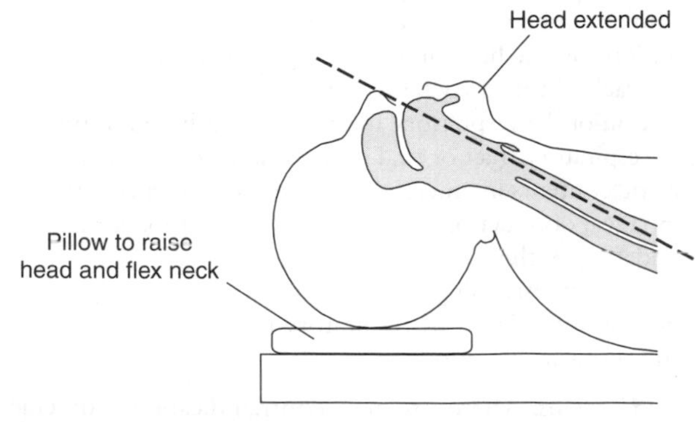

Fig. 37.4
Head position for laryngoscopy.

Conduct of intubation

After laryngeal visualization, the supraglottic area and cords may be sprayed, if required, with local anaesthetic solution (lidocaine 4%). The tracheal tube is passed from the right side of the mouth (which may be held open by the assistant's finger if necessary, permitting a clear view of the midline) and between the vocal cords into the trachea until the cuff is below the vocal cords. A semirigid stilette may be used during intubation to provide the correct degree of curvature of the tracheal tube to facilitate intubation. This is useful particularly with reinforced tubes.

The tube cuff is inflated sufficiently to abolish audible gas leaks on inflation of the lungs. The correct position of the tube must now be confirmed. If the tube has been seen clearly at laryngoscopy to pass through the vocal cords into the trachea, then equal movement of both sides of the chest during ventilation should be confirmed and auscultation in each axilla for breath sounds should be performed to ensure that the tip of the tracheal tube has not passed too far distally to enter, or occlude, one of the main bronchi (see p. 511); if there is unilateral air entry, the tube should be withdrawn slowly and carefully until air entry is equal in both lungs. If the tube has not been seen clearly to enter the trachea, or if there is any reason to suspect that its distal end is not in the trachea, then the steps outlined in Chapter 40 (p. 511) must be undertaken immediately to identify possible oesophageal intubation.

After its correct position has been determined, the tube is secured with cotton tape, bandage or sticking plaster strips. Correct fixation of the tube is important, particularly if the head is inaccessible during surgery, e.g. when the patient is in the prone position. On such occasions, extra security is gained using broad 'elastoplast' strapping over the primary fixing tape on the patient's face.

Nasal intubation

Nasal intubation may be used for dental operations, ENT operations, etc., and may be preferred for long-term intubation because it provides easier tube fixation, easier oral toilet and greater patient comfort.

A slightly smaller tube is used and is introduced preferentially into the right nostril, as the left-facing bevel of the tube favours this approach. The tube is passed along the floor of the nose and advanced *gently* into the pharynx, avoiding excessive force. Laryngoscopy takes place and the tube is advanced into the trachea by manipulation of the proximal end or by grasping the distal tip with Magill's intubating forceps to pass it between the cords.

Packing of the throat may be used after intubation, especially for oropharyngeal operations. The moist gauze pack is introduced using the laryngoscope and Magill forceps. The pharynx should be packed on each side of the tracheal tube. The pack should be applied gently to avoid abrasion of the mucosa. A 'tail' of the pack is left protruding from the mouth and the anaesthetist must accept responsibility for removal of the pack before extubation. A latex 'foam' pack may be used as an alternative to cotton gauze.

Difficult intubation

Difficult intubation may be anticipated or unanticipated. Difficulty may be anticipated from evidence sought at the preoperative visit. The unexpected case should be identified and acknowledged as such at the time of intubation and the anaesthetist should have contingency plans to overcome the situation. This subject is discussed in Chapter 40.

Complications of tracheal intubation

Complications may be mechanical, respiratory or cardiovascular and may occur early or late.

Early complications

Trauma may occur to lips and teeth or dental crowns. Jaw dislocation and dislocation of arytenoids may be produced. Trauma during intubation may result in damage to larynx and vocal cords. Nasal intubation may produce epistaxis, trauma to the pharyngeal wall or dislodgement of adenoid tissue. Obstruction or kinking of the tube can occur and carinal stimulation or bronchial intubation may take place if the tube is too long. Laryngeal trauma may produce postoperative croup, bronchospasm or laryngospasm, especially in children. Mechanical complications may be avoided with a careful technique. Broken teeth must be retrieved and the event documented. Immediate postoperative respiratory complications may be minimized by humidification of inspired gases. Cardiovascular complications of intubation include arrhythmias and hypertension, especially in untreated hypertensive patients.

Late complications

These are more common after long-term intubation. Tracheal stenosis is rare, but damage to tracheal mucosa from a cuffed tube may be related to its design; high-volume, low-pressure cuffs may be preferred for long-term intubation. Trauma to vocal cords may result in ulceration or granulomata which may require surgical removal. Cord trauma may be more common in the presence of an upper respiratory tract infection.

RELAXANT ANAESTHESIA

Indications for relaxant anaesthesia

As an alternative to deep anaesthesia with spontaneous ventilation and volatile agents leading to multisystem depression, the triad of sleep, suppression of reflexes and muscle relaxation may be provided separately with specific agents. Relaxation anaesthesia provides muscle relaxation, permitting lighter anaesthesia with less risk of cardiovascular depression. Thus the technique is appropriate for major abdominal, intraperitoneal, thoracic or intracranial operations, prolonged operations in which spontaneous ventilation would lead to respiratory depression, and operations in a position in which ventilation is impaired mechanically.

Conduct of relaxant anaesthesia

Almost universally, this involves tracheal intubation after induction of anaesthesia. This is produced either (a) after a depolarizing muscle relaxant (succinylcholine) followed, after its action has subsided, by a non-depolarizing relaxant, or (b) in the case of an elective fasting patient with normal gastric emptying and no history of hiatus hernia or regurgitation, after an intubating dose of a non-depolarizing muscle relaxant (Table 19.1) The choice of agent depends upon operative indications or the patient's condition (e.g. vecuronium and rocuronium produce little cardiovascular depression).

Controlled ventilation is commenced, first manually by compression of the reservoir bag and then by a mechanical ventilator delivering the appropriate tidal and minute volume (see Appendix VIII, p. 781). Anaesthesia and analgesia are provided by nitrous oxide/oxygen or air/oxygen, together with a volatile agent and/or i.v. analgesic. The inspired and end-expired concentrations of volatile agents should be monitored. A TIVA technique may be used (Ch. 14). Intravenous opioids, e.g. morphine, fentanyl or remifentanil, are used in small bolus doses or by continuous i.v. infusions as indicated. Analgesia may also be supplemented by opioid premedication or by use of regional or local anaesthetic techniques.

Assessment of relaxant anaesthesia

Light anaesthesia with preservation of reflexes permits the use of physical signs for the continued assessment of the adequacy of anaesthesia.

Adequacy of anaesthesia

Autonomic reflex activity with lacrimation, sweating, tachycardia, hypertension or reflex movement in response to surgery indicate 'light' anaesthesia and response to surgical stimulation, and warn that the depth of anaesthesia should be increased or further increments of i.v. analgesic given.

Awareness during anaesthesia

The possibility of conscious or unconscious awareness exists in a patient who is under the influence of a neuromuscular blocking drug if nitrous oxide/oxygen anaesthesia is unsupplemented or is supplemented by an opioid with little or no volatile agent. The anaesthetist should ensure that this possibility is avoided by constant observation of the patient for clinical signs of light anaesthesia and by use of small concentrations of a volatile agent. Up to 1% of patients may recall intraoperative events spontaneously if a mixture of nitrous oxide 67% in oxygen is administered, even with an i.v. opioid, and a proportion of these patients experience pain. Awareness during anaesthesia is now a common source of litigation. An appropriate concentration of volatile anaesthetic agent should be used routinely during elective surgery.

Adequacy of muscle relaxation

Clinical signs of return of muscle tone include retraction of the wound edges during abdominal operations and abdominal muscle, diaphragmatic or facial movement. An increase in airway pressure (with a time- or volume-cycled ventilator) may indicate a return of muscle tone. Quantitative estimation of neuromuscular status may be obtained with a peripheral nerve stimulator (see Ch. 38). Small increments (e.g. 25–35% of the original dose) of muscle relaxant may be given to maintain relaxation; alternatively, an i.v. infusion may be a more convenient method of administration, but the use of a peripheral nerve stimulator is mandatory with this technique.

Adequacy of ventilation

Clinical signs of inadequate ventilation and an increase in P_aCO_2 include venous dilatation, wound oozing, tachycardia, hypertension and attempts at spontaneous ventilation by the patient.

Measurement of airway pressure and end-expired PCO_2 with a capnograph are mandatory during relaxant anaesthesia and controlled ventilation. Monitoring expired gas volume provides useful information to adjust the degree of mechanical ventilation, and occasionally arterial PCO_2 measurement may be employed.

Reversal of relaxation

At the end of operation, residual neuromuscular block is antagonized and spontaneous ventilation should begin before the tracheal tube is removed and the patient awakened. Residual neuromuscular block is antagonized with neostigmine 2.5–5 mg (0.05–0.08 mg kg^{-1} in children). Atropine 1.2 mg or glycopyrronium 0.5 mg (in adults) counteracts the muscarinic side-effects of the anticholinesterase and may be given before, or with, neostigmine. Care should be exercised in the use of an anticholinergic agent in the presence of existing tachycardia, pyrexia, carbon dioxide retention or ischaemic heart disease.

Resumption of spontaneous ventilation should occur if normocapnic ventilation has been used and assured by monitoring the end-expired PCO_2. Tracheobronchial suction (see below) has the beneficial side-effect of stimulating respiration if used at this stage.

CONDUCT OF EXTUBATION

This may take place with the patient supine if the anaesthetist is satisfied that airway patency can be maintained by the patient in this position and there is no risk of regurgitation. In patients at risk of regurgitation and potential aspiration, the lateral position is preferred. However, it is safer to employ the lateral recovery position after extubation (Fig. 37.5). Return of respiratory reflexes is signified by coughing and resistance to the presence of the tracheal tube.

Tracheobronchial suction via the tracheal tube is carried out using a soft sterile suction catheter with an external diameter less than half the internal diameter of the tube. Preoxygenation pre-

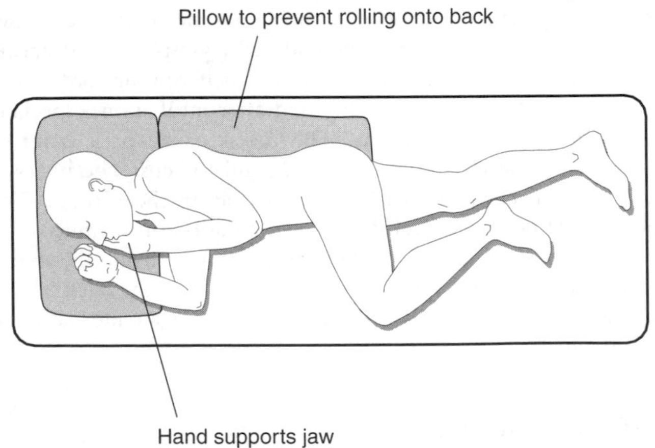

Fig. 37.5
Recovery position.

cedes suctioning, as the oxygen stores may be depleted by tracheal suction. The catheter is occluded during insertion and suction applied during withdrawal.

Pharyngeal suction is performed best under direct vision, avoiding trauma to the pharyngeal mucosa, uvula or epiglottis. This should take place before antagonism of neuromuscular block.

Oxygen 100% replaces the anaesthetic gas mixture before extubation to avoid the potential effects of diffusion hypoxia (p. 165) and to provide a pulmonary reservoir of oxygen in case breath-holding or coughing occurs.

Extubation is performed preferably during inspiration when the larynx dilates; the cuff is deflated and the tube is withdrawn along its curved axis, as careless withdrawal in a straight line may damage laryngeal structures. Some anaesthetists generate a positive pressure in the trachea during this manoeuvre by 'squeezing the bag' in order to propel secretions into the pharynx.

After extubation, the patient's ability to maintain the airway is ensured, the ability to cough and clear secretions is assessed and an oropharyngeal airway is inserted if required. Administration of oxygen is continued by face mask. Preparations are made for recovery.

Complications of tracheal extubation

Laryngeal spasm

This may follow stimulation during extubation. Extubation during deep anaesthesia and subsequent maintenance with a mask may be used. Local anaesthetic spray to the larynx may block the reflex, and pharyngeal suction before extubation removes secretions which may cause stimulation.

Regurgitation/inhalation

Aspiration via the nasogastric tube (if present) should be performed before tracheal extubation to remove gastric liquid. In emergency patients, extubation should be performed with the patient awake so that airway control is continuous. Partial incompetence of laryngeal reflexes may occur in the immediate post-extubation period, especially if local anaesthetic spray has been employed. In this event, recovery should take place with the patient in the lateral head-down position, with facilities at hand for suction, oxygenation and reintubation.

EMERGENCE AND RECOVERY

After completion of surgery anaesthetic agents are withdrawn and oxygen 100% is delivered. Following removal of the tracheal tube or LMA, the patient's airway is supported until respiratory reflexes are intact. The patient's muscle power and coordination are assessed by testing hand grip, tongue protrusion or a sustained head lift from the pillow in response to command. Return of adequate muscle power must be ensured before the patient leaves theatre. Full monitoring of the patient should not be discontinued before recovery of consciousness.

The patient is then ready for transfer from the operating table to a bed or trolley. Oxygen is delivered by face mask during transport, and further recovery takes place in a recovery area of theatre or in the recovery ward (Ch. 41).

The lateral recovery position (Fig. 37.5) is adopted unless the anaesthetist is satisfied that this is unnecessary. The patient is turned on one side, upper leg flexed and lower extended; the head is on one side and the tongue falls forward under gravity, thus avoiding airway obstruction.

FURTHER READING

Association of Anaesthetists of Great Britain and Ireland 1992 HIV and other blood borne viruses. AAGBI, London

Association of Anaesthetists of Great Britain and Ireland 1995 Suspected anaphylactic reactions associated with anaesthesia. AAGBI, London

Association of Anaesthetists of Great Britain and Ireland 1997 Checklist for anaesthetic apparatus. AAGBI, London

Brimacombe J R, Brain A I J, Berry A M 1996 The laryngeal mask airway instruction manual, 3rd edn. Intavent, Pangbourne

Latto I P, Vaughan R S 1997 Difficulties in tracheal intubation, 2nd edn. W B Saunders, London

McHardy F E, Chung F 1999 Postoperative sore throat: cause, prevention and treatment. Anaesthesia 54: 444–453

Martin J T, Warner M A 1997 Positioning in anesthesia and surgery, 3rd edn. W B Saunders, Philadelphia

38 Monitoring

The purpose of monitoring is to augment the clinical observations of anaesthetists and to help them decide on the administration of anaesthesia and any other treatments.

As anaesthesia has developed, the range and complexity of available monitors have increased rapidly. While this has brought undoubted benefits, their sophistication and complexity have brought additional problems. Before the results of any monitor are used to direct treatment, a series of questions should be asked (Table 38.1):

- *Validity – what is actually being measured?* In the case of directly measuring arterial pressure with an arterial cannula and a pressure transducer, the answer is obvious. However, in the case of 'depth of anaesthesia' monitors, for example, it is usually some physiological variable that is measured, transformed mathematically and then compared with a reference value. Unfortunately, companies usually seek to avoid disclosing the details of how the machine operates to protect their market. While this is inevitable given the complexity of the technology, the result is that users often have to trust the manufacturer and believe the information provided by the monitor.
- *What method of measurement is being used?* Any method of measurement has inherent advantages and disadvantages. The result is that externally similar pieces of equipment may produce dissimilar results.
- *Is the environment appropriate?* For example, a monitor which functions well in an operating theatre may be useless on board an ambulance or in an aircraft because of noise or vibration. The monitor may also provide additional hazards for the patient. Any potentially magnetic material taken into the vicinity of a magnetic resonance imaging (MRI) machine is likely to be accelerated by the huge magnetic field and may cause severe injuries. The magnetic field may also induce electrical currents in wires placed near the monitor, causing heating and the possibility of burning the patient. All equipment must therefore be made of non-magnetic material or moved outside the magnetic field. Several manufacturers now make specific MRI-compatible equipment.
- *Has the monitor been serviced, checked and calibrated correctly?* Most monitors have service intervals set by the manufacturer and often have components which degrade with time. Financial constraints have led to some hospitals failing to comply with manufacturers' instructions, which may lead to suboptimal performance.
- *Is the monitor appropriate for the patient?* Many pieces of equipment have been designed to be used on adults only. Their use in children and especially neonates may produce unreliable results.
- *Has the probe been applied to the correct region of the patient?* For example, a patient with aortic coarctation has markedly different arterial pressures in each arm.
- *Is the variable being measured within the range of the equipment?* For example, monitors are usually tested and validated only in relatively stable patients. Whether any monitor can function well in an infrequently encountered situation such as anaphylaxis is impossible to determine reliably. The inference is that during any anaesthetic disaster, when we need our monitors the most, they may be unreliable or even misleading.

Table 38.1 Premonitoring checks
What is being measured?
What method is being used?
Has the monitor been serviced and calibrated?
Is the environment appropriate?
Is this the correct patient?
Is this the correct range?
Can the display be read?
Have appropriate alarm limits been set?

DISPLAYS

All monitors should not only measure some aspect of the well-being of the patient, but also convey that information to the anaesthetist. Manufacturers of early monitors generally paid little attention to presentation and clinicians were presented with a collection of boxes with displays varying in colour, size, shape and legibility. In addition, the increase in the number of sensors attached to patients has led to a progressive increase in the number of boxes, with predictably confusing results. In recent years, the tendency has been towards the development of a central display unit that provides a single coordinated display. This allows a single monitor to provide a range of measurements, by adding or changing modules, and also allows faulty modules to be changed easily. While there are benefits to this approach in terms of clarity and consistency, the threat of information overload is still present. A current monitor, the Datex AS3 (Fig. 38.1), may display up to six

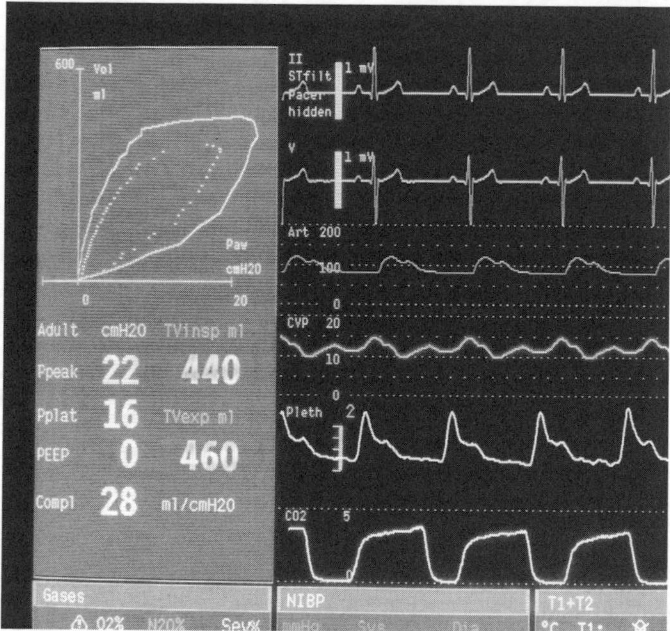

Fig. 38.1
Standard anaesthetic monitoring screen.

waveforms and associated digital values in addition to four different digital displays, with the colour and size of each display able to be altered by the operator. While the original display is clear and well designed, it is possible for an operator to make the display so complex and crowded that it is almost useless in a crisis.

Psychological tests have shown that in stressful situations, there is limited ability to absorb information and it is therefore vital that the most important information is easily seen and not obscured by a mass of interesting but non-essential data. Some manufacturers have attempted to make it easier for anaesthetists to obtain information from the monitors by using bar graphs or geometric figures which change shape with the condition of the patient, although this approach has not so far found favour with many anaesthetists.

ALARMS

The primary alarm system during any operation should obviously be the anaesthetist. In an ideal world, any change in any of the measured variables should have been noticed and corrective action taken before it moves outside the normal range. However, there are many distractions in theatre and alarms provide a useful fail-safe mechanism by which the monitors alert the anaesthetist to any abnormalities. To function, any alarm system must 'know' the 'normal range' of any variable so that it can be activated when these values are exceeded. Monitors usually have a set of default alarm limits which are activated at start-up, and some have several sets of values which can be entered by the operator for a particular procedure, e.g. for paediatric, cardiac or local anaesthesia cases. These are extremely useful as they avoid unnecessary alarms being set, e.g. for expired anaesthetic vapour concentration in an awake patient having a procedure under regional anaesthesia. Although alarms are considered a mandatory feature of monitoring equipment, they cause great difficulty if they are constantly activated. This may be caused by the anaesthetist not setting appropriate limits before starting, or the machine failing to distinguish between artefacts (caused, for example, by diathermy) and a genuine patient abnormality. Constantly sounding alarms may cause the anaesthetist to spend so much time altering the settings on the machine that he or she fails to notice that the patient needs attention. Conversely, many anaesthetists have become so used to constant alarms that their first reaction is usually to turn the alarms off and assume that it is an artefact rather than to look for a cause. Some manufacturers have attempted to address these problems by producing monitors with a series of alarms that might indicate, for example, an equipment problem, a minor physiological change, a major change or a cardiac arrest. For example, a minor change in oxygen saturation might warrant a quiet buzz, while a loss of arterial pressure would produce the equivalent of a trumpet call. Unfortunately, the lack of standardization of alarms between different manufacturers renders systems confusing.

THE CARDIOVASCULAR SYSTEM

CLINICAL

The principal aim is to ensure that the tissues of patients have an adequate oxygen supply. This is the product of cardiac output, haemoglobin concentration and haemoglobin saturation. Clinically, a patient's haemoglobin concentration and saturation may be estimated by looking at the skin, and cardiac output may be estimated by the warmth of the extremities. Therefore, observation of a good pulse, pink skin and warm fingers, especially when combined with a urine output of > 0.5 ml kg^{-1} h^{-1}, implies that there is unlikely to be a cardiovascular problem. In children, where peripheral vascular disease is rare, capillary refill time provides a valuable indication of cardiac output. Refill time is the time taken for the capillaries to refill after a digit has been exsanguinated by firm pressure. When a finger has been under pressure for 3 s, a capillary refill time of less than 1.5 s is considered normal, while a time of greater than 5 s is indicative of shock. While patients with complex problems may require more sophisticated monitors, the value of direct observation of the patient and a 'finger on the pulse' cannot be overestimated. In practice, dimmed theatre lights or surgical drapes may cause difficulties, but direct observation of the patient should always be maintained.

ELECTROCARDIOGRAPHY

The electrocardiograph (ECG) is a recording of the electrical activity of the heart usually measured at the skin surface with either three or five leads. The size of the waveform may be reduced by increased thoracic wall thickness or by poor electrode contact, often caused by poorly applied or dried out electrodes. As the changes in measured electrical potential are very small, it is very susceptible to interference from nearby electrically powered devices. Diathermy usually obliterates the ECG whenever it is used. Monitors are designed usually to withstand the large currents developed during defibrillation, so it is not necessary to remove the leads before defibrillation or cardioversion.

An audible warning is usually produced if significant arrhythmias develop. Unfortunately, this analysis is usually rendered useless during diathermy, making false alarms common. Many monitors measure the ST segment and provide a trend of its level with time. This may identify ischaemia and then provide a graphic illustration of whether or not it is responding to treatment. The position of

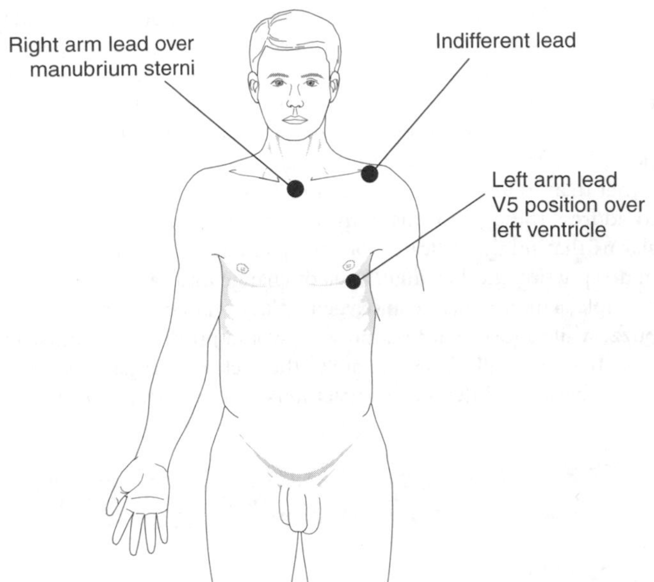

Fig. 38.2
CM5 lead configuration for electrocardiograph monitoring.

the three electrodes defines the area of myocardium that contributes to the display, so careful positioning is required. The CM5 arrangement (Fig. 38.2) is recommended for detecting ischaemia, as it 'looks' at the left ventricle.

Although the ECG has become a standard anaesthetic monitor, it only provides a measure of heart rate and rhythm. Electrical activity can still occur with no cardiac output, for example in cardiac tamponade or severe hypovolaemia. This severely limits the usefulness of the ECG as a patient monitor.

ARTERIAL PRESSURE

Palpation

Systolic pressure may be estimated easily by inflating a cuff around the upper arm to a high pressure and then detecting the return of the radial pulse as the cuff is deflated. Auscultation of arterial pressure via Korotkov sounds is also possible, although difficult in a noisy theatre. In practice, these methods are time-consuming and access to the patient may be difficult. Despite this, in situations where monitoring devices are not available or where a patient has suddenly deteriorated, estimating systolic pressure by palpation is a useful first step.

Automated oscillometer

A cuff is applied to the upper arm, or in difficult cases to the thigh or calf. The cuff is inflated automatically with a pump to above systolic pressure and then deflated progressively. Small pressure changes in the cuff caused by passage of blood underneath it are sensed by the monitor, usually via a second tube.

Automated oscillometers usually read arterial pressure in 20–50s and can be programmed to read automatically at set intervals. An example is shown in Fig. 38.3. Most anaesthetists set the machine to read once every 3–5 min during routine anaesthesia. In the event of a crisis, many monitors have a 'stat' button, which

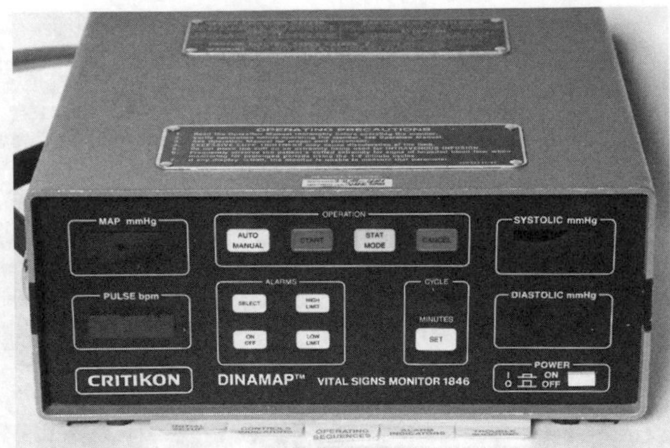

Fig. 38.3
An automated oscillometer.

repeatedly measures arterial pressure as rapidly as possible for around 5 min.

Disadvantages are shown in Table 38.2.

Finapres

This monitor uses a photoelectric probe placed on a finger. A cuff is also positioned around the same finger. The pressure in the cuff is varied automatically to eliminate changes in flow in the finger. The pressure in the cuff is then said to vary directly with arterial pressure, providing a continuous non-invasive arterial pressure measurement. As a result of doubts about its accuracy, its use has never become widespread.

Direct pressure measurement

This requires a cannula to be inserted into an artery. The radial artery or dorsalis pedis artery is usually chosen in the adult, with the femoral artery being used more often in children. In an adult, a parallel-sided 20–22G Teflon catheter is usually inserted and then connected to a pressure sensor via a length of saline-filled tubing. The entire system is connected to a bag of heparinized saline, which flushes the transducer and cannula at a rate of 1–3 ml h^{-1}. A valve is also present which allows the system to be flushed, e.g. after a sample has been obtained. The pressure transducer is set at the level of the patient's left ventricle and opened to air to obtain a zero

Table 38.2 Disadvantages of automated oscillometry
Delayed measurement with arrhythmias or patient movement
Inaccuracy if systolic pressure < 60 mmHg
Inaccurate if the wrong size of cuff is used
Discomfort in awake patients
Skin and nerve damage
Delay in drug dose reaching circulation
Backflow of blood into i.v. cannulae
Pulse oximeter on same limb malfunctions with each cuff inflation

pressure. When zeroed, the transducer then converts changes in pressure directly into changes in electrical resistance, which are measured by the monitor. A real-time waveform is usually displayed in addition to digital values of pulse rate and systolic, diastolic and mean arterial pressures. Advantages are shown in Table 38.3.

Inaccuracies may be introduced if the transducer is not zeroed correctly or if it is moved relative to the patient, usually because the patient is moved up or down on the operating table when the transducer is on a separate stand. In a few patients, there is a marked discrepancy between arterial pressure measured invasively and that measured by a non-invasive method. While the invasive pressure is more likely to be accurate, the patient's 'normal' arterial pressure is likely to have been measured non-invasively.

Damping is caused by some part of the measuring system absorbing some of the pressure changes (see Ch. 31). It may be caused by bubbles of air in the tubing, tubing which is too long or too elastic, a cannula that has become kinked or arterial spasm. Damping produces a trace with reduced amplitude and measurements of systolic and diastolic pressures that tend towards the mean pressure (Fig. 31.3).

Direct arterial pressure measurement has become standard monitoring for any high-risk patient during anaesthesia and is commonly used in patients in intensive care or high-dependency areas. Complications are shown in Table 38.4.

Before cannulating the radial artery, it is advisable to occlude both radial and ulnar arteries, then releasing the ulnar artery and observing the capillary refill to ensure that the ulnar artery is patent (Weber's test). When left in situ for more than 12 h, cannulae often malfunction, although careful insertion under aseptic conditions, firm fixation of the cannula to the surrounding skin and an operational flushing system reduce complications.

CENTRAL VENOUS PRESSURE

The pressure in the superior vena cava is usually measured to guide fluid replacement in situations such as major blood loss or where myocardial function is impaired. In normal individuals, the central venous pressure (CVP) is 0–5 cmH_2O. It is reduced in hypovolaemia and increased by heart failure, pulmonary emboli, positive pressure ventilation, cardiac tamponade and fluid overload. Ideally, the tip of any catheter should be placed just above the right atrium to ensure the desired pressure is measured. Advancing the catheter too far may cause arrhythmias and damage the myocardium. Complications are shown in Table 38.5.

There are three main routes of insertion:

Long catheters. These are inserted into a peripheral vein, via a large cannula. The approach is usually via the brachial vein in the antecubital fossa. The catheter is advanced into the superior vena cava (SVC) through the subclavian vein. Advancement of the cannula may be difficult, but abduction of the arm is sometimes helpful. The cephalic vein on the outer upper arm is less often used as it has a more tortuous route through the shoulder and success is less likely. This method is relatively easy and has a very low incidence of acute, serious complications. Unfortunately, the tip of the cannula commonly fails to reach a central vein and infection and thrombophlebitis are common if left in situ after 48 h.

Subclavian. As the subclavian vein is large and close to the SVC, a short catheter is inserted easily through the skin. The overlying clavicle affords easy fixation of the catheter to the skin and this is comfortable for patients. Unfortunately, because the needle, wire and catheter are not inserted under direct vision, accidental perforation of the adjacent subclavian artery or pleura is common. Importantly, if arterial bleeding occurs, it may not be evident and cannot be controlled by pressure because of the position of the clavicle. Damage may also be caused to the brachial plexus, which runs alongside the main vessels. Because of the incidence of major complications, subclavian cannulation is generally used only where specific advantages are evident.

Internal jugular. This route is the safest and most reliable site for cannulation, mainly because the vein is close to the skin and bleeding can be controlled by direct pressure. However, as a result of the proximity of the carotid artery, cervical spine, major nerves and the pleura, life-threatening complications are still relatively common.

It is essential first to establish a reference point, which is usually taken to be the patient's right atrium. The external markings are shown in Figure 38.4.

Table 38.3 Advantages of direct arterial pressure measurement
Accuracy of pressure measurement
Beat-by-beat observation of changes where blood pressure is variable or where vasoactive drugs are used
Accuracy at low pressures
Ability to obtain frequent blood samples

Table 38.4 Complications of arterial cannulation
Requires skill to insert
Bleeding
Arterial damage and thrombosis
Embolization
Ischaemia of tissues distal to artery
Sepsis
Inadvertent injection of drugs

Table 38.5 Complications of central venous cannulation
Acute
Arrhythmias
Bleeding
Pneumothorax
Damage to thoracic duct, oesophagus, carotid artery, stellate ganglion
Cardiac puncture
Catheter embolization
Delayed
Sepsis
Thrombosis
Cardiac rupture

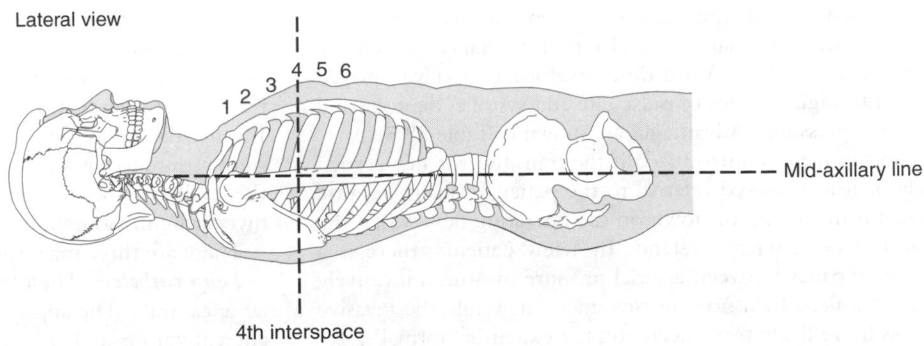

Fig. 38.4
Surface markings used to identify the position of the right atrium.

Whatever route is chosen, catheters should be inserted only where a clear indication is present; the safest route should be chosen and the catheter removed at the earliest opportunity. Careful technique and adequate observation of the patient, including a chest X-ray after insertion, are mandatory.

Measurement can be made with a simple manometer (Fig. 38.5). A vertical tube is connected to the CVP catheter and filled with intravenous fluid. The height of the patient's right atrium is then marked on the tubing as a zero point. The two are then connected and the saline allowed to flow into the patient. When the flow has stopped, the height of the column of saline above the zero point equals the CVP. Although useful on the ward and where equipment is lacking, during surgery, a less labour-intensive method with a continuous readout is needed; thus a pressure transducer is usually used.

As the normal CVP varies from 0 to 5 cmH_2O, even a small change in the relative height of the reference and measuring heights, e.g. when an operating table is moved up or down, leads to appreciable error.

In practice, a single measurement of CVP is unreliable, as the value is altered in an unpredictable manner by several factors, such as positive pressure ventilation and patient position. The response of the CVP to a fluid challenge is more valuable. In hypovolaemic patients, the CVP initially changes little with a rapid infusion of fluid. With continued infusion, the CVP increases more quickly as normovolaemia is achieved. In patients who are overloaded with fluid or who have heart failure, even small amounts of intravenous fluid causes a marked increase in the CVP. Sudden increases in CVP may also be caused by events such as pulmonary emboli, myocardial infarction or pneumothorax.

PULMONARY ARTERY PRESSURE

One of the main determinants of cardiac output, and hence oxygen delivery, is the filling pressure of the left ventricle. This usually approximates to right atrial pressure, but in ill patients, particularly in those with right ventricular failure, pulmonary oedema, mitral valve disease and those receiving positive pressure ventilation, the relationship is uncertain. Unfortunately, it is not possible to cannulate the left atrium easily. In practice, the pressure may be estimated with a pulmonary artery flotation catheter (PAFC).

These catheters usually have three lumens, and a thermistor near the tip:

- a distal lumen, which opens at the tip; this is connected to a pressure transducer and the waveform is displayed on a monitor

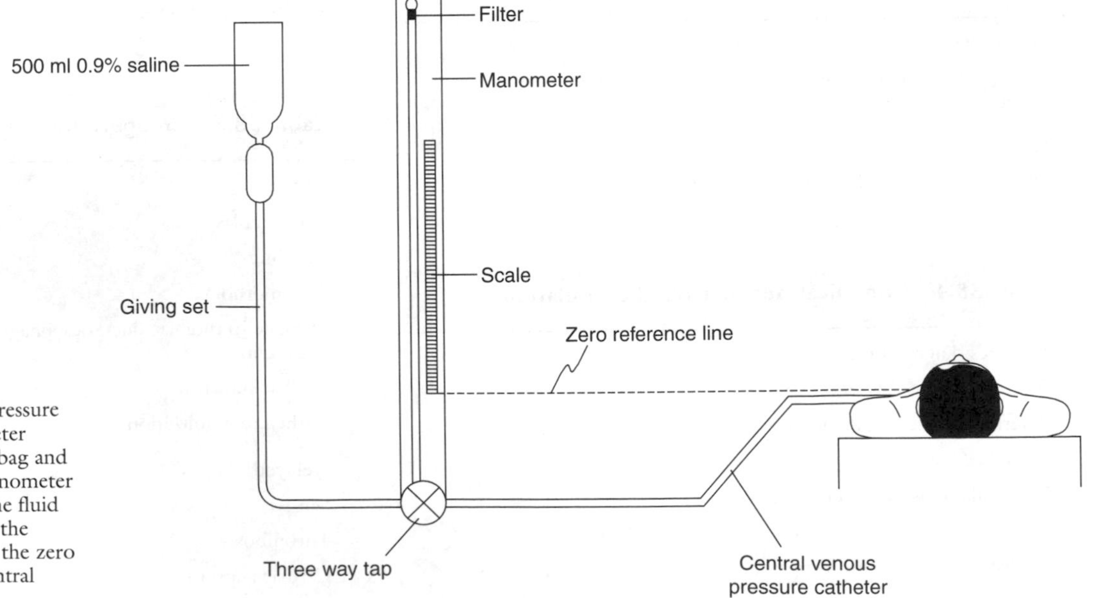

Fig. 38.5
Measurement of central venous pressure using a manometer. The manometer tubing is filled from the infusion bag and the tap turned to connect the manometer to the central venous catheter. The fluid level in the manometer falls until the height of the fluid column above the zero reference point is equal to the central venous pressure.

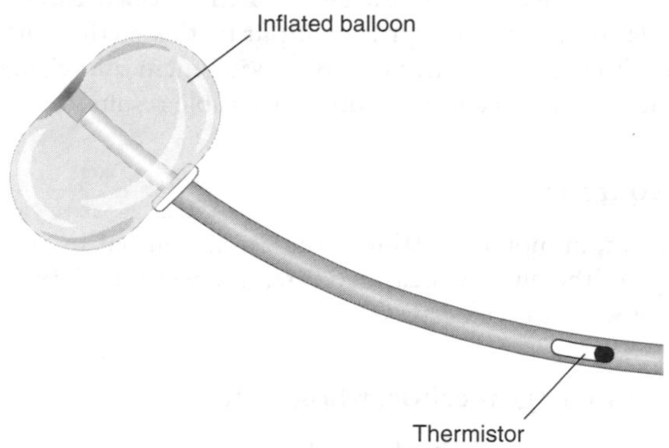

Fig. 38.6
Distal end of pulmonary artery catheter showing inflated balloon and thermistor.

- a lumen which is used to inflate a balloon, just proximal to the tip (Fig. 38.6)
- a proximal lumen which is used for cardiac output measurements (see below).

Usually, the PAFC is enclosed in a sterile sheath and then threaded through a large cannula previously inserted into a central vein. The flexible sheath allows the PAFC to be manipulated without it becoming unsterile. When the catheter is placed into the SVC, and a central venous waveform is seen on the monitor, the balloon is inflated. As the PAFC is advanced, the tip of the catheter tends to move towards the pulmonary artery as the balloon is pulled along by the blood flow. Although some manipulation may be required, it usually advances through the right atrium and right ventricle into the pulmonary artery. The corresponding changes in measured pressure can be observed as the catheter is advanced, confirming correct placement (Fig. 38.7).

If the catheter is advanced further, it eventually fills the lumen of a pulmonary artery to become 'wedged'. In this position, the tip of the catheter is isolated from the pulmonary artery by the balloon. The transducer then measures the pressure in the pulmonary capillaries, which are in continuity with the pulmonary veins and hence the left atrium. In practice, as the PAFC is advanced, at some point the measured pressure ceases to pulsate and decreases to a lower 'wedge pressure'. This is then taken as a measure of left atrial pressure. At the end of each measurement, the balloon must be deflated or pulmonary infarction may occur.

Unfortunately, the pressure varies with respiration and is influenced by a variety of factors such as pulmonary oedema and heart failure. The result is that measurements must be made very carefully. Some interpretation of the result is usually required and as with the CVP, a change in reading in response to a fluid challenge is more informative than a single reading.

In addition to the ability to estimate left atrial pressure, the PAFC also allows sampling of mixed venous blood and measurement of cardiac output.

Table 38.6 Factors leading to inaccurate cardiac output measurements

Injection of bolus is too slow
Poor mixing of injectate with the blood
Cold injectate is warmed as it passes through the heart
Ectopic heartbeats
Variability in cardiac output with each breath

CARDIAC OUTPUT

Measurement of the cardiac output has become more common as studies have shown that patients who have a low cardiac output that does not increase with treatment have greatly increased mortality. Conversely, identifying patients with low cardiac output and then increasing it, and hence oxygen delivery, has been associated with a reduction of perioperative complications in some studies.

Thermodilution method

Clinically, this is the 'gold standard' against which other methods are assessed (see Ch. 31).

In humans, a PAFC needs to be inserted and a bolus of cold water injected through the proximal lumen into the right atrium. It then passes with the blood flow into the pulmonary artery, where the decrease in temperature is measured by a thermistor at the end of the catheter. The monitor usually measures the temperature of the injectate before injection with a second thermistor. In theory, a few simple calculations result in a value for the cardiac output, but in reality many factors may lead to inaccuracies, some of which are shown in Table 38.6.

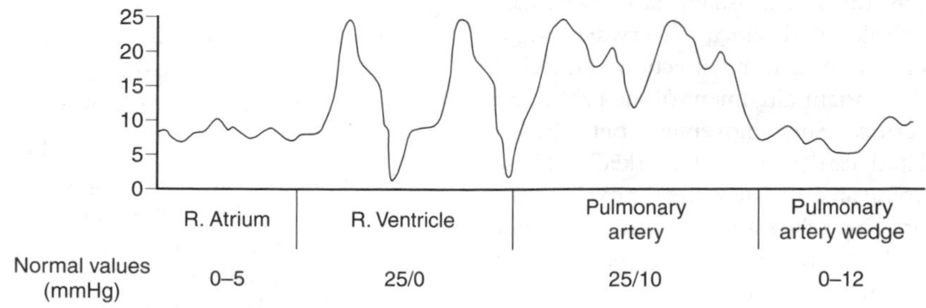

Fig. 38.7
Diagrammatic representation of pressure waveforms seen on an oscilloscope as the tip of a pulmonary artery catheter is advanced through the right artium and right ventricle to lie in the pulmonary artery. The pulmonary artery wedge waveform is seen when the balloon is inflated with the tip of the catheter in a branch of the pulmonary artery. Normal values shown represent pressures in a spontaneously breathing patient.

Table 38.7 Complications associated with pulmonary artery flotation catheters

Acute
Arrhythmias
Bleeding
Damage to lungs or large vessels
Knotting
Chronic
Sepsis
Embolization
Pulmonary infarction
Heart valve damage
Cardiac rupture

In practice, several measurements are usually taken, the most extreme results discarded and the average of three measurements used. The technique is time-consuming and accuracy is dependent on operator skill. Recent monitors have reduced these factors by incorporating a small heating coil into the PAFC, which is activated periodically, providing a bolus of heated blood, with the results again being measured with a thermistor. These monitors provide a continuous measure of cardiac output and, more importantly, demonstrate graphically changes in measurements with time.

Despite their undoubted benefits, the use of PAFCs in some studies has been associated with increased mortality, perhaps because of their complications (see Table 38.7). This has led to a search for measures of cardiac output which are safer and easier. Although no method has been found to be as reliable, several other methods are in use.

Transthoracic/transoesophageal Doppler probes

These use the principle that the frequency of a wave changes if it is reflected off a moving object. These probes are placed in the suprasternal notch or the oesophagus and emit an ultrasonic sound wave that is then reflected off red cells in the aorta. The machines then use the measured velocity and assumptions about the size of the aorta and flow patterns within it to calculate cardiac output. Estimates of stroke volume and cardiac contractility are also possible. If the descending aorta is used, then the proportion of cardiac output directed to the upper arms and head must be assumed and the calculated flow adjusted accordingly. The great advantage of these machines is that they are easy to use and provide an almost instantaneous measure of cardiac output with a very low incidence of complications. Unfortunately, the probes usually have a fairly narrow angle of detection and the calculated velocity is very dependent on the angle between the sound waves and the direction of travel of the red cells. The result is that constant alignment of the probe and the blood flow in the aorta is critical. Small movements of the probe therefore change the calculated cardiac output markedly. These monitors are unable to determine an absolute value for cardiac output reliably, but are used more to provide a trend with time. They are therefore very useful in guiding perioperative fluid management but have a limited scope in the intensive care unit.

Transthoracic impedance monitors

These monitors use the principle that as the amount of blood in the thorax varies with each heartbeat, it causes a corresponding change in the electrical conductance of the thorax. Although it is possible to measure the cardiac output by this method, in practice interference from other electrical equipment and changes in electrode conductance may produce unreliable results.

Pulse contour

Cardiac output monitors estimate the cardiac output by analysing the shape of the directly measured arterial waveform. Again, there are doubts about their accuracy.

Trans-oesophageal echocardiography

Trans-oesophageal echocardiography uses a miniaturized ultrasonic probe which is inserted into the oesophagus and which provides an image of all four cardiac chambers. It may identify malfunctioning heart valves, in addition to providing an overall picture of myocardial function. If the perfusion of areas of myocardium is compromised, these areas are observed as hypokinetic segments, before the ischaemia leads to irreversible changes. The success of therapy to reverse the ischaemia can then be observed directly. Although this technique cannot directly measure cardiac output, it may guide fluid therapy by demonstrating adequacy of cardiac filling. These monitors are expensive, provide only subjective information and require a trained and experienced operator.

PULSE OXIMETRY

Pulse oximeters measure the pulse rate and haemoglobin oxygen saturation by measuring changes in light absorption of, for example, a finger. The amount of light absorbed by a solution of haemoglobin depends on the wavelength of the incident light. When the absorption of a wide range of wavelengths is plotted out, it shows its characteristic absorption spectrum.

Each organic molecule has its own absorption spectrum and, usefully, when oxygen binds to haemoglobin, the absorption spectrum changes. At some wavelengths, termed isobestic points, there is no change with oxygenation, but at other wavelengths there are large changes in absorption. This implies that if light of the correct wavelength is chosen and passed through a solution of haemoglobin, it is possible to calculate the proportion of the haemoglobin that is oxygenated from the amount of each wavelength that is absorbed. In practice, each monitor has a probe that is placed around a part of the patient (Fig. 38.8). This is usually a finger, but other areas may be used, e.g. a toe, an ear or, in children, an arm. One side of the probe contains light-emitting diodes (LEDs) and the other side a light sensor.

The monitor then calculates the oxygen saturation and pulse rate via the steps outlined below:

1. The machine first senses the ambient light and then subtracts that amount from all subsequent measurements. Variations in the ambient light level, e.g. caused by drapes being moved, could cause errors in measurement.
2. An LED is then turned on and off rapidly. The amount of transmitted light and the way it changes over time are measured. The result is a waveform caused by an increase in absorption with each pulse as blood moves into the tissues. The frequency of this waveform is assumed to be the pulse rate. The monitor requires a series of around eight heartbeats

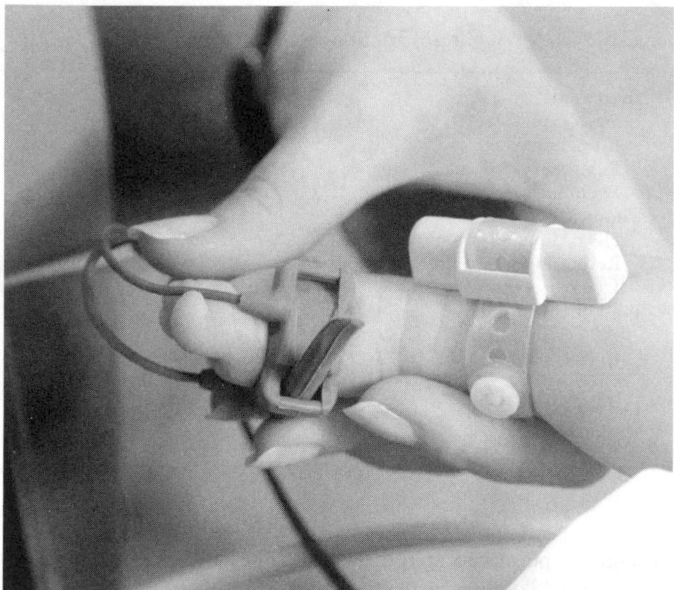

Fig. 38.8
Pulse oximeter probe on a child.

to produce a waveform and this induces a delay in measurement. Frequent ectopic beats and atrial fibrillation may also complicate results.

3. The monitor then analyses the waveform and removes the fixed component of absorption, on the assumption that it is caused by tissues such as skin, muscle and bone. The variable component is therefore assumed to result from pulsatile arterial blood. In situations where there is reduced pulsation in peripheral tissues, such as hypotension, hypovolaemia, hypothermia or cardiac bypass, the measured absorption ceases to vary with each pulse. Without the pulsatile variation, the monitor cannot determine the arterial component of absorption and saturation cannot be calculated.
4. Steps 1–3 are repeated sequentially for two or more wavelengths of light, at around 120 times a second. The results from successive beats are then averaged with a result produced about every 8 s. Comparison of the results from each wavelength allows the proportion of oxygenated haemoglobin to be calculated. These calculations are based on the assumption that only normal adult haemoglobin is present in the circulation. Results are affected if abnormal haemoglobin molecules are present. For example, carbon monoxide bound to haemoglobin is usually interpreted as oxygenated haemoglobin, giving falsely high readings. In addition, the presence of artificial pigments, whether blood markers or in the form of nail varnish, may affect results unpredictably. Lastly, inaccurate readings may result if the probe gradually moves so that some of the light bypasses the finger and enters the sensor directly.

The result is a reliable, non-invasive readout of pulse rate and saturation. Its simplicity rapidly made it one of the standard anaesthetic monitors. Its most useful applications are listed in Table 38.8.

Accuracy is around ± 2% above 70% and ± 3% between 50 and 70%. Accuracy below 50% is unknown, as it is difficult to study patients in this range ethically. Miniaturization of the circuitry has also allowed portable monitors to be developed for bedside use on general wards.

Complications are rare, but if probes are left on extremities for long periods, skin damage may occur. Unfortunately, pulse oximeters are limited in that they signal a failure of oxygenation only after the patient has become hypoxaemic, which may be several minutes after, for example, a breathing system disconnection. They are also a poor measure of ventilation. The ventilation of a patient breathing 100% oxygen may decrease enough to cause severe hypercapnia and yet cause no change in oxygen saturation.

Table 38.8 Particular uses of pulse oximetry
Dark-skinned patients
In areas of low light levels
CT and MRI scanners where access is poor
Paediatric anaesthesia
Monitoring for postoperative hypoxaemia
Diagnosing sleep apnoea

THE RESPIRATORY SYSTEM

CLINICAL

Continuous direct observation of the colour of the patient and movement of the chest and the reservoir bag in the breathing system is essential for safe anaesthesia. Both anaesthetic agents and opioids are potent depressants of respiration and hypoxic brain damage can occur in a few minutes. In cases where the patient is breathing spontaneously, constant observation is needed to detect tracheal tug, paradoxical chest movement and failure of the reservoir bag to move, indicating partial or complete airway obstruction. Free passage of air may also be confirmed by listening for the gentle sigh of clear airflow or feeling the warmth of expired air. Snoring, rattles or complete silence indicate impending or actual airway obstruction. Maintaining a clear airway in an anaesthetized patient is a skill requiring much practice, constant attention to detail and strong forearm muscles. Periodic auscultation of the chest confirms the position of a tracheal tube, detects any cumulation of secretions and detects bronchospasm.

Oesophageal stethoscopes

These consist of a small balloon-tipped probe that may be inserted into the oesophagus and connected to either a standard stethoscope headpiece or a moulded earpiece. When the length has been adjusted so the balloon is next to the heart, it provides constant monitoring of the heartbeat and breath sounds. It is especially useful in children and may detect air embolism by the characteristic, millwheel murmur. It is cheap, informative and has the advantage of ensuring that the anaesthetist stays in close contact with the patient. Complications are exceptionally rare.

Respiratory rate

Respiratory rate may be timed clinically or obtained from the capnograph. Some monitors incorporating ECG electrodes may also use these to measure the patient's respiratory rate. A very small, high-frequency current is passed across the patient's chest and the electrical impedance (i.e. the resistance to flow of an alternating current) is measured. The cyclical changes in impedance with respiration are measured and the rate displayed.

Airway pressure

This must be measured in all patients receiving positive pressure ventilation, as high airway pressure may cause damage to the alveoli, reduce cardiac output, and may predispose to pneumothorax. Causes of changes in airway pressure are shown in Table 38.9.

Many operating theatre ventilators incorporate simple mechanical pressure gauges. However, where narrow tracheal tubes are used, in extended breathing systems, and when the respiratory rates are high, the gauge may not accurately reflect airway pressure.

Table 38.9 Changes in airway pressure

Increased
Lung compliance
Bronchospasm
Pulmonary oedema
Pneumothorax
Thoracic compliance
Head-down position
Reversal of neuromuscular block
Laparoscopy
Equipment problems
Plug of sputum
Kinked tracheal tube
Decreased
Disconnection

Tidal volume

This should also needs to be measured, both as a confirmation that the patient is still undergoing ventilation and to allow ventilator settings to be optimized. Spirometers have been used for many years and consist of a housing to direct airflow, containing a small drum with vanes around its sides (Fig. 31.7). As gas passes through the device, the drum is made to rotate and the volume of gas is proportional to the movement of the drum. Although these devices are small and accurate, water vapour causes inaccuracies. Their weight dictates mounting at the machine end of a system, restricting their use mainly to circle systems when expired gas is measured. In addition, because of the inertia of the drum they tend to under-read at low tidal volumes and over-read at high volumes.

Datex monitors use a small plastic connector (Fig. 38.9), which is inserted into the airway. The connector contains a slight constriction and two carefully placed orifices. Two tubes lead from the airway connector to pressure sensors in the body of the main monitor. Measurement of the small differential pressure changes between the two tubes allows the calculation of airway pressure and the direction and amount of gas flow. The sensor is small enough to be placed at the tracheal tube, allowing inspired and expired tidal volumes to be measured.

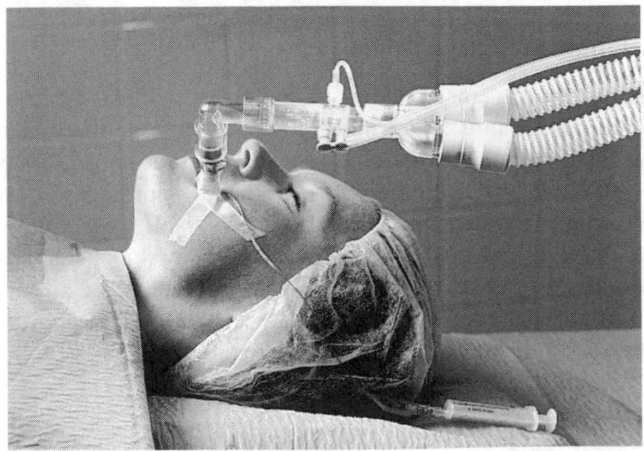

Fig. 38.9
Datex D lite connector.

Lastly, a hot wire anemometer uses a wire placed across the airflow. Any airflow cools the wire and decreases its electrical resistance. The device is simple and reliable, but delicate enough to need protection within a monitor or ventilator. It is therefore commonly used in anaesthetic machines that have integrated circuits and ventilators

Most monitors now have the facility to integrate the measurement of pressure, flow and time to produce real-time measurement of compliance in addition to flow–volume loops (see Fig. 38.1) and pressure–volume loops. These displays may be useful in patients whose lungs are difficult to ventilate or where there are rapid changes in compliance, e.g. during one-lung anaesthesia.

DISCONNECTION ALARM

Although the above monitors usually incorporate alarms that can be set to detect sudden unexpected changes in ventilation, patients undergoing mechanical ventilation should also be connected to a disconnection alarm (Fig. 38.10). This is because most breathing systems have connectors that are dislodged easily, causing failure of ventilation. The alarms are usually battery-powered and detect the cyclical changes in airway pressure. Some need to have the alarm limits set manually, but most automatically detect the normal range and then alarm if any significant change in rate or pressure occurs. They may also alarm if high airway pressures are sensed.

TISSUE OXYGENATION

It is desirable to have a constant measure of the oxygenation of the patient's tissues. This is possible in neonates by a sensor placed on the patient's skin. These transcutaneous oxygen sensors incorporate heating elements that increase the skin blood flow by localized heating to around 42°C. These probes also contain carbon dioxide sensors which are more reliable and provide values close to arterial levels, but are not suitable for routine use (Table 38.10).

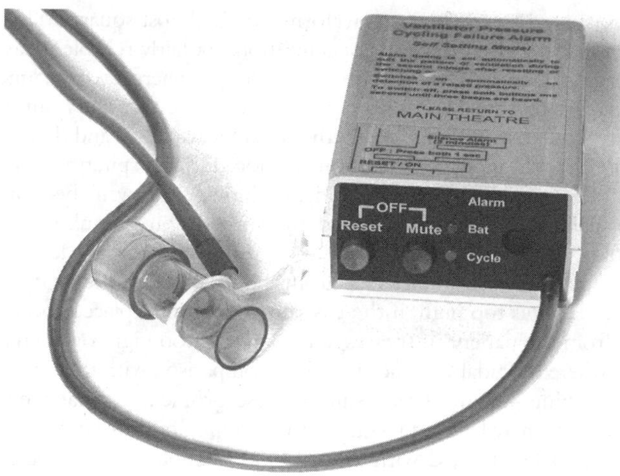

Fig. 38.10
A ventilator disconnection alarm.

Table 38.10 Problems with transcutaneous gas measurement
Probe takes time to heat up and equilibrate
Heat from probe may damage skin
Oxygen levels are much lower than arterial
Increased temperature alters the measured partial pressure
Thick skin of adults and children makes readings unreliable

Table 38.11 Oxygen delivery safety features
Visible and audible oxygen supply failure alarm
Spare oxygen cylinder is always present
Safety interlock on anaesthetic machine to prevent the setting of a hypoxic mixture
Oxygen analyser is always used in circuit

MONITORING GAS DELIVERY AND EXCRETION

During all forms of anaesthesia, it is mandatory constantly to analyse the gases inspired by the patient, to ensure hypoxic mixtures are not used and to confirm the concentration of anaesthetic agents being delivered. The delivery of adequate amounts of oxygen is so crucial to safe anaesthesia that multiple safety systems are considered mandatory (Table 38.11).

OXYGEN CONCENTRATION

Most monitors have a paramagnetic sensor that uses the tendency of oxygen to be weakly attracted to a magnetic field. Most other anaesthetic gases are diamagnetic, i.e. weakly repelled by a magnetic field. The monitor uses small spheres filled with nitrogen and suspended on a bar that is free to rotate within a strong magnetic field. When exposed to normal air, the bar finds a position where the force exerted on the spheres by the magnetic field is balanced by the torsion of the suspending wire. If the concentration of oxygen in the measuring chamber is increased, the oxygen is attracted towards the magnetic field. This inward movement tends to displace the spheres and causes the bar to rotate. The very small twisting movement is measured and amplified. When calibrated, the oxygen concentration in the chamber may then be calculated easily from the position of the bar. Although the sensor is initially expensive, it is reliable, fast and does not have any components that need replacement on a regular basis.

Other monitors use a fuel cell (Fig. 38.11), which is described in Chapter 31 (p. 369). The fuel cell measures the partial pressure of oxygen. Accuracy is usually around ± 2% with a response time of < 10 s. If the pressure of gas is increased, e.g. by putting the sensor in the supply to a Manley ventilator, the displayed values of concentration are increased.

An oxygen analyser should always be used during anaesthesia to ensure that a hypoxic mixture of gases is not delivered to the patient. Before each use, the analyser should be calibrated by exposure to air and 100% oxygen.

CARBON DIOXIDE

Measurement is vital to confirm tracheal intubation and subsequent continued ventilation. Other uses are shown in Table 38.12. Analysis of end-tidal, expired gas also provides an estimate of the concentration of carbon dioxide and anaesthetic agents in the alveoli and hence in arterial blood. As gases mix rapidly, measurements need to be rapid and occur as close to the alveoli as possible. In mainstream systems, the sensor is placed around the breathing system itself, resulting in quick, accurate measurements.

Unfortunately, the sensor may make the breathing system bulky and make the sensor vulnerable to accidental damage. Sidestream systems constantly draw a sample of around 150 ml min^{-1}, via fine-gauge tubing, out of the circuit. The sensors may therefore be housed in the main monitor and made more reliable and less liable to accidental damage. The disadvantage of a sidestream system is that, if the tubing leading from the circuit is too long or too wide, it introduces a delay before changes in carbon dioxide concentration are detected; mixing of gases within the tube may also lead to

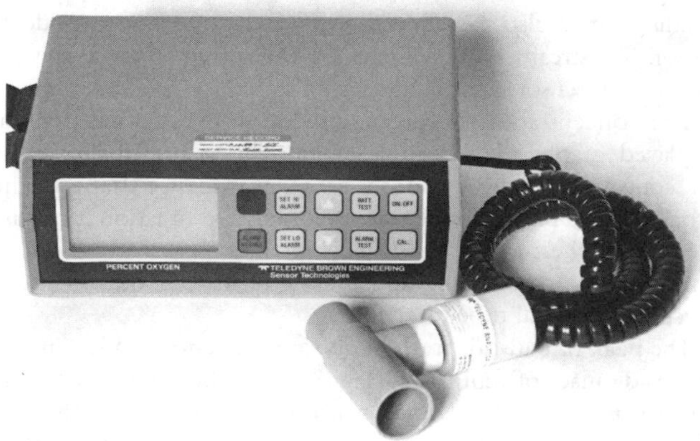

Fig. 38.11
Fuel cell oxygen analyser.

Table 38.12 Uses of capnography

Confirm tracheal intubation
Confirm continued ventilation
Confirm adequacy of ventilation
Detect rebreathing
Detect malignant hyperthermia
Detect pulmonary emboli

inaccurate readings. In circumstances such as paediatric anaesthesia, where removal of gas from the circuit may affect ventilation, most monitors incorporate the facility for the measured gas to be returned to the circuit.

Monitors measure carbon dioxide concentration by measuring the absorption of infrared light. Fortunately, each of the common anaesthetic gases and vapours has a characteristic pattern of light absorption, so that the wavelength of the light can be chosen to maximiz ¡479 e the absorption by carbon dioxide and minimize the absorption by other gases.

The basic principle is that a light of appropriate wavelength is shone across a small chamber and the amount of light passing through the chamber is measured at the other side. If a mixture of gases is passed through the chamber, the amount of light absorbed is proportional to the concentration of carbon dioxide in the mixture. To ensure accuracy, most monitors modify the principle in several ways. The beam is usually turned on and off up to 4000 times per minute to provide a zero light reference. The light from a single source of infrared light is usually split and passed through two identical chambers: one contains the gas mixture to be analysed and the other is empty. The absorption by carbon dioxide is then calculated by comparing the two beams. Lastly, each beam may be reflected through the chamber several times by a series of mirrors to increase the amount of absorption and make it more easy to measure. Because of molecular interactions, the presence of nitrous oxide could alter the measurements made by early monitors that relied on measurements at a single wavelength. Modern monitors use several wavelengths of infrared light and are therefore able automatically to detect which gases are present and in what concentration. Accuracy is around ± 2% with a response time of around 0.5 s. Correction factors may therefore be made automatically. Monitors may still be confused if other vapours are present in large concentrations; ethanol, for example, can be a problem in patients who present for emergency surgery after consuming large quantities of alcohol. Readings may also be affected by water condensing inside the sensor. Sidestream systems include a water trap to avoid this, and mainstream sensors are usually heated to reduce condensation.

The concentration of carbon dioxide in exhaled gas is usually displayed graphically (a capnograph). This is principally because the continuity of the waveform provides evidence that a tracheal tube has been placed in the trachea and that ventilation is continuing. Three chest inflations producing three peaks of expired carbon dioxide on a capnograph usually provide good evidence of successful tracheal tube insertion.

The peak or end-tidal carbon dioxide concentration is a measure of the adequacy of ventilation (Fig. 38.12). This is because the end-tidal gas is usually alveolar gas, which is in equilibrium with arterial blood. Carbon dioxide levels are zero during inspiration and expiration of dead space gas. Then, when alveolar gas starts to be excreted, the carbon dioxide concentration increases rapidly to the end-tidal level to produce a waveform that is almost square. While the end-tidal carbon dioxide concentration is a fairly reliable measure of arterial levels in those with healthy lungs, where gas exchange is impaired, end-tidal levels do not reach arterial levels. The result is that in patients with lung disease, the square wave is lost and there is a more gradual increase in carbon dioxide during expiration. The same effect may be observed suddenly during surgery if there are abnormalities of perfusion caused by hypotension or pulmonary embolus. Inaccurate readings are also produced if the gas leaving the patient is diluted by fresh gas from the circuit. This occurs if the fresh gas flow is too high, if the gas sampling point is placed too far away from the patient, if the respiratory rate is too high, or in children, where the tidal volume is small in comparison with the size of the breathing system. The result of these problems is that while capnography may be used to guide ventilation in healthy adults, any values must be checked with arterial blood samples in more complex situations. These may include patients with pulmonary disease or cases where accurate control of arterial carbon dioxide levels are critical, such as in head-injured patients.

Disposable devices have been developed which include a CO_2-sensitive chemical that may be attached to a tracheal tube. A cyclical change in colour indicates the presence of carbon dioxide and correct tube placement. They may be useful in situations where capnography is not available.

Transcutaneous measurement of carbon dioxide levels has already been mentioned (p. 370).

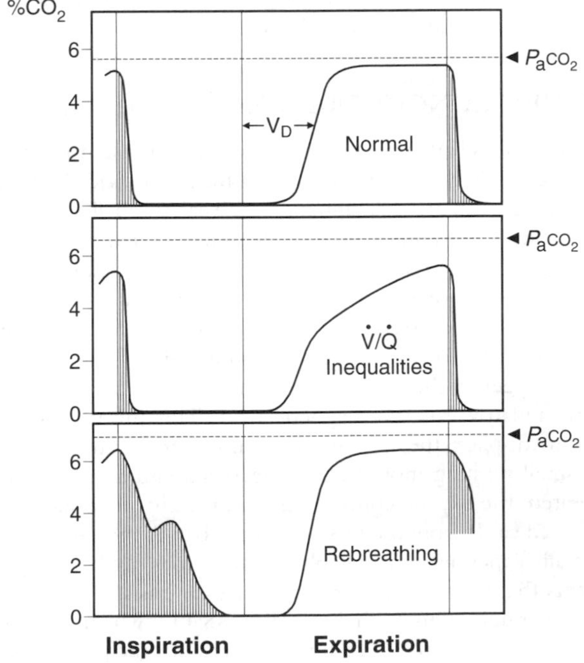

Fig. 38.12
Carbon dioxide traces recorded from the connector of the tracheal tube to illustrate the altered pattern of alveolar plateau in a patient with ventilation/perfusion ($\dot{V}/\dot{Q}$) inequalities. The bottom trace shows the presence of carbon dioxide in inspired gas during spontaneous ventilation with a Bain breathing system supplied with an inadequate flow rate of fresh gas. P_aCO_2 = Arterial carbon dioxide tension.

ANAESTHETIC AGENT MONITORING

Infrared absorption

This is used by most monitors and uses the same principles as for carbon dioxide measurement (p. 367), with the same problems. The advantages are rapid, accurate analysis, with identification of each gas present.

Quartz crystal oscillators

These oscillators use a tiny crystal coated with a layer of oil. The monitor vibrates and determines its resonant frequency. When the crystal is exposed to a mixture of gases containing an anaesthetic agent, the anaesthetic agents dissolve in the oil. This increases the mass of the crystal and changes its resonant frequency. The monitor measures the change in resonant frequency and calculates the concentration of the agent in the sample gas. As nitrous oxide, oxygen and carbon dioxide are relatively non-soluble in oil, changing their concentration in the sample gas has little effect on the result. These monitors are robust and accurate, but calibration is required for each agent . If the incorrect agent is selected or a mixture of agents is present, readings are unreliable.

Mass spectrometers

Mass spectrometers take a small sample of gas, strip the electrons from the molecules and then accelerate them into a strong magnetic field. The magnetic field then causes the molecules to move in a curved path, depending on their size and charge. They are very sensitive and accurate, but are also bulky and expensive. They are used to calibrate other monitors and may be sited centrally within a theatre complex.

Photoacoustic spectroscopic analysers

These analysers intermittently shine a powerful beam of infrared light at the sample gas. If the light is absorbed, the sample gas expands rapidly. The rapid expansion causes a very small noise – in effect a minute explosion that can be detected with a miniature microphone. Monitors may be used to measure the concentration of a variety of gases using several different wavelengths of light. They are very sensitive, but too complex for routine use.

Raman scattering analysers

In these analysers, a powerful laser light is shone at a gas sample. Raman scattering implies that a very small proportion of the light interacts with the gas, causing the wavelength of the light to be altered and scattered sideways; the wavelength of scattered light is determined by the molecular structure of the gas. The monitors analyse the scattered light and calculate the composition of the gas. The analysers are fast, accurate and relatively compact, but the powerful laser needed can make them noisy.

THE NERVOUS SYSTEM

ASSESSMENT OF CONSCIOUSNESS

Awareness, with or without pain, is an important complication of general anaesthesia and may result in litigation. It is important, therefore, that an anaesthetist strives to maintain unconsciousness. Unfortunately, at present, there is no reliable monitor and the anaesthetist relies upon administering an adequate dose of anaesthetic whilst observing for signs of light anaesthesia (excess sympathetic activity manifest as sweating, tachycardia, hypertension, dilatation of pupils and pallor). Recently, considerable attention has been directed to developing monitors of electrical function of the brain which are thought to vary with consciousness. Other uses are shown in Table 38.13.

Table 38.13 Uses of monitors of cerebral function

Avoidance of awareness during anaesthesia
Controlling sedation
Carotid artery surgery
Hypotensive anaesthesia
Treatment of epilepsy

Isolated forearm technique

In these studies, a tourniquet is applied to the upper arm and inflated above systolic pressure before induction of anaesthesia. The tourniquet does not affect the function of peripheral nerves, but ensures that neuromuscular blocking agents cannot reach the forearm. Awareness may then be detected by asking patients to clench their fist. Several studies have shown undoubted awareness during surgery, but usually without any postoperative recall. This demonstrates that lack of recall does not equate directly to adequate anaesthesia. This method is not suitable for routine use because it can only detect awareness when it has already occurred.

Electroencephalogram (EEG)

The EEG recorded from scalp electrodes identifies episodes of epilepsy, but is too complex to provide information perioperatively. Fortunately, the raw signal can now be simplified by fast Fourier analysis. The resulting histogram of activity versus frequency is easier to interpret.

Most anaesthetic agents produce an overall decrease in frequency with increasing depth of anaesthesia. This may be expressed as a median frequency or as a spectral edge (the frequency below which 95% of activity occurs). Problems include the delays in producing a result while the monitor analyses the raw EEG and differences between the changes produced by different agents.

Bispectral analysis

These monitors use a complex analysis of the EEG to produce a single number, or bispectral index (BIS), which varies with anaesthesia. Its usefulness is undetermined at present.

Respiratory sinus arrhythmia

This is the normal variation in heart rate with breathing. This variation is reduced by anaesthesia and may provide a measure of depth of anaesthesia. Initial results are promising, but factors such as autonomic neuropathy and anticholinergic drugs may invalidate the method.

Auditory evoked potentials

These monitors present a series of audible clicks to the patient via headphones. The EEG is then measured over the auditory cortex and averaged over time so that the cortical response to the clicks is isolated. The waveform produced is then analysed further and a value calculated (Fig. 38.13). Again, initial results have been promising, but the long processing time involved and problems with artefacts suggest that reliability is questionable.

BRAIN OXYGENATION

Transcranial Doppler

An ultrasonic probe is used to measure the speed of red cells flowing through the middle cerebral artery. The probe is placed over an acoustic 'window' in the temporal fossa. In the theatre setting, it may be used to confirm continued brain perfusion, e.g. during carotid artery surgery. In the intensive care unit, it may be used to identify vasospasm after subarachnoid haemorrhage or cessation of blood flow in severe head injury. Unfortunately, the machines require a trained operator, are expensive and variability in the measurements often results in the need for expert interpretation.

Near-infrared spectroscopy

This uses the same principles as a pulse oximeter to measure brain oxygenation, but instead of the light traversing a digit, the light passes through the skull and is then reflected. The system has the potential to directly measure brain oxygenation in real time. Unfortunately, doubts still remain about the validity of the information produced, mainly because of confusion about whether or not the results are biased by blood flow in the scalp.

Jugular venous saturation

As blood supply to the brain decreases, more oxygen is extracted from the available blood. Investigations have shown that a jugular venous saturation of less than 55% is associated with brain hypoxia. Although the technique is useful in brain-injured patients, it requires trained staff to insert and remove samples from the catheter. It also fails to detect isolated areas of hypoxia in an otherwise well oxygenated brain.

METABOLISM

TEMPERATURE

The body has an inner 'core' temperature, including the major organs, and also a 'peripheral' temperature, usually assumed to be skin temperature. These may be measured by probes in the nasopharynx or rectum (core) and skin (peripheral). Induction of general anaesthesia usually results in vasodilatation and an initial

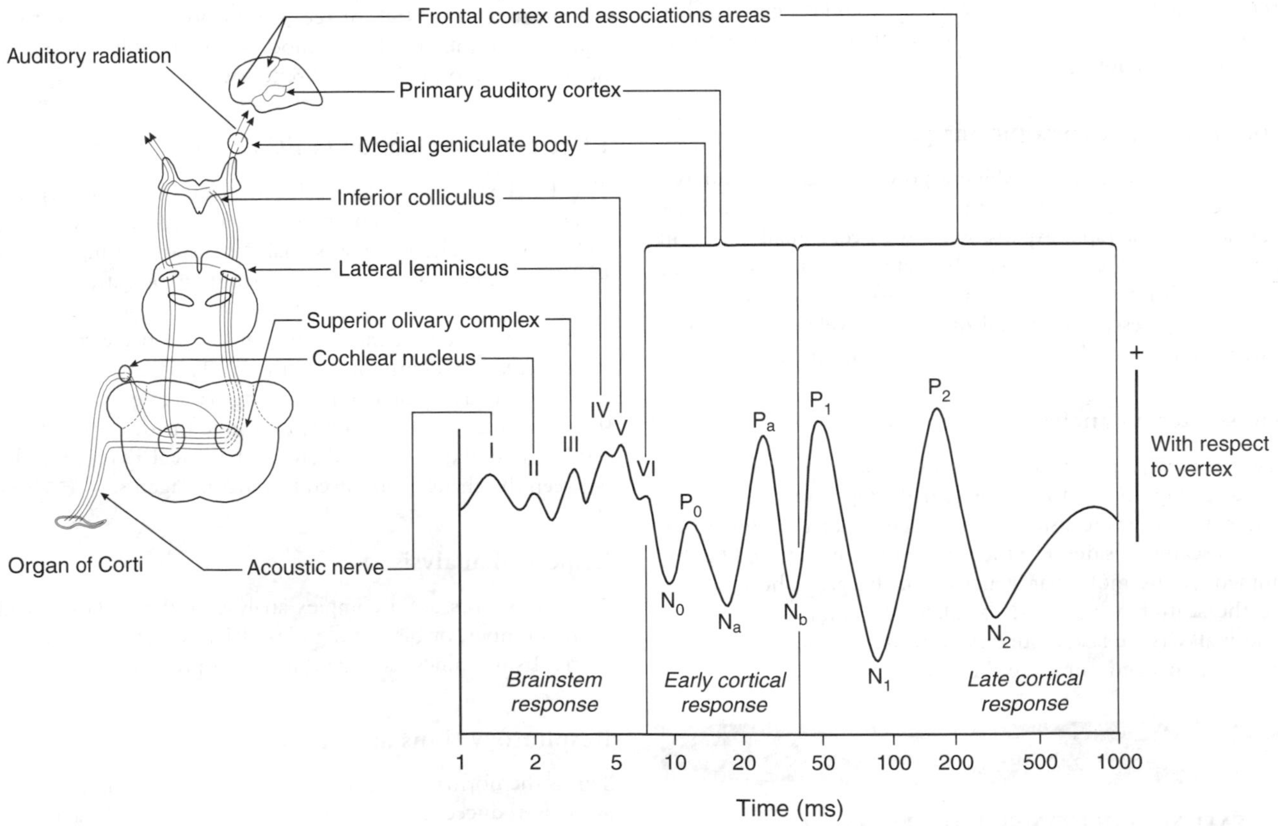

Fig. 38.13
The auditory evoked response consists of a series of waves generated from specific anatomical sites in the auditory pathway as indicated. Activity passes from the cochlea through the brainstem to the cortex.

decrease in core temperature even if no heat is lost. Low cardiac output states are characterized by a reduction in peripheral temperature as a result of vasoconstriction. A core-peripheral temperature gradient of > 2°C is indicative of low cardiac output. Hyperthermia is rare but has a variety of causes:

- over-enthusiastic heating
- sepsis
- allergic reaction
- malignant hyperthermia
- thyrotoxic crisis
- neuroleptic malignant syndrome.

Hypothermia is associated with increased perioperative morbidity (Table 38.14) and is most likely in children, elderly patients, where large parts of the patient are exposed (orthopaedics), where the abdominal cavity is opened, during long surgery and where large volumes of intravenous fluids are infused.

Temperature probes are usually made of a semiconductor whose electrical resistance decreases with temperature. The probe is usually enclosed in a smooth plastic coating to ease insertion and avoid mucosal trauma. They may either be disposable or be sterilized between cases. Care is needed to avoid trauma to mucosa during insertion, as significant blood loss may occur from the nose. Temperature measurement is a simple, cheap monitor that should be used in all but the shortest cases. Warming devices should be used in all but the shortest of cases; some of these devices are shown in Table 38.15.

In recovery areas, temperature is now commonly measured using devices which are inserted into the external auditory meatus and which measure the amount of infrared radiation emitted by the eardrum. Measurement is very simple and almost instantaneous, but measurements may be affected by, for example, ear wax.

ELECTROLYTE AND BLOOD GAS ANALYSIS

During long complex cases, regular measurement of haemoglobin, acid–base balance, electrolytes and the partial pressure of oxygen and carbon dioxide is essential to guide ventilation and the volume and type of fluids administered.

Calculated variables such as haemoglobin oxygen saturation may be provided by many automated analysers, using measurements of oxygen partial pressure, pH and bicarbonate with a standard oxygen dissociation curve held in memory. In more complex analysis, saturation, methaemoglobin and carboxyhaemoglobin may be measured directly. Electrolytes such as sodium, potassium and calcium are also commonly measured. Such analysers are often large and require regular maintenance, calibration and servicing. Traditionally, venous blood samples have been obtained and sent to the laboratory for analysis, but recent advances in technology have permitted many measurements to be made in the operating theatre. Measuring electrodes have been miniaturized and mounted on small wafers of semiconductor. For each measurement, a fresh cassette is placed in the monitor and a sample introduced into the cassette. The monitor usually self-calibrates and then measures the desired variables. The entire cassette is then discarded. This avoids the need for regular calibration and maintenance of large laboratory-type machines. Unfortunately, the cost per measurement using these systems is high (Fig. 38.14).

It is now possible to mount sensors onto probes for insertion into the patient, either directly into tissue or via a modified arterial cannula.

Table 38.14 Problems associated with hypothermia

Slow awakening
Slow metabolism of drugs
Shivering (increased oxygen consumption)
Increased systemic vascular resistance
Hypertension

Table 38.15 Commonly used warming devices

Minimal exposure, use of blankets
Airway heat and moisture exchanger
Increased theatre temperature
Plastic bags/bubble wrap around patient
Hat
Radiant heaters above patient
Warming mattress
Hot air blankets
Intravenous fluid (blood) warmer

BLOOD GLUCOSE

In diabetic patients, especially those receiving insulin infusions, blood glucose concentration should be measured regularly to avoid hypoglycaemia. Measurement of a small capillary sample is usually adequate.

BLOOD LOSS AND TRANSFUSION

During major surgery, blood loss may be a major problem. Assessing the loss is difficult because blood may be soaked up by surgical drapes, may drip onto the floor, may be sucked into a drainage bottle or soaked up by swabs. In small children, the volume of bleeding necessary to cause anaemia is very small. For example, a loss of around 20 ml in a 2 kg baby would represent a

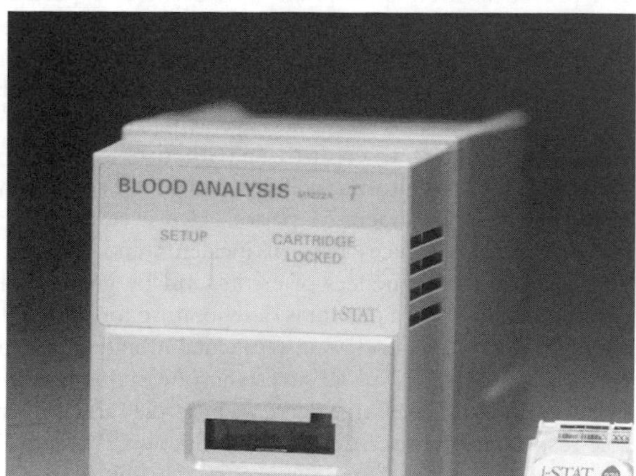

Fig. 38.14
I-stat cartridge.

major haemorrhage. The blood loss during all procedures should be assessed and recorded on the anaesthetic chart.

Red cells

Blood loss may be estimated by comparing the weight of any used swabs with a pack of clean swabs. The difference in weight is then assumed to be due to absorbed blood. This method is simple and easy, but ignores losses onto the drapes and is notoriously inaccurate. In theory, all the swabs and drapes can be washed at the end of the operation in a solution of known volume. The total amount of haemoglobin lost may then be calculated from the final haemoglobin concentration in the solution.

Clotting

Clotting abnormalities may result from a variety of factors (Table 38.16). Adequacy is usually assessed via laboratory measurement of platelet count, prothrombin time (intrinsic system), activated partial thromboplastin time (extrinsic system) and fibrinogen concentration (consumption of factors). Several systems are now available which can measure clotting in the operating theatre. A small sample of blood is obtained and mixed automatically with a standard set of reagents. The mixture is then agitated and clotting is detected by either a change in the resistance to the movement of a small bar or changes in conduction of light.

Table 38.16 Situations in which repeated assessment of clotting is useful

Massive blood loss
Perioperative anticoagulation
Reversal of heparin therapy with protamine
Liver disease
Disseminated intravascular coagulopathy

Platelets

Numbers may be measured easily in a full blood count, but this does not measure their function. Sonoclot analysis and thrombelastography are methods that measure the function of the entire coagulation system including platelet function. They measure changes in the viscoelastic properties of a sample of activated blood.

In practice, especially when blood loss is rapid, repeated arterial blood samples should be taken and the response to replacement therapy measured. Haematological advice should be sought in complex cases.

STANDARDS OF MONITORING

The presence of an appropriately trained and experienced anaesthetist is the main determinant of patient safety during anaesthesia. However, human error is inevitable, and many studies of critical incidents and mortality associated with anaesthesia have shown that adverse incidents and accidents are frequently attributable, at least in part, to error by anaesthetists.

Instrumental monitoring will not prevent all adverse incidents or accidents in the perioperative period. However, there is substantial evidence that it reduces risks of incidents and accidents both by detecting the consequences of errors, and by giving early warning that the condition of a patient is deteriorating for some other reason. The introduction of modern instrumental monitors halved the number of intraoperative cardiac arrests in one study, and the decrease was due almost entirely to a decrease in cardiac arrests from preventable respiratory causes. After the introduction of minimal monitoring standards in one American group of hospitals, the numbers of serious accidents and deaths were reduced substantially. The Australian Incident Monitoring Study found that 52% of incidents were detected first by a monitor; in more than half of these cases, the pulse oximeter or capnograph detected the first changes. It was calculated that a combination of pulse oximetry and blood pressure monitoring should detect 93% of serious incidents in the large majority of cases before organ damage occurs.

The use of pulse oximetry shortens the time to detection of critical events. The introduction of pulse oximetry decreased the number of patients admitted unexpectedly from the operating theatre to the intensive care unit. In a randomized, controlled study, the use of pulse oximetry reduced the number of episodes of hypoxaemia and the number of patients suffering myocardial ischaemia during anaesthesia and resulted in increases in the flow of oxygen used in the recovery area, the number of patients discharged to the ward with supplemental oxygen and the number of patients treated with naloxone.

There has never been a randomized, prospective study of instrumental monitoring in anaesthesia, proving conclusively that outcome is influenced. The overwhelming view is that such a study would be unethical and the circumstantial evidence that is available indicates clearly that the use of such monitoring improves the safety of patients.

The most recent recommendations of the Association of Anaesthetists of Great Britain and Ireland regarding monitoring in the perioperative period are summarized in Table 38.17, and detailed below.

It is the responsibility of the departmental head to ensure that staff are trained in the use of the monitoring equipment available.

It is the responsibility of the anaesthetist to check all equipment before use as recommended in the Association of Anaesthetists' *Checklist for Anaesthetic Apparatus.* Anaesthetists must ensure that they are familiar with all equipment that they intend to use and that they have followed any specific checking procedure recommended by individual manufacturers. During anaesthesia, it is important to monitor continuously the continuity of the oxygen supply and the correct function of the breathing system.

Oxygen supply

The use of an oxygen analyser with an audible alarm is essential during anaesthesia. It must be placed in such a position that the composition of the gas mixture delivered to the patient is monitored continuously. The positioning of the sampling port will depend on the breathing system in use. Oxygen analysers must be available whenever anaesthesia is administered.

Breathing systems

During spontaneous ventilation, observation of the reservoir bag may reveal a leak, disconnection, high pressure or abnormalities of ventilation. Carbon dioxide concentration monitoring will detect

Table 38.17 Summary of recommendations for standards of monitoring during anaesthesia and recovery. (Reproduced with permission from the Association of Anaesthetists of Great Britain and Ireland 2000)

1. The anaesthetist must be present throughout the conduct of an anaesthetic.
2. Monitoring devices must be attached before induction of anaesthesia and their use continued until the patient has recovered from the effects of anaesthesia.
3. The same standards of monitoring apply when the anaesthetist is responsible for a local anaesthetic or sedative technique for an operative procedure.
4. All information provided by monitoring devices should be recorded in the patient's notes. Trend display and printing devices are recommended as they allow the anaesthetist to concentrate on managing the patient in emergency situations.
5. The anaesthetist must check all equipment before use. All alarm limits must be set appropriately. Infusion devices and their alarm settings must be checked before use. Audible alarms must be enabled when anaesthesia commences.
6. The anaesthetist should make observations of the colour of the patient's mucosa, pupil size, response to surgical stimuli, and movements of the chest wall and reservoir bag. The pulse should be palpated and the lungs auscultated and, where appropriate, urine output and blood loss should be measured. A stethoscope must always be available.
7. Monitoring devices supplement clinical observation. The following monitoring devices are essential in every case:
   an oxygen analyser with an audible alarm
   measurement of airway pressure, with upper and lower alarm limits, when IPPV is employed
   a vapour analyser during maintenance of anaesthesia whenever a volatile anaesthetic agent is in use
   pulse oximetry
   non-invasive blood pressure measurement
   electrocardiograph
   capnograph.
8. The following devices must also be available in every case:
   a nerve stimulator whenever a muscle relaxant is used
   a means of measuring the patient's temperature.
9. Additional (mainly invasive) monitoring devices may be required for some patients or for some types of operation, e.g. invasive monitoring of vascular or intracranial pressures, cardiac output or biochemical variables.
10. When handing over to recovery staff, anaesthetists should issue clear instructions concerning monitoring during postoperative care. Monitoring of arterial oxygen saturation and non-invasive monitoring of blood pressure are essential. An electrocardiograph, nerve stimulator, capnograph and a means of measuring temperature must be immediately available.
11. Standards of care and monitoring during transfer of sedated, anaesthetized or unconscious patients should be as high as during administration of anaesthesia. Oxygen saturation, the electrocardiogram and arterial pressure should be monitored in all patients. Additional monitors may be required in some circumstances. Airway pressure, tidal volume and expired carbon dioxide concentration should be monitored continuously if the lungs are ventilated artificially.

most of these problems. Capnography is therefore an essential part of routine monitoring during anaesthesia.

Alarms

Anaesthetists must ensure that all alarms are set at appropriate values. The default settings incorporated by the manufacturer are often inappropriate and during the checking procedure the anaesthetist must review and reset the upper and lower limits as necessary. Audible alarms must be enabled when anaesthesia commences.

When intermittent positive pressure ventilation is used during anaesthesia, airway pressure alarms must also be used to detect excessive pressure within the airway and also to give warning of disconnection or leaks. The upper and lower alarm limits must be reviewed and set appropriately before anaesthesia commences.

Vapour analyser

The use of a vapour analyser is essential during maintenance of anaesthesia whenever a volatile anaesthetic agent is in use.

Infusion devices

When any component of anaesthesia (hypnotic, analgesic, muscle relaxant) is administered by infusion, the infusion device unit must be checked before use. Alarm settings and infusion limits must be verified and set to appropriate levels before commencing anaesthesia. It is essential to verify that these drugs are delivered to the patient. The infusion site should therefore be visible and must be checked regularly to ensure that extravasation does not occur.

The anaesthetist must be fully familiar with the device used before using it.

During anaesthesia, the patient's physiological state, depth of anaesthesia and function of equipment need continuous assessment. Monitoring devices supplement clinical observation in order to achieve this. The anaesthetist should make observations of the patient's mucosal colour, pupil size, response to surgical stimuli and movements of the chest wall and of the reservoir bag and should undertake palpation of the pulse, auscultation of breath sounds and, where appropriate, measurement of urine output and blood loss. A stethoscope must always be available.

Monitoring devices

The following monitoring devices are essential to the safe conduct of anaesthesia. If it is necessary to continue anaesthesia without one of these devices, the anaesthetist must clearly record the reasons in the anaesthetic record.

Induction of anaesthesia

- pulse oximeter
- non-invasive blood pressure monitor
- electrocardiograph
- capnograph.

The following must also be available:

- a nerve stimulator whenever a muscle relaxant is used
- a means of measuring the patient's temperature.

During induction of anaesthesia in children and in uncooperative adults it may not be possible to attach all monitoring devices before induction. In these circumstances, monitors must be attached as soon as possible after consciousness is lost and the reasons for delay should be recorded in the patient's notes.

For very short procedures, e.g. electro-convulsive therapy (ECT) and orthopaedic manipulations under general anaesthesia, the above monitoring standards for induction of anaesthesia will suffice under normal circumstances.

If the patient remains in the anaesthetic room for a prolonged period of time after induction of anaesthesia, for example during siting of lines, then monitoring standards must equate to those for maintenance of anaesthesia as described below.

Maintenance of anaesthesia

- pulse oximeter
- non-invasive blood pressure monitor
- electrocardiograph
- capnograph
- vapour analyser.

The following must also be immediately available:

- a nerve stimulator whenever a muscle relaxant is being used
- a means of measuring the patient's temperature.

Recovery from anaesthesia

A high standard of monitoring should be maintained until the patient is fully recovered from anaesthesia. Clinical observations must be supplemented by the following monitoring devices:

- pulse oximeter
- non-invasive blood pressure monitor.

The following must also be immediately available:

- electrocardiograph
- nerve stimulator
- means of measuring temperature
- capnograph.

If the recovery area is not immediately adjacent to the operating theatre, or if the patient's general condition is poor, adequate mobile monitoring of the above parameters will be needed during transfer. The anaesthetist is responsible for ensuring that this transfer is accomplished safely.

Regional techniques and sedation for operative procedures

Patients must have appropriate monitoring, including the following devices:

- pulse oximeter
- non-invasive blood pressure monitor
- electrocardiograph.

Additional monitoring

Some patients require additional, mainly invasive, monitoring; for example, of vascular or intracranial pressure, cardiac output or biochemical variables (see Table 38.18).

Monitoring during transfer

It is essential that the standard of care and monitoring during transfer is as high as that applied in the operating theatre and that personnel with adequate knowledge and experience accompany the patient.

The patient should be physiologically stable on departure. Appropriate monitoring must be started before transfer. The oxygen saturation, electrocardiogram and arterial pressure should be monitored in all patients. The diagnosis of arrhythmias may be very

Table 38.18 Variables which may be appropriate to monitor during anaesthesia in some patients in addition to the essential monitoring for all anaesthetised patients

Indications	Monitors
Operative duration > 3 h	Direct arterial pressure measurement
Blood loss > 10% blood volume	Central venous pressure
Operations on:	Pulmonary capillary wedge pressure
chest	Cardiac output
central nervous system	Trans-oesophageal echocardiography
cardiovascular system	Blood loss measurement
Clinically significant coexisting disease	Urine output
	Temperature
	patient
	blood warmer, mattress
	inspired gas
	Blood gas analysis
	Serum electrolyte concentrations
	Haemoglobin concentration
	Coagulation status

Table 38.19 Suggested data for inclusion on anaesthetic records (based on recommendations of the Royal College of Anaesthetists and Association of Anaesthetists of Great Britain and Ireland)

PREOPERATIVE INFORMATION	**Vital signs recording/charting**
Patient Identity	Monitors used and vital signs, recorded not less frequently than every 15 min
Name/ID No./gender	
Date of birth	**Drugs and fluids**
Assessment and risk factors	Dose, concentration, volume
Date of assessment	Cannulation
Assessor, where assessed	Injection site(s), time & route
Weight (kg), [height (m) optional]	Warmer used
Basic vital signs (BP, HR)	Blood loss, urine output
Medication, incl. contraceptive drugs	
Allergies	**Airway and breathing system**
Addiction (alcohol, tobacco, drugs)	Route, system used
Previous GAs, family history	Ventilation: type and mode
Potential airway problems	Airway type, size, cuff, shape
Prostheses, teeth, crowns	Special procedures, humidifier, filter
Investigations	Throat pack
Cardiorespiratory fitness	Difficulty
Other problems	
ASA ± comment	**Regional anaesthesia**
Urgency	Consent
Scheduled–listed on a routine list	Block performed
Urgent–resuscitated, not on a routine list	Entry site
Emergency–not fully resuscitated	Needle used, aid to location
PEROPERATIVE INFORMATION	Catheter: y/n
Checks	
Nil by mouth	**Patient position and attachments**
Consent	Thrombosis prophylaxis
Premedication, type and effect	Temperature control
Place and time	Limb positions
Place	
Date, start and end times	**POSTOPERATIVE INSTRUCTIONS**
Personnel	Drugs, fluids and doses
All anaesthetists named	Analgesic techniques
Operating surgeon	Special airway instructions, incl. oxygen
Qualified assistant present	Monitoring
Duty consultant informed	
Operation planned/performed	**Untoward Events**
Apparatus	Abnormalities
Check performed, anaesthetic room, theatre	Critical incidents
	Preop., perop., postoperative
	Context, cause, effect
	Hazard flags
	Warnings for future care

difficult, and the pulse oximeter may be inaccurate, in the presence of movement artefact. Non-invasive blood pressure measurement may also be inaccurate during movement and the use of invasive arterial pressure monitoring should be considered. In some patients, it may be necessary to monitor central venous pressure, pulmonary capillary wedge pressure and/or intracranial pressure. A monitored oxygen supply of known content sufficient to last the maximum duration of the transfer is essential. If the patient's lungs are ventilated artificially, airway pressure, tidal volume and end-tidal carbon dioxide concentration should be monitored continuously.

All monitors must be easily accessible and have clearly visible, illuminated displays. It is preferable that all monitoring functions are combined in one robust, battery-operated monitor.

ANAESTHETIC RECORD-KEEPING

It is the professional responsibility of every doctor to maintain accurate records of the treatment which patients receive, and their response to it. The anaesthetic record forms a part of a patient's medical record. The principal purpose of the anaesthetic chart is to provide details of the anaesthetic technique used, of the physiological changes which were associated with the technique and with surgery, and of complications or problems which were encountered during the procedure, as this information may assist other doctors if complications ensue, or if anaesthesia is required in the future. In addition, the anaesthetic record may be a valuable source of information if a subsequent complication results in litigation; the absence of a full record makes it difficult for an anaesthetist to demonstrate, for example, that postoperative renal failure was not attributable to unnecessary intraoperative hypotension.

The design of anaesthetic records varies widely, and is probably unimportant provided that it facilitates recording and display of all of the relevant data. Suggestions for the reasonable content of an anaesthetic record data set are shown in Table 38.19. Although the authors of these recommendations suggested that vital signs should be recorded at a minimum interval of 15 min, much greater reliance is likely to be placed on a record containing data entered at 5-min intervals.

In addition to the data set shown in Table 38.19, the anaesthetist should note, preferably on the anaesthetic record, the anaesthetic techniques which have been discussed with and agreed by the patient, and should list the risks which have been explained.

Automated records

It has been estimated that up to 20% of the anaesthetist's time is taken up with documentation. Inevitably, update from the anaesthetist's memory occurs following periods of intense activity such as induction of anaesthesia or the management of critical incidents and mishaps. This may lead to inaccuracies. In addition, it may be suggested that the anaesthetist has 'normalized' entries on the anaesthetic record, minimizing physiological change which occurred, or that the entries are fictitious.

Most monitoring systems can now be connected to an automated anaesthetic record-keeping system, which produces a continuous record of information gathered from the monitoring apparatus and the anaesthetic machine. Additional information, such as drug administration and intravenous fluid delivery, can be entered manually, and the anaesthetist can annotate events which have caused inaccurate data to be recorded.

Automated devices provide a robust, objective anaesthetic record which is less susceptible to criticism than a manual record, and from which data for audit can be obtained readily. In addition, automated systems can be interlinked with hospital information systems, so that the anaesthetic chart can include not only information about the anaesthetic, but also identification information from a central database, drug information from the pharmacy and results from the laboratory.

FURTHER READING

Association of Anaesthetists of Great Britain and Ireland 1997. Checklist for anaesthetic apparatus 2. AAGBI, London

Association of Anaesthetists of Great Britain and Ireland 1998. Risk management 1998. AAGBI, London

Association of Anaesthetists of Great Britain and Ireland 2000. Recommendations for standards of monitoring during anaesthesia and recovery 3. AAGBI, London

Sykes M K, Vickers M D, Hull C J 1991 Principles of measurement and monitoring in anaesthesia and intensive care. Blackwell Scientific Publications, Oxford

39 Fluid, electrolyte and acid–base balance

The realization that the enzyme systems and metabolic processes responsible for the maintenance of cellular function are dependent on an environment with stable electrolyte and hydrogen ion concentrations led Claude Bernard, over 100 years ago, to describe the 'milieu interieur'. Complex homeostatic mechanisms have evolved to maintain the constancy of this internal environment and thus prevent cellular dysfunction.

BASIC DEFINITIONS

Osmosis refers to the movement of *solvent* molecules across a membrane into a region in which there is a higher concentration of *solute*. This movement may be prevented by applying a pressure to the more concentrated solution – the effective osmotic pressure. This is a colligative property; the magnitude of effective osmotic pressure exerted by a solution depends on the number rather than the type of particles present.

The amounts of osmotically active particles present in solution are expressed in *osmoles*. One osmole of a substance is equal to its molecular weight in grams (1 mol) divided by the number of freely moving particles which each molecule liberates in solution. Thus, 180 g of glucose in 1 L of water represents a solution with a molar concentration of 1 mol L^{-1} and an *osmolarity* of 1 osmol L^{-1}. Sodium chloride ionizes in solution and each ion represents an osmotically active particle. Assuming complete dissociation into Na^+ and Cl^-, 58.5 g of NaCl dissolved in 1 L of water has a molar concentration of 1 mol L^{-1} and an osmolarity of 2 osmol L^{-1}. In body fluids, solute concentrations are much lower (mmol L^{-1}) and dissociation is incomplete. Consequently, a solution of NaCl containing 1 mmol L^{-1} contributes slightly less than 2 mosmol L^{-1}.

The term *osmolality* refers to the number of osmoles per unit of total weight of solvent and, unlike osmolarity, is not affected by the volume of various solutes in solution. Confusion regarding the apparently interchangeable use of the terms osmolarity (measured in osmol L^{-1}) and osmolality (measured in osmol kg^{-1}) is caused by their numerical equivalence in body fluids; plasma osmolarity is 280–310 mosmol L^{-1} and plasma osmolality is 280–310 mosmol kg^{-1}. This equivalence is explained by the almost negligible solute volume contained in biological fluids and the fact that most osmotically active particles are dissolved in water, which has a density of 1 (i.e. osmol L^{-1} = osmol kg^{-1}). As the number of osmoles in plasma is estimated by measurement of the magnitude of freezing point depression, the more accurate term in clinical practice is osmolality.

Cations (principally Na^+) and anions (Cl^- and HCO_3^-) are the major osmotically active particles in plasma. Glucose and urea make a smaller contribution. Plasma osmolality (P_{OSM}) may be estimated from the formula:

$$P_{OSM} = \underset{(\text{mmol L}^{-1})}{2\,[Na^+]} + \underset{(\text{mmol L}^{-1})}{\text{blood glucose}} + \underset{(\text{mmol L}^{-1})}{\text{blood urea}} = 290 \text{ mosmol kg}^{-1}$$

Osmolality is a chemical term and may be confused with the physiological term, *tonicity*. This term is used to describe the effective osmotic pressure of a solution relative to that of plasma. The critical difference between osmolality and tonicity is that *all* solutes contribute to osmolality, but only solutes that do not cross the cell membrane contribute to tonicity. Thus, tonicity expresses the osmolal activity of solutes restricted to the extracellular compartment, i.e. those which exert an osmotic force affecting the distribution of water between intracellular (ICF) and extracellular fluid (ECF). As urea diffuses freely across cell membranes, it does not alter the distribution of water between these two body fluid compartments and does not contribute to tonicity. Other solutes that contribute to plasma osmolality but not tonicity include ethanol and methanol, both of which distribute rapidly throughout the total body water. In contrast, mannitol and sorbitol are restricted to the ECF and contribute to both osmolality and tonicity. The tonicity of plasma may be estimated from the formula:

$$\text{Plasma tonicity} = \underset{(\text{mmol L}^{-1})}{2\,[Na^+]} + \underset{(\text{mmol L}^{-1})}{\text{blood glucose}} = 285 \text{ mosmol kg}^{-1}$$

COMPARTMENTAL DISTRIBUTION OF TOTAL BODY WATER

The volume of total body water (TBW) may be measured using radioactive dilution techniques involving either deuterium or tritium, both of which cross all membranes freely and equilibrate rapidly with hydrogen atoms in body water. Such measurements show that approximately 60% of lean body mass (LBM) is water in the average 70 kg male adult. As fat contains little water, females have proportionately less TBW (55%) relative to LBM. TBW decreases with age, falling to 45–50% in later life.

The distribution of TBW between the main body compartments is illustrated in Figure 39.1. One-third of TBW is contained in the extracellular fluid volume (ECFV) and two-thirds in the intracellular fluid volume (ICFV). The ECFV is subdivided further into the interstitial and intravascular compartments.

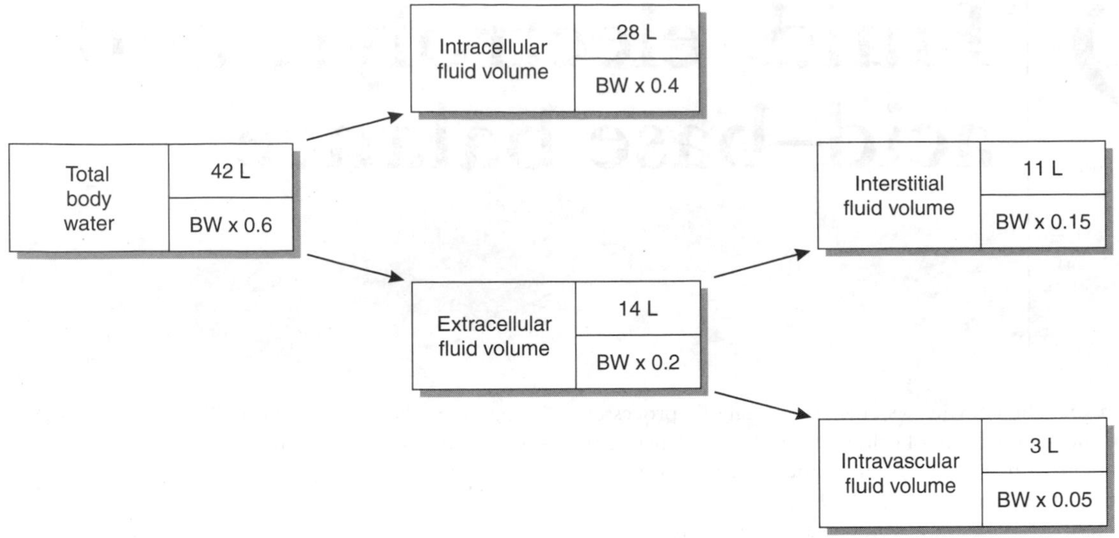

Fig. 39.1
Distribution of total body water related to body weight (BW).

In addition to the absolute volumes of each compartment, Figure 39.1 shows the relative size of each compartment compared with body weight.

SOLUTE COMPOSITION OF BODY FLUID COMPARTMENTS

Extracellular fluid

The capillary endothelium behaves as a freely permeable membrane to water, cations, anions and many soluble substances such as glucose and urea (but not protein). As a result, the solute compositions of interstitial fluid and plasma are similar. Each contains sodium as the principal cation and chloride as the principal anion. Protein behaves as a non-diffusible anion and is present in a higher concentration in plasma. The concentration of Cl^- is slightly higher in interstitial fluid in order to maintain electrical neutrality (Donnan equilibrium).

Intracellular fluid

This differs from ECF in that the principal cation is potassium and the principal anion is phosphate. In addition, there is a high protein content. In contrast to the capillary endothelium, the cell membrane is permeable *selectively* to different ions and freely permeable to water. Thus, equalization of osmotic forces occurs continuously and is achieved by the movement of water across the cell membrane. The osmolalities of ICF and ECF at equilibrium must be equal. Water moves rapidly between ICF and ECF to eliminate any induced osmolal gradient. This principle is fundamental to an understanding of fluid and electrolyte physiology.

Figure 39.2 shows the solute composition of the main body fluid compartments. Although the total concentration of intracellular ions exceeds that of extracellular ions, the numbers of osmotically active particles (and thus the osmolalities) are the same on each side of the cell membrane (290 mosmol kg^{-1} of solution).

WATER HOMEOSTASIS

Normal day-to-day fluctuations in TBW are small (< 0.2%) because of a fine balance between input, controlled by the thirst mechanisms, and output, controlled mainly by the renal–ADH system.

The principal sources of body water are ingested fluid, water present in solid food and water produced as an end-product of metabolism. Intravenous fluids are another common source in hospital patients. Actual and potential outlets for water are classified conventionally as sensible and insensible losses. Insensible losses emanate from the skin and lungs; sensible losses occur mainly from the kidneys and gastrointestinal tract. Figure 39.3 depicts the daily water balance in a 70 kg adult in whom input and output balance. It should be noted that sources of potential loss are not evident in this diagram. For example, over 5 L of fluid are secreted daily into the gut in the form of saliva, bile, gastric juices and succus entericus, yet only 100 ml of fluid is present in faeces. This illustrates the potential that exists for significant fluid loss in the presence of disease.

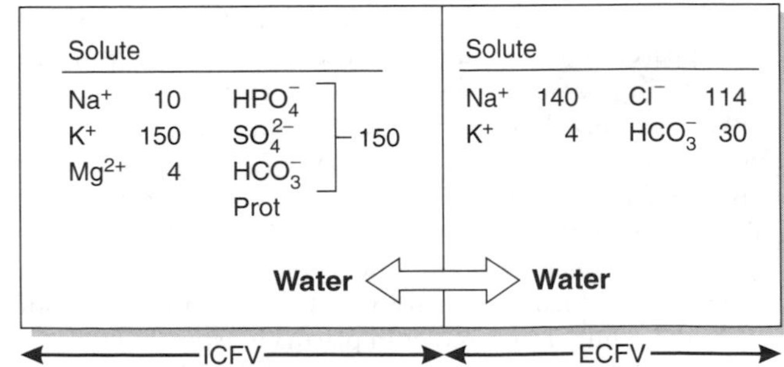

Fig. 39.2
Principal solute composition of body fluid compartments. All concentrations are expressed in mmol L^{-1}.

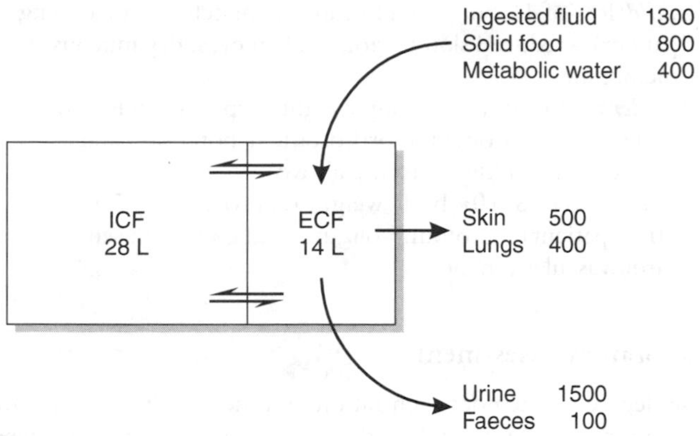

Fig. 39.3
Daily water balance. Input and output in ml.

PRACTICAL FLUID BALANCE

Calculation of the daily prescription of fluid is an arithmetic exercise to balance the input and output of water and electrolytes.

Table 39.1 shows the electrolyte contents of five intravenous solutions used commonly in the United Kingdom. These solutions are adequate for most clinical situations. Two self-evident but important generalizations may be made regarding solutions for intravenous infusion.

Rule 1

All infused Na^+ remains in the ECF; Na^+ cannot gain access to the ICF because of the sodium pump. Thus, if saline 0.9% is infused, all Na^+ remains in the ECF. As this is an isotonic solution, there is no change in ECF osmolality and therefore no water exchange occurs across the cell membrane. Thus, saline 0.9% expands ECFV only. However, if saline 0.45% is given, ECF osmolality decreases; this causes a shift of water from ECF to ICF. If saline 1.8% is administered, all Na^+ remains in the ECF, its osmolality increases and water moves from ICF to ECF to maintain osmotic equality.

Table 39.2 Compartmental expansion resulting from infusion of 1 L of saline 0.9%, saline 0.45% or glucose 5%

Intravenous infusion of 1000 ml	Change in volume (ml) ECF	ICF	Remarks
Saline 0.9%	+1000	0	Na^+ remains in ECF
Glucose 5%	+333	+666	66% of TBW is ICF
Saline 0.45%	+666	+333	33% of TBW is ECF

Rule 2

Water without sodium expands the TBW. After infusion of a solution of glucose 5%, the glucose enters cells and is metabolized. The infused water enters both ICF and ECF in proportion to their initial volumes.

Table 39.2 illustrates the results of infusion of 1 L of saline 0.9%, saline 0.45% or glucose 5% in a 70 kg adult.

Assessment of daily fluid requirements may be allocated usefully into three processes:

- normal maintenance needs
- abnormal losses resulting from the underlying pathology
- correction of pre-existing deficits.

NORMAL MAINTENANCE NEEDS

Water. Regardless of the disease process, water and electrolyte losses occur in urine and as evaporative losses from skin and lungs. It is evident from Figure 39.3 that a normothermic 70 kg patient with a normal metabolic rate may lose 2500 ml of water per day. Allowing for a gain of 400 ml from water of metabolism, this hypothetical patient needs 2000 ml day^{-1} of water. As a rule of thumb, a volume of 30–35 ml kg^{-1} day^{-1} of water is a useful estimate for daily maintenance needs.

Sodium. The normal requirement is 1 mmol kg^{-1} day^{-1} (50–80 mmol day^{-1}) for adults.

Potassium. The normal requirement is 1 mmol kg^{-1} day^{-1} (50–80 mmol day^{-1}) for adults.

Table 39.1 Electrolyte contents of commonly used intravenous fluids

Solution	Electrolyte content (mmol L^{-1})				Osmolality (mosmol kg^{-1})
Saline 0.9% ('normal saline')	Na^+	154	Cl^-	154	308
Saline 0.45% ('half-normal saline')	Na^+	77	Cl^-	77	154
Glucose 4%/saline 0.18% (glucose–saline)	Na^+	31	Cl^-	31	284
Glucose 5%		Nil			278
Compound sodium lactate (Hartmann's solution)	Na^+ K^+ Ca^{2+}	131 5 4	Cl^- HCO_3^- (as lactate)	112 29	281

Thus, a 70 kg patient requires daily provision of 2000–2500 ml of water and approximately 70 mmol each of Na^+ and K^+. This could be administered as one of the following:

- 2000 ml of glucose 5% + 500 ml of saline 0.9%
- 2500 ml of glucose 4%/saline 0.18%; plus potassium as KCl, 1 g (13 mmol) added to each 500 ml of fluid.

ABNORMAL LOSSES

These are common in surgical patients. They may be sensible or insensible and either overt or covert.

Losses from the gut are common, e.g. nasogastric suction, diarrhoea and vomiting or sequestration of fluid within the gut lumen (e.g. intestinal obstruction). Although the composition of gastrointestinal secretions is variable, replacement should be with saline 0.9% with 13–26 mmol L^{-1} of potassium as KCl. If losses are considerable (> 1000 ml day^{-1}), a sample of the appropriate fluid should be sent for biochemical analysis so that electrolyte replacement may be rationalized.

Increased insensible losses from the skin and lungs occur in the presence of fever or hyperventilation. The usual insensible loss of 0.5 ml kg^{-1} h^{-1} increases by 12% for each degree Celsius rise in body temperature.

Sequestration of fluid at the site of operative trauma is a form of fluid loss which is common in surgical patients. Plasma-like fluid is sequestered in any area of tissue injury; its volume is proportional to the extent of trauma. This fluid is frequently referred to as 'third space' loss because it ceases to take part in normal metabolic processes. However, it is not contained in an anatomically separate compartment; it represents an expansion of ECFV. Third-space losses are not measured easily. Sequestered fluid is reabsorbed after 48–72 h.

EXISTING DEFICITS

These occur preoperatively and arise primarily from the gut. The difficulty in correcting these deficits relates to an inability to quantify their magnitude accurately. Fluid and electrolyte deficits occur directly from the ECF. If the fluid lost is isotonic, only ECFV is reduced; however, if water alone or hypotonic fluid is lost, redistribution of the remaining TBW occurs from ICF to ECF to equalize osmotic forces.

Dehydration with accompanying salt loss is a common disorder in the acute surgical patient.

Assessment of dehydration

This is a clinical assessment based upon the following:

History. How long has the patient had abnormal loss of fluid? How much has occurred, e.g. frequency of vomiting?

Examination. Specific features are thirst, dryness of mucous membranes, loss of skin turgor, orthostatic hypotension or tachycardia, reduced jugular venous pressure (JVP) or central venous pressure (CVP) and decreased urine output. In the presence of normal renal function, dehydration is associated usually with a urine output of less than 0.5 ml kg^{-1} h^{-1}. The severity of dehydration may be described clinically as mild, moderate or severe and each category is associated with the following water loss relative to body weight:

- *mild:* loss of 4% body weight (approximately 3 L in a 70 kg patient) – reduced skin turgor, sunken eyes, dry mucous membranes
- *moderate:* loss of 5–8% body weight (approximately 4–6 L in a 70 kg patient) – oliguria, orthostatic hypotension and tachycardia in addition to the above
- *severe:* loss of 8–10% body weight (approximately 7 L in a 70 kg patient) – profound oliguria and compromised cardiovascular function.

Laboratory assessment

The degree of haemoconcentration and increase in albumin concentration may be helpful in the absence of anaemia and hypoproteinaemia. Increased blood urea concentration and urine osmolality (> 650 mosmol kg^{-1}) confirm the clinical diagnosis.

PERIOPERATIVE FLUID THERAPY

In addition to normal maintenance requirements of water and electrolytes, patients may require fluid in the perioperative period to restore TBW after a period of fasting and to replace small blood losses, loss of ECF into the 'third space' and losses of water from the skin, gut and lungs.

Blood losses in excess of 15% of blood volume in the adult are usually replaced by infusion of stored blood. Smaller blood losses may be replaced by a crystalloid electrolyte solution such as compound sodium lactate; however, because these solutions are distributed throughout ECF, blood volume is maintained only if at least three times the volume of blood loss is infused. Alternatively, a colloid solution (human albumin solution or a synthetic substitute) may be infused in a volume equal to that of the estimated loss.

Third-space losses are usually replaced as compound sodium lactate. In abdominal surgery (e.g. cholecystectomy), a volume of 5 ml kg^{-1} h^{-1} during operation, in addition to normal maintenance requirements (approximately 1.5 ml kg^{-1} h^{-1}) and blood loss replacement, is usually sufficient. Larger volumes may be required in more major procedures, but should be guided by measurement of CVP.

In the postoperative period, normal maintenance fluids should be administered (see above). Additional fluid (given as saline 0.9% or compound sodium lactate) may be required in the following circumstances:

- if blood or serum is lost from drains (colloid solutions should be used if losses exceed 500 ml)
- if gastrointestinal losses continue, e.g. from a nasogastric tube or a fistula
- after major surgery (e.g. total gastrectomy, repair of aortic aneurysm), when additional water and electrolytes may be required for 24–48 h to replace continuing third-space losses
- during rewarming if the patient has become hypothermic during surgery.

Normally, potassium is not administered in the first 24 h after surgery as endogenous release of potassium from tissue trauma and catabolism warrants restriction. The postoperative patient differs from the 'normal' patient in that the stress reaction modifies homeostatic mechanisms; stress-induced release of ADH, aldosterone and cortisol causes retention of Na^+ and water and increased renal excretion of potassium. However, restriction of fluid and sodium in the postoperative period is inappropriate because of increased losses by evaporation and into the 'third space'.

This syndrome of inappropriate ADH secretion may persist for several days in elderly patients, who are at risk of symptomatic hyponatraemia if given hypotonic fluids in the postoperative period. Elderly, orthopaedic patients taking long-term thiazide diuretics are especially at risk if given 5% dextrose postoperatively. Such patients can develop water intoxication and permanent brain damage as a result of relatively modest reductions in serum sodium.

After major surgery, assessment of fluid and electrolyte requirements is achieved best by measurement of CVP and serum electrolyte concentrations. Fluid and electrolyte requirements in infants and small children differ from those in the adult (see Ch. 53).

Patients with renal failure require fluid replacement for abnormal losses, although the total volume of fluid infused should be reduced to a degree determined by the urine output.

SODIUM AND POTASSIUM

SODIUM BALANCE

Daily ingestion amounts to 50–300 mmol. Losses in sweat and faeces are minimal (approximately 10 mmol day^{-1}) and final adjustments are made by the kidney. Urine sodium excretion may be as little as 2 mmol day^{-1} during salt restriction or may exceed 700 mmol day^{-1} after salt loading. Sodium balance is related intimately to ECFV and water balance.

DISORDERS OF SODIUM/WATER BALANCE

Hypernatraemia

Hypernatraemia is defined as a plasma sodium concentration of more than 150 mmol L^{-1} and may result from pure water loss, hypotonic fluid loss or salt gain. In the first two conditions, ECFV is reduced, whereas salt gain is associated with an expanded ECFV. For this reason, the clinical assessment of volaemic status is important in the diagnosis and management of hypernatraemic states. The common causes of hypernatraemia are summarized in Table 39.3. The abnormality common to all hypernatraemic states is intracellular dehydration secondary to ECF hyperosmolality. Primary water loss resulting in hypernatraemia may occur during prolonged fever, hyperventilation or severe exercise in hot, dry climates. However, a more common cause is the renal water loss that occurs when there is a defect in either the production or release of ADH (cranial diabetes insipidus) or an abnormality in response to ADH (nephrogenic diabetes insipidus).

The administration of osmotic diuretics results temporarily in plasma hyperosmolality. An osmotic diuresis may occur also in hyperglycaemia. During an osmotic diuresis, the solute causing the diuresis (e.g. glucose, mannitol) constitutes a significant fraction of urine solute, and the sodium content of the urine becomes hypotonic relative to plasma sodium. Thus, osmotic diuretics cause hypotonic urine losses which may result in hypernatraemic dehydration.

Table 39.3 Causes of hypernatraemia

Pure water depletion	
Extrarenal loss	Failure of water intake (coma, elderly, postoperative) Mucocutaneous loss Fever, hyperventilation, thyrotoxicosis
Renal loss	Diabetes insipidus (cranial, nephrogenic) Chronic renal failure
Hypotonic fluid loss	
Extrarenal loss	Gastrointestinal (vomiting, diarrhoea) Skin (excessive sweating)
Renal loss	Osmotic diuresis (glucose, urea, mannitol)
Salt gain	Iatrogenic ($NaHCO_3$, hypertonic saline) Salt ingestion Steroid excess

Hypertonic dehydration may occur also in paediatric practice. Diarrhoea, vomiting and anorexia lead to loss of water in excess of solute (hypotonic loss). Concomitant fever, hyperventilation and the use of high-solute feeds may combine to exaggerate the problem. ECFV is maintained by movement of water from ICF to ECF to equalize osmolality, and clinical evidence of dehydration may not be apparent until 10–15% of body weight has been lost. Rehydration must be undertaken gradually to prevent the development of cerebral oedema.

Measurement of urine and plasma osmolalities and assessment of urine output help in the diagnosis of hypernatraemic, volume-depleted states. If urine output is low and urine osmolality exceeds 800 mosmol kg^{-1}, then both ADH secretion and the renal response to ADH are present: The most likely causes are extrarenal water loss (e.g. diarrhoea, vomiting or evaporation) or insufficient intake. High urine output and high urine osmolality suggest an osmotic diuresis. If urine osmolality is less than plasma osmolality, reduced ADH secretion or impairment of the renal response to ADH should be suspected; in both cases, urine output is high.

Usually, hypernatraemia caused by salt gain is iatrogenic in origin. It occurs when excessive amounts of hypertonic sodium bicarbonate are administered during resuscitation or when isotonic fluids are given to patients who have only insensible losses. Treatment comprises induction of a diuresis with a loop diuretic if renal function is normal; urine output is replaced in part with glucose 5%. Dialysis or haemofiltration is necessary in patients with renal dysfunction.

Consequences of hypernatraemia

The major clinical manifestations of hypernatraemia involve the central nervous system. Severity depends on the rapidity with which hyperosmolality develops. Acute hypernatraemia is associated with a prompt osmotic shift of water from the intracellular compartment, causing a reduction in cell volume and water content of the brain. This results in increased permeability and even rupture of the capillaries in the brain and subarachnoid space. The patient may present with pyrexia (a manifestation of impaired thermoregulation), nausea, vomiting, convulsions, coma and virtually any type of focal neurological syndrome. The mortality and long-term morbidity of sustained hypernatraemia ($Na^+ > 160$ mmol L^{-1} for over 48 h) is high, irrespective of the underlying aetiology. In many cases, the development of hypernatraemia can be anticipated and prevented, e.g. cranial diabetes insipidus associated with head injury, but in situations where preventative strategies have failed, treatment should be instituted without hesitation.

Treatment of hypernatraemia

The magnitude of the water deficit can be estimated from the measured plasma sodium concentration and calculated total body water:

$$\text{Water deficit} = (\text{measured } [Na^+]/140 \times TBW) - TBW$$

Thus in a 75 kg patient with a serum sodium of 170 mmol L^{-1}:

$$\begin{aligned}\text{Water deficit} &= (170/140 \times 0.6 \times 75) - (0.6 \times 75)\\ &= 54.6 - 45\\ &= 9.6 \text{ L}\end{aligned}$$

For hypernatraemic patients *without* volume depletion, 5% glucose is sufficient to correct the water deficit. However, the majority of hypernatraemic patients are frankly hypovolaemic and intravenous fluids should be prescribed to repair both the sodium and the water deficit. Regardless of the severity of the condition, isotonic saline is the initial treatment of choice in the volume-depleted, hypernatraemic patient, as even this fluid is *relatively* hypotonic in patients with severe hypernatraemia. Once volume depletion has been corrected, further repair of any water deficit can be accomplished with hypotonic fluids. Fluid therapy should be prescribed with the intention of correcting hypernatraemia over a period of 48–72 h to prevent the onset of cerebral oedema.

Hyponatraemia

This is defined as a plasma sodium concentration of less than 135 mmol L^{-1}. Hyponatraemia is a common finding in hospital patients. It may occur as a result of water retention, sodium loss or both; consequently, it may be associated with an expanded, normal or contracted ECFV. As in hypernatraemia, the state of ECFV is important in determining the cause of the electrolyte imbalance.

As plasma osmolality decreases, an osmolal gradient is created across the cell membrane and results in movement of water into the ICF. The resulting expansion of brain cells is responsible for the symptomatology of hyponatraemia or 'water intoxication': nausea, vomiting, lethargy, weakness and obtundation. In severe cases (plasma $Na^+ < 115$ mmol L^{-1}), seizures and coma may result.

A scheme depicting the causes of hyponatraemia is shown in Figure 39.4. True hyponatraemia must be distinguished from pseudohyponatraemia. Sodium ions are present only in plasma water, which constitutes 93% of normal plasma. In the laboratory, the concentration of sodium in plasma is measured in an aliquot of whole plasma and the concentration is expressed in terms of plasma volume (mmol L^{-1} of whole plasma). If the percentage of water present in plasma is decreased, as in hyperlipidaemia or hyperproteinaemia, the amount of Na^+ in each aliquot of plasma is also decreased, even if its concentration in plasma water is normal. A clue to this cause of hyponatraemia is the finding of a normal plasma osmolality. Pseudohyponatraemia is not encountered when plasma sodium concentration is measured by increasingly employed ion-specific electrodes, because this method assesses directly the sodium concentration in the aqueous phase of plasma.

True hyponatraemic states may be classified conveniently into *depletional* and *dilutional* types. Depletional hyponatraemia occurs when a deficit in TBW is associated with an even greater deficit of total body sodium. Assessment of volaemic status reveals hypovolaemia. Losses may be *renal* or *extrarenal*. Excessive renal loss of sodium occurs in Addison's disease, diuretic administration, renal tubular acidosis and salt-losing nephropathies; usually, urine sodium concentration exceeds 20 mmol L^{-1}. Extrarenal losses occur usually from the gastrointestinal tract (e.g. diarrhoea, vomiting) or from sequestration into the 'third space' (e.g. peritonitis, surgery). Normal kidneys respond by conserving sodium and water to produce a urine that is hyperosmolal and low in sodium. In both situations, treatment should be directed at expanding the ECFV with saline 0.9%.

Dilutional hyponatraemic states may be associated with hypervolaemia and oedema or with normovolaemia. Again, assessment of volaemic status is important. If oedema is present, there is an excess of total body sodium with a proportionately greater excess of TBW. This is seen in congestive heart failure, cirrhosis and the nephrotic syndrome and is caused by secondary hyperaldosteronism. Treatment comprises salt and water restriction and spironolactone.

In normovolaemic hyponatraemia, there is a modest excess of TBW and a modest increase in ECFV associated with a normal total body sodium. Pseudohyponatraemia is excluded by finding high protein or lipid levels and a normal plasma osmolality. True normovolaemic hyponatraemia is commonly iatrogenic in origin. The syndrome of inappropriate intravenous therapy (SIIVT) is caused usually by administration of intravenous fluids with a low sodium content to patients with isotonic losses.

A more chronic water overload may occur in patients with hypothyroidism and in conditions associated with an inappropriately elevated level of ADH. The syndrome of inappropriate ADH secretion (SIADH) is characterized by hyponatraemia, low plasma osmolality and an inappropriate antidiuresis, i.e. a urine osmolality higher than anticipated for the degree of hyponatraemia. It occurs in the presence of malignant tumours which produce ADH-like substances (e.g. lung, prostate, pancreas), in neurological disorders (e.g. head injury, tumours, infections) and in some severe pneumonias. A number of drugs are associated with increased ADH secretion or potentiate the effects of ADH (Table 39.4). In patients with SIADH, the urine is concentrated in spite of hyponatraemia. Management comprises restriction of fluid intake to encourage a negative fluid balance. In severe or refractory cases, demeclocycline or lithium may result in improvement. Both drugs induce a state of functional diabetes insipidus and have been used effectively in SIADH if the primary disease cannot be treated.

Consequences of hyponatraemia

Symptoms vary with the underlying aetiology, the magnitude of the reduction of plasma sodium and the rapidity with which the

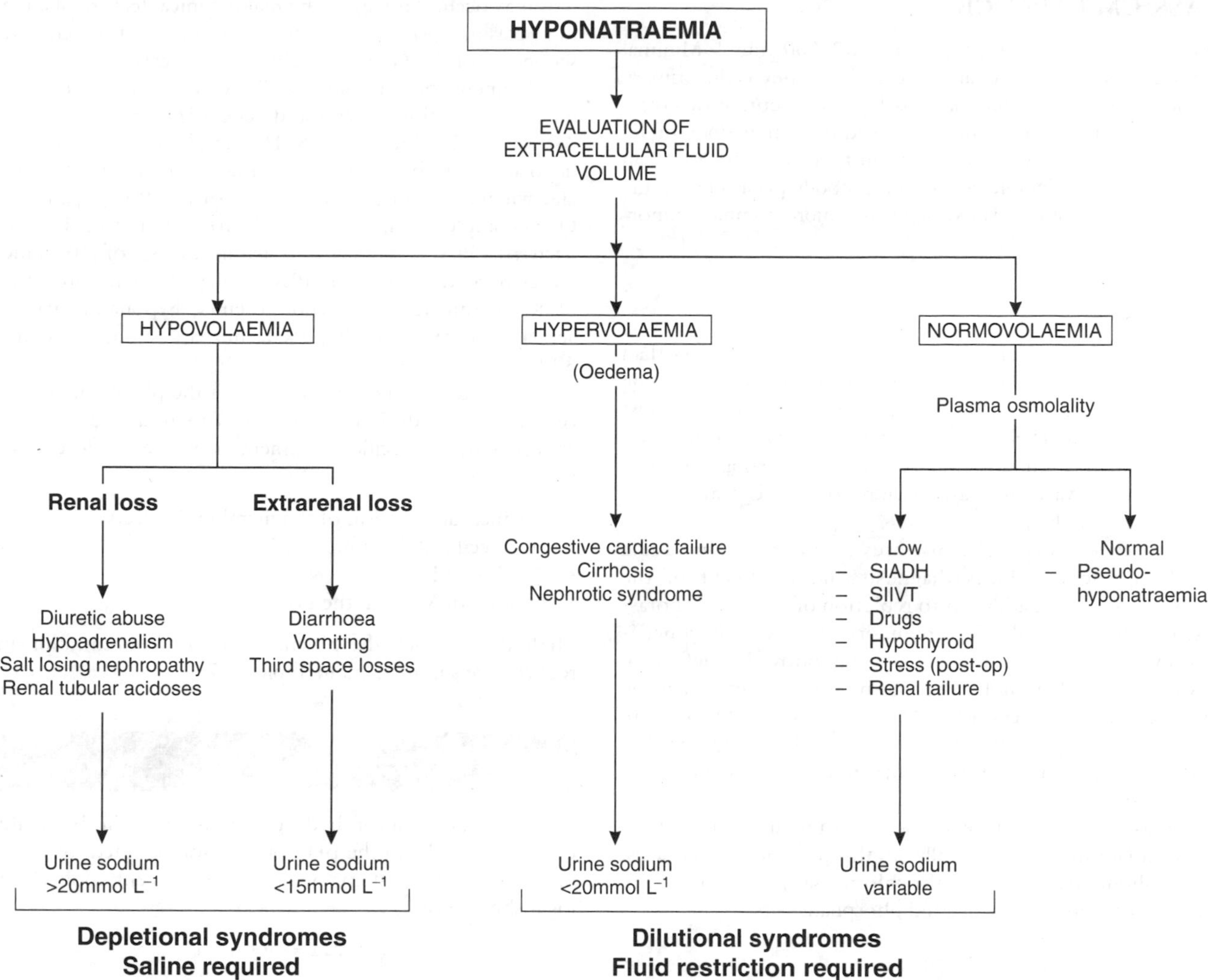

Fig. 39.4
Causes of hyponatraemia.

plasma sodium concentration decreases. Serious consequences involve the central nervous system and result from intracellular overhydration, cerebral oedema and raised intracranial pressure. Nausea, vomiting, delirium, convulsions and coma result.

Table 39.4 Drugs associated with antidiuresis and hyponatraemia

Increased ADH secretion
Hypnotics – barbiturates
Analgesics – opioids
Hypoglycaemics – chlorpropamide, tolbutamide
Anticonvulsants – carbamazepine
Miscellaneous – phenothiazines, tricyclics
Potentiation of ADH at distal tubule
Paracetamol
Indomethacin
Chlorpropamide

Treatment of hyponatraemia

Acute symptomatic hyponatraemia is a medical emergency and requires prompt intervention using hypertonic saline. The rapidity with which hyponatraemia should be corrected is the subject of controversy because of observations that rapid correction may cause central pontine myelinolysis, a disorder characterized by paralysis, coma and death. As a causal relationship between this syndrome and the rate of increase of plasma sodium has not been established and it is clear that there is a prohibitive mortality associated with inadequately treated water intoxication, rapid correction of the symptomatic hyponatraemic state is warranted. Sufficient sodium should be given to return the plasma concentration to 125 mmol L^{-1} only and this should be administered over a period of no less than 12 h. The amount of sodium needed to cause the desired correction in the plasma sodium can be calculated as follows:

$$Na^+ \text{ required (mmol)} = \text{TBW} \times (\text{desired } [Na^+] - \text{measured } [Na^+])$$

Hypertonic saline (3%) contains 514 mmol L^{-1} of Na^+ and administration poses the risk of pulmonary oedema, especially in oedematous patients in whom renal dialysis is preferable.

POTASSIUM BALANCE

The normal daily intake of potassium is 50–200 mmol. Minimal amounts are lost via the skin and faeces; the kidney is the primary regulator. However, the mechanisms for the retention of potassium are less efficient than those for sodium. In periods of K^+ depletion, daily urinary excretion cannot decrease to less than 5–10 mmol. A considerable deficit of total body potassium occurs if intake is not restored. Hypokalaemia is a more common abnormality than hyperkalaemia.

Hypokalaemia

This is defined as a plasma potassium concentration of less than 3.5 mmol L^{-1}. Non-specific symptoms of hypokalaemia include anorexia and nausea, effects on skeletal and smooth muscle (muscle weakness, paralytic ileus) and abnormal cardiac conduction (delayed repolarization with ST-segment depression, reduced height of the T wave, increased height of the U wave and a widened QRS complex).

The causes of hypokalaemia are summarized in Table 39.5. Management includes diagnosis and treatment of the underlying disorder in addition to repletion of total body potassium stores. As a general rule, a reduction in plasma K^+ concentration by 1 mmol L^{-1} reflects a total body K^+ deficit of approximately 100 mmol. Potassium supplements may be given orally or intravenously. The maximum infusion rate should not exceed 0.5 mmol kg^{-1} h^{-1} to allow equilibration with the intracellular compartment; much slower rates are employed usually.

The potassium salt used for replacement therapy is important. In most situations, and especially in the presence of alkalosis, potassium should be replaced as the chloride salt. Supplements are available also as the bicarbonate and phosphate salts.

Hyperkalaemia

This is defined as a plasma potassium concentration exceeding 5 mmol L^{-1}. Vague muscle weakness progressing to flaccid paralysis may occur. However, the major clinical feature of an increasing plasma potassium concentration is the characteristic sequence of ECG abnormalities. The earliest change is the development of tall, peaked T waves and a shortened QT interval, reflecting more rapid repolarization (6–7 mmol L^{-1}). As plasma K^+ increases (8–10 mmol L^{-1}), abnormalities in depolarization become manifest as widened QRS complexes and widening, and eventually loss, of the P wave; the widened QRS complexes merge finally into the T waves (*sine wave pattern*). Plasma concentrations in excess of 10 mmol L^{-1} are associated with ventricular fibrillation. The cardiac toxicity of K^+ is enhanced by hypocalcaemia, hyponatraemia or acidaemia. The causes of hyperkalaemia are summarized in Table 39.6.

Immediate treatment is necessary if the plasma potassium concentration exceeds 7 mmol L^{-1} or if there are any serious ECG abnormalities. Specific treatment may be achieved by four mechanisms:

- chemical antagonism of the membrane effects
- enhanced cellular uptake of K^+
- dilution of ECF
- removal of K^+ from the body.

Methods by which the plasma potassium concentration may be reduced are summarized in Table 39.7.

ACID–BASE BALANCE

The concentration of hydrogen ions (H^+) in body fluids is extremely small and the pH notation was adopted for the sake of practicality. This system expresses H^+ concentration $[H^+]$ on a logarithmic scale:

$$pH = -\log_{10}[H^+]$$

Table 39.5 Causes of hypokalaemia

Cause	Comments
Reduced intake	Usually only contributory
Tissue redistribution	Insulin therapy, alkalaemia, β_2-adrenergic agonists, familial periodic paralysis, vitamin B_{12} therapy
Increased loss	
Gastrointestinal (urine $K^+ < 20$ mmol L^{-1})	Diarrhoea, vomiting, fistulae, nasogastric suction, colonic villous adenoma
Renal	Diuretic therapy, primary or secondary hyperaldosteronism, malignant hypertension, renal artery stenosis (high renin), renal tubular acidosis, hypomagnesaemia, renal failure (diuretic phase)

Table 39.6 Causes of hyperkalaemia

Factitious (pseudohyperkalaemia)
In vitro haemolysis
Thrombocytosis
Leucocytosis
Tourniquet
Exercise

Impaired excretion
Renal failure
Acute or chronic hyperaldosteronism
Addison's disease
K^+-sparing diuretics
Indomethacin

Tissue redistribution
Tissue damage (burns, trauma)
Rhabdomyolysis
Tumour necrosis
Hyperkalaemic periodic paralysis
Massive intravascular haemolysis
Succinylcholine

Excessive intake
Blood transfusion
Excessive i.v. administration

A more logical arithmetic convention which expresses $[H^+]$ in nmol L^{-1} is gaining popularity. Table 39.8 compares values of $[H^+]$ expressed as pH and nmol L^{-1} and reveals a number of disadvantages of the pH notation. The most obvious disadvantage is that it moves in the opposite direction to $[H^+]$; a decrease in pH is associated with increased $[H^+]$ and vice versa. It is also apparent that the logarithmic scale distorts the quantitative estimate of change in $[H^+]$; for example, twice as many hydrogen ions are required to reduce pH from 7.1 to 7.0 as are needed to reduce it from 7.4 to 7.3. The pH scale gives the false impression that there is relatively little difference in the sensitivity of biological systems to an equivalent increase or decrease in $[H^+]$. However, when $[H^+]$ is expressed in nmol L^{-1}, it becomes apparent that tolerance is limited to a reduction in $[H^+]$ of only 24 nmol L^{-1} from normal, but to an increase of up to 120 nmol L^{-1}. Nevertheless, the pH notation remains the most widely used system and is employed in the remainder of this chapter.

BASIC DEFINITIONS

An *acid* is a substance that dissociates in water to produce H^+; a *base* is a substance that can accept H^+. Strong acids dissociate completely in aqueous solution, whereas weak acids (e.g. carbonic acid, H_2CO_3) dissociate only partially. The *conjugate base* of an acid is its dissociated anionic product. For example, bicarbonate ion (HCO_3^-) is the conjugate base of carbonic acid:

$$H_2CO_3 \rightleftharpoons H^+ + HCO_3^-$$

A *buffer* is a combination of a weak acid and its conjugate base (usually as a salt) which acts to minimize any change in $[H^+]$ that would occur if a strong acid or base were added to it. Buffers in body fluids represent an important defence against $[H^+]$ change. The carbonic acid/bicarbonate system is an important buffer in blood. The pH of a buffer system may be determined from the Henderson–Hasselbalch equation which, for the carbonic acid/bicarbonate system, relates pH, $[H_2CO_3]$ and $[HCO_3^-]$:

$$pH = pK + \log_{10}([HCO_3^-]/[H_2CO_3])$$

where K = dissociation constant and $pK = -\log_{10}K$.

This equation shows that $[H^+]$ in body fluids is a function of the *ratio* of base to acid. For the bicarbonate buffer system, pK is 6.1. As most of the carbonic acid pool exists as dissolved CO_2, the equation may be rewritten:

$$pH = 6.1 + \log_{10}\{[HCO_3^-]/(0.225 \times PCO_2)\}$$

The value 0.225 represents the solubility coefficient of CO_2 in blood (ml kPa^{-1}). Normally, $[HCO_3^-]$ is 24 mmol L^{-1} and P_aCO_2 is 5.3 kPa. Thus:

$$pH = 6.1 + \log_{10}[24/(0.225 \times 5.3)] = 7.4$$

Most acid–base disorders may be formulated in terms of the Henderson–Hasselbalch equation. The pH of plasma is kept remarkably constant at 7.36–7.44, i.e. a hydrogen ion concentration of 40 ± 5 nmol L^{-1}. This is achieved by:

- regulation of H^+ excretion and bicarbonate regeneration by the kidney
- regulation of CO_2 by the alveolar ventilation of the lungs.

Cellular metabolism poses a constant threat to buffer systems by the production of 'volatile acid', i.e. CO_2, from cellular respiration and the formation of 'fixed' or 'non-volatile' acids by intermediary metabolism. Thus, the acid–base status of body fluids reflects the metabolism of both H^+ and CO_2.

Table 39.7 Treatment of hyperkalaemia

Calcium gluconate 10% i.v. (0.5 ml kg^{-1} to maximum of 20 ml) given over 5 min. No change in plasma $[K^+]$. Effect immediate but transient
Glucose 50 g (0.5–1.0 g kg^{-1}) plus insulin 20 units (0.3 unit kg^{-1}) as single i.v. bolus dose. Then infusion of glucose 20%, plus insulin 6–20 units h^{-1} (depending on blood glucose)
Sodium bicarbonate 1.5–2.0 mmol kg^{-1} i.v. over 5–10 min
Calcium resonium 15 g p.o. or 30 g p.r. 8-hourly
Peritoneal or haemodialysis

Table 39.8 Comparison of logarithmic and arithmetic methods of expressing hydrogen ion concentration in the range of blood $[H^+]$ compatible with life

pH	$[H^+]$ (nmol L^{-1})	
7.8	16	
7.7	20	
7.6	25	*Alkalaemia*
7.5	32	
7.4	**40**	*Normal*
7.3	50	
7.2	63	
7.1	80	
7.0	100	*Acidaemia*
6.9	125	
6.8	160	

ACID–BASE DISORDERS

The normal pH of body fluids is 7.36–7.44. Conventional acid–base nomenclature involves the following definitions:

- *acidosis* – a process that causes acid to accumulate
- *acidaemia* – this is present if pH < 7.36
- *alkalosis* – a process that causes base to accumulate
- *alkalaemia* – this is present if pH > 7.44.

Simple acid–base disorders are common in clinical practice and their successful management requires logical analysis of pH, $[HCO_3^-]$ and P_aCO_2. The first step involves diagnosis of the primary disorder; this is followed by an assessment of the extent and appropriateness of any compensation.

Primary acid–base disorders are either *respiratory* or *metabolic*. The disorder is respiratory if the primary disturbance involves

CO_2, and metabolic if it involves HCO_3^-. Thus, four potential primary disturbances exist (Table 39.9) and each may be identified by analysis of pH, [HCO_3^-] and P_aCO_2. Both pH and P_aCO_2 are measured directly by the blood gas machine. [HCO_3^-] is measured directly on the electrolyte profile but is derived in most blood gas machines. Other derived parameters include *standard bicarbonate* and *base excess*. The standard bicarbonate is not the actual bicarbonate of the sample but an estimate of bicarbonate concentration after elimination of any abnormal respiratory contribution to [HCO_3^-], i.e. an estimate of [HCO_3^-] at a P_aCO_2 of 5.3 kPa. The base excess (in alkalosis) or base deficit (in acidosis) is the amount of acid or base (in mmol) required to return the pH of 1 L of blood to normal at a P_aCO_2 of 5.3 kPa; it is a measure of the magnitude of the metabolic component of the acid–base disorder.

After the primary disorder has been identified, it is necessary to consider if it is acute or chronic and if any compensation has occurred. The body defends itself against changes in pH by compensatory mechanisms which *tend* to return pH towards normal. Primary respiratory disorders are compensated by a metabolic mechanism and vice versa. For example, a primary respiratory acidosis is compensated for by renal retention of HCO_3^-, whereas a primary metabolic acidosis is compensated for by hyperventilation and a decrease in P_aCO_2. Thus, in each case, the *acidaemia* produced by the primary acidosis is reduced by a compensatory alkalosis. The response to a respiratory alkalosis is increased renal elimination of HCO_3^-, and a metabolic alkalosis results in hypoventilation and increased P_aCO_2, pH being restored towards normal by the compensatory respiratory acidosis. In each case, the efficiency of compensatory mechanisms is limited; compensation is usually only partial and rarely complete. Overcompensation does not occur.

Metabolic acidosis

The cardinal features of a metabolic acidosis are a decreased [HCO_3^-], a low pH, and an appropriately low P_aCO_2. The extent of the acidaemia depends upon the nature, severity and duration of the initiating pathology in addition to the efficiency of compensatory mechanisms. The magnitude of the compensatory response is proportional to the fall in [HCO_3]. The lower limit of the respiratory response is a P_aCO_2 of 1.3kPa. In a steady state:

$$\text{predicted } P_aCO_2 = (0.02 \times \text{observed bicarbonate}) + 1.1 \text{ (kPa)}$$

If the observed P_aCO_2 differs from the predicted value then an independent respiratory disturbance is present.

In most instances, establishing the presence and the cause of a metabolic acidosis is straightforward. In difficult cases, an important clue to the nature of the abnormality is given by the measurement of the ***anion gap*** in plasma:

$$\text{anion gap} = ([Na^+] + [K^+]) - ([Cl^-] + [HCO_3^-])$$

In reality, the numbers of cations and anions in plasma are the same and an anion gap exists because negatively charged proteins, together with phosphate, lactate and organic anions (which maintain electrical neutrality), are not measured. The normal anion gap is 12–18 mmol L^{-1}.

Clinically, it is useful to divide the metabolic acidoses into those associated with a normal anion gap and those with an increased anion gap. The former are caused by loss of HCO_3^- from the body and replacement with chloride. In acidoses associated with an increased anion gap, HCO_3^- has been titrated by either endogenous, e.g. lactic, or exogenous acids, thus increasing the number of unmeasured plasma anions without altering the plasma chloride concentration (Table 39.10).

Clinical effects and treatment

Metabolic acidosis results in widespread physiological disturbances, including reduced cardiac output, pulmonary hypertension, arrhythmias, Kussmaul respiration and hyperkalaemia; the severity of the disturbances is related to the extent of the *acidaemia*. Treatment should be directed initially at identifying and reversing the cause. If acidaemia is considered to be life-threatening (pH < 7.2, [HCO_3^-] < 10 mmol L^{-1}), measures may be required to restore blood pH to normal. Overzealous use of sodium bicarbonate may lead to rapid correction of blood pH, with the risks of tetany and convulsions in the short term and volume overload and hypernatraemia in the longer term. The required quantity of bicarbonate should be calculated:

$$\text{bicarbonate requirement (mmol)} = \text{body weight (kg)} \times \text{base deficit (mmol } L^{-1}) \times 0.3$$

Table 39.9 Compensatory mechanisms in acid–base disturbances. ↓↓ or ↑↑ denotes the primary abnormality. The final pH depends on the degree of compensation. Respiratory compensation for metabolic disorders is rapid; renal compensation for respiratory disorders is slow

Primary disorder	pH	HCO_3^-	P_aCO_2	Compensation
Metabolic acidosis	↓	↓↓		Hyperventilation ↓ P_aCO_2
Metabolic alkalosis	↑	↑↑		Hypoventilation ↑ P_aCO_2
Respiratory acidosis	↓		↑↑	Renal retention of HCO_3^-
Respiratory alkalosis	↑		↓↓	Renal elimination of HCO_3^-

Table 39.10 Types and causes of metabolic acidosis

High anion gap	
Overproduction of acid	Diabetic ketoacidosis Lactic acidosis type A (hypoxia, shock) or type B (biguanides) Starvation
Exogenous acid	Salicylates Methanol Ethylene glycol
Reduced excretion	Renal failure
Normal anion gap	
Bicarbonate loss	*Extrarenal* Diarrhoea Biliary/pancreatic fistula Ileostomy Ureterosigmoidostomy
	Renal Renal tubular acidosis Carbonic anhydrase inhibitors
Addition of acid (with chloride)	HCl, NH_4Cl, arginine or lysine hydrochloride

Administration of sodium bicarbonate should be followed by repeated measurements of plasma [HCO_3^-] and pH. Sodium bicarbonate is available as isotonic (1.4%; 163 mmol L^{-1}) and hypertonic (8.4%; 1000 mmol L^{-1}) solutions. Slow infusion of the hypertonic solution is advisable to minimize adverse effects.

When considering the use of sodium bicarbonate in the context of metabolic acidaemia, it is important to realize that carbon dioxide is generated during the buffering process. This may result in a superimposed respiratory acidosis, especially in those patients with impaired ventilatory reserve or at the limit of compensation. It is also important to distinguish those acidoses associated with tissue hypoxia (e.g. cardiac arrest, septic shock) from those where tissue hypoxia is not a factor. It appears that therapy with sodium bicarbonate often exacerbates the acidosis if tissue hypoxia is present. For example, in patients with type A lactic acidosis, $NaHCO_3$ increases mixed venous P_aCO_2, which rapidly crosses cell membranes resulting in an intracellular acidosis, particularly in cardiac and hepatic cells. Theoretically, this could result in decreased myocardial contractility and cardiac output and decreased lactate extraction by the liver, aggravating the lactic acidosis. Current guidelines for the management of cardiopulmonary arrest no longer recommend the routine use of sodium bicarbonate. However, if the acidosis is not associated with tissue hypoxia (e.g. uraemic acidosis) then the use of sodium bicarbonate will result in a potentially beneficial increase in arterial pH.

Metabolic alkalosis

The cardinal features of a metabolic alkalosis are an increased plasma [HCO_3^-], a high pH and an appropriately raised P_aCO_2. The compensatory response of hypoventilation is limited and not very effective. For diagnostic and therapeutic reasons, it is usual to subdivide metabolic alkalosis into the chloride-responsive and chloride-resistant varieties (Table 39.11). The differential diagnosis of metabolic alkalosis, and in particular the separation of patients on the basis of the urinary chloride concentration, is important because of the differences in treatment of the two groups. In chloride-responsive alkalosis, the administration of saline causes volume expansion and results in the excretion of excess bicarbonate; if potassium is required, it should be given as the chloride salt. In patients in whom volume administration is contraindicated, the use of acetazolamide results in renal loss of HCO_3^- and an improvement in pH. H_2-receptor antagonists may be helpful if nasogastric suction is contributing to hydrogen ion loss.

Severe alkalaemia with compensatory hypoventilation may result in seizures or CNS depression. In life-threatening metabolic alkalosis, rapid correction is necessary and may be achieved by administration of hydrogen ions in the form of dilute hydrochloric acid. Acid administration requires central vein cannulation, as peripheral infusion causes sclerosis of veins. Acid is given as 0.1 normal HCl in glucose 5% at a rate no greater than 0.2 mmol kg^{-1} h^{-1}.

Respiratory acidosis

The cardinal features of a respiratory acidosis are a primary increase in P_aCO_2, a low pH and an appropriate rise in plasma bicarbonate. The extent of the acidaemia is proportional to the degree of hypercapnia. Buffering processes are activated rapidly in acute hypercapnia and may remove enough H^+ from the extracellular fluid to result in a secondary increase in plasma HCO_3^-.

Usually, hypoxaemia and the manifestations of the underlying disease dominate the clinical picture, but hypercapnia *per se* may result in coma, raised intracranial pressure and a hyperdynamic cardiovascular system (tachycardia, vasodilatation, ventricular arrhythmias) resulting from release of catecholamines.

There are many causes of respiratory acidosis, the most important of which are classified in Table 39.12. Treatment consists of reversing the underlying pathology if possible and mechanical ventilatory support if required.

Table 39.11 Types and causes of metabolic alkalosis

Chloride-responsive (urine chloride < 20 mmol L^{-1})
Loss of acid
Vomiting
Nasogastric suction
Gastrocolic fistula
Chloride depletion
Diarrhoea
Diuretic abuse
Excessive alkali
$NaHCO_3$ administration
Antacid abuse
Chloride-resistant (urine chloride > 20 mmol L^{-1})
Primary or secondary hyperaldosteronism
Cushing's syndrome
Severe hypokalaemia
Carbenoxolone

Table 39.12 Causes of respiratory acidosis

Central nervous system
Drug overdose
Trauma
Tumour
Degeneration or infection
Cerebrovascular accident
Cervical cord trauma

Peripheral nervous system
Polyneuropathy
Myasthenia gravis
Poliomyelitis
Botulism
Tetanus
Organophosphorus poisoning

Primary pulmonary disease
Airway obstruction
- Asthma
- Laryngospasm
- Chronic obstructive airways disease

Parenchymal disease
- ARDS
- Pneumonia
- Severe pulmonary oedema
- Chronic obstructive airways disease

Loss of mechanical integrity
- Flail chest

Table 39.13 Causes of respiratory alkalosis

Supratentorial
Voluntary/hysterical hyperventilation
Pain, anxiety

Specific conditions
CNS disease
- Meningitis/encephalitis
- Cerebrovascular accident
- Tumour
- Trauma

Respiratory disease
- Pneumonia
- Pulmonary embolism
- Early pulmonary oedema or ARDS
- High altitude

Shock
- Cardiogenic
- Hypovolaemic
- Septic

Miscellaneous
- Cirrhosis
- Gram-negative septicaemia
- Pregnancy
- IPPV

Drugs/hormones
- Salicylates
- Aminophylline
- Progesterone

Respiratory alkalosis

The cardinal features of respiratory alkalosis are a primary decrease in P_aCO_2 (alveolar ventilation in excess of metabolic needs), an increase in pH and an appropriate fall in plasma bicarbonate concentration. Usually, hypocapnia indicates a disturbance of ventilatory control (in patients not receiving mechanical ventilation). As in respiratory acidosis, the manifestations of the underlying disease usually dominate the clinical picture. Acute hypocapnia results in cerebral vasoconstriction and reduced cerebral blood flow and may cause light-headedness, confusion and, in severe cases, seizures. Circumoral paraesthesia, hyperreflexia and tetany are common. Cardiovascular manifestations include tachycardia and ventricular arrhythmias secondary to the alkalaemia.

The causes of respiratory alkalosis are summarized in Table 39.13. Treatment comprises correction of the underlying cause and thus differential diagnosis is important.

FURTHER READING

Arieff A I 1991 Indications for the use of bicarbonate in patients with metabolic acidosis. British Journal of Anaesthesia 67: 165–178

Askanazi J. Starker P M, Weissman C (eds) 1986 Fluid and electrolyte balance in critical care. Butterworths, Boston

Lane N, Allen K 1999 Hyponatraemia after orthopaedic surgery. British Medical Journal 318: 1363–1364

Swales J D 1991 Management of hyponatraemia. British Journal of Anaesthesia 67: 146–154

Thomson W S T, Adams J F, Cowan R A 1997 Clinical acid–base balance. Oxford University Press, Oxford

Walmsley R N, Guerin M D 1984 Disorders of fluid and electrolyte balance. Wright, Bristol

40 Complications during anaesthesia

Most intraoperative complications involve the patient, although staff are also at risk (see Ch. 33). Information about the type, incidence and outcome of complications is provided by studies of anaesthetic morbidity, mortality and critical incidents. At least one intraoperative complication occurs in 9% of all patients undergoing surgery. The risk increases with the duration of surgery and is higher in the morbidly obese, patients at the extremes of age and those undergoing emergency or obstetric anaesthesia.

The most frequent complications during anaesthesia are arrhythmia, hypotension, adverse drug effects and inadequate ventilation of the lungs. Inadequate ventilation is commonly caused by unrecognized oesophageal intubation, poorly managed or difficult tracheal intubation, pulmonary aspiration of gastric contents, breathing system disconnections or gas supply failure. These complications are also the major causes of anaesthetic mortality, preventable intraoperative cardiac arrest and permanent neurological damage. In particular, hypotension and hypoxaemia are implicated consistently in studies of adverse outcome from anaesthesia. The source of most anaesthetic complications is human error, often in association with poor monitoring, equipment malfunction and organizational failure.

There are important implications for the anaesthetist. Continuing staff education and maintenance of appropriate anaesthetic skills are an important part of any risk management strategy. This may include a role for training using a simulator. As most complications are preventable, meticulous preparation of both the patient and anaesthetic equipment is essential to minimize the risk of an adverse event. Should an intraoperative complication occur, the anaesthetist must be able to recognize the problem rapidly and manage it effectively. This demands constant vigilance, the use of appropriate monitoring and a well-rehearsed and effective plan of action. The use of specific protocols for managing critical incidents is recommended.

CARDIOVASCULAR SYSTEM

Perfusion of vital organs must be maintained during anaesthesia and surgery. Uninterrupted intraoperative surveillance for changes in cardiovascular variables is therefore essential to ensure an adequate cardiac output and to maintain organ perfusion. Most intraoperative changes in heart rate and blood pressure are caused by pharmacological or physiological alterations in autonomic tone and are therefore potentially avoidable or easily treated by correcting the precipitating factor.

CHANGES IN HEART RATE AND RHYTHM

Bradycardia

During anaesthesia, bradycardia may be defined as any cardiac rhythm with a rate less than 60 beats min^{-1}.

Aetiology

Sinus bradycardia originates from the sinoatrial node. It is common during anaesthesia in healthy patients and is associated with the use of opioids or deep levels of anaesthesia. Surgical manipulations such as eyeball traction, cervical dilatation and peritoneal traction can increase vagal tone, producing bradycardia and occasionally sinus arrest. Drugs are a common cause of bradycardia. Succinylcholine can produce a profound decrease in heart rate, especially following repeat doses. Bradycardia occurs in some patients after intravenous injection of rapidly acting opioid analgesics such as remifentanil, alfentanil and fentanyl. There have been several reports of profound bradycardia in association with the use of propofol.

Inhalation anaesthetic agents can influence heart rate by altering sinus node or autonomic activity. Halothane and, to a lesser extent, enflurane cause dose-dependent suppression of sinus node automaticity. This may produce bradycardia and emergence of an ectopic pacemaker, often as a wandering atrial pacemaker or junctional escape rhythm (junctional bradycardia). Both halothane and enflurane also depress atrioventricular conduction; calcium channel blockers, β-blockers and digoxin potentiate this effect.

Drugs without sympathomimetic activity, such as atracurium and vecuronium, can be associated with bradycardia if used concurrently with opioids or β-blocking agents. Hypothermia and hypothyroidism are additional causes of bradycardia.

Management

Healthy patients usually tolerate a decrease in heart rate to 40 beats min^{-1}. Bradycardia becomes clinically significant if associated with an escape rhythm or a decrease in cardiac output. This can be treated with an anticholinergic agent such as glycopyrrolate or atropine, with the choice and dose depending on the clinical urgency. If bradycardia is refractory to treatment, intravenous isoprenaline or cardiac pacing may be indicated. An anticholinergic drug may be given prophylactically where surgical stimulation increases the risk of bradycardia (e.g. ophthalmic surgery) or before a second dose of succinylcholine.

Tachycardia

During anaesthesia, tachycardia may be defined as any cardiac rhythm with a rate greater than 100 beats min^{-1}.

Aetiology

Sinus tachycardia is a normal physiological response to stimulation of the sympathetic nervous system. It is observed in most patients at some time during the perioperative period. Sympathetic tone is increased by hypoxaemia, hypercapnia, inadequate anaesthesia and/or analgesia, hypovolaemia, hypotension and airway manipulations such as laryngoscopy and tracheal intubation. Other signs of sympathetic nervous activity may be present, including hypertension and ventricular ectopy. Tachycardia is also associated with an increase in metabolic rate (fever, sepsis, burns, hyperthyroidism, malignant hyperthermia), or the administration of vagolytic drugs (e.g. atropine, pancuronium) or sympathomimetic drugs (e.g. ephedrine, epinephrine). Isoflurane and desflurane may also increase heart rate. Tachycardia reduces the duration of diastolic coronary artery filling and simultaneously increases myocardial work. This may precipitate myocardial ischaemia in patients with coronary artery or hypertensive heart disease.

Management

The cause of the tachycardia should be determined and treated. This may include providing additional analgesia, deepening anaesthesia or giving intravenous fluids for hypovolaemia. Sinus tachycardia may be associated with myocardial ischaemia despite exclusion or treatment of other causes. In this situation, the tachycardia may be controlled by careful intravenous titration of a β-blocker such as esmolol.

Arrhythmia

Arrhythmia is the most frequently reported critical incident. Table 40.1 lists the commonest causes of arrhythmia during anaesthesia.

Extracellular potassium concentration has a profound effect on myocardial electrical activity. Intraoperative abnormalities of extracellular potassium are most likely to occur in patients with preoperative potassium, fluid or acid–base imbalance, especially if treated inadequately prior to anaesthesia. Hypokalaemia increases ventricular irritability and the risks of ventricular ectopy and ventricular tachycardia/fibrillation. This effect is potentiated in patients with ischaemic heart disease and in those receiving digoxin. Hyperventilation alters acid–base balance, with acute transmembrane redistribution of potassium. Serum potassium concentration can decrease by 0.5 mmol L^{-1} for every 1.3 kPa decrease in P_aCO_2. Life-threatening hyperkalaemia with atrioventricular conduction block or ventricular fibrillation can occur if succinylcholine is used in patients with burns or denervating injuries. Electrolyte disorders are discussed further in Chapter 39.

General management

Preoperative correction of fluid, electrolyte and acid–base imbalance is essential. Continuous intraoperative ECG monitoring is mandatory because arrhythmias are so common. Lead II best demonstrates atrial activity and its use is recommended for routine ECG monitoring. As the ECG gives no indication of cardiac output or tissue perfusion, the detection of an abnormal cardiac rhythm should be followed by rapid assessment of the circulation. An absent pulse, severe hypotension or ventricular tachycardia or fibrillation should be treated as a cardiac arrest.

The anaesthetist should always exclude hypoxaemia, hypotension, inadequate analgesia and light anaesthesia as possible causes of arrhythmia. Correction of the precipitating factor is often the only treatment required. If the arrhythmia persists and causes a significant decrease in cardiac output, if it is associated with myocardial ischaemia or if it predisposes to ventricular tachycardia or fibrillation, intervention with a specific antiarrhythmic agent or cardioversion is indicated.

Table 40.1 Commonest causes of arrhythmia during anaesthesia

Cardiorespiratory	Hypoxaemia Hypotension Hypo/hypercapnia Myocardial ischaemia		
Metabolic	Catecholamines	Endogenous	Inadequate analgesia Inadequate anaesthesia Airway manipulation Hyperthyroidism
		Exogenous	Sympathomimetics
	Hypo/hyperkalaemia Malignant hyperthermia		
Surgical	Increased vagal tone (eye surgery, anal stretch, mesenteric traction) Direct cardiac stimulation (chest surgery, CVP cannulae) Dental surgery		
Drugs	Vagolytics (e.g. atropine, pancuronium) Sympathomimetics (e.g. epinephrine, ephedrine) Halothane, enflurane Digoxin		

Serum potassium concentration should be measured if ventricular arrhythmias occur, especially if the patient is receiving digoxin.

Atrial arrhythmias

These can reduce the atrial contribution to left ventricular filling, resulting in a decrease in cardiac output. Premature atrial contractions are common and of little importance.

Junctional rhythm. This bradycardia is associated usually with the use of halothane. A reduction in concentration and/or a change of volatile agent are indicated. An anticholinergic drug may be required to restore sinus rhythm.

Accelerated nodal rhythm. This may be precipitated by an increase in sympathetic tone in the presence of a sensitizing volatile anaesthetic agent. Adjusting the depth of anaesthesia and/or changing the anaesthetic agent is appropriate treatment.

Supraventricular tachycardia (SVT) can occur at any time during the perioperative period in susceptible patients, such as those with Wolff–Parkinson–White or other 'pre-excitation' syndromes. If attempts to increase vagal tone and terminate the SVT by carotid sinus massage are unsuccessful, the treatment of choice is adenosine by fast intravenous injection. This is safe and effective during haemodynamic instability because adenosine has a duration of action of less than 60 s. It blocks atrioventricular conduction without compromising ventricular function. Adenosine should not be given to patients with asthma or atrioventricular conduction block. If adenosine is unavailable and the patient is normotensive, intravenous verapamil can be given in increments of 1–2 mg up to 10 mg. However, verapamil can cause prolonged hypotension and depression of ventricular function, especially in the presence of anaesthetic agents which cause myocardial depression. Cardioversion is indicated if the SVT is associated with hypotension and adenosine is unavailable.

Atrial flutter/fibrillation. These arrhythmias are most commonly observed during anaesthesia as a paroxysmal increase in ventricular rate in patients with pre-existing atrial flutter/fibrillation. After correcting any precipitating factors, digoxin by slow intravenous injection is the treatment of choice. Alternative therapy with amiodarone or a β-blocker may be necessary to control the ventricular rate in patients receiving digoxin preoperatively. Immediate cardioversion should be considered if the ventricular rate is fast with a clinically significant reduction in cardiac output.

Ventricular arrhythmias

Premature ventricular contractions (PVCs) are common in healthy patients and may be present preoperatively. If associated with a slow atrial rate (escape beats), increasing the sinus rate with an anticholinergic drug should abolish them. In other situations, an underlying cause should be sought before antiarrhythmic agents are considered, as PVCs rarely progress to more serious arrhythmias unless there is underlying myocardial ischaemia or hypoxaemia. Halothane lowers the threshold for catecholamine-induced ventricular arrhythmias; this effect is exacerbated by hypercapnia. Halothane should be used with care in patients receiving sympathomimetic drugs (including those undergoing tissue infiltration with local anaesthetics containing epinephrine) and in patients taking aminophylline or drugs which block norepinephrine re-uptake, such as tricyclic or other antidepressants. The maximum recommended dose of epinephrine for infiltration in the presence of halothane is 100 μg (10 ml of 1 in 100 000 concentration) during any 10 min period, although the rate of absorption depends on the site of injection. Although the use of enflurane or isoflurane has a lower risk, sevoflurane has an even lower potential to cause myocardial sensitization to catecholamines.

Frequent, multifocal PVCs during myocardial ischaemia may herald a more serious arrhythmia.

Other ventricular arrhythmias such as ventricular tachycardia or fibrillation are uncommon. They should be treated as a cardiac arrest.

Heart block

This is discussed in Chapter 35 (p. 435).

HYPOTENSION

In healthy patients, hypotension during anaesthesia may be defined as a mean arterial pressure less than 60 mmHg. A systolic blood pressure 25% less than the patient's preoperative value also indicates hypotension, especially in patients with pre-existing hypertension. Hypotension is clinically significant if vital organ perfusion is compromised (e.g. myocardial ischaemia or oliguria). As left ventricular coronary blood flow occurs predominantly in diastole, the value of diastolic blood pressure is particularly important in patients with coronary artery disease.

Aetiology

Hypotension is caused by a decrease in cardiac output and/or systemic vascular resistance (vasodilatation). Table 40.2 classifies the common causes of hypotension during anaesthesia. Hypotension is usually multifactorial, with hypovolaemia a frequent underlying factor (see below). Inhalation anaesthetic agents decrease arterial pressure, by reducing either cardiac output (sevoflurane and isoflurane being the least potent in this regard) or systemic vascular resistance (isoflurane and sevoflurane being the most potent), or both. Other anaesthetic agents have similar effects. Therefore, a relative overdose of anaesthetic drug can cause significant hypotension, especially in hypovolaemic or elderly patients. The hypotensive effects of anaesthetic agents are potentiated by calcium channel blockers, β-blockers, angiotensin-converting enzyme (ACE) inhibitors and other antihypertensive drugs.

Other drugs may result in vasodilatation from a direct action on blood vessels or indirectly by histamine release or 'chemical sympathectomy' (central neural blockade with local anaesthetic).

Management

The causes of decreased cardiac output (reduced preload, changes in heart rate and rhythm, and reduced myocardial contractility) and decreased systemic vascular resistance should be considered systematically. Preoperative correction of hypovolaemia is essential. The anaesthetist should anticipate the cardiovascular effects of anaesthetic agents (potentiated by antihypertensive therapy); appropriate doses of drugs should be used and intravenous fluid preloading before induction of anaesthesia should be considered. Patients receiving ACE inhibitors should omit the dose on the day of major surgery.

If intraoperative hypotension occurs and the measurement is validated, ensure adequate oxygenation, increase cardiac preload (venous return) using intravenous fluids, raising the legs or using head-down tilt if appropriate, and decrease the concentration or infusion rate of anaesthetic agents. Care must be taken to ensure delivery of sufficient anaesthetic agent to avoid awareness.

This treatment will be effective in most patients. If hypotension persists and the cause is not obvious, consider drug hypersensitivity and exclude factors that decrease venous return, especially concealed haemorrhage and pneumothorax. Examine the ECG to exclude arrhythmias and myocardial ischaemia.

Hypotension from profound vasodilatation requires further fluid administration and the use of a vasoconstrictor such as ephedrine or phenylephrine. If cardiac output remains low, careful fluid loading is indicated, using central venous pressure (CVP) as a guide. Pulmonary arterial catheter insertion and inotropic support with dobutamine should also be considered.

Hypovolaemia

Hypovolaemia is a common cause of hypotension. It refers to a fluid deficit with reduced intravascular volume (Table 40.3). Hypovolaemia occurs most often in the emergency patient. The clinical picture depends on the rate, volume and type of fluid loss and may include thirst, dryness of mucous membranes, reduced tissue turgor, tachycardia and postural or absolute hypotension. Inhaled anaesthetic agents may impair baroreceptor-mediated heart rate responses to hypovolaemia. β-Blocking drugs can also prevent compensatory tachycardia. Vasoconstriction reduces peripheral tissue perfusion, causing cool limbs and an increase in the skin–core temperature difference. Oliguria (urine output less than 0.5 ml kg^{-1} h^{-1}) and evidence of haemoconcentration or anaemia may be present. Hypokalaemia and other electrolyte abnormalities are often associated with fluid deficits, particularly when there have been gastrointestinal losses.

It is essential to assess intravascular fluid volume and fluid balance preoperatively in all patients undergoing non-elective surgery. Fluid deficit and replacement are easily underestimated, especially in patients with intestinal obstruction or concealed haemorrhage. Unless immediately life-saving, surgery should be

Table 40.3 Causes of hypovolaemia and fluid loss

Preoperative	
Haemorrhage	Trauma Obstetric Gastrointestinal Major vessel rupture (aortic aneurysm)
Gastrointestinal	Vomiting Obstruction Fistulae Diarrhoea
Other	Fasting Diuretics Fever Burns
Intraoperative	Haemorrhage Insensible loss (evaporation) Drainage of stomach, bowel, or ascites 'Third space' loss – tissue sequestration

Table 40.2 Causes of hypotension during anaesthesia

Decreased cardiac output		
Decreased preload/ venous return	Hypovolaemia	Inadequate preoperative resuscitation Gastrointestinal fluid loss Haemorrhage
	Obstruction	Pulmonary embolus Aorta/caval compression (surgery, pregnancy, tumour) Pericardial effusion/tamponade
	Increased intrathoracic pressure	IPPV/PEEP Pneumothorax
	Head-up position	
Myocardial	Reduced contractility	Drugs (most anaesthetic agents, β-blockers, calcium antagonists) Acidosis Ischaemia/infarction
	Arrhythmias Pericardial tamponade	
Decreased afterload/vasodilatation		
Drugs	Relative/absolute overdose (most anaesthetic agents, antihypertensives) Central regional blockade (local anaesthetics) Hypersensitivity (drugs, colloids, blood) Direct histamine release (morphine)	
Septicaemia		

delayed to allow adequate fluid resuscitation and restoration of intravascular volume. The response of the CVP to fluid challenges is a useful guide when assessing and treating patients with significant hypovolaemia.

As most anaesthetic agents decrease compensatory vasoconstriction and cause myocardial depression, relative overdosage is likely to reveal hypovolaemia and inadequate fluid resuscitation, resulting in hypotension and sometimes cardiovascular collapse. These effects are exaggerated in the elderly and in patients with decreased cardiac reserve or pre-existing hypertension. The risk of hypotension at induction can be reduced by giving a fluid preload and carefully titrating the induction agent to effect. Etomidate produces less cardiovascular depression than do other induction agents. Ketamine can be used for induction in patients with severe hypovolaemia where immediate operation may be life-saving.

The anaesthetist must monitor fluid balance closely during surgery. Adequate intraoperative fluid replacement must account for maintenance requirements, evaporative loss, 'third space' tissue sequestration and blood loss. For example, during abdominal operations, up to 5 ml kg^{-1} h^{-1} may be required to replace evaporative and third space losses in addition to maintenance requirements.

Haemorrhage

Adults who have lost 15% of circulating blood volume may require red blood cell transfusion to maintain oxygen-carrying capacity. Blood loss can be estimated by weighing swabs, measuring the volume of blood in suction bottles and assessing the clinical response to fluid therapy. Estimation is often difficult where large volumes of irrigation fluid have been used, e.g. during transurethral resection of the prostate. Intraoperative measurement of haemoglobin concentration may aid estimation of blood loss and guide therapy. With severe or ongoing haemorrhage, maintenance of intravascular volume is essential. An effective fluid warming device should be used when giving any cold fluid and is advisable when giving any infusion rapidly. The problems of massive transfusion are discussed on page 627.

HYPERTENSION

Intraoperative hypertension may be defined as a systolic blood pressure 25% greater than the patient's preoperative value. Hypertension increases myocardial work by increasing afterload and left ventricular wall tension. It is often associated with tachycardia. This is particularly undesirable in patients with ischaemic heart disease or left ventricular hypertrophy, in whom the myocardial oxygen supply/demand balance is easily compromised. The subendocardium is most susceptible to ischaemia in these situations. Hypertension also increases the risk of ischaemia, infarction and haemorrhage in other organs, such as the brain.

Aetiology

Table 40.4 shows the common causes of hypertension during anaesthesia. Hypertension is most often caused by increases in sympathetic tone and systemic vascular resistance. This can be a physiological response to light anaesthesia, pain, airway manipulation or surgery, or a pharmacological response (e.g. sympathomimetic drug overdose). Tachycardia and arrhythmias are associated signs of sympathetic nervous stimulation. The anaesthetist should be aware of the less common causes of hypertension such as phaeochromocytoma and malignant hyperthermia.

Table 40.4 Causes of hypertension during anaesthesia

Pre-existing	Undiagnosed or poorly controlled hypertension Pregnancy-induced hypertension Withdrawal of antihypertensive medication
Increased sympathetic tone	Inadequate analgesia Inadequate anaesthesia Hypoxaemia Airway manipulation (laryngoscopy, extubation) Hypercapnia
Drug overdose	Epinephrine Ephedrine Ketamine Ergometrine
Other	Hypervolaemia Aortic cross-clamping Phaeochromocytoma Malignant hyperthermia

Management

Preoperative control of hypertension is essential. Patients with poorly controlled or labile preoperative hypertension exhibit exaggerated vascular responses during anaesthesia and may suffer greater intraoperative and postoperative morbidity and mortality from arrhythmias and myocardial ischaemia. Where possible, surgery should be postponed until adequate control is achieved (e.g. arterial pressure less than 180/100 mmHg) and target organ function (e.g. heart and kidney) assessed. Premedication may be indicated to reduce anxiety. The use of perioperative β-blockade should be considered in susceptible patients as this may reduce the risk of cardiac morbidity.

The anaesthetist should anticipate the anaesthetic and surgical events that increase sympathetic tone. The pressor response to laryngoscopy can be obtunded by the use of an adequate dose of short-acting opioid such as alfentanil. In patients in whom the sympathetic response to extubation is undesirable, extubation can be performed during deep anaesthesia or after giving intravenous lidocaine 1–1.5 mg kg^{-1}. The response to aortic cross-clamping may be controlled by careful use of a volatile anaesthetic agent and/or nitrate infusion. Remifentanil can provide excellent control of cardiovascular responses during anaesthesia and surgery. The use of ketamine should be avoided in hypertensive patients.

If hypertension occurs in other clinical situations, ensure adequate oxygenation, depth of anaesthesia and analgesia. The use of an antihypertensive agent such as labetalol or hydralazine may then be indicated for persistent hypertension. As the effect of these drugs is potentiated by anaesthetic agents, careful titration is required.

HYPERVOLAEMIA

Hypervolaemia is fluid excess with an overfilled intravascular compartment.

Clinical features

Hypervolaemia is caused usually by excessive transfusion with blood or other intravenous fluids. Significant fluid overload produces tachycardia, elevated JVP/CVP, added heart sounds and lung crepitations. Severe overloading may cause pulmonary oedema with raised pulmonary inflation pressures, hypoxaemia, hypotension and oedema fluid in the airway.

Fluid absorption occurs during operations in which continuous irrigation is used. The volume absorbed is proportional to the duration of irrigation and can be rapid. If the fluid is hypotonic, dilutional hyponatraemia can develop. Classically, this occurs during transurethral resection of the prostate. Reduced serum osmolality promotes extravascular fluid shifts and increases the risk of pulmonary and cerebral oedema. Elderly patients and those with cardiac disease, renal disease or hypoproteinaemia are most susceptible. Hyponatraemia is associated with arrhythmias and widening of the QRS complex on the ECG. In the past, the use of irrigation fluid containing citrate was associated with metabolic alkalosis, which was sometimes severe and life-threatening.

Management

Careful monitoring of preoperative and intraoperative fluid balance is essential. If signs of hypervolaemia develop, intravenous infusions and surgical irrigation should be stopped, the inspired oxygen concentration increased and the operation terminated as soon as possible. Serum biochemistry and arterial blood gas analysis will identify associated electrolyte or acid–base disorders. Fluid restriction and administration of a loop diuretic are indicated in mild cases, with postoperative monitoring of serum electrolytes and cardiorespiratory function. In severe cases with evidence of pulmonary or cerebral oedema, tracheal intubation and ventilation may be necessary to protect the airway and enable control of arterial blood gas tensions. Inotropic support with dobutamine, invasive cardiovascular monitoring and haemofiltration should be considered.

MYOCARDIAL ISCHAEMIA

Aetiology

Myocardial ischaemia occurs when myocardial oxygen demand exceeds supply. The subendocardium is particularly vulnerable. Hypertension increases myocardial afterload and therefore oxygen demand. Hypotension can reduce oxygen supply by reducing coronary blood flow. However, tachycardia is the most important determinant of the myocardial oxygen supply/demand ratio because the duration of diastolic coronary filling is reduced simultaneously with an increase in myocardial work. In addition, it is the heart rate that determines the level of hypotension or hypertension which precipitates ischaemia: the higher the heart rate, the higher the ischaemic threshold. However, up to 50% of patients with intraoperative ischaemia have no significant haemodynamic changes at the time, and the ischaemia in some of these patients may be the result of vasospasm.

Clinical features

Patients with coronary artery disease are most at risk. The rate–pressure product (product of systolic blood pressure and heart rate) has been used as a crude index of myocardial oxygen demand, but correlates poorly with ischaemia during anaesthesia. Intraoperative myocardial ischaemia may manifest clinically as arrhythmia, hypotension or pulmonary oedema. It is diagnosed by ECG ST-segment changes (usually depression), although these are not always detected reliably without computer-assisted analysis. The use of the V5 electrode is recommended for ECG monitoring in susceptible patients (e.g. the CM5 configuration; see Ch. 38) because it is the most sensitive ECG lead for the detection of left ventricular ischaemia. When used alone, it may detect up to 85% of the ST abnormalities on a standard 12-lead ECG.

An increase in left ventricular end-diastolic pressure may precede ECG changes and is detected by an increase in the pulmonary capillary wedge pressure if a pulmonary arterial catheter is in situ. Trans-oesophageal echocardiography can detect abnormal myocardial wall motion, a sensitive indicator of ischaemia. This finding may be associated with increased perioperative morbidity. Regional wall dysfunction often persists into the postoperative period without clinical signs. Increased myocardial work during this period, e.g. from pain, can precipitate further ischaemia or infarction in susceptible patients although the risk of infarction in the general surgical population is low.

Management

The aims of management are prevention of ischaemia by the use of an appropriate anaesthetic technique and early detection in susceptible patients by the use of appropriate monitoring. If ischaemia is detected, ensure adequate arterial oxygenation, normocapnia, analgesia and depth of anaesthesia. Significant hypertension, hypotension or tachycardia can then be controlled pharmacologically. If signs of myocardial ischaemia persist, the use of a coronary vasodilator such as glyceryl trinitrate by intravenous infusion should be considered.

CARDIAC ARREST

This is discussed in Chapter 62.

EMBOLISM

Gas

Aetiology

Gas embolism describes the entry of gas bubbles into the circulation, usually via the venous route. Embolism of room air is possible if atmospheric pressure is greater than intravenous pressure at the site of an open vein. This is most likely when the surgical site is above the level of the right atrium, e.g. during head and neck operations in the head-up position. Vascular catheters are another potential route for air entry. Gas embolism, usually carbon dioxide, can also occur during insufflation procedures such as laparoscopy. Table 40.5 lists procedures associated with gas embolism.

Clinical features

The clinical presentation varies with the volume and rate of gas entry into the circulation. An entry rate of 0.5 ml kg^{-1} min^{-1} or

Table 40.5 Procedures associated with gas embolism

Head and neck surgery	ENT surgery (sinus, mastoid) Neurosurgery (posterior fossa, sitting position)
Insufflation techniques	Laparoscopy Hysteroscopy Arthroscopy Thoracoscopy
Orthopaedic surgery	Arthrography Hip and spinal surgery
Chest surgery	Breast and open cardiac operations
Other	Intravascular cannulae (venous, arterial) Epidural injection

greater has been reported to produce clinical signs. If a significant volume of gas enters the right side of the heart, blood flow is obstructed, reducing cardiac output and arterial pressure. A 'mill wheel' murmur may be auscultated via a precordial or oesophageal stethoscope. The sudden decrease in cardiac output results in a rapid decrease in end-tidal carbon dioxide concentration. The magnitude of the decrease may give an estimate of the volume of gas embolus. Hypoxaemia, tachycardia, ECG changes (including arrhythmia) and an increase in pulmonary artery pressure follow. In extreme cases, cardiac pumping is ineffective with severe hypotension and asphyxia; this occurs because gas in the right ventricle is compressed rather than ejected during systole.

Trans-oesophageal echocardiography and precordial Doppler ultrasound are the most sensitive monitors for gas passing through the heart. Clinical and ECG signs alone have a low sensitivity for detection of gas embolism. As the foramen ovale is potentially patent in more than 25% of the population, an increase in right heart pressure can open the foramen in these patients. Paradoxical gas embolism via this route or across the pulmonary capillary bed to the coronary or cerebral circulations can cause myocardial ischaemia or convulsions.

Management

If air embolism is detected, further air entry should be prevented by flooding the operative site with saline and covering it with wet gauze. During head and neck procedures, the venous pressure at the surgical site should be elevated by compressing the jugular veins, lowering the operative site where possible and applying continuous positive airway pressure (CPAP). During insufflation procedures, the surgeon must be told to allow all gas to escape from the body cavity. The lungs should be ventilated with 100% oxygen (nitrous oxide should be discontinued to avoid expansion of gas bubbles). Gas can sometimes be aspirated from the right heart if a right atrial catheter is already present, but otherwise insertion of a catheter is usually impractical and time-consuming. Expansion of the intravascular fluid volume, inotropic support of the circulation and internal or external cardiac massage may be necessary.

Gas embolism during insufflation procedures often results in massive haemorrhage within the body cavity because the raised venous pressure caused by gas embolism causes bleeding from the veins through which the gas originally entered the circulation; consequently, the surgeon should take steps to inspect the body cavity, either by cautious endoscopy or by open operation.

Thrombus

Pulmonary embolism during anaesthesia is uncommon. It is often preceded by a period of immobilization; trauma patients are therefore a high-risk group. During anaesthesia, pulmonary embolism may present with tachycardia, hypoxaemia, arrhythmia, hypotension, difficulty with ventilation, an acute decrease in the end-tidal carbon dioxide concentration or cardiovascular collapse. Other causes of these signs should be excluded before making this diagnosis.

Aetiology

Risk factors for venous thromboembolism include immobility, malignancy, smoking, trauma, pelvic and limb surgery, medication with the contraceptive pill and a past history of venous thromboembolism. Thrombosis is usually sited in the deep venous system of the lower limbs or in the pelvis. There is a high risk of thrombus formation in susceptible patients during the intraoperative period. Venous stasis in the lower limbs is produced by direct venous compression, hypovolaemia, hypotension, hypothermia and the use of tourniquets and head-up positioning. Veins can sustain trauma during positioning and surgery. Increased blood coagulability is a consequence of the stress response to surgery.

Management

The risk of thromboembolism can be classified as low, moderate or high. Low risk refers to patients undergoing minor surgery of less than 30 min duration with no other risk factors, or major surgery in patients aged less than 40 years with no other risk factors. All other patients have a moderate or high risk. Thromboprophylaxis must begin preoperatively for maximum benefit. This includes correction of risk factors where possible. For example, the oral contraceptive pill should be stopped at least 6 weeks prior to surgery in moderate- and high-risk patients. These patients should be managed with prophylactic subcutaneous heparin and leg compression stockings. During the intraoperative period, venous stasis in the lower limbs can be reduced by raising the legs, avoiding leg trauma and using apparatus for pneumatic leg compression or electrical calf muscle stimulation. A good anaesthetic and surgical technique ensures adequate fluid therapy and minimizes heat loss and tourniquet times. The use of subarachnoid or epidural anaesthesia is associated with a lower incidence of early postoperative venous thromboembolism.

If intraoperative pulmonary embolism is diagnosed, ventilate the lungs with 100% oxygen and consider bronchodilator therapy, fluid loading and inotropic support of the circulation. In extreme presentations, cardiac arrest protocols should be used. After management of the initial haemodynamic disturbance, thrombolytic therapy (if not contraindicated), anticoagulation and rarely surgical removal of the embolus may be indicated.

Other

Air or clot may embolize via arterial cannulae and produce distal ischaemia. Fat embolism to the lungs may occur in patients with fractures. There should be a high index of suspicion if unexpected haemodynamic or hypoxaemic events occur in patients undergoing surgery for pelvic or lower limb fractures. Tumour fragments can embolize during cancer surgery. Amniotic fluid embolus can occur in obstetric patients.

RESPIRATORY

HYPOXAEMIA

Hypoxaemia refers to arterial haemoglobin desaturation or reduced arterial oxygen tension; hypoxia is oxygen deficiency at the tissue level.

Aetiology

A practical classification of the causes of hypoxaemia is given in Table 40.6. Equipment problems such as leaks and disconnections are common. $\dot{V}/\dot{Q}$ mismatch can result from either inadequate ventilation or reduced pulmonary perfusion. Unless hypoxaemia is promptly recognized and treated, the consequences can be disastrous.

Clinical features

Hypoxaemia is a common perioperative event. Cyanosis is an unreliable sign of hypoxaemia, especially in the operating theatre environment. Hypoxaemia produces tachycardia, sweating, hypertension and arrhythmias, although bradycardia is the usual response to hypoxaemia in children. Tachypnoea occurs in spontaneously breathing patients. There may be clinical signs associated with the cause. As arterial desaturation progresses, bradycardia, hypotension and cardiac arrest follow.

Management

The complications of hypoxaemia are preventable. Cyanosis should seldom be witnessed by the vigilant anaesthetist because the routine use of pulse oximetry allows early detection and treatment of hypoxaemia. If hypoxaemia is detected, the following plan should be instituted.

1. Palpate the carotid pulse. Simultaneously assess the ECG and cardiac rhythm. Treat as for cardiac arrest if there is inadequate cardiac output or ventricular tachycardia/fibrillation.
2. Exclude delivery of a hypoxic gas mixture using an oxygen analyser. Increase the inspired oxygen concentration to 100%.
3. Test the integrity of the breathing system by manual ventilation of the lungs and confirm bilateral chest movement and breath sounds. Blow down the tracheal tube if necessary. Confirm the position and patency of the tracheal tube by assessing the capnograph, passing a suction catheter through the tracheal tube and auscultating the chest.
4. Search for clinical evidence of the causes of $\dot{V}/\dot{Q}$ mismatch with early exclusion of pneumothorax. If atelectasis or reduced FRC is contributory, gentle hyperinflation of the lungs should improve oxygenation. Lung volumes can be maintained by applying CPAP or PEEP.
5. If the diagnosis is difficult, measure core temperature and consider arterial blood gas analysis and chest X-ray examination.

HYPERCAPNIA

Hypercapnia refers to carbon dioxide accumulation in the blood. During anaesthesia, this is indicated by an arterial carbon dioxide tension (kPa) or end-tidal carbon dioxide concentration (%) greater than 6.0.

Table 40.6 Causes of hypoxaemia during anaesthesia

Hypoxic inspired gas mixture		
Equipment	Oxygen supply (cylinder/pipeline failure, misconnection) Flowmeters (inaccurate settings, leak) Breathing system (obstruction, leak)	
Hypoventilation		
Equipment	Ventilator failure, inadequate minute volume Breathing system (obstruction, leak, disconnection) Tracheal tube (obstruction, oesophageal intubation)	
Patient	Respiratory depression in spontaneously breathing patients Obstruction (see Table 40.7)	
$\dot{V}/\dot{Q}$ mismatch		
Patient	Inadequate ventilation	Endobronchial intubation Secretions Atelectasis Pneumothorax Bronchospasm Pulmonary aspiration Pulmonary oedema
	Inadequate perfusion	Embolus (gas, thrombus, amniotic fluid) Low cardiac output (see Table 40.2)
Other	Methaemoglobinaemia Malignant hyperthermia	

Aetiology

Intraoperative hypercapnia is caused by inadequate carbon dioxide removal or excessive carbon dioxide production. Inadequate carbon dioxide removal is most commonly caused by hypoventilation (Table 40.6) or increased alveolar dead space, but may also result from inadequate fresh gas flow and exhausted soda lime. Carbon dioxide production rises with the metabolic rate during fever, sepsis, malignant hyperthermia, drug reactions, hyperthyroidism and shivering. Inadvertent or excessive carbon dioxide delivery from the anaesthetic machine and the absorption of carbon dioxide during laparoscopic procedures are other causes of hypercapnia.

Clinical features

Progressive hypercapnia stimulates sympathetic nervous activity and may result in tachycardia, sweating and arrhythmias. Increased cerebral blood flow and alterations in blood pressure may occur. As anaesthesia suppresses autonomic responses, these signs may not occur until carbon dioxide tension is markedly increased. Acute respiratory acidosis produces an increase in serum potassium concentration. Increased carbon dioxide production in the spontaneously breathing patient stimulates tachypnoea.

Management

This is directed at the underlying cause. Mild degrees of hypercapnia are usually well tolerated in spontaneously breathing patients unless there is a contraindication such as head injury. If signs of hypercapnia occur, the anaesthetist should control ventilation.

HYPOCAPNIA

Hypocapnia refers to a carbon dioxide deficit in the blood. During anaesthesia, this is indicated by an arterial carbon dioxide tension (kPa) or end-tidal carbon dioxide concentration (%) less than 4.0. Unintentional hyperventilation in association with decreased carbon dioxide production is the usual cause during anaesthesia. Hypocapnia produces respiratory alkalosis with a decrease in serum potassium concentration. There are reductions in cerebral blood flow, cardiac output and tissue oxygen delivery. There may also be a delay in onset of spontaneous ventilation at the conclusion of anaesthesia. Decreasing the ventilatory minute volume or increasing the breathing system dead space reduces carbon dioxide removal.

RESPIRATORY OBSTRUCTION

Aetiology

Table 40.7 shows causes of respiratory obstruction. It is a common and potentially hazardous anaesthetic complication. The tracheal tube is a frequent site of obstruction, although problems can occur at any point in the breathing system or airway. Inadequate ventilation can lead to hypercapnia, hypoxaemia and reduced uptake of volatile anaesthetic agent. Total obstruction rapidly produces hypoxaemia.

Clinical features

Spontaneously breathing patients

Partial obstruction is indicated by noisy breathing or stridor, whereas complete obstruction is silent. Tracheal tug, paradoxical chest and abdominal movement ('see-saw' ventilation) and inad-

Table 40.7 Causes of respiratory obstruction during anaesthesia

Equipment	
Breathing system	Valve malfunction, kinking
Tracheal tube	External compression (surgical gag/manipulation, kinking) Occlusion of lumen (secretions, blood) Cuff (overinflation, herniation) Oesophageal or endobronchial intubation
Patient	
Oropharynx	Soft tissue (oedema from trauma/infection, reduced muscle tone) Secretions (blood, surgical packs) Tumour
Larynx	Laryngospasm Recurrent laryngeal nerve palsy Oedema (drug hypersensitivity, pre-eclampsia, infection) Tumour
Trachea	Laryngotracheobronchitis External compression (surgical manipulation, haemorrhage, thyroid tumour) Stricture (radiotherapy)
Bronchi	Secretions Pneumothorax Bronchospasm Tumour Surgical manipulation

equate reservoir bag movement are other signs. The generation of large negative intrathoracic pressures during progressively stronger attempts to breathe in when the airway is completely obstructed can precipitate pulmonary oedema in some patients, particularly young adults.

Ventilated patients

Respiratory obstruction can be associated with increased inflation pressures, a prolonged expiratory phase, hypercapnia and alteration of the end-tidal carbon dioxide waveform. Hypoxaemia may be the first sign.

Management

Early detection and prevention of hypoxaemia are essential.

Spontaneously breathing patients

Reduced muscle tone with apposition of the tongue and pharyngeal soft tissue is a common cause of upper airway obstruction. This is usually overcome by jaw lift and use of an oral or nasopharyngeal airway. Suction will remove accumulated secretions, but care is required because laryngospasm may be precipitated by the use of a suction catheter in the pharynx during light anaesthesia. If obstruction persists, ventilate the lungs manually with 100% oxygen and exclude the breathing system as the site of obstruction. Confirm the presence of bilateral chest movement and breath sounds and exclude other causes of obstruction such as laryngospasm, bronchospasm, aspiration and pneumothorax. If airway maintenance is difficult, insertion of a laryngeal mask airway or tracheal intubation should be considered.

Ventilated patients (including patients with an artificial airway)

Systematically exclude causes of obstruction in the breathing system and patient. Complete obstruction suggests an equipment problem. The easy passage of a suction catheter throughout the length of the tracheal tube confirms its patency. The distal orifice of the tracheal tube can be obstructed by the tracheal wall or a herniated cuff. This is unlikely if the tracheal tube has a Murphy eye. Surgical manipulations during neck and thoracic surgery easily distort tracheal and bronchial anatomy and can displace the tracheal tube, especially endobronchial tubes. If obstruction persists and no obvious cause is identified, assume that the tracheal tube or laryngeal mask is the site of obstruction. Immediately replace it, using manual ventilation with 100% oxygen by mask to prevent hypoxaemia.

The management of specific lower airway problems is discussed below.

Laryngospasm

Aetiology

Laryngospasm is a reflex, prolonged closure of the vocal cords in response to a trigger, usually airway stimulation during light anaesthesia. Therefore, laryngospasm is most common during induction and emergence, often precipitated by premature insertion of an oral airway, the presence of pharyngeal secretions or blood, or airway irritation by a volatile anaesthetic agent. Laryngospasm can also be produced by surgical and visceral stimuli such as incision, peritoneal traction, anal stretch and cervical dilatation. Children are particularly prone to laryngospasm. The use of intravenous barbiturates disinhibits laryngeal reflexes and increases the risk of laryngospasm in comparison with propofol. Poor management of laryngospasm can lead to inadequate ventilation with hypoxaemia, hypercapnia and reduced depth of anaesthesia. Crowing inspiratory noises with signs of respiratory obstruction suggest partial laryngospasm. Complete laryngospasm is silent.

Management

Where possible, avoid airway and surgical stimulation during light anaesthesia and use the lateral position for control of secretions during extubation and transfer. Surgical stimuli should be anticipated, and anaesthetic depth should be adjusted accordingly. If laryngospasm occurs, hypoxaemia must be prevented. The anaesthetist should remove the offending stimulus, give 100% oxygen and provide a clear airway using an oral or pharyngeal airway and gentle pharyngeal suction. Unnecessary airway manipulation can exacerbate laryngospasm. Where appropriate, anaesthetic depth may be increased with an intravenous agent and the lungs ventilated manually with care, applying CPAP to prevent hypoxaemia. Most episodes of laryngospasm respond to this treatment. If laryngospasm persists and hypoxaemia ensues, a small dose of succinylcholine (e.g. 25 mg in adults) relaxes the vocal cords and allows manual ventilation and oxygenation. A full dose of succinylcholine can be given if tracheal intubation is indicated, but is usually unnecessary. Doxapram has also been used successfully in the treatment of laryngospasm.

Bronchospasm

Aetiology

General anaesthesia can alter airway resistance by influencing bronchomotor tone, lung volumes and bronchial secretions. Patients with increased airway reactivity from recent respiratory infection, asthma, atopy or smoking are more susceptible to bronchospasm during anaesthesia. Bronchospasm may be precipitated by insertion of an artificial airway during light anaesthesia, by stimulation of the carina or bronchi by a tracheal tube or by drugs causing β-blockade or release of histamine. Drug hypersensitivity, pulmonary aspiration and foreign bodies in the lower airway can also present as bronchospasm.

Clinical features

Bronchospasm can cause expiratory wheeze, a prolonged expiratory phase, increased inflation pressures and an upwardly sloping end-tidal carbon dioxide plateau. Wheezing may occur with other causes of respiratory obstruction and these should be excluded. If bronchospasm is severe, ventilation may be quiet, with signs of hypoxaemia.

Management

Management must prevent hypoxaemia and should aim to resolve the bronchospasm. Initially, give 100% oxygen, deepen anaesthesia if appropriate and remove any precipitating factors (e.g. reposition the tracheal tube, stop the operation). If further treatment is necessary, give a bronchodilator in increments according to the response. Recommended drugs include intravenous aminophylline (up to 6 mg kg^{-1}) or salbutamol (up to 3 μg kg^{-1}). Volatile anaesthetic agents and ketamine are also effective bronchodilators. Epinephrine is indicated in life-threatening situations. Consider tracheal intubation and artificial ventilation if hypoxaemia develops in the spontaneously breathing patient. In patients receiving IPPV, ventilation should be adjusted to minimize peak airway pressure and allow sufficient expiratory time. Steroids and H_1-receptor antagonists have no immediate effect but may be indicated in the later management of severe cases of bronchospasm.

Anaesthesia for asthmatic patients

Elective surgery should proceed only if symptoms are optimally controlled. Premedication with the patient's usual bronchodilator therapy or an inhaled β_2-agonist is recommended and the use of an anxiolytic should be considered. If regional anaesthesia is contraindicated, use a general anaesthetic technique with minimal airway stimulation. If possible, avoid using drugs which release histamine and give all drugs slowly and after dilution. If tracheal intubation is necessary, ensure an adequate depth of anaesthesia. The provision of postoperative oxygen and maintenance bronchodilator therapy is essential.

PNEUMOTHORAX

Aetiology

The causes of pneumothorax during anaesthesia are listed in Table 40.8. Peak inspiratory airway pressures greater than 60 cmH_2O increase the risk of pulmonary barotrauma. Patients with recent chest trauma, asthma and chronic lung disease with bullae are most at risk, especially during IPPV. Air in the pleural space reduces ipsilateral lung ventilation. Nitrous oxide diffuses into air-filled spaces and causes a pneumothorax to expand. IPPV forces gas into the pleural space, with a rapid increase in the size of the pneumothorax; increasing $\dot{V}/\dot{Q}$ mismatch and hypoxaemia follow. If the pneumothorax is under tension, hypoxaemia, mediastinal shift, reduced venous return and impairment of cardiac output can be life-threatening.

Clinical features

A pneumothorax should be excluded if unexplained tachycardia, hypotension, hypoxaemia, cyanosis, difficulty with ventilation or high inflation pressures occur intraoperatively. Examination may demonstrate unequal air entry and/or chest movement, bronchospasm, surgical emphysema or mediastinal shift. Chest X-ray examination provides a definitive diagnosis (caution below).

Table 40.8 Causes of pneumothorax during anaesthesia

Traumatic	Chest injury (rib fracture, flail, penetrating injury)
Iatrogenic	Subclavian/internal jugular venous cannulae Brachial plexus block, intercostal nerve block Cervical/thoracic surgery Barotrauma
Spontaneous	Bullae, emphysema, asthma Congenital cystic pulmonary disease Marfan's syndrome Rapid decompression of divers

Management

Prior to anaesthesia, it is desirable to exclude a pneumothorax by X-ray examination in all patients who have suffered recent chest trauma and in those in whom a central venous catheter has recently been inserted. However, this does not preclude later development of a pneumothorax during the perioperative period, and a high index of suspicion is advisable in these patients. In patients with recent chest trauma, including rib fractures, regional analgesia or a technique using spontaneous ventilation is advised where possible. If tracheal intubation and IPPV are indicated, a chest drain should be inserted prior to anaesthesia.

If a pneumothorax is suspected intraoperatively, *treatment should not be delayed to confirm the diagnosis by chest X-ray examination.* Nitrous oxide should be discontinued and the lungs ventilated with 100% oxygen. The presence of air in the pleural space can be confirmed by careful needle aspiration on the suspected side via the second intercostal space in the midclavicular line and/or the fifth space in the mid-axillary line. If the pneumothorax is under tension, there may be a gush of air. Temporary decompression using one or more large-bore intravenous cannulae may be life-saving. If a pneumothorax is confirmed, the intravenous cannula should be left in place while a formal chest drain is inserted.

The presence of a bronchopleural fistula with substantial air leak can make ventilation ineffective. In this situation, the affected lung can be isolated by insertion of a double-lumen tube or gas exchange improved by the use of high-frequency ventilation.

INTUBATION PROBLEMS

Unintentional endobronchial intubation

Unintentional endobronchial intubation causes one-lung ventilation, resulting in a large intrapulmonary shunt, hypoxaemia, decreased uptake of volatile anaesthetic agent and, eventually, collapse of the contralateral lung. Inadvertent intubation of the right main bronchus is more common. The likelihood of this complication is reduced by cutting the tracheal tube to an appropriate length prior to intubation and confirmation of its position by auscultation after intubation and after changes in position of the patient on the operating table.

Oesophageal intubation

Unrecognized oesophageal intubation is an important and preventable cause of anaesthetic mortality and serious morbidity. Direct visual confirmation of the tracheal tube passing into the larynx anterior to the arytenoid cartilages confirms correct placement, although the tracheal tube may subsequently be displaced. If direct vision is not possible, evidence of tracheal placement must be sought actively. Auscultation of breath sounds and chest or abdominal movement with ventilation are misleading indicators of tracheal tube placement. Furthermore, preoxygenation delays the onset of arterial oxygen desaturation after oesophageal intubation; therefore neither clinical signs nor the use of pulse oximetry can be relied upon to confirm correct tracheal tube placement. A persistent and normal expired carbon dioxide waveform confirms placement of the tracheal tube, and therefore the early use of capnography after intubation is recommended strongly.

Mechanical devices such as the Wee oesophageal detector can also be used reliably to confirm the correct position of the tracheal tube. These devices use a large syringe or rubber evacuator bulb to aspirate air from the tracheal tube after intubation and prior to ventilation. Free aspiration of air indicates tracheal placement because the cartilaginous tracheal rings maintain patency, whereas the oesophageal walls collapse and cause a resistance to aspiration. Disposable chemical indicators that detect expired carbon dioxide, and transtracheal illumination via the tracheal tube with a special lighted stilette, are alternative methods to confirm tracheal intubation.

The use of fibreoptic bronchoscopy to visualize the trachea and bronchi directly via the tracheal tube gives a certain diagnosis, but is impractical in most clinical situations. If there is doubt regarding the position of the tracheal tube or if hypoxaemia occurs, removal of the tracheal tube and ventilation by mask may be life-saving.

Difficult intubation

The reported incidence of difficult intubation is one in every 65 patients. In most instances, the cause is difficulty with laryngoscopy. Poor management of difficult intubation is a significant cause of anaesthetic morbidity and mortality. Sequelae include dental and airway trauma, pulmonary aspiration and hypoxaemia.

Aetiology

Table 40.9 shows the common causes of difficult intubation. The single most important cause is an inexperienced or inadequately prepared anaesthetist, and the difficulty is often compounded by equipment malfunction.

There are numerous causes of difficult laryngoscopy related to patients. The anatomical features associated with difficult laryngoscopy are listed in Table 40.10. Of these, the atlanto-occipital distance is the best predictor of difficulty but requires an X-ray examination. Many of these factors are normal anatomical variations, but extreme abnormalities do occur and may be congenital or acquired.

Congenital. Many syndromes are associated with multiple anatomical abnormalities such as a small mouth, large tongue and cleft palate. Patients with encephalocoele, cystic hygroma or

Table 40.9 Causes of difficult intubation

Anaesthetist		
Inadequate preoperative assessment		
Inadequate equipment preparation		
Inexperience		
Poor technique		
Equipment		
Malfunction		
Unavailability		
No trained assistance		
Patient		
Congenital	Syndromes (Down's, Pierre–Robin, Treacher–Collins, Marfan's)	
	Achondroplasia	
	Cystic hygroma	
	Encephalocoele	
Acquired	Reduced jaw movement	Trismus (abscess/infection, fracture, tetanus)
		Fibrosis (post-infection/radiotherapy/trauma)
		Rheumatoid arthritis, ankylosing spondylitis
		Tumours
		Jaw wiring
	Reduced neck movement	Rheumatoid/osteoarthritis
		Ankylosing spondylitis
		Cervical fracture/instability/fusion
	Airway	Oedema (abscess/infection, trauma, angio-oedema, burns)
		Compression (goitre, surgical haemorrhage)
		Scarring (radiotherapy, infection, burns)
		Tumours/polyps
		Foreign body
		Nerve palsy
	Others	Morbid obesity
		Pregnancy
		Acromegaly

Table 40.10 Anatomical factors associated with difficult laryngoscopy

Short, muscular neck
Protruding incisors (buck teeth)
Long, high arched palate
Receding lower jaw
Poor mobility of the mandible
Increased anterior depth of mandible
Increased posterior depth of mandible (reduces jaw opening, requires X-ray)
Decreased atlanto-occipital distance (reduces neck extension, requires X-ray)

hydrocephalus may have restricted head or jaw movement. Morquio's and Down's syndromes are associated with instability of the cervical spine.

Acquired. Acquired factors can affect jaw opening, neck movement or the airway itself. Reduced jaw movement is a common cause of difficult laryngoscopy. Trauma and infection can cause reflex spasm of the masseter and medial pterygoid muscles (trismus). This occurs typically in association with dental abscess or fractured mandible and is usually relaxed by anaesthetic agents. In contrast, the reduced jaw movement associated with temporomandibular joint fibrosis is usually fixed; this can complicate chronic infection, rheumatoid arthritis, ankylosing spondylitis or radiotherapy. Any local soft tissue swelling or mass can also reduce jaw movement.

Reduced head movement is another important cause of difficult laryngoscopy; optimal positioning for laryngoscopy requires extension of the head at the atlanto-occipital joint. This joint may be damaged in patients with rheumatoid arthritis, osteoarthritis or ankylosing spondylitis. Cervical spine movement can also be reduced by surgical fusion, fibrosis or soft tissue swellings of the head and neck. Cervical spine instability (e.g. fracture, tumour, rheumatoid arthritis) makes neck movement undesirable.

Disorders of the airway itself may pose a serious threat to ventilation in addition to preventing normal laryngoscopy. Soft tissue oedema of the face/upper airway from dental abscess, other infections, drug hypersensitivity, burns or trauma can cause considerable anatomical distortion with life-threatening airway obstruction. Foreign bodies, tumours and scarring after infection, burns or radiotherapy can also cause difficult laryngoscopy. Vocal cord apposition from recurrent laryngeal nerve palsy can hinder passage of the tracheal tube through the larynx. Positioning of the tracheal tube in the trachea can be difficult if there is compression or deviation caused by a thyroid tumour, haematoma (traumatic, surgical) and thymic or lymph node tumours. Other rare disorders include vascular rings and laryngomalacia of the trachea. In clinical practice, the cause of difficult laryngoscopy is often multifactorial, e.g. in a patient with morbid obesity, pregnancy and rheumatoid arthritis.

Management

Preoperative assessment. Preoperative examination of the airway (Table 40.11) is essential. Identification of patients with a potentially difficult airway (Tables 40.9 and 40.10) before anaesthesia allows time to plan an appropriate anaesthetic technique. Previous anaesthetic records should always be consulted. However, a past record of normal tracheal intubation is no guarantee against difficulty on subsequent occasions as airway anatomy can be altered, e.g. by pregnancy or the development of disease of the cervical spine. The presence of stridor or hoarse voice are warning signs for the anaesthetist. As it is impossible to identify all patients with a difficult airway during preoperative assessment, the anaesthetist must be prepared to manage the unexpected difficult laryngoscopy.

Many additional clinical tests to predict difficult laryngoscopy have been described. None of these tests is totally reliable, but their use may complement routine examination of the airway. The 'Mallampati' test is a widely used and simple classification of the pharyngeal view obtained during maximal mouth opening and tongue protrusion (Fig. 40.1). In practice, this test suggests a higher incidence of difficult laryngoscopy if the posterior pharyngeal wall is not visualized. The predictive value of this test may be strengthened if the thyromental distance (the distance between the thyroid cartilage prominence and the bony point of the chin during full head extension) is less than 6.5 cm. The Mallampati classification correlates with the view obtained at laryngoscopy (Fig. 40.2). The difficulty associated with a 'grade 3' laryngoscopy can usually be overcome by posterior laryngeal displacement and/or the use of a gum elastic bougie. A patient whose epiglottis is not visible at laryngoscopy ('grade 4') usually has obvious preoperative anatomical abnormalities. Management of these patients requires the use of special techniques such as fibreoptic laryngoscopy.

Preoperative preparation. Premedication with an antisialagogue reduces airway secretions. This is advantageous prior to inhalation induction and essential for awake fibreoptic laryngoscopy to maximize the effectiveness of topical local anaesthesia. An anxiolytic can also be given but is contraindicated in patients with airway obstruction. The presence of a trained assistant is essential and the availability of an experienced anaesthetist and a special 'difficult intubation' trolley with a range of equipment such as gum elastic bougies, a variety of laryngoscopes and tracheal tubes, and cricothyrotomy needles is desirable.

Regional anaesthesia. This should be used if appropriate in patients with a difficult airway, although the patient, anaesthetist and equipment must be prepared for general anaesthesia in case a complication arises.

General anaesthesia. Unless tracheal intubation is essential for airway protection or to enable muscle relaxation and ventilation, the use of an artificial airway such as the laryngeal mask with spontaneous ventilation is a safe technique. If intubation is essential, the appropriate anaesthetic technique depends on the anticipated degree of difficulty, the presence of airway obstruction and the risk of regurgitation and aspiration. There is no place for the use of a long-acting muscle relaxant to facilitate intubation if difficulty is anticipated. Correct positioning of the head and neck is essential

Table 40.11 Preoperative assessment of the airway

General appearance of the neck, face, maxilla and mandible
Jaw movement
Head extension and neck movement
The teeth and oropharynx
The soft tissues of the neck
Recent chest and cervical spine X-rays
Previous anaesthetic records

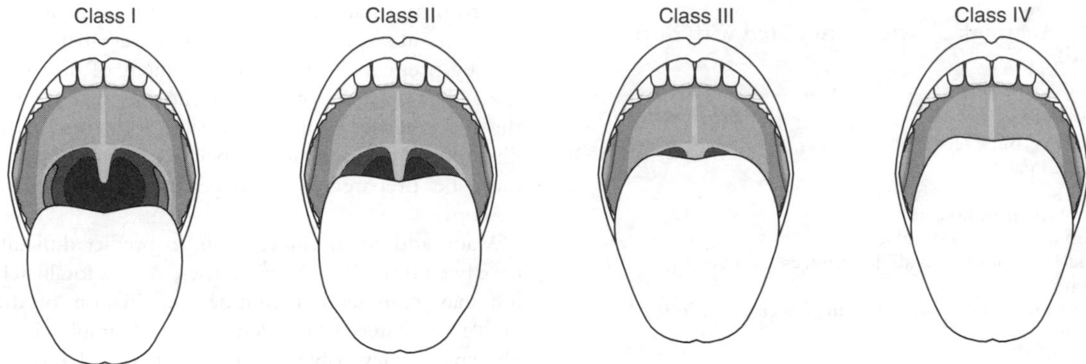

Fig. 40.1
Classification of the pharyngeal view when performing the modified Mallampati test. The patient must fully extend the tongue during maximal mouth opening. Class I, pharyngeal pillars, soft palate, uvula visible; class II, only soft palate, uvula visible; class III, only soft palate visible; class IV, soft palate not visible.

and the lungs should be preoxygenated after establishing intravenous access and appropriate monitoring. The safest anaesthetic technique can usually be chosen from the following clinical examples.

Patients with an increased risk of regurgitation and aspiration (e.g. full stomach, intra-abdominal pathology, pregnancy). An inhalation induction is inappropriate in these patients. Regional anaesthesia is preferable in the parturient (see Ch. 52). Preoxygenation and a rapid-sequence induction with succinylcholine may be used if there is little anticipated difficulty. If intubation is unsuccessful, no further doses of muscle relaxant should be used; the patient should be allowed to awaken and senior assistance should be sought. If there is a high degree of anticipated difficulty, an awake technique is recommended (see below).

Patients with little anticipated difficulty and no airway obstruction (e.g. mild reduction of jaw or neck movement). After either intravenous or inhalation induction and confirmation of the ability to ventilate the lungs manually by mask, succinylcholine may be given to provide the best conditions for tracheal intubation. If difficulty is encountered, the patient is allowed to awaken and the procedure is replanned. Where appropriate, anaesthesia can be deepened by spontaneous ventilation using a volatile anaesthetic agent and alternative techniques used to facilitate tracheal intubation (see below).

Patients with severe anticipated difficulty and no airway obstruction (e.g. severe reduction of jaw or neck movement). Appropriate techniques include inhalation induction with halothane or sevoflurane, or the use of fibreoptic laryngoscopy either awake or after inhalation induction. A muscle relaxant must not be used until the ability to ventilate the lungs manually and view the vocal cords is confirmed.

Patients with airway obstruction (e.g. burns, infection, trauma). An inhalation induction may be used, but an awake technique should be considered. Muscle relaxants should not be used until tracheal intubation is confirmed.

Extreme clinical situations. Tracheostomy performed under local anaesthesia may be the safest technique.

Inhalation induction

Premedication with an antisialagogue is desirable. Depth of anaesthesia is increased carefully by spontaneous ventilation of increasing concentrations of a volatile anaesthetic agent in 100% oxygen until laryngoscopy can be performed safely. Sevoflurane gives the best conditions for this purpose. If the larynx is viewed easily, intubation can be performed with or without succinylcholine. If the view is limited, the use of a gum elastic bougie assists passage of the tracheal tube through the larynx. Correct insertion of the bougie in the trachea may be confirmed by detecting tracheal rings, or resistance when the smaller bronchi are encountered. The tracheal tube is then 'railroaded' over the bougie into the trachea, with conventional tracheal tubes; this manoeuvre is often made easier by rotating the tracheal tube through 90° in an anticlockwise direction to align the bevel as it passes through the larynx. If this is unsuccessful, anaesthesia may be maintained and the use of fibreoptic laryngoscopy, blind nasal intubation or a retrograde technique considered. The last technique involves passage of an epidural catheter via a Tuohy needle through the cricothyroid

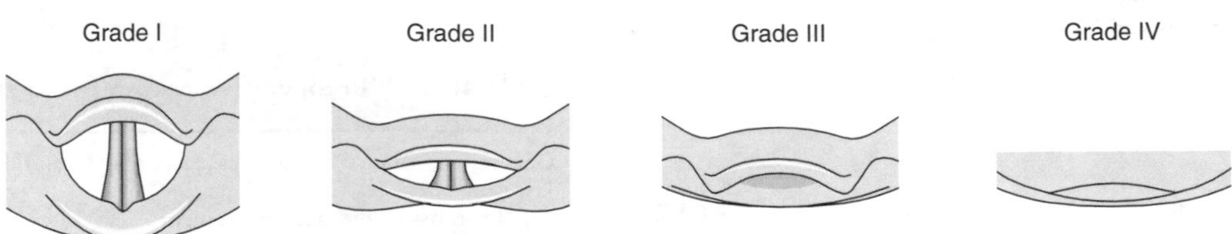

Fig. 40.2
Grading of the view at laryngoscopy. Grade I, vocal cords visible; grade II, arytenoid cartilages and posterior part of vocal cords visible; grade III, epiglottis visible; grade IV, epiglottis not visible. *Note*: the pharyngeal view (Fig. 40.1) is a clinical guide to the likely view at laryngoscopy.

membrane into the mouth and 'railroading' of the tracheal tube over the catheter into the trachea. The position of the tracheal tube must be confirmed using the methods described earlier. Trauma and bleeding may complicate this procedure, and other methods are probably safer in inexperienced hands.

Awake intubation

Fibreoptic laryngoscopy and intubation require special equipment, skill and time. The procedure may be performed by the nasal or oral route after topical anaesthesia has been achieved by spraying the nasal and oropharyngeal mucosa and/or gargling viscous preparations of local anaesthetic. The injection of 3–5 ml of lidocaine 2% through the cricothyroid membrane induces coughing and anaesthetizes the tracheal and laryngeal mucosa. Conventional laryngoscopy can also be performed in awake patients. After cricothyroid injection of lidocaine, laryngoscopy is performed in stages. The oropharynx is progressively anaesthetized with lidocaine spray until the patient tolerates deep insertion of the laryngoscope, enabling the larynx to be viewed.

Failed intubation

The incidence of failed tracheal intubation is approximately 1 in 2000 in general surgical patients but 1 in 300 in obstetric patients. However, failed intubation in obstetric patients is now a rare event because of the very high percentage of obstetric surgical patients who receive regional anaesthesia.

Poor management of failed intubation is a significant cause of anaesthetic morbidity and mortality. The aims of management are to maintain oxygenation and prevent aspiration of gastric contents. The 'failed intubation drill' is now established as an important skill for safe anaesthetic practice. An early decision to use a failed intubation protocol and call for assistance is essential, because continued attempts at tracheal intubation may result in trauma to the airway, pulmonary aspiration or hypoxaemia. Figure 40.3 shows one protocol for managing failed intubation. The obstetric patient is a special case and is considered in Chapter 52.

If the airway is obstructed and ventilation is inadequate during management of a failed intubation, there are several useful and potentially life-saving pieces of anaesthetic equipment available for use. The laryngeal mask is an essential piece of emergency airway equipment. It has been used successfully to provide an airway and allow ventilation when attempts to intubate the trachea and ventilate the lungs by other means have failed. It is also possible to pass a small diameter tracheal tube or a bougie through the laryngeal mask into the trachea. A variant of the laryngeal mask is designed specifically to allow tracheal intubation. The laryngeal mask should not be regarded as protection against pulmonary aspiration. The oesophageal obturator airway and similar devices are alternatives in an emergency, but there are doubts about their efficacy and reports of misplacement and oesophageal rupture associated with their use.

In extreme situations, transtracheal ventilation can be life-saving. The cricothyroid membrane (CTM) is punctured using a large-bore needle or intravenous cannula. Aspiration of air confirms tracheal placement. High-pressure 'jet' ventilation from a Sanders injector or the high-pressure oxygen outlet on the anaesthetic machine is delivered via the cannula. This should allow oxygenation until the patient awakens. The laryngeal inlet must be patent to allow expiration, otherwise additional cannulae must be sited in the CTM. Seldinger-type tracheostomy devices or surgical cricothyroidotomy can also be used to gain access to the tracheal lumen during emergency situations. These techniques can produce tissue injury and barotrauma.

If surgery is essential, the decision to continue anaesthesia should be made by an experienced anaesthetist. It is safe practice to maintain oxygenation, protect the airway and allow the patient to awaken.

ASPIRATION OF GASTRIC CONTENTS

Undetected regurgitation of gastric contents into the pharynx is not uncommon during anaesthesia. Pulmonary aspiration is less common but remains an important and usually preventable cause of death associated with anaesthesia. Mortality is high after major aspiration.

Aetiology

Regurgitation and pulmonary aspiration of gastric contents are more likely to occur in patients with intra-abdominal pathology, delayed gastric emptying (e.g. resulting from pain, trauma or alcohol) or inadequate gastro-oesophageal sphincter function (e.g. hiatus hernia, raised intra-abdominal pressure). Patients with reduced laryngeal reflexes, such as the elderly or sedated, are also at risk. Aspiration is more common during difficult intubation and therefore in emergency, obese or obstetric patients. Bronchospasm may be the first sign of pulmonary aspiration. If a large quantity of gastric material is aspirated, respiratory obstruction, ventilation–perfusion mismatch and intrapulmonary shunting may produce severe hypoxaemia, with chemical pneumonitis and subsequent infection.

Management

The aims of preoperative management in at-risk patients are to reduce the volume and particularly the acidity of gastric contents (see Ch. 20). If general anaesthesia is essential, the airway must be protected using a rapid-sequence induction with cricoid pressure and tracheal intubation. During emergence, extubation should not be performed until protective airway reflexes are regained. If aspiration occurs during anaesthesia, further regurgitation should be prevented by immediate application or maintenance of cricoid pressure, and the patient should be placed in a head-down position. In all but mild cases, the trachea should be intubated to facilitate removal of the aspirate and particulate matter by suction prior to the use of positive pressure ventilation. However, ventilation should not be delayed if significant hypoxaemia is imminent. Bronchodilator therapy may be required, the inspired oxygen concentration may be increased, and PEEP (or CPAP) may be employed if hypoxaemia ensues. Surgery should be postponed or abandoned as soon as possible. Bronchoscopy permits removal of solid matter and a chest X-ray and arterial blood gas measurement help in the assessment of the severity of injury. The patient should be transferred to the intensive care unit for further monitoring and respiratory care.

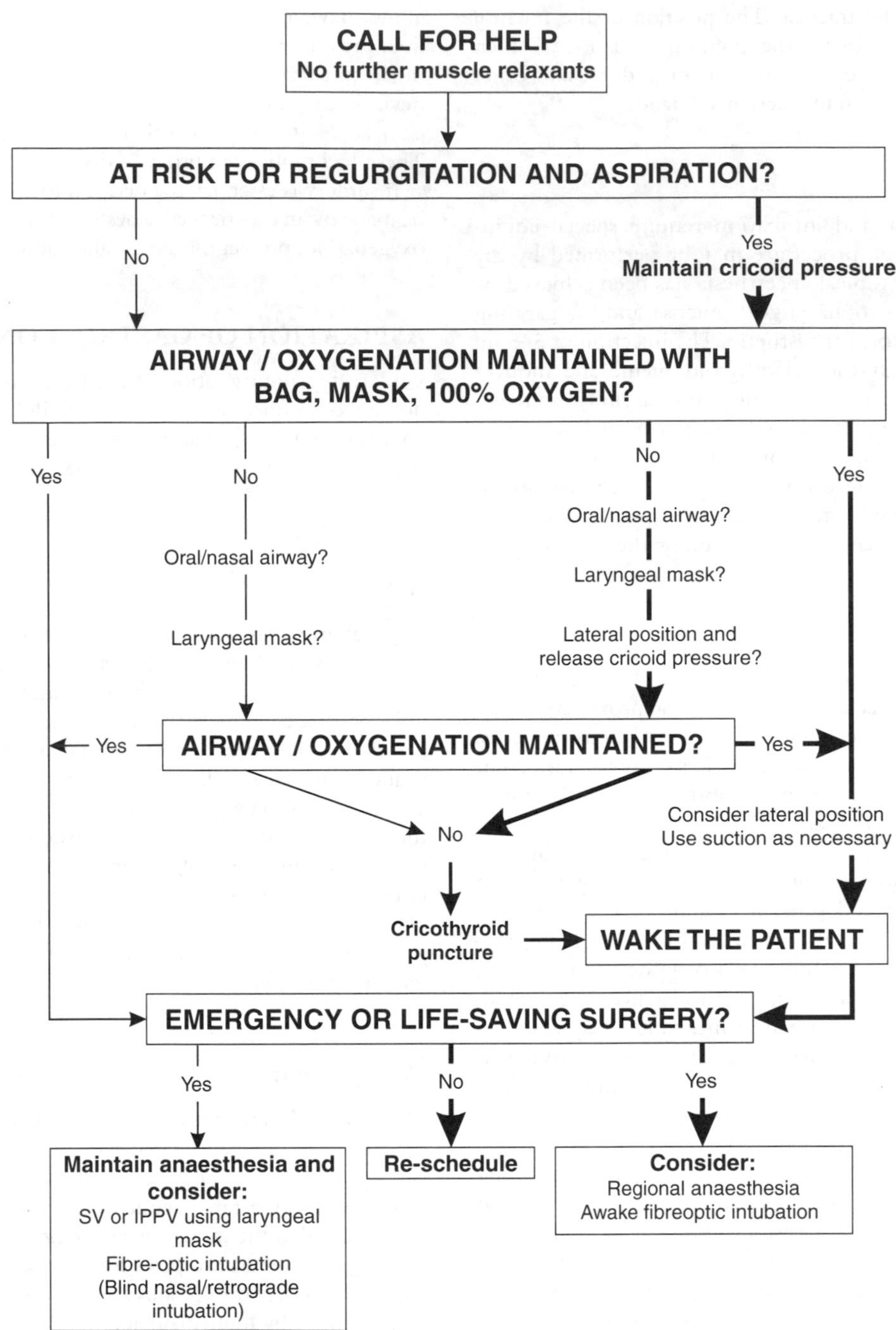

Fig. 40.3
A failed intubation protocol. Make an early decision to enter the protocol. Basic monitoring, optimal head positioning, use of bougie/stilette assumed. NOT APPLICABLE TO OBSTETRIC PATIENTS.

HICCUPS

Uncoordinated, spasmodic diaphragmatic movements may occur during induction of anaesthesia with intravenous agents such as etomidate and methohexital or in association with vagal stimulation during light anaesthesia. Anticholinergic premedication reduces the incidence of hiccups. Although difficult to treat, hiccups are of little consequence unless surgery, or rarely oxygenation, is compromised. Persistent hiccups may be abolished by deepening anaesthesia, stimulating the nasopharynx with a suction catheter or administering metoclopramide or droperidol. Profound muscle relaxation may be justified to stop all diaphragmatic movement if hiccups are causing surgical difficulty.

CENTRAL NERVOUS SYSTEM

AWARENESS

Aetiology

Awareness during anaesthesia refers to a patient experiencing an intraoperative event. As the brain is capable of processing information and memory function during anaesthesia, there is probably a spectrum of awareness that correlates with depth of anaesthesia. Of clinical importance is the patient who recalls the event postoperatively. Although awareness is often said to be most likely to occur in obstetric patients undergoing emergency caesarean section under general anaesthesia, all patients undergoing general anaesthesia are at risk. The reported incidence in non-obstetric anaesthesia is about 2 per 1000. Awareness is often said to be associated with a poor anaesthetic technique, the use of low concentrations of volatile anaesthetic agents (either inappropriately or during a hypotensive episode) and equipment problems such as breathing system disconnections and leaks. Significant degrees of intraoperative awareness occur only in patients who have received a muscle relaxant.

Management

Reducing the risk of awareness by meticulous preparation of equipment and the use of an appropriate anaesthetic technique is essential. Continuous measurement of end-tidal inhalation agent concentrations is necessary to be certain that sufficient agent has been delivered to the patient. Delivery of 0.8 MAC inhalation agent (in total) is the minimum necessary to avoid awareness.

Assessment of the depth of anaesthesia is difficult in the paralysed patient. It has been based traditionally on activity of the autonomic nervous system (e.g. tachycardia, hypertension, sweating), but these signs provide an unreliable indication of anaesthetic depth. The isolated forearm technique and monitoring of lower oesophageal motility are other unreliable techniques for assessing the depth of anaesthesia. The processed electroencephalogram (EEG) has greater application. The EEG can be analysed by computer to provide a number of indices that monitor depth of anaesthesia. Changes in the auditory evoked potential with anaesthesia also correlate with anaesthetic depth. Monitoring equipment using these principles is available for routine clinical use.

If a patient enquires about awareness at the preoperative visit, the risks and causes of awareness should be discussed to allay anxiety. It may also be appropriate electively to discuss the topic with patients planning to have caesarean section under general anaesthesia.

If a patient complains of intraoperative awareness in the postoperative period, the anaesthetist should be informed and should visit the patient forthwith, preferably with a senior colleague. The anaesthetist should establish the perioperative timing of the episode and distinguish between dreaming and awareness. If there is genuine awareness and a clear anaesthetic error, then honest admission and apology are advisable. All details should be recorded in the case notes. Although the majority of recalled events are not painful (up to 90% of patients with awareness have not experienced pain), awareness is a traumatic experience for the patient and may have psychological sequelae including insomnia, depression and fear of death. The situation is exacerbated if staff disbelieve or ignore the patient. It is essential to offer follow-up counselling for the patient and to inform the patient's general practitioner.

ISCHAEMIA OF THE CENTRAL NERVOUS SYSTEM

Ischaemic injury to the central nervous system varies from minimal, focal dysfunction to stroke or death. The mechanism is related usually to hypoxaemia and/or hypotension. The risk of ischaemic brain damage related to hypotension is increased if the patient has been positioned head-up during surgery. Rarely, intracerebral haemorrhage occurs during anaesthesia. Although the risk is increased if blood pressure has been very high, there have been reports of intracerebral haemorrhage during anaesthesia which were entirely coincidental.

The cervical spinal cord can be damaged during tracheal intubation and positioning in patients with cervical spine instability from fractures, rheumatoid arthritis and some congenital conditions such as Down's syndrome. Extreme positions of the head and neck may cause cerebral ischaemia due to vertebrobasilar insufficiency in susceptible patients. Ischaemic spinal cord injury can occur during major vascular and spinal surgery.

TEMPERATURE

HYPOTHERMIA

Hypothermia during anaesthesia may be defined as a core body temperature less than 36.0°C. Although common during anaesthesia and surgery, hypothermia can cause physiological derangement in the operating theatre and recovery area, and may increase perioperative morbidity such as infection in some patients.

Aetiology

Heat loss exceeds production in anaesthetized patients. Heat production falls as anaesthetic agents alter hypothalamic function, reduce metabolic rate, abolish the behavioural response to heat loss and reduce the ability to shiver. Many factors increase heat loss. During the first hour of anaesthesia, vasodilatation redistributes body heat to the periphery, causing a rapid decrease of core temperature followed by a slower but steady decline. Over 50% of heat loss is from radiation. This is exacerbated when the ambient temperature is less than 24°C, during surgery with open body cavities and during transfer with inadequate covering. Evaporative heat loss is increased by ventilation of the lungs with dry, cold anaesthetic gases, the use of wet packs, sweating and operations with open body cavities. High theatre air flow rates promote convective and evaporative heat loss. Irrigation or intravenous infusion with cold fluids and prolonged surgery are associated with increased heat loss. The risk of hypothermia is greatest in neonates, patients with a low metabolic rate such as the elderly, and patients with burns.

The effects of hypothermia are proportional to the change in temperature. Metabolic rate is reduced by up to 10% for every 1°C fall in body temperature. There is a decrease in cardiac output and an increase in haemoglobin oxygen affinity. These lead to a reduction in tissue oxygen delivery. Significant hypothermia is associated with metabolic acidosis, oliguria, altered platelet and clotting function, and reduced hepatic blood flow with slower drug metabolism. The MAC of volatile agents is reduced and muscle relaxants have a longer duration of effect. Postoperative shivering increases oxygen consumption and myocardial work.

Management

Measures to minimize heat loss (Table 40.12) should begin when the patient leaves the ward for theatre. Patients are particularly vulnerable during transfers and the first hour of anaesthesia.

Induced hypothermia is used occasionally in some centres for highly specialized paediatric neurological or cardiac operations where circulatory arrest provides optimal operating conditions. Lowering the metabolic rate reduces tissue oxygen consumption and allows a short time of deliberate circulatory arrest. Hypothermia reduces intracranial pressure and is occasionally induced in the management of children with severe head injury.

HYPERTHERMIA

Hyperthermia during anaesthesia may be defined as a core body temperature greater than 37.5°C or an increase in temperature of greater than 2°C h^{-1}.

Aetiology

Hyperthermia is usually caused by an increase in heat production. Causes include sepsis, drug reactions, excessive catecholamine secretion (phaeochromocytoma, thyroid storm) and malignant hyperthermia. Elevated metabolic rate and oxygen consumption increase cardiac output and minute ventilation and may lead to acidosis. Without treatment, sweating and vasodilatation produce hypovolaemia. Extreme hyperthermia results in seizures and central nervous system damage.

Table 40.12 Measures to reduce heat loss

Environment
Increase the ambient temperature and humidity
Patient
Cover patient during transfers and induction of anaesthesia
Warm all irrigation, intravenous fluids and blood
Insulate patient with plastic wrap, swaddling (limbs, head)
Warming blanket (more effective on top of patient)
Enclose exposed viscera in plastic bags
Warm and humidify inspired gases

Management

General measures include exposure of the body surface, application of ice packs, the use of fans and administration of cooled intravenous fluids. Specific measures depend on the cause. The management of malignant hyperthermia is discussed on page 521.

ADVERSE DRUG EFFECTS

Table 40.13 shows a classification of drug-related complications. Although uncommon, hypersensitivity (allergy) and idiosyncratic reactions are potentially disastrous without early recognition and effective management. In contrast, drug interactions and the incorrect use of drugs are common problems. These are usually predictable, preventable and the result of human error. The risk of an adverse reaction increases in a non-linear fashion with the number of drugs given to a patient. Therefore, as polypharmacy is usual during anaesthesia, there is a substantial risk of a drug reaction.

HYPERSENSITIVITY

Aetiology

True hypersensitivity describes an enhanced immunological reaction. Hypersensitivity reactions may be either anaphylactic or anaphylactoid. These reactions differ from direct, drug-induced histamine release, which does not have an immunological basis. The reported incidence of hypersensitivity (anaphylaxis) in anaesthetic practice varies from about 1:10 000 to 1:20 000. Most reactions during general anaesthesia follow intravenous drug administration.

Anaphylaxis (immediate hypersensitivity or Gell and Coombs type 1 reaction). This is an antibody-mediated reaction to an antigen, characterized by a sudden, life-threatening, generalized pathophysiological response involving the cutaneous, respiratory or cardiovascular systems. Primary antigen exposure stimulates the production of specific IgE antibodies which bind to mast cells. Re-exposure with antigen bridging of these IgE antibodies stimulates mast cell degranulation and systemic release of the mediators of anaphylaxis. Mediators include histamine, prostaglandins, platelet-activating factor and leukotrienes. Anaphylaxis has been reported in patients without apparent previous exposure to the specific antigen, probably due to immunological cross-reactivity; this is true particularly of reactions to muscle relaxants.

Anaphylactoid reactions. These are not IgE-mediated although the clinical presentation resembles anaphylaxis. The precise

Table 40.13 Drug complications

Hypersensitivity	Allergic	Mostly unpreventable, uncommon
Idiosyncratic	Genetic	
Interactions	Pharmacokinetic Pharmacodynamic	Predictable, preventable, common
Other	Incorrect choice, dose, route Other unwanted effects	

immunological mechanism is not always evident, although many reactions involve complement, kinin and coagulation pathway activation.

Non-immunological histamine release. This is caused by the direct action of a drug on mast cells. The clinical response depends on both the drug dose and the rate of delivery but is usually benign and confined to the skin. Anaesthetic drugs which release histamine directly include *d*-tubocurarine, atracurium, doxacurium, mivacurium (all of similar chemical derivation), morphine and pethidine. Clinical evidence of histamine release, usually cutaneous, occurs in up to 30% of patients during anaesthesia.

Important agents in anaesthetic practice

Most drugs are capable of precipitating a hypersensitivity reaction.

Intravenous induction agents. The incidence of severe reactions to thiopental has been reported as about 1: 14 000. Methohexital is associated with a higher reported incidence of hypersensitivity and there is cross-reactivity among barbiturates. Barbiturates may also cause direct histamine release. Propofol has caused anaphylaxis. Drugs solubilized in Cremophor EL are associated with a high incidence of anaphylactoid reactions. For this reason, Althesin and propanidid are no longer available for use in human anaesthetic practice. Hypersensitivity to benzodiazepines and etomidate is rare and these drugs do not cause direct histamine release.

Muscle relaxants. These are the most common cause of hypersensitivity in anaesthetic practice, with an overall incidence of about 1: 5000. Succinylcholine is the most immunogenic, although reactions to vecuronium, atracurium, alcuronium, gallamine and *d*-tubocurarine are well documented. The majority of reactions are IgE-mediated. There is significant cross-reactivity between muscle relaxants and other drugs having quaternary ammonium molecules. Pancuronium appears to be the least likely drug in this group to cause anaphylaxis.

Opioids. Anaphylaxis has been reported with most opioids. Fentanyl is a rare cause of anaphylaxis and does not lead to significant direct histamine release. Morphine, codeine and pethidine may cause dose-dependent, non-immunological, cutaneous histamine release.

Local anaesthetics. Hypersensitivity to local anaesthetics is rare. Reactions are more likely to be the result of dose-related toxicity, sensitivity to the effects of added vasoconstrictor or a reaction to preservatives such as paraben and benzoates. Amide local anaesthetic agents are considered safer than esters in patients with a previous history of sensitivity.

Colloid solutions. The overall reported incidence of hypersensitivity is about 3–4 per 10 000 anaesthetics, with plasma protein and gelatin solutions presenting the lowest and highest risks, respectively. The mechanism of reaction is often uncertain, although gelatin solutions may cause both direct histamine release and anaphylaxis. All hyperosmolar solutions can release histamine directly. These solutions (e.g. mannitol) should be infused slowly.

Antibiotics. The anaesthetist is often asked to give antibiotics around the time of induction of anaesthesia for prophylaxis of wound infection. Penicillins are most often implicated in hypersensitivity reactions. There is some cross-reactivity with cephalosporin antibiotics.

Radiocontrast media. Hypersensitivity reactions have been reported in up to 3% of patients, although vasomotor symptoms such as flushing, warmth, nausea and cutaneous phenomena are more common. Reactions may be severe, and most occur within minutes of administration. The risk of a reaction is markedly increased if the patient has suffered a previous reaction. Newer agents are associated with a lower risk.

Blood products. See Chapter 23.

Latex allergy. This is now recognized as an important cause of hypersensitivity. The reaction usually starts from 30–60 min after the start of surgery, often abdominal and gynaecological surgery. There is often a history of cross-reactivity to some foods, including banana and avocado.

Others. Protamine, streptokinase, aprotinin, atropine, bone cement and latex-containing products are just a few of the many substances that may cause severe reactions during the perioperative period.

Clinical features (Table 40.14)

As the patient is unable to volunteer symptoms during general anaesthesia, drug hypersensitivity should be considered in the differential diagnosis of any major cardiorespiratory problem. Reactions are more common in females, with a history

Table 40.14 Clinical features of drug hypersensitivity. Note that the condition may present with any feature alone, or any combination of features

Skin	
Symptoms	Pruritus, burning
Signs	Erythema, urticaria, oedema (head/neck/airway/generalized)
Respiratory	
Symptoms	Shortness of breath, wheeze
Signs	Cough, laryngospasm, bronchospasm, increased inflation pressure, pulmonary oedema
Cardiovascular	
Symptoms	Feeling faint
Signs	Syncope, tachycardia, hypotension, absent peripheral pulses, arrhythmia, cyanosis, cardiovascular collapse/arrest
Gastrointestinal	
Symptoms	Abdominal cramps, nausea, vomiting, diarrhoea

of allergy, atopy or previous exposure to anaesthetic agents, and over 90% of reactions occur immediately after induction of anaesthesia. There is a clinical spectrum of severity related to the degree of mast cell degranulation and host response.

Coughing, skin erythema, difficulty with ventilation or loss of a palpable pulse are often the first signs in severe reactions. Cardiovascular collapse, bronchospasm and angio-oedema are the most common clinical features. Reactions involving major involvement of a single physiological system are common, e.g. bradycardia and profound hypotension with no evidence of bronchospasm or angio-oedema. Erythema of the skin may be short-lived or absent because cyanosis from poor tissue perfusion and hypoxaemia may be profound. The awake patient may experience a sense of impending doom, dyspnoea, nausea and vomiting. The differential diagnosis should include anaesthetic drug overdose and other causes of bronchospasm, hypotension or hypoxaemia.

Management

Emergency management

Early recognition and effective action are essential because mortality increases if treatment is delayed. Death results from inadequate cardiorespiratory function. The aims of management are to prevent or correct hypoxaemia, to maintain cerebral and tissue perfusion and to stop mediator release. A specific management 'drill' should be used. Table 40.15 shows such a drill for the emergency management of anaphylaxis during general anaesthesia. *The use of intravenous epinephrine is essential treatment in the management of anaphylaxis.* It is life-saving if given early because it produces peripheral vasoconstriction, increased cardiac output, mast cell stabilization and bronchodilation. Corticosteroids and H_1-receptor antagonists have a delayed onset of action and therefore have a role only in later management.

Later management

After stabilization, the patient should be transferred to the intensive care unit. Progressive oedema involving the airway often develops rapidly. Tracheal intubation and mechanical ventilation are recommended until the patient is clinically stable and airway patency may be guaranteed after a period of observation. Sequential venous blood sampling over a 24 h period should be performed. The most important sample is at 1 h after the beginning of the reaction. The sample should be separated and stored at −20°C for subsequent measurement of serum tryptase concentration; if the concentration is elevated, this indicates mast cell degranulation. A negative test does not exclude a hypersensitivity reaction. Blood coagulation should also be monitored. The patient should be reviewed after discharge by an appropriate clinician and further investigations performed. Intradermal or skin prick tests are recommended. A Medicalert bracelet or other form of hazard alert should be carried by the patient. The details of the reaction must be recorded in the medical records and reported to the appropriate adverse drug reactions body. The patient's general practitioner must be informed.

Table 40.15 Guideline for management of an adult patient with suspected anaphylaxis during anaesthesia (Reproduced with permission from AAGBI 1995)

Initial therapy

1. Stop administration of drug(s) likely to have caused the anaphylaxis.
2. Maintain airway: give 100% oxygen.
3. Lay patient flat with feet elevated.
4. Give epinephrine. This may be given intramuscularly in a dose of 0.5–1 mg (0.5–1.0 ml of 1:1000 solution) and may be repeated every 10 min according to the arterial pressure and pulse until improvement occurs.

   Alternatively, 50–100 μg intravenously over 1 min has been recommended (0.5–1.0 ml of 1:10 000 solution) for hypotension, with titration of further doses as required.

   In a patient with cardiovascular collapse, 0.5–1 mg (5–10 ml of 1:10 000) may be required intravenously in divided doses by titration. This should be given at a rate of 0.1 mg min^{-1}, stopping when a response has been obtained.
5. Start intravascular volume expansion with crystalloid or colloid.

Secondary therapy

1. Antihistamines (chlorpheniramine 10–20 mg by slow i.v. infusion).
2. Corticosteroids (100–300 mg hydrocortisone i.v.).
3. Catecholamine infusions (starting doses: epinephrine 4–8 μg min^{-1} [0.05–0.1 μg kg^{-1} min^{-1}]; norepinephrine 4–8 μg min^{-1} [0.05–0.1 μg kg^{-1} min^{-1}]; isoproterenol 0.05–0.1 μg min^{-1}).
4. Consider bicarbonate (0.5–1.0 mmol kg^{-1} i.v.) for acidosis.
5. Airway evaluation (before extubation).
6. Bronchodilators may be required for persistent bronchospasm.

Anaesthesia in the susceptible patient

Regional anaesthesia should be used if possible. In patients who require general anaesthesia, the preoperative use of sodium cromoglycate, nebulized bronchodilators, corticosteroids and H_1- and H_2-receptor antagonists should be considered. A safe technique avoids re-exposure to implicated agents and uses drugs with a low potential for hypersensitivity and direct histamine release. These include volatile agents, etomidate, fentanyl, pancuronium and benzodiazepines. All drugs should be given slowly in diluted form. Full resuscitation facilities must be immediately available.

IDIOSYNCRATIC REACTIONS

An idiosyncratic drug reaction is a qualitatively abnormal and harmful drug effect which occurs in a small number of individuals and is precipitated usually by small drug doses. There is often an associated genetic defect and the reaction may be fatal. Succinylcholine sensitivity (see Ch. 19), malignant hyperthermia and acute intermittent porphyria are important examples of drug idiosyncrasy in anaesthetic practice.

Malignant hyperthermia

Malignant hyperthermia (MH) is an inherited myopathic disorder characterized by a marked increase in metabolic rate. The reported incidence varies considerably but is approximately 1 in 50 000. Rapid and effective treatment is essential to avoid mortality; over the last 30 years, the fatality rate has fallen from 70 to about 5%.

Aetiology

MH is an inherited disorder. The genetics of MH are complex. Mutations in the human ryanodine receptor in skeletal muscle (a calcium release channel with a role in excitation–contraction coupling) are apparent in some families. Predisposition to MH has been defined in only three rare clinical myopathies. Inheritance of the MH gene (which may have various chromosomal locations) and contact with specific agents can trigger abnormal calcium release from the sarcoplasmic reticulum into the cytoplasm. This leads to myofibrillar contraction, depletion of high-energy muscle phosphate stores, accelerated metabolic rate, increased carbon dioxide and heat production, increased oxygen consumption and metabolic acidosis. The usual triggering agents are succinylcholine or any volatile anaesthetic agent.

Clinical features

The MH syndrome may present at any time during the perioperative period. The clinical features and their severity vary considerably. The most consistent early sign is unexplained and progressive tachycardia. Spontaneously breathing patients may present with tachypnoea. MH should be considered in any anaesthetized patient if there is a progressive increase in end-tidal carbon dioxide concentration despite a normally adequate minute volume, or if the patient's body temperature increases during anaesthesia. Classically the temperature rises by more than 2°C h^{-1} and may exceed 40°C in some patients, although this is not a universal feature. Muscle rigidity is common and often involves the limbs. Without treatment, the full MH syndrome can develop, with progressive deterioration and cardiovascular collapse. The syndrome is characterized by sweating, cyanosis, mottled skin, hypoxaemia, ventricular arrhythmias and severe metabolic and respiratory acidosis. Muscle injury can cause significant potassium release, with ECG signs of hyperkalaemia. Coagulopathy, hypocalcaemia, elevated serum creatine kinase concentration, oliguria, myoglobinuria and acute renal failure are other sequelae.

An alternative presentation of MH is masseter spasm shortly after the administration of succinylcholine for tracheal intubation. Less than 10% of patients with this presentation progress to the full MH syndrome.

Management

Administration of volatile anaesthetic agent should be discontinued immediately and the lungs hyperventilated with 100% oxygen. If end-tidal carbon dioxide monitoring is not available, use at least twice the predicted minute volume. The trachea should be intubated at the earliest opportunity if a tracheal tube is not already in place. Experienced help should be obtained in both the operating theatre and the laboratory, and the operation must be abandoned as soon as possible.

Intravenous dantrolene is indicated specifically and should be given in doses of 1–2 mg kg^{-1} every 5 min until the rise in arterial carbon dioxide tension is controlled and decreasing. The mean and maximum doses used are 2.5 and 10 mg kg^{-1}, respectively. Dantrolene is packaged as a powder that requires several minutes to reconstitute, forming an alkaline solution. It is a skeletal muscle relaxant and causes muscle weakness if a large dose is given.

MH is associated with severe, life-threatening acidosis which can develop rapidly. Consequently, the early use of intravenous sodium bicarbonate should be considered, and large amounts may be necessary.

The patient should be cooled actively with ice packs to the axillae and groins and chilled intravenous saline should be infused. If necessary, gastric and rectal lavage with iced saline can be performed. Peritoneal dialysis and cardiopulmonary bypass have also been used to cool patients with MH.

If possible, substitute the anaesthetic breathing system with an unused system. Monitor core temperature, CVP, direct arterial pressure and urine output. Early and serial blood samples should be collected for analysis of acid–base status, arterial blood gas tensions, coagulation and serum electrolyte concentrations, especially potassium and glucose. Hyperkalaemia should be treated with intravenous insulin and glucose. Arrhythmias usually resolve after treatment of hyperkalaemia and acidosis, but specific antiarrhythmic drugs may be required.

A urine output greater than 1 ml kg^{-1} h^{-1} should be encouraged by ensuring an adequate circulating blood volume, and using intravenous mannitol if necessary. Haemofiltration may be indicated in the management of biochemical abnormalities and/or renal dysfunction. The patient must be managed in an intensive care unit for at least 48 h because the syndrome can recur during this time. Treatment with oral dantrolene is recommended for 48 h.

Any patient who experiences a clinical episode resembling MH, as well as the first-degree relatives of patients with confirmed MH, should be referred to a specialist centre for further assessment. The tests used to identify individuals with MH susceptibility vary between centres. The most common test is halothane- and caffeine-induced contracture of a muscle specimen. Less invasive genetic tests are being developed.

Anaesthesia in the susceptible patient

This should be a planned in-patient procedure with the facility for extended postoperative monitoring. The aim of management is to prevent contact with volatile agents and succinylcholine. A 'clean' anaesthetic machine can be prepared by flushing the machine overnight with 100% oxygen and using a new breathing system. The use of anticholinergic premedication is not advisable because it interferes with thermoregulation. Full resuscitation facilities and dantrolene should be immediately available. Regional anaesthesia should be used if possible. Safe drugs for use in susceptible patients include barbiturates, propofol, etomidate, benzodiazepines, non-depolarizing muscle relaxants, opioids and local anaesthetic agents. Total intravenous anaesthesia with propofol is one recommended technique. Monitoring of end-tidal carbon dioxide concentration, ECG, arterial pressure, oxygen saturation and continuous core temperature is mandatory.

Acute intermittent porphyria

Acute intermittent porphyria (AIP) is a rare but serious metabolic disorder caused by an inherited deficiency of an enzyme required for haem synthesis. This allows potential accumulation of porphyrin precursors in the pathway. The hepatic synthesis of these porphyrin precursors is controlled by the enzyme δ-amino laevulinic acid synthetase. Induction of this enzyme by barbiturates and many other drugs causes accumulation of precursors and manifests clinically as acute neuropathy, abdominal pain and delirium. On occasions, the abdominal pain can mimic an 'acute abdomen', leading to surgical intervention. If an at-risk patient is identified, porphyrinogenic drugs including barbiturates must be avoided because AIP can be fatal. Drugs considered safe for use in patients with AIP include propofol, midazolam, succinylcholine, vecuronium, nitrous oxide, morphine, fentanyl, neostigmine and atropine.

DRUG INTERACTIONS

Pharmacokinetic

This describes modification of the absorption, distribution, metabolism or excretion of one drug by another. Examples include the reduction in clearance of warfarin and lidocaine by cimetidine and the effect of opioids on the absorption of orally administered drugs by increasing gastric emptying time.

Pharmacodynamic

This describes interactions in which the pharmacological response to a drug is changed by the presence of another. Examples include potentiation of the myocardial depressant effect of volatile agents and intravenous induction agents in patients receiving a β-blocker or calcium antagonist, and the enhancement of neuromuscular blockade by aminoglycoside antibiotics.

Other drug complications

The incorrect choices of a drug, its dose or route of administration are common, preventable complications. The risk of errors involving ampoule and syringe identification can be minimized by a sound anaesthetic technique including the use of labels. Inappropriate mixing of incompatible drugs can cause precipitation due to a change in pH, most often caused by mixing acidic and alkaline drugs. Absolute or relative overdosage is a frequent event and can be disastrous. Excessively rapid drug administration can also cause complications such as histamine release (e.g. mivacurium).

Most drugs have undesirable side-effects. For example, etomidate inhibits cortisol synthesis and can increase mortality in critically ill patients when used continuously for sedation. Nitrous oxide interferes with methionine synthesis and haemopoiesis. In addition nitrous oxide diffuses into gas-filled spaces. For example, the use of 70% nitrous oxide for 2 h doubles the volume of bowel gas and may compromise gut blood supply, reduce surgical access and increases the incidence of postoperative nausea and vomiting. Nitrous oxide also increases the size and/or pressure in gas-filled spaces such as a pneumothorax.

INJURY

Most intraoperative injuries are sustained as a result of poor positioning or tracheal intubation. Nerve, dental and ophthalmic injuries are common causes of litigation, although most are preventable. Thermal and electrical injuries are less common but potentially disastrous. Neurological deficits present during the postoperative period although these are usually sustained intra-operatively.

PERIPHERAL NERVE

The reported incidence of peripheral nerve injury is about 1 in every 1000 anaesthetics. Poor positioning is a common underlying factor. The brachial plexus and superficial nerves of the limbs (ulnar, radial and common peroneal) are the most frequently affected nerves. The usual mechanism of injury to superficial nerves is ischaemia from compression of the vasa vasorum by surgical retractors, leg stirrups or contact with other equipment. Nerve injury can be part of a compartment syndrome of a limb after ischaemia from poor positioning. Ischaemic injury is more likely to occur during periods of poor peripheral perfusion associated with hypotension or hypothermia. Nerves can also be injured by traction, e.g. the brachial plexus during excessive shoulder abduction. Needlestick or chemical injury can also occur during regional anaesthesia.

Meticulous care is necessary when positioning the patient. Padding should be used beneath tourniquets and to protect pressure points. Extreme joint positions should be avoided. Close surveillance of tourniquet ischaemia times is essential. Although most injuries recover within several months, all patients with a peripheral nerve injury must be referred to a neurologist for continuing care. Many ulnar nerve palsies occur in patients with an anatomical predisposition, which may be deduced from a history of numbness after sleep or as a result of posture at work. In these patients, the elbows should not be placed in flexion during surgery.

DENTAL

Dental damage is the most frequently reported anaesthetic injury and is usually sustained during difficult laryngoscopy. The injury varies from chipping or scratching teeth to fracture and avulsion, most often involving the upper incisors. Preoperative assessment and documentation of dentition are essential. If a tooth is accidentally avulsed, it should be reimplanted in its socket with minimal interference and a dental surgeon consulted at the earliest opportunity.

OPHTHALMIC

Corneal abrasions are associated with inadequate eye protection, especially during transfer or use of the prone position. The use of adhesive tape to close the eyelids is also a risk factor. Lubricated dressings such as sterile paraffin gauze may be a preferable method of securing the eyelids. Mechanical pressure to the globes should be avoided at all times, because of the risk of retinal ischaemia and permanent blindness. Retinal detachment has been reported with extreme Trendelenburg positioning and as a result of pressure exerted on the eye in patients placed in the prone position.

THERMAL AND ELECTRICAL

The high-density electrical current used with surgical diathermy is a potential source of injury. If the return current path is interrupted by incorrect application of the diathermy pad, then the ECG electrodes or other points of contact between skin and metal can provide an alternative electrical path, producing serious burns. Failure of thermostatic control of warming devices is a source of thermal injury.

EQUIPMENT PROBLEMS

About a third of all critical incidents are related to equipment failure and most are preventable. Most equipment problems have implications for the patient and some have been described above (e.g. leaks and disconnections involving the anaesthetic machine and gas delivery system).

MONITORING APPARATUS

The equipment used for monitoring can provide inaccurate data and mislead the inexperienced anaesthetist. For example, non-invasive blood pressure equipment can be unreliable at extremes of low or high blood pressure and pulse oximeters can fail to provide data in patients with poor peripheral perfusion. Ultimately, the anaesthetist must rely on clinical skills during the conduct of anaesthesia. Invasive monitoring is a further source of complications. Central venous and pulmonary arterial catheterization are associated with numerous problems, including thrombosis, sepsis, pneumothorax and damage to deep structures. The use of arterial and peripheral venous cannulae can lead to thrombophlebitis, sepsis, air embolism and tissue damage from extravasation of fluids or drugs.

TOURNIQUETS

The incorrect use of tourniquets and bandages can traumatize skin, dislodge deep venous thrombi and produce nerve and muscle ischaemia. Deflation of a tourniquet after a period of limb ischaemia is associated with translocation of acidotic blood to the circulation. Hypercapnia, acidosis and depression of cardiac function may be clinically significant in patients with poor cardiorespiratory function. Limb tourniquets are contraindicated in patients with sickle cell disease, peripheral neuropathy, limb infections or peripheral vascular disease, including deep venous thrombosis. The tourniquet should be applied with adequate padding to the proximal limb, and avoiding bony prominences. The correct pressure for arm and leg tourniquet inflation is 50 and 100 mmHg, respectively, above systolic blood pressure. The duration of limb ischaemia in healthy patients should not exceed 2 h without a reperfusion time of at least 20 min.

FURTHER READING

Association of Anaesthetists of Great Britain and Ireland 1995 Suspected anaphylactic reactions associated with anaesthesia 2. AAGBI, London

King T A, Adams A P 1990 Failed tracheal intubation. British Journal of Anaesthesia 65: 400–414

Taylor T H 1992 Editorial: avoiding iatrogenic injuries in theatre. British Medical Journal 305: 595–596

Taylor T H, Major E (eds) 1993 Hazards and complications of anaesthesia, 2nd edn. Churchill Livingstone, London

41 Postoperative care

In modern anaesthetic practice, the patient is monitored and supervised closely and continuously during induction and throughout the operative procedure. However, many problems associated with anaesthesia and surgery may occur in the immediate postoperative period, and it is essential that supervision by adequately trained and experienced personnel is continued during the recovery period. In addition, some major and minor complications of anaesthesia and surgery may occur at any time in the first few days after operation.

THE EARLY RECOVERY PERIOD

Most hospitals have a recovery ward in close proximity to the operating theatre suite (see Ch. 33). The Association of Anaesthetists of Great Britain and Ireland recommends that fully staffed recovery facilities must be available at all times in hospitals with an emergency surgical service. Some anaesthetizing locations (e.g. the X-ray department) may not have a recovery ward. This section describes common problems which occur in the immediate postoperative period and refers specifically to their management in a recovery ward; however, the same principles are applicable to recovery in other locations.

The recovery period starts as soon as the patient leaves the operating table and the direct supervision of the anaesthetist. All the complications listed below may occur at any time, including the period of transfer from operating theatre to recovery ward; in some operating theatre suites, the transfer to the recovery ward may last for several minutes, and it is essential that the standard of observation does not diminish during the journey. The patient must be supervised and monitored closely *at all times.*

SYSTEMS AFFECTED

Central nervous system

Consciousness may not return for several minutes after the end of general anaesthesia and may be impaired for a longer period of time. During this period, a patent airway must be maintained. There is a risk of aspiration into the lungs of any material, e.g. gastric content or blood, which is present in the pharynx. Consciousness may also be depressed in patients who have received sedation to facilitate endoscopy or regional anaesthesia.

Excitement and confusion may occur during recovery and may result in injury. Pain may be severe if long-acting analgesics have not been given during surgery.

Cardiovascular system

Peripheral resistance and cardiac output may be reduced because of residual effects of anaesthetic drugs in the absence of surgical stimulation. Hypovolaemia may be present because of inadequate fluid replacement during surgery, continued bleeding postoperatively or expansion of capacitance of the vascular system as a result of rewarming. Cardiac output may also be reduced as a result of arrhythmias or pre-existing disease. Hypertension may occur as a result of increased sympathoadrenal activity after restoration of consciousness, especially if analgesia is inadequate.

Respiratory system

Hypoventilation occurs commonly, usually as a result of residual effects of anaesthetic drugs or incomplete antagonism of neuromuscular blocking drugs. Hypoxaemia may result from hypoventilation, ventilation/perfusion imbalance or increased oxygen consumption produced by restlessness or shivering.

Gastrointestinal

Nausea and vomiting are common in the immediate postoperative period.

STAFF, EQUIPMENT AND MONITORING

The recovery ward should be staffed by trained and experienced nurses. One nurse must remain with each patient at all times until consciousness and airway reflexes return. The responsibility for the patient's welfare remains with the anaesthetist. In many hospitals, an anaesthetist is designated to be available immediately to treat complications detected by the nursing staff in the recovery ward.

The patient is nursed in a bed if a prolonged stay is anticipated, but more commonly on a trolley (Fig. 41.1). All beds and trolleys must have the facility to be tipped head-down. Suction apparatus, including catheters, an oxygen supply with appropriate face mask, a self-inflating resuscitation bag and anaesthetic mask, a pulse oximeter and an automated oscillometer (or at least a sphygmomanometer), must be available for each patient. In addition, there should be a complete range of resuscitation equipment within the recovery area; this includes an anaesthetic machine, a range of laryngoscopes, tracheal tubes, bougies, intravenous (i.v.) cannulae, fluids, emergency drugs, electrocardiogram (ECG)

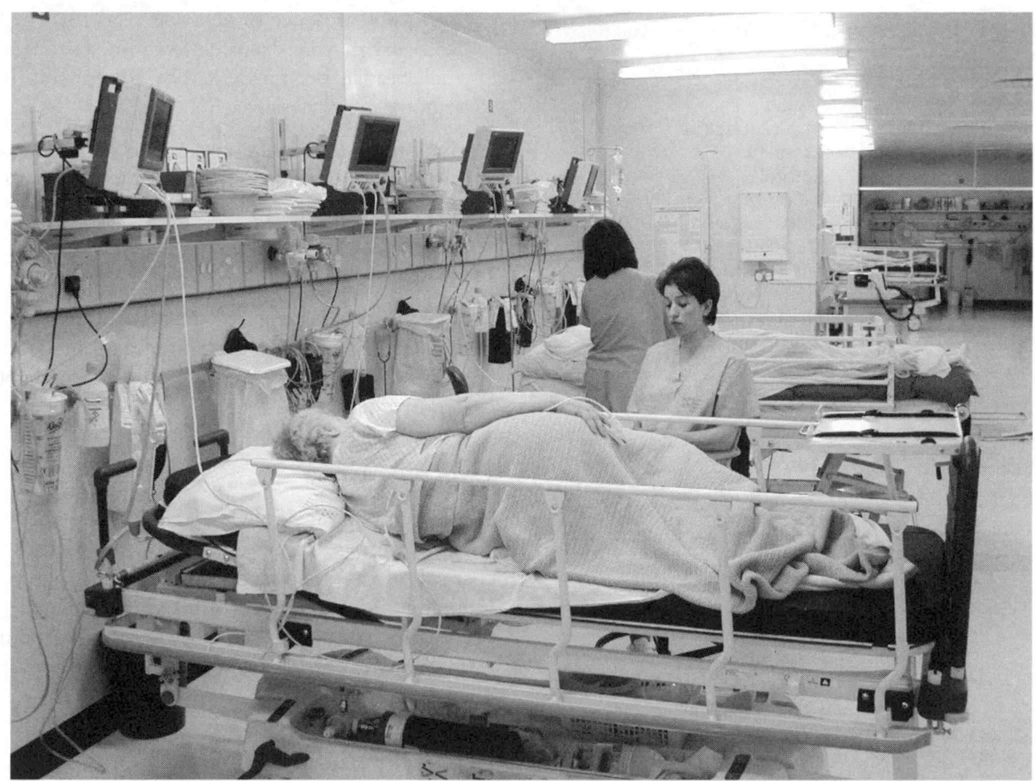

Fig. 41.1
Part of a recovery ward. Many patients are nursed on a trolley, but a bed is used for those who have undergone major surgery and those who need to stay for several hours.

monitor and defibrillator. Facilities for cricothyroid cannulation, e.g. minitracheotomy set, and for formal tracheostomy should also be available.

A wide range of drugs should be stored in the recovery area for the treatment of common complications and also emergency events (Table 41.1).

All patients should be monitored by measurement of pulse rate, arterial pressure, arterial oxygen saturation and respiratory rate and by assessment of level of consciousness, peripheral circulation and adequacy of ventilation; in some circumstances, minute volume may be measured using a respirometer (e.g. Wright's). Depending on the nature of work undertaken in the theatre suite, a proportion of bed stations should have the facility for monitoring ECG, systemic and pulmonary arterial pressures and central venous pressure (CVP) continuously; this may be required in high-risk patients or those who have undergone major surgery. Capnography should be available for use in patients who require tracheal intubation. At least one mechanical ventilator should be available. Urine output should be measured routinely in patients who have undergone major surgery. Wounds and surgical drains should be inspected regularly for signs of bleeding.

A record should be made of pulse rate, arterial pressure and arterial oxygen saturation, respiratory rate, level of consciousness, pain score, sensory level (if regional anaesthesia has been used), and any other relevant information (such as complications, and drug and fluid administration) obtained while the patient is in the recovery area. In most units, recordings of physiological measurements are made every 5 min, at least until consciousness has returned.

The patient should not be discharged to the surgical ward until the following criteria have been met:

- Consciousness has returned fully, a patent airway can be maintained and protective reflexes are present.
- Ventilation and oxygenation are satisfactory.
- The cardiovascular system is stable with no unexplained cardiac irregularity or persistent bleeding. Consecutive measurements of pulse rate and arterial pressure should approximate to the patient's normal preoperative values or be at an acceptable level commensurate with the planned postoperative care. Peripheral perfusion should be adequate.
- Pain and nausea are controlled.
- Temperature is within acceptable limits.

High-risk patients or those who have undergone major surgery should stay in the recovery ward for up to 24 h. If this is not feasible, or if instability persists for longer than 24 h, the patient should be transferred to a high-dependency or intensive care unit.

Although the recovery room nurse undertakes the direct care of the patient, the responsibility for the patient remains with the anaesthetist. Patients must only be discharged to the ward with the anaesthetist's consent.

The remainder of this chapter is devoted to the diagnosis and management of common problems which occur in the postoperative period. Some of these occur most frequently in the immediate recovery period, while others may occur at any time during the

Table 41.1 Drugs which should be available in the recovery room

Adenosine	Insulin
Alfentanil	Isoprenaline (isoproterenol)
Aminophyilline	Ketamine
Antibiotics	Ketorolac
Aprotinin	Labetalol
Aspirin	Lidocaine
Atracurium	Metaraminol
Atropine	Methoxamine
Bupivacaine	Methylprednisolone
Calcium chloride	Metoclopramide
Calcium gluconate	Midazolam
Calcium heparin	Morphine
Chlorphenamine (chlorpheniramine)	Naloxone
Co-proxamol	Neostigmine
Cyclizine	Nifedipine
Dexamethasone	Norepinephrine
Diazepam	Ondansetron
Diclofenac	Papaverine
Digoxin	Paracetamol
Dobutamine	Pethidine
Dopamine	Phentolamine
Doxapram	Phenytoin
Edrophonium	Phytomenadione
Ephedrine	Potassium chloride
Epinephrine	Procainamide
Fentanyl	Prochlorperazine
Flumazenil	Propranolol
Furosemide	Protamine
Glucose	Ranitidine
Glyceryl trinitrate	Salbutamol
Glycopyrronium	Sodium citrate
Hyaluronidase	Sodium nitroprusside
Hydralazine	Succinylcholine
Hydrocortisone	Tranexamic acid
Hyoscine	Verapamil

patient's convalescence from surgery. Some surgical procedures are associated with specific complications.

CENTRAL NERVOUS SYSTEM

CONSCIOUS LEVEL

Many patients are unconscious on arrival in the recovery ward because of residual effects of anaesthetic drugs. The duration of impaired consciousness depends on:

- *The drugs used.* Recovery of consciousness may be delayed if the following agents have been used:
  - volatile anaesthetics with a high blood/gas solubility coefficient
  - barbiturates, particularly if large total doses have been given
  - benzodiazepines
  - opioids with a long duration of action, including large doses of fentanyl.
- *The timing of drug use.* Delayed recovery may occur if a long-acting i.v. anaesthetic or analgesic drug has been given towards the end of the procedure, or if the more soluble volatile agents have been continued until the end of surgery.
- *Pain.* The presence of pain speeds recovery of consciousness. Recovery may be delayed after minor procedures or if potent analgesia has been provided by administration of opioids or by regional anaesthesia.

Undue prolongation of consciousness should not be attributed to these factors alone. Other causes should be considered, as their early recognition may prevent serious sequelae.

Hypoglycaemia

This occurs most commonly in diabetic patients treated with oral hypoglycaemic agents or insulin and an inadequate intake of glucose. The perioperative management of the diabetic patient is discussed in Chapter 35.

Hyperglycaemia

Hyperglycaemia in known diabetics may occur as a result of inadequate provision of insulin or injudicious infusion of glucose. However, coma is unusual in acute hyperglycaemia. Undiagnosed diabetics with hyperglycaemia and ketosis may present for surgery because of abdominal pain, and prolonged postoperative coma may occur unless the metabolic defect is diagnosed and treated.

Cerebral pathology

Consciousness may be impaired by functional or structural cerebral damage. Possible causes include:

- episodes of cerebral ischaemia (e.g. carotid artery surgery, profound hypotension) or hypoxia during anaesthesia
- intracranial haemorrhage, thrombosis or infarction – these may occur fortuitously or may have been associated with intraoperative hypertension, hypotension or arrhythmias
- pre-existing cerebral lesions, e.g. tumour, trauma – anaesthetic techniques which increase intracranial pressure are likely to impair cerebral function
- epilepsy – convulsions may have been masked by anaesthesia or neuromuscular blocking drugs
- air embolism
- intracranial spread of local anaesthetic solution after subarachnoid injection – introduction into the subarachnoid space may be accidental, e.g. during epidural block or, rarely, interscalene brachial plexus block; unconsciousness is almost always accompanied by apnoea.

Other causes

- *Hypoxaemia.* In the presence of an adequate circulation, coma occurs only if profound hypoxaemia is present.
- *Hypercapnia.* Unconsciousness may occur if arterial carbon dioxide tension (P_aCO_2) exceeds 9–10 kPa.
- *Hypotension.*
- *Hypothermia.*
- *Hypo-osmolar or TURP syndrome.* This results most commonly from absorption of water from the bladder during transurethral resection of the prostate (TURP). The investigation and management of this condition are described on page 579.
- *Hypothyroidism.*
- *Hepatic or renal failure.*

CONFUSION AND AGITATION

These occur occasionally during emergence from an otherwise uncomplicated anaesthetic. They are more common in elderly patients, particularly if hyoscine has been given as a premedicant. Atropine also crosses the blood–brain barrier and may result in the central anticholinergic syndrome, characterized by restlessness and confusion, together with obvious antimuscarinic effects. Glycopyrronium does not cross the blood–brain barrier and is preferable to atropine for antagonism of the muscarinic effects of neostigmine in elderly patients; in addition to its lack of central effects, it produces less tachycardia and antagonizes the effects of neostigmine for a longer period.

All the factors listed above as causes of prolonged coma may also result in confusion and agitation. Pain may also contribute, although it is seldom responsible alone. Emergence delirium is associated particularly with the use of ketamine and may occur after the administration of etomidate. Septicaemia may result in confusion, as may distension of the stomach or bladder.

A lightly sedated, conscious patient with inadequate antagonism of neuromuscular blocking drugs may appear to the inexperienced observer to be agitated and confused. Movements are uncoordinated. The condition is distressing to the patient and is an indication of a poor anaesthetic technique. It should never be allowed to develop.

PAIN

This subject is discussed fully in Chapter 42. The effects of pain should be differentiated from those of hypercapnia and hypovolaemia (Table 41.2).

RESPIRATORY SYSTEM

HYPOVENTILATION

Common causes of hypoventilation in the immediate postoperative period are listed in Table 41.3. Hypoventilation results in an increase in P_aCO_2 (Fig. 41.2) and a decrease in alveolar oxygen tension (P_AO_2), and thus hypoxaemia, which may be corrected by increasing the inspired concentration of oxygen.

Airway obstruction

Airway obstruction caused by the tongue, by indrawing of the pharyngeal muscles or by blood or secretions in the pharynx is ameliorated by placing the patient in the lateral or recovery position (see Fig. 37.5, p. 468). This position should be used for all unconscious patients who have undergone oral or ear, nose and throat surgery, and for patients at risk of gastric aspiration.

Partial obstruction of the airway is characterized by noisy ventilation. As the obstruction increases, tracheal tug and indrawing of the supraclavicular area occur during inspiration. Total obstruction is signalled by absent sounds of breathing and paradoxical movement of the chest wall and abdomen.

In many patients, a clear airway is maintained only by displacing the mandible anteriorly and extending the head. In some, it is necessary also to insert an oropharyngeal airway, although this may

Table 41.2 Common problems in the recovery room: symptoms and signs

	Pain	Hypercapnia	Hypovolaemia
Conscious level	May be restless May be quiescent if severe pain	Comatose	Restless or quiescent depending on extent of analgesia and residual anaesthesia
Periphery	Vasoconstriction, pallor ± sweating	Warm, flushed with bounding pulse (if normovolaemic)	Vasoconstriction, pallor ± sweating
Heart rate	Tachycardia	Tachycardia	Tachycardia
Arterial pressure	Systolic ↑ Diastolic ↑ Pulse pressure normal	Systolic ↑ Diastolic ↑ ↓ Pulse pressure ↑	Systolic and diastolic may be normal until marked reduction in stroke volume, then ↓ Pulse pressure ↓

Table 41.3 Causes of postoperative hypoventilation

Factors affecting airway	Factors affecting ventilatory drive	Peripheral factors
Upper airway obstruction: Tongue Laryngospasm Oedema Foreign body Tumour Bronchospasm	Respiratory depressant drugs Preoperative CNS pathology Intra- or postoperative cerebrovascular accident Hypothermia Recent hyperventilation (P_aCO_2 low)	Muscle weakness: Residual neuromuscular block Preoperative neuromuscular disease Electrolyte abnormalities Pain Abdominal distension Obesity Tight dressings Pneumo-/haemothorax

CNS, central nervous system; P_aCO_2, arterial carbon dioxide tension.

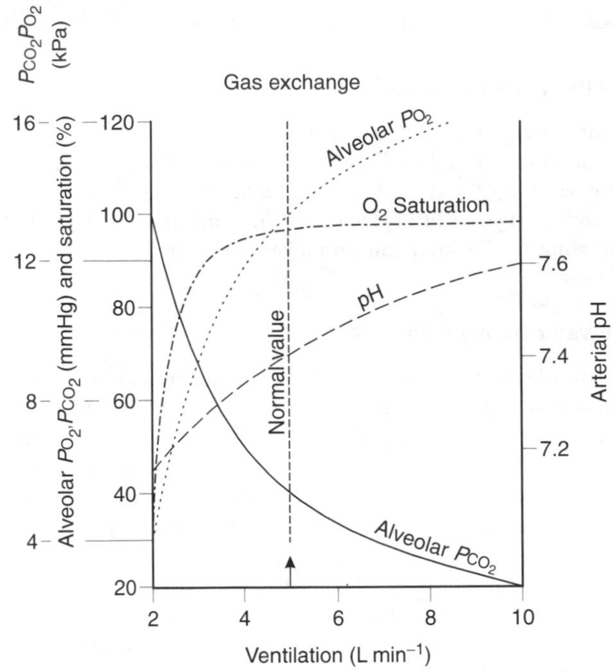

Fig. 41.2
Gas exchange during hypoventilation. Note the relatively rapid increase in alveolar partial pressure of carbon dioxide (P_{CO_2}) compared with the slow decrease in arterial oxygen saturation. P_{O_2}, partial pressure of oxygen.

stimulate coughing, gagging and laryngospasm during recovery of consciousness. A nasopharyngeal airway is often tolerated better, but there is a risk of causing haemorrhage from the nasopharyngeal mucosa. Occasionally, insertion of a laryngeal mask airway is necessary to maintain the airway until consciousness has returned fully; very occasionally, tracheal intubation is required.

Blood, oral secretions or regurgitated gastric fluid which have accumulated in the pharynx should be aspirated and the patient placed in the recovery position to allow any further fluid to drain anteriorly.

Foreign bodies, such as dentures (particularly partial dentures) or throat packs, may cause airway obstruction. It may be difficult to maintain a patent airway in unconscious patients with an oral, pharyngeal or laryngeal tumour.

Obstruction of the upper airway occurs intermittently after recovery from anaesthesia. Obstructive sleep apnoea is common in the postoperative period and may result in decreases of arterial oxyhaemoglobin saturation (S_aO_2) to less than 75%. Episodes occur with the greatest frequency in the first 4 h after anaesthesia and are more common and severe in patients who receive opioids for postoperative analgesia than in those in whom analgesia is provided by a regional technique.

Airway obstruction may result from haemorrhage after surgery to the neck, including thyroid surgery; the wound should be opened urgently, and the haematoma drained. Occasionally, tracheal collapse occurs after thyroidectomy in patients who have developed chondromalacia of the cartilaginous rings of the trachea caused by pressure from a large goitre. Inspiratory stridor may be present or there may be total obstruction during inspiration; the trachea must be reintubated immediately.

Laryngeal spasm

This complication is relatively common after general anaesthesia. It may be partial or complete and is usually caused by direct stimulation of the cords by secretions or blood, or of the epiglottis by an oropharyngeal airway or laryngeal mask. It may follow extubation of the trachea in the semiconscious patient. It may be difficult to differentiate this condition from airway obstruction caused by the pharyngeal wall; if airway obstruction persists despite implementation of the measures described above, laryngoscopy should be undertaken.

Any obvious foreign material causing laryngospasm should be removed by aspiration, and oxygen 100% administered. If obstruction is complete, positive pressure ventilation by mask may force some oxygen through the cords to maintain arterial oxygenation until the spasm has subsided; there is a significant risk of inflating the stomach with oxygen during this procedure. If attempts to oxygenate the lungs fail, succinylcholine should be administered, and the lungs ventilated with oxygen when the spasm is relieved. When satisfactory oxygenation has been achieved, it may be advisable to intubate the trachea to reduce the risk of regurgitation of gastric contents, as the stomach may have been inflated with oxygen, and to administer 60–65% nitrous oxide in oxygen to minimize the risk of awareness if the patient regains consciousness before muscle power returns. When the effects of succinylcholine have terminated, oxygen 100% is administered and the trachea is extubated when the patient regains consciousness.

Rarely, laryngeal obstruction occurs after thyroid surgery if both recurrent laryngeal nerves have been traumatized.

Laryngeal oedema

This occurs occasionally after tracheal intubation and may result in severe obstruction, particularly in a child. Treatment depends on the severity of the obstruction; immediate reintubation may be required if obstruction is complete, but partial obstruction may subside if the patient is treated with heated humidified gases. Dexamethasone may hasten resolution of the oedema.

Bronchospasm

This may result from stimulation of the airway by inhaled material. It is commoner in asthmatic or bronchitic patients and in smokers. It may result directly from intrinsic asthma or may be part of an anaphylactic reaction. Several drugs used in anaesthetic practice may precipitate bronchospasm either by a direct effect on bronchial muscle or by releasing histamine; these include barbiturates, *d*-tubocurarine, morphine, mivacurium and atracurium. Treatment comprises the removal of any predisposing factor and the administration of oxygen and bronchodilators.

Ventilatory drive

There are several possible causes of reduced ventilatory drive during recovery from anaesthesia (Table 41.3). The presence of intracranial pathology, e.g. tumour, trauma or haemorrhage, may affect ventilatory drive in the postoperative period. Ventilation is reduced in the presence of hypothermia, although it is usually appropriate for the metabolic needs of the body. Hypoventilation occurs in the hypocapnic patient, e.g. after a period of hyperventilation until P_aCO_2 is restored to normal, and in the presence of primary metabolic alkalosis.

The most important cause of reduced ventilatory drive during recovery is the effect of drugs administered by the anaesthetist in the perioperative period. All the volatile and i.v. anaesthetic agents – with the exception of ketamine – depress the respiratory centre; significant concentrations of these drugs remain in the brain stem during the early postoperative period.

All opioid analgesics depress ventilation. With most opioids, the effect is dose-dependent, although the agonist-antagonist agents are claimed to have a ceiling effect. In the majority of patients, opioids do not produce apnoea, but result in decreased ventilatory drive and an increase in P_aCO_2, which plateaus at an elevated value. The elderly are particularly sensitive to drug-induced ventilatory depression. The treatment of postoperative pain begins in the recovery area, often by administration of i.v. opioids by the medical or nursing staff, and ventilation must be monitored carefully after each dose.

Spinal (intrathecal or epidural) opioids, particularly lipid-insoluble agents such as morphine, may produce ventilatory depression some hours after administration. Patients who have received subarachnoid or epidural opioids should remain in the recovery ward or in a high-dependency unit for at least 12 h after administration of the last dose of spinal morphine, or at least 3 h after fentanyl, unless protocols and training programmes for surgical ward nurses have been implemented.

Reduced ventilatory drive is easy to diagnose if the ventilatory rate or tidal volume is clearly reduced. However, lesser degrees of hypoventilation may be difficult to detect, and the signs of moderate hypercapnia, e.g. hypertension and tachycardia, may be masked by the residual effects of anaesthetic agents, or misdiagnosed as pain-induced (Table 41.2).

Mild hypoventilation is acceptable provided that oxygenation remains adequate; this can easily be achieved by a modest increase in fractional concentration of oxygen (F_IO_2; see below). If ventilatory drive is reduced excessively by opioids, resulting in an increasing P_aCO_2 or delayed recovery of consciousness, naloxone in increments of 1.5–3 μg kg^{-1} should be administered every 2–3 min until improvement occurs. Administration of excessive doses of naloxone reverses the analgesia induced by systemic (but not to the same extent by spinal) opioids; large doses may cause severe hypertension and have been associated with cardiac arrest on rare occasions. The effects of i.v. naloxone last only for 20–30 min; in order to prevent recurrence of reduced ventilation after long-acting opioids, an additional dose (50% of the effective i.v. dose) may be administered intramuscularly or an i.v. infusion instituted.

Peripheral factors

The commonest peripheral factor associated with hypoventilation is residual neuromuscular blockade. This may be exaggerated by disease of the neuromuscular junction, e.g. myasthenia gravis, or by electrolyte disturbances. Inadequate reversal of neuromuscular blockade is usually associated with uncoordinated, jerky movements, although these may occur occasionally during recovery of consciousness in patients with normal neuromuscular function. Measurement of tidal volume is not a reliable guide to adequacy of reversal of neuromuscular blockade; a normal tidal volume may be achieved with only 20% return of diaphragmatic power, but the ability to cough remains severely impaired. If the patient is able to lift the head from the trolley for 5 s or maintain a good hand grip, it is likely that there is sufficient return of neuromuscular function for adequate ventilation and maintenance of the airway. Some more objective means of assessment are listed in Table 41.4, but these require the cooperation of the patient. In the unconscious or uncooperative patient, nerve stimulation (see Ch. 19) provides the best means of assessing neuromuscular function, although there are differences among the non-depolarizing relaxants in the relationship between their actions in the forearm and diaphragm.

If residual non-depolarizing blockade is confirmed, further doses of neostigmine may be administered (with atropine or glycopyrronium) up to a total of 5 mg; in higher doses, neostigmine can worsen neuromuscular function. If the block persists, artificial ventilation must be maintained while the cause is sought.

Factors responsible most commonly for difficulty in antagonism of neuromuscular block include overdosage with muscle relaxant, too short an interval between administration of the drug and the antagonist, hypokalaemia, respiratory or metabolic acidosis, administration of aminoglycoside antibiotics, local anaesthetic agents, diseases affecting neuromuscular transmission and muscle disease.

Delayed elimination of all of the non-depolarizing muscle relaxants (except atracurium and cis-atracurium) has been reported, and causes prolonged neuromuscular block. Delayed elimination occurs most frequently in the presence of renal or hepatic insufficiency, or in dehydrated patients with low urine output. Muscle paralysis may recur 30–60 min after administration of neostigmine if elimination of the relaxant is inadequate, even if antagonism appears to be satisfactory initially. A similar phenomenon may occur if acidosis develops, or when patients who have been hypothermic are rewarmed.

Prolonged neuromuscular block after succinylcholine or mivacurium occurs in the presence of atypical plasma cholinesterase or a low concentration of normal plasma cholinesterase. Paralysis after succinylcholine may persist for up to 8 h, although in most instances recovery occurs within 20–120 min. Neostigmine should not be administered if prolonged neuromuscular block occurs after administration of succinylcholine.

Artificial ventilation of the lungs must be maintained or resumed in any patient who has inadequate neuromuscular function. Anaesthesia should be provided to prevent awareness; this is achieved most easily with nitrous oxide and a low concentration of a volatile anaesthetic agent.

Hypoventilation may be caused also by restriction of diaphragmatic movement resulting from abdominal distension, obesity,

Table 41.4 Clinical assessment of the adequacy of antagonism of neuromuscular block

Subjective
Grip strength
Adequate cough
Objective
Ability to sustain head lift for at least 5 s
Ability to produce vital capacity of at least 10 ml kg^{-1}

tight dressings or abdominal binders. Pain, particularly from thoracic or upper abdominal wounds, may cause reduced ventilation.

The presence of air or fluid in the pleural cavity may result in hypoventilation. Pneumothorax may occur during intermittent positive pressure ventilation (IPPV). It is an occasional complication in healthy patients, but is a particular risk in those with chronic obstructive airways disease, especially if bullae are present, and after chest trauma. It may complicate brachial plexus nerve block, central venous cannulation or surgery involving the kidney or neck. Haemothorax may result from chest trauma or central venous cannulation. Hydrothorax may be caused by pleural effusions or inadvertent infusion of fluids through a misplaced central venous catheter. These rapidly remediable causes of hypoventilation are often overlooked.

Treatment

This consists primarily of treatment of the cause. Mild or moderate hypoventilation resulting from residual effects of anaesthetic drugs may respond to a bolus dose or infusion of doxapram. Artificial ventilation should be reinstituted if severe hypercapnia is present or P_aCO_2 continues to rise, or if the clinical condition of the patient is deteriorating.

HYPOXAEMIA

A functional classification of causes of hypoxaemia in the early recovery period is shown in Table 41.5. An inspired oxygen concentration of less than 21% should never occur, although P_aO_2 is decreased when air is breathed at high altitudes.

Ventilation–perfusion abnormalities

These are the commonest cause of hypoxaemia in the recovery room. Cardiac output and pulmonary arterial pressure may be reduced after general or regional anaesthesia, causing impaired perfusion of some areas of the lungs. Functional residual capacity (FRC) is reduced during and immediately after anaesthesia, and closing capacity (see p. 111) may encroach on the tidal breathing range, resulting in reduced ventilation of some lung units, particularly those in dependent alveoli. Thus the scatter of ventilation/perfusion (V/Q) ratios is increased. Areas of lung with increased ratios constitute physiological dead space; unless there is central depression of ventilation, an increase in dead space is usually followed by an increase in minute volume. Areas of lung with low V/Q ratios increase venous admixture, which results in hypoxaemia unless the inspired oxygen concentration is increased.

Table 41.5 Functional classification of the causes of hypoxaemia in the postoperative period

Reduced inspired oxygen concentration
Ventilation–perfusion abnormalities
Shunting
Hypoventilation
Diffusion deficits
Diffusion hypoxia after nitrous oxide anaesthesia

Shunt

Physiological shunt may be increased in the immediate postoperative period if small airways closure has been extreme. Shunting may be present also in patients with pulmonary oedema of any aetiology, or if there is consolidation in the lung. Shunt may be increased in the later postoperative period as a result of retention of secretions and underventilation of the lung bases because of pain; these changes lead to alveolar consolidation and collapse.

Hypoventilation

This has been discussed in detail above. Moderate hypoventilation, with some elevation of P_aCO_2, leads to a modest reduction in P_aO_2 (Fig. 41.3). Obstructive sleep apnoea may produce profound transient but repeated decreases in arterial oxygenation. S_aO_2 may decrease to less than 75%, corresponding to a P_aO_2 of less than 5 kPa (40 mmHg). These repeated episodes of hypoxaemia cause temporary, and possibly permanent, defects in cognitive function in elderly patients and may contribute to perioperative myocardial infarction. Obstructive sleep apnoea is exacerbated by opioid analgesics, and patients who are known to suffer from this condition should be monitored carefully in the postoperative period, preferably in a high-dependency unit. Patients who normally use a continuous positive airways pressure (CPAP) mask to reduce obstructive sleep apnoeic episodes should use the mask at night throughout the postoperative period.

Diffusion defects

Interstitial oedema produced by overtransfusion of fluids or by left ventricular dysfunction may cause hypoxaemia by impairment of oxygen transfer across the alveolar–capillary membrane.

Diffusion hypoxia

Nitrous oxide is 40 times more soluble than nitrogen in blood. When administration of nitrous oxide is discontinued at the end of anaesthesia, nitrous oxide diffuses out of blood into the alveoli in larger volumes than nitrogen diffuses in the opposite direction. Consequently, the alveolar concentrations of other gases are diluted. P_aO_2 is reduced and arterial oxygenation impaired if the patient breathes air; P_aCO_2 is also reduced, causing hypoventilation. S_aO_2 is reduced to values as low as 90% for several minutes in normal individuals after breathing 50% nitrous oxide in oxygen. Arterial desaturation is greater in elderly patients, if higher concentrations of nitrous oxide have been used, or if P_aCO_2 is initially low because of hyperventilation during anaesthesia.

Diffusion hypoxia is avoided by the administration of oxygen for 10 min after discontinuation of nitrous oxide anaesthesia.

Reduced venous oxygen content

Assuming that oxygen consumption remains unchanged, anaemia or reduced cardiac output results in increased oxygen extraction from circulating arterial blood, and consequently in a reduction in mixed venous oxygen content. In the presence of increased V/Q scatter or intrapulmonary shunt, this causes a variable degree of arterial hypoxaemia. Similarly, if cardiac output remains constant, increased oxygen utilization by the tissues (as may occur during

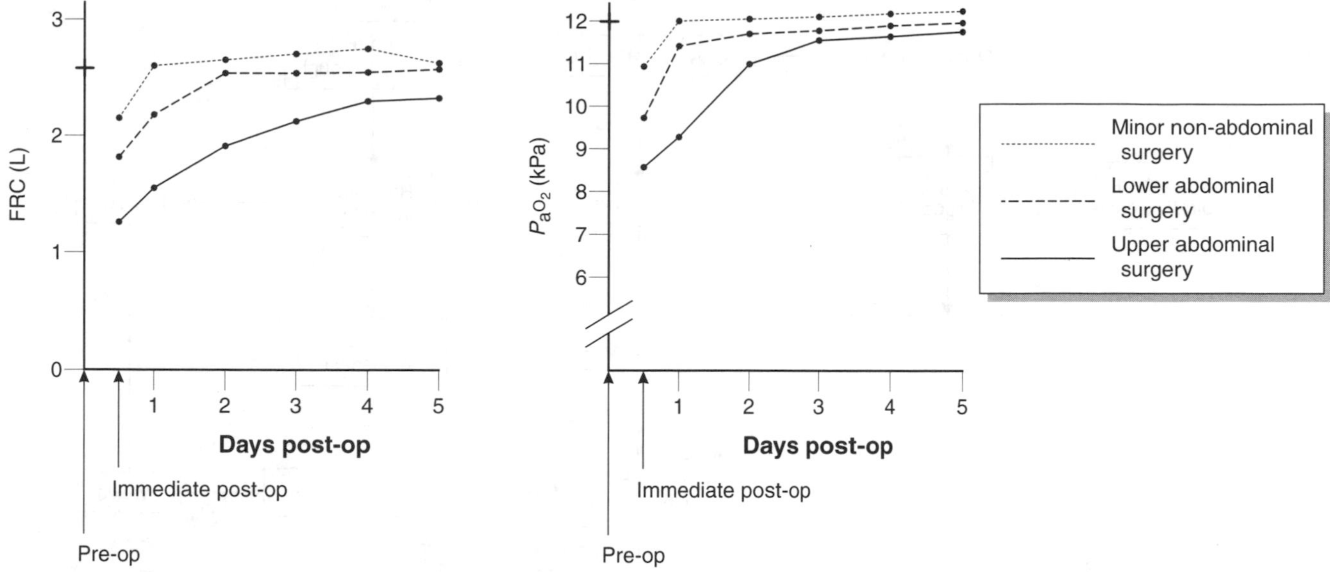

Fig. 41.3
Changes in functional residual capacity (FRC) and arterial oxygen tension (P_aO_2) postoperatively.

shivering, restlessness or malignant hyperthermia) causes a reduction in mixed venous oxygen content and a worsening of arterial hypoxaemia if any shunt is present.

Tissue hypoxia

Oxygenation of the tissues is a function of arterial oxygenation, oxygen carriage in blood, delivery of blood to the tissues and transfer of oxygen from the blood. It may be impaired by respiratory or cardiovascular dysfunction, by severe anaemia or by a leftward shift of the oxyhaemoglobin dissociation curve (reduced P_{50}).

PULMONARY CHANGES AFTER ABDOMINAL SURGERY

Patients with previously normal lungs suffer impairment of oxygenation for at least 48 h after abdominal surgery. The extent of this impairment is related to the site of operation. It is less marked after lower abdominal surgery, more severe if there has been a large incision in the upper abdomen and worst after thoracoabdominal procedures. In these circumstances, the differences between pre- and postoperative P_aO_2 may be as much as 4 kPa.

Impairment of oxygenation in the postoperative period is related to a reduction in FRC. After induction of anaesthesia, there is an abrupt decrease in FRC. The magnitude of the decrease is similar for anaesthetic techniques in which the patient breathes spontaneously and those in which IPPV is employed. Postoperatively, this decrease is maintained by wound pain, which causes spasm of the expiratory muscles, and abdominal distension, which leads to diaphragmatic splinting. This is also influenced by the site of surgical incision; the greatest reduction follows thoracic or upper abdominal surgery. The supine position also reduces FRC.

The reduction in FRC may lead to closing capacity impinging upon the tidal breathing range. This results in small airways closure during normal tidal ventilation. Gas trapping occurs in the affected airways and subsequent absorption of air may lead to the development of small, discrete areas of atelectasis which are not visible on chest X-ray. This occurs mainly in the dependent parts of the lung and may be demonstrated by CT scan very soon after induction of anaesthesia. The result is an increase in the number of areas of low V/Q ratio within the lungs. The relationship between changes in FRC and P_aO_2 postoperatively is shown in Figure 41.3.

In most patients, these abnormalities return towards normal by the fifth or sixth postoperative day. However, if the changes have been marked, the areas of low V/Q ratio may become a focus for infection, particularly in the presence of retained secretions. The following factors contribute to retention of secretions after surgery:

- *Inability to cough.* This results mostly from wound pain. However, excessive sedation may contribute also. Postoperative electrolyte imbalance, especially hypokalaemia or hypophosphataemia, may compound the situation by interfering with muscle function.
- *Suppression of bronchial mucosal ciliary activity.* This results from the use of unhumidified anaesthetic gases.
- *Antisialagogue drugs.* When antisialagogue premedicants have been used, the secretions become more viscid. The dry mucosa itself is more prone to inflammatory reaction. If this occurs, the exudate produced increases the problem still further.
- *Infection.* If pulmonary infection supervenes, impairment of oxygenation may contribute to a lack of cooperation in clearing secretions.

A combination of these factors may result in retention of secretions, leading to areas of visible pulmonary collapse on chest X-ray and an increase in the work of breathing. Ultimately, oxygenation of the blood may become inadequate despite oxygen therapy, or carbon dioxide retention may occur. The sequence of events that culminate in ventilatory failure is shown in Figure 41.4.

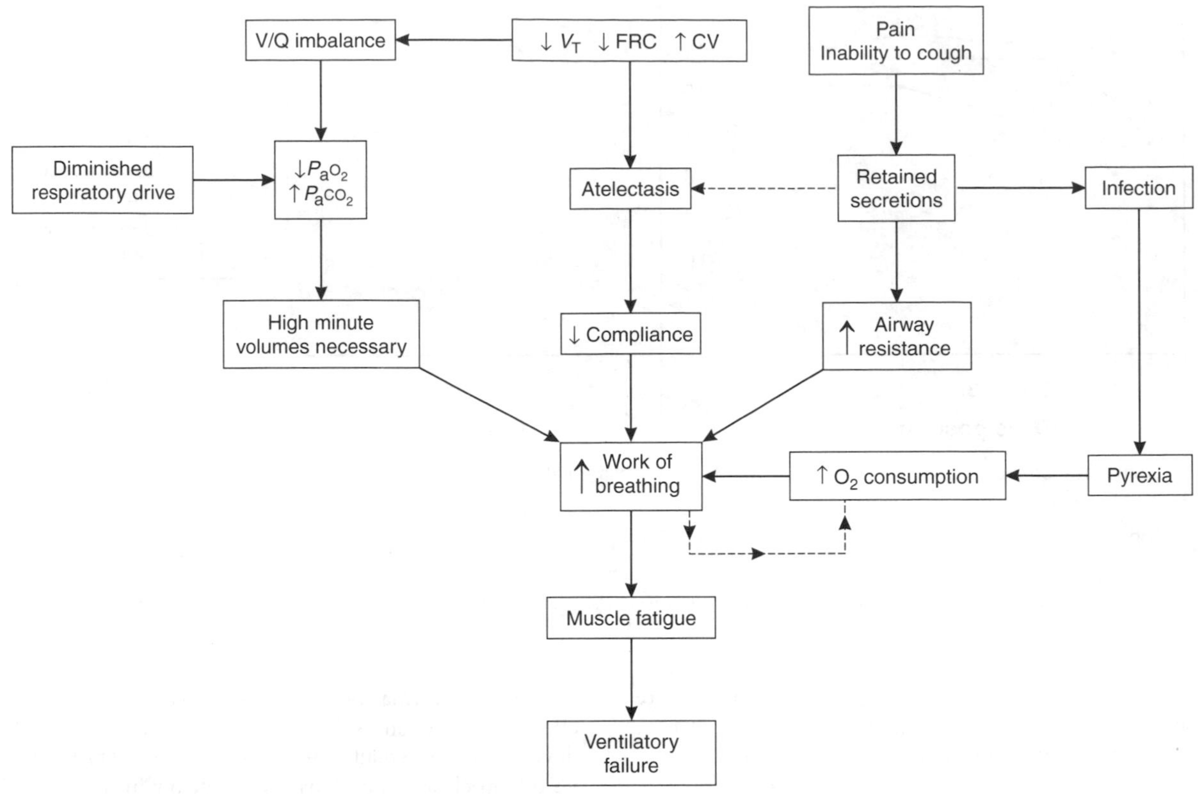

Fig. 41.4
Diagrammatic representation of events that result in postoperative ventilatory failure. V_T, tidal volume; FRC, functional residual capacity; CV, closing volume; *V/Q*, ventilation/perfusion; P_aO_2, arterial oxygen tension; P_aCO_2, arterial carbon dioxide tension.

Predisposing factors

- *Site of surgery.* Pulmonary complications occur more commonly after upper abdominal or thoracic surgery than after lower abdominal operations.
- *Pre-existing respiratory disease* increases the complication rate. This is particularly so in the presence of concurrent infection or excessive secretions.
- *Smokers* have an increased incidence of pulmonary complications compared with non-smokers.
- *Obesity* is associated with a high incidence of pulmonary complications. Obese patients have a low FRC and increased work of breathing postoperatively.

The anaesthetic technique has little effect on the incidence of postoperative pulmonary complications.

Clinical findings

Collapse of lung units

In patients who develop clinical symptoms, the first signs of atelectasis are usually seen within 24 h of operation. The triad of pyrexia, tachycardia and tachypnoea is often present. Temperature is usually in the range of 38–39°C. There is often a productive cough. If atelectasis is extensive, the patient is cyanosed. On physical examination, localizing signs are uncommon unless the area of involvement is large. Chest X-ray reveals patchy areas of atelectasis.

Pneumonia

Lobar pneumonia is rarely seen postoperatively. Bronchopneumonia is more common, especially in the elderly. The onset of symptoms is not as rapid as in atelectasis. There is usually fever and associated tachycardia, with an increase in the ventilatory rate. Physical examination usually reveals areas of consolidation, predominantly at the lung bases, which are evident on chest X-ray.

Treatment

If a pulmonary complication is suspected, a sputum sample should be sent to the laboratory for bacteriological analysis. Appropriate antibiotic therapy may then be started. Intensive physiotherapy should be prescribed in an attempt to remove secretions and re-expand atelectatic areas of the lung.

Patients with pulmonary collapse are usually hypoxaemic, but P_aCO_2 remains normal or may be low as a result of tachypnoea, at least in the early stages. Usually, oxygen in moderate concentrations (30–40%) is sufficient to correct hypoxaemia, but this should be confirmed by blood gas analysis. If the patient fails to respond to these measures, signs of respiratory distress develop. The patient becomes drowsy and ventilation is laboured, with rapid shallow breathing involving the accessory muscles. P_aCO_2 increases and arterial oxygenation deteriorates despite oxygen therapy. The presence of continued deterioration in blood gases is an indication for ventilatory support.

REDUCING PULMONARY COMPLICATIONS

Preoperative

Measures to reduce pulmonary complications should begin preoperatively. Upper and lower respiratory tract infections should be treated before surgery. Dental sepsis and sinus infections should be eradicated. Pre-existing chronic respiratory disorders should be treated so that the patient is in optimal condition before surgery. Spirometry is useful to monitor such treatment, but arterial blood gas analysis is the only assessment which has been demonstrated to correlate well with the need for postoperative ventilatory support. Smoking should be discouraged and weight loss encouraged where indicated. In patients with increased risk factors, heavy premedication should be avoided to ensure minimal ventilatory depression at the end of the procedure.

Intraoperative

At induction, care should be taken not to introduce infection by contaminated equipment. During prolonged procedures, the anaesthetic gases should be humidified. If neuromuscular blocking agents are used, particular care should be taken to ensure that antagonism is adequate.

Postoperative

Analgesia should be optimal to ensure adequate coughing and cooperation during physiotherapy, which should be started as soon as possible after operation.

OXYGEN THERAPY

Hypoxaemia may occur to some degree in any patient during the early recovery period as a result of one or more of the mechanisms described above. Consequently, *all* patients should receive additional oxygen for the first 10 min after general anaesthesia has been discontinued. Oxygen therapy should be continued for a longer period in the presence of any of the conditions listed in Table 41.6.

Oxygen therapy is particularly beneficial in treating hypoxaemia caused by hypoventilation; P_aO_2 is substantially increased by a modest increase in F_IO_2. In contrast, higher concentrations are required in the presence of a shunt fraction in excess of 0.1–0.15 (Fig. 41.5). Known concentrations of oxygen may be administered by a tightly fitting mask supplied with metered flows of air and oxygen via either an anaesthetic breathing system or a CPAP system (see Ch. 60). In small children, an oxygen tent or headbox may be used. However, oxygen is usually administered by less cumbersome disposable equipment.

Oxygen therapy devices

The characteristics of oxygen face masks depend predominantly on their volume, the flow rate of gas supplied and the presence of holes in the side of the mask. If no gas is supplied, face masks act as increased dead space and result in hypercapnia unless minute volume is increased; the increase in dead space is proportional to the volume of the mask. If the mask contains holes, air is entrained readily during inspiration.

When oxygen is supplied, the inspired oxygen concentration increases, but to an extent which depends upon the relationship between the oxygen flow rate and the ventilatory pattern. If there is a pause between expiration and inspiration, the mask fills with oxygen and a high concentration is available at the start of inspiration; during inspiration, the inspired oxygen is diluted by air drawn in through the holes when the inspiratory flow rate exceeds the flow rate of oxygen. During normal tidal ventilation, the peak inspiratory flow rate (PIFR) is 20–30 L min^{-1}, but is considerably higher during deep inspiration or in the hyperventilating patient. If there is no expiratory pause, alveolar gas may be rebreathed from the mask at the start of inspiration; this occurs especially when the oxygen flow rate is low or when no holes are present in the mask. A predictable and constant inspired oxygen concentra-

Table 41.6 Conditions in which prolonged oxygen therapy is required after operation

Hypotension
Ischaemic heart disease
Reduced cardiac output
Anaemia
Obesity
Shivering
Hypothermia
Hyperthermia
Pulmonary oedema
Airway obstruction
After major surgery

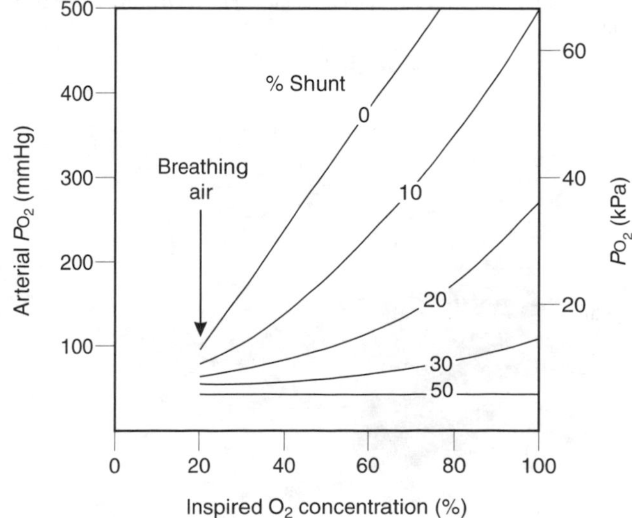

Fig. 41.5
Response of arterial partial pressure of oxygen (P_{O_2}) to increased inspired oxygen concentrations in the presence of various degrees of shunt. Note that, in the presence of shunt, arterial P_{O_2} remains well below the normal value when 100% oxygen is breathed. Nevertheless, useful increases in arterial oxygenation occur with a shunt of up to 30%.

tion may be achieved only if the total gas flow to the mask exceeds the patient's PIFR.

Fixed-performance devices

These masks, also termed high air flow oxygen enrichment (HAFOE) devices, provide a constant and predictable inspired oxygen concentration irrespective of the patient's ventilatory pattern. This is achieved by supplying the mask with oxygen and air at a high total flow rate. Oxygen is passed through a jet which entrains air (Fig. 41.6). The mask is designed in such a way that the total flow rate of gas to the mask exceeds the expected PIFR of most patients who require oxygen therapy. For example, if a jet designed to supply 28% oxygen is supplied with an oxygen flow rate of 4 L min^{-1}, approximately 41 L min^{-1} of air is entrained and a total flow of 45 L min^{-1} passes to the patient's face.

Various types of HAFOE device are available; an example is shown in Figure 41.7. Ventimasks are the most accurate, but a different mask is required for each of the range of oxygen concentrations available. Some manufacturers produce masks in which the jet device can be changed by the user, so that the oxygen concentration may be adjusted as appropriate.

The air-entraining jets of HAFOE devices provide a relatively constant oxygen concentration irrespective of the flow rate of oxygen. The recommended oxygen flow rates are larger when jets providing a high concentration are used (e.g. 8 L min^{-1} for 40%, 15 L min^{-1} for 60%) so that the total flow rate supplied to the mask remains adequate despite the smaller proportion of air entrained. The total flow rates through masks which deliver more than 28% oxygen are between 20 and 30 L min^{-1} when the recommended oxygen flow rates are provided; higher flow rates of oxygen may be used in patients who are thought to have an increased PIFR.

Because of the high fresh gas flow rate, expired gas is rapidly flushed from the mask. Thus, rebreathing does not occur, i.e. fixed-performance devices do not act as an additional dead space.

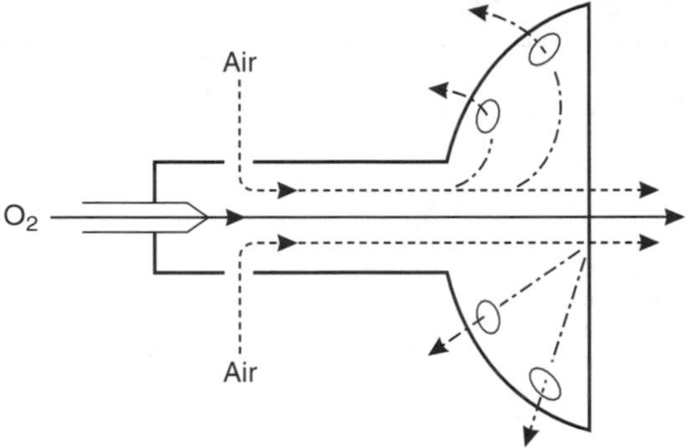

Fig. 41.6
Diagram of high air flow oxygen enrichment (HAFOE) mask (see text for details).

Variable-performance devices

All other disposable oxygen masks and nasal cannulae provide an oxygen concentration which varies with the oxygen flow rate and the patient's ventilatory pattern. Although there is no increase in dead space when nasal cannulae are used, all variable-performance disposable face masks add dead space, the magnitude of which depends on the patient's pattern of ventilation. Table 41.7 gives an indication of the range of oxygen concentrations achieved with a number of commonly used variable-performance devices; an example is are shown in Figure 41.8.

Oxygen therapy in the recovery ward

The large majority of patients recovering after anaesthesia require only a modest increase in $F_{I}O_2$ to overcome the combined effects of mild hypoventilation, diffusion hypoxia and some degree of increased V/Q scatter. Usually, an inspired concentration of 30% is adequate and this may be achieved in most instances by supplying an oxygen flow rate of 4 L min^{-1} to any of the variable perform-

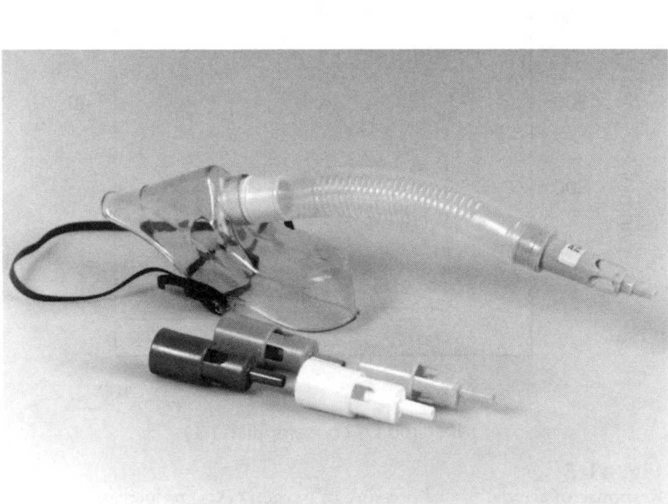

Fig. 41.7
A high air flow oxygen enrichment (HAFOE) face mask.

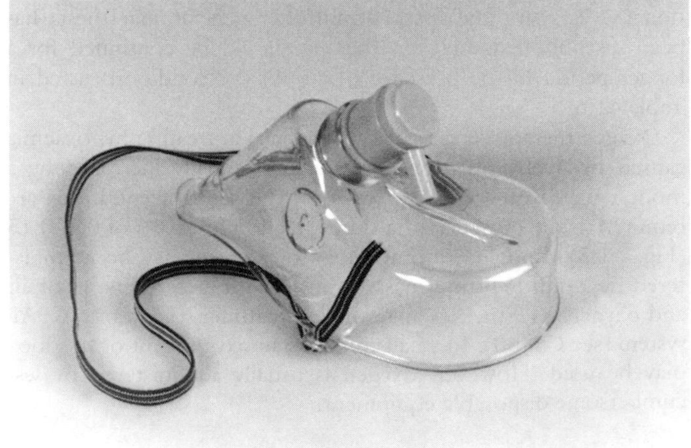

Fig. 41.8
A variable performance oxygen face mask.

Table 41.7 Oxygen masks, flow rates and approximate oxygen concentration delivered

Type of mask	Oxygen flow ($L\ min^{-1}$)	Oxygen concentration (%)
Edinburgh	1	24–29
	2	29–36
	4	33–39
Nasal cannulae	1	25–29
	2	29–35
	4	32–39
Hudson	2	24–38
	4	35–45
	6	51–61
	8	57–67
	10	61–73
MC	2	28–50
	4	41–70
	6	53–74
	8	60–77
	10	67–81

ance devices (Table 41.7). However, in a small proportion of patients, it is necessary to control the $F_{I}O_2$ more strictly.

Controlled oxygen therapy

This is required in two categories of patient:

- Some patients with chronic bronchitis develop chronic hypercapnia, and ventilatory drive is produced largely by hypoxaemia. If P_aO_2 increases above the level which stimulates breathing, ventilatory depression may occur. However, these patients may become dangerously hypoxaemic after anaesthesia, and oxygen therapy is required so that adequate oxygenation of the tissues is maintained. The aim of oxygen therapy in these circumstances is to increase arterial oxygen content without an excessive increase in P_aO_2. This is achieved by a modest increase in $F_{I}O_2$. In the hypoxaemic patient, the relationship between arterial oxygen tension and saturation (and therefore oxygen content) is represented by the steep portion of the oxyhaemoglobin dissociation curve, and a small increase in oxygen tension results in significant increases in saturation and oxygen content (Fig. 41.9).
  The use of a variable-performance device in these patients is unsatisfactory, as an unacceptably high $F_{I}O_2$ may be delivered. A fixed-performance device delivering 24% oxygen should be used initially, and the response assessed. If the patient remains clinically well, and the P_aCO_2 does not increase by more than 1–1.5 kPa, 28% oxygen – and subsequently higher concentrations – may be administered if further increases in P_aO_2 are desirable.
  Most patients with chronic bronchitis do not depend on hypoxaemia for respiratory drive and should not be denied adequate inspired concentrations of oxygen. Patients at risk can usually be detected preoperatively by the presence of central cyanosis; hypoxaemia and hypercapnia are confirmed by blood gas analysis.
- Patients with increased shunt, e.g. those with acute respiratory distress syndrome (ARDS), pulmonary oedema or pulmonary consolidation, may require a high inspired oxygen concentration (Fig. 41.5), which cannot be guaranteed if a variable-performance device is used. In addition, serial blood gas analysis is normally used to assess improvement or

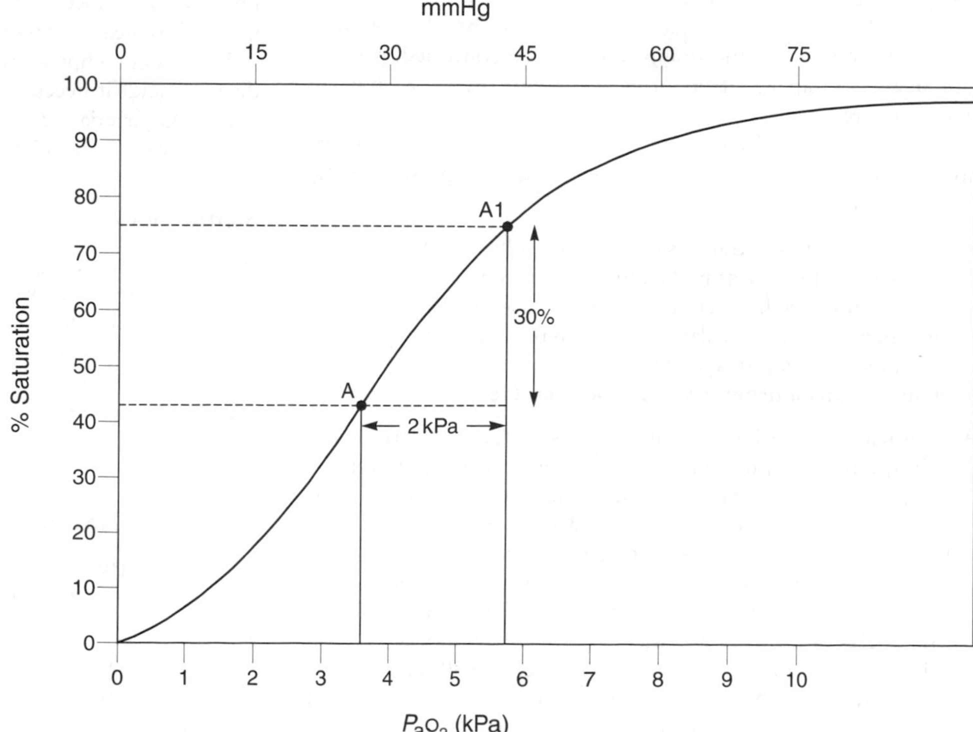

Fig. 41.9
Effect of controlled oxygen therapy on oxygen saturation in a hypoxaemic chronic bronchitic patient. A small increase in inspired oxygen concentration produces a modest increase in arterial oxygen tension (P_aO_2) but a substantial increase in arterial oxygen saturation.

deterioration in their condition. Changes in $P_{a}O_2$ and the degree of shunt may be interpreted accurately only if the $F_{I}O_2$ is known. Thus, controlled oxygen therapy should be employed, using a fixed-performance device which delivers 40% oxygen or more.

CARDIOVASCULAR SYSTEM

HYPOTENSION

Residual effects of anaesthetic drugs

Hypotension may result from the residual vasodilator effect of i.v. or inhalation anaesthetic drugs, particularly in patients who are experiencing little pain. Subarachnoid or epidural nerve block may also cause hypotension which persists into the postoperative period. Heart rate is seldom elevated, and the peripheries are warm if anaesthetic drugs or regional anaesthesia are the cause of hypotension. A systolic arterial pressure of 80–90 mmHg is tolerated well except by the elderly or patients with myocardial disease. No treatment is required in most patients. Elevation of the legs often increases arterial pressure by increasing venous return. Intravenous infusion of 7–10 ml kg^{-1} of colloid solution is usually effective in restoring normotension if there is concern; infusion should be undertaken cautiously in elderly patients and in those with cardiovascular disease.

Other causes of hypotension in the recovery period are more sinister and must be excluded before it may be assumed that residual anaesthesia is responsible.

Hypovolaemia

This may result from inadequate or inappropriate replacement of preoperative or intraoperative fluid and blood losses, or from postoperative haemorrhage. Surgical bleeding may be obvious from inspection of wounds and drains, but may be concealed, particularly in the abdomen, retroperitoneal space or thorax, even when drains are present.

Inadequate surgical haemostasis is the usual cause of postoperative bleeding, but coagulation disorders may be present in the following circumstances:

- after massive blood transfusion, which results in decreased concentrations of clotting factors and reduced platelet numbers
- pre-existing bleeding tendency, e.g. haemophilia
- disseminated intravascular coagulation produced by sepsis, amniotic fluid embolism, etc.
- if anticoagulant drugs have been administered.

A coagulation disorder is frequently associated with prolonged bleeding after venepuncture, oozing from the wound and the development of petechiae or bruises. The investigation and management of coagulation disorders are discussed in Chapter 23.

Hypotension caused by hypovolaemia is accompanied by signs of poor peripheral perfusion, e.g. cold, clammy extremities and pallor. Tachycardia may be present but is masked, not infrequently, by the effects of drugs (e.g. anticholinesterases, β-blockers). CVP may be low or normal. Urine output is reduced (< 30 ml h^{-1}). The effects of hypovolaemia on arterial pressure are more pronounced in the presence of vasodilatation or reduced myocardial contractility resulting from the effects of residual anaesthetic drugs, or antihypertensive, calcium channel or β-blocker therapy. In patients who have undergone prolonged surgery, and particularly if the core temperature is below normal, vasoconstriction may be profound and hypovolaemia may be unmasked at a relatively late stage, as normal vasomotor tone returns with rewarming.

Treatment comprises elevation of the legs and administration of appropriate crystalloid or colloid solutions; in elderly or high-risk patients, or if hypovolaemia is profound, administration of fluids should be monitored by measurement of CVP. Clotting factors or platelets should be administered if appropriate, and surgical bleeding treated by re-operation if necessary.

Arrhythmias

These are discussed below (p. 537).

Ventricular failure

Left or right ventricular failure may cause hypotension. Right ventricular failure is uncommon in the postoperative period and is secondary usually to acute pulmonary disease, e.g. ARDS.

Left ventricular failure in the postoperative period is associated most commonly with perioperative myocardial infarction or overtransfusion. The peripheral circulation is poor. Usually, tachycardia is present and there is clinical and radiological evidence of pulmonary oedema. Jugular venous pulse and CVP are usually elevated, but they may remain normal despite a substantial increase in left atrial pressure, particularly if right ventricular hypertrophy is present. Thus, left ventricular failure may be misdiagnosed as hypovolaemia in some patients, and in some instances the two conditions coexist. If there is doubt about the diagnosis, a small fluid load may be administered (no more than 200 ml) and the response of arterial pressure and CVP monitored; if the diagnosis remains uncertain, a pulmonary artery catheter should be inserted to measure pulmonary artery and left atrial pressures.

Treatment comprises administration of oxygen, fluid restriction, diuretics and, if necessary, inotropic support or vasodilator therapy. ECG, arterial pressure and CVP should be monitored. The possibility of myocardial infarction should be investigated.

Septic shock

In this condition, hypotension is accompanied by raised cardiac output and peripheral vasodilatation in the early stages, followed by vasoconstriction and reduced cardiac output caused partly by loss of fluid from the circulation. CVP monitoring is essential and a pulmonary artery catheter is desirable. Treatment includes infusion of appropriate volumes of colloid solutions, inotropic support, antibiotic therapy and, if necessary, surgical treatment of the source.

HYPERTENSION

Arterial hypertension is a common complication in the early postoperative period. The causes include the following:

- pain
- pre-existing hypertension, particularly if controlled inadequately
- hypoxaemia

- hypercapnia
- administration of vasopressor drugs
- after aortic surgery, as a result partly of increased plasma concentration of renin.

A combination of these causes may be present. Hypertension results in increased cardiac work and myocardial oxygen consumption, and may result in myocardial ischaemia or infarction, left ventricular failure or cerebral haemorrhage. The cause should be elicited rapidly and treated if possible. Oxygen should be administered. If no remediable cause is found, vasodilatation with hydralazine, sodium nitroprusside or glyceryl trinitrate should be started. Alternatively, labetalol may be used, particularly if there is a degree of tachycardia. Such treatment may unmask hypovolaemia (see above) and additional i.v. fluids may be required.

ARRHYTHMIAS (see also p. 434).

These are common during and immediately after anaesthesia. The majority are benign and require no treatment. However, the cause should be sought and their effect on the circulation assessed. Common causes include the following:

- residual anaesthetic agents
- hypercapnia
- hypoxaemia
- electrolyte or acid–base disturbance
- vagal stimulation, e.g. by tracheal tube or suction catheters
- myocardial ischaemia or infarction
- pain.

Sinus tachycardia is common and may be a reflex response to hypovolaemia or hypotension. It also occurs in the presence of hypercapnia, anaemia or hypoxaemia, and if the metabolic rate is elevated by fever, shivering, restlessness or malignant hyperthermia. The commonest cause is pain. Tachycardia increases myocardial oxygen consumption and decreases coronary artery perfusion by reducing diastolic time. The combination of arterial hypertension and tachycardia is dangerous in the presence of ischaemic heart disease and should *not* be allowed to persist, as it may result in myocardial infarction. Sinus tachycardia should be treated specifically only if it persists after therapy for underlying causes has been given; a small i.v. dose of a cardioselective β-blocker (e.g. metoprolol 1–2 mg) should be administered slowly. The EGG must be monitored.

Sinus bradycardia may result from inadequate antagonism by atropine or vagal stimulation by neostigmine, pharyngeal stimulation during suction or the residual effects of volatile anaesthetic agents. Other causes include hypoxaemia (especially in neonates and infants), raised intracranial pressure, myocardial infarction and some cardiac drugs, e.g. β-blockers, digoxin. Oxygen should be administered. Intravenous atropine is usually effective and should be given in a dose of 0.4–0.6 mg in adults if the heart rate is less than 45 beats min^{-1} or if there is associated hypotension. In the presence of severe bradycardia, external cardiac massage is necessary to increase cardiac output.

Bradycardia may also occur as a result of complete heart block.

Supraventricular arrhythmias, including atrial fibrillation, flutter or supraventricular tachycardia, are treated as in other circumstances. Rapid arrhythmias are best treated by cardioversion, but may require pharmacological therapy to prevent recurrence. Nodal rhythm with a normal heart rate is common in the perioperative period, particularly when volatile anaesthetic agents have been used. Supraventricular arrhythmias may cause moderate hypotension because of the loss of synchronization between atrial and ventricular contractions.

Ventricular arrhythmias. Premature ventricular contractions (PVCs) may require treatment with i.v. lidocaine 1–1.5 mg kg^{-1} if they are frequent (< 5 min^{-1}), multifocal or occur close to the preceding T wave; however, most cardiologists regard PVCs as benign if cardiac output is adequate. Ventricular tachycardia requires immediate treatment with lidocaine or cardioversion. The management of ventricular fibrillation and asystole are discussed in Chapter 35.

CONDUCTION DEFECTS

In the perioperative period, these usually occur in patients with pre-existing heart disease (see p. 435). Heart rate and cardiac output in complete heart block may increase in response to isoproterenol, but electrical pacing should be started as soon as possible. Patients who develop second-degree heart block during anaesthesia or in the recovery ward should be transferred to a coronary care or intensive therapy unit for an appropriate period of observation.

MYOCARDIAL ISCHAEMIA

This occurs most commonly in patients with pre-existing coronary artery disease, and most often in the presence of hypoxaemia, hypotension, hypertension or tachycardia. The ECG should be monitored throughout the recovery period in patients known to be at risk, and precipitating factors should be avoided. Angina occurring during the recovery period should be treated by elimination of any predisposing factor and administration of glyceryl trinitrate sublingually or intravenously.

MYOCARDIAL INFARCTION

The average incidence of myocardial infarction (MI) is 1–2% in unselected patients over 40 years of age undergoing major noncardiac surgery. Pre-existing coronary artery disease and, in particular, evidence of a previous MI result in a higher risk. Mortality in patients who suffer a perioperative MI may be as high as 60%. Perioperative MI occurs most commonly on the third postoperative day, but may happen at any time during or after surgery.

A number of factors which may be detected during preoperative assessment are known to increase the likelihood of perioperative MI. The most important of these is the time interval between surgery and a previous MI. One extensive study of risk factors which might predict major cardiac complications (including, but not exclusively, MI) showed that preoperative evidence of cardiac failure, arrhythmias (of any type) or aortic stenosis, and age were also associated with a high risk. In addition, there is evidence that pre-existing uncontrolled hypertension is associated with increased risk. These problems are discussed more fully in Chapter 34.

The incidence of perioperative MI is related also to intraoperative and postoperative factors. The magnitude of surgery is an important determinant; in patients with a history of previous MI, the incidence of perioperative reinfarction associated with major vascular surgery is considerably higher than when surgery is performed outside the thorax and abdomen. In patients with ischaemic heart disease, postoperative MI is more likely if there is evidence of ischaemic changes on ECG during operation. Such changes are associated most commonly with episodes of intraoperative hypotension, hypertension or tachycardia; the last two occur most frequently in response to noxious stimuli, e.g. tracheal intubation, surgical incision. The drugs used and the manner in which they are employed by the anaesthetist influence the incidences of both intraoperative ischaemia and perioperative MI. Regional anaesthesia is not associated with a reduction in risk when major surgery is undertaken.

Reduction of risk

The incidence of perioperative MI may be reduced by the following:

Identification of patients at risk. Elective surgery should be postponed if possible until at least 3 months after a previous MI.

Treatment of risk factors. Cardiac failure, hypertension and arrhythmias should be controlled before surgery. If necessary, the operation should be postponed until control is achieved. Coronary artery bypass grafting or aortic valve replacement may be required in patients with severe coronary artery disease or aortic stenosis, respectively, before other major abdominal or thoracic surgery is undertaken.

Avoidance of ischaemia. The anaesthetic technique and postoperative management should ensure adequate oxygenation of the myocardium and should minimize myocardial oxygen demand (see Ch. 35).

Monitoring. ECG must be monitored throughout anaesthesia, including induction, in all patients at risk; the CM5 electrode configuration (see Fig. 38.2) is suitable for detection of ischaemic changes. Arterial pressure should be monitored regularly, and continuously in patients undergoing major surgery. Monitoring of right and left atrial pressures by central venous and pulmonary artery catheterization, and prompt treatment of abnormalities which occur during operation and in the early postoperative period reduce the incidence of perioperative MI.

Diagnosis

Perioperative MI may be difficult to diagnose. It occurs most commonly on the third postoperative day. The classic distribution of pain is present in only 25% of patients.

The diagnosis should be considered in any patient at risk who develops an arrhythmia or becomes hypotensive in the postoperative period. Premature ventricular contractions occur in 90% of patients who experience an MI; sinus bradycardia and the development of any degree of atrioventricular conduction defect are also common. There is often a pyrexia of up to 39°C. The diagnosis is confirmed by changes in serial ECG recordings and/or cardiac enzymes.

OTHER MAJOR POSTOPERATIVE COMPLICATIONS

DEEP VENOUS THROMBOSIS (DVT)

The main factors postulated by Virchow as contributing to the formation of venous thrombi are:

- changes in the composition of blood
- damage to walls of blood vessels
- decreased blood flow.

However, the exact trigger mechanism which initiates thrombosis remains unknown.

Risk factors

A higher incidence of DVT has been reported in patients with:

- extensive trauma
- infection
- heart failure
- blood dyscrasias
- malignancy
- metabolic disorders.

DVT is commoner after hip, pelvic and abdominal surgery than after other types of surgery. There is a well-established association between spontaneous DVT and oestrogen, and DVT may occur in women who take some types of oral contraceptive pill. The number of women who develop this complication is small. However, the incidence increases if surgery is performed while the patient is currently taking the drug. The risk is reduced but not abolished if a low-oestrogen (50 µg or less) preparation is used. Women who take hormone replacement therapy are also at increased risk.

Diagnosis

Approximately 70% of patients with a DVT have neither symptoms nor signs. Fifty per cent of patients with calf pain and tenderness on dorsiflexion of the foot do not have a DVT. Often there is mild pyrexia.

Investigations

Venography

This is an effective method for demonstrating most thrombi of clinical importance.

Radioactive fibrinogen uptake

Iodine-labelled fibrinogen is taken up preferentially by a growing thrombus. The investigation is quick to perform and may detect small thrombi in the calf vessels. Its main disadvantage is that it cannot be used to detect iliac and pelvic vein thrombi, although most thrombi in surgical patients occur in the calf. It does not correlate well with either venography or the development of pulmonary embolism and is associated with a high incidence of false-positive results.

Ultrasonography

This is non-invasive and simple to perform. However, it is insensitive and is useful only for confirming the diagnosis of a major thrombus.

Prophylaxis

Elimination of stasis

The efficacy of early ambulation after operation in reducing the incidence of DVT is not clear. Attempts directed at preventing stasis, including physiotherapy, elastic stockings and elevation of the feet, may reduce the incidence of DVT but have not been shown to influence the incidence of pulmonary embolism.

Two methods are currently used for increasing venous return from the lower limbs during surgery:

- *Electrical stimulation of the calf muscles.* A low-voltage current is applied across the calf to contract the muscles every 2–4 s.
- *Pneumatic compression of the calves.* The legs are encased in an envelope of plastic material, which is inflated and deflated rhythmically, thus squeezing the calves intermittently. This technique may be continued postoperatively.

Although the incidence of DVT is substantially reduced by these techniques, there is no reduction in the incidence of, or mortality from, pulmonary embolism.

Alteration of blood coagulability

Platelet aggregation

Various drugs which interfere with different aspects of platelet function have been investigated. These include dextran 70, dipyridamole, aspirin and chloroquine. There is no evidence to suggest that dipyridamole or aspirin prevents DVT. Infusion of dextran during and after surgery may reduce the incidence of fatal postoperative pulmonary embolism but its role in the prevention of peripheral venous thrombosis is undetermined.

The coagulation mechanism

Oral anticoagulant instituted before operation is the only well-substantiated method of reducing venous thrombosis. However, there is a risk of increased surgical haemorrhage. Low-dose heparin, 5000 units subcutaneously 2 h before operation and subsequently at 8 or 12 h intervals until the patient is mobile, reduces the risk of DVT and carries little risk of major haemorrhage. If DVT does occur, it is more likely to be confined to the calf if heparin has been given. Subcutaneous heparin reduces the incidence of fatal pulmonary embolism. There is evidence that low-molecular-weight heparins (dalteparin, enoxaparin and tinzaparin) are more effective antithrombotics than standard heparin in orthopaedic surgery, and they are as effective and safe in other types of surgery. They have a longer duration of action and are therefore more convenient.

PULMONARY EMBOLISM

This term covers a range of events from sudden circulatory collapse and death, through minor episodes of pleurisy and haemoptysis, to the long-standing disability of patients with chronic thromboembolic pulmonary hypertension. The acute forms of pulmonary embolism are encountered after anaesthesia and surgery. In the elderly, multiple small pulmonary emboli may be misdiagnosed as bronchopneumonia.

The common sites of origin for thrombi which result in pulmonary embolus are the veins of the pelvis and lower extremities. The most common time for presentation of a postoperative pulmonary embolism is during the second week. In some patients, predisposing factors may have existed preoperatively for some time, and the whole time-scale of events may be shifted; the embolus may occur at the time of, or shortly after, surgery.

Diagnosis

Presenting features

The principal features are circulatory collapse and sudden dyspnoea, often associated with chest pain. If the embolus is large, the pulmonary artery outflow is blocked and sudden death results. If the embolus involves more than 50% of the main pulmonary arteries, it is termed massive.

Physical signs

A low cardiac output state develops. Tachypnoea and central cyanosis are usual. There is arterial hypotension, sinus tachycardia and a constricted peripheral circulation. The jugular venous pressure is elevated. A fourth heart sound is usually present on auscultation.

Investigations

ECG (Fig. 41.10). This reflects acute right ventricular strain, with features that often include right axis deviation, T-wave inversion in leads V_1–V_4 and sometimes right bundle branch block. The classic S1–Q3–T3 pattern is less common.

Chest X-ray. This is often unremarkable but may show areas of oligaemia reflecting pulmonary vascular obstruction.

Arterial blood gases. There is usually hypoxaemia because of ventilation–perfusion imbalance, and hypocapnia resulting from hyperventilation.

Perfusion and ventilation lung scans. The perfusion scan shows uneven circulation, with perfusion defects delineating the emboli. A simultaneous ventilation scan is usually normal.

Pulmonary angiography. This provides a definitive diagnosis of major obstruction in the pulmonary circulation. This investigation is particularly useful if the patient is critically ill and the diagnosis is in doubt, and is essential if pulmonary embolectomy is planned. However, it is invasive and normally requires transfer of the patient to the X-ray department.

Treatment

DVT

The mainstay of therapy is anticoagulation. Initially, i.v. heparin is infused in a dose of 40 000 units day^{-1}. At the same time, oral anticoagulant therapy is started. Warfarin is used most commonly. Heparin may be discontinued after 48 h. Oral anticoagulants are continued for at least 3 months.

Pulmonary embolism

Immediate treatment consists of administration of oxygen in a high concentration and i.v. heparin. Digoxin is often useful. Sometimes it is necessary to use additional inotropic support for the circulation. Heparin is continued for 5–6 days. Oral anticoagulant therapy is started as soon as possible and is continued for at least 6 months.

Massive pulmonary embolus which does not respond to the above measures may warrant the use of thrombolytic agents, e.g.

streptokinase. The risk of haemorrhage with these agents is considerably higher than with heparin. If the cardiovascular effects of the embolism are life-threatening, open pulmonary embolectomy under cardiopulmonary bypass may be considered.

POSTOPERATIVE RENAL DYSFUNCTION

The kidney is vulnerable to a wide range of drugs and chemicals. It is particularly susceptible to toxic substances for the following reasons:

- large blood flow per unit mass
- high oxygen consumption
- non-resorbable substances concentrated by tubules
- permeability of tubular cells.

All anaesthetic techniques depress renal blood flow and, secondary to this, interfere with renal function. Provided that prolonged hypotension is avoided, the effects are temporary. However, there is the potential for some anaesthetic agents to produce permanent renal damage.

The administration of the volatile anaesthetic agent methoxyflurane was associated with a relatively high incidence of renal dysfunction. Clinically, the defect was characterized by failure of the concentrating ability of the kidney. In certain instances, this progressed to high-output renal failure. The nephrotoxicity of methoxyflurane was dose-dependent and was caused by inorganic fluoride ions produced during its metabolism. Administration of methoxyflurane in combination with other nephrotoxic drugs, e.g. aminoglycosides, was particularly hazardous.

Large quantities of fluoride ion are also produced during metabolism of enflurane and sevoflurane, although a much smaller proportion of these drugs (2–3%) is metabolized in comparison to methoxyflurane (45%). Concentrations of fluoride ion in blood following administration of sevoflurane may exceed the value associated with renal impairment after anaesthesia with methoxyflurane. However, there has been no evidence to suggest that either enflurane or sevoflurane is associated with renal impairment related to the production of fluoride ions. The reason is probably related to the fact that the very soluble methoxyflurane continues to be metabolized for some days, resulting in prolonged production of fluoride ions, whereas the peak concentrations associated with the use of enflurane and sevoflurane are of short duration because of their relative insolubility in tissues.

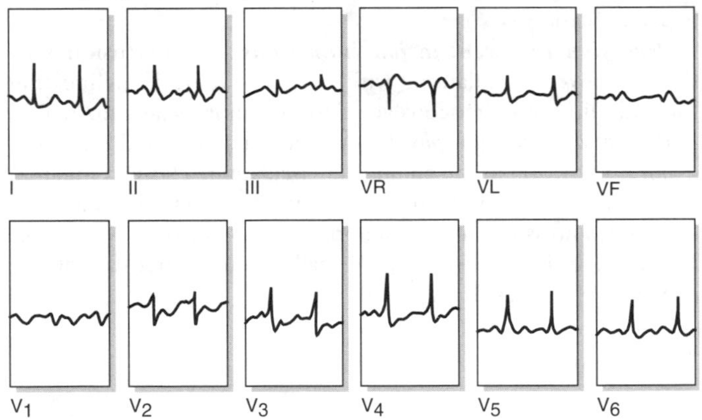

Fig 41.10
Typical electrocardiogram changes in plumonary embolism.

POSTOPERATIVE HEPATIC DYSFUNCTION

There are many causes of postoperative hepatic dysfunction (Table 41.8). Most patients show no evidence of hepatic damage after anaesthesia and surgery. If it occurs, it is usually attributable to one of the causes shown in Table 41.8. However, if other causes are excluded, consideration should be given to the possibility of hepatotoxicity from anaesthetic drugs.

Chloroform was the first anaesthetic agent to be suspected of causing hepatic damage. In large doses, chloroform is a direct hepatotoxin, and after anaesthesia a hepatitis-like syndrome, with histological evidence of centrilobular hepatic necrosis, occurred occasionally. Methoxyflurane was also associated with hepatic damage, causing a syndrome clinically similar to viral hepatitis. Two of the volatile agents in current use have been implicated in cases of postoperative hepatic dysfunction.

Halothane

Attention was first focused on halothane-associated hepatitis in the early 1960s. Numerous case reports prompted institution in 1969 of the largest retrospective anaesthetic study ever undertaken (United States National Halothane Study). The incidence and causes of fatal hepatic necrosis occurring within 6 days of anaesthesia were reviewed. The overall incidence was 1 in 10 000; that associated with halothane was 1 in 35 000 and was no greater than the incidence associated with other anaesthetic agents. However, it is believed at present that there is a small number of patients who develop post-anaesthetic jaundice in which halothane is the aetiological agent.

The histological picture of halothane-associated hepatitis is similar to that seen in type A viral hepatitis. Clinically, there is hepato-

Table 41.8 Causes of postoperative hepatic dysfunction

Increased bilirubin load	Hepatocellular damage	Extrahepatic biliary obstruction
Blood transfusion	Pre-existing liver disease	Gallstones
Haemolysis and haemolytic disease	Viral hepatitis	Ascending cholangitis
Abnormalities of bilirubin metabolism	Sepsis Hypotension/hypoxia Drug-induced hepatitis Congestive heart failure	Pancreatitis Surgical misadventure

cellular jaundice, with elevation of the aminotransferase enzymes. The exact mechanism of liver damage is not known. At present, there are two main hypotheses:

- Metabolites of reductive halothane metabolism bind covalently to hepatocyte macromolecules, causing hepato cellular damage.
- Halothane or its metabolites react with hepatocyte proteins to form antigenic compounds, against which the body mounts an immune response that results in hepatocellular damage.

Antibodies to halothane have been demonstrated in patients who have suffered hepatic damage after administration of the drug. At present, this is the most promising method for evaluating the aetiology of a condition which has been a source of great controversy.

The following groups of patients are believed to be at the greatest risk of developing hepatic dysfunction after halothane anaesthesia:

- patients subjected to repeated halothane anaesthetics, especially within a 3-month period
- patients who have developed unexplained pyrexia or jaundice after a previous halothane anaesthetic
- obese patients, particularly women.

Enflurane

Several causes of unexplained jaundice have been reported after the use of enflurane.

OTHER COMPLICATIONS (Table 41.9)

LOCAL VASCULAR COMPLICATIONS

Haematoma formation is probably the commonest complication of i.v. injection. This usually results from inadequate pressure at the injection site after removal of the needle. Phlebitis, thrombosis or thrombophlebitis may occur after intravenous injections. Most drugs used currently by anaesthetists are associated with low incidences of these complications; intravenous diazepam is a potent cause of phlebitis, although the formulation of diazepam in a fat emulsion (Diazemuls) has overcome this problem.

Intravenous infusions commonly cause thrombophlebitis. The incidence is related to the duration of infusion, and this is more important than the type of cannula used. Thrombophlebitis is rare if the infusion site is changed every 12 h. If it is changed every 72 h, the incidence of thrombophlebitis is 70%. Cannulae constructed from polytetrafluorethylene (Teflon) appear to be the least thrombogenic of those available.

Arterial cannulation is commonly performed to permit continuous monitoring of systemic arterial pressure during major surgery. Unfortunately, it is not without adverse sequelae. Intimal damage may lead to thrombosis and occasionally aneurysm formation. Recannulation of the vessel generally occurs, even when the vessel has been completely occluded. Nevertheless, gangrene of the extremities is an occasional complication, particularly if the brachial artery is used rather than the radial artery. Ischaemia of the hand or fingers may occur after radial artery cannulation if there is inadequate collateral circulation.

It has been suggested that a modified Allen's test should be performed to assess the adequacy of the collateral circulation through the ulnar artery before radial artery cannulation. The patient is asked to clench the fist, and radial and ulnar arteries are compressed by the examiner. The patient is subsequently instructed to unclench the fist; the examiner releases the ulnar artery and observes the palm of the hand. If there is adequate collateral flow, prompt return of colour to the palm is seen; if there is little or no return of colour within 15 s, the collateral flow is poor. However, there is some doubt about the relationship between the results of Allen's test and the incidence of ischaemic episodes after radial artery cannulation. After an arterial cannula has been inserted, regular checks should be made to ensure that there is no evidence of ischaemia in the area supplied by the artery; if detected at an early stage, permanent damage can be avoided.

The incidence of thrombosis after arterial cannulation is reduced by the use of a cannula made of Teflon and of a diameter that is small relative to the size of the artery. A 20-gauge cannula is appropriate in the adult, and a 22- or 24-gauge cannula in children. Arterial damage is also reduced by avoiding multiple punctures of the artery during cannulation. The incidence of radial artery thrombosis is highest in the presence of sepsis, low cardiac output states and when the duration of cannulation is prolonged beyond 24 h.

NAUSEA AND VOMITING

Although often regarded by medical and nursing staff as only a minor complication of anaesthesia and surgery, nausea and vomiting are frequently the cause of great distress to patients. Many studies have been undertaken to investigate nausea and vomiting after anaesthesia and surgery. The incidence varies from 14 to 82%, the wide range resulting partly from differences in design of studies. Many factors contribute to the aetiology of postoperative nausea and vomiting and these are discussed in detail in Chapter 21.

Prevention and treatment

The incidence of postoperative vomiting may be reduced by careful selection of drugs in the perioperative period, and the prophylactic use of antiemetic agents (see Ch. 21).

Table 41.9 Minor morbidity resulting from anaesthesia
Nausea and vomiting
Related to operation site
Females > males
Sore throat
Up to 70% of patients
Hoarseness
Laryngeal granulomata
Headache
Up to 60% of patients
Backache
Discomfort from catheters, drains, nasogastric tubes
Anxiety
Muscle pains
Up to 100% of those who receive succinylcholine
Shivering
Drowsiness
Anorexia
Disorientation
Thrombophlebitis at injection site
Bruised or cut lip
Chipped teeth
Corneal abrasions

HEADACHE

The reported incidence of severe headache after anaesthesia and surgery ranges from 12 to 35%, but up to 60% of patients complain of some headache. Individuals who are susceptible to headaches caused by stress, etc. are more likely to complain of postoperative headache. Most investigations have failed to identify any single agent as being responsible for postoperative headache after general anaesthesia. Severe postural headache may occur after dural puncture (see p. 563).

SORE THROAT

Up to 80% of patients complain of sore throat after anaesthesia and surgery. Some of the common causes include:

- *Trauma during tracheal intubation.* Damage to the pharynx and tonsillar fauces may be caused by the laryngoscope blade.
- *Trauma to the larynx.* This is more likely if a red rubber tracheal rube is used rather than a plastic disposable tube, or if the tube has been forced through the vocal cords. A poorly stabilized tube causes more frictional damage to the larynx than one which is securely stabilized.
- *Trauma to the pharynx.* This may occur during passage of a nasogastric tube or insertion of an oropharyngeal or laryngeal mask airway, and is particularly common when a throat pack has been used. Occasionally, the pharynx or upper oesophagus may be perforated during insertion of a nasogastric tube, or during difficult tracheal intubation, and severe pain in the throat is often the first symptom. Sore throat is likely if a nasogastric tube remains in situ during the postoperative period.
- *Other factors.* The mucous membranes of the mouth, pharynx and upper airway are sensitive to the effects of unhumidified gases; the drying effect of anaesthetic gases may cause postoperative sore throat. The antisialagogue effect of anticholinergic drugs may also contribute to this symptom.

The use of topical local anaesthetics does not reduce the incidence of sore throat. Lubrication of the tracheal tube is effective in reducing the incidence, although there is no difference in this respect between plain or local anaesthetic jellies. However, there is little difference in the incidence of sore throat between an anaesthetic technique in which tracheal intubation is employed and one in which only an oropharyngeal or laryngeal mask airway is used.

In the absence of a nasogastric tube, postoperative sore throat is usually of short duration; most patients are symptom-free within 48 h.

HOARSENESS

This should not be confused with sore throat. It is almost always associated with tracheal intubation and is caused predominantly by prolonged abduction of, and pressure on, the vocal cords. However, traumatic tracheal intubation can cause direct trauma to the vocal cords, resulting in prolonged hoarseness.

LARYNGEAL GRANULOMATA

These may occur after tracheal intubation, and arise from areas of ulceration, usually on the posterior aspect of the vocal cords. The ulcers are caused by pressure and consequent ischaemia. Granulomata are reported most frequently after thyroidectomy.

If hoarseness persists for longer than 1 week, indirect laryngoscopy should be performed. If ulceration is present, complete voice rest is indicated. Any granulomata present should be excised; untreated granulomata may grow to such a size as to obstruct the airway.

DENTAL TRAUMA

This is the commonest cause of litigation against anaesthetists. Damage usually occurs during laryngoscopy, especially if tracheal intubation is difficult. Loose teeth, crowns, caps and bridges are particularly susceptible to damage. Preoperative enquiry and examination should alert the anaesthetist to the possibility of damage.

OCULAR COMPLICATIONS

Carelessness is the commonest cause of damage to the eyes; corneal abrasion is the most frequent lesion. The eyes are often allowed to remain open during anaesthesia. The cornea is thus exposed and vulnerable to the irritant effects of skin preparations, dust and surgical drapes. This type of damage is easily prevented by securing the eyelids in a closed position with adhesive tape.

Retinal infarction has occurred on rare occasions as a result of pressure on the eyeball from a face mask. It can also occur if patients are placed in the prone position in such a way that pressure is exerted on the eye, e.g. by a horseshoe head rest.

MUSCLES

Problems associated with inadequate reversal of neuromuscular blocking drugs are discussed above. The detection and treatment of malignant hyperthermia are described on p. 521; it is important to appreciate that this condition may present during recovery.

Shivering

This is a common complication in the recovery room. It may occur in patients who are hypothermic as a result of prolonged surgery, or during injection of local anaesthetic solution into the epidural space. However, in most patients, the onset of shivering is not related to body temperature, and there is evidence from electromyography that the characteristics of postoperative (or post-anaesthetic) shivering differ from those of thermoregulatory shivering. The incidence and severity of shivering are increased in patients who have received an anticholinergic premedication, and women are more likely to shiver in the luteal than in the follicular phase of the menstrual cycle.

Shivering increases oxygen consumption and carbon dioxide production and may result in hypoxaemia and hypercapnia if the response of the respiratory centre to carbon dioxide is impaired by drugs. Oxygen should be administered. A small dose of pethidine is frequently effective in aborting postoperative shivering.

Succinylcholine pains

Muscle pains after succinylcholine are very common, occurring in at least 50% of patients who receive the drug. The muscles involved most frequently are those of the shoulder girdle, neck and thorax. The pain is similar in nature to that caused by viral-related myositis. The incidence is influenced by the following factors:

- *Age.* Succinylcholine pains are unusual in young children and the elderly.
- *Gender.* Women are more susceptible than men. The incidence is reduced during pregnancy.
- *Type of surgery.* There is an increased incidence after minor procedures, when early ambulation is likely.
- *Physical fitness.* The incidence is higher in individuals who are physically fit.
- *Repeated doses.* The incidence is increased if repeated doses of succinylcholine are administered.

The exact cause of muscle pains after succinylcholine is unknown, although it is thought that fasciculations produced by depolarization of the motor nerve end-plate are involved in the pathogenesis. However, the visible extent of fasciculations does not correlate with the severity of subsequent pain. Myoglobinuria occurs after administration of succinylcholine, demonstrating that muscle cell injury does occur.

After minor surgery, the patient may be disturbed by the muscle pains to a greater extent than the discomfort caused by the operative procedure.

It is possible to reduce, but not to eliminate, the incidence of succinylcholine pains by pretreatment with one of the following agents:

- a small dose of non-depolarizing muscle relaxant (usually 10% of the normal dose) 2–3 min before induction of anaesthesia
- a small dose of succinylcholine (0.1 mg kg^{-1})
- lidocaine 1 mg kg^{-1}
- diazepam 0.15 mg kg^{-1} i.v. before induction of anaesthesia
- dantrolene 2 h preoperatively.

SURGICAL CONSIDERATIONS

During the recovery period, several surgical complications may occur. These include haemorrhage, blockage of drains or catheters and soiling of dressings. Prosthetic arterial grafts may block, resulting in ischaemia of the limbs. Recovery ward nurses and anaesthetists must be aware of potential surgical complications, as rapid surgical intervention may be required.

The recovery period may also be used to institute orthopaedic traction before the patient returns to the ward.

FURTHER READING

Association of Anaesthetists of Great Britain and Ireland 1993 Immediate postanaesthetic recovery. AAGBI, London

Frost E A M 1996 Postanaesthesia care. In: Aitkenhead A R, Jones R M (eds) Clinical anaesthesia. Churchill Livingstone, Edinburgh, p 619–635

Frost E A M, Goldiner P L 1990 Postanesthetic care. Appleton & Lange, Norwalk, CT

42 Postoperative pain

Pain is an extraordinarily complex sensation which is difficult to define and equally difficult to measure in an accurate objective manner. It has been defined as the sensory appreciation of afferent nociceptive stimulation which elicits an affective (or autonomic) component; both are subjected to rational interpretation by the patient. It may be represented as a Venn diagram (Fig. 42.1), the shaded area of which represents the quantum of suffering experienced by the patient. The advantage of describing pain by means of the Venn diagram is that it may be seen instantly that the sensation of pain differs among individual patients; the emotional component may vary according to the patient's psychological composition and the rational component varies with the patient's previous experience, insight and motivation.

Postoperative pain differs from other types of pain in that it is usually transitory, with progressive improvement over a relatively short time-course. Typically, the affective component tends towards an anxiety state associated with diagnosis of the condition and fear of delay in provision of analgesic therapy by attendants. In contrast, chronic pain is persistent, frequently with fluctuating intensity, and the affective component contains a greater depressive element. Thus, acute pain is more easily amenable to therapy than chronic pain. Despite this, a recent survey showed that most adults still expect to have significant postoperative pain after surgery, and that this is their primary concern before surgery. Such concern may be justified, because traditional management of postoperative pain, using intramuscular opioid administration given on demand, often fails to produce good analgesia.

The traditional management of postoperative pain comprises the prescription of a standard dose of an opioid, to be given on demand by a nurse when the patient's pain threshold has been exceeded. This leads to poor control of postoperative pain for the following reasons:

- Responsibility for management of pain is delegated to the nursing staff who err on the side of caution in the administration of opioids. They tend to give too small a dose of drug too infrequently because of unwarranted fears of producing ventilatory depression or addiction.
- Because the administration of drugs is left entirely to the discretion of the nursing staff, the degree of empathy between nurse and patient affects analgesic administration. This explains the common observation that the mean dosage of morphine given for a standard operation varies among hospitals and even among wards in the same hospital.
- Because the measurement of pain is difficult, it is seldom possible to adjust the dosage of drug to match the extent of pain.

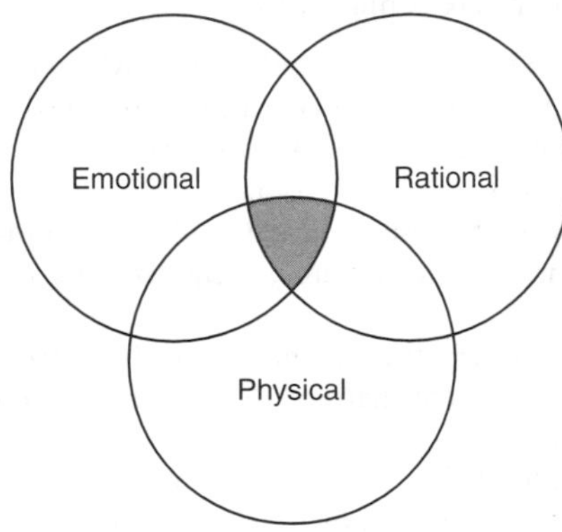

Fig. 42.1
The interrelationship between emotional, rational and physical components of pain. Perceived pain is represented by the area of intersection of all three components.

- There are enormous variations in the extent of analgesic requirements depending upon the type of surgery, pharmacokinetic variability, pharmacodynamic variability, etc.

These inadequacies in the traditional management of postoperative pain have been confirmed by a survey of ethical problems nurses face, which showed that they regard pain management to be a significant problem in their clinical practice.

The physiology of acute pain is no longer considered to be a simple 'hard-wired' system with a pure 'stimulus–response' relationship (see Ch. 17). Changes occur within the nervous system following any prolonged, noxious stimulus, as in the postoperative period where the surgical wound sends afferent neuronal information to the central nervous system for some time. Both 'peripheral' and 'central' sensitization occur and alter the body's response to further peripheral sensory input. Moreover, surgery generates a catabolic state by changes in endocrine hormonal control with increased secretion of catabolic hormones and decreased secretion of anabolic hormones. The results include pain; nausea, vomiting and intestinal stasis; alterations in blood flow, coagulation and fibrinolysis; alterations in substrate metabolism; alterations in water and electrolyte handling by the body; and increased demands on the cardiovascular and respiratory systems.

New principles of pain management have been developed to improve analgesia after surgery in the light of our new understanding of the processes involved. These include the recognition of the adverse effects of unrelieved pain, the need for an experienced and flexible approach to the problem by medical and nursing staff, and the necessity of informing the patient about the pain relief process. It is best to make plans for analgesia before surgery takes place, and this is especially important in short stay surgery where the patient is discharged home soon after the operation. The safety and efficacy of postoperative pain management may be improved by frequent assessment of the patient, good education of the staff and patients about the techniques and drugs used, preparation of protocols and guidelines for staff to follow, and regular evaluation by quality assurance programmes.

CAUSES OF VARIATION IN ANALGESIC REQUIREMENTS

Using patient-controlled analgesic apparatus (see below), it has been shown that there is marked interindividual variation in analgesic requirements. Thus, after cholecystectomy, some patients may require no morphine within the first 24 h, whereas others may require as much as 120 mg. Unfortunately, there is no way of predicting in advance the extent of opioid requirements of an individual patient. In clinical practice, requirements are assessed on a trial-and-error basis; anaesthetists are therefore in an ideal position to be involved in prescribing postoperative analgesia, as they obtain a 'feel' for dose requirements during management of anaesthesia.

Site and type of surgery

In general, upper abdominal surgery produces greater pain than lower abdominal surgery, which in turn is associated with greater pain than peripheral surgery. This generalization is not entirely accurate; operations on the richly innervated digits may be associated with quite severe pain.

The type of pain may differ with different types of surgery. Operations on joints are associated with sharp pain; in contrast, abdominal surgery is associated with two types of pain: a continuous dull nauseating ache (which responds well to morphine) and sharper pain induced by coughing and movement (which responds poorly to morphine). Pain associated with surgery on the digits may respond relatively poorly to opioids but well to non-steroidal anti-inflammatory drugs. There is some evidence that minimally invasive, laparoscopic, surgery produces less postoperative pain than do traditional techniques, but there has been little research in this area to date.

Table 42.1 provides an approximate guide to the duration and severity of postoperative pain.

Age, gender and body weight

The analgesic requirements of males and females are identical for similar types of surgery. However, there is a reduction in analgesic requirements with advancing age. Consequently, it is essential that the anaesthetist reduces the dosage of opioid drugs in elderly patients. For example, reasonable starting doses for intramuscular (or subcutaneous) postoperative morphine administration would be from 7.5 to 12.5 mg for patients aged 20–39 years, but the dose should be reduced to only 2.5–5.0 mg for 70- to 85-year-old patients.

The established anaesthetic practice of prescribing the potent opioid drugs on a mg or μg per body weight basis lacks scientific validity. There is no evidence to suggest that variations in body weight in the adult population affect opioid requirements.

Psychological factors (Table 42.2)

The patient's personality affects pain perception and response to analgesic drugs. Thus, patients with a low anxiety and low neuroticism score on a personality scale exhibit less postoperative pain and require smaller doses of opioid than patients who rate highly on these scales. Patients with high scores may exhibit a higher incidence of postoperative chest complications.

The extent of a patient's anxiety also affects pain perception; increased anxiety results in a greater degree of perceived postoperative pain and increased opioid requirements.

These psychological factors help to explain the efficacy of preoperative psychotherapy. Anxiety and postoperative analgesic requirements are reduced if the preoperative assessment by the anaesthetist includes an explanation of forthcoming perioperative events and details regarding the provision of pain relief.

Pharmacokinetic variability

After the intramuscular injection of an opioid, there is a three- to sevenfold difference between patients in the rate at which peak plasma concentrations of the drug occur and a two- to fivefold difference in the peak plasma concentration achieved. This is illustrated in Figure 42.2, which shows the mean change in plasma concentration after the first and second, and seventh and eighth injections. The variability in the plasma concentration is reflected by the large standard deviation of the mean. In addition, average concentrations increase after each of the first few injections; oscil-

Table 42.1 Duration and severity of postoperative pain

Site of operation	Duration of opioid use (h)	Severity of pain (0–4)
Abdominal		
Upper	48–72	3
Lower	Up to 48	2
Inguinal	Up to 36	1
Thoracotomy	72–96	4
Limbs	24–36	2
Faciomaxillary	Up to 48	2
Body wall	Up to 24	1
Perineal	24–48	2
Hip surgery	Up to 48	2

Table 42.2 Psychological factors which influence postoperative analgesic requirements

Personality
– more pain if high neuroticism/extroversion
Social background
Culture
Motivation
Preoperative psychotherapy

lation around a steady mean concentration does not occur until after approximately the fourth injection.

This pharmacokinetic variability helps to explain the relatively poor response to a single intramuscular injection given in the postoperative period.

Pharmacodynamic variability

Although there are widespread pharmacokinetic variations between patients in response to administration of opioids, the major reason for variation in opioid sensitivity is pharmacodynamic, i.e. a difference in the inherent sensitivity of opioid receptors.

Using continuous infusions of opioids to achieve equilibrium between receptor drug concentration and plasma concentration, it is possible to define a steady-state plasma concentration of opioid at which analgesia is produced. This is termed the minimum effective analgesic concentration (MEAC); values of MEAC for the commonly available opioids are shown in Table 42.3. MEAC levels vary four- to fivefold between individual patients and are affected by age and differences in psychological profile.

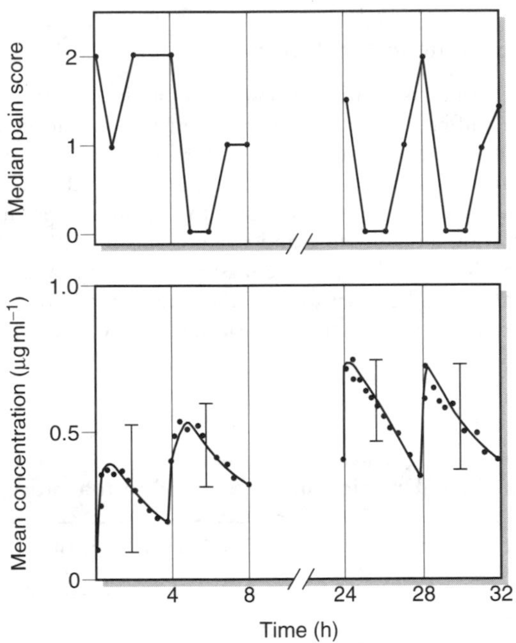

Fig. 42.2
Blood concentrations of pethidine and pain score after surgery; a pain score of 0 indicates no pain. Doses of pethidine 100mg have been given 4-hourly. Mean blood concentration of pethidine continues to rise for 24 h before a plateau is reached. Little pain relief is provided by the first dose. Even after 24 h, significant pain is present 3 and 4 h after each injection, as blood concentrations decline.

Table 42.3 Minimum effective analgesic concentration (MEAC) in blood for a number of analgesic drugs. Note the wide range of values for each agent

Drug	MEAC (ng ml^{-1})
Fentanyl	1–3
Alfentanil	100–300
Pethidine	300–650
Morphine	12–24
Methadone	30–70

Table 42.4 Methods of treating postoperative pain

Conventional administration of opioid
Intramuscular or subcutaneous on-demand bolus

Opioid agonist/antagonist drugs

Parenteral administration of opioid
Bolus intravenous administration
Continuous intravenous infusion
Patient-controlled analgesia
- Bolus } intravenous
- Bolus + infusion } subcutaneous/extradural

Non-parenteral administration of opioid
Sublingual
Oral
Transmucosal
Rectal
Transdermal
Nasal
Inhalation
Intra-articular opioids

Local anaesthetic techniques

Spinal/extradural opioids

Entonox

Non-steroidal anti-inflammatory drug (NSAIDs)

Paracetamol

NMDA antagonists

α_2-Adrenergic agonists
Systemically
Extradurally

Non-pharmacological methods
Cryotherapy
Transcutaneous electrical nerve stimulation (TENS)
Acupuncture
Psychological methods

METHODS OF TREATING POSTOPERATIVE PAIN (Table 42.4)

CONVENTIONAL ADMINISTRATION OF OPIOIDS

Intramuscular administration of opioids on a *pro re nata* (p.r.n.; as required) basis is the method used most commonly for prescribing postoperative analgesia. However, for the reasons noted above, this leads frequently to inadequate pain relief. Almost 60% of patients report dissatisfaction with the quality of postoperative analgesia administered in this way.

Intramuscular injection results in variable absorption, particularly in patients with hypothermia, hypovolaemia or hypotension. In addition, there is inevitably a considerable delay between request for analgesia and subsequent administration while controlled drugs are checked and drawn into a syringe. Although it is customary to prescribe opioids on a 4-hourly p.r.n. basis, there are frequently much longer periods between injections and this may lead to considerable 'breakthrough' pain.

The commonest cause of postoperative nausea and vomiting is the administration of opioids either intraoperatively or in the postoperative period. It should therefore be standard practice to prescribe antiemetic drugs regularly for administration with opioids.

Regular administration of intramuscular opioids provides improved analgesia, although care must be taken to avoid overdosage in debilitated patients and those at the extremes of age.

The advantages and disadvantages of repeated p.r.n. administration of opioids are listed in Table 42.5. Drugs used commonly for postoperative pain and antiemesis are listed in Table 42.6; their pharmacological properties are discussed fully in Chapters 18 and 21.

SUBCUTANEOUS ADMINISTRATION OF OPIOIDS

Morphine can be given subcutaneously, and patients prefer this to intramuscular injections. Small gauge cannulae can be placed subcutaneously and left in place for two to three days, avoiding the need for repeated skin punctures. Absorption of morphine from the subcutaneous route is comparable to absorption from the intramuscular route.

Table 42.5 Advantages and disadvantages of intramuscular p.r.n. administration of opioids

Advantages	Disadvantages
Familiar practice	Fixed dose not related to pharmacovariability
Gradual onset of side-effects	i.m. Administration causes profound pharmacovariability
Nursing assessment before administration	Painful injections
Inexpensive	Fluctuating plasma concentrations
	Delayed onset of analgesia

Table 42.6 Drugs used systemically for postoperative pain relief and antiemesis

Drug	Dose i.m. or s.c. (healthy adult)
Opioids	
Morphine	10 mg 4-hourly
Pethidine	100 mg 3-hourly
Buprenorphine (sublingual)	0.4 mg 6-hourly
Moderate analgesics	
Ketorolac	10–30 mg 6-hourly
Dihydrocodeine	50 mg 4-hourly
Antiemetics	
Prochlorperazine	12.5 mg 6-hourly
Perphenazine	5 mg 6-hourly
Cyclizine	50 mg 6-hourly
Metoclopramide	10 mg 6-hourly
Ondansetron	4 mg i.v. 6-hourly

ALGORITHMS FOR OPIOID ADMINISTRATION

Various acute pain services have constructed algorithms for postoperative intramuscular or subcutaneous opioid administration that other less experienced members of staff can then follow to provide safe and effective pain relief for their patients. Figure 42.3 is an example of this. An important aspect of such algorithms is the frequent assessment of the patient to ensure safety and efficacy of the treatment. Clinical assessments include pain (at rest and upon movement) and sedation scores, respiratory rate and arterial blood pressure. The algorithm includes a description of recommended doses and instructions on how to treat recognized side-effects such as respiratory depression. An important feature of such algorithms is that they permit more frequent opioid administration, e.g. '2-hourly p.r.n.'.

Sites of action and properties of morphine and morphine-like drugs

Opioids act supraspinally (nucleus raphe magnus, periaqueductal and periventricular grey areas), in the spinal cord (around C-fibre terminals in lamina I and the substantia gelatinosa, lamina II), and peripherally (opioid receptors are transported peripherally in axons, and are expressed by immune cells at the site of tissue damage). The actions of morphine are:

- Analgesia – morphine produces analgesia by binding with opioid receptors which are present in high concentrations in the periaqueductal area and limbic system of the brain and in the region of the substantia gelatinosa of the spinal cord
- Ventilatory depression
- Sedation
- Cough suppression
- Vasodilatation
- Release of histamine
- Constipation
- Nausea and vomiting
- Pupillary constriction
- Biliary spasm
- Urine retention
- Tolerance
- Physical dependence (addiction to opioids is rare when they are used for the relief of acute postoperative pain).

The most important side-effects of morphine are ventilatory depression and nausea and vomiting. (As significant hypoxaemia may occur for several days postoperatively, supplemental oxygen is recommended for at least the first 48–72 h following major surgery, and in the elderly or high-risk patient regardless of the analgesic method used.) Morphine should not be administered to patients with biliary or renal colic (occasionally it may precipitate pain in patients with gall bladder disease when administered as premedication) and should be avoided in patients with head injury and perhaps in asthmatics. Alternative drugs are described in Chapter 18. Tramadol is an interesting synthetic analgesic as it has both opioid and non-opioid mechanisms of action and may produce analgesia with less respiratory depression, sedation, gastrointestinal stasis and abuse potential. Unfortunately, as with morphine, the use of tramadol is associated with nausea and vomiting.

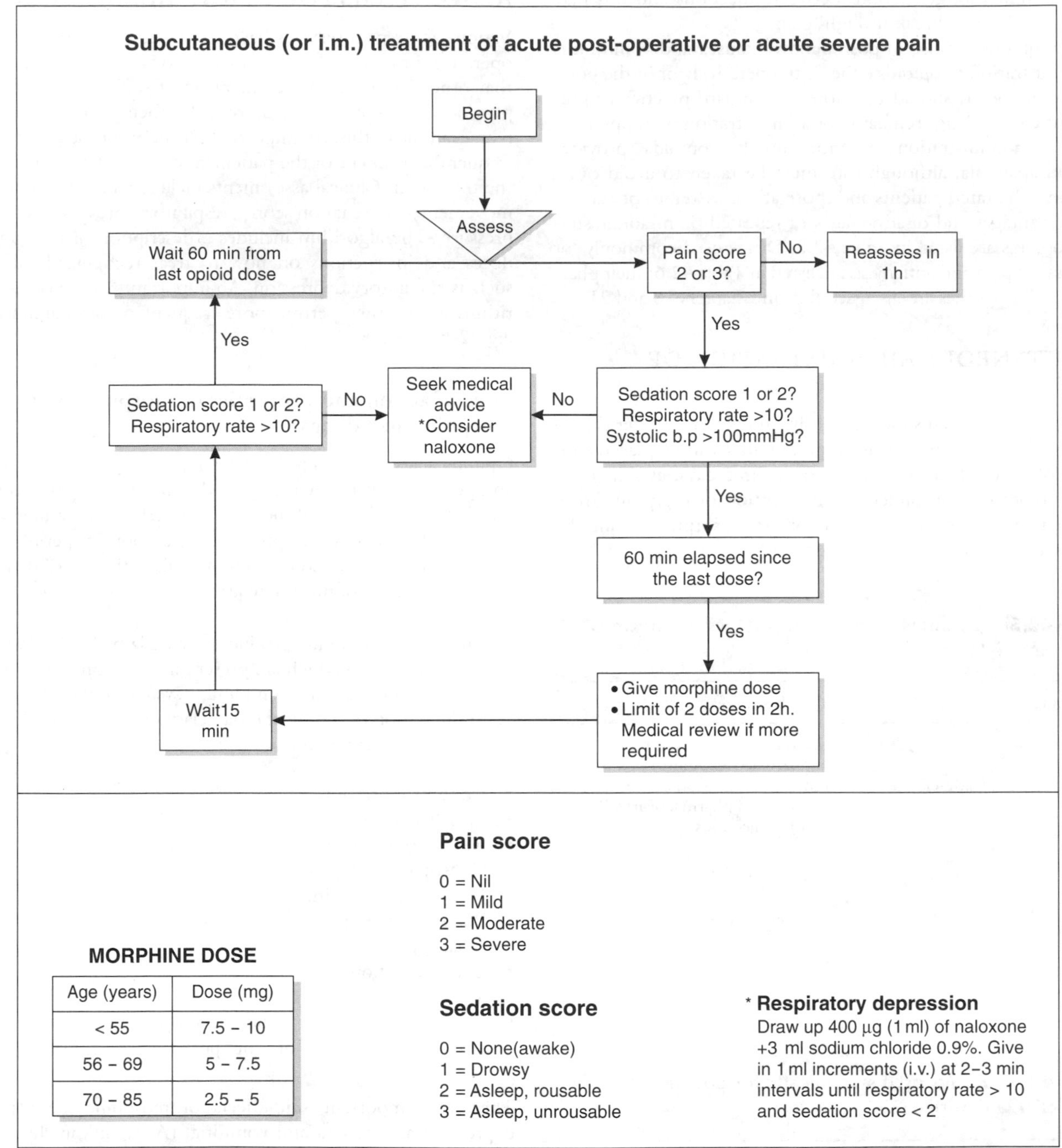
Subcutaneous (or i.m.) treatment of acute post-operative or acute severe pain
Begin
Assess
Wait 60 min from last opioid dose
Pain score 2 or 3?
No
Reassess in 1 h
Yes
Yes
Sedation score 1 or 2? Respiratory rate >10?
No
Seek medical advice *Consider naloxone
No
Sedation score 1 or 2? Respiratory rate >10? Systolic b.p >100mmHg?
Yes
60 min elapsed since the last dose?
Yes
• Give morphine dose
• Limit of 2 doses in 2h. Medical review if more required
Wait15 min
Pain score
0 = Nil
1 = Mild
2 = Moderate
3 = Severe
MORPHINE DOSE
Sedation score
0 = None(awake)
1 = Drowsy
2 = Asleep, rousable
3 = Asleep, unrousable
* Respiratory depression
Draw up 400 µg (1 ml) of naloxone +3 ml sodium chloride 0.9%. Give in 1 ml increments (i.v.) at 2–3 min intervals until respiratory rate > 10 and sedation score < 2

Age (years)	Dose (mg)
< 55	7.5 – 10
56 – 69	5 – 7.5
70 – 85	2.5 – 5

Fig. 42.3
Subcutaneous (or intramuscular) treatment of acute postoperative or acute severe pain.

PARENTERAL ROUTES OF OPIOID ADMINISTRATION

Bolus i.v. administration

It is possible to improve the quality of analgesia in the postoperative period by giving small incremental doses of opioid i.v. when required. However, this carries the risk of rapid induction of ventilatory depression and in many hospitals cannot be undertaken by nursing staff in the wards. In general, this technique is employed only by anaesthetists and experienced nursing staff in the immediate recovery period.

Continuous i.v. infusion (Table 42.7)

This technique is employed to provide analgesia in patients receiving artificial ventilation in ITU. An infusion rate designed to exceed MEAC in all patients is clearly safe and ventilatory depression is an advantage in this situation.

Continuous infusions have been used in general surgical wards for the provision of postoperative analgesia in spontaneously breathing patients. The dosage rate is determined by the medical attendant on a trial-and-error basis and a fixed infusion rate prescribed. However, this carries great risks of producing ventilatory depression and cannot be recommended in spontaneously breathing patients outside a high-dependency or intensive therapy unit.

Patient-controlled analgesia (PCA)

The main problem with continuous i.v. infusion is that there is no way of predicting an individual patient's MEAC. With PCA, the patient determines the rate of i.v. administration of the drug, thereby providing feedback control.

PCA equipment comprises an accurate source of infusion, coupled to an i.v. cannula and controlled by a patient–machine interface device. Safety features are incorporated to limit the preset dose, the number of doses which may be administered and the 'lockout' period between doses. Advantages and disadvantages of PCA are listed in Table 42.8.

The drug that has been used most commonly with PCA is morphine. The size of the demand dose is usually 1–2 mg with a lockout period of between 5 and 10 min. Fentanyl (10–20 μg), pethidine (10 mg) and hydromorphone (0.2 mg) can also be used for intravenous PCA. Although there may be some theoretical advantage in the use of a continuous low-dose infusion on which the patient may superimpose demand bolus administrations, in practice several clinical investigations have failed to reveal any advantage. Because of the slightly increased risk of overdosage, therefore, it is generally recommended that PCA apparatus be used in the 'bolus alone' mode.

Intravenous PCA is now a standard method of providing postoperative analgesia in many hospitals worldwide. It provides better pain relief than conventional intermittent intramuscular administration. It is essential that monitoring of the patient is not reduced, as respiratory depression may occur with this technique and many patient will require antiemetics for nausea. If the pump is being used to deliver morphine via an intravenous infusion, it is essential that a one-way valve be incorporated between the PCA equipment and the infusion giving set in order to prevent morphine collecting in the giving set which may then be delivered as a large bolus at a later time, with possible lethal effects.

The effective and safe use of PCA requires frequent monitoring of the patient by nurses who have had in-service training and accreditation in the use of the drugs and devices. There is evidence that PCA is more effective when it is overseen by an acute pain service involving pain nursing staff and pharmacists. Standard PCA prescription orders and drug dilutions may minimize complications. PCA may also be used to deliver opioids subcutaneously or epidurally.

Table 42.7 Advantages and disadvantages of continuous i.v. infusions

Advantages	Disadvantages
Rapid onset of analgesia	Fixed dose not related to pharmacodynamic variability
Steady-state plasma concentrations	Errors may be fatal
Painless	Expensive fail-safe equipment required
	May result in less frequent assessment by nursing staff

Table 42.8 Advantages and disadvantages of patient controlled analgesia (PCA)

Advantages	Disadvantages
Dose matches patient's requirements and therefore compensates for pharmacodynamic variability	Technical errors may be fatal
	Expensive equipment
Doses given are small and therefore fluctuations in plasma concentrations are reduced	Requires ability to cooperate and understand
Reduces nurses' workload	
Painless	
Placebo effect from patient autonomy	

NON-PARENTERAL OPIOID ADMINISTRATION

Sublingual opioids

Sublingual administration requires cooperation. With buprenorphine, good analgesia can be provided without the need for painful injections, making this route popular with patients and convenient for nursing staff.

This route is confined largely to buprenorphine. Combination with morphine may result in dysphoria and withdrawal phenomena. If this route is chosen, it is preferable to use buprenorphine as the sole opioid in the perioperative period, although, as it is a partial opioid agonist, it has a ceiling effect for analgesia.

Oral route

All the opioids undergo extensive metabolism in the gut wall and liver (first-pass metabolism) and therefore the bioavailability is relatively low (e.g. 20–30% for morphine). In the immediate postoperative period, there is invariably a reduction in the rate of gastric emptying (caused mainly by the intraoperative or preoperative use of opioids). For this reason, care should be taken if opioids are used orally for pain relief in the postoperative period because:

- absorption may be delayed, with poor analgesia
- if opioids have been given orally on a regular basis, there is a danger of a large dose being dumped into the upper gastrointestinal tract when gastric motility returns to normal, resulting in overdosage and ventilatory depression.

If normal gastric emptying has resumed, then oral opioids can be used safely and effectively after surgery to provide analgesia without the need for injections.

Transmucosal

Oral transmucosal fentanyl citrate has been prepared as a palatable solid matrix (presented as a lollipop) for use as a pre-anaesthetic medication in children. The time to the onset of pain relief is of the order of 9 min, and both transmucosal (buccal) and gastric routes contribute to the absorption of fentanyl. Side-effects include nausea and vomiting, and hypoxaemia. At present, the preparation is not available in the UK or in Australia.

The rectal route

The rectal route may be used as a means of delivering morphine but there is marked variability in the plasma concentrations achieved. Venous blood from the lower part of the rectum drains directly into the systemic circulation, but the upper part drains into the portal circulation. Thus, bioavailability varies according to the site of a suppository within the rectum. However, this route avoids the problems of reduced gastrointestinal motility. Probably the best indication for the rectal route is the treatment of chronic intractable pain, particularly where there is dysphagia.

Inhaled/intranasal

Intranasal spray devices for fentanyl are now available in some countries. Inhaled opioid preparations are being developed that have metered inhalers with improved pulmonary drug delivery systems and lockout times, and in the future they may allow non-invasive PCA administration.

Transdermal

Because of the high lipid solubility and high potency of fentanyl, this drug may be absorbed across the skin in sufficient quantities to produce effective plasma concentrations. Transdermal fentanyl patches are available with delivery rates from 25 to 100 μg h^{-1}. Because of the difficulty in matching transdermal patches of differing strengths to the pharmacodynamic variability between different patients, this technique is not suitable for management of acute pain, but is used for the relief of cancer pain. Drug delivery systems are being developed that use iontophoresis to improve transdermal opioid absorption.

LOCAL ANAESTHETIC TECHNIQUES

Many local anaesthetic techniques, administered for the purpose of operative surgery or during the course of general anaesthesia, may provide excellent analgesia in the early postoperative period. However, it is usually necessary for the anaesthetist to administer an opioid to the patient before the block regresses, to reduce the likelihood of severe pain when the block wears off.

Many local anaesthetic techniques may be used for the primary purpose of providing analgesia in the early postoperative period. However, a major disadvantage is that the duration of blockade with a 'single-shot' technique is relatively short. Bupivacaine (0.25 or 0.5%) has been the drug of choice and may produce peripheral nerve blockade lasting for 8–12 h and occasionally for as long as 18 h. The duration of action for epidural nerve block is 4–6 h. Ropivacaine has similar local anaesthetic characteristics to bupivacaine, but with less cardiac toxicity. Ropivacaine is available as 2, 7.5 and 10 mg mL^{-1} preparations; motor blockade is less at low doses than with bupivacaine.

Epinephrine may be added to a local anaesthetic solution to prolong the block, although this produces relatively little effect on the duration of analgesia produced by bupivacaine or ropivacaine. The most effective means of prolonging the block is by the use of a catheter to permit either repeated bolus doses or a continuous infusion of local anaesthetic to be administered.

Local anaesthetic blocks in common use are described in Chapter 43. The following blocks represent those which are employed most usefully for postoperative analgesia.

Spinal nerve block

Subarachnoid analgesia rarely lasts more than 3–4 h with the drugs currently available and is therefore of limited use for postoperative analgesia, although there is evidence that intrathecal analgesia can modify the physiological changes associated with surgery. Although the insertion of a catheter into the subarachnoid space is employed in the USA, this is not a popular manoeuvre in the UK or Australia.

Epidural block

Epidural block is popular for postoperative analgesia because of familiarity with the technique and ease of insertion of a catheter. Epidural analgesic techniques can provide superior postoperative analgesia and modify the physiological changes associated with some forms of surgery. Postoperative epidural analgesia can reduce the incidence of pulmonary morbidity. However, epidural techniques also have uncommon but serious risks attached to catheter insertion and removal (e.g. epidural haematoma) and so the risk–benefit ratio for each patient must be considered. Repeated injections may be made through the catheter or a dilute solution of local anaesthetic infused continuously. Initially, bupivacaine produces analgesia lasting up to 4 h, but by 24–48 h some tolerance develops and single-bolus administrations may last for only 2 h. Ropivacaine, in low doses, may offer the advantage of producing similar sensory block with less motor impairment.

Bupivacaine 0.25% injected at L2/3 provides good analgesia after lower abdominal or perineal surgery, e.g. hysterectomy or transurethral resection of prostate. Upper abdominal procedures require a higher block; 15 ml of bupivacaine 0.5% produces analgesia up to T7.

For thoracic surgery, an epidural catheter may be inserted in the thoracic region between T6 and T8, and volumes of bupivacaine of 6–12 ml may provide excellent postoperative analgesia.

In general, it is recommended that epidural catheter techniques should be used only when the patient is nursed in a high-dependency unit, because of the risks of hypotension after epidural injections and total spinal block if the catheter migrates into the subarachnoid space. However, in some institutions, continuous infusion epidural techniques are managed on general wards, but only with the benefit of adequate medical and nursing staff experience, and the existence of clear protocols for monitoring and the early detection of side-effects.

Some potential advantages of epidural analgesia

- Improve postoperative respiratory function.

- Reduces the stress response to surgery after lower abdominal and lower limb surgery (minimal effect after upper abdominal or thoracic surgery).
- Minimize the hypercoagulable state after major surgery; there is a reduction in deep venous thrombosis and pulmonary embolism after hip surgery.
- Reduced intraoperative blood loss during surgery on the lower part of the body.
- Improves postoperative gut function, facilitating early enteral nutrition.

Some potential complications of epidural analgesia

- Dural puncture (0.6–1.3%).
- Epidural haematoma – the risk is increased by impaired haemostasis when the catheter is placed or removed. Guidelines must be followed for concomitant prophylactic low-molecular-weight heparin and low-dose heparin therapy.
- Epidural abscess, meningitis and direct neurological damage.
- Systemic local anaesthetic toxicity, total spinal analgesia.
- Sympathetic blockade (haemodynamic effects), urinary retention and motor block.

Caudal block

Caudal administration of local anaesthetic drugs is useful for child day-case surgery, e.g. circumcision, or in patients undergoing anal or perineal surgery. It is customary to administer only a single dose of local anaesthetic; catheter techniques are unpopular in the UK because of the risk of infection. Suitable dosages of local anaesthetic solution for use by the caudal route are shown in Table 42.9.

Other regional blocks used for postoperative analgesia

Intercostal nerve blockade. Blocks from T4 to T8 or 9 provide satisfactory analgesia for pain relief after subcostal incision for cholecystectomy. Intercostal blocks may be repeated at regular intervals; catheters have been used for repeated administration. Bilateral blockade should not be carried out because of the risk of pneumothorax.

Paravertebral block. This may be used to provide analgesia after thoracic or abdominal surgery. Local anaesthetic solution is injected into the region of the paravertebral space to block the dorsal sensory nerve roots as they emerge from the vertebral foramina. This technique may be performed using single or repeated injections or with an indwelling catheter.

Table 42.9 Doses of bupivacaine (0.25% plain) for caudal analgesia

Adult	Child
0.3–0.4 ml kg^{-1}	0.5–0.7 ml kg^{-1} (or 0.1 ml year^{-1} for each segment to be blocked)

N.B. Dosage of bupivacaine should *never* exceed 2 mg kg^{-1}.

Interpleural analgesia may be used to provide unilateral analgesia after thoracotomy, breast surgery, open cholecystectomy and renal surgery. The use of interpleural analgesia can improve postoperative respiratory function, although the presence of intercostal chest drains or haemothorax may diminish the effectiveness of this procedure.

Brachial plexus analgesia, using a catheter placed close to the plexus and a continuous infusion of local anaesthetic, covers almost all of the upper limb and produces a sympathetic block that may be beneficial following plastic surgery.

Femoral nerve block, using a continuous infusion technique, is useful for relief of pain after knee surgery and may facilitate recovery after knee arthroplasty.

Combined ilioinguinal and iliohypogastric nerve block is a safe and effective regional technique for postoperative pain control after inguinal hernia repair.

Wound infiltration after minor or paediatric surgery is an established analgesic technique for pain relief, but the benefit after major surgery is not clear.

SPINAL AND EPIDURAL OPIOIDS

In recent years, there has been great interest in the use of opioids by the subarachnoid or epidural routes. After injection of opioid into the cerebrospinal fluid (CSF), drug is taken up in the region of the substantia gelatinosa within the dorsal horn. It is thought that opioids act predominantly on the presynaptic enkephalin receptors, although opioid is absorbed from the CSF into the circulation. After epidural administration of opioids, the drug diffuses through the dura into CSF and produces analgesia by the same mechanism as that associated with subarachnoid injection. However, there is more rapid uptake of opioid into the circulation via the rich network of blood vessels in the epidural space. Consequently, there is a rapid increase in both CSF and blood concentrations of the drug after epidural administration.

Uptake into the dorsal horn, and rate of passage through the dura are dependent upon lipid solubility. Thus the more highly lipid-soluble drugs (e.g. fentanyl) have a more rapid onset and a shorter duration of action. The less lipid-soluble drugs (e.g. morphine) have a slower rate of onset of action; in addition there is a greater dispersion within the CSF because of reduced uptake into spinal cord and the drug may reach the medulla to cause delayed ventilatory depression.

Subarachnoid opioids

This route is less popular than the epidural route of administration for opioids because of the production of spinal headache. However, smaller doses are required than with the epidural route and therefore systemic concentrations are lower. The quality of analgesia is not as good as that achieved with subarachnoid local anaesthetic drugs.

Epidural opioids

The administration of epidural opioids is more popular because spinal headache is avoided and a catheter technique may be used. It is possible to achieve analgesia without the motor or autonomic block produced by local anaesthetic injected into the epidural space. Thus, postural hypotension and changes in heart rate do not occur. Early ventilatory depression may occur as a result of systemic absorption (e.g. within the first 1–2 h), but late ventilatory depression (8–20 h) is a result of rostral spread of opioid within the CSF to the medulla. Prolonged duration of action of analgesia is produced by a single injection (up to 24 h).

Side-effects of epidural opioids

- Early ventilatory depression – occurs more commonly with lipid-soluble agents.
- Late ventilatory depression – occurs more commonly with agents of lower lipophilicity.
- Coma – occurs relatively late, usually in association with late ventilatory depression and can be reversed by naloxone.
- Urinary retention.
- Itching – this is reversed only partially by naloxone.
- Nausea and vomiting.

Epidural opioids are more effective when used in combination with local anaesthetics to produce a synergistic analgesic action. This reduces the necessary dose and the side-effects that would be associated with the local anaesthetic or the opioid alone. For example, continuous epidural infusions of combined solutions of low concentrations of bupivacaine (or ropivacaine) with fentanyl provide good postoperative analgesia with minimal side-effects.

INHALATION OF VOLATILE OR GASEOUS ANAESTHETICS

Although volatile anaesthetics were used in the past, the only agent in current use is N_2O. This is administered in the form of Entonox (premixed 50% N_2O, 50% O_2) usually via a demand valve and face mask. Entonox is used extensively in obstetric analgesia, in the field situation (e.g. by ambulance personnel to provide analgesia at the site of an accident) or occasionally in the wards during change of surgical dressings.

NON-STEROIDAL ANTI-INFLAMMATORY DRUGS (NSAIDs)

The use of NSAIDs (cyclooxygenase inhibitors) for postoperative pain relief is now routine practice. NSAIDs may be given orally, rectally (e.g. diclofenac 100 mg) or intravenously (e.g. ketorolac 10 mg). NSAIDs produce pain relief without sedation, respiratory depression or nausea and vomiting, but their use is limited by gastric, renal and platelet side-effects. A recent authoritative and extensive review of the published literature concerning NSAIDs drew the following conclusions:

- NSAIDs are not sufficiently effective as the sole analgesic agent after major surgery.
- NSAIDs are often effective after minor or outpatient surgery.
- NSAIDs often decrease opioid requirement. Significant reduction in opioid side-effects has been noted in a few studies only.
- The quality of opioid-based analgesia is often enhanced by NSAIDs.
- NSAIDs increase bleeding time and some studies have shown increased blood loss after surgery.

The major adverse effects of NSAIDs for surgical patients are those involving the gastrointestinal system, renal and platelet function, and aspirin-induced asthma in susceptible patients. The adverse effects of NSAIDs are serious, and contraindications (e.g. peptic ulceration, bleeding diathesis, renal impairment, aspirin-sensitive asthma) must be respected. The incidence and severity of NSAID-related adverse effects are greater in elderly patients. Aspirin is contraindicated in children less than 12 years old. There have been case reports of sudden renal dysfunction in patients given NSAIDs perioperatively; risk factors for this may include nephrotoxic antibiotics (e.g. gentamicin), raised intra-abdominal pressure during laparoscopy, hypovolaemia and age greater than 65 years.

New drugs have been developed that selectively inhibit the inducible cyclooxygenase enzyme, COX-2, and spare the constitutive, COX-1, enzyme. Most conventional NSAIDs in clinical use are non-specific inhibitors of COX-1 and COX-2, and many of the side-effects of the older drugs may be by COX-1 inhibition and disruption of physiological prostaglandin production. COX-2 is induced by tissue damage and inflammation, and selective inhibitors of this enzyme may produce analgesia with fewer side-effects. For example, at normal doses, COX-2 inhibitors do not affect platelet function. The COX-2 inhibitors available at present include meloxicam, nimesulide, celecoxib and rofecoxib. There is encouraging evidence that COX-2 inhibitors have less gastrointestinal side-effects, but renal toxicity and the effect on individuals with aspirin-senstive asthma are not clear. More studies are required to confirm the analgesic efficacy of COX-2 inhibitors in surgical patients.

PARACETAMOL

Paracetamol is a useful adjunct to opioids in the treatment of postoperative pain, with fewer contraindications than the NSAIDs. It is analgesic and antipyretic, but not anti-inflammatory. The mechanism of action is unclear, but may involve the selective inhibition of prostaglandin synthesis in the central nervous system. In adults with normal hepatic and renal function, the recommended dose is 500–1000 mg orally or rectally every 3–6 h when necessary, with a maximum daily dose of 6 g day^{-1} for acute use and 4 g day^{-1} for chronic use (care must be taken to avoid inadvertent paracetamol overdosage and resultant hepatic and renal toxicity). An intravenous preparation, propacetamol, is available in some European countries and has been shown to be an effective postoperative analgesic.

NMDA ANTAGONISTS

The activation by excitatory amino acids (glutamate) of spinal cord dorsal horn *N*-methyl-D-aspartate (NMDA) receptors is essential for the development of central sensitization (see Ch. 17). The anaesthetic agent ketamine is a potent NMDA receptor antagonist. Low-dose subcutaneous or intravenous ketamine infusions (5–15 mg h^{-1}) produce significant pain relief after surgery. Unfortunately, the side-effects of ketamine, including hallucinations, limit the use of this agent. Dextromethorphan is an alternative NMDA receptor antagonist which has been shown to reduce opioid requirements following oral surgery and during abdominal surgery.

NON-PHARMACOLOGICAL METHODS

Cryotherapy

This may be applied to intercostal nerves exposed during a thoracotomy. The nerve is surrounded by an iceball produced by intense sub-zero temperatures at the end of a probe. The neuronal disruption produced by this method is temporary and sensation returns after some months, although it may be accompanied by unpleasant paraesthesiae and occasionally by persistent neuralgia.

Transcutaneous electrical stimulation

A small alternating current is passed between two surface electrodes at low voltage and at a frequency between 0.2 and 200 Hz. It is thought that the technique acts by increasing CNS concentrations of endorphins. Acupuncture may work in a similar manner. The technique produces only moderate analgesia.

Acupuncture

Acupuncture has been assessed as a technique for pain relief after surgery. There is evidence that acupuncture reduces pain and analgesic consumption after dental and abdominal surgery, although there is some variability in the method of administration.

PRE-EMPTIVE ANALGESIA

The importance of peripheral and central sensitization in amplifying pain perception has directed research towards preventing these processes. Experimentally, it has been shown that nociceptive stimulation from the periphery causes functional changes in the spinal cord which lead to enhancement and prolongation of the sensation of pain. It has also been shown that prior administration of analgesics may inhibit the development of the hyperexcitability within the spinal cord. Unfortunately, however, in clinical practice, prior administration of analgesics (pre-emptive analgesia) has not been shown to have an important effect on postoperative pain. Further studies are being performed on pre-emptive analgesia, incorporating additional strategies to modulate the prolonged neuronal input to the spinal cord from the peripheral tissue inflammatory process.

BALANCED (MULTIMODAL) ANALGESIA

The concept of balanced analgesia is analogous to that of balanced anaesthesia. It is possible to block the development of pain by the use of a combination of different drugs acting at different sites: peripherally, on somatic and sympathetic nerves, at spinal cord level, and centrally. The benefit of this technique is that not only may superior analgesia be achieved by a combination of drugs but their individual doses may be reduced, thereby decreasing the incidence of side-effects. For example, after thoracotomy, the addition of an NSAID to a regimen based on intercostal nerve blocks and PCA morphine significantly improves analgesia.

Pain transmission may be blocked clinically at the following sites:

- inhibition of peripheral nociceptor mechanisms using NSAIDs, steroids or opioids
- blockade of afferent neuronal transmission using peripheral, epidural or spinal local anaesthetic administration
- interference at both spinal cord level and higher centres using spinal and systemic opioids.

The use of non-opioid analgesics in multimodal analgesia minimizes opioid side-effects including gastrointestinal stasis. After bowel surgery, multimodal analgesia (an epidural infusion of a low-dose local anaesthetic and opioid mixture, and systemic NSAID) produces excellent pain relief, avoids the need for systemic opioids, and speeds the recovery of gastrointestinal function. This facilitates early mobilization of the patient and a more rapid return to enteral nutrition.

Typically, for minor surgery, e.g. hernia repair on a day-case basis, the anaesthetist may employ multimodal or balanced analgesia in the form of:

- preoperative administration of a mild oral analgesic, e.g. paracetamol or an NSAID
- administration of fentanyl intraoperatively +/− tramadol
- local anaesthetic block using ilioinguinal and iliohypogastric nerve blocks and wound infiltration
- the use of NSAIDs in the form of a diclofenac suppository 100 mg.

With this technique, patients frequently do not require supplementary opioids postoperatively and may be managed on a day-case basis using simple oral analgesics in the postoperative period, e.g. paracetamol. Oral tramadol may be useful if stronger postoperative analgesia is required.

NEUROPATHIC PAIN IN THE POSTOPERATIVE PERIOD

The possibility of the development of neuropathic pain should be borne in mind after surgery, as it is often missed in patients with acute pain and may require specific therapy (see Ch. 61 for the management of chronic pain). A useful definition of neuropathic pain is 'pain associated with injury, disease or surgical section of the peripheral or central nervous system'. One diagnostic clue after surgery is an unexpected increase in opioid consumption, as neuropathic pain often responds poorly to opioids. Features suggestive of neuropathic pain include:

- pain without ongoing tissue damage
- sensory loss
- allodynia (pain in response to non-painful stimuli)
- hyperalgesia (increased pain in response to painful stimuli)
- dysaesthesiae (unpleasant abnormal sensations)
- burning, stabbing or shooting pain
- a delay in onset after injury.

ACUTE PAIN SERVICES

The supervision of postoperative pain relief has been allocated in many hospitals to acute pain services, often staffed by anaesthetists and nurses. The establishment of an acute pain service in a hospital has been shown to improve postoperative pain management. Acute pain services have various roles:

- continuing staff education about pain
- standardization of orders of analgesic prescription and monitoring of patients
- the provision of new or specialized methods of pain relief
- audit and clinical research.

In the future, acute pain services may be better integrated with surgical and other staff, to form perioperative care services that can direct all aspects of multimodal analgesia, perioperative nutrition and postoperative mobilization to facilitate the rapid recovery of the patient after surgery.

FURTHER READING

McQuay H, Moore A (eds) 1998 An evidence-based resource for pain relief. Oxford University Press, Oxford

National Health and Medical Research Council of Australia 1999 Acute pain management: scientific evidence. Commonwealth of Australia, Canberra

Ogilvy A J, Smith G 1994 Postoperative pain. In: Nimmo W S, Rowbotham D J, Smith G (eds) Anaesthesia, 2nd edn. Blackwell Scientific Publications, Oxford

Royal College of Anaesthetists 1998 Guidelines for the use of non-steroidal anti-inflammatory drugs in the perioperative period. RCA, London

43 Local anaesthetic techniques

The efficacy and use of local anaesthetic techniques is increasing. This is as a result of advances in drugs, equipment and the anatomical approaches to nerve blocks, together with a greater understanding of the relationships between the doses, concentrations and subsequent effects of the local anaesthetic agents employed. This chapter outlines the basic principles of patient management and the methods employed in the performance of a variety of blocks which are commonly undertaken by the trainee anaesthetist.

Regional techniques for obstetrics and dental surgery are described in other chapters.

FEATURES OF LOCAL ANAESTHESIA

In some circumstances, regional anaesthesia may have distinct advantages over general anaesthesia, e.g. in the use of axillary block for hand surgery in a respiratory cripple. However, rather than view a local anaesthetic technique as a rival to general anaesthesia, it is more useful to consider it as part of an individually selected technique which may include the use of sedative or centrally acting anaesthetic drugs. Although the trainee may consider local anaesthesia as having advantages and disadvantages, it becomes apparent with experience that an advantage in one situation may be a disadvantage in another.

Preservation of consciousness is often considered to be an advantage of regional anaesthesia. For example, the patient undergoing caesarean section is able to protect her own airway and experience the birth of the child. However, patients who require other forms of surgery may be unhappy at the prospect of being awake; in this situation the combination of a regional block and light general anaesthesia may be valuable.

One benefit of a regional block is the quality of early postoperative analgesia, but this may carry disadvantages. Some patients are distressed by the accompanying numbness, although correct preoperative explanation should minimize this concern; in addition, it is important that nursing staff are aware of the risk of trauma to the blocked segments.

Other features of regional anaesthesia include simplicity of administration, sympathetic blockade, attenuation of the stress response and minimal depression of ventilation. Some studies have suggested that the net effect of these features may be a reduction in the incidence of major postoperative complications, but this remains controversial.

COMPLICATIONS OF LOCAL ANAESTHESIA

The incidence of complications may be minimized by ensuring adequate supervision and training in local anaesthetic techniques, and by exercising care in the performance of each block. Sufficient expertise and equipment must always be available to deal with potential complications. Complications common to many techniques are discussed in this section; more specific problems are considered later.

LOCAL ANAESTHETIC TOXICITY

This usually results from accidental intravascular injection, an excessive dose of local anaesthetic or faulty technique, particularly during performance of Bier's block.

Features and treatment

These are described in Chapter 15.

Prevention

Correct technique, careful and repeated aspiration and the use of a test dose are important, but the main safety measure is *slow injection* of the local anaesthetic. This prevents rapid production of very high plasma concentrations even if the injection is intravascular. By this means, toxicity may be diagnosed early, the injection discontinued and a major reaction avoided. Fast injection of local anaesthetic is not necessary for the performance of any block.

Test dose

This may be used before administration of the main dose of local anaesthetic drug. It is particularly indicated for epidural block, where it should be capable of demonstrating inadvertent intravenous (i.v.) or subarachnoid injection. A test dose of 4 ml of 2% plain lidocaine is sufficient to cause mild symptoms in most patients after accidental i.v. injection, and any features of local anaesthetic blockade 2 min after injection are good evidence of accidental subarachnoid block. No test dose is infallible; slow administration of the main dose is the most important factor in avoiding local anaesthetic toxicity.

HYPOTENSION

There are several possible mechanisms by which a local anaesthetic technique may cause hypotension. The anaesthetist must always remember that surgical factors may be responsible.

Sympathetic blockade

A limited sympathetic block may be produced by peripheral nerve anaesthesia, but only central blocks are likely to produce hypotension by this mechanism.

Total spinal blockade

This is discussed on page 567. It occasionally occurs during subarachnoid block if excessive spread of local anaesthetic solution occurs, and is a recognized complication of epidural block if the dura has been penetrated. Apnoea may occur if local anaesthetic solution reaches the cerebrospinal fluid (CSF) during interscalene brachial plexus block, or the ventricular system during retrobulbar nerve block.

Vasovagal attack

This is particularly likely to occur in an anxious patient with a rapidly ascending spinal block. Pallor, nausea and bradycardia are associated with the hypotension. The supine position is no guarantee against this complication. Rapid resolution results from placing the patient head-down and the administration of i.v. ephedrine 5–6 mg. Cautious i.v. sedation (e.g. midazolam 1–2 mg) may be helpful.

Anaphylactoid reaction

This is very rare with amide local anaesthetics.

Local anaesthetic toxicity

This is considered above and in Chapter 15.

MOTOR BLOCKADE

To avoid unnecessary distress, patients must be warned of the possibility of limb weakness or paralysis which may persist for some time after operation.

PNEUMOTHORAX

This is a potential hazard of supraclavicular brachial plexus, intercostal and paravertebral blocks. The possibility of its occurrence is an absolute contraindication to the use of these techniques in outpatients and also to the performance of these blocks bilaterally.

URINARY RETENTION

This may follow the use of central blocks. It is important to avoid overhydration, as bladder distension may require catheterization. The use of large volumes of crystalloid in the treatment of hypotension often has a very transient effect and predisposes patients to urinary retention, or worse pulmonary oedema, when the block regresses.

NEUROLOGICAL COMPLICATIONS

Carefully performed blocks rarely result in neurological complications.

Neuritis with persisting sensory changes and/or weakness may result from trauma to the nerve, intraneural injection or bacterial, chemical or particulate contamination of the injected solution. Injection of the incorrect solution has caused some of the most severe neurological complications. To avoid this serious error, all drugs must be checked personally by the anaesthetist immediately before injection.

Anterior spinal artery syndrome may follow an episode of prolonged, severe hypotension and results in painless permanent paraplegia. *Adhesive arachnoiditis* has been described after subarachnoid and epidural blockade and may lead to permanent pain, weakness and bladder or bowel dysfunction. It is suspected that this complication results from injection of the incorrect solution. *Haematoma* or *abscess* formation in the spinal canal after subarachnoid or epidural anaesthesia results in weakness and sensory loss below the level of spinal cord compression. It is associated with intense back pain and is a neurosurgical emergency which demands immediate decompression to avoid permanent disability.

EQUIPMENT PROBLEMS

Needles are most likely to break at the junction with the hub and therefore should never be inserted fully. Catheters may also break, but exploratory surgery to find small pieces of catheter is inappropriate, as complications are very unlikely.

GENERAL MANAGEMENT

PATIENT ASSESSMENT AND SELECTION

Careful preoperative evaluation is as important before a local anaesthetic as it is before general anaesthesia, and the same principles of preoperative management apply. Therapy to improve the patient's condition before surgery should be instituted if appropriate. It is inappropriate to proceed with surgery under local anaesthesia for the sake of convenience in the poorly prepared patient. A decision on the need for immediate surgical intervention should be made before the anaesthetic technique is chosen.

The preoperative visit should be used to establish rapport with the patient. A clear description of the proposed anaesthetic should be given in simple terms, but there is rarely a need for excessive detail. Occasionally patients require some explanation of the reasons for selecting a regional technique before accepting it, but there should be no attempt at coercion.

Potential problems related to the intended block should be sought. Anatomical deformities may render some blocks impractical. A history of allergy to amide local anaesthetics is rare, but is an absolute contraindication, as is infection at the site of needle insertion. For most blocks, anticoagulant therapy and bleeding diatheses are also absolute contraindications, and the use of major blocks in patients with distant infection or receiving low-dose subcutaneous (s.c.) heparin, especially low molecular weight heparin, requires careful consideration. Sympathetic blockade with consequent vasodilatation may lead to profound hypotension in patients with aortic or mitral stenosis because of the relatively constant cardiac output. Hypovolaemia must be corrected before contemplating subarachnoid or epidural anaesthesia.

There is no evidence that neuromuscular disorders or multiple sclerosis are adversely affected by local anaesthetic techniques, but most anaesthetists use regional anaesthesia in such patients only if there are obvious benefits to be gained; any perioperative deterioration in the neurological condition is often associated by the patient with the local anaesthetic procedure. Raised intracranial pressure is a contraindication to central blockade.

SELECTION OF TECHNIQUE

Local anaesthetic drugs may be administered by:

- single dose
- intermittent bolus:
  — repeated injections
  — indwelling catheter for repeat administration
- continuous infusion (with optional bolus doses) via a catheter.

If regional anaesthesia has been selected primarily to provide analgesia during and after surgery under general anaesthesia, a distal technique is appropriate and is associated with the fewest complications.

Because a local anaesthetic technique renders only part of the body insensible, it is essential that the method employed is tailored to, and sufficient for, the planned surgery. Account must be taken of the duration of surgery, its site (which may be multiple, e.g. the need to obtain bone grafting material from the iliac crest), and the likelihood of a change of procedure in mid-operation. The problem of multiple sites of surgery may be met by one block which covers both sites, or by more than one regional procedure. The duration of anaesthesia may be tailored to the anticipated duration of surgery by selection of an appropriate local anaesthetic agent, or may require the use of a technique which allows further administration of drug.

PREMEDICATION

Manipulation of fractures and other short emergency procedures are often carried out using a local anaesthetic technique in the unpremedicated patient, as rapid recovery is desirable. However, premedication is helpful before in-patient elective or emergency surgery. An oral benzodiazepine allays anxiety, but an opioid (e.g. morphine) alleviates the discomfort of prolonged immobility which may be required during a long procedure. Preoperative analgesia may be required before definitive fixation. A nerve block may be useful in these circumstances, e.g. to alleviate the pain from a fractured femur, but often the administration of opioids, preferably i.v. in a controlled manner, is more appropriate at this time.

Patients should be fasted for all but the most minor peripheral nerve blocks.

TIMING

It is essential that sufficient time is allowed to perform the block without undue haste on the part of the anaesthetist. This is largely a matter of organization, and the experienced practitioner seldom causes delay to an operating list. Any preoperative delay is compensated for by the ability to return the patient to bed immediately after completion of surgery.

RESUSCITATION EQUIPMENT

A full range of resuscitation equipment must be in working order and immediately available. This includes:

- an anaesthetic breathing system through which oxygen may be administered under pressure via a face mask or tracheal tube
- a laryngoscope with two sizes of blade, a range of tracheal tubes and an introducer
- a table which can rapidly be tilted head-down
- suction apparatus
- intravenous cannulae and fluids
- thiopental to control convulsions
- drugs to treat hypotension, especially atropine, ephedrine and either methoxamine or phenylephrine.

A cannula must be inserted intravenously before any local anaesthetic block is performed in case emergency therapy is required.

REGIONAL BLOCK EQUIPMENT

Regional anaesthesia may be used with basic equipment, but some special items increase the success rate and reduce the risk of complications.

Needles

Very fine spinal needles (26G) have significantly reduced the incidence of post-spinal headache. 29G needles are now readily available, but confident and successful use of these needles requires greater expertise than is needed for the use of larger needles.

Pencil-point 24G needles are associated with a reduced incidence of post-spinal headache. Disposable prepacked spinal and epidural needles ease preparation and ensure sterility. Short-bevelled needles (Fig. 43.1) reduce the likelihood of nerve damage and are recommended for plexus and peripheral nerve blockade. Sheathed needles are valuable for use with nerve stimulators.

Immobile needle technique

For plexus and major nerve blocks, local anaesthetic drug is drawn into labelled syringes and connected to the block needle by a short length of tubing (see Fig. 43.2, p. 558). This allows the anaesthetist to hold the needle steady while aspiration tests are performed and syringes changed. The system must be primed to avoid air embolism.

Catheters

Continuous administration of local anaesthetic drugs has been made possible by the development of high-quality catheters, which are introduced through a needle and can be left in position for hours or even days. Careful fixation is essential to maintain the position of the catheter in the postoperative period.

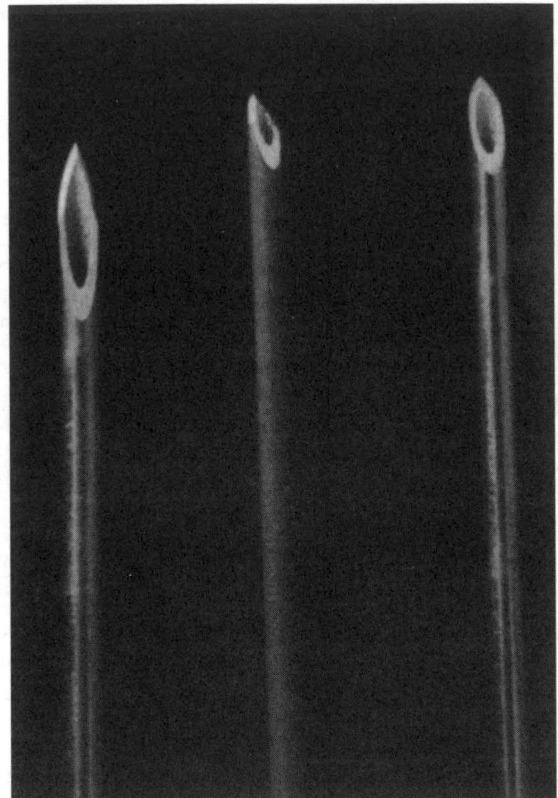

Fig. 43.1
Left to right : standard-bevelled, sheathed and unsheathed short-bevelled needles.

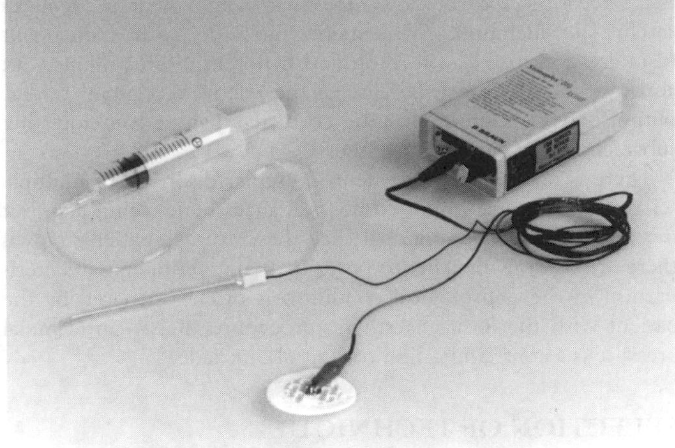

Fig. 43.2
Nerve stimulator and insulated stimulating needle.

Nerve stimulators

Many anaesthetists prefer to elicit paraesthesiae when performing a major nerve block. However, a nerve stimulator (Fig. 43.2) is a useful aid, especially for the beginner. It is important to explain to the patient the sensation elicited by stimulation.

Stimulators that deliver a constant current and give a digital display of the current used are readily available. One lead is attached to an electrocardiogram (ECG) electrode on the patient's skin, and the other to the shaft of the needle. After skin puncture, the stimulator is set to a frequency of 1 Hz and an initial current of 3 mA. As the nerve is approached, motor fibre stimulation causes muscle movement. This procedure is not painful unless the nerve is touched, when paraesthesiae result.

The current is gradually reduced until movement is still present at a current of, optimally, less than 1 mA. At this point, an aspiration test is performed and 2 ml of local anaesthetic solution injected. Movement should cease immediately. If it does not, and an unsheathed needle is being used, the tip may be beyond the nerve; the needle should be withdrawn slightly and the procedure repeated. Severe pain on injection suggests intraneural injection, in which case the needle should be repositioned. When the correct position has been found, the remainder of the anaesthetic solution should be injected slowly with repeated aspiration tests.

ASEPSIS

A 'no-touch' technique is essential. Drapes should be used for all major blocks and gloves and gown should be worn by the beginner. Gown, gloves, hat and mask are recommended for all central blocks even with a no-touch technique, especially when a catheter is inserted. Good practice is fostered by taking precautions seriously.

MONITORING

It is essential that the anaesthetist remains with the patient. Monitoring equipment should be appropriate to the anaesthetic and surgical procedure.

SUPPLEMENTARY TECHNIQUES

A local anaesthetic may be the only drug administered to the patient, or it may form part of a balanced anaesthetic technique. During surgery, patients may be awake, or sedated by i.v. or inhalational means. Propofol, midazolam or low concentrations of nitrous oxide are commonly employed. General anaesthesia may be used as a planned part of the procedure. Experienced anaesthetists use a combination of regional and general anaesthesia to obtain advantages from both.

When a surgical tourniquet is used, the chosen block must extend to the tourniquet site unless the procedure is brief. Discomfort from prolonged immobility on a hard table is relieved by the administration of an opioid either as a premedicant or i.v. during surgery; this type of discomfort is not relieved by sedative drugs, which often result in the patient becoming confused and uncooperative.

AFTER-CARE

Clear instructions should be given to the nurses caring for the patient.

After day-case surgery, the patient must be in a safe condition at the time of discharge. Plexus blockade with a long-acting agent is inappropriate because of the risk of the patient injuring the anaesthetized limb, but is suitable for postoperative pain relief in supervised inpatients. Patients who have received central blockade should have routine nursing observations at least until the block has worn off.

Continuous infusion techniques are suitable for use only by experienced anaesthetists. When used correctly, administration by infusion is safer than repeated bolus injection of drug, but regular observations are essential and the nursing staff must have an adequate level of knowledge to appreciate possible complications. An anaesthetist must be available within the hospital at all times.

INTRAVENOUS REGIONAL ANAESTHESIA (IVRA)

Ideally, IVRA (Bier's block) should be the first local anaesthetic technique learnt by a trainee, because its technical simplicity allows the trainee to concentrate on acquiring the skills of patient management. Bier's block is simple, safe and effective when performed correctly using an appropriate drug in correct dosage. Deaths from IVRA have resulted from incorrect selection of drug and dosage, incorrect technique and the performance of the block by personnel unable to treat toxic reactions. The drug involved in these deaths, bupivacaine, was not the most suitable agent and is no longer recommended. The lessons to be learned from these deaths are applicable to all local anaesthetic techniques, and emphasize that expert guidance is essential even when learning the most basic blocks.

INDICATIONS

IVRA is suitable for short procedures when postoperative pain is not marked, e.g. manipulation of Colles' fracture or carpal tunnel decompression. Recovery is rapid, and the technique is appropriate for outpatient surgery. Premedication may delay patient discharge and a reassuring visit preoperatively from the anaesthetist is usually sufficient in these circumstances.

METHOD (Fig. 43.3)

IVRA involves isolating an exsanguinated limb from the general circulation by means of an arterial tourniquet and then injecting local anaesthetic solution intravenously. Analgesia and weakness occur rapidly and result predominantly from local anaesthetic action on peripheral nerve endings.

An orthopaedic tourniquet of the correct size is applied over padding on the upper arm. All connections must lock, and the pressure gauge should be calibrated regularly. A cannula is inserted intravenously in the contralateral arm in case administration of emergency drugs is required. An indwelling cannula is inserted into a vein of the limb to be anaesthetized; scalp vein needles are best avoided as they are liable to penetrate the vein during exsanguination. A vein on the dorsum of the hand is preferred; injection into proximal veins reduces the quality of the block and increases the risk of toxicity. Exsanguination by means of an Esmarch bandage improves the quality of the block and increases the safety of the technique by reducing the venous pressure developed during injection. In patients with a painful lesion (e.g. Colles' fracture), elevation combined with brachial artery compression is adequate. The tourniquet should be inflated to a pressure 100 mmHg above systolic arterial pressure.

In an adult, 40 ml of prilocaine 0.5% is injected over 2 min with careful observation that the tourniquet remains inflated. Analgesia is complete within 10 min, but it is important to inform the patient that the feeling of touch is often retained at this time. The anaesthetist must be ready to deal with toxicity or tourniquet pain throughout the surgical procedure. The tourniquet should not be released until at least 20 min after injection, even if surgery is completed. This delay allows for diffusion of drug into the tissues so that plasma concentrations do not reach toxic levels after release of the tourniquet. The technique of repeated reinflation and deflation of the cuff during release has little effect on plasma concentrations and is not necessary.

Reinstitution of the block within 30 min of tourniquet release is possible using 50% of the initial dose, because some drug is retained within the limb. Bilateral blocks may be performed without exceeding the maximum recommended doses, but it is preferable to do this consecutively rather than concurrently.

Tourniquet pain

This may be troublesome if the cuff remains inflated for longer than 30–40 min. It is sometimes alleviated by inflating a separate tourniquet below the first on an area already rendered analgesic by the block; the first cuff is then deflated. Failing this, light general anaesthesia is preferable to administration of large and often ineffective doses of opioids and sedatives.

CHOICE OF DRUG

The agent of choice for this procedure is prilocaine 0.5% plain. It has an impressive safety record with no major reactions reported after its use, although minor side-effects such as transient lightheadedness after release of the tourniquet are not uncommon. The drug has distinct pharmacokinetic advantages in IVRA (see Ch. 15). Methaemoglobinaemia does not result from the doses used for IVRA.

LOWER LIMB

IVRA of the foot may be produced using the same dose of prilocaine and a calf tourniquet positioned carefully to avoid compression of the common peroneal nerve on the neck of the fibula.

CENTRAL NERVE BLOCKS

Spinal anaesthesia is a term that may be used to denote all forms of central blockade, although it usually refers to intrathecal administration of local anaesthetic. The term subarachnoid block (SAB) avoids ambiguity. The technique of SAB is basically that of lumbar puncture, but a knowledge of factors which affect the extent and duration of anaesthesia, and experience in patient management are essential. Epidural nerve block may be performed in the sacral (caudal block), lumbar, thoracic or cervical regions, although lumbar block is used most commonly. Local anaesthetic solution is injected through a needle after the tip has been introduced into the epidural space, or may be injected through a catheter placed in the space.

PHYSIOLOGICAL EFFECTS OF SAB

Differential nerve blockade

Local anaesthetic solution injected into the cerebrospinal fluid (CSF) spreads away from the site of injection and the concentration of the solution decreases as mixing occurs. A differential blockade of fibres occurs because small fibres are blocked by weaker concentrations of local anaesthetic solution. Sympathetic fibres are blocked to a level approximately two segments higher than the upper segmental level of sensory blockade. Motor blockade may be several segments caudal to the upper level of sensory block. A sensory level to T3 with SAB may be associated with total blockade of the T1–L2 sympathetic outflow.

Respiratory system

Low SAB has no effect on the respiratory system and the technique is an important part of the anaesthetist's armamentarium for patients with severe respiratory disease.

Motor blockade extending to the roots of the phrenic nerves (C3–5) causes apnoea.

Blocks which reach the thoracic level cause loss of intercostal muscle activity. This has little effect on tidal volume (because of diaphragmatic compensation), but there is a marked decrease in vital capacity resulting from a significant decrease in expiratory reserve volume. The patient may experience dyspnoea, difficulty in taking a maximal inspiration or in coughing effectively. A thoracic block may lead to a reduction in cardiac output and pulmonary artery pressure and increased ventilation/perfusion imbalance, resulting in a decrease in arterial oxygen tension ($P_{a}O_2$). Awake patients with a high spinal block should always be given oxygen-enriched air to breathe.

Cardiovascular system

The cardiovascular effects are proportional to the height of the block and result from denervation of the sympathetic outflow tracts (T1–L2). This produces dilatation of resistance and capacitance vessels and results in hypotension. In awake patients, compensatory vasoconstriction above the height of the block may compensate almost completely for these changes, thereby maintaining arterial pressure, but general anaesthetic agents may reduce this compensatory response, with consequent profound hypotension.

Hypotension is augmented by:

- the use of head-up posture
- any degree of hypovolaemia – pre-existing or induced by surgery.

Prevention of hypotension

Both the incidence and the degree of hypotension are reduced by limiting the height of the block and, in particular, by keeping it below the sympathetic supply to the heart (T1–5). Many authorities advise that all patients who receive subarachnoid or epidural block should be placed in a slight head-down position (5–10°) throughout the procedure. This small degree of tilt has little effect on distribution of block, but has a significant effect on venous return.

It is common practice to attempt to minimize hypotension during SAB or epidural anaesthesia by preloading the patient with 500–1000 ml of crystalloid solution i.v. before or during the institution of the block. These volumes are usually ineffective even in the short term, may risk the development of pulmonary oedema in susceptible individuals either during the procedure or when the block wears off, and may lead to postoperative urinary retention. Appropriate fluid should be given to replace blood and fluid losses and prevent dehydration.

Bradycardia may occur because of:

- neurogenic factors, particularly in awake patients, i.e. vasovagal syndrome
- block of the cardiac sympathetic fibres (T1–4).

Careful patient positioning, maintenance of a normal circulating volume and the use of pharmacological agents (see later), if required, should minimize the incidence of hypotension.

SAB has no direct effect on the liver or kidneys, but reductions in hepatic and renal blood flow occur in the presence of hypotension associated with high spinal blocks.

Gastrointestinal system

The vagus nerve supplies parasympathetic fibres to the whole of the gut as far as the transverse colon. Spinal blockade causes sympathetic denervation (proportional to height of block), and unopposed parasympathetic action leads to a constricted gut with increased peristaltic activity. This is regarded by some as advantageous for surgery.

Nausea, retching or vomiting may occur in the awake patient and are often the first symptoms of impending or established hypotension.

If nausea or retching occurs, the anaesthetist must measure arterial pressure and heart rate immediately and take appropriate measures.

PHYSIOLOGICAL EFFECTS OF EPIDURAL BLOCK

The physiological effects of epidural blockade are similar to those following SAB, but may develop more slowly. Additional effects may occur from the much larger volumes of anaesthetic solutions used, as there may be appreciable systemic absorption of local anaesthetic and epinephrine if an epinephrine-containing solution is used.

INDICATIONS FOR SAB

Blockade is produced more consistently and with a lower dose of drug by the subarachnoid route than by epidural injection. It is not customary in the UK to use a catheter in the subarachnoid space and the duration of analgesia is therefore limited to 2–4 h. SAB is most suited to surgery below the umbilicus and in this situation the patient may remain awake. Surgery above the umbilicus using SAB is less appropriate and would necessitate a general anaesthetic in addition, in order to abolish unpleasant sensations from visceral manipulation resulting from afferent impulses transmitted by the vagus nerves.

Types of surgery

Urology

Subarachnoid block is very appropriate for urological procedures such as transurethral prostatectomy, but it should be remembered that a block to T10 is required for surgery involving bladder distension. Perineal and penile operations may be carried out more conveniently under peripheral blockade or caudal anaesthesia.

Gynaecology

Minor procedures such as dilatation and curettage may be performed reliably with a block to T10. For major intra-abdominal gynaecological procedures and for diagnostic laparoscopy, light general anaesthesia is usually necessary in addition.

Obstetrics

The rapid onset of SAB may be advantageous in some circumstances, but this should be weighed against the high incidence of post-lumbar-puncture headache in this group of patients. The introduction of the pencil-point spinal needle with a reduction in the incidence of post-lumbar-puncture headache has led to an increased use of SAB in obstetric practice.

Any surgical procedure on the lower limbs or perineum

For patients with medical problems, low SAB may be the anaesthetic technique of choice:

Metabolic disease. Diabetes mellitus.

Respiratory disease. Low SAB has no effect on ventilation and obviates the requirement for anaesthetic drugs with depressant properties. There is some evidence that SAB may reduce the incidence of chest infection.

Cardiovascular disease. Low SAB may be valuable in patients with ischaemic heart disease or congestive cardiac failure, in whom a small reduction in preload and afterload may be beneficial. SAB is effective in preventing cardiovascular responses to surgery (e.g. hypertension, tachycardia) which are undesirable, particularly in patients with ischaemic heart disease.

INDICATIONS FOR EPIDURAL BLOCKADE

The indications for epidural anaesthesia are widespread, because it is an extremely versatile technique which can be tailored to suit a variety of situations. The duration of analgesia may be prolonged as necessary by means of an indwelling catheter and the use of intermittent top-ups or a continuous infusion. Bupivacaine is the drug of choice when one of these continuous techniques is used. The pharmacokinetic properties of bupivacaine are such that, with the doses necessary to maintain adequate blockade, systemic accumulation of the drug is slow and the risk of toxicity is small. Either local anaesthetic drugs or opioids may be used epidurally, but the latter are most suited to provision of postoperative analgesia and are inadequate for surgery in most circumstances. Almost all opioids have been tried by the epidural route with success.

CONTRAINDICATIONS TO SAB AND EPIDURAL ANAESTHESIA

Most contraindications are relative, but are best regarded as absolute by the trainee:

- bleeding diathesis
- hypovolaemia
- sepsis – local or systemic
- severe stenotic valvular heart disease – the patient may be unable to compensate for vasodilatation because of a fixed cardiac output
- pre-eclamptic toxaemia – epidural block has been used with great benefit in this condition, but a platelet count of less than 100×10^9 L^{-1} usually precludes epidural or subarachnoid anaesthesia
- acute neurological diseases/raised intracranial pressure
- lack of patient consent.

PERFORMANCE OF SAB

Intravenous access

An intravenous infusion must be given before lumbar puncture is performed.

Positioning the patient (Table 43.1)

Lumbar puncture for SAB may be performed with the patient sitting or in the lateral decubitus position (Fig. 43.3). If it is anticipated that lumbar puncture may be difficult, the midline is usually more discernible with the patient in the sitting position, but the risk of hypotension in the sedated patient or following institution of the block is increased. The technique of lumbar puncture for the patient in the lateral position is described in the next section.

Technique of lumbar puncture

For the right-handed anaesthetist, the patient is positioned on the operating table in the left lateral position. The patient's back should lie along the edge of the table and must be vertical. A curled position opens the spaces between the lumbar spinous processes. An assistant stands in front of the patient to assist with positioning and to reassure the patient. The anaesthetist must inform the patient before performing each part of the procedure.

A line between the iliac crests lies on the fourth lumbar spinous process or the L 4/5 interspace; lumbar puncture should be performed at the L 3/4 or L 4/5 space. A full sterile technique (with gown, gloves and surgical drapes) is adopted. All drugs should be drawn into syringes directly from sterile ampoules using a filter needle to prevent the injection of glass particles into the subarachnoid space. A selection of spinal needles (22–26 gauge) should be available.

The skin and subcutaneous tissues are infiltrated with local anaesthetic using a small needle. The spinal needle is inserted in the midline, midway between two spinous processes. In the well-positioned patient, the needle is directed at right angles to the skin. Passage through the interspinous ligament and ligamentum flavum into the spinal canal is appreciated easily with a 22-gauge needle (Fig. 43.4A). With some practice, these structures are usually discernible with a 26-gauge needle or 24g pencil-point needle, which all anaesthetists should aspire to use. The use of an introducer (19-gauge needle) is advisable to brace the 26-gauge needle, which is very flexible. When the needle tip has entered the spinal canal, the stilette is withdrawn from the needle and the hub is observed for flow of CSF; a needle with a transparent hub makes this easier. A gentle aspiration test should be performed if a free flow of CSF is not observed.

The three most common reasons for difficulty are poor patient position, failure to insert the needle in the midline and directing the needle laterally (Fig. 43.4B). This last fault is seen most easily from one side and is usually apparent to onlookers, but not to the anaesthetist, who looks only along the line of the needle.

When CSF is obtained, the syringe containing the local anaesthetic solution should be firmly attached to the needle. Gentle aspiration confirms the needle position and the solution is injected at a rate of 1 ml every 5–10 s. Aspiration after injection confirms that the needle tip has remained in the correct place. Needle and introducer are withdrawn and the patient placed supine.

Table 43.1 Techniques of subarachnoid block

Type of block	Upper level of analgesia	Position during lumbar puncture	Volume of solution
Saddle block	S1	Sitting 5 min	1 ml hyperbaric solution
Low thoracic	T10–12	Sitting/lateral decubitus	3–4 ml*
High thoracic	T4–6	Lateral decubitus Sitting (immediately supine)	2–3 ml hyperbaric solution
Unilateral	Not possible with hyperbaric solutions which eventually affect both sides after the patient is placed supine. Hypobaric solutions, e.g. tetracaine in water, may be used when the patient can remain with the operative side uppermost throughout, e.g. hip replacement surgery		

* Plain bupivacaine is slightly hypobaric at body temperature and the eventual block height is difficult to predict. Plain tetracaine, available in some countries, is truly isobaric, gives a more predictable height of block and is often used in volumes of 2 ml to achieve low thoracic blockade.

Factors affecting spread (Table 43.2)

The most important factor which affects the height of block in SAB is the baricity of the solution, which may be made hyperbaric (i.e. denser than CSF) by the addition of glucose. The specific gravity (SG) of CSF is 1.004. The addition of glucose 5 or 6% to a local anaesthetic produces a solution with SG of 1.024 or greater. A patient who assumes the sitting position for 5 min after injection of 1 ml of hyperbaric solution develops a saddle block which

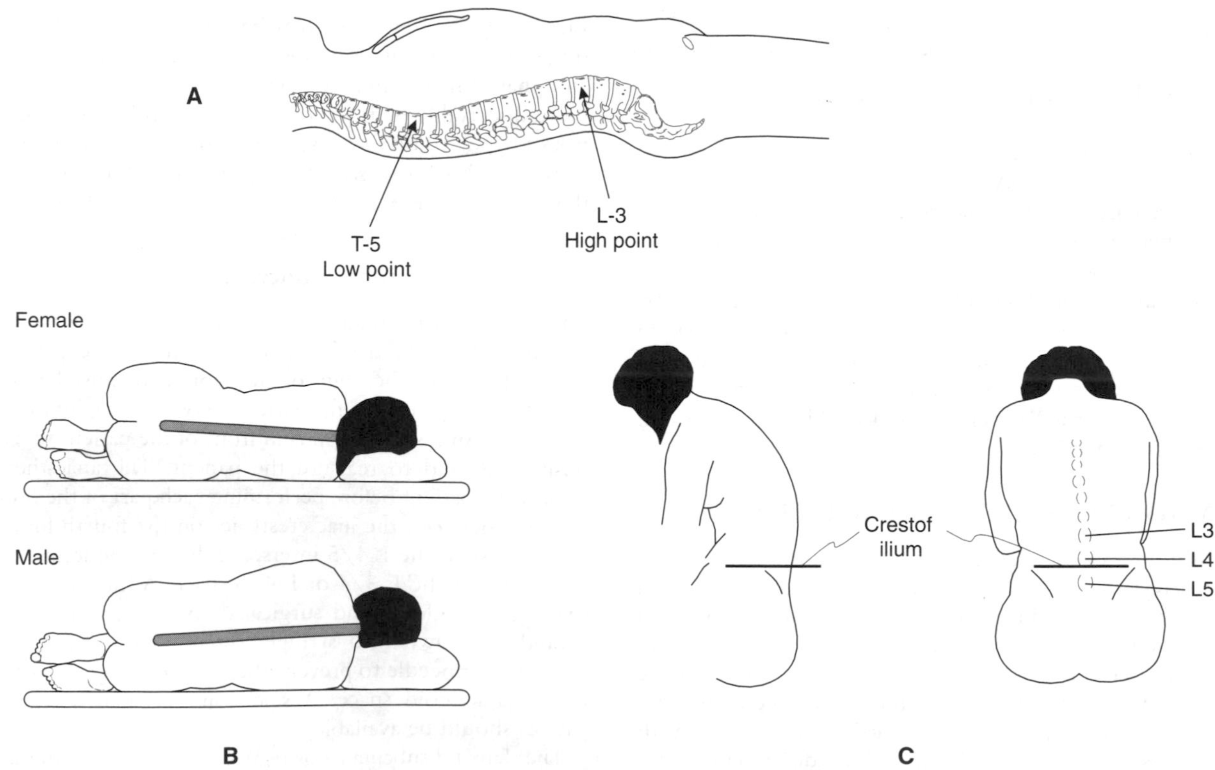

Fig. 43.3
Spinal curvature. **A.** Supine position. **B.** Lateral position. **C.** Sitting position.

affects the perineum only. Conversely, a patient placed supine immediately after injection develops a block to the mid-thoracic region. Slightly larger volumes are advisable to ensure spread above the lumbar curvature (Fig. 43.3).

Within the range normally used for SAB (2–4 ml), the volume of solution has only a minor effect on spread. Obesity, pregnancy and a high site of injection are minor factors which increase the height of the block; lower volumes may be desirable in these situations. Barbotage and rapid injection may produce high blocks, but increase the unpredictability of spread.

Factors affecting duration

The duration of anaesthesia depends on the drug used and the dose of drug employed. Vasoconstrictors added to the local anaesthetic solution significantly increase the duration of action of tetracaine, which is widely used in the USA, but this is not so for other agents.

Agents

Only three agents are readily available for SAB in the UK. Plain bupivacaine 0.5% is slightly hypobaric at body temperature and may very occasionally have an unpredictable spread and produce an inadequate block. It is used in volumes of 3–4 ml and lasts 2–3 h. Hyperbaric bupivacaine 0.5% is much more predictable and consistently produces a block to the umbilicus (and usually to T5) in supine patients. As with all hyperbaric solutions, hypotension is encountered more frequently because of higher levels of sympathetic blockade. Volumes of 2–3 ml are used and a duration of 2–3 h is usually assured. Plain lidocaine 2% usually provides analgesia of the lower limbs and perineum. Volumes of 3–4 ml are used and duration is approximately 1 h.

Complications

Acute

Hypotension. Significant hypotension should be anticipated with SAB. Changes in position, e.g. turning the patient from the supine to the prone position, may result in a sudden increase in the height of block, with consequent extension of sympathetic blockade. This may occur even after 15–20 min. Treatment (Table 43.3) may not be necessary; moderate hypotension may help to reduce operative blood loss and is tolerated well by most patients. Severe or unwanted hypotension may be treated by i.v. fluids or drugs. The use of large volumes of crystalloid or colloid in this situation is not recommended, as urinary retention may occur postoperatively or circulatory overload may result when the block wears off. However, it is essential that operative blood losses are replaced promptly, and when blood losses are expected (e.g. caesarean section) it is wise to administer fluid in advance of the loss. Hypotension is associated commonly with bradycardia, and ephedrine 5–6 mg i.v. is the most appropriate treatment. Atropine may be useful, but sympathomimetic drugs are usually more effective than vagolytics.

Oversedation. This may occur when sedative drugs have been administered before performance of SAB. When the block is established, the previously satisfactory level of sedation may become excessive, with the attendant risks of respiratory obstruction or aspiration. Some reports of cardiac arrest associated with SAB may be related to hypoxaemia produced in this manner.

Table 43.2 Factors influencing spread of hyperbaric spinal solutions

Factor	Effect
Position of patient	Sitting position produces perineal block only, provided that small volumes are used
Spinal curvature	With standard volumes (2–3 ml) the block often spreads to T4. With small volumes (1 ml) the block may affect only the perineum even when the patient is placed supine immediately
Dose of drug	Within the range of volumes usually employed (2–4 ml), increasing the dose of drug increases the duration of anaesthesia rather than the height of the block
Interspace	Minor factor affecting height of block
Obesity	Minor factor affecting height of block. Obese patients tend to develop higher blocks
Speed of injection	Rapid injection makes the height of block more variable
Barbotage	No longer employed. Makes the height of block more variable

Postoperative

Headache. This is more common in young adults and particularly in obstetric patients. It may present up to 2–7 days after lumbar puncture, and may persist for up to 6 weeks. Characteristically, it is worse on sitting, occipital in distribution and very disabling. The incidence is reduced by using small-gauge or pencil-point needles and ensuring that the bevel of the needle penetrates the dura in a sagittal plane. Simple analgesics may be the only treatment required, but occasionally an epidural blood patch is necessary. The incidence of post-spinal headache is not reduced by keeping the patient supine for 24 h; the patient should remain supine only until the anaesthetic has worn off and the risk of postural hypotension is minimal. If headache is severe and persistent, an epidural blood patch may be performed by removing 20 ml of the patient's own blood under aseptic conditions and injecting it epidurally at the same interspace as SAB was performed. Injection should be stopped if discomfort is experienced. This is 70–80% effective for lumbar puncture headache and appears to be remarkably free from adverse effects.

Other complications include:

- Urinary retention – this may be associated with the surgical procedure. Large volumes of i.v. fluids may increase the frequency of this complication.
- Labyrinthine disturbances.

Table 43.3 Management of hypotension

5^0 Head-down tilt	
Maintain blood volume	
Heart rate:	
< 60 beat min^{-1}	Atropine 0.3 mg
60–80 beat min^{-1}	Ephedrine 3 mg
> 80 beat min^{-1}	Methoxamine 2 mg

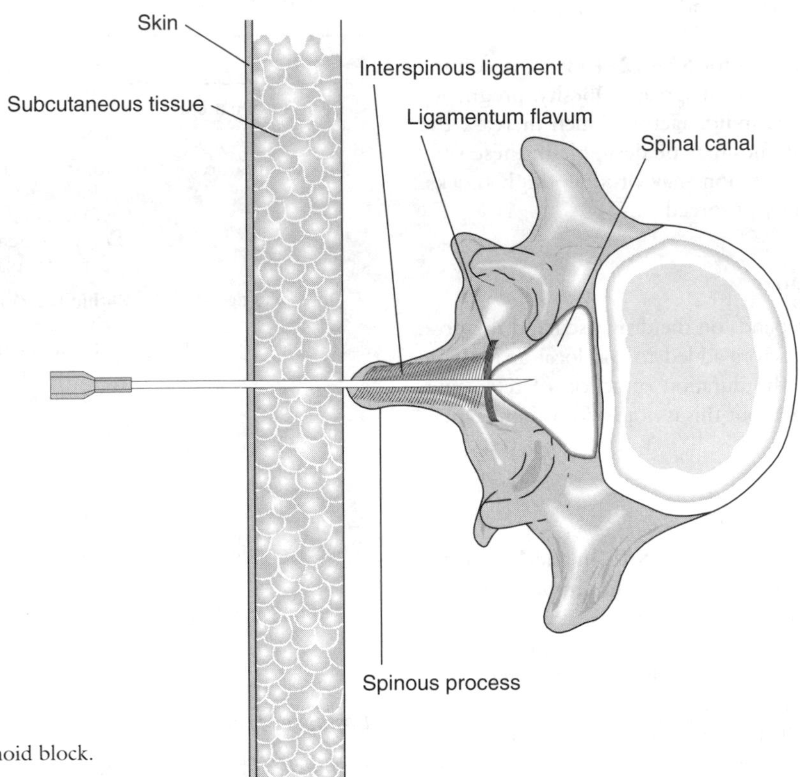

Fig. 43.4a
Midline approach for subarachnoid block.
A. Correctly angled.

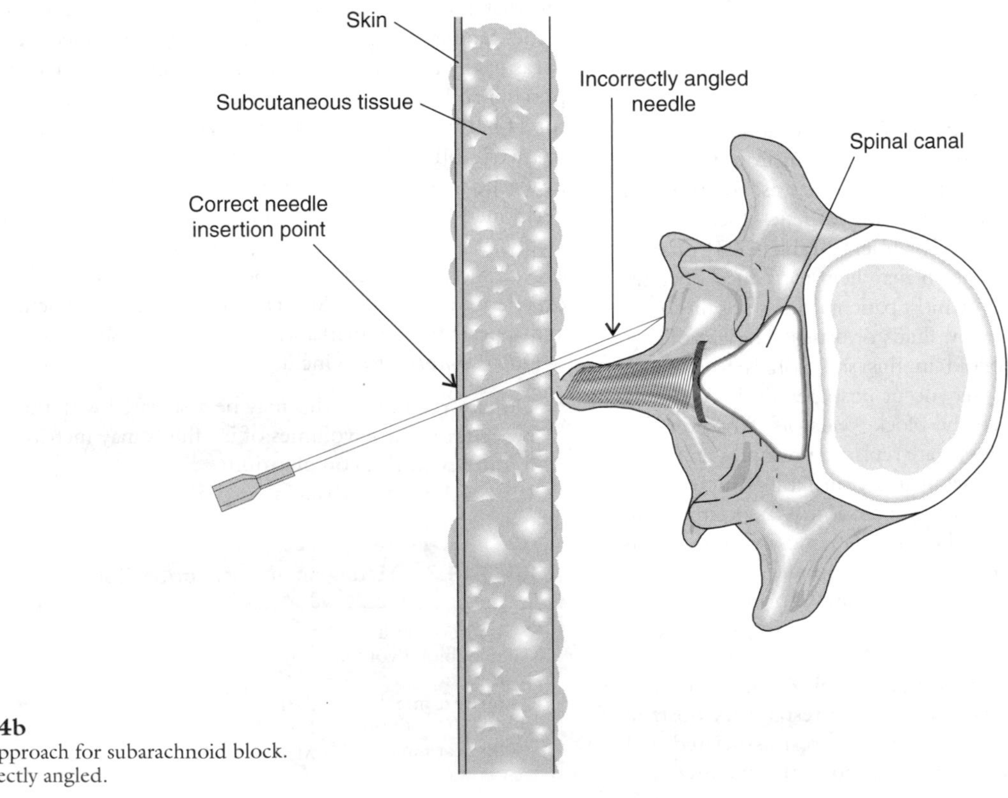

Fig. 43.4b
Midline approach for subarachnoid block.
B. Incorrectly angled.

- Cranial nerve palsy – sixth nerve palsy may occur and is usually temporary. This complication is more common with larger needles.
- Meningitis and meningism.
- Spinal cord trauma caused by inserting the needle at too high an interspace – fortunately these conditions, giving rise to permanent neurological damage or paraplegia, are extremely rare.

PERFORMANCE OF EPIDURAL BLOCK

By virtue of its great versatility, epidural analgesia is probably the most widely used regional technique in the UK. It may be used for procedures from the neck downwards and the duration of analgesia can be tailored to meet the needs of surgery and postoperative pain relief by using a catheter system.

The major differences between SAB and epidural block are summarized in Table 43.4. Further expansion of the technique has taken place with the advent of epidural administration of opioids (see Ch. 17), and other agents such as clonidine or ketamine may have a place in providing postoperative epidural analgesia.

Equipment

Epidural anaesthesia is usually performed using a Tuohy needle (Fig. 43.5). The needle is marked at 1 cm intervals and has a Huber point which allows a catheter to be directed along the long axis of the epidural space. Disposable catheters are available with a single end-hole or with a sealed tip and three side-holes distally.

Table 43.4 Differences between subarachnoid and extradural block

	Subarachnoid	Epidural
Dose of drug used	Small: minimal risk of systemic toxicity	Large: possibility of systemic toxicity after intravascular injection or total spinal blockade after subarachnoid injection
Rate of onset	Fast: 2–5 min for initial effect 20 min for maximum effect	Slow: 5–15 min for initial effect 30–45 min for maximum effect
Intensity of block	Usually complete anaesthesia	Often not complete anaesthesia for all segments
Pattern of block	May be dermatomal for first few minutes, but rapidly develops appearance of cord transection	Dermatomal
Addition of vasoconstrictor	Reliably prolongs block with tetracaine, but not with other drugs	Reliably prolongs block with lidocaine. May prolong block with bupivacaine, but not in all patients

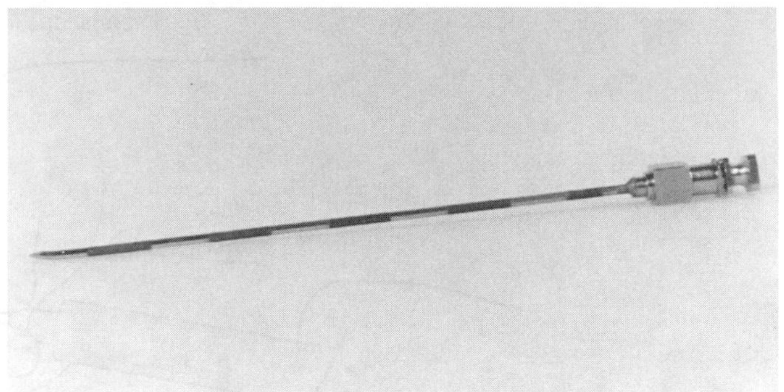

Fig. 43.5
16-Gauge Tuohy extradural needle.

Technique

Epidural block may be performed at any level of the vertebral column to provide segmental analgesia over an area that can be predetermined with reasonable success. Initial experience should be gained in the lumbar region before progressing to sites above the termination of the spinal cord.

The pressure in the epidural space is usually subatmospheric, particularly in the thoracic region, because of communications by valveless veins between the epidural and intrathoracic spaces. Some older methods of identifying the epidural space (e.g. Odom's indicator, Macintosh's balloon) relied on detection of the subatmospheric pressure in the epidural space. However, methods which depend on loss of resistance to injection of air or saline as the tip of the needle penetrates the ligamentum flavum and enters the epidural space have become more popular. A midline approach is described here, using loss of resistance to saline to detect the epidural space.

The patient is positioned as for SAB and the vertebral level is identified from the iliac crests. The skin and subcutaneous tissues of the third lumbar interspace are infiltrated with local anaesthetic solution in the midline. A sharp needle is used to puncture the skin and the Tuohy, round-ended epidural needle is introduced through the skin puncture, subcutaneous tissue and supraspinous ligament. The common reasons for difficulty are the same as those for SAB. When inserted into the interspinous ligament, the unsupported needle remains steady. The stilette is withdrawn and a 10 or 20 ml plastic syringe filled with saline is attached and advanced using firm but gentle pressure on the plunger. The needle must be gripped tightly at all times (Fig. 43.6) to prevent sudden forward movement. When the needle penetrates the ligamentum flavum, there is a sudden loss of resistance to pressure on the plunger, but the needle must not be allowed to advance further. The needle must not be rotated after its tip has entered the epidural space, as this increases the risk of penetration of the dura.

Single-dose technique

The syringe containing local anaesthetic is connected to the epidural needle, and after aspiration a test dose is administered to detect intravascular or subarachnoid placement. After an appropriate pause, the remainder of the solution is injected at a rate not exceeding 10 ml min^{-1} while verbal contact is maintained with the patient.

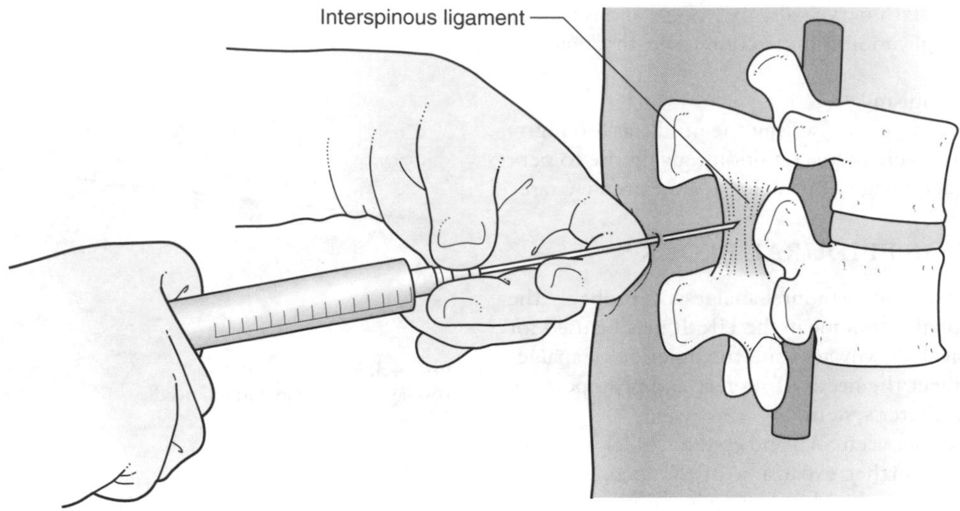

Fig. 43.6
Loss of resistance technique to identify the extradural space. See text for details.

Catheter insertion

An epidural catheter should pass freely through the needle into the epidural space. If the catheter does not thread easily, the needle should be repositioned, as forcing the catheter into the epidural space makes intravascular placement more likely. When a sufficient length of catheter (2–3 cm) is in the space, the needle is carefully withdrawn over the catheter. After ensuring that there is no flow of blood or CSF down the catheter, the hub is attached and an aspiration test performed; if blood or CSF is obtained, the catheter should be reinserted in an adjacent space. A filter is connected and a test dose given. If this is satisfactory, the catheter is fixed to the patient's back with adhesive strapping and the main dose is administered.

Factors affecting spread

Epidural spread is variable and the initial dose depends on the clinical situation. The volume of solution has a relatively minor effect on spread, and increasing the dose of local anaesthetic is more likely to prolong the duration of the block than to increase spread. Posture has a minimal effect on spread, but patients who are pregnant or aged over 60 years may have an increased likelihood of a high block with a given dose of local anaesthetic.

Factors affecting onset

Onset time is reduced by increasing the concentration of the local anaesthetic and by the addition of epinephrine 1:200 000.

Factors affecting duration

The choice of local anaesthetic agent has a major effect on the duration of anaesthesia. The concentration of the drug also has an effect; the higher concentrations of bupivacaine produce a more prolonged block. To some extent this is a reflection of increased dose, which is known to increase the duration of anaesthesia. The addition of epinephrine 1:200 000 to lidocaine increases duration.

Agents

Lidocaine

This drug is used in concentrations of 1.5–2% with or without epinephrine 1:200 000. Without epinephrine, the duration of action is approximately 1 h; a duration of approximately 2–2.5 h may be expected when solutions containing epinephrine are used.

Bupivacaine

This agent is available in concentrations of 0.25, 0.5 and 0.75%. The 0.75% concentration is no longer recommended for obstetric use. Increasing the concentration results in a faster onset, a denser block, more profound motor block (and therefore muscle relaxation) and increased duration of anaesthesia. A block lasting more than 4 h may be achieved with 0.75% solution. The addition of epinephrine 1:200 000 prolongs analgesia with 0.75% bupivacaine; the block may last for 6–8 h.

Ropivacaine

This long-acting agent is less cardiotoxic than bupivacaine and may produce less motor block for a similar degree of sensory blockade. It is less potent than bupivacaine and slightly higher concentrations/doses are used.

Complications

Intraoperative

Dural tap. The incidence should be less than 0.5% in experienced hands. It usually occurs with the needle rather than the catheter and is immediately obvious because of the free flow of CSF. Puncture of the dura with a large epidural needle leads to a high incidence of headache. If this occurs, epidural block should be produced at an adjacent space, and 0.9% saline 40 ml h^{-1} should be infused epidurally for 36 h after surgery or labour to reduce the likelihood of headache. Simple analgesics may suffice if headache occurs; if not, an epidural blood patch should be performed.

Accidental total spinal anaesthesia (see below) is rare because the dural tap is usually obvious.

Total spinal anaesthesia. This may occur if the large volume of solution used for epidural anaesthesia is injected into the subarachnoid space. The consequences may be:

- profound hypotension
- apnoea, unconsciousness and dilated pupils secondary to local anaesthetic action on the brain stem.

Paralysis of the legs should alert the physician to the possibility of subarachnoid injection. When using a test dose, motor function should be tested by asking the patient to raise the whole leg and not merely to wiggle the toes; movement of the toes may not be abolished for 20 min after SAB, if at all. It should be noted that relatively large volumes of local anaesthetic solution, e.g. 10 ml of bupivacaine 0.25%, may be injected into the subarachnoid space without total spinal anaesthesia occurring.

Provided that skilled resuscitation is undertaken rapidly, a total spinal should be followed by complete recovery. Appropriate personnel and equipment should be present before epidural analgesia is undertaken and whenever top-up injections are administered.

Massive epidural block and subdural block. A very high block may occur in the absence of subarachnoid injection. This may be associated with Horner's syndrome.

Other complications include:

- intravenous toxicity (see Ch. 15)
- hypotension
- urinary retention
- shivering
- nausea/vomiting – this may result from hypotension or visceral manipulation in the awake patient.

Postoperative

- *Headache* following dural tap.
- *Epidural haematoma.* The spinal canal acts as a rigid box, and an expanding haematoma within the canal compresses the spinal cord, resulting in loss of neurological function unless the compression is relieved surgically at a very early stage. Decompression within 6 h is completely effective in virtually all patients, but after 12 h it is almost totally ineffective.
- *Epidural abscess*
- *Other neurological complications,* e.g. damage to a single nerve root or paraplegia following accidental administration of potassium chloride.

ANTICOAGULANTS AND SAB OR EPIDURAL ANAESTHESIA

Oral anticoagulants

Anticoagulation should be stopped at an appropriate time before surgery if SAB or epidural anaesthesia is planned. The degree of anticoagulation most appropriate for the patient depends on a balance between the risk of withholding anticoagulation and the nature of the surgery, in particular the associated risk of bleeding.

Platelets

The platelet count should ideally be in excess of 150×10^9 L^{-1}.

Table 43.5 Guidelines for the insertion and removal of epidural catheters in association with low-molecular-weight heparins (LMWH)

1. Patients who need DVT prophylaxis before theatre, should receive LMWH the day before at approximately 18.00 h.
2. LMWH should not be given on the day of surgery – this allows 12 h before catheter placement; although the LMWH is providing DVT prophylaxis at this time, plasma concentrations are below peak activity and therefore less likely to create a problem.
3. LMWH may be given 2 h after placement of an epidural catheter.
4. The epidural catheter should be removed 12 h after the last dose of LWMH and the next dose cannot be given until 2 h have elapsed.
5. Antiplatelet drugs and anticoagulant drugs should not be used concurrently with LMWH.
6. The smallest effective dose of LMWH should be used.
7. Patients should have regular (every 4 h) neurological examination after removal of the epidural catheter. This should include sensation, power and reflexes.
8. In cases of traumatic or repeated epidural puncture, administration of LMWH should be delayed for more than 24 h; an alternative method of DVT prophylaxis should be used.
9. Epidural mixtures should contain a low concentration of bupivacaine so that motor function may be assessed.
10. If the patient develops a neurological abnormality either during epidural infusion or within 48 h of epidural catheter removal, an urgent MRI scan is required and a neurosurgical opinion should be obtained.

Heparin

The half-life of heparin given i.v. is 50–160 min, depending on dose. When given s.c., blood concentrations vary widely; in some patients plasma concentrations are in the anticoagulant range. At present, it is regarded as imprudent to use SAB or epidural analgesia when subcutaneous heparin has already been given, especially the low-molecular-weight variety. Removal of an epidural catheter should be timed to precede, rather than follow, administration of a further dose of subcutaneous heparin.

Guidelines for the use of low-molecular-weight heparin and epidural anaesthesia are given in Table 43.5.

Intraoperative heparinization

Epidural analgesia and SAB offer advantages for major vascular surgery, but the routine use of heparin introduces the theoretical risk of haemorrhage if an epidural catheter is in place. The precise risk is unknown, as prospective trials would require in excess of 10 000 cases. Some large series (3000 patients) have been conducted under epidural analgesia without haematoma formation.

CAUDAL ANAESTHESIA

Caudal block involves injection of local anaesthetic into the epidural space through the sacral hiatus to obtain anaesthesia of sacral and coccygeal nerve roots. Injection of very large volumes to obtain anaesthesia of lumbar and thoracic roots is seldom practised in adults because there is a high incidence of side-effects and failure to achieve a sufficiently high block. With appropriate volumes, caudal blockade affects the lower limbs infrequently, does not cause sympathetic blockade and has a low risk of dural puncture. The anatomy is variable and difficulty is experienced in approximately 5% of subjects.

Indications

Caudal anaesthesia is suitable for perineal operations, e.g. haemorrhoidectomy. Regional anaesthesia for circumcision is better achieved with a penile block.

Method

Caudal blockade may be performed with the patient in the prone position, but the left lateral position is usually more acceptable to the patient. Palpation down the sacral spine leads to the depression of the sacral hiatus at S5, flanked by the sacral cornua, through which the needle is inserted. A 21-gauge hypodermic needle is introduced through skin and sacrococcygeal ligament in a cephalad direction at 45° to the skin (Fig. 43.7). When the membrane is penetrated, the needle hub is depressed toward the natal cleft, and the needle inserted 2–3 mm along the sacral canal; it must be remembered that the dura may extend to S3. Lidocaine 2%, with or without epinephrine, and bupivacaine 0.5% are suitable agents. In an adult, 10 ml of solution blocks anal sensation consistently.

In conjunction with light general anaesthesia, caudal anaesthesia provides smooth operating conditions and good postoperative analgesia. With this combined technique, the advantages of performing caudal block before induction of general anaesthesia are as follows:

- The patient does not need to be repositioned while anaesthetized.
- Subperiosteal injection is reported by the patient.
- Accidental i.v. injection may be detected before the full dose is given.

For patients undergoing haemorrhoidectomy, many surgeons rely on the tone in the anal sphincter to identify it accurately and avoid damage. In these patients, light general anaesthesia may be supplemented by a short-acting opioid such as alfentanil for the intraoperative period, and caudal anaesthesia given following the procedure. Extremely effective postoperative analgesia lasting several hours is provided. If there is doubt about needle position, 2 ml of air should be injected before the local anaesthetic solution. Correct positioning of the needle is confirmed by listening over the lower thoracic spine using a stethoscope. A characteristic 'whoosh' should be heard.

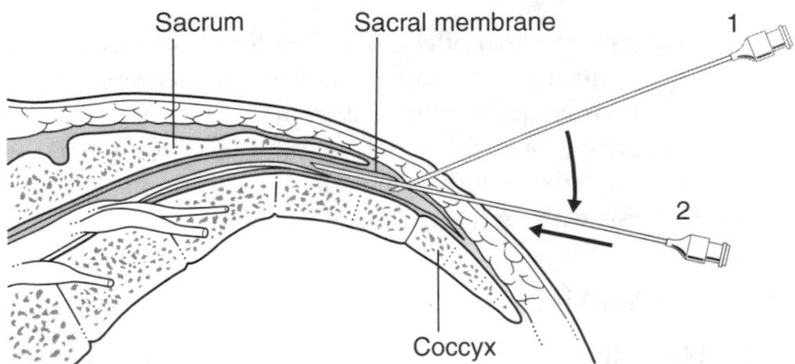

Fig. 43.7
Needle position for caudal anaesthesia.

Complications

Misplaced needle. Injection into subcutaneous tissue causes a swelling with fluid, or surgical emphysema with 2–3 ml of air. Intraosseous or subperiosteal injection results in marked resistance to injection. Penetration of rectum and fetal head (in obstetric practice) have been reported but should not occur if the technique is performed carefully.

Dural tap. This is rare, but the procedure should be abandoned if CSF is aspirated.

PERIPHERAL BLOCKS

HEAD AND NECK BLOCKS

These are mostly specialized blocks which are used in ophthalmic and plastic surgery. Only the technique of local anaesthesia for awake intubation is described here. Blocks used in ophthalmic surgery are discussed in Chapter 47.

Awake intubation

This may be the safest option in a patient with upper airway obstruction or a history which suggests difficulty with intubation. Sedation with midazolam or a combination of fentanyl and droperidol is desirable if this is not likely to exacerbate airway obstruction. A fibreoptic or rigid technique of laryngoscopy may be employed, but considerable experience is necessary with the former.

The patient sucks a benzocaine lozenge, or the mouth and pharynx are sprayed with lidocaine 1%. The laryngoscope blade and tube are smeared with 4% lidocaine gel. This may suffice in sick patients, but in robust subjects a cricothyroid injection is necessary. A 25-gauge needle is advanced through the cricothyroid membrane (Fig. 43.8a+b) and air is aspirated to confirm the posi-

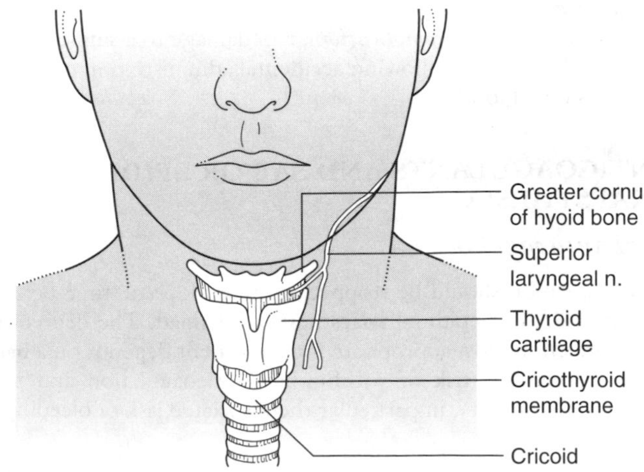

Fig. 43.8a
Cricothyroid injection.

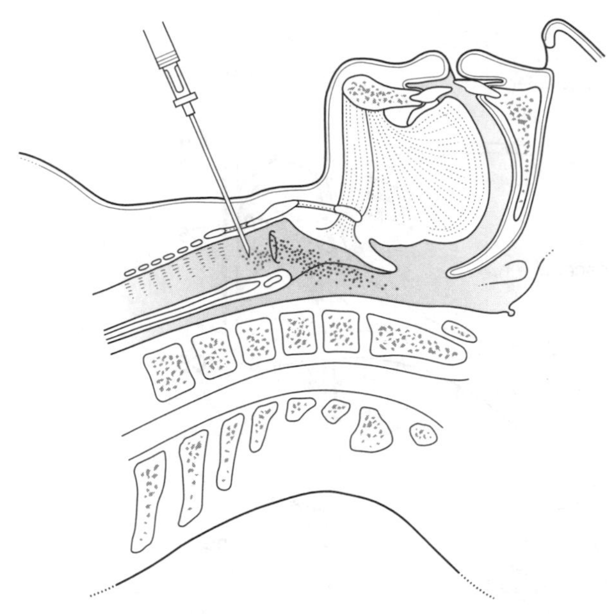

Fig. 43.8b

tion. Two millilitres of lidocaine 2% are injected and the needle is withdrawn immediately. A vigorous cough results and spreads the solution. The total dose of lidocaine must be kept as low as possible because absorption from mucous membranes is rapid.

UPPER LIMB BLOCKS

The upper limb is well suited to local anaesthetic techniques, as it is possible to block almost the whole arm with a single injection. Percutaneous approaches to the brachial plexus were first described in 1911, but approaches based on the concept of a sheath surrounding the brachial plexus are more effective.

Anatomy of the brachial plexus

The nerve supply of the upper limb is mainly derived from the brachial plexus, which is formed from the anterior primary rami of the fifth to eighth cervical and first thoracic nerve roots. The roots of the plexus divide repeatedly and recombine to form trunks, divisions, cords and terminal nerves (Fig. 43.9). The roots emerge from the intervertebral foramina and combine into three trunks above the first rib. Each trunk separates above the clavicle into anterior and posterior divisions; anterior divisions supply the flexor structures of the arm and posterior divisions the extensor structures. The divisions recombine into three cords, which surround the second part of the axillary artery behind the pectoralis minor and then form the terminal nerves (Fig. 43.10).

The roots lie between the anterior and middle scalene muscles and are invested in a sheath, derived from the prevertebral fascia, which splits to enclose the scalene muscles. This fascial covering extends into the axilla and causes solution injected anywhere within the sheath to spread along the line of the plexus. The cutaneous and deep nerve supplies of the upper limb are depicted in Figure 43.11.

Part of the cutaneous nerve supply of the upper limb is not derived from the brachial plexus; the upper medial part of the arm is supplied by the intercostobrachial nerve (T2) and has to be blocked separately if a tourniquet is to be used for a prolonged period. The reader is referred to standard texts for a more detailed anatomical description.

Axillary block

Positioning

The patient lies supine with the arm to be blocked abducted to no more than 90° and the elbow bent to 90° (Fig. 43.12). Further abduction with the hand placed behind the head is convenient, but the axillary vessels become stretched and distorted, and performance of the block is more difficult.

Method

The axillary artery is palpated and followed as far medially as possible. A skin wheal is raised with local anaesthetic at this point just above the palpating finger. A short-bevelled block needle is introduced through this wheal after puncturing the skin with a standard 19-gauge needle. A nerve stimulator is attached and the needle is directed towards the apex of the axilla at an angle which places it alongside, but not penetrating, the axillary artery. A click may be felt as the needle enters the sheath. Stimulation causes flexion or extension at the wrist or elbow. When this is produced by a suitably low current, the local anaesthetic is injected.

Forty millilitres of solution are required in an adult to achieve consistent blockade of the musculocutaneous and axillary nerves which leave the sheath at the level of the coracoid process. Digital pressure should be applied just distal to the needle during and immediately after injection to promote proximal flow of solution; a venous tourniquet is ineffective for this purpose. After completion of injection, the arm should be returned to the patient's side and digital pressure maintained. This manoeuvre may allow further spread of local anaesthetic beyond the humeral head.

The intercostobrachial nerve is blocked using 5 ml of solution. This can be performed without further skin puncture by redirecting the needle in the subcutaneous tissues around the medial side of the arm.

Disadvantages and complications

The onset time may be as long as 30–40 min. If the musculocutaneous nerve is not blocked, there is no analgesia on the lateral border of the arm. Puncture of the axillary artery is rarely a problem, but may lead to haematoma formation or inadvertent intravascular injection. The block should not be abandoned if the axillary artery is punctured; indeed the transarterial approach of axillary block is well described. Local anaesthetic solution is injected after penetrating the posterior wall of the artery and performing a careful aspiration test. Nerve damage occurs rarely and usually results from malposition of the anaesthetized limb or failure to recognize a compression syndrome postoperatively.

Supraclavicular block

Supraclavicular approaches to the brachial plexus are favoured by many anaesthetists and the relatively recent description by Winnie (1984) of the subclavian perivascular approach has increased the safety of this technique.

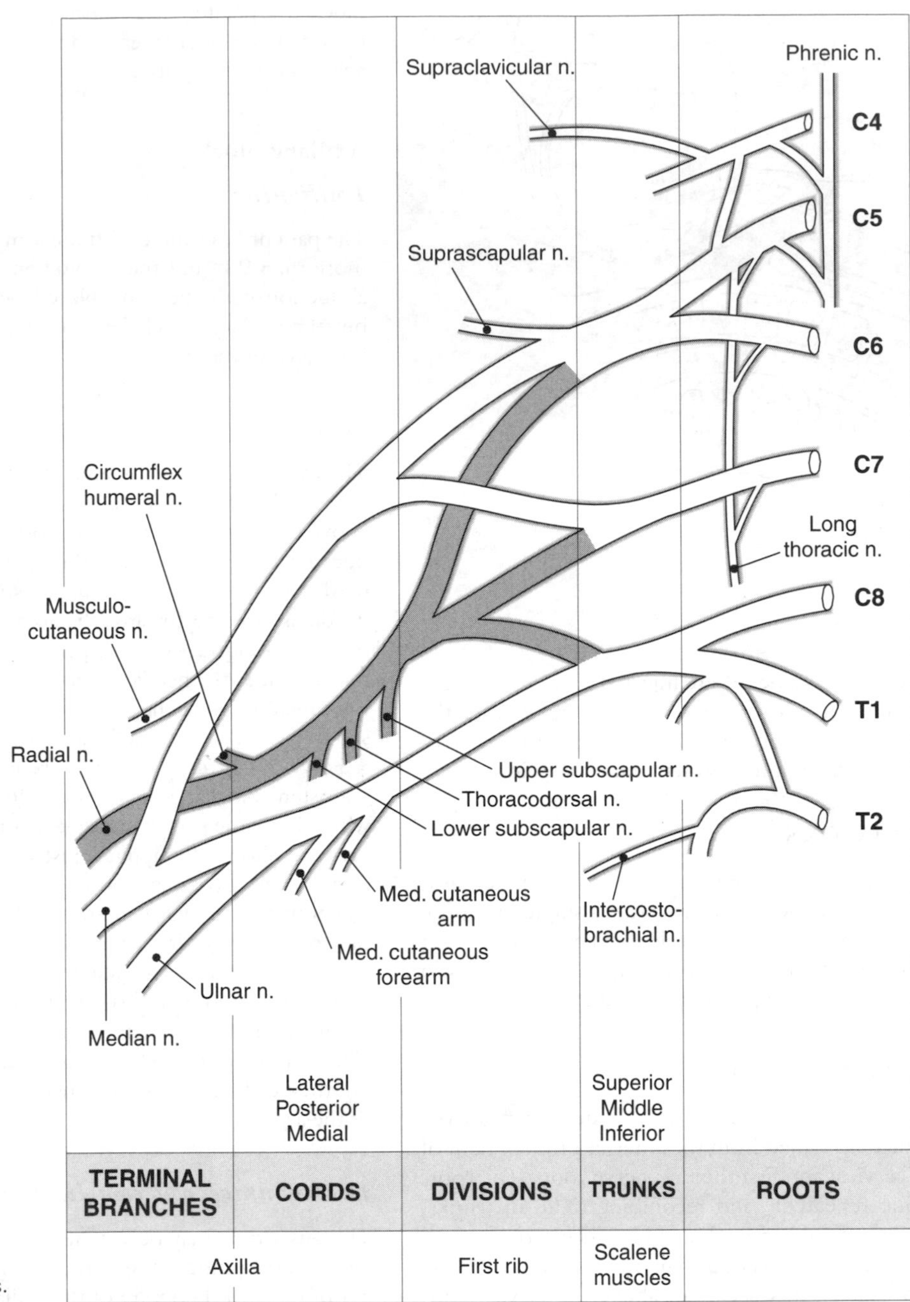

Fig. 43.9
Formation of the brachial plexus.

Advantages

Onset time may be as short as 10–15 min, analgesia of the whole arm is more likely and 25–30 ml of solution is sufficient in an adult.

Disadvantages

The risk of pneumothorax is always present, but is very small in experienced hands. Phrenic nerve paralysis is probably common, but is usually asymptomatic. However, axillary block is the method of choice if there is diminished respiratory reserve. If bilateral blocks are intended, one should be performed by the axillary route. Recurrent laryngeal nerve block may result in hoarseness. Sympathetic block is relatively common and results in Horner's syndrome. Subarachnoid or epidural spread of local anaesthetic solution is possible, but rare.

Interscalene block

This is the highest approach to the brachial plexus and may be the most suitable block for proximal procedures on the arm. Block of the C8 and T1 roots may prove difficult, and this approach is therefore less suitable for hand surgery. Complications are similar

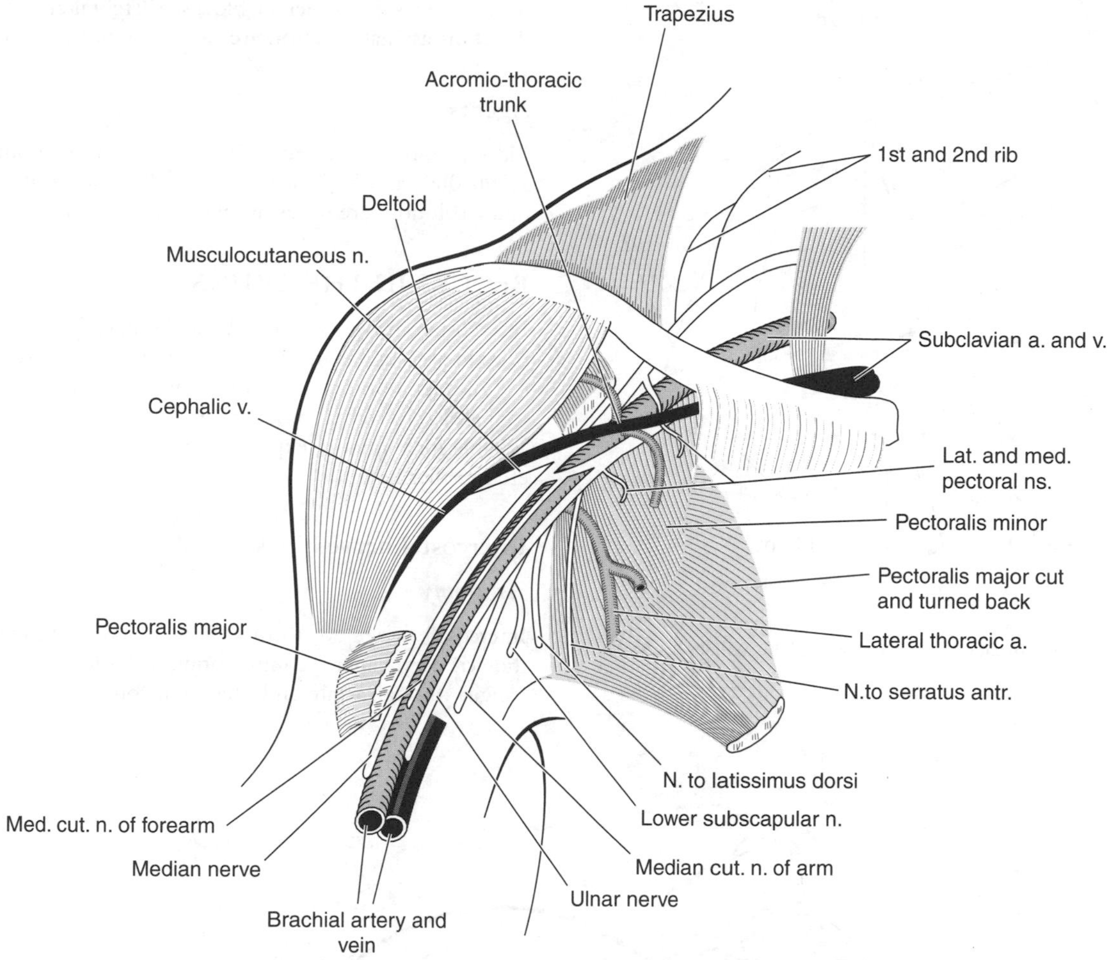

Fig. 43.10
Relationship of the brachial plexus to adjacent structures.

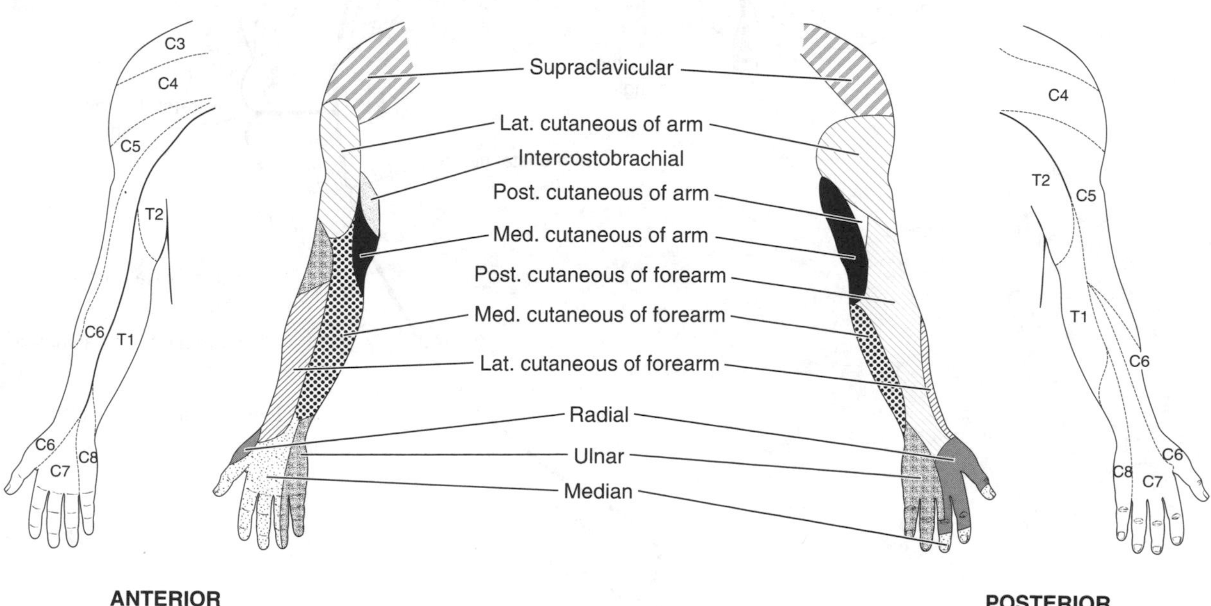

Fig. 43.11
Innervation of the upper limb: outer, dermatomal innervation of the skin; inner, cutaneous nerve supply to the upper limb.

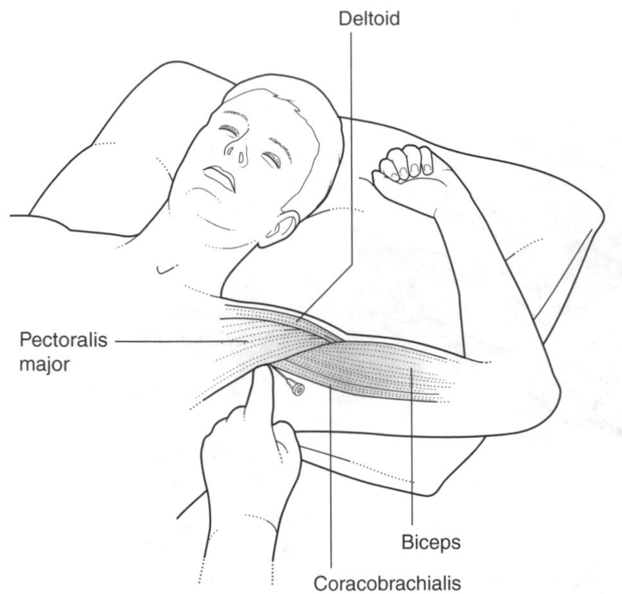

Fig. 43.12
Correct position and approach for axillary block. The axillary artery is palpated by the finger.

to those for supraclavicular blocks. Vertebral artery puncture and direct intraspinal injection are also possibilities.

Agents

Lidocaine or prilocaine 1.5–2%, with or without epinephrine 1:200 000, and bupivacaine 0.375–0.5% are suitable. The more dilute solutions are necessary when larger volumes are required.

BLOCKS IN THE TRUNK

Intercostal and paravertebral blocks have potentially important roles in abdominal and thoracic surgery, but there is a significant risk of pneumothorax when they are performed by unskilled personnel. Paravertebral block is a relatively difficult procedure, only suitable for the more experienced anaesthetist, and is not considered further here.

Intercostal nerve block

Anatomy

Intercostal nerves are formed from the ventral rami of segmental thoracic nerves after communicating with the associated sympathetic ganglia through white and grey rami communicantes (Fig. 43.13).

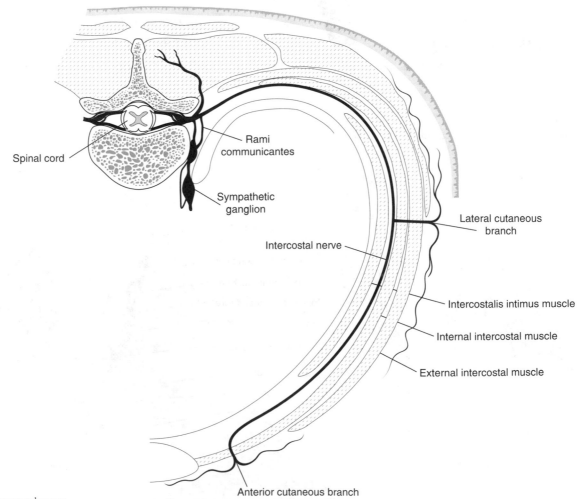

Fig. 43.13
Anatomy of the intercostal nerve.

An intercostal nerve has three main branches: the lateral cutaneous branch divides into anterior and posterior branches; the anterior terminal branch supplies the anterior thorax, rectus muscle and overlying skin; and a collateral branch arises from most nerves in the posterior intercostal space. This may rejoin the main nerve or form a separate anterior cutaneous nerve. Fibres from T1 join the brachial plexus, T2 and T3 supply fibres to form the intercostobrachial nerve, and T12, together with L1, contribute to the iliohypogastric, ilioinguinal and genitofemoral nerves.

Method

The optimal place to block the intercostal nerve is proximal to the formation of the lateral cutaneous branch, posterior to the mid-axillary line. With the patient in the lateral position, nerve blocks may be conveniently performed immediately following surgery for unilateral procedures such as open biliary and gall bladder surgery. In awake patients, a sitting position with the patient leaning forward to abduct the scapulae is often convenient. A 23 gauge needle is inserted perpendicular to the skin to make contact with an appropriate rib. The needle is then 'walked' caudally until it can be inserted under the lower border of the rib. After passing through the external intercostal muscle, up to 5 ml of local anaesthetic solution should be injected freely following a negative aspiration test. Rapid absorption of local anaesthetic solution may produce high systemic concentrations after multiple intercostal nerve blocks and the dose and concentration of drug need to be chosen carefully; 0.25–0.5% bupivacaine with 1:200 000 epinephrine is recommended, depending on the number of intercostal nerves being blocked. Pneumothorax and haemorrhage are the most likely complications after intercostal nerve block, but total spinal and profound sympathetic blockade have been reported and the anaesthetist must be prepared to deal with such severe complications.

Field block for inguinal hernia repair

The main nerves which supply the groin are the subcostal (T12), iliohypogastric (L1) and ilioinguinal (L1). Their blockade produces good postoperative analgesia, but supplementary infiltration, especially around the internal ring and hernial sac, is usually necessary during surgery if this is the only anaesthetic employed.

A needle is inserted 1.5 cm medial and inferior to the anterior superior iliac spine. Using a regional block needle, the external oblique aponeurosis is readily appreciated as the needle is advanced. Fifteen millilitres of local anaesthetic are injected deep to the aponeurosis, down to the inner surface of the ilium between the abdominal muscle layers. Another 5 ml of solution are deposited superficial to the external oblique aponeurosis medially from this point. Bupivacaine 0.5% is a suitable agent for postoperative analgesia.

Local infiltration is employed routinely as the sole anaesthetic in some centres and may be the method of choice in the unfit patient or in the day-case unit, but only when surgeons are experienced with this technique.

Penile block

The dorsal nerves to the penis are derived from the pudendal nerves and are blocked with 5–10 ml of local anaesthetic solution injected inferior to the symphysis pubis in the midline at a depth of 3–4 cm. Care must be taken to avoid intravascular injection in this area and vasoconstrictors *must not* be used. Plain bupivacaine 0.5% is suitable. The base of the penis is innervated by the genital branch of the genitofemoral nerve, which may be blocked if necessary by s.c. infiltration around the penis.

Penile block is quick and simple, produces a limited effect and is the block of choice for circumcision or other minor penile surgery such as meatotomy. It is commonly used in combination with light general anaesthesia and provides good postoperative pain relief. However, a simpler technique is to smear lidocaine jelly over the wound on a regular 4- to 6-hourly basis in the postoperative period.

LOWER LIMB BLOCKS

Lower limb blocks are practised less frequently than upper limb blocks for three reasons:

- It is not possible to block the whole of the lower limb with one injection.
- Subarachnoid or epidural anaesthesia may prove simpler.
- There is an impression among anaesthetists that lower limb blocks are difficult and unreliable.

However, new approaches to the peripheral nerves of the lower limb have simplified the subject and the blocks considered below are appropriate for the junior anaesthetist.

Sciatic nerve block

Anatomy

The sciatic nerve (L4, 5, S1–3) arises from the sacral plexus, passes through the great sciatic foramen and descends in the posterior thigh to the popliteal fossa, where it divides into the tibial and common peroneal nerves. In the thigh, it supplies muscles and the hip joint. The posterior cutaneous nerve of the thigh (S1–3) may run with the sciatic nerve or separate from it proximally; this nerve supplies the skin of the posterior thigh and upper calf. The tibial and common peroneal nerves, together with the saphenous nerve, supply all structures below the knee.

Method

There are four approaches to the sciatic nerve; the supine approach described by Raj is the most straightforward. After leaving the pelvis, the sciatic nerve lies in a groove between the greater trochanter and the ischial tuberosity covered only by skin, subcutaneous tissue and gluteus maximus. The patient lies supine with both the hip and knee flexed to 90°. This manoeuvre stretches the nerve and holds it firmly in the groove while making the gluteus maximus thinner. After infiltration of the skin, a short-bevelled 3 in (7.5 cm) needle is inserted midway between the greater trochanter and the ischial tuberosity, at right angles to the skin. A nerve stimulator simplifies this technique; stimulation should cause plantar or dorsiflexion of the foot.

This block has a high success rate with few complications. In combination with femoral nerve block, it is suitable for operations below the knee. The posterior cutaneous nerve is not blocked if it does not run with the sciatic.

Lidocaine 1.5–2% with or without epinephrine 1:200 000, prilocaine 1.5–2% and bupivacaine 0.375–0.5% are suitable agents.

Fifteen to 20 ml of solution are necessary. The more dilute solutions are required when other blocks are performed concurrently.

Femoral nerve block

Anatomy

The femoral nerve (L2–4) arises from the lumbar plexus and runs between psoas and iliacus to enter the thigh beneath the inguinal ligament, 2–3 cm lateral to the femoral artery and at a slightly greater depth. Branches of the anterior division include the intermediate and medial cutaneous nerves of the thigh and the supply to the sartorius. The posterior division supplies the quadriceps and the hip and knee joints and terminates as the saphenous nerve, which supplies the skin of the medial side of the calf as far as the medial malleolus and sometimes the medial side of the dorsum of the foot.

Method

The patient lies supine and the inguinal ligament and femoral artery are identified. The skin is anaesthetized just lateral to the femoral artery, 1 cm below the inguinal ligament. A short-bevelled needle is inserted parallel to the artery in a slightly cephalad direction (Fig. 43.14). Patellar twitching is observed when the femoral nerve is stimulated. Care should be taken not to confuse this movement with the movement obtained by direct stimulation of the sartorius. Ten to 15 ml of solution are required.

Femoral nerve block is usually combined with sciatic block for operative procedures. Analgesia after femoral fracture or knee surgery may be satisfactory with femoral nerve block alone.

The inguinal perivascular technique of lumbar plexus anaesthesia (three-in-one block) provides anaesthesia in the distribution of the femoral, lateral cutaneous and obturator nerves from a single injection and is an extension of the femoral nerve block technique. Twenty to 30 ml of solution are necessary and digital pressure is

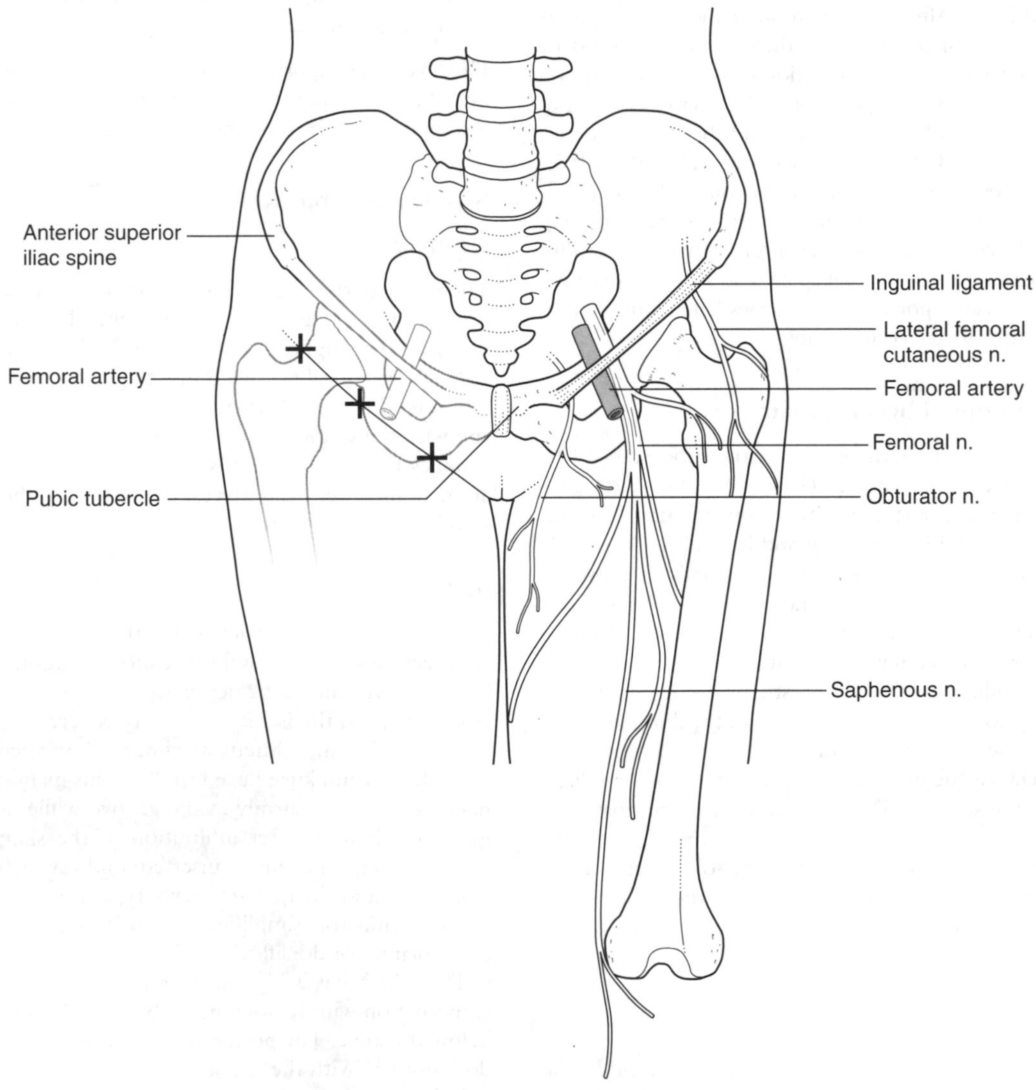

Fig. 43.14
Position and approach for femoral nerve block. The anterior superior iliac spine and femoral artery are marked.

applied below the needle to encourage cephalad spread of the solution between iliacus and psoas.

Suitable local anaesthetic agents for femoral or three-in-one block are the same as for sciatic nerve block.

Mid-tarsal block

In comparison with the traditional ankle block, mid-tarsal block has the advantages of clear landmarks, a supine position and reliability. If performed after induction of light general anaesthesia, it provides good postoperative analgesia and is ideal for operations such as removal of metatarsal heads.

Anatomy

Five nerves supply the forefoot. The medial and lateral plantar nerves are the terminal branches of the tibial nerve and enter the foot posterior to the medial malleolus; they supply deep structures within the foot and all of the sole. The common peroneal nerve divides into deep and superficial branches; the deep peroneal nerve supplies the web space between first and second toes, and the superficial branch supplies the dorsum of the foot. The saphenous nerve may supply a variable area of skin on the medial side of the dorsum of the foot. The sural nerve is a branch of the tibial nerve; it runs posterior to the lateral malleolus and supplies skin over the lateral side of the foot and fifth toe.

Method

The posterior tibial artery is palpated as far distally as possible. Injection of 3 ml of local anaesthetic to each side of it, below deep fascia, blocks medial and lateral plantar nerves. Injection of 2 ml of local anaesthetic to each side of the dorsalis pedis artery, below deep fascia, blocks the deep peroneal nerve. The saphenous, superficial peroneal and sural nerves are blocked by s.c. infiltration at the level of the ankle joint in a line extending from a point anterior to the medial malleolus to a point posterior to the lateral malleolus as for a classic ankle block. A complete block of the foot requires 15 ml of solution; bupivacaine 0.375–0.5% is most suitable for postoperative analgesia. It is probably advisable to avoid this block when the circulation to the foot is impaired.

SPECIAL SITUATIONS

Paediatric techniques

Most blocks used in adult practice are suitable for use in children, but because of the nature of most paediatric surgery and the understandable difficulties that may be experienced with patient cooperation, only a limited number of techniques are commonly used. Many of these are used for postoperative analgesia and are performed after induction of light general anaesthesia; they should only be performed by experienced anaesthetists.

The disposition of local anaesthetic agents in children differs from that in adults. Recent work suggests that, in children of less than 1 year of age, and particularly in the neonate, very high plasma concentrations of local anaesthetic may ensue after standard doses based on weight. In children over 1 year of age, plasma concentrations are consistently lower than would be expected from adult data.

Agents and doses for paediatric blocks are shown in Table 43.6.

Table 43.6 Agents and doses of local anaesthetics used in paediatric practice

Caudal anaesthesia	
0.25% Bupivacaine	
0.5 ml kg^{-1}	Sacral block
1.0 ml kg^{-1}	Low thoracic block
0.19% Bupivacaine (three parts bupivacaine 0.25%: one part saline)	
1.25 ml kg^{-1}	Mid-thoracic block
Penile block	
0.5% Bupivacaine *plain*	
Body weight	Dose
2.5 kg	0.5 ml
10 kg	1.0 ml
20 kg	2.0 ml
40 kg	4.0 ml
Axillary block	
0.25% Bupivacaine	
Body weight	Dose
10 kg	6 ml
20 kg	12 ml
30 kg	18 ml
40 kg	24 ml

Topical anaesthesia

The introduction of EMLA (eutectic mixture of local anaesthetics) cream allows anaesthesia of intact skin. The cream must remain in contact with the skin for at least 1 h and is held in place with an occlusive dressing. This technique is particularly useful before venepuncture in children.

FURTHER READING

Cousins M J, Bridenbaugh P O 1998 Neural blockade in clinical anesthesia and management of pain, 3rd edn. Lippincott, Philadelphia

Ellis H, Feldman S 1983 Anatomy for anaesthetists, 4th edn. Blackwell Scientific Publications, Oxford

Eriksson E 1979 Illustrated handbook in local anaesthesia. Lloyd-Luke, London

Horlocker T T 1998 Spinal and epidural blockade and perioperative low molecular weight heparin: smooth sailing on the Titanic (editorial). Anesthesia and Analgesia 86: 1153–1156

Murphy T M, Fitzgibbon D 1996 Local anaesthesia techniques. In: Aitkenhead A R, Jones R M (eds) Clinical anaesthesia. Churchill Livingstone, Edinburgh, p 557–593

Wildsmith J A W, Armitage E N 1993 Principles and practice of regional anaesthesia, 2nd edn. Churchill Livingstone, Edinburgh

Winnie A P 1984 Plexus anesthesia, vol I. Perivascular techniques of brachial plexus block. Churchill Livingstone, New York

44 Anaesthesia for gynaecological and genitourinary surgery

Gynaecological and genitourinary surgery have much in common. Both include frequently performed 'minor' procedures. Modern narrow-gauge fibreoptic telescopes allow some to be performed at outpatient clinics, with topical anaesthesia administered by the operator. Others need general anaesthesia, which is best provided on a day-care basis. Although patients undergoing gynaecological surgery tend to be young, many presenting in the urology service are elderly and have concurrent disease. Being treated as a day-care patient might need different, but not less, anaesthetic assessment (including appropriate investigations) even though the visits may be very frequent for some patients.

POSITIONING THE PATIENT

Many procedures are carried out with the patient in the lithotomy position. Care is needed to avoid damage to the common peroneal nerve because the legs may press against the lithotomy poles. The Lloyd-Davies position provides a variant of the lithotomy position. It is traditionally used for those with osteoarthritis of the hips or the lumbar spine. Before placing anaesthetized patients in these positions, they should be adequately anaesthetized, with good airway control, because it is impossible to turn them rapidly onto the side should they regurgitate or vomit stomach contents. During positioning, the patient's head must be supported, and the arms prevented from falling. The anaesthetic breathing tubes must be free to move and monitoring apparatus connected without unnecessary delay. These positions increase the pressure of the abdominal contents on the diaphragm, making spontaneous respiration more difficult and causing closure of basal alveoli. This may lead to a decrease in oxygen saturation, most marked in the obese when head-down tilt is used. The combination of respiratory obstruction, if allowed to develop, with the expiratory effort of the lower abdominal muscles commonly seen during anaesthesia results in extensive movement with respiration, making the view through endoscopic instruments difficult and occasionally too dangerous to allow more extensive surgery.

After surgery the legs are lowered, resulting in a reduction in venous return and cardiac output. This is exacerbated by some cardiovascular drugs, spinal or epidural anaesthesia and blood loss. The legs should be lowered before recovery from anaesthesia, so that the patient can be turned to the lateral position if necessary.

MINIMALLY INVASIVE SURGERY

Many of these operations are 'laparoscopic procedures', including clipping of the Fallopian tubes, ovarian cystectomy, emergency surgery for ectopic pregnancy, nephrectomy, adrenalectomy, vaginal hysterectomy and iliac lymph node dissection. For laparoscopic surgery the surgeon creates a pneumoperitoneum, most commonly by insufflating the peritoneal cavity with carbon dioxide. As carbon dioxide is soluble in blood, the risk of gas embolus is reduced. It is also inexpensive and non-flammable. Increased pressure and duration of pneumoperitoneum decrease the patient's tolerance of this procedure during surgery.

PHYSIOLOGICAL CHANGES

Respiration

The pneumoperitoneum increases intra-abdominal pressure and reduces both chest wall and lung compliance, and also functional residual capacity. These effects are more marked for patients undergoing surgery in the lithotomy posture. Hypoventilation ensues and intrapulmonary shunt is increased. A decrease in the cardiac output increases the ventilation/perfusion ratio and alveolar dead space.

Cardiovascular system

Bradycardia commonly occurs after peritoneal insufflation, whereas asystole is rare. Both decreases and marked increases in arterial pressure may occur during laparoscopic surgery. The increased intra-abdominal pressure decreases venous return, leading to a reduction in cardiac index, but sometimes a compensatory increase in systemic vascular resistance (SVR) maintains systolic arterial pressure. Increases in arterial pressure are caused by increased levels of arginine vasopressin release during pneumoperitoneum, causing increases in SVR. Reduction in insufflating pressure raises arterial pressure lowers a rapid return to normal levels occurs after release of the pneumoperitoneum.

COMPLICATIONS OF LAPAROSCOPIC SURGERY

- If the Verres needle is not inserted fully into the peritoneal cavity, carbon dioxide is forced subcutaneously, leading to surgical emphysema.
- Blood vessels may be punctured by the Verres needle in the abdominal wall, in the peritoneal cavity or retroperitoneally. Blood loss in the abdominal wall and retroperitoneal space may be considerable before detection.
- Abdominal viscera may be perforated during surgery, causing leakage of intestinal contents, peritonitis and septicaemia.
- If the pressure used to inflate the peritoneum is too high, carbon dioxide may be forced through congenital foramina in the

diaphragm, causing pneumomediastinum, pneumothorax or pneumopericardium. Increased ventilating pressures may also lead to pneumothorax by rupturing emphysematous bullae.

- It is possible for insufflating gas to cause gas embolism. The Verres needle or trocar may be sited in a vessel, or gas may be forced into open venous sinuses by high intra-abdominal pressures. When the carbon dioxide embolus reaches the heart, cardiac output decreases abruptly, less blood is delivered to the lungs and the end-tidal carbon dioxide suddenly decreases.

ANAESTHETIC IMPLICATIONS OF LAPAROSCOPIC SURGERY

An appropriate vein should be cannulated with a large-gauge cannula. The choice of induction and maintenance agent is not important. As there is a risk of severe bradycardia, some anaesthetists give glycopyrrolate 0.2 mg or atropine 0.3 mg at induction. There is a high incidence of postoperative nausea and vomiting (PONV) after laparoscopy, especially following gynaecological procedures. An antiemetic should be given prophylactically.

In several studies of short laparoscopic procedures, there have been no incidents of regurgitation and inhalation in spontaneously breathing patients, either with a face mask or laryngeal mask airway (LMA). The use of face masks or LMAs with spontaneous ventilation should be considered only for quick procedures (up to about 10 min pneumoperitoneum) in healthy, slim patients. Carbon dioxide is absorbed through the peritoneum and increases the carbon dioxide load to be excreted, and longer procedures involve increased work of breathing over a considerable time. In addition, carbon dioxide absorbed through the peritoneum increases respiratory drive, making tracheal intubation and artificial ventilation necessary. Intubation and intermittent positive pressure ventilation (IPPV) are also necessary in patients who have pre-existing respiratory and cardiovascular disease or those who are obese. An intra-arterial cannula is useful for carbon dioxide measurement in patients with respiratory disease undergoing prolonged laparoscopic procedures; there is a greater difference than usual between the partial pressure of carbon dioxide in arterial blood and alveoli.

There is more rapid recovery of respiratory function, decreased postoperative pain and consequent smoother recovery after laparoscopic surgery than after open operations. Pain after laparoscopy is caused by the stretching of the peritoneum (which produces an inflammatory response), residual gas, the effects of the surgery and the 'portholes' or any skin incisions. Pain is treated optimally with local anaesthetic, paracetamol, non-steroidal anti-inflammatory drugs (NSAIDs) and opioids if required. The longer the pneumoperitoneum and the higher the pressure used, the more severe is postoperative pain.

Laparoscopic sterilization

This produces additional pain from tubal ischaemia. Many methods of local anaesthesia have been used: instillation of local anaesthetic through the uterus to the inside of the Fallopian tubes, injection of local anaesthetic into the mesosalpinx, dipping Filshie clips in local anaesthetic jelly, and instillation of local anaesthetic into the Pouch of Douglas via an epidural catheter inserted through the abdominal wall. None of these is always effective, and some patients may still require an opioid. One or two doses of intravenous fentanyl may be sufficient. In some centres, patient-controlled analgesia (PCA) with alfentanil is used. Other patients need morphine.

The ischaemic pain diminishes after 2 or 3 h and pain may then be managed with NSAIDs, paracetamol and weak oral opioids, such as dihydrocodeine, codeine or tramadol. Patients who have received opioid drugs and who then travel home are particularly likely to be nauseated. Prophylactic antiemetics are justified.

SURGERY FOR MALIGNANCY

OPEN PELVIC SURGERY

Some urological and gynaecological operations have the same basic anaesthetic requirements. Wertheim's hysterectomy, total cystectomy and radical prostatectomy have a duration of 2–4 h. During these operations, there is often extensive blood loss, the patient's temperature decreases and there is considerable postoperative pain. Patients undergoing radical prostatectomy and cystectomy are frequently elderly and have concomitant disease. Full assessment is essential, including history, examination and relevant investigations to ascertain the extent of any respiratory or cardiovascular disease. The choice of induction agent is dependent on the patient's condition, whilst the choice of volatile agent is not important. Tracheal intubation and ventilation are necessary. Epidural analgesia or opioid drugs provide intraoperative analgesia. Epidural analgesia provides cardiovascular stability, imparts some protection against deep venous thrombosis, reduces blood loss and decreases some elements of the stress response to surgery. However, there may be precipitate decreases in arterial pressure if bleeding occurs and measurement of central venous pressure (CVP) is useful to ensure the patient's circulation remains well filled. Monitoring of intra-arterial blood pressure and temperature is also advisable. The patient should be kept warm by maintaining a warm environment, minimizing his or her exposure, especially during insertion of cannulae/catheters, the use of warmed intravenous fluids, warming blankets and warm humidified gases. A high-dependency area is ideal for continuing epidural or other analgesia, supervision of fluid balance and rewarming of the patient. Younger and more healthy patients may have to be managed in a general surgical ward, with PCA or other techniques. In patients undergoing cystectomy, the ureters are diverted into a loop of small bowel and the resulting ileus may be prolonged by opioid analgesia.

RADICAL VULVECTOMY AND TOTAL AMPUTATION OF PENIS

Both these operations are performed with the patient in Lloyd-Davies or lithotomy positions. There is often marked blood loss and heat loss. Intubation and ventilation are advisable in all but the very healthy and slim. The use of invasive monitoring is dependent upon the patient's state of health and the extent and difficulty of the surgery. Temperature should be monitored and the patient kept warm as for open pelvic surgery. Epidural analgesia intra- and postoperatively is ideal for these patients. If this is not possible, PCA may be used in the postoperative period.

NEPHRECTOMY

Renal tumour is a common reason for nephrectomy. Other causes include hydronephrotic non-functioning kidney and live donor nephrectomy for transplant. There are other operations performed via the same incision, such as pyeloplasty, which have similar anaesthetic implications. Full assessment of the patient is required with particular reference to renal function and arterial pressure. Anaemia may accompany impaired renal function or chronic infection of the hydronephrotic kidney. The report of the computerized tomography (CT) of a renal tumour indicates if there is extension along the renal vessels and the inferior and superior venae cava. The extent of the tumour and its proximity to vessels provide information on the likely duration of surgery and the potential blood loss. Patients require tracheal intubation and ventilation of the lungs, to allow surgical access, because of the position and the risk of pneumothorax during surgery. Central venous and direct arterial pressure measurement may be required if extensive blood loss is anticipated or if the patient has significant cardiovascular disease. Temperature should be monitored and the patient kept warm. The patient is placed in the lateral position with the flank raised to open the space between the ribs and the pelvis for surgical access. Attention must be paid to the position of upper and lower limbs. The arm must not be abducted excessively at the shoulder and all areas of the body in contact with supports must be well padded. After positioning the patient, correct placement of the tracheal tube should be checked in case inadvertent endobronchial intubation has occurred. As the legs are dependent, there is a risk of decreased venous return. This may be exacerbated by kinking of the inferior vena cava as a result of the position of the trunk.

There is a risk of pneumothorax intraoperatively from perforation of the pleura by the surgeon. The hole is generally small, so the use of positive pressure ventilation and manually inflating the lung before closure of the pleura generally help to prevent postoperative problems. A chest drain may be inserted before the end of surgery. The incision used for these operations is very painful and various methods of local analgesia are used. Thoracic epidural block provides good analgesia. Intercostal blocks may be used but they have a short duration of action and carry a risk of pneumothorax, as does interpleural analgesia. PCA may be the best available method. If there is renal impairment and morphine is used, a reduced dose or a longer lockout period may be necessary, as morphine-6-glucuronide is a renally excreted active metabolite of morphine. The addition of paracetamol and NSAIDs to the analgesic regimen reduces opioid requirement. NSAIDs may be used only if there are no contraindications, the remaining kidney is functioning well and the patient is kept well hydrated.

TUMOURS

Testicular tumours

Orchidectomy may be undertaken through the scrotum or inguinal region. There are no special anaesthetic requirements for this surgery. Assessment of the patient determines if a regional technique, e.g. spinal anaesthetic, or a general anaesthetic is most suitable. In the case of general anaesthesia, the patient's condition determines if intubation and ventilation, laryngeal mask airway or face mask is required. In cases of advanced testicular cancer, dissection of the para-aortic nodes is undertaken; this is a major operation, and the same type of anaesthetic technique as that used for major pelvic surgery is suitable.

Cervical tumours

Many procedures are undertaken involving diathermy to the cervix. If there is no contraindication, general anaesthesia via a face mask or LMA is satisfactory. Postoperative pain is not usually a problem.

Bladder tumours

These are often removed repeatedly by diathermy or loop excision. Some destruction by laser can be carried out without a general anaesthetic. Patients may attend regularly for general anaesthesia, as a day case, for several years. It is essential to carry out appropriate preoperative assessment each time, as these are frequently elderly individuals with declining general health. The lithotomy position is used. These procedures may be carried out with spinal anaesthesia. However, they are frequently rapid and unless there is a contraindication, general anaesthesia with a face mask or LMA is suitable. Occasionally there is rapid blood loss, so a large-gauge cannula should be used. The bladder is irrigated continuously and this makes blood loss difficult to estimate. During diathermy, the obturator nerve is often directly stimulated; this leads to excessive jerking movements of the leg, surgery is made more difficult and there is a risk of perforation of the bladder. Paralysis and ventilation may therefore be required to prevent perforation. If the bladder is perforated, irrigating fluid is absorbed into the perivesical space and can cause TURP syndrome (see below).

There is often postoperative pain which may require opioid analgesia.

SURGERY FOR RENAL TRACT STONES

Renal stones are frequently idiopathic but may be caused by hypercalciuria arising from sarcoidosis, malignancy, renal tubular acidosis, hyperparathyroidism, Cushing's syndrome or administration of adrenal corticosteroids. All these diseases may have anaesthetic implications and should be investigated at preoperative assessment. Patients with recurrent urinary tract infection related to bladder malfunction, e.g. neurological diseases or congenital abnormalities, form stones. This type of stone may be large and grow to become a staghorn calculus in the renal pelvis.

Many renal tract stones are removed by extracorporeal shock wave lithotripsy. This uses ultrasound to disintegrate the stone and the procedure may take an hour. Patients are usually awake, experience pain and require analgesia. Occasionally the procedure is not tolerated and general anaesthesia is required. Administering general anaesthesia in unfamiliar surroundings can be hazardous. The anaesthetist must insist on skilled assistance, adequate lighting and monitoring of arterial pressure, oxygen saturation, ECG and capnography.

PERCUTANEOUS LITHOTRIPSY

This procedure may be undertaken when extracorporeal shock wave lithotripsy has failed. The patients include those with staghorn calculi and associated infection. The procedure takes place in the X-ray department – a hazardous area for patient and anaesthetist alike. It is unfamiliar, often cramped, and it is essential for the anaesthetist to have a trained and experienced assistant. It is usually best to anaesthetize the patient on a trolley as X-ray tables may not tip head-down quickly.

Procedure

First of all a balloon-tipped ureteric catheter is passed through a cystoscope. The balloon is dilated just below the kidney to enable distension of the renal pelvis. This also prevents stone fragments from passing into the ureter. The patient is then placed in the prone position, a nephrostomy track is created and a nephroscope is passed. The stone may then be removed with forceps or fragmented with an ultrasonic probe. Continuous flushing of the pelvis with normal saline clears fragments of stone, distends the renal pelvis, washes away blood and cools the ultrasonic probe. Normal saline is used to prevent hyponatraemia.

Possible problems

Fluid in retroperitoneal space. This may occur if the renal pelvis is ruptured. A check should be kept on the fluid input and collection. If a deficit of more than 2 L occurs, the procedure may need to be terminated.

Sepsis. Many patients have chronic urinary infection. Bacteria may be flushed into the venous system of the kidney if the pressure from the irrigation is too great. All patients should receive appropriate intravenous antibiotics, but signs of cardiovascular collapse may suggest Gram-negative septicaemia.

Cooling. Heat loss may be a major problem; in addition to routine methods of maintaining normothermia, the irrigating fluid should be warm, and waterproof drapes applied.

Bleeding. In addition to bleeding sustained at the nephrostomy site, large vessels, spleen and liver may be punctured. A large retroperitoneal haematoma may collect and is difficult to diagnose. All bleeding is harder to detect in the environment of the X-ray department.

Pneumothorax. This may occur whilst performing the nephrostomy.

Electrical hazards. Irrigating fluid may cause electrical equipment to 'short circuit'.

Anaesthetic technique

Regional anaesthesia

Epidural blockade should extend to reach the sixth thoracic level. The operation may last up to 3 h and therefore a catheter technique is required. Patients become very uncomfortable lying prone for this length of time.

General anaesthesia

As the patient is prone, intubation and ventilation are recommended. Attention must be paid to positioning of the head, padding of the eyes, and of the limbs at vulnerable points. The choice of induction, neuromuscular blocking and maintenance agents is less important than good monitoring, particularly of heat loss.

ENDOSCOPIC SURGERY

TRANSURETHRAL RESECTION OF THE PROSTATE GLAND

This is a common operation, performed in the lithotomy position. Continuous irrigation with glycine is used to allow vision of the operative site. Glycine has reasonable optical properties, does not conduct electricity, but is hypotonic. Chippings are cut from the prostate gland with a wire loop. When enough tissue has been cut away, diathermy is used to stop any further bleeding. A catheter, usually a three-way irrigating type, is inserted after surgery.

Possible problems

Haemorrhage

This is difficult to quantify as blood is mixed with the irrigation fluid. Suggestions for measuring blood loss include assaying the haemoglobin concentration of the collected irrigating fluid and, from the known volume, calculating the quantity of haemoglobin lost. This is not very practical. A sample of the total irrigating fluid and blood may be placed in a test tube and compared with standard concentrations of haemoglobin; again, knowing the total volume of fluid, the amount of haemoglobin lost can be estimated.

The total weight of prostate chippings is a guide to the amount of blood lost. More than 40–50 g should alert the anaesthetist to the possibility of large blood loss. Blood loss is proportional to the time spent resecting. Assiduous monitoring of heart rate and arterial pressure can help to identify bleeding, although this may be a late sign. In practical terms, the decision to transfuse is often made by assessment of the patient's clinical condition rather than as a result of measuring blood loss.

TURP syndrome

This is a complex syndrome which may encompass hypo-osmolality, hyponatraemia, hyperglycinaemia, hyperammonaemia and intravascular fluid shifts. These changes are caused by absorption of irrigating fluid through open prostatic veins, and later by its absorption from pooled irrigation fluid in the retroperitoneal and perivesical spaces. Hyperammonaemia is caused by metabolism of absorbed glycine.

Massive haemolysis may occur from hypo-osmolality. Haemoglobinaemia from the haemolysis, in combination with hypotension, may lead to acute renal failure.

Symptoms of TURP syndrome include hyper- or hypotension, pulmonary oedema, confusion, convulsions and visual disturbance. These may occur from as early as 15 min into the resection up to 12 h after operation. The incidence of this syndrome may be decreased by maintaining the height difference between the bladder and the bag of irrigating fluid at 80 cm or less to decrease intravesical pressure. Continuous irrigating resectoscopes also result in lower intravesical pressure. Restricting the resection time to 1 h decreases the incidence of TURP syndrome. Surgery must be abandoned as soon as possible if TURP syndrome is suspected.

Various methods may be used to estimate fluid absorption. Addition of ethanol to the irrigating fluid followed by measurement of alcohol in expired gas gives an indication of the quantity of fluid absorbed. Measurements of serum sodium concentration or osmolality are also good guides.

Treatment depends on careful assessment and consists of mannitol, hypertonic saline or loop diuretics. Mannitol does not cause as great a loss of sodium through renal excretion as do loop diuretics. Supportive management, including ventilation, is often required until electrolyte abnormalities are corrected.

Anaesthetic technique

TURP is frequently performed in very elderly men. These patients have a high incidence of concomitant disease, especially of the respiratory tract and cardiovascular system. There is a risk of septicaemia in those patients with urinary tract infection, stones in the bladder or an indwelling catheter. These patients should have intravenous antibiotics, as should any patient with a joint prosthesis or valvular heart disease.

Spinal anaesthesia is useful particularly for patients with significant respiratory disease, although coughing during the procedure makes surgery difficult. An additional advantage of spinal anaesthesia is postoperative analgesia. Frequently, the worst discomfort has settled by the time the anaesthesia has regressed.

One of the biggest concerns with spinal anaesthesia is hypotension caused by sympathetic blockade, as blood loss may result in precipitate decreases in arterial pressure because of lack of compensatory vasoconstriction. There is often additional hypotension when the legs are lowered at the end of surgery. Reductions in arterial pressure may be treated by fluid or vasoconstrictors; ephedrine is commonly used, but produces tachycardia.

Spinal anaesthesia has traditionally not been used for patients with ischaemic heart disease. However, the incidence of silent myocardial ischaemia is the same whether general anaesthesia or spinal anaesthesia is used. It appears to be related to the severity of the pre-existing cardiac disease. There is some evidence that the increase in cardiac pre- and afterload when the spinal anaesthetic regresses can induce ischaemia.

A dose of heavy bupivacaine 0.5%, sufficient to produce a block to the eighth thoracic nerve, is needed; this is generally about 2.7–3 ml. Postdural puncture headache is less common in elderly men than in other groups of patients. The incidence is least with the use of pencil-point needles. The choice between spinal and general anaesthesia depends on the patient's preoperative condition and the preferences of both the patient and the anaesthetist. The usual absolute contraindications to spinal analgesia (anticoagulants, clotting disorders and local sepsis) apply. Any method of general anaesthesia is suitable, depending on the patient's medical condition. A caudal injection of local anaesthetic may be useful for postoperative pain.

Careful monitoring of arterial pressure and drainage from the catheter is necessary after surgery and the possibility of TURP syndrome should be borne in mind for 12 h or so, especially if the resection was prolonged.

LASER DESTRUCTION OF THE PROSTATE

This is a much less invasive operation than TURP. It is quicker and there is minimal blood loss. It is thought not to produce as reliable results as TURP, but with refinement of technique it may become more common.

ENDOMETRIAL ABLATION

This operation is undertaken to remove endometrium in women with menorrhagia. Continuous irrigation is used, so detection of bleeding is difficult and there is a risk of absorption of the glycine used as irrigating fluid. This risk is generally regarded as less than with TURP in men. A regional or general anaesthetic technique is suitable. Postoperative pain may be managed with paracetamol, NSAIDs and/or opioid drugs as required. Prophylactic antiemetics are advisable.

INCONTINENCE SURGERY

PROCEDURES FOR THE IRRITABLE BLADDER

Helmstein's procedure

An expandable bag is placed in the bladder at cystoscopy and filled to a pressure just below mean arterial pressure for 6 h with the aim of increasing bladder capacity. The distension is very painful and an epidural infusion of bupivacaine and an opioid is used.

Clam cystoplasty

In this procedure, a segment of small bowel is resected, opened out and used to create a 'patch' in the bladder. The interruption of the bladder by the bowel patch stops transmission of irritable contractions and avoids premature voiding. Muscle relaxation, tracheal intubation and IPPV are required. The choice of anaesthetic drugs depends on the patient's general health. Postoperative pain may be treated with an epidural or PCA. There is often postoperative ileus, which may be made worse by opioids.

PROCEDURES FOR STRESS INCONTINENCE

Burch colposuspension

This is performed through a Pfannensteil incision. If there are no contraindications, a spontaneously breathing technique can be used. Some surgeons perform these operations laparoscopically, as this results in less pain and earlier mobility. If a laparoscopic technique is used, it is sensible to intubate the trachea and ventilate the lungs. If sensible is of the open type, postoperative analgesia with opioid drugs is needed.

Tension-free vaginal tape

This is a relatively new procedure. Two curved needles, joined by a strip of 'tape', are passed through the vaginal vault and out on to the skin of the abdomen, one on each side. The needles are removed and the tape is held at the skin. The tape passes round the bladder neck between the two attachments. It is tightened at the abdominal skin until it is just tight enough to prevent leakage of urine with coughing, but slack enough to allow voiding of urine. The patient is required to be awake, cooperative and able to give a good cough for the second part of the procedure, which is not painful. It is essential that the patient is given a full explanation of the proceedings. The first part of the procedure is conducted using local anaesthesia. A large volume is required (about 100 ml), for infiltration. Sedation is useful during this first phase. Target-controlled propofol infusion, which provides a variable level of sedation, is useful. Midazolam and fentanyl may be used, but there is a danger of rendering the patient apnoeic or heavily sedated and uncooperative. It is possible to give a general anaesthetic with sevoflurane for the first part of the procedure, although a longer period elapses before the patient is able to give a deep cough. It is not possible to use a regional technique, as this relaxes the pelvic floor muscles and the correct tension is not obtained.

HYSTERECTOMY

This can be performed abdominally or vaginally, for menorrhagia or malignancy. It is essential to check for anaemia. Both these operations can be performed with spinal or epidural anaesthesia, which decreases blood loss. For abdominal hysterectomy, the spinal or epidural is usually combined with a general anaesthetic. Vaginal hysterectomy is performed in the lithotomy position, and if patients have epidural or spinal anaesthesia, they may be allowed to breathe spontaneously if there are no contraindications.

Without regional analgesia, opioid analgesia is required intra-operatively. There is a high incidence of postoperative nausea and vomiting, so prophylactic antiemetics should be given. Postoperative analgesia may be provided by an epidural or opioid drugs via PCA, with paracetamol and NSAIDs as supplements.

EMBOLIZATION OF FIBROIDS

This procedure is undertaken with an awake patient, in the X-ray department. Catheters are passed through the femoral arteries to the uterine artery and into the vessels supplying the fibroids, and the vessels are embolized. Pain is experienced as the fibroid tissue becomes ischaemic. Administration of regular NSAIDs and paracetamol is advisable both before and after the procedure. A bolus dose of opioid drug is often required after embolization. Severe pain may last for several hours and a PCA may be needed for 1 or 2 days.

SUCTION VAGINAL TERMINATION OF PREGNANCY

This is undertaken before 12 weeks of gestation. The operation is performed in the lithotomy position. All volatile agents cause relaxation of the uterus, so many anaesthetists use an infusion or intermittent boluses of propofol, supplemented with fentanyl or alfentanil. Other anaesthetists use 0.5 of the minimum alveolar concentration (MAC) of a volatile agent with nitrous oxide. Dilatation of the cervix is very stimulating and if the patient is not anaesthetized adequately, laryngospasm may occur. Alfentanil is useful to prevent this response, as high concentrations of volatile agent are not advisable.

Syntocinon may be given to encourage contraction of the uterus and this may cause a transient decrease in arterial pressure. There is little postoperative pain. The procedure is usually performed as a day case and paracetamol or an NSAID is suitable for analgesia at home.

GYNAECOLOGICAL AND UROLOGICAL EMERGENCIES

UROLOGICAL

There are not many true urological emergencies: torsion of the testes is the most important. The anaesthetic requirements for this procedure are dictated by the general health of the patient.

GYNAECOLOGICAL

Ectopic pregnancy

This often presents as abdominal pain with a positive pregnancy test. If there is not extensive bleeding, some gynaecologists remove the ectopic pregnancy laparoscopically. The anaesthetic implications of laparoscopy are described earlier in this chapter. A rapid sequence induction may be required if the patient has a full stomach. If the ectopic pregnancy is bleeding, an open operation is performed. The degree of hypovolaemia should be assessed carefully before surgery. It is essential to resuscitate the patient fully during preparation for surgery. Great care is needed at induction to avoid a precipitate decrease in blood pressure. If there is excessive bleeding, a clotting screen should be performed and any deficiencies corrected. Postoperative analgesia with PCA and supplementary analgesics is required. Epidural analgesia is not used as the patient is usually hypovolaemic and may develop deranged clotting.

Evacuation of retained products of conception

This is an extremely common emergency procedure, which is usually very brief (5–10 min). Surgery is performed in the lithotomy position. There is occasionally excessive bleeding, necessitating immediate surgery. Often the operation may be performed at a time when the patient has an empty stomach, thus avoiding tracheal intubation.

Because volatile anaesthetic agents may cause some degree of uterine relaxation, many anaesthetists use an infusion or intermittent boluses of propofol, supplemented with alfentanil or fentanyl. Syntocinon is often required. The cervix is often already open, so that dilatation is not necessary. Postoperative pain can be managed with oral analgesics.

FURTHER READING

Alexander J I 1997 Pain after laparoscopy. British Journal of Anaesthesia 79: 369–378

Brichant J F 1995 Anaesthesia for minimally invasive abdominal surgery. In: Adams A P, Cashman J N (eds) Recent advances in anaesthesia and analgesia, 19. Churchill Livingstone, Edinburgh, ch 3

Edwards N D, Callaghan L C, White T, Reilly C S 1995 Perioperative myocardial ischaemia in patients undergoing transurethral surgery: a pilot study comparing general with spinal anaesthesia. British Journal of Anaesthesia 74: 368–372

Gravenstein D 1997 Transurethral resection of the prostate (TURP) syndrome: a review of the pathophysiology and management. Anesthesia and Analgesia 84: 438–446

Naef M M, Mitchell A 1994 Anaesthesia for laparoscopy. In: Kaufman L, Ginsburg R (eds) Anaesthesia review, 11. Churchill Livingstone, Edinburgh, ch 3

Windsor A, French G W G, Sear J W, Foex P, Millett S V, Howell S J 1996 Silent myocardial ischaemia in patients undergoing transurethral prostatectomy. A study to evaluate risk scoring and anaesthetic technique with outcome. Anaesthesia 51: 728–732

Wong D H, Hagar J M, Mootz J et al 1996 Incidence of perioperative myocardial ischaemia in TURP patients. Journal of Clinical Anesthesia 8: 627–630

45 Anaesthesia for orthopaedic surgery

ßAbout 17% of all operations in the UK are for orthopaedic, spinal or trauma surgery. Aspects of trauma and spinal surgery are dealt with in Chapters 51 and 57, respectively. This chapter gives a framework for the conduct of anaesthesia for orthopaedic surgery.

THE PATIENT'S CONDITION

Many orthopaedic patients are young and healthy. Risks of serious complications from anaesthesia are small, but seemingly minor side-effects such as postoperative nausea and vomiting or succinylcholine pains, or apparently minor complications such as peripheral nerve damage associated with the use of nerve blocks may cause considerable distress.

Older patients often accept higher risks of anaesthesia and surgery to improve the quality of their remaining years. Medical conditions that may affect any surgical patient are described in Chapter 35, but several conditions and treatment regimens are more specific to orthopaedic patients.

RHEUMATOID ARTHRITIS

Patients with rheumatoid arthritis may present for synovectomy, arthrodesis, major joint replacement or soft tissue procedures such as nerve decompression or tendon surgery. Any affected joint may be painful and special care is needed during i.v. cannulation when the disease involves joints in the hand. It may be an ordeal for the patient to lie still under prolonged regional anaesthesia for surgery on one joint because of pain in other joints.

The disease affects the cervical spine in up to 80% of patients. About a quarter of these have instability or subluxation, with a risk of dislocation. Neck movements, particularly those likely to be required during tracheal intubation and positioning, should be assessed. Recent X-rays of the neck in flexion and extension (with 'through the mouth' views) or magnetic resonance images should be examined for evidence of separation of the odontoid peg from the atlas, or subluxation of any cervical vertebrae. These images are not easy to interpret; a radiologist should advise (Fig. 45.1). Patients with an unstable neck should be managed by an experienced anaesthetist, especially if tracheal intubation is planned. Tracheal intubation is even more difficult if movement of the temporomandibular joint is restricted. The need for tracheal intubation should be considered. For many procedures, the use of a laryngeal mask airway is a suitable and potentially less traumatic alternative. If tracheal intubation is required, intubation aids such as the intubating laryngeal mask airway or fibreoptic-guided intubation may be safer than insertion of a tracheal tube using direct laryngoscopy.

Although many other features of rheumatoid arthritis have a limited effect on the conduct of anaesthesia, the heart, lungs and kidneys may be involved. Both normochromic normocytic and iron-deficiency anaemias are common; the latter is often associated with gastric bleeding caused by non-steroidal anti-inflammatory drugs (NSAIDs) (Table 45.1).

OTHER SYSTEMIC DISEASE

Ankylosing spondylitis may also present problems with tracheal intubation, but these result from rigidity of the cervical spine rather than instability. The use of the laryngeal mask airway is a suitable option for many procedures. If tracheal intubation is necessary, it may be difficult or impossible to obtain a view of the larynx by direct laryngoscopy. In many patients, tracheal intubation may be undertaken with the aid of a gum elastic bougie, but in some it is necessary to resort to the use of the intubating laryngeal mask airway or fibreoptic intubation.

Kyphosis and limitation of chest expansion develop in some patients, with evidence of restrictive lung disease. Aortic regurgitation and atrioventricular conduction defects are rarer complica-

Table 45.1 Anaesthesia and rheumatoid arthritis

Feature	Anaesthetic implication
Cervical spine	Assess movements and plan intubation
Temporomandibular joint	Restricted movement
Wrist	Care during i.v. cannulation
Polyarticular involvement	Difficulty lying still for long procedures
Anaemia	Normochromic common; iron deficiency – NSAIDs likely cause
NSAIDs	Assess gastric ulceration risk Check urea and electrolytes; avoid hypovolaemia
Disease-modifying drugs	Check leucocyte count – clean anaesthetic technique
Corticosteroids	Care with skin Cover with physiological dose
Pain relief	Care with NSAIDs; assess ability to cope with PCA

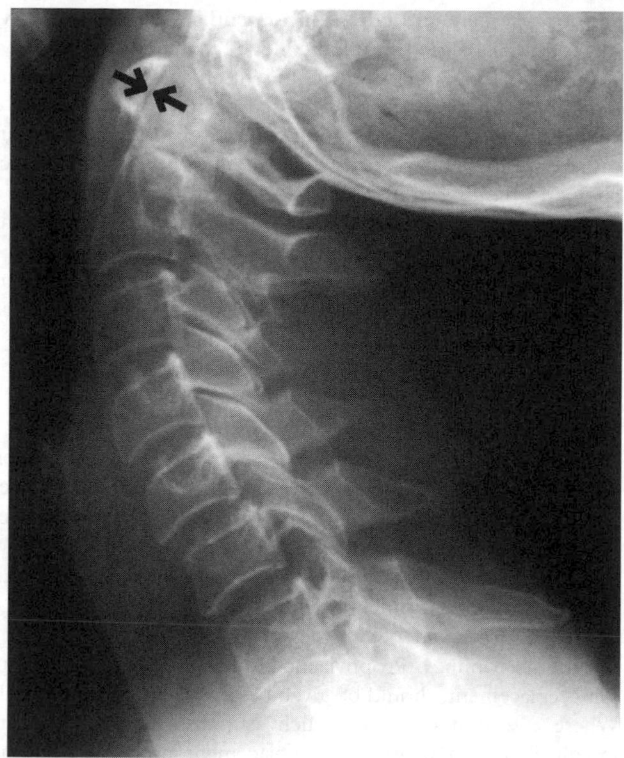

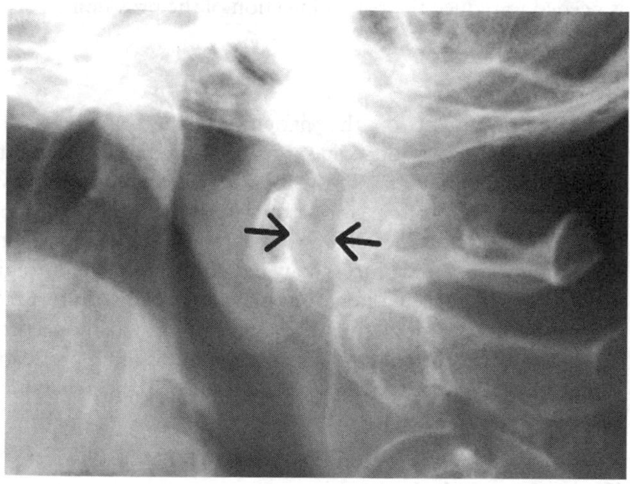

Fig. 45.1
Cervical spine: rheumatoid arthritis. The normal apposition of the anterior arch of the atlas in the extension view **(A)** widens in flexion **(B)** to show atlantoaxial subluxation.

tions. Total hip replacement may be required in patients who have developed avascular necrosis of the femoral head as a result of alcoholism or sickle cell disease (Table 45.2). In addition to the precautions detailed in Chapter 23 for patients with sickle cell disease, a plan for blood transfusion management should be agreed with a haematologist. The use of a limb tourniquet is contraindicated, even for patients suffering from sickle cell trait.

Table 45.2 Anaesthesia and non-rheumatoid arthropathies

Arthropathy	Anaesthetic note
Ankylosing spondylitis	Cervical immobility: plan intubation Restrictive lung disease Aortic regurgitation: atrioventricular condition defects
Alcoholism	May need hip replacement Anticipate postoperative delirium
Sickle cell haemoglobinopathy	May need hip replacement or peripheral surgery Planned transfusion (and other i.v. fluid) policy Maintain normothermia Avoid tourniquet Oxygen after surgery

DRUG THERAPY

Some drugs used to control pain or retard inflammatory arthropathy influence anaesthetic care.

NON-STEROIDAL ANTI-INFLAMMATORY DRUGS

If paracetamol fails, NSAIDs often succeed in controlling pain. Many patients who present for orthopaedic surgery already take NSAIDs. After minor operations, these drugs are often satisfactory in the management of postoperative pain. They are usually inadequate alone in controlling pain after major procedures, but their use reduces the dose requirements, and thus the side-effects, of opioid analgesics.

Thromboxane A_2 and prostaglandin endoperoxide synthesis, needed for the haemostatic function of platelets, are reduced by NSAIDs, which inhibit the cyclo-oxygenase (COX) enzyme systems required for their formation from arachidonic acid. There are two COX isoforms; COX-1 is needed to synthesize prostaglandins which protect the gastric mucosa, and COX-2 is involved with inflammatory responses. Inhibition of these systems ceases rapidly when NSAIDs are stopped. Aspirin also inhibits COX enzyme systems, but inhibition persists for up to 10 days after treatment with aspirin is stopped.

Although NSAIDs taken up to the time of surgery increase surgical blood loss, this does not imply that preoperative administration should be avoided. NSAIDs are valuable in providing analgesia pre- and postoperatively, and increased surgical blood loss is usually modest. Of more concern is gastroduodenal ulceration, of which the first symptom can be life-threatening upper gastrointestinal haemorrhage. The risk of ulceration is dose-related, commoner as age advances and even commoner if corticosteroids are also used to control inflammation. NSAIDs should be avoided in patients who have a history suggestive of gastrointestinal ulceration or bleeding.

Although the mode of action of low-dose heparin differs from that of NSAIDs, two drugs which may increase gastrointestinal blood loss should not be given simultaneously to patients at risk of gastric bleeding.

The use of NSAIDs can impair renal function and can lead to postoperative renal failure. NSAIDs should be avoided if there is any overt evidence of renal impairment or hypovolaemia. Patients who are elderly or diabetic, and those receiving ACE inhibitors, β-blockers or immunosuppressives are at special risk.

DRUGS USED TO MODIFY THE PROGRESS OF DISEASE

Methotrexate modifies the disease process of rheumatoid arthritis, but affects both liver function and leucocyte production. Both methotrexate and steroids reduce immune competence, and sterile techniques for invasive anaesthetic procedures should be used. Patients who take steroids regularly to control inflammatory conditions may be unable to increase endogenous steroid production in the postoperative period because of suppressed adrenocortical function. Partly because of unwanted effects, including delayed wound healing and gastrointestinal ulceration, the current approach for perioperative steroid therapy is to use small 'physiological' doses. Regimens start at induction and continue during the postoperative period with hydrocortisone 25 mg four times daily until the patient's regular regimen can be resumed. Cover is not usually needed in patients who have not taken regular steroids in the 3 months before surgery, or for adults who take less than 10 mg prednisolone daily.

OTHER ASPECTS OF PERIOPERATIVE CARE

Table 45.3 summarizes the key points.

Pain relief

Rapid mobilization is helped by good pain relief, which should be tailored for each patient and each operation.

Regional techniques should not result in motor blockade for longer than the normal period of enforced bed rest. Continuous epidural analgesia with local anaesthetic may result in hypotension and, occasionally, in depression of ventilation. Patients in whom this technique is used should be nursed in a high-dependency area or intensive care unit. Urinary retention may be precipitated in older men; a urinary catheter passed prophylactically in the clean environment of the operating theatre is better than urgent catheterization in the ward when retention occurs. Intrathecal or epidural opioids can also be used to provide postoperative analgesia, but the doses used should be as low as possible to minimize the risk of depression of ventilation.

Patient-controlled analgesia is a very effective technique in the postoperative period, but is inappropriate if, because of arthritis of the hands, the patient cannot press the delivery button.

Table 45.3 Perioperative care and orthopaedic surgery

Aspect	Anaesthetic implication
Regional techniques	Consider postoperative mobilization Risk–benefit analysis for epidural and subarachnoid anaesthesia Consider sedation for long procedures
Infection risk	Comply with local policies Clean techniques Antibiotic prophylaxis
Posture	Care with movement and pressure points Secure i.v. and airway access
Thromboprophylaxis	Identify risk category before deciding
Temperature control	Apply forced air heating early
Postoperative fluids	Avoid 'top-up' transfusion Avoid excess 5% glucose

Asepsis

An infected prosthetic joint, caused most commonly by staphylococcal infection, is a personal and economic disaster. There is a trend towards abandonment of face masks by operating theatre staff in patients undergoing general or gynaecological surgery. However, this policy may not be followed in the orthopaedic theatre. Surgery is often carried out under a laminar flow hood, which blows clean filtered air downwards, with the anaesthetist and the patient's head outside its confines. Prophylactic antibiotics, prescribed for major joint replacement, should be given before any tourniquet is inflated. Where a second operation, such as transurethral prostatectomy, rapidly follows a major joint replacement procedure, the anaesthetist and surgeons should consider whether antibiotic prophylaxis is needed to reduce the risk of infection of the prosthesis.

Posture

Forceful movement of the patient by the surgeon is often inevitable during orthopaedic surgery. Where there is firm attachment to the table, such as in the modified lateral position in which hip replacement is often carried out, careful checking of pressure points and of i.v. and airway access should precede draping. Although some procedures may be performed under regional anaesthesia alone, long operations may result in discomfort related to posture. In addition, the noises generated by orthopaedic surgeons may cause distress to the patient and it is often preferable to supplement regional blocks with sedation or light general anaesthesia.

Thromboprophylaxis

Deep venous thrombosis (DVT) may complicate any operation, but is associated particularly with surgery on the pelvis, hip or knee. Pulmonary embolism (PE) may be fatal and accounts for about half of all deaths after hip replacement. Although infusions of dextran have been shown to reduce the incidence of PE after surgery, there is a relatively high risk of anaphylaxis associated with the administration of dextran, and low-dose heparin regimens have become the norm. There is evidence that heparin reduces the incidence of fatal PE in high-risk groups, including patients who undergo surgery on the pelvis, hip or knee. Compared with unfractionated heparins (UFHs), low molecular-weight heparins (LMWHs) inhibit the coagulation enzyme Xa and bind antithrombin 3 to a similar extent, but bind less to thrombin. The use of LMWH might be expected to result in less surgical bleeding than when UFH is used. LMWH probably protects better against DVT after hip replacement, but the evidence for better prophylaxis against PE is less firm. The simplicity of once-daily administration of LMWH is an added advantage compared with UFH.

Epidural anaesthesia reduces fibrinolysis and activation of clotting factors, reduces the risk of DVT and may reduce the risk of PE. These advantages, and the very small risk of epidural haematoma in patients who have received heparin, must be considered in an overall risk–benefit assessment of epidural anaesthesia or analgesia during and after surgery.

Correctly applied, graduated stockings and intermittent calf compression devices reduce the incident of DVT, but there may be no extra benefit for patients who receive heparin.

Temperature loss

Heat is redistributed from core to periphery, with a reduction of temperature of about 1°C in the first hour of anaesthesia, and at a slower rate thereafter. For some orthopaedic procedures, much of this first hour is spent in the anaesthetic room. Elderly patients who receive i.v. fluids at room temperature, and those with large evaporative losses from surgical wounds, are at particular risk. After surgery, normal core temperature is restored more slowly in patients who have received local anaesthetics intrathecally or epidurally because of residual vasodilatation in skin. During hip replacement, hypothermia is known to be associated with increased blood loss, because of the narrow temperature range in which enzyme-dependent systems work, and perhaps because of platelet sequestration in the spleen. The most effective way of avoiding excessive heat loss is by forced air warming systems, although heating i.v. and surgical fluids and the use of impermeable surgical drapes to reduce heat loss by evaporation are also of value.

Tourniquets

Effective venous exsanguination, either by elevation of the limb or by winding a rubber bandage around it, followed by rapid application of a tourniquet cuff to a pressure sufficient to occlude the arterial supply, produces a bloodless surgical field (Table 45.4). The cuff should be about 20% wider than the diameter of the limb. To avoid damage by shearing and compression of skin, nerves and other tissues, the tourniquet should be lined with fabric and applied over muscle bulk. To avoid injury from chemical burns, entry of spirit cleansing lotions under the cuff must be prevented.

The tourniquet is maintained above systolic arterial pressure, commonly by up to 100 mmHg for the arm and 200 mmHg for the leg. These rather wide margins are used for two reasons. First, the pressure on the measuring gauge is not the same as the effective tourniquet pressure; the narrower the cuff, the greater is the difference. Second, blood pressure commonly increases about 30 min after the tourniquet is inflated. This is not caused by the alteration in the balance between blood volume and circulatory capacity resulting from exsanguination of the limb and inflation of the tourniquet, but results probably from activation of C 'slow' pain fibres by ischaemia. The pain that accompanies this is difficult to relieve, and the conscious patient who can no longer tolerate it may require general anaesthesia. Subarachnoid anaesthesia prevents tourniquet pain in the leg; the denser the block, the better the prevention, and the addition of an opioid to the local anaesthetic prolongs toleration of the tourniquet. General anaesthesia does not always stop the relentless increase in arterial pressure.

Electromyographical and histological changes that follow prolonged application of a tourniquet reverse after deflation, although the maximum period of safe ischaemia is not known. Lasting damage is unlikely if a tourniquet time of 90–120 min is not exceeded.

When the tourniquet is deflated, the products of anaerobic metabolism in the limb are released and a bolus of acidaemic, hypercapnic blood is returned to the abruptly increased capacity of the circulation. This can result in transient cardiovascular changes, including cardiac arrhythmias and changes in arterial pressure. There may also be an increase in intracranial pressure (which is of importance in patients with reduced intracranial compliance, e.g. as a result of recent head injury). Bleeding may also occur. Tourniquets on more than one limb should not be deflated (or inflated) simultaneously.

Tourniquets are contraindicated to differing degrees in patients with poor peripheral circulation, crush injuries, infection and sickle cell disease or trait.

Table 45.4 Tourniquets

Precautions

Cuff width 120% of limb diameter
Apply cuff over muscle bulk
Gauge pressure greater than effective pressure
Prevent spirit access under cuff
Pain and hypertension after 30 min
Check BP after deflation
Contraindications – poor peripheral circulation, crush injury, heart failure, sickle cell disease or trait

Blood loss and fluid replacement

Orthopaedic operations are opportunities to avoid autologous blood transfusion. Strategies include pre-deposit donation of blood by the patient, and acute normovolaemic haemodilution immediately before surgery. Blood loss may be reduced by discontinuing NSAIDs for 24–48 h before surgery or avoiding administration of aspirin for 10 days.

Posture, maintenance of normothermia and surgical technique also contribute to reductions in blood loss. Epidural and spinal anaesthesia reduce venous pressure and therefore blood loss. Cell salvage with retransfusion can be used during and after surgery, and 'top-up' transfusion to 'normal' haemoglobin levels should be resisted; iron supplements are safer.

Despite these measures, autologous transfusion cannot always be avoided. Patients undergoing hip replacement, and particularly revision procedures, often bleed heavily, especially when the femur is being reamed. During knee replacement, a substantial volume of blood may be lost at the end of the operation when the tourniquet is removed. Despite the use of wound drains, some blood is lost into deeper tissues.

Fluid and electrolyte replacement is discussed in detail in Chapter 39. Hyponatraemia sometimes occurs after orthopaedic surgery.

MAJOR JOINT REPLACEMENT

Table 45.5 summarizes key differences between types of joint replacement.

HIP REPLACEMENT

Most hip prostheses are of the 'cemented' variety. The operation may be performed in either a supine or a modified lateral position. The femoral head is removed, and the new cup and femoral components are fixed to prepared bone with polymethylmethacrylate cement. Application and hardening of the cement, particularly after its insertion into the femoral shaft, are sometimes accompanied by sudden reductions in end-tidal CO_2 concentration and blood pressure. Although attributable in part to toxic monomers released as the cement polymerizes, the high incidences of these changes which were reported when the technique was relatively new were probably related to a high frequency of air embolism; air trapped under the cement was forced into the circulation as the prosthesis was pushed into the femoral shaft. Techniques such as filling the shaft from the bottom upwards have reduced the incidence of adverse events, but insertion may still cause embolism of marrow, fat or blood clots. This is not the only time of danger. If the intramedullary pressure increases above venous pressure, embolization of air is a risk; intramedullary pressure reaches its highest values when intact bone is first opened and reamed.

Although hip replacement procedures can be performed under regional anaesthesia alone, sedation or light anaesthesia is usually necessary in addition (see above). More commonly, 'balanced' anaesthesia is used. Surges in venous pressure compromise the effectiveness of the bond between the hardening cement and bone, and may be prevented by epidural or lumbar plexus anaesthesia or by the administration of an appropriate concentration of a volatile anaesthetic agent. Paradoxically, many anaesthetists increase the rate of fluid replacement at this stage, anticipating a decrease in arterial pressure.

To reduce the risk of dislocation of the new joint, the effects of non-depolarizing muscle relaxant drugs should not be reversed until after the patient has been placed in bed after the insertion of an abduction splint. A risk of dislocation remains if the patient is rolled in bed or placed in the sitting position during the early recovery period.

Elderly patients, particularly those who have relied on NSAIDs for long periods of time, require surprisingly little analgesia after hip replacement, provided that the quality of pain control in the immediate postoperative period is good. A combination of opioids, NSAIDs and regular paracetamol minimizes the dose requirements of each, and thus the risks of side-effects.

Revision of hip replacement may take several hours. 'Balanced' anaesthesia, often including an epidural block, is usually used. In addition to the precautions for primary hip replacement, central venous and invasive arterial pressure monitoring should be considered and a bladder catheter should be inserted to monitor urine output. Fresh frozen plasma may be required to correct abnormalities of coagulation if major blood loss occurs.

Dislocation of a prosthetic hip needs manipulation and reduction to relieve pain and is more urgent if posterior dislocation threatens the sciatic nerve. This is more likely after trauma. Usually a brief anaesthetic without paralysis suffices; if reduction is difficult, muscle relaxation may be required. It is often unrealistic to move the patient from the bed before inducing anaesthesia, but precautions against regurgitation and aspiration of gastric fluid, including antacids and rapid sequence induction, may be indicated if urgent reduction is required or if the patient has been receiving systemic opioid analgesics (which delay gastric emptying). Usually, the patient wakes up with less pain than before manipulation.

KNEE REPLACEMENT

General anaesthesia with opioid analgesia is an appropriate technique for this operation. Knee replacement is performed with the patient in the supine position, and subarachnoid or epidural block with sedation is a realistic alternative. Pain after knee replacement is much more severe than after other major joint replacements. After general anaesthesia, pain relief for up to 36 h can be achieved by combined sciatic and 'three-in-one' femoral sheath blocks. If there is no contraindication to its use, a NSAID, together with paracetamol and an opioid, can be used to minimize the risks of side-effects of systemic analgesia. If subarachnoid anaesthesia has been used at operation, analgesia lasting for up to 24 h after surgery can be achieved by adding morphine to the local anaesthetic; a dose of morphine 100 μg usually achieves effective analgesia with little risk of depression of ventilation.

Thromboembolism is less of a risk after knee replacement than after other major joint replacements because a tourniquet is used. However, significant blood loss may occur when the tourniquet is deflated and it may be necessary to reassess fluid and blood transfusion needs in the early recovery period.

Manipulation under anaesthesia is sometimes needed in the postoperative period. Muscle relaxants are not required. Depending on the extent of manipulation, i.v. opioid analgesia may be required to control pain, especially in the first hour after the procedure.

Table 45.5 Anaesthesia and joint replacement

Joint	Posture	Embolic problems	Blood loss	Pain
Hip	Lateral or supine	PE (high risk), fat, air, marrow, monomers	Significant	Moderate
Knee	Supine	PE (medium–high risk)	Tourniquet postpones	Severe
Shoulder	Deckchair	Air, fat, marrow	Often slight	Moderate

PE, pulmonary blood clot embolus.

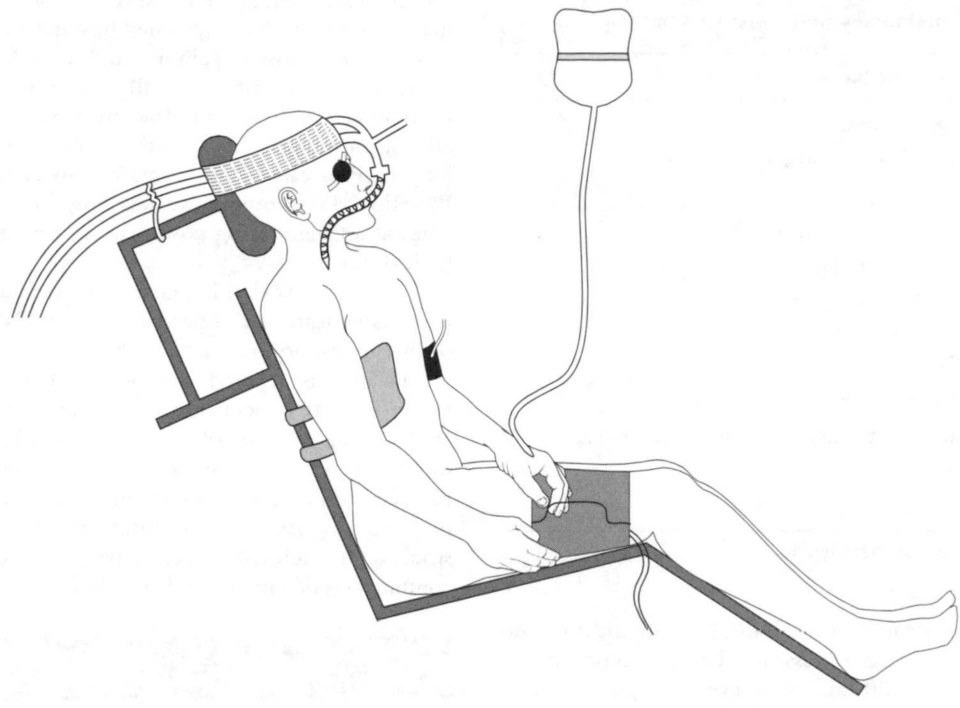

Fig. 45.2
Deckchair position for shoulder surgery.

SHOULDER REPLACEMENT

Patients undergoing shoulder replacement are often younger than those who require hip or knee joint replacements. They usually mobilize more rapidly in the postoperative period and rarely require prolonged infusion of i.v. fluids or blood transfusion. During surgery, the patient is placed in a 'deckchair' position (Fig. 45.2). A 'fail-safe' technique includes tracheal intubation with a reinforced tube. Surgery often involves vigorous manipulation of the arm, so the head needs to be fixed firmly to the operating table. To avoid sudden hypotension, elevation to the deckchair position should be undertaken with a free-running i.v. infusion, and with a vasopressor readily available. Because the shoulder is above the heart during surgery, air embolism is a risk. Interscalene block provides effective analgesia after surgery; transient neuropraxia may be blamed on these blocks but is more likely to be caused by the surgical procedure.

Table 45.5 shows key differences between different joint replacements. The same general precautions apply to other procedures on the shoulder, except that when no prosthesis is inserted and infection risk is less important, intermittent injections of local anaesthetic through a subacromial catheter inserted at the end of surgery are an option for pain relief.

OTHER ORTHOPAEDIC OPERATIONS

Many peripheral orthopaedic operations need only a simple inhalation technique, combined with local anaesthesia. At the end of many procedures, a plaster of Paris cast is applied. If anaesthesia ends before the plaster hardens, the patient may move, break the cast and need to be re-anaesthetized. Table 45.6 lists points specific to several specific procedures.

REGIONAL ANAESTHESIA AND ORTHOPAEDIC SURGERY

Regional anaesthesia, either alone or in combination with general anaesthesia, is well suited to orthopaedic surgery. Table 45.7 shows local anaesthesia blocks suitable for operations at a number of sites. Some of these blocks are suitable as the sole anaesthetic for short procedures. Apart from subarachnoid, epidural and

Table 45.6 Anaesthetic implications of specific operations

Operation	Anaesthetic implications
Elbow arthrodesis	Sometimes severe pain after surgery
Ganglion excision	Infiltration unsuitable – regional or GA needed
Wrist arthroscopy	Persistent pain after surgery – try NSAIDs
Excision of trapezium	Sometimes severe pain after surgery
Tibial osteotomy	Sometimes severe pain after surgery
Long bone fractures	Fat embolism frequent
Soft tissue trauma	Often relatively pain-free after surgery
Compound fractures	Need urgent surgery
Arthroscopy	Light anaesthesia risks damage to instrument or patient

Table 45.7 Regional anaesthesia and analgesia

Site of surgery	Suitable blocks
Shoulder	Interscalene
Arm	Interscalene ± intercostobrachial
Forearm	Axillary, IVRA
Hand	Axillary, IVRA, wrist
Fingers	Metacarpal, digital
Hip	Epidural, subarachnoid, lumbar plexus, femoral 'three-in-one' ± sciatic
Long bone fractures	Femoral ± sciatic
Knee	Femoral 'three-in-one' ± sciatic
Knee arthroscopy	Intracavity and infiltration of entry portals
Foot	Ankle
Toes	Digital

IVRA, intravenous regional anaesthesia.

interscalene blocks, regional blocks with local anaesthetic drugs do not relieve tourniquet pain. Progress may become impossible in the conscious patient after 30 min or so, even though the site of surgery may still be pain-free. Often the only solution in this situation is general anaesthesia.

Bone grafts to limbs easily anaesthetized by regional techniques may need to be taken from other parts of the body, e.g. the iliac crest. Consequently, it may be more appropriate to use general anaesthesia when bone grafting is planned.

Intravenous regional anaesthesia

Intravenous regional anaesthesia (IVRA) in the arm is suitable for manipulation of wrist fractures and brief operations on the distal arm and hand. It is easy to perform, but can be fatal unless properly performed. Death is caused by a bolus of local anaesthetic solution reaching the heart. Before performing IVRA, it is essential to understand how the risk of complications can be minimized and how they can be treated if they materialize. Details of the technique and safety precautions are described in Chapter 43.

DAY-CARE ORTHOPAEDIC PROCEDURES

Principles of anaesthesia for day-care surgery are discussed in detail in Chapter 50. They include prompt pain relief and treatment of nausea and vomiting to allow early discharge. As with many procedures, the occasional day-case anaesthetist or surgeon is well advised to adopt the techniques of the more experienced.

For orthopaedic procedures, postoperative pain is minimized if a local or regional anaesthetic block is used intraoperatively, with or without sedation or general anaesthesia. Blocks which interfere least with motor function are best; femoral nerve block is particularly unsuitable for knee arthroscopy, because the patient is expected to walk out of the day-case unit. Instillation of bupivacaine into the cavity of the knee joint and infiltration of the entry incisions are more suitable methods for providing postoperative analgesia. Brief arthroscopy causes less pain than a prolonged procedure; if the operation lasts more than 30 min, postoperative pain may be so severe that unplanned hospital admission is required.

Severe but transient pain may follow deflation of a limb tourniquet; maintaining anaesthesia for a few minutes after release of the tourniquet often prevents the problem. Severe, persistent pain after arthroscopy is likely only if the procedure has been prolonged. Pain caused by haemarthrosis is relieved by aspiration. Elevation of the limb reduces swelling and is a simple and effective method for minimizing postoperative pain and the need for analgesic drugs.

If a regional block is impractical, then an appropriate alternative is the administration of paracetamol or a NSAID before surgery, or by suppository during anaesthesia. If it is anticipated that opioid analgesia is required, the sooner the drug is given, the better. Prophylactic treatment of nausea and vomiting should be considered, particularly if opioid analgesics are likely to be administered or if the patient is female. Other risk factors which may justify prophylactic administration of an antiemetic are a previous history of postoperative nausea and vomiting and a susceptibility to motion sickness. In high-risk patients, prophylactic administration of a combination of antiemetic drugs should be considered.

FRACTURED NECK OF FEMUR

This condition is becoming more common as the proportion of elderly patients in the community increases. Patients are usually female and often frail. In addition to the need to reduce and fix the fracture, surgery aims to relieve pain and to minimize the complications associated with prolonged bed rest. Surgery should not be postponed longer than is necessary to treat concurrent conditions which are clinically important and amenable to treatment. For example, rapid atrial fibrillation should be corrected and treatment for heart failure initiated. To postpone surgery to treat intercurrent chest infection may be counterproductive because it prolongs immobility. After relief of pain, physical examination and laboratory investigations have been completed, surgery should follow as soon as possible. Patients might not have drunk for hours, or even days, and an i.v. infusion to correct dehydration or to treat overt anaemia by blood transfusion may be required. None of these need delay surgery unduly.

The fracture may be repaired by 'screws' or 'pin and plate', or a prosthetic femoral head may be inserted, with or without cement. If these procedures are performed with the patient in the supine position, a modified operating table allows X-ray screening.

The immediate mortality after repair of fractured neck of femur is less when subarachnoid anaesthesia rather than general anaesthesia is used during surgery, probably because of a reduction in thromboembolic complications. However, the mortality after 28 days is not influenced by the choice of anaesthetic technique. Thus, choice of technique can be made by considering other aspects of the patient's condition, pain relief after surgery, individual preferences of the anaesthetist, and the preference of the patient.

Subarachnoid anaesthesia is an effective technique for repair of fractured neck of femur and is usually a better choice than epidural block. However, it is necessary to place the patient in the lateral position in order to perform lumbar puncture, which can cause considerable discomfort. It is best to position the patient with the injured femur uppermost. Small doses of an intravenous sedative or short-acting opioid analgesic may be used to relieve distress during positioning and insertion of the spinal needle; it is essential that the patient's condition is monitored appropriately while the block is performed. Up to 2.5 ml of hyperbaric bupivacaine 0.5% is injected at the L3/4 or L4/5 interspace, either in the midline or using a paramedian approach. Successful block provides sudden relief from pain, in addition to satisfactory surgical anaesthesia.

When general anaesthesia is selected, intravenous administration of a small dose of thiopental or inhalation of sevoflurane are particularly appropriate techniques for induction. In most centres, it is usual to intubate the trachea and ventilate the lungs mechanically during the procedure. Elderly patients, particularly those with impaired renal or hepatic function, may be sensitive to the effects of non-depolarizing muscle relaxants and opioid analgesics, and it is prudent to use reduced doses, at least initially.

Maintenance of oxygen delivery is particularly important in this group of patients, who may be acutely or chronically anaemic, who may recently have been hypothermic, and who may already be confused. During surgery, steps should be taken to maintain body temperature and a satisfactory arterial pressure, with infusion of fluid and/or blood, and administration of a vasopressor if indicated.

Following repair of fractured neck of femur, the patient is usually more comfortable than before operation and analgesia should be prescribed with a view to early mobilization.

FURTHER READING

Anonymous 1998 Low molecular weight heparins for venous thromboembolism. Drug and Therapeutics Bulletin 36: 25–28

Gielen M J M, Sienstra R 1991 Tourniquet hypertension and its prevention: a review. Regional Anesthesia 16: 191–194

Lane N, Allen K 1999 Hyponatraemia after orthopaedic surgery (editorial). British Medical Journal 318: 1363–1364

Loach A (ed) 1994 Orthopaedic anaesthesia, 2nd edn. Edward Arnold, London

Nicholson G, Burrin J M, Hall G M 1998 Peri-operative steroid supplementation. Anaesthesia 53: 1091–1104

Pinnock C A, Fischer H B J, Jones R P 1998 Peripheral nerve blockade. Churchill Livingstone, Edinburgh

Wedel D J (ed) 1993 Orthopedic anesthesia. Churchill Livingstone, New York

46 Anaesthesia for ENT surgery

Two hundred and seventy thousand ear, nose and throat operations are performed in the UK each year, accounting for approximately 5% of the workload of an anaesthetic department. Patients are usually young and healthy and the average hospital stay is short (less than 3 days). Many operations are performed as day cases, thereby reducing the need for in-patient admission.

Children and young adults are frequently apprehensive and require reassurance. Some may have an atopic history which influences the anaesthetic technique. Older patients may have hypertension or ischaemic heart disease and require careful preoperative assessment.

Smooth anaesthesia and a clear airway are essential, as coughing and straining result in venous congestion which may persist during surgery and cause increased bleeding. Partial obstruction of the airway may lead to hypoxaemia, hypercapnia and unduly light anaesthesia.

The patient's eyes should be protected from corneal abrasions in all ENT procedures by taping the eyelids shut, except for procedures where the periorbital fat may be accessed e.g. nasal polypectomy.

THE SHARED AIRWAY

Special problems are caused when the airway is shared by both anaesthetist and surgeon. If bleeding is anticipated, the airway *must* be protected and the oropharynx packed to avoid contamination of the larynx with blood, pus and other debris. Techniques which rely on insufflation of anaesthetic vapours to an unintubated, unprotected trachea are no longer in common use and are not described here.

During tonsillectomy, the Boyle Davis gag sometimes compresses the tracheal tube and causes partial airway obstruction. During IPPV, this is detected by a decrease in compliance and increased inflation pressure and, in the spontaneously breathing patient, by decreased movement of the reservoir bag.

At the end of the procedure, the pack must be removed and the pharynx cleared of blood and debris before the trachea is extubated with the patient in a head-down lateral position.

THE LARYNGEAL MASK AIRWAY

The laryngeal mask airway (LMA) has been used for all types of ENT anaesthesia. To justify its use, the anaesthetist must be able to demonstrate that it conveys an advantage over the traditional use of an endotracheal tube.

TONSILLECTOMY

Each year 80 000 adenotonsillectomies are performed in the UK, with a rate of 8 per 1000 children under the age of 15. This frequency is 40% of that 15 years ago. In 1968 there were six deaths, a mortality rate of 1 in 28 000, but this has now been reduced to less than 1 in 100 000.

Most children attend for surgery on the day of operation and premedication is often not practical for these children. If premedication is required before tonsillectomy, it is administered most conveniently to the younger child as a syrup (trimeprazine 1.5 mg kg^{-1} or diazepam 0.2 mg kg^{-1}). Some anaesthetists combine this with atropine 20 μg kg^{-1} to a maximum of 600 μg given orally (except in hot weather) to decrease secretions intraoperatively.

Most children are given an i.v. induction of anaesthesia after the application of a patch of EMLA cream; some children, however, may prefer an inhalation induction and this is necessary in the child with poor venous access. Oral intubation is facilitated by succinylcholine or performed under deep inhalation anaesthesia; on occasions it may be difficult to maintain a patent airway because of respiratory obstruction produced by the enlarged tonsils.

Analgesia is given during surgery, but good control of postoperative pain still eludes us. Tracheal extubation is performed with the patient slightly head-down in a lateral position after suction has ensured that the pharynx is free from blood. The trachea may be extubated either under deep anaesthesia or when fully awake; with 'deep extubation' the anaesthetist must continue to take responsibility for protecting the airway. Postoperative vomiting is a significant problem (50% of children vomit at least once) and therefore antiemetics should be prescribed.

Blood loss during tonsillectomy is not usually measured but may be deceptively large. Increasing numbers of children under 3 years of age (15 kg) are presenting for tonsillectomy for sleep apnoea syndrome. Particular care is required in this group as blood transfusion is necessary after 100 ml blood loss. Many of these children should have an intravenous infusion until they are ready to take oral fluids.

The reinforced LMA is frequently used for tonsillectomy; however, the Boyle Davis gag is more difficult to place and obstruction to the airway occurs more frequently.

THE POSTOPERATIVE BLEEDING TONSIL

These patients fall into two separate groups; those with an acute bleed in the immediate postoperative period (usually in the recovery area) and those who ooze blood slowly from the tonsil bed. This latter group are usually diagnosed on the ward, on the basis of the clinical signs of hypovolaemia – tachycardia, pallor and sweating. Swallowing is not uncommon, followed by vomiting of a large quantity of blood. Anaesthesia for these children is difficult and the assistance of an experienced anaesthetist must be sought. An i.v. infusion is essential and blood transfusion may be required.

The group with an acute bleed present a particularly difficult problem in that there is active bleeding in the airway. They require an inhalation induction of anaesthesia (isoflurane in oxygen) in the left lateral position with Trendelenburg tilt and frequent pharyngeal suction. Intubation of the trachea is undertaken under deep anaesthesia.

The second group present with the problems of hypovolaemia and a full stomach; after resuscitation, the patient is placed head-down in a lateral position and suction apparatus is positioned within grasp. After preoxygenation, a small dose of thiopental (2–3 mg kg^{-1}) is given followed by succinylcholine 1 mg kg^{-1} and cricoid pressure is applied, although this may make laryngoscopy difficult.

When bleeding has been controlled surgically, the stomach is emptied with a nasogastric tube, and the trachea is extubated with the patient in the lateral position.

It should be emphasized that induction of anaesthesia with thiopental or propofol must never be attempted before adequate resuscitation has been undertaken and the intravascular volume restored.

ADENOIDECTOMY

Adenoidectomy is often combined with either tonsillectomy or examination of the ears under anaesthesia. Anaesthesia is induced either by inhalation or via the i.v. route. Oral tracheal intubation is advisable either under deep anaesthesia or facilitated by succinylcholine. A Boyle Davis gag is inserted, the adenoids are curetted and the postnasal space is packed to achieve haemostasis. After 3 min, this pack is removed, the patient is turned into the lateral position and the trachea is extubated.

Increasingly, adenoidectomy in the absence of tonsillectomy is being performed as a day-case procedure. For these patients, rectal paracetamol may be an appropriate analgesic.

MICROLARYNGOSCOPY

The operating microscope revolutionized the treatment of laryngeal disorders. The Kleinsasser laryngoscope is supported on the chest by rests and the operating microscope allows detailed examination and assessment of the larynx.

Premedication with pethidine and promethazine has been suggested if there is no evidence of airway obstruction. The most popular anaesthetic technique uses a Coplan's microlaryngoscopy tube (5 mm ID, 31 cm long, constructed from soft plastic, with a 10 ml cuff volume). Anaesthesia is induced with an i.v. induction agent followed by a non-depolarizing muscle relaxant; the vocal cords are sprayed with 3 ml lidocaine 4% to assist smooth anaesthesia and to minimize the possibility of postextubation laryngospasm. Alternatively, the cords may be 'painted' with 3% cocaine at the end of the procedure, which has the added advantage of reducing bleeding from biopsy sites. The Coplan's tube is passed either orally or nasally. The lungs are ventilated artificially with 66% N_2O in O_2 supplemented with a volatile agent and analgesic drug. The small-diameter tube does not impede the surgeon's view and allows good access to the larynx. The cuff prevents contamination of the trachea with blood or debris.

At the end of the procedure, the pharynx is cleared with suction under direct vision, muscle relaxants are antagonized and tracheal extubation is performed in a lateral position. Oxygen is administered to minimize the risk of hypoxaemia if laryngeal stridor occurs.

Other techniques used for microlaryngoscopy include:

- topical analgesia to the larynx with insufflation of N_2O/O_2 and halothane via a fine catheter
- neuroleptanalgesia combined with topical analgesia
- Venturi ventilation with O_2 using a catheter and a Sanders injector. Hypnosis is maintained with increments of a rapidly metabolized induction agent.

In children, microlaryngoscopy is performed using spontaneous ventilation via an oral tracheal tube one size smaller than would be used normally. The larynx should be sprayed with a measured quantity of lidocaine in an attempt to prevent postoperative laryngospasm. Occasionally the surgeon requests to observe the larynx without a tracheal tube in situ; in these circumstances the tube is removed during deep anaesthesia, allowing examination to take place during emergence or during Venturi ventilation via the operating laryngoscope.

LARYNGECTOMY

The incidence of carcinoma of the larynx is 3–4 per 100 000 population. Many tumours may be treated with radiotherapy and therefore surgery is relatively uncommon for this condition. Airway obstruction by tumour is the major anaesthetic problem; alcohol and smoking are aetiological factors which may influence anaesthesia.

Respiratory function should be assessed preoperatively, although this is difficult to measure accurately if there is airway obstruction. Chest physiotherapy should always be prescribed as it aids clearance of secretions pre- and postoperatively.

When respiratory obstruction is suspected, opioid or sedative premedication should be avoided. All patients presenting for laryngectomy undergo flexible nasal endoscopy to assess the larynx; the findings of this investigation are of great importance to the conduct of the anaesthetic. If there is a risk of mechanical obstruction on induction of anaesthesia, an inhalation technique should be used; if this results in severe respiratory obstruction, awake intubation may be required. A selection of non-cuffed tracheal tubes should be available as the lumen of the trachea may be narrowed at the level of the cords or subglottically. Laryngoscopy and intubation may be more difficult if preoperative radiotherapy has reduced the mobility of the floor of the mouth.

In the absence of respiratory obstruction, an i.v. induction agent may be used; it should be given slowly in minimal dosage until consciousness is lost. If subsequently the patient's lungs can be inflated using a face mask, succinylcholine may be given to facilitate tracheal intubation; if not, anaesthesia is deepened slowly with nitrous oxide and halothane in oxygen until laryngoscopy is possible. If there is any doubt regarding the patient's ability to maintain a patent airway after loss of consciousness, the anaesthetist must *not* use an i.v. induction agent.

Monitoring of ECG and arterial pressure must be commenced in the anaesthetic room before induction of anaesthesia, which is maintained using controlled ventilation with nitrous oxide in oxygen supplemented by a volatile agent and opioid analgesic. Induced hypotension is often used to facilitate dissection of the neck (see Ch. 36). When the larynx has been dissected free, it is important to check that a sterile tracheal tube and compatible connections are available before the trachea is divided. The patient's lungs are ventilated with 100% oxygen for 2 min, the tracheal tube is withdrawn into the larynx and disconnected, the trachea is divided and a second tracheal tube is placed rapidly into the open end of the trachea, connected to the anaesthetic circuit and secured firmly. This tube should be positioned carefully within the shortened trachea to prevent inadvertent one-lung anaesthesia.

At the end of surgery, residual neuromuscular block is antagonized and the tracheal tube changed for a tracheostomy tube. Adequate humidification is essential postoperatively. Enteral nutrition is provided via a nasogastric tube.

PHARYNGOLARYNGO-OESOPHAGECTOMY

Pharyngolaryngo-oesophagectomy is performed for tumours of the postcricoid region. The pharynx and larynx are removed and the stomach mobilized and anastomosed in the neck behind the tracheostomy. There are two surgical approaches: in one, after initial laparotomy, the stomach is passed through a mediastinal tract which is formed by blunt dissection; in the other more common procedure, the stomach is mobilized via a thoraco-abdominal incision to be anastomosed in the neck. Thus several problems may arise:

- difficulty in intubation
- temperature loss resulting from a large surgical incision, a prolonged operative procedure and extensive blood loss
- pneumothorax if the pleura is damaged during dissection
- rupture of the trachea causing difficulty in ventilation and mediastinal emphysema.

LASER SURGERY

The laser is used to strip polyps or tumours from the vocal cords accurately and with immediate control of bleeding. There are two anaesthetic problems:

- *Damage to the tracheal tube.* It has been found that in the presence of oxygen PVC microlaryngoscopy tubes may be ignited by the intensity of the laser beam. The use of an aluminized PVC tube does not remove this threat completely. The introduction of cuffed flexible stainless steel tubes for nasal or oral use has essentially solved this problem. For added safety, the cuffs should be filled with water.
- *Retinal damage.* The DOH recommends that all personnel wear protective spectacles to prevent retinal damage. Anaesthetists are particularly at risk as they are unable to retire behind the operating microscope during the laser procedure.

NASAL OPERATIONS

PREPARATION OF THE NOSE WITH LOCAL ANAESTHETIC

In 1942, Moffatt described a method of topical anaesthesia of the nose using cocaine as an alternative to spraying or packing the nose. There were three advantages of his method: minimal patient discomfort during preparation, a low risk of cocaine toxicity and a bloodless surgical field.

In 1952, Curtiss simplified Moffatt's method as follows; the patient lies supine with his or her head extended fully over the end of a trolley and supported by an assistant. A round-ended angulated needle is inserted with its tip directed along the floor of the nose. When the angle of the needle is reached, the tip is directed towards the roof of the nose and 2 ml of solution deposited when the tip has made contact. The procedure is repeated in the second nostril. The patient remains in this position for 10 min and is advised not to swallow any solution which may have trickled into the pharynx. The patient then sits upright and spits out any residual solution.

Analgesia is produced by accumulation of cocaine in the region of the sphenopalatine ganglion, thereby blocking most of the sensory supply to the nose, including the anterior ethmoidal nerve. The columella is not affected and requires a separate injection. Arterial blood supply to the nose accompanies the nerve supply and is therefore constricted by the cocaine, producing good haemostasis.

Preparation of the nose in this manner enables any operation to be performed and dispenses with the need to use hypotensive techniques to control surgical bleeding.

In the anaesthetized patient, Moffatt's prescription can be further modified by diluting it into 20 ml of solution: 10 ml is instilled into each nostril with the head extended, after placement of a gauze throat pack. The pack holds the solution in the nose for maximum effect. This method has the advantage of requiring less precise placement of the solution.

ANAESTHETIC TECHNIQUE FOR NASAL OPERATIONS

Anaesthesia for nasal surgery has been revolutionized by the introduction of the LMA. Difficulties in maintaining a patent airway in the presence of surgical nasal packing are almost completely eliminated by leaving the LMA in place postoperatively until the patient rejects it in the recovery room.

Anaesthesia for nasal surgery may be maintained using either spontaneous or controlled ventilation, depending on the duration of surgery. The pharynx should be packed with 2-inch ribbon gauze so that blood, pus or debris does not contaminate the larynx. The presence of the pack should be marked in writing on the strapping which secures the tube (or LMA) to remind the anaesthetist to remove it at the end of the operation.

The patient is positioned 10° head-up and all breathing system connections are checked before surgery begins. When surgery has been completed, the pack is removed, the pharynx is cleared and the patient is turned into a lateral position.

If an endotracheal tube is used, a Guedel airway should be placed in position before the tracheal tube is removed to provide a patent airway in the presence of surgical nasal packing. The advent of cannulated nasal packs has improved the patient's airway, but not all procedures are suitable for these packs.

EPISTAXIS

Surgical intervention may be necessary to control bleeding from the nose and may involve packing the nose or postnasal space or ligation of the maxillary artery.

The patient is often elderly and may be hypertensive. It is essential that the blood volume is restored before induction of anaesthesia. The problems inherent in haemorrhage from the upper airway and a stomach containing swallowed blood are similar to those of the bleeding tonsil and the anaesthetic technique used is similar.

THE SINUSES

Bacterial infection of the paranasal sinuses occurs when the self-cleansing mechanism becomes impaired and mucus accumulates and stagnates. Antral washouts and intranasal antrostomies are performed to aid restoration of normal mucosal activity. In a Caldwell Luc operation, radical antrostomy is performed via a buccal incision above the canine tooth.

In all these procedures, the airway is protected by means of an oral tracheal or LMA and pharyngeal pack. Ethmoidectomy may require hypotensive anaesthesia.

MAXILLECTOMY

Excision of the maxilla for tumour is a major procedure and hypotensive anaesthesia is used to reduce bleeding; ECG monitoring using a CM5 lead is advisable. Accurate measurement of arterial pressure requires radial artery cannulation. A pack or obturator is inserted into the maxillectomy cavity at the end of surgery; first a mould is fashioned from a rapidly setting plastic compound in situ and additional debris may be deposited in the pharynx as a result. Usually, the patient is anaesthetized on a second occasion 1 week later to insert the permanent prosthesis.

EARS

MYRINGOTOMY

Examination of the ears together with myringotomy and insertion of grommets is carried out commonly in children who have secretory otitis media. This operation is usually performed as a day case. Either inhalation or i.v. induction, following the application of EMLA cream, may be used and anaesthesia is maintained with spontaneous ventilation via a face mask for myringotomy alone; if adenoidectomy is performed also, oral tracheal intubation is required. The use of nitrous oxide increases middle ear pressure significantly, especially when combined with IPPV, and this may alter the appearance of the tympanic membrane.

MIDDLE EAR SURGERY

Relative hypotension is required to minimize haemorrhage in the field of the microscope. Smooth anaesthesia is essential for operations on the middle ear. Coughing, straining or bucking increases venous pressure and produces oozing which may persist for some time. Premedication may be given orally. After induction of anaesthesia with thiopental, succinylcholine is used to facilitate intubation with a non-kinking oral tracheal tube; the trachea and larynx are sprayed with lidocaine to aid tolerance of the tube. The hypertensive response to intubation may be attenuated with alfentanil. Often, sufficient reduction in arterial pressure is obtained using nitrous oxide in oxygen with halothane, enflurane or isoflurane in combination with a non-depolarizing muscle relaxant, opioid and IPPV. Small doses of a β-blocker to reduce heart rate are often effective adjuvants. A 10° head-up tilt aids venous drainage. When induced hypotension is used, ECG and accurate arterial pressure monitoring are essential. Labetalol, glyceryl trinitrate or sodium nitroprusside can be used as infusions for relative hypotension. A 25% reduction in mean arterial blood pressure is usually adequate to produce a good surgical field.

The middle ear is a closed cavity and nitrous oxide diffuses rapidly into it, causing an increase in pressure. The maximum pressure is reached approximately 40 min after induction. There is concern that this may cause grafts to become dislodged. Such complications have led some authors to suggest that O_2/N_2 should be used in place of O_2/N_2O gas mixtures. Surgical techniques have improved and been modified over the years so that an increase in middle ear pressure is no longer a significant surgical problem. It is therefore no longer necessary to turn off the nitrous oxide before the end of the procedure.

Bandaging the ear at the end of surgery involves movement of the head. This should be anticipated and supervised by the anaesthetist to prevent undue movement which may lead to gagging on the tracheal tube. If labyrinthine function is disturbed, an antiemetic may be necessary to control postoperative vertigo and vomiting.

The LMA is used in major ear surgery, but the anaesthetist must be aware that if the airway is lost during the procedure, as a result of movement of the head, the operation may have to be abandoned.

FURTHER READING

Chambers W A 1994 ENT anaesthesia. In: Nimmo W S, Rowbotham D J, Smith G (eds) Anaesthesia, 2nd edn. Blackwell Scientific Publications, Oxford

Hospital Inpatient Inquiry Series MB4, 27. DHSS Office of Population Censuses and Surveys, Welsh Office, ENT Microfiches 24, 25

Puttick N, Van der Walt J H 1987 The effect of premedication on the incidence of postoperative vomiting in children after ENT surgery. Anaesthesia and Intensive Care 15: 158

Van der Spek A L, Spargs P M, Norton M L 1988. The physics of lasers and implications for their use during airway surgery. British Journal of Anaesthesia 60: 709

47 Anaesthesia for ophthalmic surgery

Patients who present for eye surgery are frequently at the extreme ends of age. Both neonatal and geriatric anaesthesia present special problems. Some eye surgery may last many hours and repeated anaesthetics at short intervals are often necessary. The anaesthetic technique may influence intraocular pressure (IOP), and skilled administration of either local or general anaesthesia contributes directly to the successful outcome of the surgery. Close co-operation and clear understanding between surgeon and anaesthetist are essential. Risks and benefits must be assessed carefully and the anaesthetic technique selected accordingly.

Ophthalmic surgery can be classified into subspecialities and intraocular or extraocular procedures may be performed (Table 47.1); each has different anaesthetic requirements.

Table 47.1 Categorization of ophthalmic surgery
Ophthalmology subspecialities
Paediatric
Oculoplastic
Retinovitreous
Anterior segment
Glaucoma
Neuro-ophthalmology
Extraocular operations
Globe and orbit
Eyebrow and eyelid
Lacrimal system
Muscles
Conjunctiva
Cornea, surface
Intraocular operations
Iris and anterior chamber
Lens and cataracts
Vitreous
Retina
Cornea, full thickness

CHOICE OF ANAESTHESIA

Ophthalmic surgery can be carried out under either local or general anaesthesia. The type of surgery, planned duration, age and fitness of the patient influence the choice (Table 47.2). Usually, local anaesthesia is preferred for older patients, as the stress response to surgery is diminished and complications such as post-operative confusion, nausea, vomiting and urinary retention are mostly eliminated. Younger patients are often too anxious for local anaesthesia and are usually managed with general anaesthesia.

Table 47.2 Preferred anaesthetic technique for common surgical procedures in ophthalmology
Local anaesthesia
Cataract
Glaucoma techniques
Minor extraocular plastic surgery
Laser dacrocystorhinostomy
Minor anterior segment procedures
General anaesthesia
Paediatric surgery
Squint surgery
Major oculoplastic surgery
Dacrocystorhinostomy
Perforating keratoplasty
Orbital trauma repair
Perforating eye injuries
Retinovitreous surgery

CONDITIONS FOR INTRAOCULAR SURGERY

For most intraocular operations, the eye must be immobile and pain-free. Except for glaucoma surgery, the pupil should be dilated and intraocular pressure reduced.

Widespread use of the operating microscope has enabled the surgeon to place finer and stronger sutures with more precision than previously. The risk of wound dehiscence following postoperative Valsalva-type manoeuvres has been reduced.

INTRAOCULAR PRESSURE (IOP)

There is a diurnal variation in IOP, but a mean pressure of 15 mmHg above atmospheric pressure is normal. Resting pressure greater than 22 mmHg is considered abnormal.

EXPULSIVE HAEMORRHAGE

In the presence of raised IOP, sudden reduction in pressure on incision of the globe may lead to the expression of the contents. The balance between venous and intraocular pressure is crucial. An increase in venous pressure causes fluid to pool in the choroid and may progress to cause rupture of the ciliary artery with prolapse of the iris. On rare occasions, disastrous expulsive haemorrhage may result in the loss of the entire contents of the eyeball.

CONTROL OF INTRAOCULAR PRESSURE

Factors controlling IOP are similar to those that influence intracranial pressure, as both involve manipulation of a volume contained in a semirigid container. These factors include external pressure, volume of arterial and venous vasculature (choroidal volume) and the volumes of the aqueous and vitreous humour (Fig. 47.1).

External pressure

Pressure from squeezing the eyes closed or the injection of a volume of local anaesthetic into the orbit is transmitted to the eyeball and increases the IOP. During general anaesthesia, pressure from the anaesthetic mask, retractors, etc. should be avoided.

Venous pressure

Venous congestion increases vascular volume within the eye and reduces aqueous drainage through the canal of Schlemm, causing an increase in IOP. During anaesthesia, venous pressure is influenced mainly by posture and transmitted intrathoracic pressure. A 15° head-up tilt causes a significant decrease in IOP.

Raised arterial pressure, anxiety, restlessness, full bladder, coughing, retching and airway obstruction cause an increase in venous pressure which is reflected immediately in the IOP. Intermittent positive pressure ventilation (IPPV) produces a small increase in venous pressure secondary to the increase in mean intrathoracic pressure, but is compensated for by control of arterial $P\text{CO}_2$.

Arterial blood gas tensions

Arterial $P\text{CO}_2$ is an important determinant of choroidal vascular volume and IOP. A reduction in $P_a\text{CO}_2$ constricts the choroidal vessels and reduces IOP. Elevation of $P_a\text{CO}_2$ results in a proportional and linear increase in IOP. Increases in $P_a\text{CO}_2$ may also increase central venous pressure. Hypoxaemia produces intraocular vasodilatation and an increase in IOP.

Arterial pressure

Stable values of arterial pressure within the physiological range maintain normal IOP. Sudden increases in systolic arterial pressure above the normal autoregulatory range increase choroidal blood volume and consequently IOP. Reduction in arterial pressure below normal physiological levels reduces IOP, but the response is unpredictable in old age when arterial capacitance is reduced.

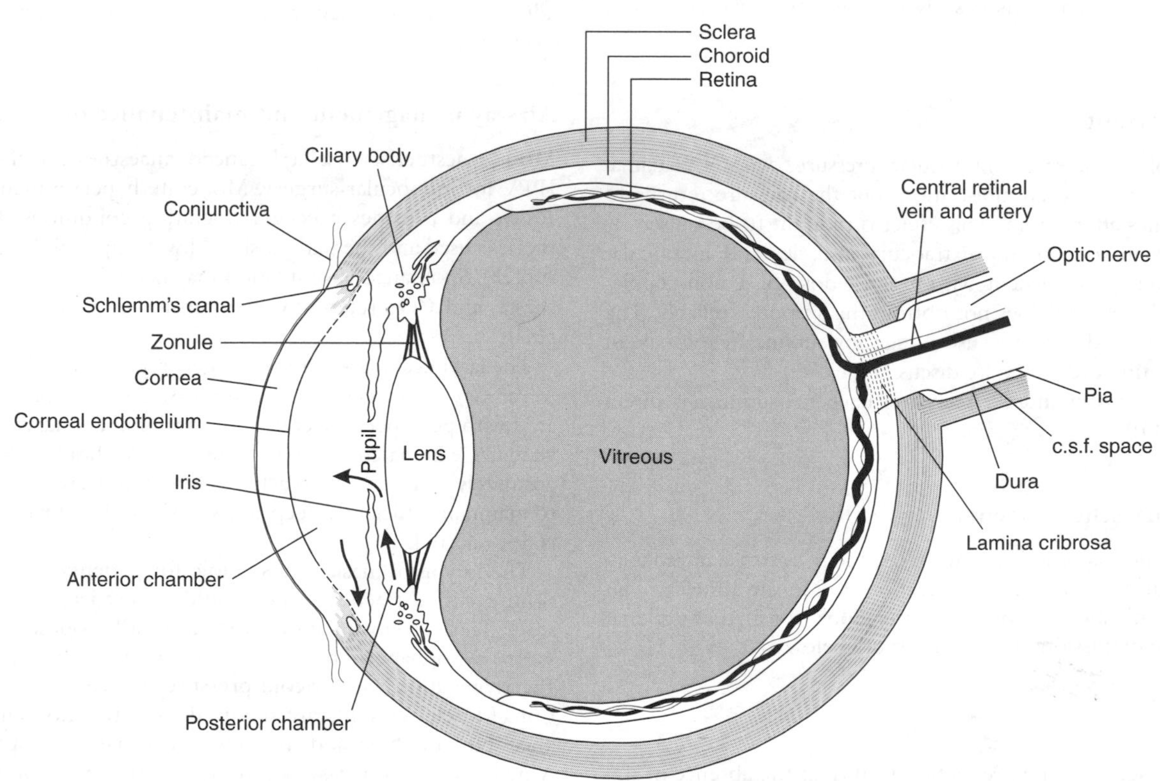

Fig. 47.1
Cross-section through eye and optic nerve. Heavy arrows indicate flow of aqueous.

Aqueous and vitreous volumes

A decrease in either aqueous or vitreous volume reduces IOP. Osmotic diuretics are sometimes used to reduce aqueous and vitreous volume. Acetazolamide reduces the production of aqueous.

Haelon (sodium hyaluronate)

Sodium hyaluronate is used as a soft viscous retractor during surgery. It can augment the effect of general anaesthesia by controlling vitreous bulge and compensates for small changes in IOP. Sodium hyaluronate is a large-molecular-weight, clear viscoelastic polysaccharide. The manufactured product is injected by the surgeon at the time of incision and helps to maintain the shape of the anterior chamber and the work space.

EFFECT OF ANAESTHETIC DRUGS ON IOP

Premedication

Drugs used for premedication have little effect on intraocular pressure, and the commonly used anxiolytic and antiemetic drugs may be used as preferred.

Induction agents

Most of the intravenous induction agents, with the exception of ketamine, reduce intraocular pressure and may be used as indicated clinically. Ketamine is best avoided if intraocular surgery is planned.

Muscle relaxants

Succinylcholine increases intraocular pressure, with a maximal effect 2 min after i.v. administration, but the pressure returns to baseline values after 5 min. This effect is thought to be caused by the increase in tone of the extraocular muscles and intraocular vasodilatation. Pretreatment with a small dose of a non-depolarizing muscle relaxant does not obtund this response reliably. The problems involved with the use of succinylcholine in the patient with penetrating eye injury are discussed below.

Non-depolarizing muscle relaxants have no significant direct effects on IOP.

Volatile anaesthetic agents

All the volatile anaesthetic agents in use today decrease intraocular pressure. Nitrous oxide has no effect on IOP in the absence of air or a therapeutic inert gas bubble in the globe (for further explanation, see the discussion on retinal surgery below).

Opioids

Opioids cause a moderate reduction in IOP in the absence of significant ventilatory depression. They contribute to postoperative nausea and vomiting and are not usually required for postoperative analgesia following eye surgery.

TECHNIQUES OF GENERAL ANAESTHESIA

Premedication

Premedication administration on the ward is not now used routinely for eye surgery. A short-acting benzodiazepine such as temazepam may be given orally as premedication to anxious patients. These drugs should be used with caution in the elderly as they may result in confusion. Premedication by injection is not necessary. Anticholinergic agents cause a dry mouth and discomfort and do not need to be given with premedication. They are more likely to be needed in strabismus or retinal surgery, but may be given intravenously after induction if necessary.

Induction

The synergistic effects of midazolam with short-acting opioid analgesics such as fentanyl or alfentanil may precede induction. These drugs reduce dose requirements of induction and maintenance agents and modify the cardiovascular response to airway manipulation. This combination should be administered with caution in the elderly who easily become apnoeic with small doses. Propofol is used widely because of its short duration of action, pleasant induction and reduced postoperative nausea. Etomidate is useful in elderly or unfit patients because of its cardiostability, reduction in IOP and rapid recovery. Frequent pain on injection and involuntary movements offset these advantages. Thiopental is still a satisfactory alternative for induction in both adults and children. Inhalation induction with sevoflurane is another alternative and has largely superseded halothane for gaseous induction in children. It may be used in needle-phobic adults or as a cost-effective alternative to propofol induction and maintenance.

Airway management and maintenance of anaesthesia

Most anaesthetists use a balanced anaesthesia technique with IPPV for intraocular surgery. Moderate hyperventilation reduces P_aCO_2 and provides excellent operating conditions. Less anaesthetic is used and the patient should wake up rapidly at the end of surgery. Spontaneous ventilation may need deeper levels of anaesthesia, and CO_2 retention, hypotension and slow recovery may result.

The laryngeal mask has now largely replaced tracheal intubation for intraocular surgery. Insertion is easier and the problems associated with postoperative coughing, straining and laryngospasm are virtually eliminated. The laryngeal mask should be positioned accurately to give unobstructed ventilation. Care should be taken to maintain sufficiently deep anaesthesia so that the laryngeal mask is not rejected.

The laryngeal mask is unsuitable for patients at risk of aspiration; a cuffed tracheal tube should be used to protect the airway. This group includes the morbidly obese, those with gastro-oesophageal reflux and patients with hiatus hernia. Preoxygenation with cricoid pressure reduces the risk of aspiration. Muscle relaxants are required for intubation and maintenance, but coughing and straining at extubation are problems for which there is no easy solution. Continuation of the volatile agent until reversal of residual neuromuscular blockade, or the use of i.v. lidocaine, has been recommended to overcome this problem.

PENETRATING EYE INJURY

The anaesthetic management of the patient with a penetrating eye injury and a full stomach creates a dilemma. Rapid sequence induction with tracheal intubation is advisable, but the use of succinylcholine is theoretically contraindicated as it produces an increase in IOP which could expel the ocular contents. It may be possible to delay surgery for a few hours, but following trauma, gastric emptying is not assured in the usual time-scale. Drugs which facilitate gastric emptying such as metoclopramide may help. In choosing a muscle relaxant for tracheal intubation, the risks of further damage to the eye must be weighed against the life-threatening dangers of pulmonary aspiration. If it is anticipated that tracheal intubation will be uneventful, a large dose of non-depolarizing muscle relaxant (rocuronium may be the most appropriate for this purpose) can be substituted for succinylcholine in the usual rapid sequence technique. Care should be taken not to exert pressure on the injured eye with the face mask during preoxygenation. If intubation is difficult and ventilation with a face mask is not efficient, the resulting hypoxaemia and hypercapnia may cause more damage to the eye than a single dose of succinylcholine.

Anaesthetic management during surgery conforms to the pattern used for other intraocular procedures. Extubation should be performed with the patient in the lateral position and almost awake.

RETINAL SURGERY

General anaesthesia is used for most retinal surgery. Patients are often in younger age groups and the procedures may take longer than anterior segment surgery. Patients are liable to become uncomfortable and restless if required to lie still on a hard operating table for too long. Local anaesthesia is an option which should be considered in the medically compromised patient or for retinal procedures of short duration. Careful monitoring is needed as the oculocardiac reflex is not blocked reliably by local anaesthetic. The surgeon can readily top up the local anaesthetic if it starts to wear off.

As fundal examination, vitrectomy and laser therapy are carried out in the dark, the anaesthetist must ensure that there is sufficient lighting to conduct anaesthesia safely. Goggles *must* be worn by all theatre staff during laser therapy.

Towards the end of a retinal detachment procedure, the surgeon often injects a bubble of sulphur hexafluoride (SF_6) or perfluoropropane (C_3F_8) into the eye to tamponade the retina. Some minutes before this is done, the anaesthetist must discontinue administration of nitrous oxide but continue to maintain anaesthesia with air, oxygen and additional volatile agent. The use of a continuous intravenous propofol technique is a suitable alternative. If the nitrous oxide is not eliminated beforehand, it equilibrates with the tamponading gas during the operation, but at the end of the anaesthetic the nitrous oxide diffuses out and reduces the pressure in the gas bubble. The inhaled anaesthetic gas mixture at the time of injection of SF_6 or C_3F_8 should approximate as nearly as possible to normal room air. As soon as there is sufficient recovery from anaesthesia, the patient is turned to the prone position so that the bubble exerts upward pressure on the area of the retinal detachment.

Silicone oil may be used for a similar effect. These patients have to return at a later date for removal of the oil under anaesthesia. If it stays in the eye too long it can emulsify and obscure vision or block the drainage of the anterior chamber causing an increase in the IOP. Patients with intraocular tamponading gas bubbles are in danger from the bubble expanding if subsequent nitrous oxide anaesthesia is administered for purposes other than surgery on the same eye. The ophthalmologist should be consulted beforehand.

LOCAL ANAESTHESIA

Serious reactions to local orbital anaesthesia are rare but have been well documented. The need to monitor patients closely is now well recognized. Better quality of patient care, quicker turnaround times and excellent operating conditions can be achieved by the skilled anaesthetist trained in local orbital anaesthesia techniques. A detailed knowledge of the anatomy of the eye is a prerequisite (Fig. 47.2).

APPLIED ANATOMY OF THE ORBIT

The orbit is a four-sided bony pyramid with its base pointing anteriorly and its apex posteromedially. The medial walls of the right and left orbits are parallel to each other (see Figs 47.3 and 47.4). The mean distance from the inferior orbital margin to the apex is 55 mm. This has important implications when injections are made into the orbit. The deeper the injection, the narrower is the space, and the greater the chance of causing damage to the structures within. The inferotemporal quadrant is relatively avascular and is probably the safest approach for orbital injections.

Squeezing and closing of the eyelids are controlled by the zygomatic branch of the facial nerve (VII), which supplies the motor innervation to the orbicularis oculi muscle. This nerve emerges from the foramen spinosum at the base of the skull, anterior to the mastoid and behind the earlobe. It passes through the parotid gland before crossing the condyle of the mandible, then passes superficial to the zygoma and malar bone before its terminal fibres ramify to supply the deep surface of the orbicularis oculi. The facial nerve also supplies secretomotor parasympathetic fibres to the lacrimal glands, and glands of the nasal and palatine mucosa.

Movement of the globe is controlled by the six extraocular muscles. The motor nerves which control these muscles emerge from the skull through the superior orbital fissure. The common tendinous ring forms the fibrous origin of the four rectus muscles at the apex of the orbital cone. The trochlear nerve (IV) emerges through the superior orbital fissure *outside* the common tendinous ring and supplies the superior oblique muscle. All the other motor nerves to the extraocular muscles pass *inside* the common tendinous ring and are situated inside the cone. The ophthalmic division of the oculomotor nerve (III) divides into superior and inferior branches before emerging from the superior orbital fissure. The superior branch supplies the superior rectus and the levator palpebrae superioris muscles. The inferior branch divides into three to supply the medial rectus, the inferior rectus and the inferior oblique muscles. The abducent nerve (VI) emerges from the superior orbital fissure beneath the inferior branch of the oculomotor nerve to supply the lateral rectus muscle.

Sensation to the eyeball is supplied through the ophthalmic division of the trigeminal nerve (V). Just before entering the orbit, it divides into three branches: lacrimal, frontal and nasociliary. The nasociliary nerve is sensory to the entire eyeball. It emerges

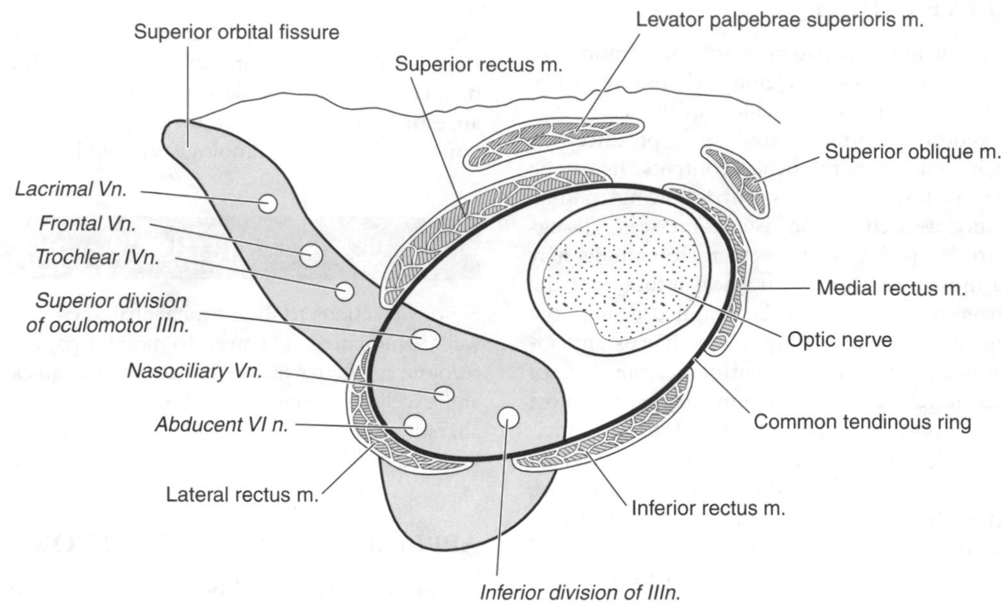

Fig. 47.2
Anatomy of the right orbit: relationship of the four rectus muscles and the apex of the cone to the orbital nerve supply.

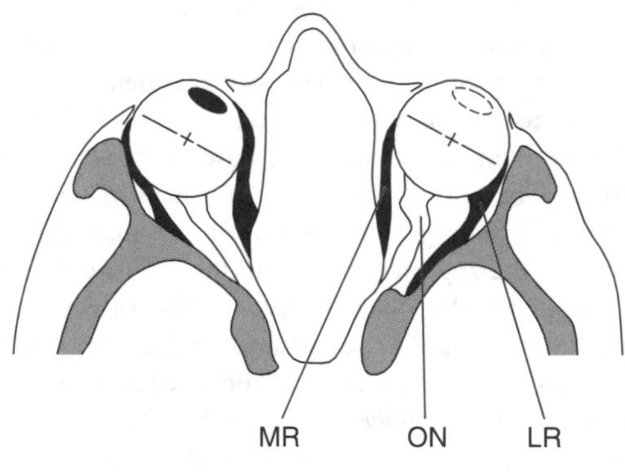

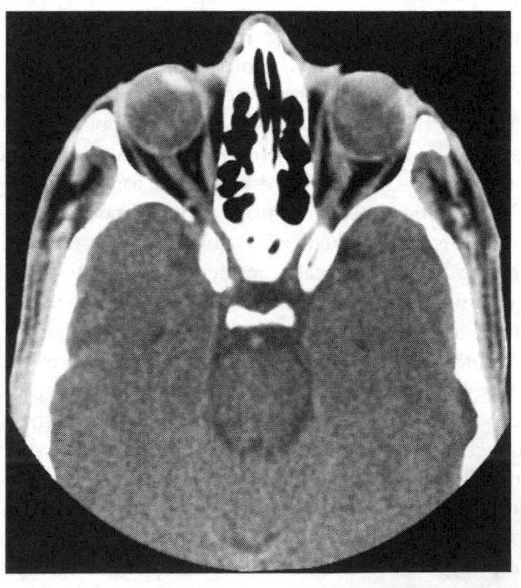

Fig. 47.3
CT scan of orbits taken in coronal view with the subject looking to the right. Note the almost parallel sides of the medial orbital walls; optic nerve movement to left; the optic nerve canal and optic nerve chiasma; the proximity of the midbrain; that the cataract has been removed from the right eye. MR, medial rectus muscle; LR, lateral rectus muscle; ON, optic nerve.

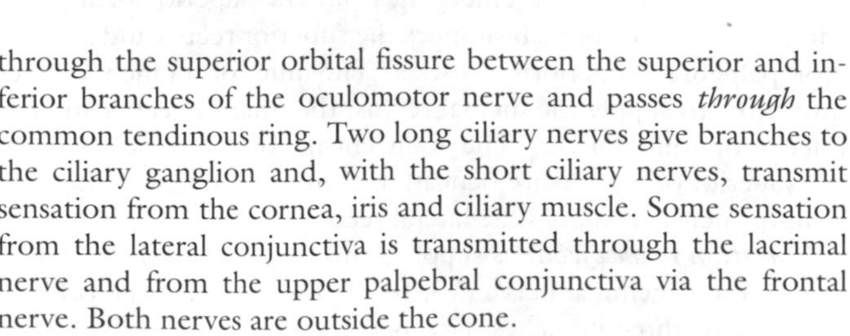
through the superior orbital fissure between the superior and inferior branches of the oculomotor nerve and passes *through* the common tendinous ring. Two long ciliary nerves give branches to the ciliary ganglion and, with the short ciliary nerves, transmit sensation from the cornea, iris and ciliary muscle. Some sensation from the lateral conjunctiva is transmitted through the lacrimal nerve and from the upper palpebral conjunctiva via the frontal nerve. Both nerves are outside the cone.

The cone is the area between the four rectus muscles and the posterior surface of the globe. The muscles arise from a fibrous ring which bridges over the superior orbital fissure. Through this common tendinous ring pass the optic nerve, the ophthalmic artery, the two divisions of the oculomotor nerve, the nasociliary nerve and the abducent nerve. The superior and inferior ophthalmic veins may also pass through the ring. Tenon's capsule or bulbar fascia is a thin membrane that envelops the eyeball from the

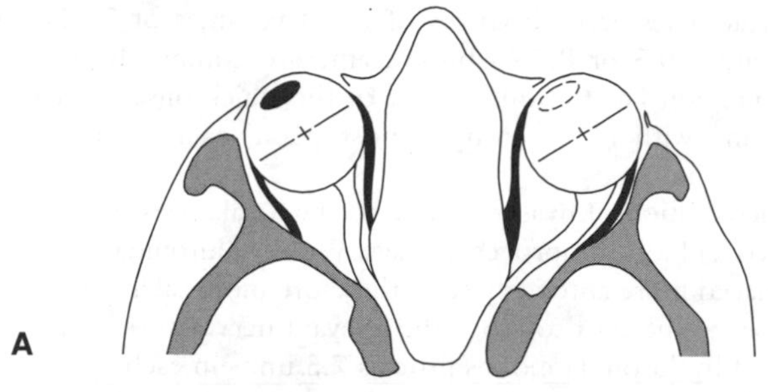

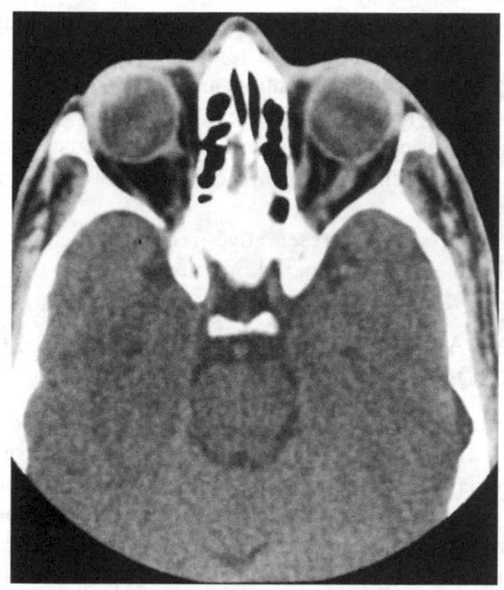

Fig. 47.4
CAT scan of the same patient as in Fig. 47.3, now looking to the left. Note the optic nerve movement to the right.

optic nerve to the sclerocorneal junction, separating it from the orbital fat and forming a socket in which it moves. The sheaths of the rectus muscles interconnect in the perimysium in a complex and variable manner and form the walls of the cone. Well-defined expansions laterally and medially form the check ligaments, and inferiorly a hammock-like expansion forms the suspensory Lockwood's ligament.

SELECTION OF PATIENTS FOR LOCAL ANAESTHESIA

Local anaesthesia is the normal choice for older people undergoing cataract surgery. This preferred type of anaesthetic should be discussed by the ophthalmologist when he first sees the patient. The young, the mentally unstable and those with physical disabilities that prevent them from lying still are usually unsuitable. Warfarin therapy is not considered an absolute contraindication to local anaesthesia provided that preoperative INR values are in the therapeutic target range. There are some patients whose chronic illness poses too severe a risk for general anaesthesia, but whose quality of life may be improved by the proposed surgery. The chance of having surgery under local anaesthesia need not be denied to this group. Operating conditions may not be ideal. Surgery of brief duration may have to proceed with the patient semi-sitting and the surgeon standing.

Premedication is not usually necessary, but if needed may be given intravenously just before the local anaesthetic block is inserted. Caution should be exercised with the dose of benzodiazepines in the elderly. There is a danger that the oversedated patient may fall asleep during the surgery, only to wake up suddenly and, in confusion, try to sit up. Very small increments of propofol (10 mg or less) may be given to anxious patients; midazolam in small doses (1 mg) or the two in combination may be very effective. If the patient is sufficiently relaxed at the time of injection of the local anaesthetic, the chances of complications such as orbital haemorrhage may be reduced.

AXIAL LENGTH AND EYE MOVEMENTS

It is good practice at the time of the preoperative visit to check the axial length of the eyeball. All patients scheduled for fitting of an intraocular lens will have an ultrasound scan and this measurement will have been recorded. There is an increased danger of global perforation in the high myope and patients with an axial length in excess of 25 mm should be treated with caution (see Figs 47.5 and 47.6). Patients scheduled for glaucoma surgery are not usually scanned preoperatively, but rarely have a long axial length. The extraocular movements and facial nerve function should be checked and recorded. It is not unknown for a patient with a pre-

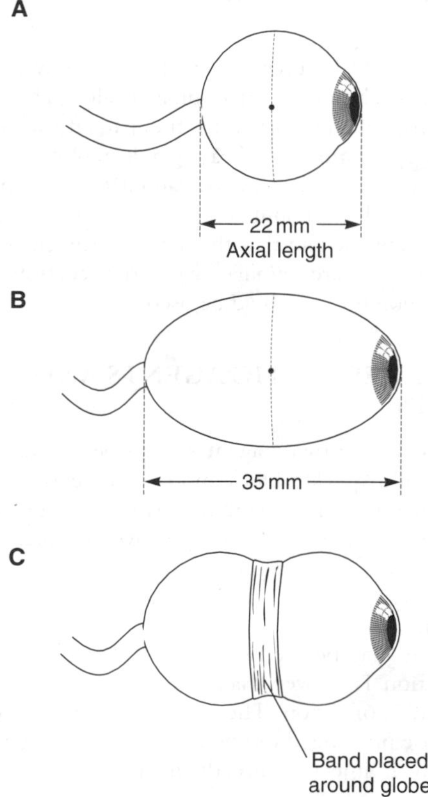

Fig. 47.5
Eyeballs of various shapes. **A.** Normal eyeball. **B.** High myope. **C.** Scleral buckle applied after surgery for retinal detachment.

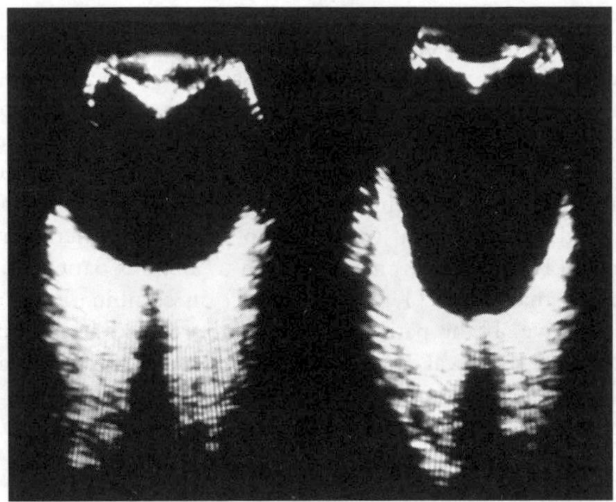

Fig. 47.6
Ultrasound scans of a normal eyeball (left) and a high myope.

existing Bell's palsy to try to implicate a subsequent facial nerve block. Myopathy of one or more of the extraocular muscles following the inadvertent injection of local anaesthetic into the muscle has been recorded. This complication is more likely to occur if the more concentrated long-acting local anaesthetic agents are used.

CONDITIONS FOR PERFORMING LOCAL EYE BLOCKS

The patient should be prepared in the same way as for general anaesthesia and should be in optimal health. The staff should establish a friendly rapport with the patient, who should be allowed to keep dentures and hearing aids in place.

A suitable vein should always by cannulated in all patients. It is essential that full cardiopulmonary resuscitation equipment is immediately available and that the medical personnel who undertake these blocks are familiar with resuscitation techniques. Appropriate monitoring should be used.

LOCAL ANAESTHETIC AGENTS AND ADJUNCTS

The ideal local anaesthetic agent should be safe and painless to inject. It should quickly block motor and sensory nerves. The duration should be long enough to perform the operation but not so long as to cause persistent postoperative diplopia.

Lidocaine 2% is safe and produces effective motor and sensory blocks, but even with the addition of epinephrine may last less than 90 min.

Bupivacaine may be used in 0.5 or 0.75% concentrations. Its onset of action is slower than that of lidocaine but it has a longer duration of action. The more concentrated solutions are liable to cause prolonged diplopia on the morning after surgery, or myopathy if injected directly into one of the extraocular muscles.

Prilocaine 2–4% has a rapid onset of action, few side-effects and a duration of action comparable with that of bupivacaine. Ropivacaine 1% has been shown to be effective.

Local anaesthetic mixtures of equal volumes of 2% lidocaine and either 0.5 or 0.75% bupivacaine are commonly used. This combination has the dual effect of the quick onset of action of lidocaine with the prolonged postoperative analgesic effect of bupivacaine.

The addition of hyaluronidase to the local anaesthetic used for intraconal blocks improves efficacy. With hyaluronidase, an injectate placed more anteriorly (and therefore more safely) in the orbit diffuses to the apex to block the relevant nerves as they emerge. A dose of hyaluronidase of as little as 7.5 units in each 1 ml of local anaesthetic is optimal. The advantage of using hyaluronidase in extraconal anaesthesia has not been clearly shown.

Vasoconstrictors such as epinephrine and felypressin may be added to the injectate. They improve the solidity and duration of the block and may reduce the incidence of haemorrhage. There is a small risk that retinal circulation may be impaired by the vasconstrictor action on the ophthalmic artery.

pH adjustment of bupivacaine and lidocaine by the addition of sodium bicarbonate allows more of the local anaesthetic solution to exist in the uncharged form, facilitating faster onset and less discomfort.

Freshly prepared, preservative-free anaesthetic mixtures are preferable to the pre-prepared mixtures.

LOCAL ANAESTHESIA TECHNIQUES FOR INTRAOCULAR SURGERY

Ophthalmic regional anaesthesia should provide conditions appropriate for the surgeon's needs and planned surgery. Topical anaesthesia with 1% tetracaine, 0.4% oxybuprocaine eyedrops or other topical local anaesthetic may be used for minor surgery to the conjunctiva if akinesia of the globe is not necessary. Some surgeons are using topical anaesthesia for phacoemulsification of cataracts. A small incision which does not require sutures is made so that the ultrasound probe may be inserted. The globe is then held in position by the probe and a hook inserted through another small incision as there is no akinesia. This is inevitably associated with some discomfort but avoids other potential complications.

EXTRACONAL, INTRACONAL OR SUB-TENON'S ANAESTHESIA

Many different techniques and ingredients may be used to achieve the aims of akinesia, analgesia and a soft eyeball. The anaesthetist must learn a suitable technique under the supervision of an experienced practitioner.

Three different methods are practised: extraconal (peribulbar), intraconal (retrobulbar) and sub-Tenon's anaesthesia.

Intraconal anaesthesia places the injectate in the fatty compartment which surrounds the nerve to be blocked, whereas extraconal techniques rely on variable diffusion across connective tissue septa. Periconal techniques were introduced more recently in the expectation that the incidence of complications would be reduced, but this expectation has not been realized. Periconal anaesthesia takes longer to achieve the same degree of akinesia and analgesia than intraconal anaesthesia. Sub-Tenon's injections involve a minor surgical procedure, and although avoiding some of the complications of the two other techniques, have their own problems.

All orbital blocks should be performed with the patient looking straight ahead in the primary gaze position. This ensures that the optic nerve is slack and out of the direct line of approaching needles (see Figs 47.7–47.9).

The gauge of needle should be the finest that can be used comfortably. In practice, this would be a 25 or 27 gauge needle, as finer needles are difficult to manipulate and larger needles may cause more pain and damage. Sharp needles are used because blunt needles are painful to insert and cause vasovagal syncope. The operator should consistently use the same volume syringe with the same gauge needle, as it is then possible to feel and judge the resistance to injection. A correctly placed injection has minimal resistance.

Following orbital injection, gentle digital pressure and massage help to disperse the anaesthetic and reduce IOP. Extraocular volume is reduced further by application of a pressure-reducing device such as Honan's balloon. It is important that this is applied for a period of at least 20 min and at a pressure of no greater than 35 mmHg. At this pressure, blood supply to the eyeball is assured. The balloon should be removed just before surgery. The low IOP facilitates surgery but the effect lasts for only a short time.

Extraconal (peribulbar) anaesthesia

These techniques rely on the placement of relatively large volumes and high concentrations of local anaesthetic outside the cone. The anaesthetic mixture takes time to diffuse through the connective tissue layers of the cone. Spread of the anaesthetic superficially ensures that the terminal fibres of the facial nerve are blocked as they enter the orbicularis oculi. Most peribulbar methods require two initial injections, each of about 5 ml of local anaesthetic. The volume injected depends on the shape of the orbit. The inferotemporal injection should be made to a depth of no more than 30 mm from the infraorbital margin using a fine 25 gauge or smaller needle. The safest sites for the injections are in the inferotemporal quadrant and just medial to the medial canthus. The inferotemporal injection can be perconjunctival or percutaneous. Topical local anaesthetic drops should be applied to the conjunctiva before injecting. The superonasal quadrant should be avoided, as injection at this site may damage the trochlear apparatus or cause haemorrhage. After the injections, a pressure-reducing device should be applied to the eye for 10 min before checking again for akinesia. Additional injections may be necessary.

Intraconal (retrobulbar) anaesthesia

Intraconal injection

The intraconal injection may be inserted (Fig. 47.8) with the patient looking straight ahead. The anaesthetist uses one index finger to palpate the groove between the eyeball and the inferolateral orbital margin and gently displaces the eyeball superiorly. A fine retrobulbar needle on a 5 ml syringe of local anaesthetic is inserted perpendicularly until the point is safely past the equator of the globe. The point is then directed superomedially and floats into the cone with minimal resistance. After aspiration, 2–4 ml of local anaesthetic are injected very slowly. The syringe and needle are then withdrawn in the reverse direction to which they were

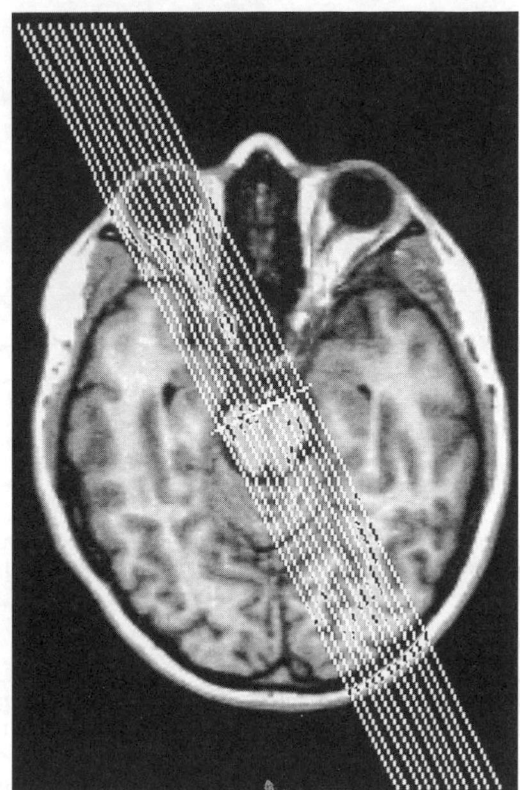

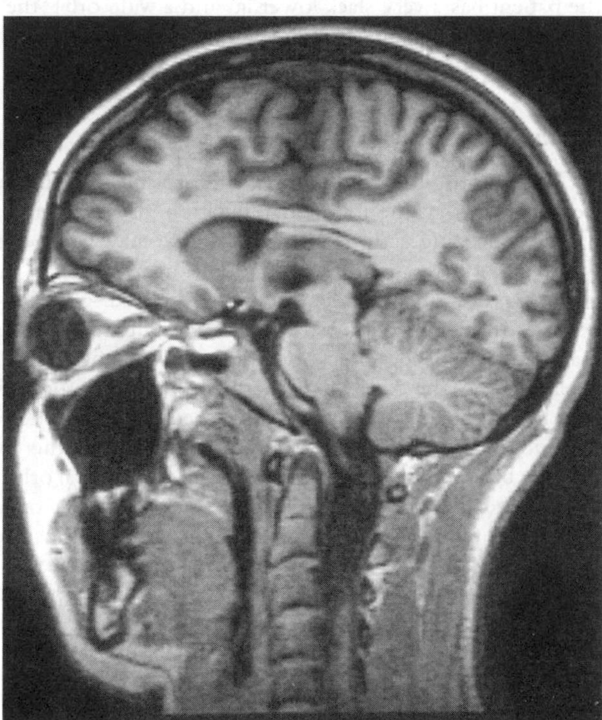

Fig. 47.7
MRI scan of the left orbit. **A.** Note the oblique angle of scan needed to visualize the optic nerve. **B.** Note the slackness of the optic nerve with the eyeball in the neutral gaze position.

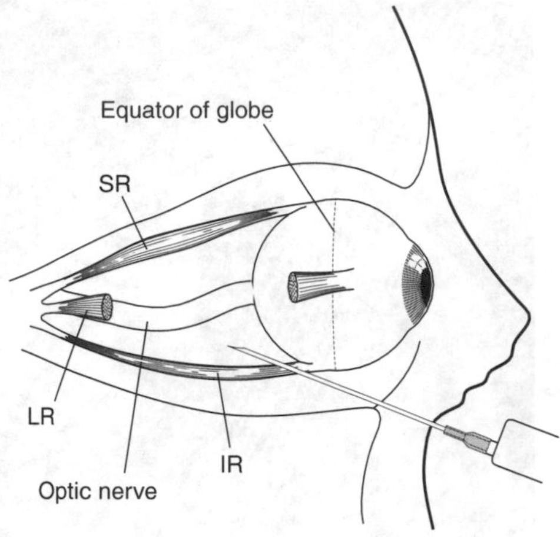

Fig. 47.8
Intraconal injection is placed between the inferior border of the lateral rectus and the inferior rectus. SR, superior rectus; LR, lateral rectus; IR, inferior rectus.

inserted. The last 1–3 ml of local anaesthetic are injected just under the orbicularis oculi muscle, where it spreads to block the terminal fibres of the facial nerve and enhance the facial nerve block. A single-shot local anaesthetic with intraconal and sub-orbicularis injection is effective in patients who do not have marked blepharospasm. With marked blepharospasm, a separate facial nerve block may be needed first (see below). Alternatively, if the patient has a very slack lower lid and a wide orbit, the infero-temporal intraconal injection may be made perconjunctivally after prior application of topical anaesthesia.

Facial nerve block

By blocking the facial nerve first, the orbicularis oculi muscle is weakened so that the intraconal injection may be inserted without its squeezing action. The facial nerve may be blocked anywhere along its course to the orbit and many different methods have been described. Nadbath described blocking the nerve as it emerges from the stylomastoid foramen, but this technique has many unwanted side-effects. O'Brien blocked the facial nerve as it passed over the condyle of the mandible. Atkinson infiltrated over the zygoma, and Van Lint infiltrated the orbit. The simplest method is to use the most prominent part of the zygoma, midway between the tragus of the ear and the lateral orbital margin, as the landmark. A 25 gauge 30 mm needle on a 5 ml syringe containing the local anaesthetic mixture is inserted perpendicularly down to the zygoma, withdrawn from the periosteum and aspirated. A volume of 3–5 ml is injected lateral to the lateral orbital margin. Gentle massage to the wheal that is raised helps to spread the local anaesthetic and ensures that there is no bleeding.

Sub-Tenon's anaesthesia

This procedure requires a certain amount of surgical dexterity and a cooperative patient. Its popularity with anaesthetists has increased. Topical anaesthetic drops are applied to the conjunctiva

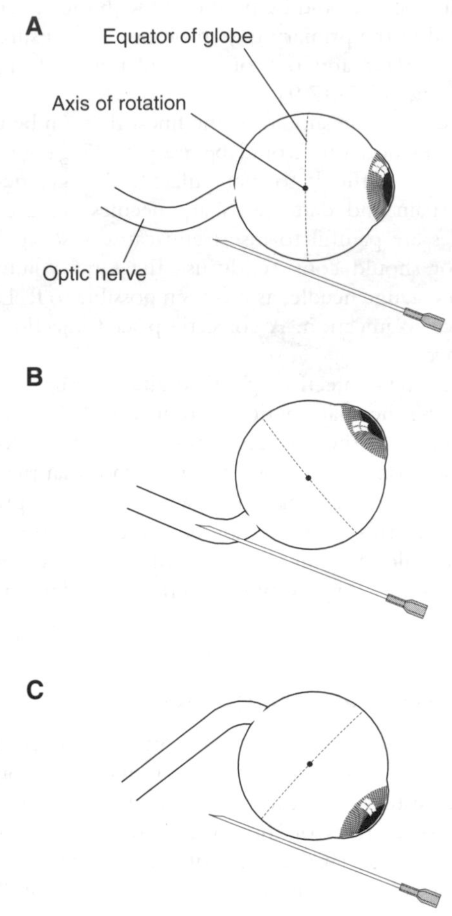

Fig. 47.9
Movements of the optic nerve in relation to eyeball movement when the needle is introduced into the cone from the inferotemporal quadrant. **A**. Primary gaze. **B**. Upwards and inwards. **C**. Downwards and outwards.

and a speculum inserted. Using forceps and a blunt pointed pair of scissors, a small incision is made in the infero-medical conjunctiva. A special curved, blunt pointed cannula is then passed into the sub-Tenon's space and 1–3ml of anaesthetic are introduced. This method reduces the risk of CNS spread, optic nerve damage and global puncture but may be more likely to cause superficial haemorrhage. Akinesia is often poor.

COMPLICATIONS OF LOCAL ANAESTHESIA

Haemorrhage

Haemorrhage is a serious complication of both intraconal and extraconal anaesthesia and occurs with a frequency of between 0.1 and 3%. It is more likely to occur in patients who have acquired vascular disease. Despite this, eventual visual outcome after surgery is not significantly worse than in patients who have uncomplicated anaesthesia. The haemorrhage may be either venous or arterial in origin and may be concealed or revealed. Extravasation of blood into the periorbital tissues increases the tissue volume and pressure. This is transmitted to the globe, raising the intraocular tension and creating difficult and dangerous conditions for intraocular surgery (see Fig. 47.10).

Venous haemorrhage usually presents as markedly bloodstained chemosis and raised IOP. It may be possible to reduce the IOP by digital massage and the cautious application of an IOP-reducing device to such an extent that surgery can proceed safely. Before the decision is made to proceed with surgery or postpone it for a few days, it is advisable to measure and record IOP.

Arterial haemorrhage is a more serious complication and urgent measures must be taken to stop the haemorrhage and reduce the seriously elevated IOP. Firm digital pressure usually stops the bleeding and, when it has been arrested, consideration must be given to reducing the IOP so that the blood supply to the retina is not jeopardized. Lateral canthotomy, intravenous acetazolamide, intravenous mannitol or even paracentesis may need to be considered in consultation with the ophthalmologist.

Prevention of haemorrhage

Patients with hypertension are more likely to bleed and optimal control of arterial pressure should be achieved before surgery is attempted. The fewer injections that are made into the orbit, the less is the chance of damaging a blood vessel. Cutting and slicing movements at the needle tip should be avoided. Fine needles are less traumatic than thicker ones. Deep intraorbital injections are more likely to cause haemorrhage than are shallow injections. The inferotemporal quadrant has fewer blood vessels and is less hazardous. Blunt Atkinson-type needles have been recommended but are painful to insert, cause vasovagal syncope and may still damage blood vessels. A technique of producing, by slow injection, a liquid stilette of local anaesthetic in front of the advancing needle also has its advocates. The addition of epinephrine to the injectate may reduce the incidence of haemorrhage. It is advisable to apply firm digital pressure to the orbit as soon as the needle is withdrawn after any intraorbital injection, as this reduces any tendency to ooze.

Central spread

Mechanism

The cerebral dura mater provides a tubular sheath for the optic nerve as it passes through the optic foramen. This sheath fuses to the epineurium of the optic nerve and is continuous with the sclera, providing a potential conduit for local anaesthetic to pass subdurally to the brain. Central spread occurs if the needle tip has perforated the optic nerve sheath and injection is made. Even a tiny volume injected under the optic nerve sheath may pass to the central nervous system and/or cross the optic chiasma to the opposite eye and may cause life-threatening sequelae. The time of onset of symptoms is variable, but any major sequelae develop usually in the first 15 min after the injection. It is advisable that the patient's face is not covered up on the operating table for at least this interval after the block has been inserted.

Another mechanism for central spread may occur on rare occasions if an orbital artery is cannulated by the needle tip. The local anaesthetic is injected in a retrograde fashion up the artery until it meets a branch, where it can then flow in a cephalad direction. The onset of central nervous system toxicity is almost instantaneous if this mechanism is invoked; in addition, orbital haemorrhage can be expected.

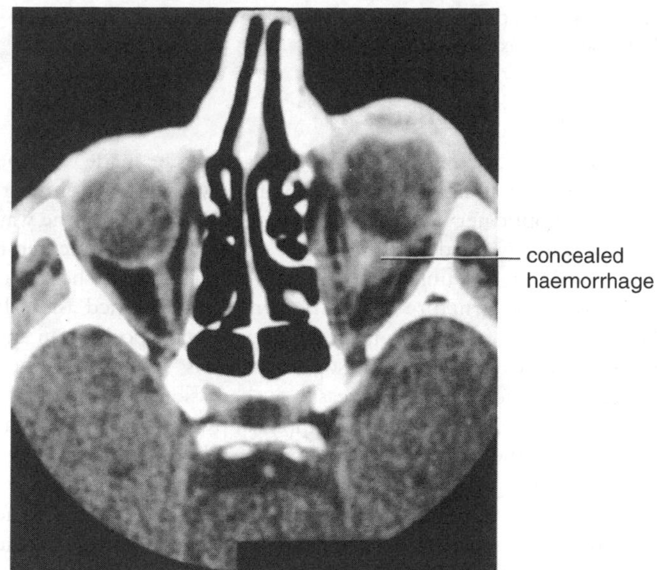

Fig. 47.10
CT scan taken in coronal section of a patient following an intraconal haemorrhage. Note the marked proptosis of the right eye and the confined space occupied by the haemorrhage. This was a concealed haemorrhage as, despite elevated intraocular pressure and proptosis, no signs of bleeding or bruising were evident until the next day.

Signs and symptoms of central spread

The symptomatology of central spread is varied and depends upon which part of the central nervous system is affected by the local anaesthetic. As a result of the anatomical proximity of the optic nerve to the midbrain (see Fig. 47.3) it is usual for this area to be involved. A range of different signs and symptoms has been described, involving the cardiovascular and respiratory systems, temperature regulation, vomiting, temporary hemiplegia, aphasia and generalized convulsions. Palsy of the contralateral oculomotor and trochlear nerves with amaurosis (loss of vision) is pathognomonic of central nervous system spread and should be sought in any patient whose response to questions following block are not as crisp as they were beforehand.

Treatment of central spread

The treatment is symptomatic throughout the duration of effect of the local anaesthetic drug. With longer-acting local anaesthetic agents, treatment may be required for 60–90 min. The patient must be monitored intensively. Bradycardia requires treatment with an anticholinergic drug. Asystole has been reported rarely, but if it occurs, intravenous epinephrine and sustained cardiac massage are required. Respiratory depression or apnoea necessitates ventilatory support and administration of supplementary oxygen. Convulsions are treated conveniently with intravenous sodium thiopental and conversion to general anaesthesia. When vital signs are stable, it may be feasible to continue with the proposed surgery under general anaesthesia in the knowledge that the patient needs continuing intensive support until the local anaesthetic action has worn off.

Prevention of central spread

Intraconal or extraconal injections should always be made with the patient looking straight ahead in the primary gaze position (Fig. 47.9). The optic nerve is then slack (Fig 47.8) and out of the way of the advancing needle. If the needle encounters the optic nerve in this position, it is unlikely to damage or perforate its sheath, as slackness in the structure allows the nerve to be pushed aside. If the eyeball is directed away from the primary gaze position in any other extreme direction, the optic nerve is stretched. When stretched, the nerve cannot be easily pushed aside. The most dangerous position is when the patient looks upwards and inwards, as this presents the stretched nerve to a needle directed from the inferotemporal quadrant. As in the prevention of haemorrhage, injections should not be made too deeply into the orbit where the optic nerve is tethered to its sheaths as it emerges through the optic foramen. It is good practice to withdraw the needle by 1 mm from its maximum depth before injection is made. If the tip had been resting against the optic nerve sheath, this manoeuvre withdraws the tip to a safer position.

Puncture of the eyeball

Global puncture is a serious complication of local anaesthesia for eye surgery. It has been reported following both intraconal and extraconal injections and even following local anaesthesia for more minor procedures such as eyelid surgery. With appropriate care, it should be a very rare complication. The sclera is a tough structure and in most cases is not perforated easily.

Puncture of the eyeball is most likely to occur in patients with high myopia, previous retinal banding, posterior staphyloma or a deep sunken eye with a narrow orbit (Fig. 47.5).

Not all eyeballs are the same length and not all orbits are the same shape. In most patients who present for cataract surgery, an ultrasound measure is made of the axial length of the eyeball to calculate the power of the intraocular lens. Normal eyeballs have an axial length of 20–24 mm. High myopes have much longer axial lengths of 25–35 mm and extreme caution should be exercised in these patients. The axial length in patients for glaucoma surgery is not usually measured.

Global puncture is often a double puncture of the posterior segment of the eyeball; the tip of the needle is in the orbit at the time of injection and the local anaesthetic block may be good. Puncture is usually recognized at the time of surgery and presents as an exceptionally soft eye. In cataract surgery, if the block is good, the surgeon should be encouraged to proceed with the lensectomy but to stitch up the eye with twice as many sutures as normal. Without lensectomy, it may not be possible to observe the damage to the posterior segment of the eye. It can be expected that the needle track through the vitreous will form a band of scar tissue. If this is not excised, it contracts and detaches the retina, sometimes causing sudden total blindness in the affected eye.

Optic nerve damage

Fortunately, this is a rare complication which results usually from obstruction of the central retinal artery. This artery is the first and smallest branch of the ophthalmic artery, arising from that vessel as it lies below the optic nerve. It runs for a short distance within the dural sheath of the optic nerve and about 35 mm from the orbital margin, pierces the nerve and runs forward in the centre of the nerve to the retina. Damage to the artery may cause bleeding into the confined space of the optic nerve sheath, compressing and obstructing blood flow. If the complication is recognized soon enough, it may be possible to perform surgical decompression of the optic nerve.

Myopathy of the extraocular muscles

The inadvertent injection of a long-acting local anaesthetic into any extraocular muscle body may result in prolonged weakness of the muscle. An injection site some distance away from these muscles should be selected.

Vasovagal syncope

This is more likely to occur in young and anxious patients when eye blocks are administered. Painful injection with a blunt Atkinson needle may cause this response. It is important that a vein is cannulated before any block is given. Treatment is symptomatic and should include administration of oxygen, intravenous injection of an anticholinergic agent and appropriate positioning. Differentiation from central spread should be made by testing vision and extraocular movements in the opposite eye.

EXTRAOCULAR PROCEDURES

ANAESTHESIA FOR STRABISMUS SURGERY

The commonest procedure in paediatric ophthalmic surgery is correction of squint. The eye should be immobile with absent muscle tone. The use of a non-depolarizing muscle relaxant may be preferred as this prevents variation in muscle tone which may occur with an imbalance between the depth of anaesthesia and the applied surgical stimulus. Succinylcholine must be avoided. In patients who have had previous strabismus surgery or orbital trauma, the surgeon may need to differentiate between paretic and restricted eye movement by performing a forced duction test. Absence of muscle tone is necessary for this test to be performed accurately. If the surgeon is repairing the strabismus with an adjustable suture technique, it is also important that all traces of muscle relaxant have been eliminated by the time the suture is adjusted.

Squint and ptosis are presenting signs of the progressive external ophthalmoplegia syndrome (PEO). Patients with this syndrome may have marked cardiac and respiratory decompensation and pose a significant hazard for anaesthesia. Preoperative pulmonary function testing is advisable. Myasthenia gravis may also present with ptosis and strabismus.

Botulinum toxin is occasionally administered in the treatment of strabismus and blepharospasm. Ketamine is a suitable anaesthetic for children scheduled to undergo this procedure, as it does not reduce muscle power; the surgeon tests muscle power intraoperatively.

There is a rare association between malignant hyperthermia and strabismus.

Oculocardiac reflex

This reflex may be triggered by extraorbital muscle traction, causing severe bradycardia or even cardiac arrest. It is more pronounced in young people. Some anaesthetists give prophylactic atropine or glycopyrrolate at induction. When it occurs, the surgical stimulus must be suspended until the heart rate has recovered, and if necessary anticholinergic drugs given. A heart rate monitor which the surgeon can hear is useful.

Postoperative nausea and vomiting

The incidence of postoperative nausea and vomiting following squint is high. Various antiemetic drugs and techniques are commonly used. As most of these operations are carried out as a day surgery procedure under general anaesthesia, it is important to avoid preparations which cause excessive sedation.

EXAMINATION UNDER ANAESTHESIA

Children may require repeated examinations under anaesthesia (EUAs). If the purpose of the EUA is to measure IOP, as may be the case in neonates with congenital glaucoma, the method of anaesthesia must be discussed with the surgeon. Inhalation anaesthesia by mask is often satisfactory, but the surgeon may wish to measure IOP while the patient is still lightly anaesthetized, before IOP is reduced by the effects of anaesthetic drugs. Painless preoperative intravenous cannulation using EMLA local anaesthetic cream has made i.v. induction feasible for most children. The use of the laryngeal mask is ideal. Ketamine does not lower the IOP, but it is a long-acting anaesthetic and may cause hallucinations and nightmares postoperatively; it should be reserved for special cases.

DACROCYSTORHINOSTOMY (DCR)

Open DCR is carried out usually under general anaesthesia because the operation is frequently bilateral and may be complicated by haemorrhage. It is necessary to use a tracheal tube and throat pack because blood may trickle down the nasopharynx. The nostril(s) should be packed with cocaine paste or another suitable vasoconstrictor before operation. The operation site may be infiltrated with epinephrine by the surgeon and caution is necessary with the use of halothane.

The use of lasers for DCR has largely eliminated haemorrhage and local anaesthesia is preferable if open surgery is not planned.

DRUG INTERACTIONS

Patients with eye disease often use systemic or topical medications which may pose potential problems for the anaesthetist. Systemic absorption of potent eyedrops is reduced if the lacrimal puncta are occluded digitally while the drops are being inserted.

Cyclopentolate is an antimuscarinic with an action of up to 24 h; 1% drops are used to dilate the pupil and paralyse the ciliary muscle before surgery. Excessive systemic absorption causes toxic effects similar to those associated with an overdose of atropine. The young and the very old are particularly susceptible.

Phenylephrine is a direct-acting α-adrenergic stimulant and has weak β-effects; 2.5% or 10% drops are used to dilate the pupil. Systemic effects may cause an increase in myocardial irritability and hypertension. Dangerous interactions with monoamine oxidase inhibitors may occur.

Epinephrine is used intraoperatively in a dilute solution by the surgeon to reduce excessive bleeding. Systemic absorption may be significant. Caution is necessary with halothane.

Timolol or other β-blocking agents are used topically to treat glaucoma. Systemic absorption may be significant. Asthma and chronic obstructive airways disease may be exacerbated. Precautions should be observed as for systemic β-adrenergic blocking drugs.

Ecothiopate iodide (phospholine iodide) is a potent anticholinesterase and is used rarely in the treatment of glaucoma. It depletes pseudocholinesterase and thus prolongs the action of succinylcholine.

Botulinum toxin A is an effective treatment in a variety of neuromuscular conditions including strabismus. It causes a decrease in skeletal muscle power by binding irreversibly to receptor sites on the cholinergic nerve terminal. Function does not return until new motor end-plates have formed. When injected locally into the extraocular muscle(s), the toxin binds rapidly and firmly to the tissue; in the doses used normally, it should not cause systemic side-effects.

Mannitol is an osmotic diuretic which reduces the volume of the vitreous humour. Infusions in doses of up to 1.5 g kg^{-1} are given before surgery over a period of 30–45 min. There is an initial increase in circulating blood volume followed by a diuresis and decrease in blood volume. When combined with the induction of general anaesthesia, haemodynamic instability may occur. Particular caution must be exercised in patients with cardiovascular disease. A urinary catheter should be inserted preoperatively if patients are to receive mannitol in this way.

Acetazolamide, a carbonic anhydrase inhibitor, is used in the medical treatment of glaucoma. Its main actions are to reduce the production of aqueous humour and to facilitate drainage. It is of questionable value during surgery because it results in increased intrachoroidal vascular volume. Congenital glaucoma is treated with acetazolamide and repeated surgery. Metabolic acidosis may be a serious consequence of this treatment and the neonate presenting for anaesthesia for glaucoma surgery must be treated with special care. Any respiratory depression caused by sedatives, opioids or anaesthesia reduces the compensatory respiratory alkalosis. It may be advisable to perform blood gas analysis before anaesthesia.

FURTHER READING

Barry Smith G, Hamilton R C, Carr C A 1996 Ophthalmic anaesthesia: a practical handbook, 2nd edn. Arnold, London

Todd J G 1994 Anaesthesia for ophthalmic surgery. In: Nimmo W S, Rowbotham D J, Smith G (eds) Anaesthesia, 2nd edn. Blackwell Scientific Publications, London

48 Anaesthesia for radiology and radiotherapy

General anaesthesia outside the operating theatre may be challenging for the anaesthetist, as specialized environments pose unique problems. The anaesthetist must attempt to provide a service with standards, safety and comfort for patients that are equal to those in the main operating department.

GENERAL CONSIDERATIONS AND PRINCIPLES

In many hospitals, radiology and radiotherapy departments have not been designed with anaesthetic requirements in mind. Anaesthetic apparatus often competes for space with bulky equipment and, in general, conditions are less than optimal. For example:

- Monitoring capabilities and anaesthetic equipment should be of a standard similar to that used in the operating department. In reality, such equipment may not be readily available and the equipment used is often the oldest in the hospital. The anaesthetist who is unfamiliar with the environment should spend time becoming accustomed to the layout and equipment. Access to the patient may be difficult and this places more reliance on sophisticated monitors. Clinical observation may be limited by poor lighting.
- Preparation of the patient may be inadequate because the patient comes from a ward in which staff are unfamiliar with preoperative protocols.
- Anaesthetic assistance and maintenance of anaesthetic equipment may be less than ideal. Consequently, the anaesthetist must be particularly vigilant in checking the anaesthetic machine, especially as it may be disconnected and moved when not in use. Empty gas cylinders need to be replaced in older suites without piped gases and also the anaesthetist must ensure the presence of drugs, spare laryngoscope and batteries, suction and other routine equipment.
- Communication between radiologist, radiotherapist and the anaesthetist may be poor. This may lead to failure in recognizing the other's requirements.
- Recovery facilities are often non-existent. The anaesthetists may have to recover their own patients in the suite. Consequently, they must be familiar with the location of recovery equipment, including suction, supplementary oxygen and resuscitation equipment. Alternatively, patients may be transferred to the main hospital recovery area. This requires the use of routine transfer equipment such as monitoring and oxygen.

ANAESTHESIA FOR RADIOLOGICAL PROCEDURES

In most hospitals, the anaesthetic department is called upon to anaesthetize patients for diagnostic and therapeutic radiological procedures. These procedures include angiography, computed tomography (CT) scanning and magnetic resonance imaging (MRI). The major requirement of all these imaging techniques is that the patient remains almost motionless. Thus, anaesthesia may be necessary when these investigations are performed in children, the critically ill or the uncooperative patient. The presence of pain or lengthy procedures may also be an indication for anaesthesia.

Radiological studies may require administration of conscious sedation. This is where medication, often given by a non-anaesthetist, is used to alter perceptions of painful and anxiety-provoking stimuli while maintaining protective airway responses and the ability to respond appropriately to verbal command. Medical personnel responsible for the sedation should be familiar with the effects of the medication and skilled in resuscitation. There should be easy access to a resuscitation kit. A single operator for the radiological procedure and the administration of sedation is at risk of distraction and therefore of missing side-effects. Ideally, different individuals should be responsible for each of these tasks. Guidelines for prescribing, evaluating and monitoring sedation should be readily available.

Intravascular contrast agents are used routinely during angiographic and other radiological investigations. The anaesthetist must always be aware of the risk of adverse reaction to contrast dyes. Over recent years, low-osmolarity contrast media have been introduced. These cause less pain and have fewer toxic effects than the older contrast agents, but are more expensive. Factors contributing to the development of adverse reactions include speed of injection and type and dose of contrast used.

Coronary and cerebral angiography are associated with a high risk of reaction. Other major risk factors are patients with allergies, asthma, extremes of age (under 1 and over 60 years), cardiovascular disease and a history of previous contrast medium reaction. Fatal reactions are rare, occurring in about 1 in 100 000 procedures. Nausea and vomiting are common (consider prophylactic antiemetic), which may progress to urticaria, hypotension and bronchospasm. Adequate hydration is important, as patients undergoing contrast dye procedures usually have an induced osmotic diuresis which can exacerbate pre-existing renal dysfunction. A urinary catheter may be useful for patients undergoing long procedures.

Treatment of allergic reactions depends on the severity of the reaction. This usually consists of general supportive methods such as fluids, oxygen and careful monitoring. Drugs such as epinephrine, atropine, steroids and antihistamines should be readily available.

Healthcare workers are exposed to X-rays in the radiology and imaging suites. The greatest source is usually from fluoroscopy and digital subtraction angiography. Ionizing radiation from a CT scanner is relatively low because the X-rays are highly focused. Radiation intensity and exposure decrease with the square of the distance from the emitting source. The recommended distance is 1–2 m. This precaution, together with lead aprons and thyroid shields, keep exposure to a safe level.

CT SCANNING

General principles

A CT scan provides a series of tomographic axial 'slices' of the body. It is used most frequently for intracranial imaging and for studies of the thorax and abdomen. Each image is produced by computer integration of the differences in the radiation absorption coefficients between different normal tissues and between normal and abnormal tissues. The image of the structure under investigation is generated by a cathode ray tube and the brightness of each area is proportional to the absorption value.

One rotation of the gantry produces an axial slice or 'cut'. A series of cuts is made, usually at intervals of 7 mm, but this may be larger or smaller depending on the diagnostic information sought. The first-generation scanners took 4.5 min per cut, but the newest scanners take only 2–4 s.

Anaesthetic management

CT is non-invasive and painless, requiring neither sedation nor anaesthesia for most adult patients. However, patients who cannot cooperate (most frequently paediatric and head trauma patients) may need general anaesthesia to prevent movement, which degrades the image. Anaesthetists may also be asked to assist in the supervision of critically ill patients from the ITU in the CT scan room.

General anaesthesia is preferable to sedation when there are potential airway problems or when control of intracranial pressure (ICP) is critical. As the patient's head is inaccessible during the CT scan, the airway needs to be secured. In the majority of situations, tracheal intubation is more appropriate than using a laryngeal mask airway (e.g. full stomach). The scan itself requires only that the patient remains motionless and tolerates the tracheal tube. If ICP is high, controlled ventilation is essential to induce hypocapnia and decrease cerebral blood flow.

A propofol/thiopental, nitrous oxide, oxygen, volatile and relaxant technique with tracheal intubation and mild hyperventilation is acceptable. Anaesthetic complications include kinking of the tracheal tube (especially during extreme degrees of head flexion required for examination of the posterior fossa; positioning and movement of the gantry during the procedure may cause kinking or disconnection of the anaesthetic circuit), hypothermia in paediatric patients and acute brain stem compression if the head is flexed excessively in the presence of an infratentorial tumour.

If during the scan the anaesthetist is observing the patient from inside the control room, it is imperative that alarms/monitors have visual signals that can be easily seen.

Stereotactic-guided surgery is possible using CT scanners. Most procedures involve aspiration or biopsy of intracranial masses. This procedure is used because it minimizes injury to adjacent structures. Pins are used to hold a radiolucent frame around the head to ensure a motionless field inside the scanner. This allows precise localization. Access to the patient and airway with the frame attached inside the scanner is difficult.

MAGNETIC RESONANCE IMAGING

General principles

Magnetic resonance imaging (MRI) is an imaging modality that does not use ionizing radiation, but depends on magnetic fields and radiofrequency pulses for the production of its images. The imaging capabilities of MRI are superior to those of CT for examining intracranial, spinal and soft tissue lesions. MRI can differentiate clearly between white and grey matter in the brain, thus making possible the in vivo diagnosis of demyelination. It can display images in the sagittal, coronal or transverse planes and, unlike the CT scanner, is capable of detecting disease in the posterior fossa. It has the advantage that no ionizing radiation is produced.

An MRI imaging system requires a large magnet in the form of a tube which is capable of accepting the entire length of the human body. A radiofrequency transmitter coil is incorporated in the tube which surrounds the patient; the coil also acts as a receiver to detect the energy waves from which the image is constructed. In the presence of the magnetic field, protons in the body align with the magnetic field in the longitudinal axis of the patient. Additional perpendicular magnetic pulses are applied by the radiofrequency coil; these cause the protons to rotate into the transverse plane. When the pulse is discontinued, the nuclei relax back to their original orientation and emit energy waves which are detected by the coil. The magnet is over 2 m in length and weighs approximately 500 kg. The magnetic field is constantly applied even in the absence of a patient. It can take several days to establish the magnetic field if removed and this is only done in an emergency.

Anaesthetic management

The indications for general anaesthesia during MRI are similar to those for CT. In addition, the scanner is very noisy and the patient lies on a long thin table in a dark confined space within the tube. This can cause claustrophobia or anxiety-related problems which may require sedation or anaesthesia.

There are other unique problems presented by MRI. These include relative inaccessibility of the patient and the magnetic properties of the equipment. The body cylinder of the scanner surrounds the patient totally; manual control of the airway is impossible and tracheal intubation or laryngeal mask airway is essential. The patient may be observed from both ends of the tunnel and may be extracted quickly if necessary. As there is no hazard from ionizing radiation, the anaesthetist may approach the patient in safety.

The magnetic effects of MRI impose some restrictions on the selection of anaesthetic equipment. Any ferromagnetic object distorts the magnetic field sufficiently to degrade the image. It is also likely to be propelled towards the scanner and may cause a significant accident if it makes contact with the patient or staff. Of relevance to anaesthetists is any equipment that needs to be used in the

MRI room. The layout of the MRI room/suite determines if the majority of equipment needs to be inside the room and therefore MRI-compatible, or outside the room with long MRI-compatible circuits, leads and tubing to the patient. Consideration needs to be given to intravenous fluid stands, oxygen and nitrous oxide cylinders (use special aluminium cylinders), anaesthetic machine, ventilators, infusion pumps and monitoring equipment including stethoscopes and nerve stimulators. Although laryngoscopes are non-magnetic, standard batteries need to be replaced with non-magnetic lithium batteries. Laryngeal mask airways without metal springs in the pilot tube valve should be available.

Technical problems with monitors include interference with imaging signals resulting in distorted MRI pictures and radiofrequency signals from the scanner inducing currents in the monitor which may give unreliable monitor readings. Special MRI-compatible monitors are available or unshielded ferromagnetic monitors can be kept just outside the MRI room and used with long shielded or non-ferromagnetic cables (e.g. the pulse oximeter lead may be a fibreoptic cable). Heart rate and ventilatory rate may be monitored with an oesophageal stethoscope, although the sounds may be obscured by the noise of the equipment. If the patient is allowed to breathe spontaneously, movement of the reservoir bag may be used as an index of ventilation. A non-invasive automated arterial pressure monitor, in which metallic tubing connectors are replaced by nylon connectors, is useful. Distortion of the ECG may occur, which interferes with ischaemia monitoring. This needs to be considered in patients with active ischaemic heart disease.

Anaesthesia may be induced outside the MRI room where it is safe to use ferromagnetic equipment and there may be relatively more space around the patient for ease of anaesthetic administration. Most patients benefit from the use of short-acting drugs associated with rapid recovery and minimal side-effects.

Bank cards, credit cards and other belongings containing electromagnetic strips become demagnetized within the vicinity of the scanner. Personal computers, pagers and calculators may also be damaged.

MRI-guided surgery is a new, highly specialized form of surgery that may continue to be developed. It offers surgeons radiological images of the tissues immediately beyond their operative field. This is made possible by the development of an open configuration scanner as opposed to the traditional closed tubular scanner. The open configuration consists of upright paired coils between which the medical staff can access the patient. The absence of ionizing radiation places less restriction on the duration of staff presence. The anaesthetic considerations are similar to those of the traditional MRI scanner except that here the anaesthetist and all the related equipment are required to be in the vicinity of the scanner and therefore compatible with a magnetic field. Surgery that has been performed in this environment includes endoscopic sinus surgery.

Hazards

The static magnetic field may prove dangerous in patients with implanted ferromagnetic devices. Patients fitted with a demand cardiac pacemaker should not be exposed to MRI because induced electrical currents may be mistaken for natural electrical activity of the heart and may inhibit pacemaker output. Metallic implants, e.g. intracranial vascular clips, may be dislodged from blood vessels. Patients with large metal implants should be monitored for implant heating. Heating of the pulse oximeter probe may result in burns.

DIAGNOSTIC AND INTERVENTIONAL ANGIOGRAPHY

General principles

Direct arteriography using percutaneous arterial catheters is used widely for the diagnosis of vascular lesions. Catheters are usually inserted by the Seldinger technique via the femoral artery in the groin. Injection of contrast medium gives images that are viewed by conventional cut film radiography or by digital subtraction angiography. New non-invasive angiographic techniques used with CT or MRI have reduced the need for direct arteriography for the diagnosis of vascular lesions. CT may demonstrate major vascular lesions such as thoracic or abdominal aneurysms. The advent of spiral and double helical CT scanners allows whole vascular territories to be mapped within 30 s and produce superior images, including three-dimensional pictures. MRI is sensitive to the detection of flow and, together with more sophisticated scanning and data collection techniques, its use for assessment of vascular structures is increasing.

Anaesthetic management

Most angiographic procedures may be carried out under local anaesthesia or with sedation if necessary during more complex investigation. Sedation to augment local anaesthesia must be avoided in the presence of intracranial hypertension, as the increased $P_{a}CO_2$ leads to vasodilatation and a further increase in ICP; in addition, vasodilatation results in poor-quality angiography. General anaesthesia is usually necessary for children and may be required for nervous patients or those unable to co-operate. The drawbacks of general anaesthesia include prolonging the time taken for the investigation and increasing the cost and risks associated with anaesthesia. Moreover, the patient is unable to react to misplaced injections and untoward reactions. A conscious patient would describe symptoms, allowing the procedure to be stopped immediately. Interventional radiological procedures are more likely to require sedation or general anaesthesia because of patient discomfort and longer duration. General anaesthesia for angiography is more comfortable for the patient and ensures complete immobility during X-ray exposures.

Adequate hydration is essential for these patients, as they are often fasted and the contrast medium causes an osmotic diuresis. All i.v. cannulae and monitor leads may require extensions to enable the anaesthetist to remain an acceptable distance from the patient to minimize exposure. This also allows the anaesthetist to remain outside the range of movement of the imaging machine.

Complications of angiography

- *Local* – haematoma and haemorrhage, vessel wall dissection, thrombosis, perivascular contrast injection, adjacent nerve damage, loss and knotting of guide wire and catheters.
- *General* – contrast reactions of varying severity, emboli from catheter clots, cholesterol and air, septicaemia and vagal inhibition.

Cerebral angiography

This may be performed to demonstrate tumours, arteriovenous malformations, aneurysms, subarachnoid haemorrhage and cerebrovascular disease. The risk of complications is generally increased in the elderly and those with pre-existing vascular disease, diabetes, stroke and transient ischaemic attacks. Many of these patients have intracranial hypertension. Therefore, control of arterial pressure and carbon dioxide tension is essential if these patients require general anaesthesia. Obtunding the pressor response to intubation and careful positioning to avoid increasing central venous pressure are necessary to prevent elevation of intracranial pressure. A relaxant/IPPV technique with moderate hyperventilation to induce hypocapnia (P_aCO_2 = 4.0–4.5 kPa) is often used. A moderate reduction in P_aCO_2 causes vasoconstriction of normal vessels, slows cerebral circulation and contrast medium transit time, and improves delineation of small vascular lesions. The failure of autoregulation within tumours increases blood flow relative to that in other areas because of an intracerebral steal phenomenon and allows better visualization of their vascularity.

Transient hypotension and bradycardia or asystole may occur during cerebral angiography with contrast dye injection. This usually responds to volume replacement and atropine. Brain damage in the past was attributed to toxic contrast agents and local damage to carotid and vertebral arteries. Nowadays, complications during interventional neuroradiology include haemorrhage from rupture of the lesion or vessel and ischaemia as a result of thromboembolism (e.g. clot forming around the catheter tip), vasospasm, embolic material or hypoperfusion. All may occur rapidly with devastating results. Occasionally, urgent craniotomy may be required.

Embolization procedures

The use of angiographic embolization continues to grow and become more sophisticated. It is undertaken for vascular malformations and fistulae, aneurysms, tumours, acute haemorrhage and ablation of function of an organ. Venous embolization is used to treat gastro-oesophageal varices, testicular varices and ablation of adrenal gland function. It may be performed as an alternative to surgery, particularly if the patient is unfit and the operation carries a high risk. Its use before surgery can help to reduce intraoperative blood loss.

Embolizations involve the injection of an embolic material to stimulate intravascular thrombosis, resulting in vessel occlusion. Embolic agents include gelatin sponge, polyvinyl alcohol particles, spiral metal coils, balloons and liquids such as ethyl alcohol. Patients must be watched carefully for disruption of flow in other vascular beds.

The anaesthetic management is similar to that for standard angiographic procedures. Sedation, local anaesthesia or general anaesthesia are administered according to the clinical situation. They can be long and painful procedures, in which case general anaesthesia would be the most pleasant option for the patient. In some cases, patient cooperation is required to help with the detection and avoidance of neurological or mechanical deficits that can arise from inadvertent occlusion of flow to vital tissues. These patients may be anaesthetized by intermittent propofol and short-acting opioids, or given midazolam sedation. Nausea and vomiting are common so prophylactic antiemetics may be given. Often a high dose of contrast medium is used and therefore adequate hydration and a urinary catheter are important to minimize the development of renal failure.

Cardiac catheterization

General anaesthesia is required mainly for children (rarely in adults as sedation is usually adequate). In children, congenital heart disease may cause abnormal circulations and intracardiac shunts, which often present with cyanosis, dyspnoea, failure to thrive and congestive heart failure. Radiological procedures include pressure and oxygen saturation measurements, balloon dilatation of stenotic lesions (e.g. pulmonary valve), balloon septostomy for transposition of the great arteries and ductal closure.

The ideal anaesthetic technique would not produce myocardial depression, would avoid hypertension and tachycardia, preserve normocapnia and maintain spontaneous respiration on air. All techniques have their limitations. Positive pressure ventilation causes changes in pulmonary haemodynamics and therefore influences measurements of flow and pressure. Spontaneous respiration with volatile agents may not be suitable for patients with significant myocardial disease. The onset of action of anaesthetic drugs will be influenced by cardiac shunts and congestive failure. Contrast medium in the coronary circulation may cause profound transient changes in the ECG. Therefore, ECG and invasive arterial pressure monitoring should be used to allow rapid assessment of arrhythmias and hypotension. Children with cyanotic heart disease may be polycythaemic, thereby predisposing them to thrombosis.

INTUSSUSCEPTION

This condition usually occurs between the ages of 6 and 18 months. Commonly, the ileum invaginates into the caecum because of small bowel lymphadenopathy. General anaesthesia or sedation may be necessary in the radiology department during attempted reduction of the intussusception by instillation of rectal barium. Insufflation with air or oxygen is also possible.

The major problems are those of anaesthetizing any young child in an unfamiliar environment. Precautions should be taken to minimize the decrease in body temperature. Hypothermia may be exacerbated if the infant lies in cold barium that has been expelled. Fluid losses are always greater than expected and crystalloids or colloids may be needed to restore circulating blood volume.

BRONCHOGRAPHY

Bronchography is an imaging technique that is no longer in regular use. Until recently, it was the definitive investigation for diagnosing bronchiectasis and assessing the extent of disease. This has been replaced by high-resolution CT. Bronchography is occasionally used to investigate recurrent haemoptysis if other investigations are negative. It may also be used to demonstrate bronchopleural fistulae and congenital lesions of the lung.

Contrast medium may be given by various approaches, including cricothyroid puncture, nasal or transoral drip and tracheal intubation. General anaesthesia is used in children. Adults tolerate unilateral bronchography with local anaesthesia, but bilateral procedures with coughing and hypoxia make general anaesthesia desirable.

Commonly, respiratory function in these patients is compromised and additional hypoxaemia is inevitable after inhalation of the oil-based contrast medium.

Intravenous or inhalation induction is followed by tracheal intubation without any local anaesthetic spray, so that the cough reflex returns rapidly at the end of the procedure. Spontaneous ventilation is preferred as it allows contrast medium to be drawn gradually into the bronchi to provide even distribution; controlled ventilation tends to disperse the dye too rapidly and delineates the bronchial tree poorly. Contrast medium is instilled through a catheter passed down the lumen of the tracheal tube. The posture of the patient is altered sequentially to fill the various lobes of the lung.

As much contrast material as possible is removed at the end of the procedure by suction. The tracheal tube remains in situ until there is an active cough reflex. Humidified oxygen should be given during the recovery period and the patient should be nursed in a head-down position with the healthier lung uppermost. Physiotherapy is given ideally before beginning the procedure and at the end after extubation.

ANAESTHESIA FOR RADIOTHERAPY

Adults may require general anaesthesia for insertion of radioactive sources locally to treat some types of tumour. The commonest tumours to be treated in this way are carcinoma of the cervix, breast or tongue. These procedures are undertaken in the operating theatre and the anaesthetic management is similar to that for any type of surgery in these anatomical sites. However, the patients may have undergone anaesthesia recently for a diagnostic procedure and may require more than one anaesthetic for radiotherapy treatment; consequently, halothane should be avoided. In addition, the anaesthetist may be exposed to radiation and appropriate precautions should be taken.

Radiotherapy is used increasingly in the management of a variety of malignant diseases which occur in childhood. These include the acute leukaemias, Wilms' tumour, retinoblastoma and central nervous system tumours. High-dose X-rays are administered by a linear accelerator, but all staff must remain outside the room to be protected from radiation.

Anaesthesia in paediatric radiotherapy presents several problems:

- Treatment is administered daily over a 4–6 week period and necessitates repeated doses of sedation or general anaesthesia.
- The patient must remain alone and motionless for short periods during treatment, but immediate access to the patient is required in an emergency.
- Monitoring is difficult as the child can be observed only on a closed-circuit television screen during treatment.
- Recovery from anaesthesia must be rapid, as treatment is organized usually on an outpatient basis and disruption of normal activities should be minimized.

Before treatment begins, the fields to be irradiated are plotted and marked so that the X-rays can be focused on the tumour without damaging surrounding structures. This procedure requires the child to remain still for 20–40 min and takes place in semi-darkness. Radiotherapy treatment is of much shorter duration; two or three fields are irradiated for 30–90 s each, but a considerably longer period of anaesthesia is required so that the child can be positioned correctly and the radiation source focused precisely. A typical treatment session lasts 20–30 min.

Anaesthetic management

A wide range of anaesthetic techniques have been used for radiotherapy. Ketamine can be given intravenously or intramuscularly but is not used widely by anaesthetists because of the following problems: excessive salivation, even if an antisialagogue is prescribed, and the risk of airway obstruction or laryngospasm. Tachyphylaxis occurs with repeated use, and sudden purposeless movements are not infrequent. The use of ketamine as a sole anaesthetic agent is unsatisfactory.

Often these children have a Hickman catheter in situ to ensure reliable i.v. access for a range of medications and blood sampling. This makes induction of anaesthesia far simpler and avoids repeated venous cannulation which may become technically difficult, but also increasingly distressing for the patient, parent and anaesthetist. The dead space volume of a Hickman catheter must always be remembered. Failure to flush these catheters immediately after administering drugs can lead to disastrous consequences when the anaesthetic drugs are flushed into the bloodstream at a later time. Inhalation induction with the child sitting on the parent's knee is an alternative technique.

When anaesthesia has been induced, the child is placed on a trolley and anaesthesia maintained with nitrous oxide, oxygen and volatile agent delivered via a laryngeal mask. No analgesia is required and tracheal intubation is generally not necessary. There is virtually no surgical stimulation and patients may be maintained at relatively light anaesthetic levels allowing for rapid emergence and recovery.

Monitoring during radiotherapy under general anaesthesia is not easy. Closed-circuit television cameras provide visual monitoring of the patient's respiratory movements. Standard monitoring should include ECG, pulse oximeter and automatic non-invasive arterial pressure. A microphone may transmit the audible ECG signal and the saturation-dictated pitch of the oximeter signal.

FURTHER READING

Fried M P, Hsu L, Topulos G P, Jolesz F A 1996 Image-guided surgery in a new magnetic resonance suite: preclinical considerations. Laryngoscope 106: 411–417

Manninen P H 1997 Anaesthesia for neuroradiology. Canadian Journal of Anaesthesia 44: R34–39

Sutton D 1998 Textbook of radiology and imaging. Churchill Livingstone, Edinburgh

Walters F J M 1993 Anaesthesia and intensive care for the neurosurgical patient. Blackwell Scientific Publications, Oxford

49 Anaesthesia and psychiatric disease

The anaesthetic management of the patient with a psychiatric illness requires specific considerations:

- Psychiatric patients are frequently depressed (with or without confusion) with little appreciation and understanding of anaesthesia.
- Patients are often being treated with psychotropic drugs with potentially serious drug interactions with anaesthetic agents.
- Patients may have associated pathology as a consequence of alcohol/drug abuse.
- Repeated anaesthesia is required for electroconvulsive therapy (ECT).

ANAESTHESIA AND ELECTROCONVULSIVE THERAPY

Electroconvulsive therapy is used widely in psychiatric practice, with over 100 000 treatments being administered to patients in England each year under general anaesthesia; ECT is therefore an important topic for anaesthetists.

ECT is a highly successful treatment for severe depression and some other psychiatric disorders. It is often quicker, safer and more effective and has fewer side-effects than drug therapy.

Originally, seizures were induced chemically and electrical stimulation was not introduced until the late 1930s. The high incidence of trauma, such as fractures and dislocations, that occurred during unmodified fits led to the use of muscle relaxants to control convulsions. The use of succinylcholine during ECT pre-dates its use in mainstream anaesthesia by a number of years. However, ECT remains a highly emotive and controversial area of psychiatric practice dreaded by the public and demonized by the media. Its adverse image has led to a failure of commitment by psychiatrists and anaesthetists such that equipment, training and supervision remain suboptimal in some units.

ADMINISTRATION OF ECT

The electrical stimulus produced by all ECT devices comprises brief pulses of current interrupted by longer periods of electrical inactivity. The electrical transmission lasts for only a fraction of the total stimulus duration and this results in a decrease in the amount of electrical energy required to provoke a generalized seizure.

The electrical stimulus is applied to the patient's head by hand-held electrodes of low impedance. Traditionally, electrodes are placed in the bifrontotemporal region for bilateral ECT, whereas both electrodes are placed over the non-dominant hemisphere to produce unilateral ECT.

INDICATIONS FOR ECT

The main indication for ECT is for the treatment of severe and drug-refractory depression. ECT also has a role in the management of some other psychiatric conditions, e.g. mania and some types of schizophrenia and catatonia.

PHYSIOLOGICAL EFFECTS OF ECT (Table 49.1)

Cardiovascular system

Activation of the autonomic nervous system is responsible for the profound cardiovascular changes during ECT. The autonomic disturbance consists of a parasympathetic–sympathetic sequence; this results in an initial bradycardia followed by tachycardia and hypertension secondary to intense sympathetic stimulation. In combination with the increased muscle activity of the convulsion, this increases myocardial oxygen demand and may result in myocardial ischaemia in susceptible individuals unless hypoxaemia is avoided by administration of supplementary oxygen during the convulsion.

Table 49.1 Physiological effects of electroconvulsive therapy

Cardiovascular effects	
Immediate	
Parasympathetic stimulation	Bradycardia Hypotension
Late (after 1 min)	
Sympathetic stimulation	Tachycardia Hypertension Arrhythmias Myocardial oxygen consumption increases
Cerebral effects	
Cerebral oxygen consumption	Increased
Cerebral blood flow	Increased
Intracranial pressure	Increased
Intraocular pressure	Increased
Intragastric pressure	Increased

Cerebrovascular system

Cerebral blood flow increases dramatically in response to the increase in cerebral oxygen consumption that accompanies the seizure. There is an associated increase in ICP which may prove hazardous in patients with a space-occupying lesion.

CONTRAINDICATIONS TO ECT (Table 49.2)

ECT is a safe procedure and there are few contraindications; however, it is best avoided in those patients with an intracranial mass lesion, recent myocardial infarction or cerebrovascular accidents. Age is no barrier to treatments. ECT may be the treatment of choice in pregnancy compared with the alternative of drug therapy.

ANAESTHETIC CONSIDERATIONS

Anaesthesia for ECT is complicated by the fact that the choice of drugs used and the conduct of the anaesthetic may directly affect the success of treatment by influencing the seizure threshold and duration. Insufficient seizure duration renders ECT ineffective, but increasing seizures augment unwanted effects such as confusion and memory impairment. A technique of modified ECT has evolved in which drugs are employed to reduce the detrimental effect of ECT without the abolition of the essential beneficial effects.

Pre-anaesthetic assessment

All patients should receive a visit and evaluation by the anaesthetist before treatment. Special attention should be paid to cardiorespiratory function, symptoms of oesophageal reflux, allergies and previous anaesthetic experiences. The presence of loose or missing teeth should also be noted.

Some antidepressant drugs delay gastric emptying and the patient should be fasted for a period of at least 8 h before anaesthesia. This may seem simple, but many of these patients are extremely unreliable and occasionally uncooperative, so that careful supervision is required to ensure that fasting does occur.

Premedication with sedatives or opioids is not required and may serve only to prolong the anaesthetic recovery time. Routine administration of atropine is no longer considered to be necessary.

Table 49.2 Contraindications to electroconvulsive therapy

Absolute
Recent myocardial infarction (< 3 months)
Recent cerebrovascular accident (< 3 months)
Intracranial mass lesion
Relative
Angina pectoris
Congestive cardiac failure
Severe pulmonary disease
Severe osteoporosis
Major bone fractures
Glaucoma
Retinal detachment
Pregnancy

Anaesthetic management

There is no clear advantage to the use of propofol for ECT, as recovery from anaesthesia is no quicker than with barbiturates. Whilst propofol does obtund some of the cardiovascular effects of ECT, it also inhibits seizures which may impair the efficacy of ECT. Randomized controlled trials of the effect of propofol on the outcome of ECT are needed. Methohexital is the induction agent used most commonly. Thiopental offers no advantages over methohexital and prolongs the recovery time. The use of muscle relaxants in ECT has virtually eliminated the risk of fractures – succinylcholine in a dose of 0.5 mg kg^{-1} is the most commonly used.

After induction of anaesthesia, hyperventilation of the patient's lungs by bag and mask before application of ECT stimulation lowers the seizure threshold and prolongs seizure duration.

When the limbs are flaccid, a rubber 'bite block' is inserted between the teeth before electrical stimulation is applied. During the seizure, artificial ventilation of the lungs with oxygen is continued to avoid arterial desaturation until adequate spontaneous ventilation has returned.

Patients should be recovered in the lateral position by trained nursing staff with equipment available immediately for treatment of any emergency.

Good record-keeping is vital so that any problems or changes to anaesthetic or electrical stimulus are known at the next treatment. Close cooperation between anaesthetist and psychiatrist is essential for optimal treatment.

MORBIDITY AFTER ECT

Modified ECT in association with skilled anaesthetic management is safe and effective. Patients may complain of headache, muscle aches and confusion for 1–2 h after treatment, but memory disturbances may persist for several weeks. The latter are minimized by unilateral ECT over the non-dominant cerebral hemisphere.

ORGANIZATION OF ANAESTHETIC SERVICES FOR ECT

Historically the provision of anaesthetic services for ECT has been a low priority for directorates. Many units have no suitably trained assistance for the anaesthetist. Standards of facilities and equipment in isolated ECT units are often inferior to those normally acceptable to an anaesthetist. For these reasons, ECT should not be left to unsupervised trainees.

Every unit should have a consultant anaesthetist responsible for ECT with an equivalent role for a psychiatrist. There should be clear departmental guidelines as to:

- Who is qualified to administer anaesthetics?
- How should they be trained?
- Who should assist the anaesthetist?
- Who should supervise recovering patients?
- What facilities and equipment should be available?

DRUG INTERACTIONS

Concomitant administration of psychotropic drugs is frequent in psychiatric patients scheduled for anaesthesia. The drugs encountered most commonly are tricyclic antidepressants, monoamine oxidase inhibitors, phenothiazines and lithium.

TRICYCLIC ANTIDEPRESSANTS

Tricyclic antidepressants inhibit the reuptake of norepinephrine into the presynaptic nerve terminals. Most of these drugs also have anticholinergic effects.

Tricyclic antidepressants may produce tachycardia and arrhythmias even in therapeutic doses and the hypertensive response to directly acting sympathomimetic amines is increased dramatically. Although it has been recommended that tricyclic antidepressants are discontinued 2 weeks before anaesthesia, this may not be possible in many psychiatric patients.

Side-effects of tricyclic therapy include sedation and anticholinergic symptoms (dry mouth, blurred vision, delayed gastric emptying, constipation, urinary retention). Centrally acting anticholinergic drugs (atropine, hyoscine) should be avoided in premedication because the additive effect may precipitate confusion, especially in the elderly.

MONOAMINE OXIDASE INHIBITORS (MAOIs)

Monoamine oxidase is responsible for the intraneuronal metabolism of sympathomimetic amines. Inhibition of this enzyme by drugs such as phenelzine and tranylcypromine is responsible for their antidepressant action. Usually, these agents are used when the response to tricyclic antidepressants has been unsatisfactory.

Tyramine, a precursor of norepinephrine, is known to precipitate hypertensive crises in the presence of MAOIs. Similarly, indirectly acting sympathomimetic amines, e.g. ephedrine, result in unpredictable changes in arterial pressure. These hypertensive responses may be eliminated by withdrawal of MAOIs 2 weeks before anaesthesia, but as with tricyclic drugs this may not always be practical in the psychiatric patient.

The interaction between MAOIs and pethidine is also important, although uncommon. Agitation, restlessness, hypertension, rigidity, convulsions and hyperpyrexia may result. Morphine appears to be safe.

PHENOTHIAZINES

Phenothiazines possess antipsychotic, antiemetic, antihistamine and sedative properties. Interactions with anaesthetic drugs are common. The central depressant actions of opioids are potentiated and opioid requirements are decreased. Central anticholinergic effects are additive with those of atropine and hyoscine, so that glycopyrrolate is the preferred antisialagogue. Moderate α-adrenoceptor blockade aggravates the hypotensive effect of anaesthetic agents.

LITHIUM

Lithium carbonate is used predominantly in the long-term treatment of mania. Its mode of action is inhibition of the release, and increased reuptake, of norepinephrine.

As lithium tends to act as an imperfect sodium ion, potentiation of both depolarizing and non-depolarizing muscle relaxants occurs and close monitoring of neuromuscular function is necessary.

Lithium is excreted by the kidneys. Toxicity may ensue in hyponatraemic states, when there is intense renal conservation of sodium and consequently lithium. The risk may be minimized by the use of a saline infusion during the perioperative period.

OTHER MENTAL DISORDERS

LEARNING DISABILITIES

Patients should be assessed in the presence of parents or a guardian. Relevant medical history can be obtained, consent for surgery given (if the patient is unable to provide this) and rapport established with the patient.

Pharmacological premedication is usually unnecessary. The interval between arrival in the anaesthetic room and induction of anaesthesia should be minimized and the presence of a reassuring parent may be invaluable. A flexible approach by the anaesthetist is required during induction of anaesthesia, which may have to be performed with the patient in the sitting position. Adequate help must be available to lift or restrain the patient if necessary. Induction of anaesthesia should be as smooth and rapid as possible; either an inhalation or i.v. technique may be used. Occasionally, i.m. ketamine is required.

Poor dental hygiene and difficulty with tracheal intubation should be anticipated.

Patients must be allowed to recover undisturbed and the presence of parents or guardians in the recovery area is to be encouraged.

DOWN'S SYNDROME

Down's syndrome is associated with a variety of medical abnormalities including congenital heart disease and duodenal or choanal atresia. Patients with this condition have a large tongue, small mandible and increased incidence of subglottic stenosis; consequently, airway management and tracheal intubation may prove difficult. Antibiotics are necessary in the prophylaxis of endocarditis. Abnormal responses to anaesthetic agents have not been substantiated.

ALCOHOL WITHDRAWAL

Denial of alcohol intake in the perioperative period may result in disturbances associated with acute withdrawal. Delirium tremens is characterized by extreme disorientation, increased psychomotor activity, hallucinations, marked autonomic activity and hyperpyrexia. Usually, the syndrome lasts for 7–10 days.

Delirium tremens should be treated by correction of fluid and electrolyte imbalance and administration of vitamins, particularly thiamine. Control is achieved most readily by i.v. sedation with 0.8% clomethiazole; barbiturates should be avoided.

A nitrous oxide, oxygen and relaxant technique with analgesic supplementation is suitable if anaesthesia is required for a surgical procedure, although maintenance of anaesthesia may require the administration of larger doses of anaesthetic agents than normal.

FURTHER READING

Editorial 1998 Anaesthesia and electroconvulsive therapy. Anaesthesia 53: 615–617

50 Day-case anaesthesia

A day-case patient is one who is admitted for investigation or operation on a planned non-resident basis. The patient occupies a bed in a ward or unit set aside for this purpose. The concept of day-case anaesthesia and surgery has existed for many years. In 1899, Ries showed that patients improved with early ambulation and suffered fewer complications. In 1900, Cushing described hernia repairs using cocaine as a local anaesthetic, and in 1909, when Nicoll reported a series of 8988 outpatient operations in children, he stressed the need for careful selection of patients.

During the last 30 years, there has been rapid expansion in the use of day-case surgery. At the inception of day-care procedures, a case was considered suitable if it took less than 90 min. Procedures that are commonly selected today are those taking less than 60 min to complete and which do not cause severe haemorrhage or produce excessive amounts of postoperative pain (Table 50.1). Increasingly complex cases are now performed as day procedures, including laparoscopic cholecystectomy.

To achieve a pain-free ambulant patient requires skilful patient selection and experienced anaesthetists and surgeons working within a day-case surgery unit. Many anaesthetists and surgeons have indicated that day surgery represents a safe, cost-effective and efficient practice.

PATIENT SELECTION

The selection of patients for day-case surgery is of vital importance if maximum use is to be made of the resources in the day-case unit and also to facilitate smooth running of the unit. The selection of patients must take into account two separate aspects: first the patient's state of health, and second his or her social circumstances. Patients should normally be ASA I or II, i.e. normal healthy people or those with minor systemic disease not interfering with normal activities, the latter including medical conditions that are well controlled with therapy, e.g. hypertension and non-insulin-dependent diabetes. An upper limit of body mass index of 30–34 (weight [kg]/height^2 [m^2]) is used in several day surgery units. An upper age limit of greater than 70 years should be judged on biological rather than chronological age. In urology, in particular, patients over this age regularly attend the day unit for check cystoscopy. A limit is also set with regard to the distance from the hospital to the patient's home, and a responsible adult must be at home with the patient during the first 24 h after surgery. An example of guidelines used for patient selection for day-case anaesthesia is shown in Table 50.2.

The selection of patients for day-case surgery is made at the time of outpatient consultation and routine measurement of pulse, BP and urine analysis and other relevant investigations (e.g. ECG, full blood count and sickle cell testing) are performed; these routine tests reduce problems when patients are admitted on the day of surgery. Careful attention to patient selection and consultation with anaesthetists involved in the provision of anaesthetic services to the day unit minimize problems. Studies have demonstrated that a simple preoperative questionnaire can be very effective in screening patients to detect common medical problems. A typical preoperative questionnaire is shown in Table 50.3.

When considering children for day-case procedures, they should be healthy, normally falling into ASA I or II groups. Premature babies who have not reached 60 weeks conceptual age should not be considered for day-case surgery and special consideration should be given to babies who have been receiving ventilatory support. The parent must be able to cope with the pre-procedure instructions and with the care of the child after treatment. The parent must agree to day treatment and be available to stay

Table 50.1 A selection of surgical procedures commonly undertaken as day cases

Gynaecology
Dilatation & curettage, laparoscopy, vaginal termination of pregnancy, colposcopy

Plastic surgery
Dupuytren's contracture release, removal of small skin lesions, nerve decompression

Ophthalmology
Strabismus correction, lacrimal duct probing, examination under anaesthesia

ENT
Adenoidectomy, tonsillectomy, myringotomy, insertion of grommets, removal of foreign body, polyp removal

Urology
Cystoscopy, circumcision, vasectomy

Orthopaedics
Arthroscopies, carpal tunnel release, ganglion removal

General surgery
Breast lumps, herniae, varicose veins, endoscopy

Paediatrics
Circumcision, orchidopexy, squint, dental extractions

Table 50.2 Guidelines for patient selection for day-case surgery under general anaesthesia

ASA I and II only
Age: 6 months – 70 years (except for repeat procedures e.g. cystoscopy)
Weight: body mass index = weight/height^2 (kg m^{-2})
  < 30: acceptable
  31–34: discuss with anaesthetic department
Generally healthy, i.e. can climb two flights of stairs

Patient exclusions
Cardiovascular
Previous MI
Hypertension: diastolic > 100 mmHg
Angina: at rest, more than three attacks per week or low exercise tolerance
Arrhythmias
Heart failure

Respiratory
Acute respiratory tract infection
Asthma requiring regular β_2-agonists or steroids
Chronic obstructive airways disease

Metabolic
Alcoholism
Insulin-dependent diabetes
Renal failure
Liver disease

Neurological/musculoskeletal
Arthritis of jaw or neck, cervical spondylosis or ankylosing spondylitis
Myopathies, muscular dystrophies or myasthenia gravis
Multiple sclerosis
Cerebrovascular accidents or transient ischaemic attacks
Epilepsy > 3 fits per year

Drugs
Steroids
Monoamine oxidase inhibitors
Anticoagulants
Antiarrhythmics
Insulin

Table 50.3 A typical preoperative questionnaire

Name	Date
DOB	Operation
Unit number	

Blood pressure (mmHg)
Pulse (bpm)
Weight (kg)
Temperature (°C)

Please answer the following questions:

	No	Yes
Have you had anything to eat or drink in the last 4 h?		
Have you had any previous operations?		
Will you go home alone?		
Will you be on your own when you get home?		
Have you, or anybody in your family, ever had any problems with general anaesthetics?		
Do you have a cough or a cold?		
Have you had any serious illnesses in the past?		
Do you suffer with heart disease or high blood pressure?		
Do your ankles swell?		
Do you get breathless or have chest pain on exercise or at night?		
Do you have asthma or bronchitis?		
Do you smoke?		
Do you have epilepsy (fits)?		
Do you have diabetes?		
Do you suffer from anaemia, bruise easily or bleed excessively?		
Have you ever had liver disease or been jaundiced?		
Do you drink excessive amounts of alcohol?		
Are you allergic to anything, including Elastoplast?		
Are you taking any drugs or medication from your GP?		
Do you have any loose or false teeth?		
Do you usually wear contact lenses?		
If female, are you pregnant?		

throughout the day, although there may be exceptions for older children who attend regularly. The facilities at home should be taken into account, as should travel conditions. After a general anaesthetic, the use of public transport is inappropriate.

Following selection of a patient for day-case surgery, the nature of the operation and the routine of management are fully explained to the patient and the consent form may be signed. Many units issue the patient with explanatory leaflets or audio cassettes explaining the procedure. A date for the operation may then be arranged and registration completed as for an in-patient admission. It is wise to book any pathological or radiological investigations that are required well in advance of the day of admission.

The patient should be given written instructions detailing the date and time of attendance at the day unit, with written instructions relating to preoperative starvation and the patient's usual medication, e.g. antihypertensives should be taken as usual but oral hypoglycaemics must be omitted on the morning of surgery. These instructions should be written clearly in plain English, and advise the patient not to eat anything from midnight for a morning list.

Recent clinical studies suggest that overnight fasting may not be justified in adults or children. Pulmonary aspiration usually occurs in emergency abdominal and obstetric procedures where there may be complicating factors such as recent food and fluid intake, trauma or administration of opioid analgesics. These factors do not normally apply to healthy elective day-case patients. The universal order of nil by mouth from midnight should only apply to solids. Clear fluids should be allowed until 3 h before the scheduled time of surgery. The effect of giving patients 150 ml clear fluid 2 h before general anaesthesia for termination of pregnancy has been studied, and the results showed that clear fluids do not increase the incidence of regurgitation or vomiting during anaesthesia and that preoperative thirst was decreased in the clear fluid group. An example of instructions for children relating to preoperative starvation is given in Table 50.4. It is advisable to ask patients who smoke to refrain from smoking for 4–6 weeks before the operation. The patients should be asked to bring with them all tablets and medicines that they take regularly.

After day-case surgery, patients should be accompanied home and should also be advised to abstain from drinking alcohol and not to drive a car or operate machinery for 24 h.

Table 50.4 Preoperative starvation instructions for children

Morning operations
Children over 4 years old
Nothing to eat or drink after midnight on the day before the operation.

Children between 2 and 4 years old
Wake the child when you go to bed and give a drink and a biscuit; after this *nothing* to eat or drink.

Children less than 2 years old
Wake the child very early on the morning of the operation and give a milk drink (up to 1/2 pint milk). This must be completed by 6 am; after this *nothing* to eat or drink.

Afternoon operations
Children of all ages
Nothing to eat or drink after a light breakfast before 9 am.

ORGANIZATION OF THE DAY-CASE UNIT

THE TYPES OF UNIT

There are three common types of day-case unit:

- A unit within a hospital complex, but with separate staff, wards and operating theatre; this is functionally the most flexible type as it may be adapted to the varying requirements of day-case patients.
- A unit with a separate ward, but using the hospital's main operating theatre complex.
- Outside the UK, it is common for a separate centre to have its own operating theatres and wards remote from a conventional hospital.

Ideally, day surgical units should not be free-standing but situated on in-patient hospital sites. The ward area should be close by the theatre, to reduce portering time, particularly when short operations are to be performed. This arrangement also enables parents to accompany their children to the anaesthetic room if this is desirable.

Preferably the unit should be near a car park and well signposted to facilitate the prompt arrival of patients and to avoid unnecessary delays.

FACILITIES AVAILABLE

The accommodation should ideally include:

- *An admission area*, which includes reception, treatment and examination rooms, a nurses' station, lavatories, a play room and a discharge area.
- *An anaesthetic room*, fully equipped and large enough to allow free access around the patient's trolley to permit the use of local or general anaesthesia. There should be good lighting, scavenging, piped gases and suction equipment, anaesthetic machine and monitoring equipment. The hazards and risks of day surgery general anaesthesia are no less than for in-patient surgery; indeed, in some respects they may be greater and the facilities provided must be comparable.
- *An operating theatre*. This should be of the same specification as the in-patient equivalent. A good operating light, air conditioning and piped services are required, in addition to the usual scrub-up, lay-up and autoclave facilities. There is always the possibility of a minor operation developing unexpectedly into a major operation and this demands that the theatre is well equipped to deal with this eventuality.
- *A fully equipped recovery room*. This must always be equipped and staffed for the safe recovery of patients after general anaesthesia. Piped gas supplies and resuscitation equipment are mandatory and the full range of monitoring and ventilation equipment must be readily available.

Other facilities that should be available include office space, equipment store, staff locker room, a staff room, a pantry to make drinks and lavatories for patients, parents and staff.

ADMISSION

Patients should be admitted to the day ward in adequate time for history-taking and examination. The results of any investigation requested as an outpatient should be available and noted. Patients should receive an identity bracelet and their names should be entered into the nursing record. The surgeon should ensure the indication for surgery is still present, e.g. presence or absence of lumps to be removed, as it may be several months since the clinic appointment; the consent form should be signed if not already done during the outpatient appointment, and the operation site marked. A pregnancy test in women of fertile age may need to be performed if there is any risk of pregnancy.

ANAESTHESIA

PREMEDICATION

Most anaesthetists do not routinely prescribe premedication for day cases, as mostly it is unnecessary. Premedication drugs that may be used include the following.

Benzodiazepines

It is thought that sedative premedication may prolong the recovery time and delay the patient's discharge from hospital. However, a double-blind study of temazepam premedication for day cases found effective anxiolysis in the groups that received 10 or 20 mg temazepam; there was no delay in recovery times as measured by memory test cards and all patients were discharged from the day unit 3 h after administration of general anaesthesia. Oral midazolam has been used as a premedicant in day surgery, but it was found that it produced delay in immediate and late recovery when compared with temazepam.

Antiemetics

If patients are at high risk of postoperative nausea and vomiting (PONV), antiemetics can be safely administered orally before operation, or via the intravenous or rectal route perioperatively.

Antacids

If there is a risk of acid reflux, H_2 antagonists are commonly prescribed as a premedication in day surgery.

Analgesics

Oral non-steroidal anti-inflammatory drugs (NSAIDs) and paracetamol may be given preoperatively if the patient declines rectal administration perioperatively. Patient satisfaction with self-administration of rectal diclofenac preoperatively has been recently reported. Tetracaine (amethocaine) has a useful role for children and nervous adults or those with a needle phobia as it acts within 20 min and it does not cause local vasoconstriction.

GENERAL AND REGIONAL ANAESTHESIA

General, local or regional anaesthesia can be administered safely to day-case patients. The choice of technique should be determined by surgical requirements, anaesthetic considerations and the patient's physical status and preference.

General anaesthesia

The choice of induction and maintenance agent depends upon the requirements of the patient and the preference of the anaesthetist. Any induction agent used in day-case anaesthesia should ensure a smooth induction, good immediate recovery with minimal postoperative sequelae and a rapid return to street fitness.

Several intravenous induction agents have been used successfully for induction of anaesthesia in day-case patients; these include methohexital, etomidate and thiopental. However, propofol is now used widely as the primary induction agent in day-case anaesthesia. One of the main advantages of propofol is the ease and rapidity with which patients recover from its effects. Patients are clear-headed and have a lower incidence of PONV.

Inhalation agents used for induction of anaesthesia include halothane and sevoflurane. Both are non-irritant to the airways, but the latter has the advantage of more rapid induction in both children and adults, minimal cardiovascular side-effects and a rapid recovery profile. However, sevoflurane causes more PONV than propofol.

Which technique should be used for maintenance of anaesthesia? Comparisons of recovery after enflurane and halothane techniques in patients undergoing day-case anaesthesia suggest that recovery is faster after enflurane. Times to awakening were reported to be not significantly different between isoflurane and enflurane in patients undergoing short surgical procedures. The use of nitrous oxide for maintenance of anaesthesia has been shown to increase the risk of PONV; however, its use does reduce the requirements for volatile agents. Newer techniques such as target-controlled infusion (TCI) of propofol with or without the ultrarapid-acting opioid remifentanil or the use of sevoflurane may confer some advantages, but these have to be balanced against the cost of these agents. TCI of propofol is an intravenous technique for maintenance of anaesthesia. It takes into account the patient's weight (kg), and the desired drug concentration in blood ($\mu g\ ml^{-1}$). An initial target concentration of 4–6 $\mu g\ ml^{-1}$ is often set and then adjusted as appropriate. The infusion rate is calculated by a computer within the pump.

A clear airway is a fundamental requirement of safe anaesthesia. In day-case anaesthesia, simple face mask anaesthesia with a Guedel airway is commonly used. The laryngeal mask is used frequently in both adults and children. Longer procedures may necessitate the use of a tracheal tube. A rapid-sequence induction technique with tracheal intubation is not a contraindication to day surgery.

The choice of muscle relaxant depends on the anticipated duration of surgery. Succinylcholine is associated with muscle pains, especially in ambulant patients, and for all but the shortest procedures is not ideal in the day-case setting. Of the non-depolarizing muscle relaxants (NDMRs) currently available, atracurium and vecuronium have a relatively short duration of action when they are used in appropriate doses and are readily antagonized after 15–30 min. Mivacurium has a short duration of action which may make it suitable for day-case anaesthesia. It undergoes rapid hydrolysis by plasma cholinesterase, but it must be remembered, as with the use of succinylcholine, that a small number of patients may suffer prolonged muscle paralysis because of plasma cholinesterase deficiency. Rocuronium may have a role as it has a more rapid onset of action than any of the other NDMRs, providing intubating conditions within 30–60 s. However, it has a duration of action similar to that of vecuronium. More recently, cisatracurium, the stereoisomer of atracurium, has been introduced with a similar duration of action to that of atracurium but without the side-effects of histamine release.

Regional anaesthesia

Spinal anaesthesia has been used for day-case anaesthesia, but its use is limited by the occurrence of an unacceptable incidence of headache especially in younger patients. Also, slow return of motor power and difficulty with micturition may delay discharge.

Local anaesthetic blocks are an excellent choice for day-case patients, because of the low incidence of PONV and the provision of good postoperative analgesia. Inguinal hernia repair is commonly performed under an ilioinguinal nerve block and local infiltration. For operations on the hand or arm, axillary brachial plexus block is preferable to the supraclavicular approach because of the risk of producing a pneumothorax, which may become apparent only after discharge. Intravenous regional anaesthesia (Bier's block) may be used successfully for hand operations.

POSTOPERATIVE CARE

Postoperative pain control should be started pre- or intraoperatively by supplementing intravenous or inhalation anaesthesia with a combination of an NSAID, paracetamol (especially in children), shorter-acting opioid analgesics, and local/regional block intraoperatively. The patient's awakening is smoother and discharge home is quicker. The most frequently used drugs to provide intraoperative analgesia are fentanyl and alfentanil; the relatively short duration of action of these drugs makes them suitable for use in day-case anaesthesia.

The provision of good postoperative analgesia is primarily the responsibility of the anaesthetist. Anaesthetists can do little to limit the number of patients requiring admission for surgical complications, but can play a major role in reducing admissions caused by pain or vomiting.

Caudal block is used to reduce pain in paediatric patients (circumcision, herniorrhaphy, hypospadias, orchidopexy), using 0.25% plain bupivacaine; this can provide excellent postoperative analgesia. Whenever a caudal block is administered for analgesia, care must be taken to ensure that motor strength is not compromised. There does not appear to be any advantage in using more concentrated solutions than 0.25% bupivacaine. Ropivacaine is reported to produce more selective sensory nerve block. Penile blocks and the application of local anaesthetic cream are also effective. Intra-articular local anaesthetics have been found to be useful following arthroscopy.

NSAIDs, e.g. diclofenac and more recently ketorolac, are useful for provision of postoperative analgesia in day-case patients. Ketorolac is a potent peripherally acting injectable analgesic associated with few central nervous system side-effects.

The factors contributing to postoperative nausea and vomiting include a previous history of PONV, gender (females are more susceptible), the use of longer-acting opioid analgesic drugs such as morphine, the choice of anaesthetic technique or agents, operative procedure, pain, sudden movement or position change, history of motion sickness, hypotension, obesity, day of menstrual cycle and high oestrogen levels. A relationship between pain and the frequency of nausea and vomiting in the postoperative period has been established. There is controversy regarding the use of opioid analgesics in the day-case patient, because they may increase PONV. Several studies have shown that if an opioid, nitrous oxide anaesthetic is given, the occurrence of PONV is increased compared with an inhalation anaesthetic. In contrast, there are studies which have demonstrated that an opioid-supplemented anaesthetic technique results in earlier ambulation and discharge.

PONV can be reduced by the use of low-dose droperidol 10–20 $\mu g\ kg^{-1}$, and the selective $5HT_3$ antagonist ondansetron appears to be an effective antiemetic without causing drowsiness or extrapyramidal symptoms.

Recovery from anaesthesia is an important aspect of day-case anaesthesia. The recovery area should be provided with monitoring equipment such as pulse oximetry and ECG. Many day surgery units in the UK now have three separate recovery areas: the first stage is for the immediate postoperative period, when patients require one-to-one nurse to patient care and monitoring; the second involves lower nursing dependency care where the patient is not attached to monitoring, but is mobilizing and usually given something to eat and drink; and the third stage is the discharge area. The overall responsibility for assessing when patients are ready to go home is that of the clinicians involved. Often, experienced nursing staff who work regularly in the day unit become very good at detecting potential problems with day-case patients.

In general, discharge of the patient should not take place until the patient is able to sit unaided, walk in a straight line and stand still without swaying. Usually patients have been able to have a drink and something to eat (this also demonstrates the absence of nausea). A responsible person should be present to escort the patient home and both the responsible person and the patient should be given both verbal and written discharge instructions. The patient should be advised to refrain from activities such as driving a car, operating machinery and drinking alcohol for 24 h. Communication with the patient's general practitioner is very important and many units are now using modern telecommunications, e.g. e-mail and fax machines, to ensure that the GP is aware of the operation performed and the requirements for postoperative follow-up. Patient hotels are a relatively new concept where patients spend their first postoperative night in a hotel near to the day surgery unit for which the hospital pays. There is a resident nurse and these have been used so far for patients who have had, for example, a tonsillectomy. Patient hotels are cheaper than an in-patient overnight stay and are useful for those patients who live too far from the day unit to be considered for day surgery under normal circumstances.

FURTHER READING

Dashfield A K, Birt D J, Thurlow J, Kestin I G, Langton J A 1998 Recovery characteristics using single breath 8% sevoflurane or propofol for induction of anaesthesia in day-case arthroscopy patients. Anaesthesia 53: 1062–1066

Hitchcock M, Ogg T W 1995 Anaesthesia for day-case surgery. British Journal of Hospital Medicine 54: 202–206

Sneyd J R, Carr A, Byrom W D, Bilski A J T 1998 A meta-analysis of nausea and vomiting following maintenance of anaesthesia with propofol or inhalational agents. European Journal of Anaesthesiology 15: 433–445

Strunin L 1993 How long should patients fast before surgery? Time for new guidelines. British Journal of Anaesthesia 70: 1–3

51 Emergency anaesthesia

Patients scheduled for elective surgery are usually in optimal physical and mental condition, with a definitive surgical diagnosis and with coexisting medical disease well controlled.

In contrast, the patient with a surgical emergency may have an uncertain diagnosis and uncontrolled coexisting medical disease, with associated cardiovascular, respiratory and/or metabolic derangements.

Thus, a major principle governing the practice of emergency anaesthesia is to be prepared for all potential complications, including vomiting and regurgitation, hypovolaemia and haemorrhage, and abnormal reactions to drugs in the presence of electrolyte disturbances and renal impairment.

PREOPERATIVE ASSESSMENT

The objective of emergency anaesthesia is to permit correction of the surgical pathology with the minimum of risk to the patient. This requires adequate and accurate preoperative evaluation of the patient's general condition, with particular attention to specific problems that may influence anaesthetic management.

It is essential to ascertain the likely surgical diagnosis, the magnitude of the proposed surgery and how urgently surgery is required, as these dictate both the extent of preoperative preparation and the method of anaesthesia.

A pertinent past medical and drug history is elicited. In particular, enquiry is made into the presence and severity of specific symptoms relevant to cardiopulmonary reserve: angina, productive cough, dyspnoea of effort, orthopnoea or nocturnal coughing bouts. The presence of such symptoms should provoke detailed enquiry into the cardiovascular and respiratory systems (see Ch. 34 on preoperative assessment).

Depending upon the urgency of surgery, physical examination may be selective to identify significant cardiopulmonary dysfunction or any abnormalities that might lead to technical difficulties during anaesthesia. Basal crepitations, triple rhythm and raised jugular venous pulse signify impaired ventricular function and limited cardiac reserve, which increase significantly the risk of anaesthesia. It is also important to exclude arrhythmias and heart sounds indicative of valvular heart disease, as these influence the patient's response to physiological change and thus anaesthetic management. Assessment of respiratory function is particularly difficult, as the patient in pain (with or without peritoneal irritation) may be unable to cooperate with pulmonary function testing.

It is important to cultivate the habit of airway evaluation if a rapid-sequence induction (see p. 622) is contemplated, as contingency plans are required for management of the patient in the event of failure to intubate the trachea. Irregular dentition, limitation of mouth opening, poor range of movement at the atlanto-occipital joint and/or reduced distance between the hyoid bone and the mental symphysis are associated with difficult laryngoscopy. A history of difficult intubation is of considerable significance.

Finally, a review of any laboratory investigations is made and urgent requests are made for additional tests, which may influence patient management.

ASSESSMENT OF VOLAEMIC STATUS

Assessment of intravascular volume is essential, as underestimated or unrecognized hypovolaemia may lead to circulatory collapse during induction of anaesthesia, which attenuates the sympathetically mediated increases in arteriolar and venous constriction. In any patient in whom fluid is sequestered or lost (e.g. peritonitis, bowel obstruction) or in whom haemorrhage has occurred (e.g. trauma), efforts should be made to quantify the blood volume or extracellular fluid volume and to correct any deficit.

INTRAVASCULAR VOLUME DEFICIT

Assessment of blood loss may be made from the history and any measured losses, but more commonly the anaesthetist has to rely on clinical evaluation of the patient's circulatory status. Profound circulatory shock with hypotension, poor peripheral perfusion, oliguria and cerebral obtundation is easy to recognize. However, recognition of the early manifestations of haemorrhage, such as tachycardia and cutaneous vasoconstriction, requires a more careful assessment. Useful indices include heart rate, arterial pressure (especially pulse pressure), the state of the peripheral circulation, central venous pressure and urine output. Table 51.1 describes approximate correlation between these clinical indices and the extent of haemorrhage, but it should be stressed that these refer to the 'ideal' patient. In young, healthy adults, arterial pressure may be an unreliable guide to volume status because compensatory mechanisms may preclude a measurable decrease in arterial pressure until over 30% of the patient's blood volume has been lost. In such patients, attention should be directed to pulse rate, skin circulation and a diminishing pulse pressure. In elderly patients with widespread arterial disease, limited cardiac reserve and a rigid vas-

Table 51.1 Clinical indices of extent of blood loss

Class of hypovolaemia	1 Minimal	2 Mild	3 Moderate	4 Severe
Percentage blood volume lost	10	20	30	Over 40
Volume lost (ml)	500	1000	1500	Over 2000
Heart rate (beat min^{-1})	Normal	100–120	120–140	Over 140
Arterial pressure (mmHg)	Normal	Orthostatic hypotension	Systolic below 100	Systolic below 80
Urinary output (ml h^{-1})	Normal (1 ml kg^{-1} h^{-1})	20–30	10–20	Nil
Sensorium	Normal	Normal	Restless	Impaired consciousness
State of peripheral circulation	Normal	Cool and pale	Cold and pale, slow capillary refill	Cold and clammy Peripheral cyanosis

cular tree (fixed total peripheral resistance), signs of severe hypovolaemia may become evident when blood volume has been reduced by as little as 15%. However, as baroreceptor sensitivity decreases with age, elderly patients may exhibit less tachycardia for any degree of volume depletion.

In general, hypovolaemia does not become apparent clinically until blood volume has been reduced by at least 1000 ml (20% of blood volume). A reduction by more than 30% of blood volume occurs before the classic 'shock syndrome' is produced, with hypotension, tachycardia, oliguria and cold, clammy extremities. Haemorrhage in excess of 40% of blood volume may be associated with loss of the compensatory mechanisms that maintain cerebral and coronary blood flow, and the patient becomes restless and agitated and eventually comatose.

In patients with major trauma, it is valuable to compare the clinical assessment of the extent of haemorrhage with the measured or assumed loss. A marked disparity between these two estimates leads not infrequently to a diagnosis of a further concealed source of haemorrhage.

Extracellular volume deficit

Assessment of extracellular fluid volume deficit is difficult, as considerable losses must occur before clinical signs are apparent. Clinical acumen and a high index of suspicion are necessary to detect the subtle signs of lesser deficits.

Guidance is obtained from the nature of the surgical condition, the duration of impaired fluid intake and the presence and severity of symptoms associated with abnormal losses (e.g. vomiting). At the time of the earliest radiological evidence of intestinal obstruction, there may be 1500 ml of fluid sequestered in the lumen of the bowel. If the obstruction is well established and vomiting has occurred, the deficit may exceed 3000 ml. At this stage, clinical signs are minimal, but evident to the skilled observer.

For convenience, extracellular fluid volume loss may be graded into four degrees of severity; in each instance, loss is expressed as the percentage of the body weight lost as a fluid. It may be seen from Table 51.2 that in minor degrees of extracellular fluid volume loss, diagnosis is dependent on two highly subjective signs: diminished skin elasticity and reduced intraocular pressure. Changes in skin turgor are difficult to assess in elderly patients in whom a natural loss of subcutaneous tissue elasticity may contribute to the impression of reduced turgor. The most reliable sites for interpreting 'tenting' of the skin as a sign of tissue dehydration are the anterior thigh, the forehead, sternum, clavicle or tibia, areas where, under normal circumstances, there is little subcutaneous fat or redundant skin. Soft eyeballs resulting from lower intraocular pressure are assessed by asking the patient to close his or her eyes and look downwards; the examiner presses lightly on the eyeballs (above the tarsal plate) with the index finger of each hand.

It should be noted that the presence of orthostatic hypotension indicates considerable deficit which, if not corrected, may lead to severe hypotension on induction of anaesthesia. Orthostatic hypotension should be elicited with caution.

Laboratory investigations may help to confirm the extent of extracellular fluid volume deficit. Haemoconcentration results in an increased haemoglobin concentration and an increased packed cell volume. As dehydration becomes more marked, renal blood flow diminishes, reducing renal clearance of urea and consequently increasing the concentration of blood urea. Patients with moderate volume contraction exhibit a pre-renal pattern of uraemia characterized by an elevation in blood urea out of proportion to any elevation in serum creatinine. Under maximal stimulation from ADH and aldosterone, conservation of sodium and water by the kidneys results in excretion of urine of low

Table 51.2 Indices of extent of loss of extracellular fluid

Percentage body weight lost as water	ml of fluid lost per 70 kg	Signs and symptoms
Over 4% (mild)	Over 2500	Thirst, reduced skin elasticity, decreased intraocular pressure, dry tongue, reduced sweating
Over 6% (mild)	Over 4200	As above, plus orthostatic hypoten sion, reduced filling of peripheral veins, oliguria, nausea, dry axillae and groins, low CVP, apathy, haemoconcentration
Over 8% (moderate)	Over 5600	As above, plus hypotension, thready pulse with cool peripheries
10–15% (severe)	7000–10 500	Coma, shock followed by death

sodium content (0–15 mmol L^{-1}) and high osmolality (800–1400 mosmol kg^{-1}).

After estimation of the extent of blood volume or extracellular fluid volume deficit, correction is accomplished with the appropriate fluid. Hartmann's solution (compound sodium lactate) and 0.9% saline are isotonic, remaining predominantly in the extracellular space, and are suitable for the replacement of extracellular fluid losses. Anaemia is treated preferably by blood transfusion, but alternative fluids may be used (see Ch. 23). The optimal time for surgical intervention is when all fluid deficits have been corrected, but if there are urgent indications for surgery (e.g. presence of gangrenous bowel), compromise is necessary. As a general rule, the demonstration of orthostatic hypotension indicates that further fluid replacement is required.

THE FULL STOMACH

Of all the hazards of emergency anaesthesia, vomiting or regurgitation of gastric contents, followed by aspiration into the tracheobronchial tree whilst protective laryngeal reflexes are obtunded, is one of the commonest and most devastating.

Vomiting is an active process that occurs in the lighter planes of anaesthesia. Consequently, it is a potential problem during induction of, or emergence from, anaesthesia, but should not occur during maintenance if anaesthesia is sufficiently deep. In light planes of anaesthesia, the presence of vomited material above the vocal cords stimulates spasm of the cords, which prevents material from entering the larynx. Apnoea may persist until severe hypoxaemia occurs, at which point the vocal cords open and ventilation resumes. Thus the presence of laryngeal reflexes provides a margin of safety provided that the anaesthetist clears the oropharynx of all debris before ventilation resumes.

In contrast, regurgitation is a passive process that may occur at any time, is often 'silent' (i.e. not apparent to the anaesthetist) and, if aspiration occurs, may have clinical consequences ranging from minor pulmonary sequelae to fulminating aspiration pneumonitis and acute respiratory distress syndrome (ARDS). Because regurgitation occurs usually in the presence of deep anaesthesia or at the onset of action of muscle relaxant drugs, laryngeal reflexes are absent and the risk of aspiration is high.

In elective surgery, patients are usually starved of food and drink overnight, or at least for 4–6 h, although the need for such absolute rules concerning clear fluids has been questioned. However, in emergency surgery, it may be necessary to induce anaesthesia urgently before an adequate period of starvation occurs. In addition, the patient's surgical condition is often accompanied by delayed gastric emptying.

The most important factors determining the extent of gastric regurgitation are the function of the lower oesophageal sphincter and the rate of gastric emptying.

THE LOWER OESOPHAGEAL SPHINCTER

The lower oesophageal sphincter (LOS) is an area (2–5 cm in length) of higher resting intraluminal pressure situated in the region of the cardia. The sphincter relaxes during oesophageal peristalsis to allow food into the stomach, but remains contracted at other times. The structure cannot be defined anatomically but may be detected using intraluminal pressure manometry.

The LOS is the main barrier preventing reflux of gastric contents into the oesophagus and many drugs used in anaesthetic practice affect its resting tone. Reflux is related not to the LOS tone *per se*, but to the difference between gastric and LOS pressures; this is termed the *barrier pressure*. Drugs that increase the barrier pressure decrease the risk of reflux. Prochlorperazine, cyclizine, anticholinesterases, α-adrenergic agonists and succinylcholine increase barrier pressure. For many years it was thought that the increase in intragastric pressure during succinylcholine-induced fasciculations predisposed to reflux. However, there is an even greater increase in LOS pressure with a consequent increase in barrier pressure.

Anticholinergic drugs, ethanol, ganglion-blocking drugs, tricyclic antidepressants, opioids and thiopental reduce LOS pressure and it is reasonable to assume that these drugs increase the tendency to gastro-oesophageal reflux.

GASTRIC EMPTYING

Under normal circumstances, peristaltic waves sweep from cardia to pylorus at a rate of approximately three per minute, although temporary inhibition of gastric motility follows recent ingestion of a meal. The rate of gastric emptying is proportional to the volume of the stomach contents, with approximately 1–3% of total gastric content reaching the duodenum per minute. Thus, emptying occurs at an exponential rate. The presence of some drugs, fat, acid or hypertonic solutions in the duodenum delays significantly the rate of emptying (the inhibitory enterogastric reflex), but both the nervous and humoral elements of this regulating mechanism are still poorly understood. Many pathological conditions are associated with a reduced rate of gastric emptying (Table 51.3). In the absence of any of these factors, it is reasonably safe

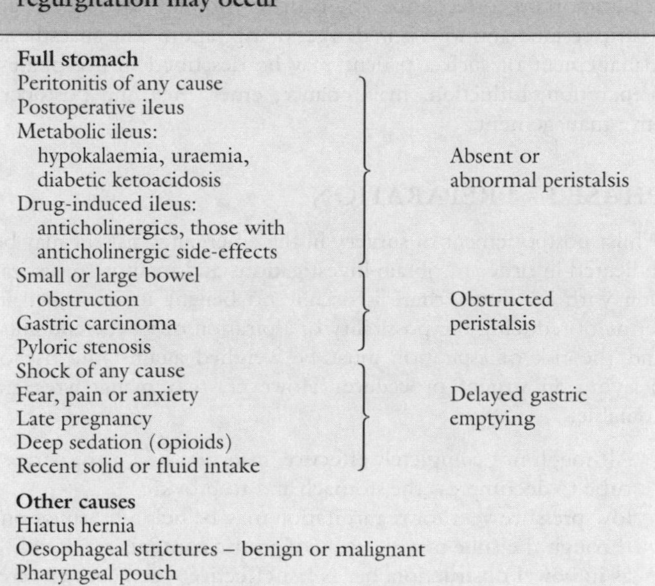

Table 51.3 Situations in which vomiting or regurgitation may occur

Full stomach	
Peritonitis of any cause Postoperative ileus Metabolic ileus: hypokalaemia, uraemia, diabetic ketoacidosis Drug-induced ileus: anticholinergics, those with anticholinergic side-effects	Absent or abnormal peristalsis
Small or large bowel obstruction Gastric carcinoma Pyloric stenosis	Obstructed peristalsis
Shock of any cause Fear, pain or anxiety Late pregnancy Deep sedation (opioids) Recent solid or fluid intake	Delayed gastric emptying
Other causes	
Hiatus hernia	
Oesophageal strictures – benign or malignant	
Pharyngeal pouch	

to assume that the stomach is empty provided that solids have not been ingested within the preceding 6 h, or fluids consumed in the preceding 2 h, and provided normal peristalsis is occurring.

Vomiting and regurgitation during induction of anaesthesia are encountered most frequently in patients with an acute abdomen or trauma. All patients with minor trauma (fractures or dislocations) must be assumed to have a full stomach; gastric emptying virtually ceases at the time of significant trauma as a result of the combined effects of fear, pain, shock and treatment with opioid analgesics. In all trauma patients, the time interval between ingestion of food and the accident is a more reliable index of the degree of gastric emptying than the period of fasting. It is not uncommon to encounter vomiting up to 24 h after ingestion of food when trauma has occurred very shortly after the meal. Thus the 4–6 h rule is quite unreliable.

Injury from the aspiration of gastric contents results from three different mechanisms: chemical pneumonitis (from acid material), mechanical obstruction from particulate material and bacterial contamination. Aspiration of liquid with a pH < 2.5 is associated with a chemical burn of the bronchial, bronchiolar and alveolar mucosa, leading to atelectasis, pulmonary oedema and reduced pulmonary compliance. Bronchospasm may also be present. The claim that patients are at risk if they have more than 25 ml of gastric residue with a pH < 2.5 is based on data from animal studies extrapolated to humans and should not be regarded as indisputable fact. Day cases often have residual gastric volumes higher than 25 ml.

If aspiration of gastric contents occurs, the first manoeuvre after the airway is secured is to suction the trachea to remove as much foreign material as possible. If particulate matter is obstructing proximal bronchi, bronchoscopy may be necessary. Hypoxaemia is managed with O_2, IPPV and PEEP. Steroids are not recommended and antibiotics should be given if the aspirated material is considered unsterile.

TECHNIQUES OF ANAESTHESIA

It is important to recognize any patient who may have significant gastric residue and who is in danger of aspiration. The anaesthetic management of such a patient may be described in five phases: preparation, induction, maintenance, emergence and postoperative management.

PHASE I – PREPARATION

Whilst postponement of surgery in the emergency patient may be indicated in order to obtain investigations and institute resuscitation with i.v. fluids, there is usually no benefit to be gained in terms of reducing the possibility of aspiration of gastric contents, and the risk of aspiration must be weighed against the risk of delaying an urgent procedure. However, two manoeuvres are available:

- Although not completely effective, insertion of a nasogastric tube to decompress the stomach and to provide a low-pressure vent for regurgitation may be helpful. Aspiration through the tube may be useful if gastric contents are liquid, as in bowel obstruction, but is less effective when contents are solid. Cricoid pressure is still effective at reducing regurgitation even with a nasogastric tube in situ.
- Clear oral antacids (e.g. sodium citrate) may be used to raise the pH of gastric contents immediately before induction. However, this also increases gastric volume. Particulate antacids should not be used, as they can be very damaging to the airway if aspirated. The preoperative administration of H_2-receptor antagonists can consistently raise gastric pH and may reduce the chance of chemical pulmonary injury occurring in the event of inhalation. Although this is standard practice in obstetric anaesthesia, few anaesthetists employ these measures for emergency general surgery. The regimens that may be used are described in Chapters 21 and 52.

PHASE II – INDUCTION

Rapid-sequence induction

This is the technique employed most frequently for the patient with a full stomach, although it contravenes one of the fundamental rules of anaesthesia, namely that muscle relaxants are not given until control of the airway is assured. The decision to employ the rapid-sequence induction technique balances the risk of losing control of the airway against the risk of aspiration. It is therefore imperative to assess carefully whether or not difficulty is likely to be encountered in performing tracheal intubation. The anaesthetist must have prepared a contingency plan for management of the patient should intubation fail. If preoperative evaluation indicates a particularly difficult airway, the anaesthetist should consider alternative methods of proceeding, e.g. local anaesthetic techniques or 'awake intubation' under local anaesthesia.

For rapid-sequence induction to be consistently safe and successful, it should be performed with meticulous attention to detail. The patient *must* be on a tipping trolley or table, preferably with an adjustable headpiece so that the degree of neck extension/flexion may be altered quickly. Ideally, the patient's head should be in the classic 'sniffing position' with the neck flexed on the shoulders and the head extended on the neck. Failure to appreciate this point increases the likelihood of difficult intubation.

The anaesthetist *must* be aided by at least one skilled assistant to perform cricoid pressure, assist in turning the patient, obtain smaller tracheal tubes, supply stilettes for tubes, etc. High volume suction apparatus *must* be functioning and the suction catheter should be within reach of the anaesthetist's hand.

As with any anaesthetic, the machine should have been checked before starting, the ventilator adjusted to appropriate settings and all drugs drawn up into labelled syringes before induction. The patient should breathe 100% O_2 for 3–5 min while appropriate monitoring devices are attached and an i.v. infusion started (if not already in place). The optimal inclination of the operating table is debatable as some authorities recommend the reverse Trendelenburg (head-up) position (to prevent regurgitation) and others the classic Trendelenburg position (to prevent aspiration of any regurgitated or vomited material). In general, the optimum position is that in which the junior anaesthetist has gained greatest experience in performing intubation.

Pre-induction measurement of heart rate, arterial pressure (and, when appropriate, central venous pressure) and inspection of the ECG are made and a skilled assistant is positioned on the patient's right side to perform Sellick's manoeuvre (cricoid pressure). It is important that the assistant can identify the cricoid cartilage, as compression of the thyroid cartilage distorts laryngeal anatomy and may render tracheal intubation very difficult. To perform Sellick's manoeuvre correctly, the thumb and forefinger of the right hand press the cricoid cartilage firmly in a posterior direction, thus compressing the oesophagus between the cricoid cartilage and the vertebral column. Because the cricoid cartilage forms a complete ring, the tracheal lumen is not distorted (Fig. 51.1).

Opinions differ with regard to the time at which cricoid pressure should be applied. Some prefer to inform the patient and apply it just before administration of the i.v. induction agent; others apply it as soon as consciousness is lost.

With the assistant in position, a predetermined sleep dose of i.v. induction agent is given (usually thiopental 4 mg kg^{-1} or less in the presence of hypovolaemia). Without waiting to assess the effect of the induction agent, a paralysing dose of succinylcholine (1.5 mg kg^{-1}) is administered immediately. As soon as the jaw begins to relax, laryngoscopy is performed and the trachea intubated. Cricoid pressure is maintained until the cuff of the tracheal tube is inflated and correct placement of the tube ascertained by auscultation of both lungs. The lungs are gently ventilated manually, as excessive increases in intrathoracic pressure may have harmful effects on circulatory dynamics. One of the main disadvantages of the rapid-sequence induction technique is the haemodynamic instability which may result if the dose of induction agent is excessive (hypotension, circulatory collapse) or inadequate (hypertension, tachycardia, arrhythmia). Unfortunately, selection of the correct dose is difficult and is dependent largely upon the experience of the anaesthetist. For thiopental, a dose of 4 mg kg^{-1} may suffice for healthy, young patients, 2 mg kg^{-1} for the elderly and less for the very frail. An alternative is etomidate 0.1–0.3 mg kg^{-1} (which, in equipotent doses, is less cardiodepressant than thiopental).

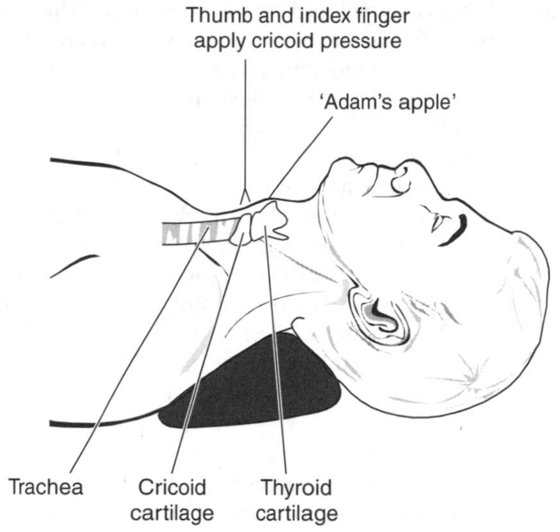

Fig. 51.1
Sellick's manoeuvre. The cricoid carilage is palpated immediately below the thyroid cartilage.

Inhalation induction

If there is reasonable doubt about the ability to perform intubation or to maintain a patent airway in a patient with a full stomach (e.g. the patient with faciomaxillary trauma or the child with epiglottitis or bleeding tonsil), an inhalation induction may be used with oxygen and halothane. When the patient has reached a deep plane of anaesthesia, laryngoscopy is performed followed by an attempt at tracheal intubation during spontaneous ventilation. Normally, the patient should be placed in the left lateral, head-down position, but if circumstances do not allow the lateral position then the supine posture with cricoid pressure may have to be accepted.

Awake intubation

Although blind nasal intubation is a valuable skill, the introduction of the narrow-bore fibreoptic intubating laryngoscope has replaced it as the technique of choice in those patients who are likely to develop unrelievable airway obstruction when loss of consciousness occurs (e.g. trismus from dental abscess or a known difficult intubation). Before embarking on awake fibreoptic nasal intubation, it is necessary to render the nasopharynx and, to a greater or lesser extent, the upper airway insensitive, so that the introduction of a tracheal tube may be tolerated. The details of the technique differ depending on the preference of the individual anaesthetist and one method that is employed commonly is described below:

1. The nasal mucosa is anaesthetized with cocaine solution 4% (maximum 2.5 ml per 70 kg) which is sprayed into the more patent nasal passage. In addition to providing surface anaesthesia, this shrinks the nasal mucosa and reduces the chance of bleeding. A well lubricated, soft nasopharyngeal airway (size 6 or 7) is then gently inserted into the nasopharynx and left in situ for 3–5 min. Lidocaine is sprayed through the nasopharyngeal airway to anaesthetize the oropharynx and supraglottic area.
2. Anaesthesia of the tracheal mucosa below the vocal cords is accomplished best by transtracheal injection of local anaesthetic. A 21 gauge needle is introduced in the midline through the cricothyroid membrane. Entry into the trachea is confirmed by aspiration of air and a bolus of 3–5 ml of lidocaine 1% is injected rapidly. Invariably this results in a bout of coughing which aids spread of the local anaesthetic over the inferior surface of the vocal cords. This procedure may be omitted if the risk of aspiration is considered high, as anaesthesia of the upper airway increases the risk of pulmonary aspiration if vomiting or regurgitation occurs.

For patients in whom there is a high risk of aspiration, it is possible with experience to perform awake nasal intubation after performing only step 1 above and employing a 'spray as you go' technique, injecting aliquots of lidocaine through the suction port of the fibreoptic laryngoscope as it is advanced.

The nasopharyngeal airway is removed and, with the patient's head in the 'sniffing the morning air' position, a well lubricated, reinforced endotracheal tube (size 6 or 7) is inserted gently into the anaesthetized nostril and advanced towards the nasopharynx. The tube should be rotated slowly between thumb and forefinger (pill-rolling movement) and a distinct 'give' is felt on entry into the nasopharynx. Whilst maintaining optimal head position, the fibreoptic laryngoscope is then advanced through the endotracheal tube and the pharynx and laryngeal aperture are visualized. As maximal vocal cord abduction occurs during inspiration, the scope is advanced slowly in small steps coordinated with inspiration. Even with good upper airway anaesthesia, entry into the larynx results frequently in a violent cough. Once through the larynx, the position of the scope is confirmed by visual recognition of tracheal rings and the endotracheal tube is railroaded gently over the scope into the trachea. Position is again confirmed by seeing tracheal rings and the scope removed.

Although considerable practice is needed in the operation of this instrument to ensure a successful outcome, attention to the details of the technique improves the chance of success.

Regional anaesthesia

Anaesthetic expertise in the use of regional anaesthesia is lacking in many UK hospitals. This is unfortunate, as local blocks are eminently suitable for emergency procedures on the extremities (e.g. to reduce fractures or dislocations).

Brachial plexus block by the axillary, supraclavicular or interscalene approach is satisfactory for orthopaedic manipulations or surgical procedures involving the upper extremity. It satisfies surgical requirements for analgesia, muscle relaxation and immobility. There is minimal effect on the cardiovascular system and there is a prolonged period of analgesia postoperatively. Similarly, i.v. regional anaesthesia is useful for orthopaedic reductions; prilocaine 0.5% plain is the drug of choice.

For regional anaesthesia of the lower extremity, techniques available include subarachnoid, epidural and sciatic/femoral blocks. Spinal and epidural blocks are contraindicated if there is doubt about the adequacy of extracellular fluid or vascular volumes, as large decreases in arterial pressure may result from the associated pharmacological sympathectomy.

It is a common surgical misconception that subarachnoid or epidural anaesthetic techniques are safer than general anaesthesia for patients in poor physical condition. It must be emphasized that for the *inexperienced* anaesthetist, these techniques are invariably more dangerous than general anaesthesia for the patient with moderate/major trauma or any intra-abdominal emergency condition.

PHASE III – MAINTENANCE OF ANAESTHESIA

In emergency anaesthesia, there are strong arguments in favour of a balanced technique of anaesthesia combining:

- anaesthesia – loss of awareness
- analgesia to attenuate autonomic reflexes in response to the painful stimulus
- muscle relaxation.

If a rapid-sequence induction has been performed, the patient's lungs are gently ventilated manually whilst heart rate and arterial pressure measurements are repeated to assess the cardiovascular effects of the drugs used and of the insult of tracheal intubation. Nitrous oxide 50–66% (dependent upon the patient's condition) in oxygen contributes to loss of patient awareness but does not ensure it and some anaesthetists advocate the use of 0.5–1% isoflurane or 0.5–1% enflurane in addition.

When there is evidence of return of neuromuscular transmission (by clinical signs or use of a nerve stimulator) as succinylcholine is degraded, a non-depolarizing myoneural blocking agent is administered. The choice is dependent upon the patient's condition and the effect of the induction of anaesthesia on the patient's cardiovascular status. Rocuronium and atracurium are both appropriate drugs for routine use. Pancuronium (dose 50–100 μg kg^{-1}) is useful in patients with hypovolaemia, as it tends to increase arterial pressure and heart rate. (The tachycardia it produces is undesirable in patients with ischaemic heart disease or valvular disease.) Atracurium has virtually no cardiovascular effects in clinical doses and is useful if renal impairment is present.

When the muscle relaxant has been administered, the tracheal tube is connected to a mechanical ventilator and minute volume adjusted to produce normo- or slight hypocapnia. There are few accurate means of estimating ventilatory requirement, but a minute volume of 100 ml kg^{-1} min^{-1} at a tidal volume of 8–12 ml kg^{-1} should be employed initially. The inspiratory flow rate should be adjusted to minimize peak airway pressure.

Before the initial surgical incision is made, analgesia may be supplemented by small incremental doses of morphine 1–5 mg or fentanyl 25–100 μg.

The use of supplemental doses of analgesic and muscle relaxant drugs is described in Chapters 10 and 11. The trainee should be aware that during emergency anaesthesia, particularly for intra-abdominal or trauma surgery, much smaller doses of drugs are usually required. As a general rule, it is safe practice to administer half the dose, which might be considered appropriate for an elective patient, and to determine further doses by assessment of the subsequent response. If there are poor or inadequate recovery room facilities, it is also a good general rule to err on the side of caution in the use of i.v. drugs.

Fluid management

During emergency intra-abdominal surgery, there may be large blood and fluid losses which exceed the patient's maintenance fluid replacement. These include evaporative losses from exposed gut and mesentery, blood loss on to swabs and into suction bottles, and the poorly defined 'third space' losses caused by sequestration of fluid in inflamed and traumatized tissue. Intraoperatively, maintenance requirements are supplied with Hartmann's solution (compound sodium lactate) at 2 ml kg^{-1} h^{-1}. An appropriate volume of replacement for third-space loss and evaporative gut loss is given in addition. This volume depends on the degree of surgical trauma but is normally in the range 2–7 ml kg^{-1} h^{-1}.

Haemorrhage in excess of 15% blood volume in adults or 10% in children is usually an indication for blood transfusion.

PHASE IV – REVERSAL AND EMERGENCE

Any volatile agent is discontinued 5 min before surgery finishes. On insertion of the last skin suture, direct pharyngoscopy is performed and secretions/debris removed from the pharynx; if a nasogastric tube is in situ, it is aspirated and left unspigoted. Glycopyrrolate and neostigmine are given in one bolus of 20 and 50 μg kg^{-1}, respectively, and ventilation is undertaken manually (with an F_IO_2 of 1.0) so that spontaneous ventilatory activity may be detected. Because the risk of aspiration of gastric contents is as great on recovery as at induction, extubation of the trachea should not be performed until protective airway reflexes are intact. To demonstrate the adequacy of reflexes, both level of consciousness and neuromuscular transmission should be assessed.

Level of consciousness

The patient should be awake and respond appropriately to verbal commands, e.g. eye opening.

Neuromuscular function

The adequacy of reversal of paralysis may be determined by observing the patient's ability to sustain a head lift for 5 s and sustain a firm grip without fade. Preferably, a nerve stimulator is used to define reversal of neuromuscular transmission (see Ch. 19).

Immediately before tracheal extubation, the patient is turned to the lateral position (if possible) and asked to take a deep inspiration while gentle positive pressure is applied to the airway. At the peak of inspiration, the cuff is deflated and the tracheal tube removed as the patient exhales, thus assisting removal of any secretions which may have accumulated above the cuff. Oxygen 100% is administered until a regular ventilatory rhythm is re-established and the patient has demonstrated an ability to cough and maintain a patent airway. Breathing 40% O_2, the patient is transported in the lateral position to the recovery room and remains there until all vital signs are stable, postoperative shivering has ceased, core temperature is normal and there is good perfusion as judged by warm extremities and good urine output.

If there is any doubt about the adequacy of ventilation after reversal of neuromuscular blockade, the patient is taken to the recovery room with the tracheal tube in situ and this is removed from the trachea only when ventilation and gas exchange are adequate.

PHASE V – POSTOPERATIVE MANAGEMENT

Postoperatively, the patient requires analgesics, e.g. morphine 0.2 mg kg^{-1} i.m. 4-hourly or as patient-controlled analgesia, if appropriate. If there is continued concern about the metabolic or volaemic state of the patient, these dosages should be reduced considerably. Fluid balance should take into account maintenance needs plus compensation for abnormal fluid loss (e.g. gastric aspirate, loss from intestinal fistulae or from surgical drains). This subject is discussed in Chapter 39.

The need for further blood replacement is assessed by regular observation of vital signs and drainage measurements and postoperative Hb or haematocrit measurements.

Prophylactic postoperative IPPV

Continuation of IPPV should be considered electively in several circumstances, some of which are listed in Table 51.4.

Table 51.4 Indications for continuation of ventilatory assistance postoperatively

Prolonged shock/hypoperfusion state of any cause
Massive sepsis (faecal peritonitis, cholangitis, septicaemia)
Severe ischaemic heart disease
Extreme obesity
Overt gastric acid aspiration
Previously severe pulmonary disease

THE ANAESTHETIST AND MAJOR TRAUMA

The management of the patient with major trauma requires a multidisciplinary team effort. Successful treatment is often dependent on the efficacy of the initial resuscitation and rapid formulation of the correct priorities. In many hospitals, the anaesthetic/ICU trainee is an integral member of the 'trauma team', which is called whenever a multiply injured patient is expected. Increasingly, trauma management is based on Advanced Trauma Life Support (ATLS) teaching and it is important that the trainee is familiar with major ATLS protocols.

The suggested scheme for trauma management is as follows:

1. *Rapid primary survey.* Recognition and treatment of any *immediately* life-threatening complications, such as airway obstruction, tension/open pneumothorax, massive haemothorax, haemoperitoneum, flail chest, cardiac tamponade or intracranial injury.
2. *Resuscitation of vital functions.* Haemorrhage control, intravenous access and volume resuscitation.
3. *Detailed secondary survey.* Recognition of any *potentially* life-threatening injuries, such as ruptured aorta, pulmonary/cardiac contusions, diaphragmatic rupture, haemoretroperitoneum and pelvic disruption.
4. *Definitive care.*

Steps 1 and 2 are performed simultaneously. The anaesthetic trainee may be involved in any or all of the above areas of management.

PRIMARY SURVEY/RESUSCITATION OF VITAL FUNCTIONS

As soon as the patient arrives in the accident and emergency department, a rapid primary survey is performed at the same time as resuscitation of vital functions. The approach is similar for all ill patients and the trainee should look for and treat:

- airway obstruction – effective airway management is paramount; hypoxaemia and hypercapnia are extremely undesirable and their avoidance must be guaranteed
- breathing difficulty due to pneumothorax or flail chest
- circulatory shock and the need for control of obvious bleeding.

Airway/breathing

The first priority for the anaesthetist when confronted with an unconscious trauma victim is to establish the patency of the patient's airway whilst assuring immobilization of the cervical spine. If upper airway obstruction is present, the pharynx is cleared of any debris and the jaw displaced forward (jaw thrust). Neck tilt and chin lift are avoided as these manoeuvres could displace an unstable cervical spine. Early establishment of a patent airway is paramount to successful resuscitation and although unstable cervical spine injuries are relatively uncommon, *all* patients should be assumed to be at risk until proven otherwise. Exclusion of this injury will require cervical spine radiography and possibly computed tomography (CT). No patient should remain even marginally hypoxaemic for the purposes of clinical assessment, but in the alert patient who is to have a semi-urgent intubation, consideration should be given to clinical exclusion of cervical spine injury, flail chest, abdominal tenderness etc.

When the airway is clear, attention is directed to the adequacy of ventilation and the need for tracheal intubation. If the patient is apnoeic, ventilation by mask with 100% oxygen is started immediately, as good oxygenation and correction of hypercapnia should be ensured before tracheal intubation is undertaken. The possibility of a cervical spine injury does not contraindicate orotracheal intubation provided it is performed with care *and* in-line immobilization of the cervical spine is maintained throughout the procedure.

In general, airway assessment reveals one of three clinical scenarios:

- *Patient is conscious, alert, talking.* Give high-flow oxygen via face mask. There is no need for immediate airway intervention and a full clinical evaluation can be done. Persisting signs of shock and/or the diagnosis of serious underlying injuries might be an indication for planned endotracheal intubation and mechanical ventilation.
- *Patient has a reduced conscious level but some degree of airway control and gag reflex still present.* If the patient is maintaining the airway and breathing adequately then there is no need for immediate intervention. Endotracheal intubation will be necessary but a clinical evaluation can be done whilst equipment is being readied.
- *Patient has a reduced conscious level, gag reflex absent.* If the patient is unable to maintain the airway or is breathing poorly, intubation and ventilation should be carried out at once.

All trauma patients are intubated via the orotracheal route using a rapid-sequence induction with in-line stabilization of the cervical spine. The dose of induction agent is judged bearing in mind the patient's cardiovascular state and the possibility of intracranial injury. If there are clinical signs suggesting a pneumothorax or surgical emphysema and/or a flail segment is apparent then a chest drain should be inserted simultaneously or before mechanical ventilation is commenced. Persistence of hypoxaemia after institution of mechanical ventilation suggests unrecognized pneumothorax, haemothorax, pulmonary contusion or poor cardiac output due to hypovolaemia, tamponade etc.

Patients with severe faciomaxillary trauma who are cooperative and awake despite their injuries may not require immediate tracheal intubation, but do need frequent and regular upper airway evaluation to assess the rate of progress of pharyngeal or laryngeal oedema which may proceed to complete airway obstruction with alarming rapidity.

When the airway is under control, ventilation is deemed adequate and any obvious external bleeding has been arrested, the next priority is evaluation of the cardiovascular system; this may be divided into assessment of blood volume status and pump function.

Circulation

This has been described earlier in this chapter. Haemorrhage is the most common cause of shock in the injured patient and virtually all patients with multiple injuries have an element of hypovolaemia. Patients with major trauma often require urgent restoration of circulating blood volume. At least two large-gauge (14-gauge) i.v. cannulae are inserted percutaneously into veins in one or two limbs and both cannulae are attached to blood warming coils. Isotonic electrolyte solutions are used for initial resuscitation and 1–2 L of Hartmann's solution is given as rapidly as possible and the patient's response is assessed. If this does not increase perfusion and arterial pressure significantly and crossmatched blood is not yet available, either plasma or a plasma substitute should be considered. Human albumin solution is very expensive and probably has little advantage over starch and gelatin solutions. Their half-life in the circulation is approximately 4 h in the normal patient, but is shorter in the presence of shock. As 85% is excreted by the kidneys, gelatin solutions promote an osmotic diuresis and may therefore preserve urine output and renal function. Up to 1500 ml may be given initially; in most circumstances this is adequate to restore circulating blood volume until crossmatched blood is available. Warmed, stored blood is administered subsequently to maintain urine output, arterial pressure and CVP. As soon as possible, a reliable CVP catheter is inserted. The right internal jugular vein is the preferred site for this purpose. Fluid is infused through the peripheral i.v. cannulae to produce a CVP of approximately 5–10 mmHg (zero reference mid-axillary line).

Whilst whole blood is the ideal fluid for restoration of blood volume in haemorrhagic shock, if the patient is exsanguinating (> 40% blood loss), a synthetic colloid (gelatin or hydroxyethylstarch) should be given immediately while crossmatching is undertaken. Type-specific blood may be given, as the chance of a reaction is less than 1% in males (over 2% in parous females), but in this situation the imperative is on the diagnosis and surgical management of the source of haemorrhage. If the breach in the circulation is large then the prime objective of resuscitation is to maintain cerebral and coronary perfusion whilst control of the source of bleeding is accomplished, *not* to restore a normal blood pressure.

Pump function

The commonest cause of pump failure in major trauma is the presence of a tension pneumothorax, but other possibilities include severe myocardial contusion and traumatic pericardial tamponade.

Tension pneumothorax causes compression of the mediastinum (heart and great vessels) and presents with extreme respiratory distress, shock, unilateral air entry, a shift of the trachea towards the normal side and distension of the veins in the neck, although the last sign may not be seen in hypovolaemic shock. It may be relieved immediately by insertion of a 14-gauge cannula through the second intercostal space in the midclavicular line, but this should be followed by standard chest drainage. If there is any suspicion of tension pneumothorax, IPPV should not be instituted until decompression has been achieved, otherwise mediastinal compression is increased. Patients with blunt chest trauma and fractured ribs may develop a tension pneumothorax rapidly when positive pressure ventilation is commenced and consideration should be given to the prophylactic insertion of chest drains in such patients.

DEFINITIVE CARE

Whenever possible, hypovolaemia should be corrected before anaesthesia is induced, but if the rate of haemorrhage is likely to exceed the rate of transfusion and continued transfusion results only in further bleeding (e.g. ruptured aorta), it is necessary to induce anaesthesia in a hypovolaemic patient.

On arrival in theatre, the patient is placed on the operating table, which is covered by a warming blanket at 37°C. One hundred per cent oxygen is given whilst at least two large-gauge cannulae are inserted (each connected to a blood warming coil), if this has not already been accomplished. In patients with major trauma, anaesthesia should be induced in theatre so that surgery can start as soon as possible. Figure 51.2 illustrates standard monitoring which is necessary for the management of major trauma. In the unconscious patient, the trachea may be intubated after administration of a paralysing dose of succinylcholine. If the patient is conscious, despite being severely hypovolaemic, a controlled rapid-sequence induction using ketamine as the i.v. induction agent is preferred. The dose of ketamine is critical and often very small doses (0.3–0.7 mg kg^{-1}) suffice. If the dose is misjudged, cardiovascular decompensation similar to that seen with other i.v. induction agents may occur. The depressant effects of i.v. induction agents are exaggerated because the *proportion* of the cardiac output going to the heart and brain is increased. In addition, the rate of redistribution and/or metabolism is decreased as a result of reduced blood flow to muscle, liver and kidneys and thus blood concentrations remain elevated for longer periods in comparison with healthy patients. Ketamine should not be used in patients with significant head injury. Etomidate (0.1–0.3 mg kg^{-1}) is an alternative for normovolaemic patients with head injury, but is more likely to attenuate compensatory mechanisms. Even a single bolus dose of etomidate may interfere with adrenal function and recommendations concerning the use of this drug must be guarded.

After tracheal intubation, the lungs are ventilated at the lowest peak airway pressure consistent with an acceptable tidal volume. Pancuronium or rocuronium is given in small incremental doses of 1 or 5 mg, respectively, to maintain relaxation. When the haemodynamic situation has stabilized and systolic arterial pressure exceeds 90 mmHg, consideration may be given to deepening anaesthesia. This should be undertaken cautiously and, in principle, agents which are rapidly reversible or rapidly excreted should be used.

In the shock state, there is very rapid uptake of inhalation agents. As a result of chemoreceptor stimulation, the patient hyperventilates, thus accelerating the rate of increase of alveolar concentration of anaesthetic gas. Similarly, reduced cardiac output and pulmonary blood flow decrease the rate of removal of anaesthetic agent from the alveoli, producing a rapid increase in alveolar concentration. Thus the MAC value is approached more rapidly than in normovolaemic patients.

Monitoring should be comprehensive in these patients (Fig. 51.2) and should be commenced before induction of anaesthesia when feasible. Blood may be sampled from the arterial line to monitor changes in acid–base state, haemoglobin concentration, coagulation and electrolyte concentrations. Requirements for further colloid replacement may be assessed from CVP measurement and urine output.

When surgical bleeding has been controlled, the patient's cardiovascular status should improve, but if hypotension persists despite apparently adequate fluid administration, other causes of haemorrhage should be sought (Table 51.5). It is important that the anaesthetist assesses the patient regularly during prolonged anaesthesia to exclude these latent complications of major trauma.

MASSIVE TRANSFUSION

One definition states that if an amount greater than 50% of the patient's blood volume is replaced rapidly, the transfusion is deemed massive, e.g. 5 units of blood in 1 h in a 70 kg adult. Stored blood is an unphysiological solution with a pH of 6.6–7.2, serum potassium concentration of 5–25 mmol L^{-1} and a temperature of 4–6°C. It contains citrate as an anticoagulant. When stored for more than 5 days, it contains insignificant amounts of 2,3-DPG; consequently the oxygen dissociation curve is shifted to the left. Blood stored for more than 24 h has no functional platelets; concentrations of factors V and VIII are approximately 10% of normal, and of factor IX 20% of normal. Effete cells and platelets clump together, forming debris that is potentially harmful when infused in sufficient quantity. However, many of these disadvantages of stored blood are not clinical problems. For example, citrate is removed by metabolic conversion in the liver (forming mostly bicarbonate), the transfused cells act as a potassium 'sink' and mop up excess potassium quickly, and the post-transfusion alkalosis (resulting from citrate metabolism) may contribute to hypokalaemia in the post-transfusion period. If the transfused blood is warmed to body temperature before transfusion and a 20 micron filter is used to remove unwanted cellular debris, the commonest problem is acute haemostatic failure.

Transfusion of bank blood in quantities approaching the patient's blood volume causes a dilutional thrombocytopenia and some degree of clotting factor deficiency, both of which affect haemostasis adversely. These abnormalities may be detected by a platelet count, prothrombin time and partial thromboplastin time, reflecting disorders of extrinsic and intrinsic systems as a result of dilutional loss of factors V and VIII. Treatment should be directed at correcting the dilutional coagulation change and consists of fresh frozen plasma (at least 1 unit for every 4 units of blood), platelet concentrate for severe thrombocytopenia (platelet count less than 30 × 10^9 L^{-1}) or milder thrombocytopenia in patients

Table 51.5 Causes of persistent hypotension

Cause	
Continued overt bleeding Continued concealed bleeding – chest, abdomen, retroperitoneal space, pelvis, soft tissues of each thigh	Surgical or medical (check platelets and clotting screen)
Pump failure – haemothorax, pneumothorax, tamponade, myocardial contusion	
Metabolic problem – acidaemia (only correct pH less than 7.1), hypothermia (largely preventable), hypocalcaemia	

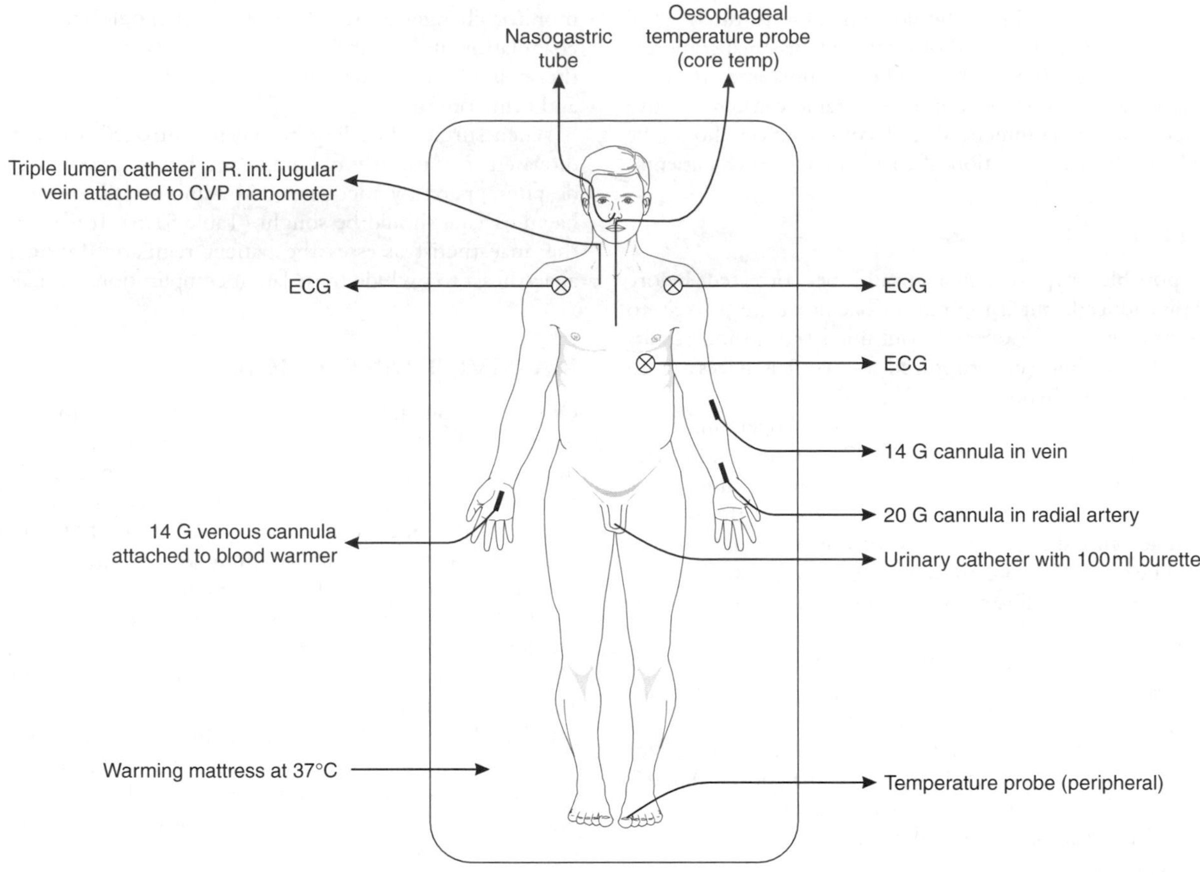

Fig. 51.2
Commonly used monitoring and resuscitation attachments in management of a patient with multiple injuries. Pulse oximetry and capnography are also used during anaesthesia.

with possible intracranial injury. Requests for these expensive blood products should be made early as there is often delay in obtaining them and it is better, if possible, to prevent the development of coagulation failure and the resulting bleeding tendency. Although diffuse pathological bleeding may be secondary to dilutional effects, it is also a manifestation of tissue hypoperfusion due to shock and inadequate or delayed resuscitation. Clinically, this microvascular bleeding produces oozing from mucosae, raw surfaces and puncture sites and may increase the extent of soft tissue and pulmonary contusions. It is difficult to treat and this underscores the importance of rapid and adequate resuscitation.

The rapid and effective restoration of an adequate circulating blood volume is crucial in the management of major haemorrhage, as mortality increases with increasing duration and severity of shock. Inadequate volume replacement is the most common complication of haemorrhagic shock. The importance of the prevention of hypothermia during massive transfusion cannot be overstated. Hypothermia causes platelet dysfunction, reduced metabolism of citrate and lactate and an increased tendency to cardiac arrhythmias, which may result in a bleeding diathesis, hypocalcaemia, metabolic acidaemia and cardiac arrest. Core temperature should be measured continuously during massive transfusion and every effort must be made to prevent heat loss. Thermally insulating plastic drapes can be used to cover the patient, who should be placed on a heated 'ripple' mattress. A heated water bath humidifier is more efficient than the disposable heat and moisture exchangers. Efficient systems for heating stored blood and allowing rapid infusion are available, but all fluids should be warmed to body temperature if possible.

FURTHER READING

American College of Surgeons 1997 Advanced trauma life support program for doctors, 6th edn. American College of Surgeons, Chicago

Horsey P J 1997 Major trauma and massive transfusion. Anaesthesia 52: 1027–1029

Nimmo W S, Rowbotham D J, Smith G (eds) 1994 Anaesthesia, 2nd edn. Blackwell Scientific Publications, London

52 Obstetric anaesthesia and analgesia

Obstetric anaesthesia and analgesia involve caring for women during childbirth in three situations:

- Provision of analgesia for labour, usually by epidural or spinal analgesic techniques.
- Anaesthesia for instrumental (e.g. forceps or Ventouse) or caesarean delivery.
- Care of the critically ill parturient.

The obstetric anaesthetist is involved in the care of the parturient as part of a multidisciplinary team, including obstetricians, midwives, health visitors and physicians. There are few other areas of anaesthetic practice where communication skills and good record-keeping are so important. Successive reports from the Confidential Enquiries into Maternal Deaths (CEMD) have highlighted the problems of women with intercurrent medical disease and the importance of the obstetric anaesthetist in their care. This has led to the establishment of obstetric anaesthetic assessment clinics in many hospitals. The education of colleagues, patients and the public about the role of obstetric anaesthetists is essential so that patients are fully informed and hence feel more comfortable about consenting to regional anaesthesia and analgesia techniques when these may be indicated.

Many anaesthetists in training approach their obstetric module with trepidation for several possible reasons: all anaesthetists have heard that mothers may die, albeit rarely, as a result of general anaesthesia and that these were previously healthy young women. In addition, they may be aware of the challenge of performing regional blocks under the scrutiny of a partner in patients who are awake.

The Obstetric Anaesthetists' Association (OAA) recommendations for modular training in obstetric anaesthesia categorize the training modules into basic and advanced. In the obstetric anaesthetic module, trainees are expected to develop communication, organizational and technical skills. The OAA core curriculum provides the framework for this chapter and it is summarized under the following headings:

- anatomy and physiology of pregnancy
- basic obstetrics
- gastrointestinal physiology and antacid therapy
- pain and pain relief in labour
- epidural and subarachnoid analgesia
- regional anaesthesia for the parturient
- general anaesthesia for the parturient
- assessment of the pregnant woman presenting for anaesthesia and analgesia
- emergencies in obstetric anaesthesia:
  - — major haemorrhage
  - — failed intubation
  - — pre-eclampsia and eclampsia
  - — total spinal or epidural block
  - — amniotic fluid embolus
  - — maternal and neonatal resuscitation
- anaesthesia for interventions other than delivery
- audit
- pharmacology of relevant drugs.

ANATOMY AND PHYSIOLOGY OF PREGNANCY

The reader is referred to Chapter 10 for an outline of the physiology of pregnancy.

PAIN PATHWAYS IN LABOUR AND CAESAREAN SECTION

The afferent nerve supply of the uterus and cervix is via Aδ and C fibres that accompany the thoracolumbar and sacral sympathetic outflows. The pain of the first stage of labour is referred to the spinal cord segments associated with the uterus and the cervix, namely T10, 11, 12 and L1. Pain of distension of the birth canal and perineum is conveyed via S2–S4 nerves (Fig. 52.1). When anaesthesia is required for caesarean section, all the layers between the skin and the uterus must be anaesthetized. It is important to remember that the most sensitive layer is the peritoneum, and therefore the block should extend up to at least T4 and also include the sacral roots (S1–S5).

ANATOMY OF THE EPIDURAL SPACE

The epidural space is the space between the periosteal lining of the vertebral canal and the spinal dura mater. It contains spinal nerve roots, lymphatics, blood vessels and a variable amount of fat (Figs 52.2 and 52.3). Its boundaries are as follows:

- *superiorly* – the foramen magnum, where the dural layers fuse with the periosteum of the cranium; hence local anaesthetic solution placed in the epidural space cannot extend higher than this
- *inferiorly* – the sacrococcygeal membrane

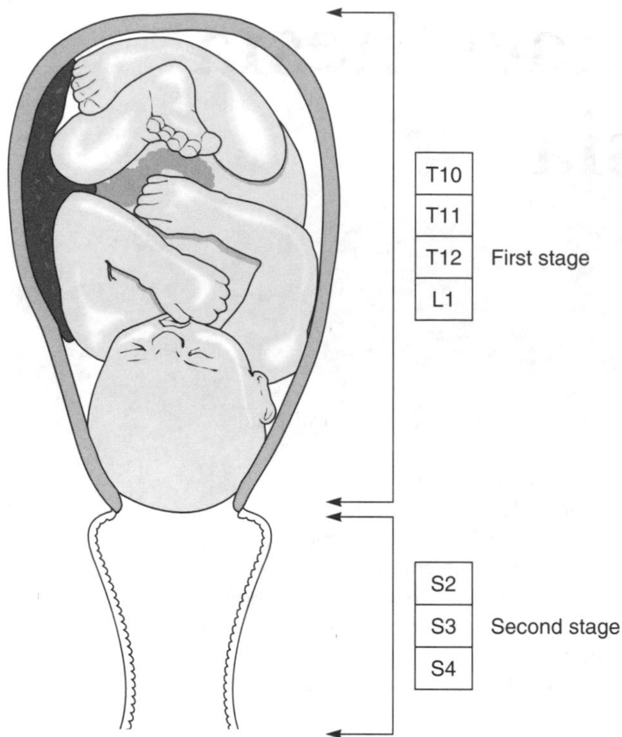

Fig. 52.1
Nerve supply to the uterus and birth canal.

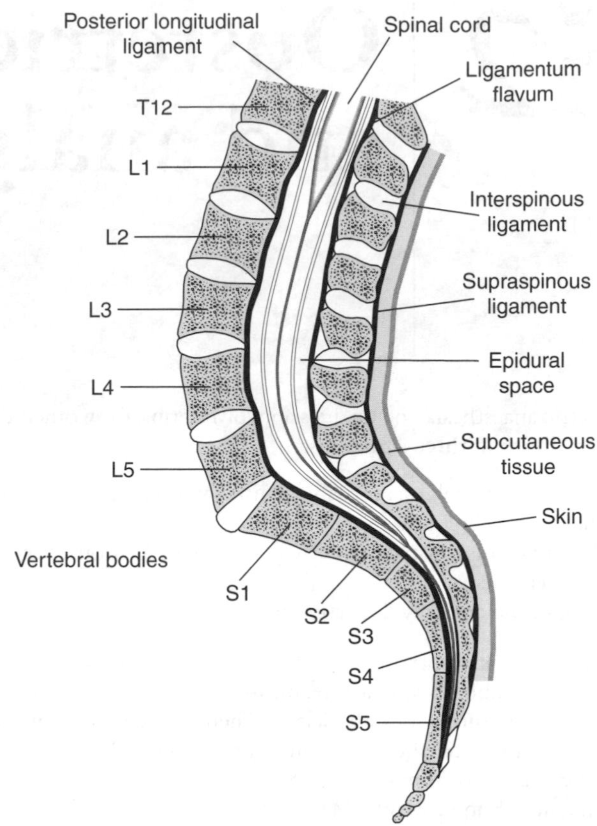

Fig. 52.2
The vertebral column. Note that the spinal cord ends at the level of L1 or L2 and that the dural sac extends to the level of S2 vertebra.

- *anteriorly* – the posterior longitudinal ligament
- *posteriorly* – the ligamentum flavum and vertebral laminae
- *laterally* – the pedicles of the vertebrae and the intervertebral foramina.

In the normal adult, the spinal cord begins at the foramen magnum and ends at the level of L1 or L2 where it becomes the cauda equina. The epidural space is a tube containing the spinal cord, the cerebrospinal fluid (CSF) and the meninges. It is crossed by 32 spinal nerves, each with a dural cuff: therefore it is a leaky tube. The subarachnoid space extends further than the cord, to the level of S2. Below this level, the dura blends with the periosteum of the coccyx. Between the dura and arachnoid is the subdural space, within which local anaesthetic solution may spread extensively.

ANATOMY AND PHYSIOLOGY OF THE AIRWAY IN PREGNANCY

The incidence of difficult intubation in term parturients is approximately 1 in 300 cases, compared with 1 in 2200 in the non-pregnant population. This is caused in part by the physiological changes of pregnancy which affect the airway (Table 52.1). These factors increase the difficulty in seeing the larynx and increase the rate at which hypoxaemia develops in an apnoeic patient.

Table 52.1 Physiological changes of pregnancy which increase the risk of hypoxaemia
Interstitial oedema of the upper airway, especially in pre-eclampsia
Enlarged tongue and epiglottis
Enlarged, heavy breasts which may impede laryngoscope introduction
Increased oxygen consumption
Restricted diaphragmatic movement, reducing FRC

BASIC OBSTETRICS

NORMAL LABOUR

A large number of pregnant women are assessed as being 'low risk' and are predicted to have a normal labour, but the diagnosis of normal labour is retrospective. The descriptors of normal labour are:

- contractions occurring every 3 min and lasting 45 s
- progressive dilatation of the cervix (approximately 1 cm h^{-1})
- progressive descent of the presenting part
- vertex presenting with the head flexed and the occiput anterior
- labour not < 4 h (precipitate) or > 18 h (prolonged)
- delivery of a live healthy baby
- delivery of a complete placenta and membranes
- no complications.

The first stage of labour

Initially, the cervix effaces (i.e. becomes thin along its vertical axis and soft in consistency) and then cervical dilatation begins. The

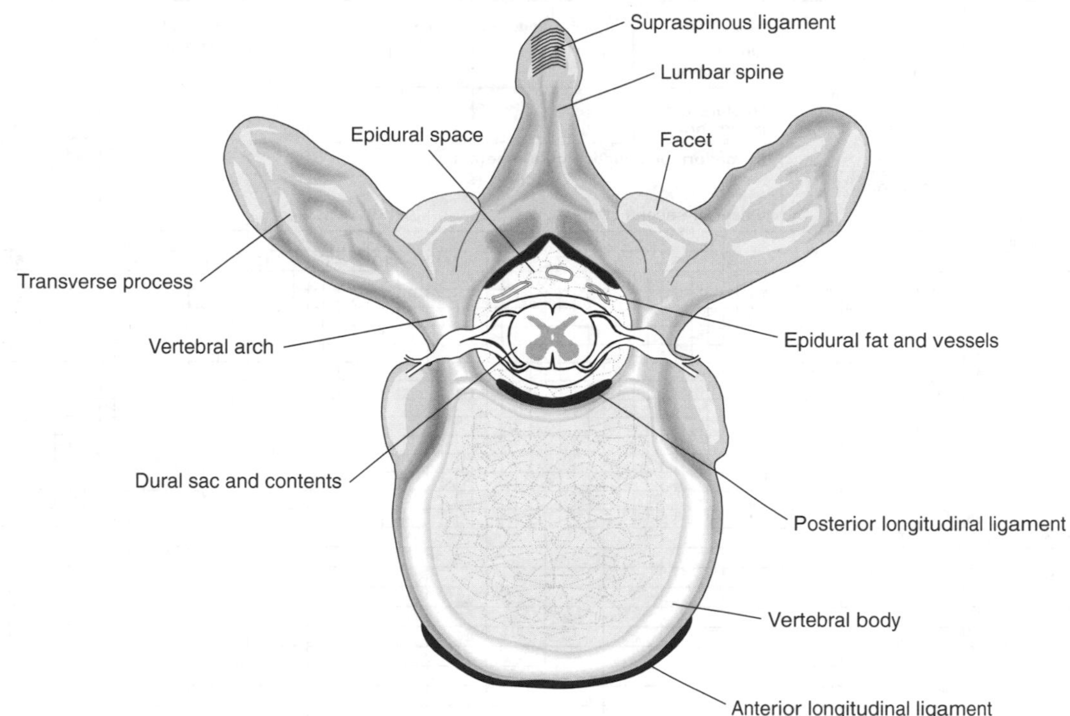

Fig. 52.3
Anatomical relations of the epidural space.

rate of cervical dilatation should be about 1 cm h^{-1} for a primiparous woman and 2 cm h^{-1} for a multigravid woman. It is standard practice to examine the woman every 4 h, or more frequently if there is cause for concern. Routine observations are made as follows and these are charted on the partogram (Fig. 52.4):

- fetal heart rate every 15 min
- maternal pulse rate half-hourly
- BP half-hourly
- temperature 4-hourly
- urinalysis at each emptying of the bladder.

The fetal heart may be monitored intermittently by auscultation using Pinard's stethoscope or by cardiotocographic monitoring. The cardiotocograph is recorded either intermittently or continuously depending on the conditions of the labour and fetus. The fetal heart may be recorded using either an abdominal transducer or a clip applied to the fetal head. Radiotelemetry is available in some units and this allows the woman to be mobile while her baby is monitored.

The second stage of labour

The second stage of labour commences at full dilatation of the cervix and terminates at the delivery of the baby. At full dilatation of the cervix, the character of the contractions changes and they become associated with a strong urge to push. In normal labour, Ferguson's reflex occurs, where there is an increase in circulating oxytocin secondary to distension of the vagina from the descending presenting part of the fetus, with consequent increased strength of uterine contractions at full dilatation. Epidural analgesia may attenuate the effect of this reflex. The second stage of labour may be classified into passive and active stages and this is particularly relevant when epidural analgesia is used. With epidural analgesia, the labouring woman does not have the normal sensation at the start of the second stage of labour produced by Ferguson's reflex, and therefore the active stage of pushing should commence only when the vertex is visible or the woman has a strong urge to push. A normal active second stage should not exceed 1 h of active pushing as the fetus may become acidotic. At the delivery of the anterior shoulder, intramuscular oxytocin is given to hasten the delivery of the placenta and to stimulate uterine contraction.

The third stage of labour

The third stage of labour is the complete delivery of the placenta, membranes and the contraction of the uterus. It is usually managed actively by administering an oxytocic to decrease the risk of a postpartum haemorrhage, but it may also be managed without an oxytocic. During the third stage of labour there is redistribution of the former placental blood flow (about 15% cardiac output). This results in an increase in circulating blood volume which is potentially dangerous to those women who have cardiac disease as it may precipitate heart failure immediately postpartum.

FETAL MONITORING

Recent developments have made it possible to assess fetal well-being in the antenatal period. An obstetric anaesthetist is often involved when a decision to deliver the baby early is made on the outcome of these assessments. The most commonly used tests are:

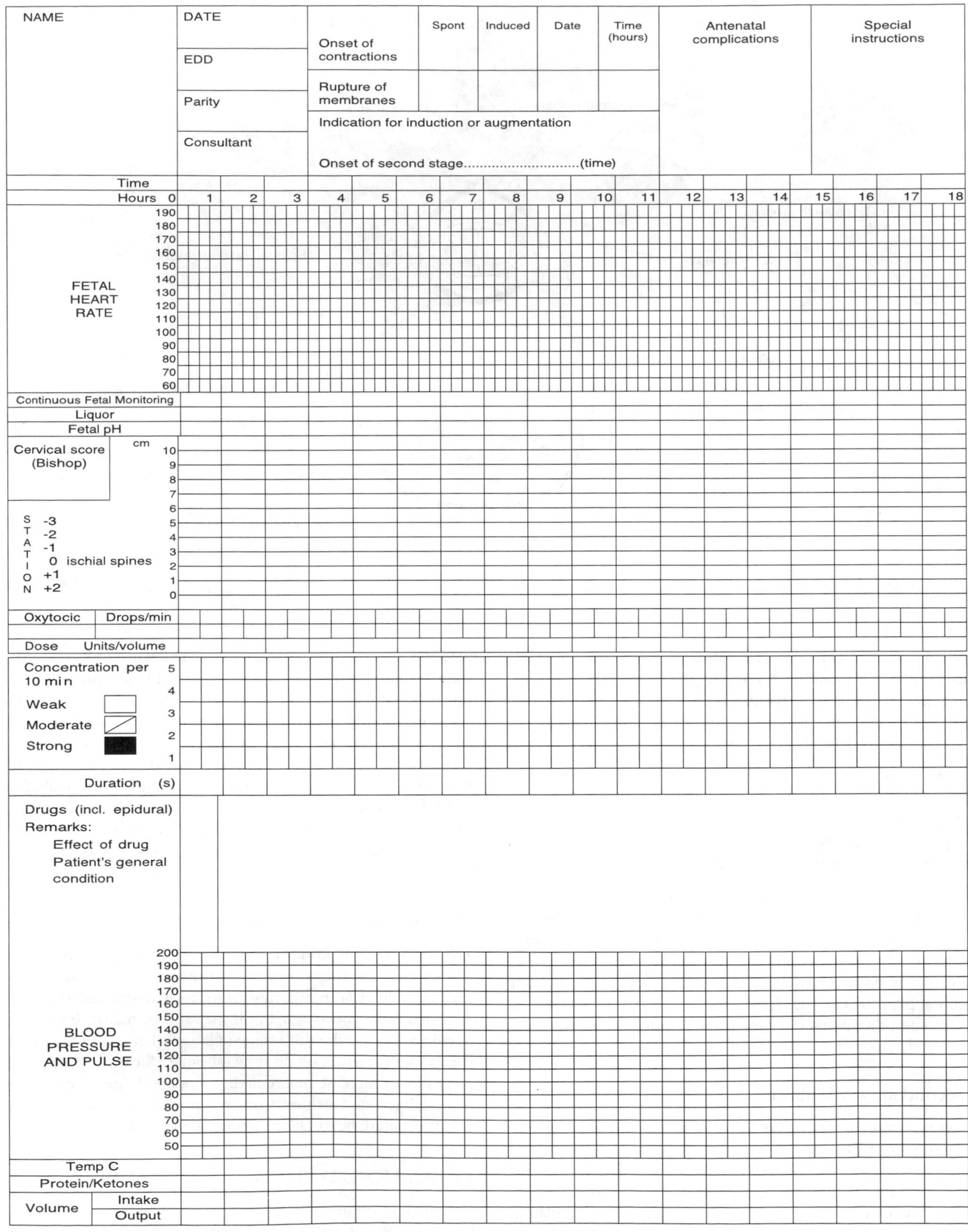
NAME
DATE
EDD
Parity
Consultant
Onset of contractions
Rupture of membranes
Spont
Induced
Date
Time (hours)
Indication for induction or augmentation
Onset of second stage.............................(time)
Antenatal complications
Special instructions
Time
Hours 0 1 2 3 4 5 6 7 8 9 10 11 12 13 14 15 16 17 18
FETAL HEART RATE
190 180 170 160 150 140 130 120 110 100 90 80 70 60
Continuous Fetal Monitoring
Liquor
Fetal pH
Cervical score (Bishop)
cm
10 9 8 7 6 5 4 3 2 1 0
STATION
-3
-2
-1
0 ischial spines
+1
+2
Oxytocic
Drops/min
Dose
Units/volume
Concentration per 10 min
5 4 3 2 1
Weak
Moderate
Strong
Duration (s)
Drugs (incl. epidural)
Remarks:
Effect of drug
Patient's general condition
BLOOD PRESSURE AND PULSE
200 190 180 170 160 150 140 130 120 110 100 90 80 70 60 50
Temp C
Protein/Ketones
Volume
Intake
Output

Fig. 52.4
Example of a partogram.

- serial ultrasonography
- serial Doppler flow studies
- cardiotocograph (CTG) monitoring.

It is important that the anaesthetist communicates with the obstetrician and understands how compromised the fetus is when asked to give analgesia or anaesthesia to these mothers. The degree of urgency for the delivery depends on the condition of the fetus.

Monitoring of the fetus is an important part of intrapartum care, as labour is a stressful event for the fetus. Fetal well-being may be monitored routinely using the following methods:

- fetal heart auscultation
- fetal heart cardiotocography
- colour of the liquor
- fetal blood sampling.

The ability of the fetus to maintain oxygenation is diminished with each uterine contraction. The normal fetus has a baseline heart rate of 110–150 beats min^{-1} and a variability of 5–20 beats min^{-1}. It may accelerate with contractions but should not decelerate. The normal CTG trace simultaneously records fetal heart and uterine contractions; it is therefore possible to monitor the effect of contractions on the fetal heart rate. Decelerations in fetal heart are classified as early, variable and late. Early decelerations are synchronous with contractions and are usually benign. Variable decelerations are variable in shape, extent and rate of occurrence and may or may not indicate hypoxaemia. Late decelerations persist after the end of the contraction and are usually pathological. Opioids or other sedative drugs may cause a flat trace with loss of beat-to-beat variability. Any trace that causes concern, especially in a high-risk pregnancy, is an indication for fetal blood sampling.

Colour of the liquor may be monitored when the membranes are ruptured. The liquor colour is observed for the presence of meconium. The appearance of new meconium may indicate fetal hypoxia, as hypoxaemia may cause the fetal anal sphincter to relax. The appearance of thick new meconium is an indication for urgent delivery. If meconium is aspirated into the lungs of the neonate, severe lung damage may ensue, and therefore a paediatrician should be present at delivery if meconium is present. When the fetus becomes hypoxic, there is an accumulation of lactic acid and a reduction in fetal pH. Fetal blood sampling allows more accurate assessment of fetal well-being than is afforded by the CTG and should be performed whenever there is anxiety about the CTG or when there is meconium in the liquor. When fetal blood sampling is performed, care must be taken to avoid maternal inferior vena caval compression, which may lead to impaired venous return from the mass of the gravid uterus on the inferior vena cava (IVC), with resultant hypotension and syncope. This is most likely to happen if the woman lies supine, and hence it is often termed the 'supine hypotension syndrome'. Parturients at or near term should always lie on their side or at a 15° tilt from horizontal.

Values for fetal pH are as follows:

- pH > 7.25: normal
- pH 7.20–7.25: borderline abnormality and sampling should be repeated 30 min later
- pH < 7.20: significant acidosis requiring urgent delivery of the baby.

Urgency of delivery is guided by the results of fetal monitoring and does not fall into the Confidential Enquiry into Perioperative Deaths (CEPOD) categorization for urgency.

There is much discussion about how the urgency of caesarean section delivery should be classified and the following four grades and definitions are proposed at present:

Grade 1.	Emergency:	immediate threat to life of woman or fetus.
Grade 2.	Urgent:	maternal or fetal compromise which is not immediately life-threatening.
Grade 3.	Scheduled:	needing early delivery but no maternal or fetal compromise.
Grade 4.	Elective:	at a time to suit the patient and the maternity team.

This should be clearer than the present three-point classification of emergency, urgent and elective. The classification applies at the time of decision to operate, e.g. an episode of fetal compromise caused by aortocaval compression responding to therapy, followed some hours later by Caesarean section for failure to progress, would be graded as 3, not 2. Similarly, a case booked as an elective procedure for malpresentation could eventually be classified as Grade 3 if the woman goes into labour before the chosen date of surgery.

GASTROINTESTINAL PHYSIOLOGY AND ANTACID THERAPY

Changes in smooth muscle tone occur early in pregnancy as a result of an increase in progesterone. This leads to a decrease in the tone of the lower oesophageal sphincter and, combined with the increased abdominal mass, results in an increased possibility of regurgitation and pulmonary aspiration of gastric contents. The pH of the gastric contents is lower, and therefore there is an increased incidence of heartburn in pregnancy. Gastric emptying is not delayed during pregnancy but is delayed in labour, especially by pain, anxiety and opioids.

Mendelson first described the syndrome of aspiration of gastric contents in 1946. He described the pathological changes seen when solid food or liquid gastric contents are inhaled during anaesthesia in pregnancy. The chemical pneumonitis that resulted from inhalation of the acid gastric contents in pregnancy prompted the following recommendations:

- Withhold oral feeding during labour and substitute parenteral administration where necessary.
- Wider use of local anaesthesia where indicated and feasible.
- Alkalinization and emptying of stomach contents before general anaesthesia.
- Competent administration of general anaesthesia, with appreciation of the dangers of aspiration during induction and recovery.
- Adequate delivery room equipment, including transparent masks, suction, laryngoscope and tilting table.
- Anaesthetist to remain with the patient until return of laryngeal reflexes.

These recommendations still hold true today and have been reiterated in successive reports of CEMD. There are still no clear guidelines for oral intake in labour, although most units allow free access to clear fluids (solid food and milk prohibited). There has been progress towards the increasing use of regional anaesthesia and there has also been an improvement in the standard of obstetric anaesthesia.

As it has been shown that acid aspiration causes chemical pneumonitis, various methods are used routinely to reduce the acidity of the stomach contents. Particulate antacids, e.g. magnesium trisilicate, were used until they themselves were implicated in causing a chemical reaction in the lungs of animals. This led to the use of non-particulate antacids of which the most popular is 0.3 mol sodium citrate 30 ml administered orally less than 30 min before general anaesthesia. In addition, H_2 antagonists have now become standard gastric acid prophylaxis. Ranitidine 150 mg may be administered orally 6-hourly throughout labour. Whether or not it should be administered to all labouring women or only those perceived to be at risk of anaesthetic intervention is controversial. It is routine practice to administer oral ranitidine before elective caesarean section, e.g. in two doses – one the night before and the second on the morning of operation. Metoclopramide 10 mg may be administered before anaesthesia to hasten gastric emptying. It may be given either orally or intravenously depending on the urgency of the situation.

PAIN AND PAIN RELIEF IN LABOUR

It is only in the last 150 years that effective methods of pain relief have been available. Queen Victoria was given chloroform by John Snow for the birth of her eighth child and this did much to popularize the use of pain relief in labour. Many women go into labour unaware that they may need pain relief, although 75% of first-time mothers experience sufficient pain for them to request pain relief. Melzack et al (1981), using the McGill pain questionnaire, found that the pain of labour is amongst the most severe in the human experience of pain, equivalent to the pain of the amputation of a digit. Several studies have tried to assess the pain of labour. Melzack (1984) found the following for primigravidae: 9.2% very mild, 29.5% mild, 37.9% moderate and 23.4% severe.

THE EFFECT OF PAIN AND ANALGESIA ON THE MOTHER AND FETUS

A long, painful labour may lead to an exhausted, frightened and hysterical mother incapable of decision-making. A traumatic labour may, in extreme circumstances, lead to a post-traumatic stress syndrome.

Figure 52.5 summarizes the effects of pain. Pain compromises placental blood flow and renders uterine contractions less effective. Increased catecholamine secretion results in increased myocardial work and arterial pressure and may also compromise blood flow to the placenta by peripheral vasoconstriction. Activation of the adrenocortical hormones may adversely affect electrolyte, carbohydrate and protein metabolism.

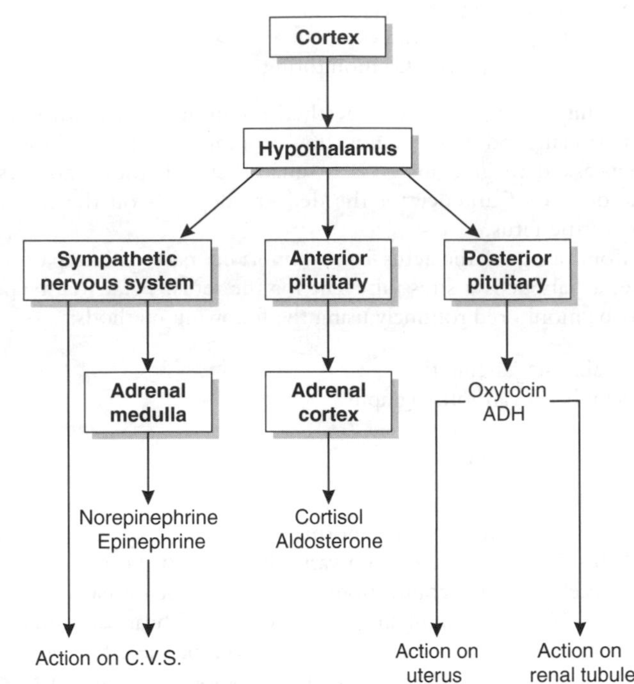

Fig. 52.5
The adverse effects of pain in labour on mother and fetus.

The ideal analgesic

The ideal analgesic for labour should provide rapid-onset excellent pain relief in both first and second stages without risk or side-effects to mother or fetus and should also retain the mother's ability to mobilize and be independent during labour. Many women do not wish complete pain relief, and therefore the analgesic should be easy to control. There is no ideal analgesic at the present time, but it is perhaps most closely approached by low-dose central neuraxial (spinal or epidural) techniques which provide effective analgesia in over 90% cases while preserving motor function to a large degree. Effective epidural (or spinal) analgesia reverses the adverse physiological effects of labour pain listed above by blocking the psychological and biochemical stress response, resulting in improved maternal well-being and placental perfusion.

LABOUR ANALGESIA

Labour analgesia may be classified broadly into the following areas:

- non-pharmacological
- parenteral
- inhalation
- regional.

Non-pharmacological analgesia

Birth preparation classes

In the 1930s, Grantly Dick-Read proposed that childbirth may be painless, as it is a normal life-event, and that society had conditioned women to believe that childbirth was painful. He proposed that education of women about the process of labour and delivery and training them in relaxation therapy would obviate any need for analgesics. Active partner participation was encouraged.

The goals of childbirth preparation are to fully inform women about what to expect in labour and to enhance their ability to cope without analgesia. Fernand Lamaze popularized the technique in North America and Frederick Leboyer modified the technique to suggest birth in quiet conditions with gentle initial handling of the newborn. Although there are few controlled studies on outcome, published observations do not indicate any benefits in terms of outcome of labour and reduced maternal morbidity from childbirth preparation.

Environment and the management of labour

Continuous support in labour is associated with shorter labours and reduced requirement for analgesia. Traditional cultures have always had the support of experienced women to be with the woman in labour. Midwifery (literally 'with woman') has its roots in this role of emotional support. Mobility in labour is helpful in maintaining the dignity and independence of the woman in labour, and while it is thought to be helpful, there are no randomized controlled trials to support the view that pain is easier to cope with when ambulant. Most would accept that a bath or shower is relaxing, although whether this should be extended to water birth is controversial.

Transcutaneous electrical nerve stimulation (TENS)

This technique is based on Melzack and Wall's 'gate control' theory of pain. It involves passage of a small electrical current through skin to reach the peripheral nervous system. Myelinated, larger-diameter nerve fibres (Aβ) have a lower threshold for stimulation by external electrical impulses than myelinated Aδ and unmyelinated C fibres, which transmit pain impulses. Selective stimulation of large-diameter fibres, transmitting touch and vibration sense, inhibits painful stimuli transmission to the substantia gelatinosa of the dorsal horn of the spinal cord. The TENS electrodes should be applied at the appropriate dermatomal levels involved with the transmission of pain in labour (see Fig. 52.1). The TENS machine then emits a low background stimulus that may be boosted with each contraction. There is little evidence that use of TENS reduces the need for analgesics, duration of labour or incidence of instrumental delivery.

Hypnosis

First used by James Braid in 1843, hypnosis involves the patient being in a state of intense concentration, where positive feelings are suggested and reinforced and negative ones played down. Clearly, this requires the continuous presence of a skilled hypnotist throughout the labour, preceded by several training sessions with that therapist before labour. While this method may provide reliable analgesia for a small number of women, it has not proved suitable on a large scale for labour analgesia.

Acupuncture

Acupuncture has only recently received attention for labouring women. In volunteer parturients, it was found to be ineffective in almost 80% of cases.

Parenteral (systemic) analgesia

Many opioids have been used to provide obstetric analgesia, but the most popular have been pethidine, morphine and diamorphine. Pethidine has become established in obstetric practice without good scientific data to support its use, and in the UK two doses of 100 mg may be prescribed for a labouring woman by a midwife. Pethidine is given by intramuscular injection and the maximum effect is seen about 1 h after administration. The analgesic effects are variable and pethidine may also cause significant side-effects, such as maternal sedation, nausea and vomiting, dysphoria and inhibition of gastric emptying. It may also have adverse effects on the fetus as it freely crosses the placenta, potentially causing CTG abnormalities and respiratory and neurobehavioural depression of the newborn. It is standard practice for paediatric staff to be available at delivery of an infant whose mother has received pethidine within 3 h of delivery. These problems are not obviated by the use of patient-controlled analgesia (PCA) with pethidine, but studies have shown that the greater control that PCA gives to the patient may reduce the overall amount of pethidine required for an acceptable level of analgesia.

Inhalation analgesia

The ideal inhalation agent should be a good analgesic in subanaesthetic doses, have a rapid onset of action and recovery; and not accumulate. Nitrous oxide is relatively insoluble in blood and has these properties. Other anaesthetic agents have been investigated, but so far only isoflurane has shown promise and it has been used as Isonox (50% nitrous oxide and 50% oxygen with 0.2% isoflurane) with some success. In the UK, nitrous oxide is supplied as Entonox, which is 50% nitrous oxide and 50% oxygen under pressure in a cylinder (see Ch. 13). Entonox is administered usually via an on-demand valve with a face mask or mouthpiece. Administration needs to be timed for the maximum analgesic effect to coincide with the peak of the contraction. Most women tend to hyperventilate while breathing Entonox, and therefore there is often an alternate phase of hyperventilation and then hypoventilation, especially if the Entonox is administered after pethidine. Although Entonox is a reasonably effective analgesic, many women feel faint and nauseated and may vomit or become out of control.

Regional analgesia for labour

This is described below.

EPIDURAL AND SUBARACHNOID ANALGESIA

This is the most effective form of analgesia in labour, with up to 90% women reporting complete or near-complete pain relief. However, it is invasive and patients require careful monitoring.

Indications for epidural analgesia

In addition to relief of pain and distress, there are several indications for which epidural analgesia may be helpful in securing a good outcome from labour. These are summarized in Table 52.2.

Contraindications to epidural analgesia in labour

Maternal refusal

There is a small number of women who, after a careful explanation of the risks and benefits of regional analgesia, refuse consent, possibly because of medical problems, e.g. complex back surgery. Ideally, discussions should take place in the antenatal period and clear notes should be made in the medical record.

Bleeding disorders

These may be acquired or congenital. The potential to cause bleeding in the epidural space varies widely. Epidural haematoma is a serious complication of an epidural and may cause spinal cord compression with resultant paraplegia. Each case needs careful assessment as to the risks and benefits of administering the regional anaesthetic. This assessment may need team planning with haematology and obstetric staff. Most units have delivery suite guidelines for the common problems, e.g. pre-eclampsia, prophylactic heparin, etc.

Sepsis in the lumbar area and systemic sepsis

Local infection in the area adjacent to the epidural site may introduce infection into the epidural space, potentially leading to the formation of an epidural abscess. The presence of systemic infection or systemic inflammatory response syndrome (SIRS) may cause the instrumentation involved in siting the epidural to become itself a focus for development of a local infection. An expert assessment of the risk–benefit ratio for siting an epidural must be made in these circumstances.

TECHNIQUE OF EPIDURAL ANALGESIA

Preparation

Consent. Information should be given to the woman about regional analgesia and anaesthesia in the antenatal period. Leaflets, videos and parentcraft classes are important in ensuring that women are well informed before labour. It is often difficult to explain the risks and benefits of epidural analgesia to a woman who is distressed and under the effects of pethidine and Entonox; under these circumstances, misunderstandings may arise.

Intravenous cannulation. A continuous infusion of crystalloid (at about 500 ml h^{-1} initially) should always be commenced before embarking on the block.

Arterial pressure. A baseline arterial pressure value is recorded.

Bladder contents. The patient should have recently emptied her bladder.

Clothing. The patient should be wearing suitable clothing.

Positioning. The position of the patient is the same for epidural, spinal or combined spinal-epidural (CSE) block: either the lateral or the sitting position. There is no evidence that any position is superior, but the lateral position minimizes the risk of aortocaval compression, while the sitting position may enable bony landmarks to be palpated more easily and may be more comfortable for the patient. There is evidence that the lateral position is associated with less hypotension than the sitting position during induction of spinal and CSE blocks. These positions are compared in Table 52.3.

Normal labour

In the lateral position, the knees and hips are fully flexed and the neck is flexed onto the chest in order to maximize the intervertebral distance. In both positions, the iliac crests are palpated and a line drawn between them bisects either the spin-

Table 52.2 Indications for epidural analgesia

- Maternal request
- Occipitoposterior presentation
- Pregnancy-induced hypertension or pre-eclampsia
- Prematurity or IUGR
- Intrauterine death
- Induction or oxytocin augmentation of labour
- Instrumental or caesarean delivery likely
- Previous caesarean delivery
- Presence of significant concurrent disease (e.g. heart disease, diabetes, hypertension)
- Twin pregnancy

Table 52.3 Comparison of sitting and lateral positions for performing spinal or epidural procedures

Sitting	Lying (left lateral)
Advantages	
Midline easier to identify in obese women	Can be left unattended without risk of fainting
Obese patients may find this position more comfortable	No orthostatic hypotension
	Utero-placental blood flow not reduced (particularly important in the stressed fetus)
Disadvantages	
Uteroplacental blood flow decreased	May be more difficult to find the midline in obese patient
Orthostatic hypotension may occur	
Increased risk of orthostatic hypotension if Entonox and pethidine have been administered	
Patient sitting on edge of bed may be too far away from a small anaesthetist for good manual dexterity	
Assistant (or partner) needed to support patient	

ous process of L4 or the L4/5 intervertebral space (see Fig 52.6).

Conduct of the epidural

1. Epidural, spinal and CSE blocks are performed in a strictly aseptic manner. After cleaning the area with iodine or chlorhexidine, it is important to ensure that there is no contamination of the epidural equipment by the skin preparation and that the skin is dry before the epidural is sited.
2. Cover the back with sterile drapes.
3. Identify the bony landmarks. For labour analgesia, intervertebral spaces L2–5 are the positions of choice. The L4 spinous process is palpated and the desired space identified.
4. A skin wheal of local anaesthetic (1% lidocaine) is raised at the intended point of insertion of the Tuohy needle and the superficial ligaments in the path of the epidural needle are infiltrated.
5. With the bevel cephalad, the Tuohy needle is advanced firmly through the skin, supraspinous and infraspinous ligaments until it becomes anchored in the ligamentum flavum.
6. The methods of identifying the epidural space are:
   — tactile, with loss of resistance to either air or saline
   — visual, using a hanging-drop technique.
   With the loss-of-resistance technique, the stilette is removed and a loss-of-resistance syringe containing saline or air is attached to the Tuohy needle. This is a tactile technique, whereby there is a loss of resistance to the gradually advancing needle as it passes through the ligamentum flavum (Table 52.4).
7. As the anaesthetist advances the Tuohy needle with the fingers and thumb of the left hand on the Tuohy needle wings, the dorsum of the hand should be resting on the patient's back in order to control the advance of the needle using either intermittent or continuous pressure on the piston of the loss-of-resistance syringe. The epidural space is identified by loss of resistance. The advantages and disadvantages of air or saline use for loss of resistance are summarized in Table 52.4.
8. When loss of resistance is confirmed, the distance from the skin at which the epidural space lies is noted.
9. The plastic catheter introducer is placed on the end of the Tuohy needle and the catheter is advanced to 15–20 cm, at the same time warning the patient that she may feel pins and needles in one of her legs or her back. The catheter should never be withdrawn back through the Tuohy needle, as a part of it may be sheared off and left inside the patient's epidural space. If withdrawal of the catheter is necessary, the needle and catheter are removed together.
10. The Tuohy needle is withdrawn, having first noted the distance from skin to epidural space, ensuring the catheter stays in position. Ensure that 3–4 cm of catheter is within the epidural space.
11. The filter is attached and the catheter is checked to ensure that no blood or CSF flows back using gravity. A test dose may now be given.
12. The epidural catheter is fixed.

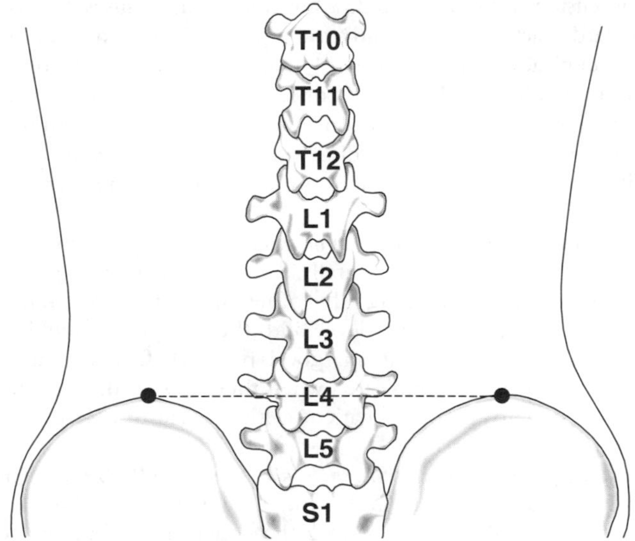

Fig. 52.6
The lumbar spine. A line drawn between the iliac crests crosses either the spinous process of the L4 vertebra or the L4–L5 intervertebral space.

Test dose

This involves administration of a small dose of local anaesthetic (e.g. 2 ml 2% lidocaine or 3 ml 0.5% bupivacaine) to check for inadvertent intrathecal or vascular placement. Hypotension or

Table 52.4 Comparison of air and saline for loss-of-resistance technique

Saline	Air
Advantages	
May give a better end point for loss of resistance	If fluid appears during insertion it can be assumed to be CSF until proved otherwise
May push the dura away from the point of the needle, thus reducing the chances of dural puncture	No filter is required
	No dilutional effect; the small amount of air used does not usually distort the tissues
	No possibility of confusion with other substances
Disadvantages	
May be confused with CSF	More difficult to define the point of loss of resistance with air than with saline
Must be filtered to avoid introduction of minute glass particles	
Dilutes the local anaesthetic which is put into the epidural space	
Another ampoule is opened, thus providing a possibility for user error	
Preservative-free saline must be used	

marked motor block within 5 min of such a test dose suggests intrathecal placement. If an inadvertent intravascular injection occurs, the early signs are circumoral tingling and pallor and possibly a metallic taste in the mouth. The current use of dilute concentrations of local anaesthetics with the opioid fentanyl has led to a change of practice in some centres regarding the test dose. With ambulatory or 'walking' epidurals, a CSE technique or an epidural with 0.1% bupivacaine/fentanyl 2 μg ml^{-1} may be used. A 15 ml bolus is commonly given to commence ambulatory epidural analgesia, amounting to 15 mg bupivacaine in total. This dose is increasingly being given without a preceding test dose in order to spare the amount of bupivacaine given and hence minimize motor block. This 15 mg dose is equivalent to a test dose of 3 ml 0.5% bupivacaine; hence, even if it were given intrathecally, it would not cause a higher spinal than the standard test dose.

CSE for labour and the 'walking' epidural

In 1993, anaesthetists in Queen Charlotte's Hospital in London described combined spinal-epidural (CSE) technique for labour analgesia; this minimized motor block to the extent that a large proportion of their patients walked around the delivery suite.

Technique

The Tuohy needle is advanced to identify loss of resistance in the lumbar region (as for an epidural). Then, a 25–27 gauge 120 mm long pencil-point (Whitacre or Sprotte) needle is advanced through the Tuohy to puncture the dura, and an intrathecal injection of 1 ml 0.25% bupivacaine with 25 μg fentanyl is given. The spinal needle is withdrawn and the epidural catheter is passed and left in place as before. The intrathecal injection usually produces rapid-onset analgesia (< 5 min) and approximately 70% of patients have normal or near-normal leg power such that they may walk. The intrathecal injection has an analgesic duration of the order of 90 min, after which the epidural component of the CSE is used, usually commencing with a 15 ml bolus of bupivacaine 0.1% with fentanyl 2 μg ml^{-1}, without a test dose, as described above.

Assessment

The preservation of motor function and reduced need for bladder catheterization have increased maternal satisfaction with epidural analgesia, although there have been concerns that proprioception may be affected even with this low dose of local anaesthetic, potentially making walking hazardous. The medicolegal position of the anaesthetist in the event of a fall of a parturient during a walking epidural is unclear. Nonetheless, if visual and vestibular function is intact, proprioceptive impairment seems to have a minimal effect on walking. Many parturients do not wish to walk and, moreover, clinical trials to date have not shown that walking significantly alters outcome of labour.

MANAGEMENT OF THE LABOURING WOMAN WITH EPIDURAL ANALGESIA

Posture

A labouring woman should be positioned with at least a 15° left lateral tilt to prevent aortocaval compression (supine hypotension syndrome). The weight of the gravid uterus compresses the vena cava and aorta against the vertebral bodies, thereby restricting blood flow. The reduction in systemic vascular resistance in women with epidural analgesia decreases the ability of the woman to maintain her arterial pressure, and therefore she is more likely to faint. In addition, the lumbosacral spine should be supported, as the epidural may allow unnatural positions to be adopted, which would usually produce back discomfort. Prolonged abnormal posture may contribute to low back pain after the epidural has worn off; in the past this has been ascribed incorrectly to the epidural itself.

Monitoring of mother and baby

A partogram is a chart upon which the progress of mother and baby is documented. It records arterial pressure, temperature, uterine contractions, fetal heart rate, cervical dilation in relation to time in labour, intravenous fluids, urinary output and drugs given (Fig 52.4).

Analgesia for the first stage of labour requires a sensory block extending from T10 to L1, while for the second stage, S2–S5 block is desirable. The aim is to provide effective analgesia with minimal side-effects. Local anaesthetics injected into the epidural space affect all nerves to some degree in the following order: sympathetic fibres, pain fibres, proprioception fibres and finally motor fibres. The volume of local anaesthetic solution governs the spread of the block, whereas the concentration of local anaesthetic governs the density of block with an increased risk of motor block.

Maintenance of analgesia

Epidural analgesia for labour may be maintained by the following:

Repeated bolus administration. After the first dose has been given by the anaesthetist, boluses are usually administered as required by a midwife trained in the use of epidural analgesia. The volume and concentration need to be great enough to provide adequate analgesia, but large volumes may cause too great a spread of block, with attendant hypotension, toxicity and hypotension. Bupivacaine 0.25% given in 10 ml boluses has been standard practice until recently when more dilute mixtures using 0.1% bupivacaine and 2 μg ml^{-1} fentanyl in 10–15 ml boluses have been adopted. The lower concentration of local anaesthetic reduces the incidence of hypotension and increases the ability of the woman to mobilize. The disadvantage of boluses is the possibility of intermittent pain if top-ups are not administered at appropriate intervals.

Continuous infusion by syringe pump. Local anaesthetic/fentanyl mixture is infused epidurally at a constant rate (e.g. 0.1% bupivacaine containing 2 μg ml^{-1} of fentanyl infused at a rate of 10 ml h^{-1}). The sensory level and the analgesia should be checked regularly to maintain good pain relief. The infusion method is particularly indicated when there is a need for cardiovascular stability (e.g. the patient with cardiac disease or pre-eclampsia).

Patient-controlled epidural analgesia (PCEA). This involves establishing analgesia with an initial bolus dose and maintaining analgesia by allowing the patient to self-administer boluses of analgesic solution as required by depressing a button on a special computer-controlled volumetric syringe. There may or may not be a low-dose background infusion. The advantage of this method is that it gives more control to the patient and studies have shown that total analgesic consumption is reduced using PCEA.

Problems maintaining epidural analgesia

Epidural is not effective. If the epidural is not providing good analgesia within 15–20 min with 15 ml 0.1% bupivacaine/fentanyl 2 μg ml^{-1} or 10 ml of 0.25% bupivacaine, the catheter is probably not in the epidural space and it should be withdrawn and re-sited.

Missed segment or unilateral block. Groin pain is the most common manifestation of a missed segment, i.e. L1, and it is important to ensure that the bladder is empty and the block is not unilateral. A bolus of dilute bupivacaine and fentanyl or a small bolus, e.g. 5 ml of 0.25% bupivacaine, often gives analgesia. If there is persistent groin pain present between contractions, the possibility of uterine dehiscence should be excluded.

Hypotension. If the patient feels faint or her arterial pressure decreases, she should be turned onto her side to exclude aortocaval compression. Intravenous fluids and oxygen should be administered while extensive regional block is excluded. Catheter migration may occur and an accidental spinal may manifest itself at any stage of the epidural. If the hypotension persists, ephedrine should be administered.

REGIONAL ANAESTHESIA FOR THE PARTURIENT

The common indications for anaesthesia for parturients are caesarean section, forceps delivery, retained placenta and suturing of trauma to the birth canal. Regional anaesthesia is the technique of choice. Anaesthesia is discussed under the following headings:

- elective caesarean section
- emergency caesarean section
- forceps and Ventouse delivery
- retained placenta
- trauma to the birth canal
- post-delivery analgesia
- complications of regional anaesthesia and analgesia in obstetrics.

ELECTIVE CAESAREAN SECTION

Regional anaesthesia is the technique of choice for elective caesarean section. Although most women presenting for elective caesarean section expect to be awake for the delivery of their baby, they still need careful preoperative explanation of the procedure with explanation of the risks. As many hospitals admit women on the day of surgery, it may be difficult to give sufficient time to the preoperative visit, and therefore it is advisable to have an information sheet for the woman before admission to hospital. The woman should be warned about hypotension (and associated nausea and vomiting), post-dural puncture headache and the possibility of an imperfect block. The techniques available are as follows:

- spinal anaesthesia
- epidural anaesthesia
- combined spinal-epidural anaesthesia.

Spinal anaesthesia is the most popular choice for elective caesarean section with increasing popularity of the combined spinal-epidural (CSE) technique.

Spinal anaesthesia

Most spinal anaesthetics are performed with the patient on the operating table as this reduces the need to move. The following points are mandatory:

- routine pre-anaesthetic equipment check
- monitoring of arterial pressure, ECG and oximetry
- intravenous infusion of crystalloid, initially at a rate of 500 ml h^{-1}
- vasopressor available, e.g. ephedrine
- aseptic technique.

Ensure that drugs are available for the administration of general anaesthesia.

Spinal anaesthesia may be performed with the patient in either the sitting or the lateral position, curled up as for siting an epidural. The choice of needle is important so as to minimize the incidence of post-dural puncture headache; it is generally accepted that the conical tip or pencil-point needle is best, although a small Quincke tip needle may be used if the others are unavailable. It is important to remember that the spinal cord ends around L2 in a normal adult, so the spinal needle should be inserted at L3/4 or below. When the interspace has been chosen, local anaesthetic is injected along the proposed line of insertion of the spinal needle. The spinal needle introducer is then inserted, followed by the spinal needle, and the chosen local anaesthetic is injected when free flow of CSF is identified. If a spinal nerve is touched, the patient experiences excruciating pain radiating along the route of that nerve. The spinal needle must be removed and the patient reassured. Local anaesthetic must not be injected if there is any possibility of it being given into a nerve as this may cause permanent neurological damage.

Hyperbaric bupivacaine 0.5% is the drug of choice and 2.5 ml is usually sufficient. An opioid may be added to the local anaesthetic as this may improve the quality of anaesthesia and provide postoperative analgesia. Fentanyl 25–50 μg or morphine 0.1–0.2 mg may be used. All drugs injected into the epidural space or the CSF should be in preservative-free solution. Arterial pressure should be measured at 1 min intervals and the patient placed horizontal, ensuring that aortocaval compression is prevented by lateral tilt. The block should be tested for loss of sensation to cold or pinprick. It is good practice to test the block from the sacral roots to the thoracic dermatomes, even though it is unusual for a spinal block to be patchy or to miss the sacral roots. The height of the block should be T4 bilaterally. Hypotension is treated with ephedrine in boluses of 3 mg or as an infusion, although there is increasing popularity for the use of prophylactic ephedrine to avoid the development of hypotension. Phenylephrine 0.05–0.1 mg boluses are also safe and effective for hypotension. The patient should be carefully observed at all times.

Surgery may start when the anaesthetist is happy that there is good anaesthesia. Peritoneal traction and the swabbing of the paracolic gutters are the most stimulating parts of the operation and the times when pain or discomfort are most likely to be experienced. Exteriorization of the uterus is to be discouraged as this is challenging even to the most perfect block. Pain or discomfort should be treated promptly. Nitrous oxide and/or small doses of intravenous opioids, e.g. fentanyl or alfentanil, are useful. If the pain is severe, general anaesthesia should be offered and administered if appropriate. Syntocinon 5–10 units are normally administered intravenously after the delivery of the baby to assist myometrial contraction. Routine postoperative care should take place in a well-equipped recovery area.

Epidural anaesthesia

Epidural anaesthesia was the regional anaesthetic of choice until pencil-point spinal needles were introduced. The disadvantages of epidural anaesthesia are that the onset of the block is longer than that for spinal anaesthesia and that the spread of the block may be patchy, often giving poor anaesthesia of the sacral roots. The cardiovascular stability that can be achieved with an epidural is excellent and this implies that the technique may be considered the anaesthetic of choice in some patients with heart disease or pre-eclampsia. When the epidural catheter is in place, anaesthesia can be achieved by local anaesthetic often combined with an opioid.

The following are standard prescriptions for an epidural anaesthetic:

- bupivacaine 0.5% 15–20 ml with 1 in 200 000 epinephrine (freshly added) – this should be given in divided doses
- lidocaine 2% 15–20 ml with 1 in 200 000 epinephrine (freshly added) – this should be given in divided doses
- fentanyl 50 µg or diamorphine 2.5 mg may be administered in addition to the local anaesthetic and has been shown to improve the quality of the anaesthesia.

It is essential to test the block thoroughly from the thoracic level down to the sacral roots to ensure that good anaesthesia has been produced before surgery starts.

CSE

There are various techniques for this, although the 'needle through needle' technique described above is probably the most popular. A full description of the other techniques is outside the remit of this chapter. The CSE allows increased flexibility by combining an epidural and a spinal. The spinal anaesthetic is a single-shot technique and while most of the time this is no problem, delay in starting surgery, a difficult, long operation or failure of the block may occur. The epidural may not achieve such profound or rapid anaesthesia, although it has the advantages of flexibility and cardiovascular stability.

In the CSE technique, the spinal is usually conducted using the same dose of drugs as listed in the spinal section and the epidural, although placed as an 'insurance', is often used only for postoperative pain relief. The CSE may also be used as a sequential block, with a smaller intrathecal dose of local anaesthetic being given, followed by an epidural top-up to achieve full anaesthesia. This method provides greater cardiovascular stability as the onset of the block is slower, while an excellent sacral block is achieved with the spinal anaesthetic. This technique has extended the use of regional anaesthesia in pre-eclampsia.

EMERGENCY CAESAREAN SECTION

Regional anaesthesia has increased in frequency for emergency caesarean section partly because of the increased use of spinal anaesthesia and also because of the increase in use of epidural analgesia in labour.

Topping up an existing epidural

A labour epidural may be topped up to achieve anaesthesia within 10–20 min using either lidocaine 2% with 1 in 200 000 epinephrine or bupivacaine 0.5% with 1 in 200 000 epinephrine. Sodium bicarbonate may be added to each of these solutions (e.g. 1–2 ml of 8.4% sodium bicarbonate) to increase the pH and increase the speed of onset of anaesthesia. The epidural should be topped up incrementally while the patient is monitored continuously. Between 10 and 20 ml of local anaesthetic solution are usually needed. While the epidural is being topped up, it is important to explain what is going to happen and to ensure that the woman understands what she is likely to feel and that help is available if pain or discomfort is experienced.

Spinal anaesthesia for an emergency

Spinal anaesthesia is to be encouraged for the woman who has no epidural in situ and who requires an emergency caesarean section. There are times when general anaesthesia is indicated, but these decrease as experience with spinal anaesthesia increases. Spinal anaesthesia may be used in the same manner as for an elective caesarean section; however, it is important to explain the procedure to the woman as fully as possible in the time available and to be present after the caesarean section to describe events slowly. Follow-up is particularly important in the emergency situation.

FORCEPS AND VENTOUSE DELIVERY

Surgical anaesthesia is required for any operative delivery, except for a simple 'lift-out' by forceps or Ventouse. For a simple lift-out, the labour epidural should be well topped up. Ideally, time to achieve good perineal anaesthesia should be allowed before the woman is placed in the lithotomy position for the assisted delivery. Bupivacaine 0.5% or lidocaine 2% in a dose of around 10 ml is appropriate. If the delivery is more complex than a simple lift-out, surgical anaesthesia is required. It is preferable to deliver such patients in the operating theatre where caesarean section may be performed if there is any doubt about the ability to deliver the baby vaginally. In these situations, the anaesthetist should have prepared the anaesthetic as if for caesarean section using any of the prescriptions for caesarean delivery mentioned above.

RETAINED PLACENTA

Regional anaesthesia may be used for manual removal of retained placenta after a careful assessment of blood loss. It is easy to underestimate the blood loss if there has been a continuous trickle of blood for some time. If the woman is not significantly hypovolaemic, the anaesthetic of choice is a spinal, unless there is an epidural in situ. Both techniques should provide good surgical anaesthesia with a block extending from at least T10 to the sacral roots.

TRAUMA TO THE BIRTH CANAL

The anaesthetist is often asked to provide anaesthesia for the repair of birth trauma. The full extent of the damage may not be known as it may not be possible to examine the woman without anaesthesia. The trauma may be extensive and involve disruption of the anal sphincter, which is classified as a third-degree tear. There may be considerable blood loss and it is important to assess this before performing regional anaesthesia. If there is an epidural in situ, this may be topped up for the repair. If there is no epidural, then a spinal anaesthetic is the technique of choice. Hyperbaric bupivacaine 0.5% in a volume of 1.5 ml provides good sacral analgesia.

POST-DELIVERY ANALGESIA

The anaesthetist is usually involved in the continuing care of the woman post-delivery and this includes the provision of pain relief for:

- normal delivery
- tears
- forceps and Ventouse
- caesarean section.

Normal delivery

The pain experienced after a normal delivery is caused mainly by uterine contractions and also bruising of the perineum. Simple analgesia in the form of paracetamol is usually adequate, although if there is severe bruising of the perineum, NSAIDs are helpful, e.g. diclofenac suppositories.

Tears and episiotomy

After the repair of an episiotomy or tear there may be considerable pain which needs more than simple analgesia. NSAIDs provide excellent analgesia for most women. If the woman has had a third-degree tear repaired, she will often have had a regional anaesthetic for the repair, and the use of epidural or intrathecal opioids provides good postoperative analgesia, particularly if combined with rectal diclofenac.

Forceps and Ventouse delivery

An episiotomy is usually performed to facilitate the forceps or Ventouse delivery and this may be extensive; therefore pain management as above is appropriate.

Caesarean section

The extensive use of regional anaesthesia for caesarean section has led to intrathecal and epidural opioid analgesia being routine practice in most units. Combined with NSAIDs, paracetamol and other simple analgesics, this enables women to mobilize early after caesarean section. It is prudent to have clear postoperative guidelines for the care of women in the postoperative period and these should include sedation scores. Those women who are unable to have NSAIDs do not have such good pain control and continuing epidural opioid analgesia may be needed. Those women who have had their caesarean section under general anaesthesia may be managed with PCA using morphine in the same way as other postoperative patients. This is combined with NSAIDs where appropriate.

COMPLICATIONS OF REGIONAL ANAESTHESIA AND ANALGESIA IN OBSTETRICS

Although regional anaesthesia is now very safe and effective, all procedures have potential complications.

Shearing of the epidural catheter

An epidural catheter should not be withdrawn through a needle as this may damage or shear the catheter. Any sheared portion of catheter is inert and sterile and thus unlikely to cause a problem, but a full account should be made in the medical record.

Post-dural puncture headache (PDPH)

The incidence of PDPH is 0.5–1% and is often higher in teaching hospitals. It may occur at the time of epidural insertion or be caused later by catheter migration into the intrathecal space. The clinical presentation is of an occipital headache which may radiate anteriorly, aggravated by sitting and possibly associated with nausea, photophobia and, rarely, diplopia resulting from stretching of the VIth cranial nerve as it passes through the dura. The differential diagnosis of meningitis, subarachnoid haemorrhage or even cerebral space-occupying lesions should be considered and excluded by history and simple clinical examination.

Management of PDPH

- Bed rest is still recommended, although it is worthless in terms of reducing leak of CSF.
- Infusion of epidural normal saline 60 ml before the epidural catheter is removed may reduce the incidence of PDPH by 20%, as may infusion, under gravity, of normal saline for 12–24 h postpartum.
- Give i.v. and oral fluids to prevent dehydration.
- Give simple analgesics, e.g. paracetamol, 500 mg 4-hourly.
- Caffeine 0.5% infusion may produce cerebral vasoconstriction.
- Antidiuretic hormone may also relieve symptoms by an unknown mechanism.
- Blood patch – a sample of the patient's own venous blood is collected under aseptic conditions and injected into the same or an adjacent epidural space to seal the CSF leak. It is 90% effective. It is not usually recommended as a first-line treatment because it carries complications such as infection, arachnoiditis and potential problems with subsequent epidurals.

Backache

Backache is common after childbirth, 50% of women suffering at some stage in pregnancy. An anaesthetist is often called to assess patients with backache if they have received an epidural. Certainly, insertion of epidural anaesthesia may contribute to short-term acute back pain if it causes:

- an epidural haematoma
- an epidural infection causing abscess or meningitis
- mild local bruising from poor technique.

However, long-term backache is not caused by epidural anaesthesia, as has been clearly shown in two prospective studies of over 1000 women giving birth, followed up the day after delivery and 3 months later. The incidence of new-onset backache was of the order of 40–50%, but there was no difference in the incidence of backache at 3 months between those who had received an epidural and those who had not. There was a trend towards a slightly higher chance of back pain on day 1, explained by minor local trauma.

Epidural haematoma

This is a very rare but potentially disastrous complication. Only 38 cases of true epidural haematoma (requiring neurosurgical intervention) from spinal anaesthesia and eight cases following epidural anaesthesia have been described in the literature. The estimated incidence is thus less than 1/250 000. The signs of an epidural haematoma are:

- new-onset, severe, back pain
- prolonged, profound motor weakness > 6 h after the last top-up or cessation of an infusion
- sudden onset of incontinence.

Immediate CT or MRI scan is warranted to confirm the diagnosis, and neurosurgical evacuation of the haematoma within 8 h of the onset of symptoms results in a good outcome.

Epidural abscess or meningitis

These conditions are rare. An abscess, as with a haematoma, may give rise to a space-occupying lesion in the epidural space, resulting in compression of the spinal cord and its nutrient arteries, leading to paraplegia. Meningitis may occur as a complication of regional techniques and may be bacterial, viral or chemical. It is essential that a good aseptic technique is used when regional blocks are sited and that meningitis is excluded in the differential diagnosis of headache.

Systemic toxic reaction

This is a result of high blood concentration of local anaesthetic, caused either by a total dose greater than the body's ability to metabolize it or by too rapid administration (bolus or infusion). Local anaesthetic toxicity is described in Chapter 15.

Hypotension

Hypotension is usually defined as a 25% decrease in systolic or mean arterial pressure or an absolute decrease of 40 mmHg. Small decreases in pressure are insignificant and may be associated with improved uteroplacental blood flow. Rapidly developing hypotension after spinal anaesthesia may cause unpleasant dizziness and nausea in about 50% of patients and should be treated with vasopressors, e.g. ephedrine, until arterial pressure is restored, while at the same time maintaining normovolaemia and ensuring that there is no aortocaval compression.

Neurological deficit

Neurological deficit may be caused by the drugs used for the procedure or by trauma from the needles or catheter. The incidence of dysaesthesiae and persistent numbness or weakness of more than 1 week's duration resulting from an epidural is approximately 1:150 000. Where a particular nerve root has been bruised by the epidural needle or catheter, reassurance may be given that these symptoms resolve over 3–6 months, but patients should be followed up on an outpatient basis. Several peripheral nerves may be injured during delivery and falsely attributed to the epidural:

- lateral popliteal nerve – by stirrups, causing foot drop
- lateral cutaneous nerve of the thigh – by groin pressure from the lithotomy position, causing anterolateral thigh numbness
- femoral nerve or sciatic nerve – by the lithotomy position, causing weak quadriceps with loss of knee reflex or back of the leg pain with loss of ankle reflex, respectively
- sacral plexus and obturator nerves – these cross the pelvic brim and rarely may be damaged by occipital presentation or forceps delivery.

Arachnoiditis

Inflammation of the arachnoid membrane, caused by chemical toxins (wrong substance injected) or infection, usually presents as intractable back pain, potentially leading to permanent neurological damage. It is extremely rare.

As any complications may have medicolegal implications, it is important to:

- document the problem at the time
- explain the problem to the patient and relatives
- ensure consultant involvement.

GENERAL ANAESTHESIA FOR THE PARTURIENT

Since the 1960s, a triennial report termed the Confidential Enquiry into Maternal Deaths (CEMD) has provided an audit of obstetric and anaesthetic practice. In the most recent triennium (1996–98), there was only one death caused by anaesthesia, while in previous reports there were larger numbers. The increasing safety of anaesthesia in obstetrics is the result of many factors:

- increasing use of epidural analgesia in labour
- increasing use of regional anaesthesia for operative delivery
- increase in dedicated consultant obstetric anaesthetic sessions
- improved teaching of obstetric anaesthesia
- improved assistance for the anaesthetist.

Deaths caused by anaesthesia generally result from hypoxaemia and/or acid aspiration associated with a failure to intubate the trachea and difficulty in maintaining the airway during general anaesthesia (GA).

GA continues to be required in the following situations:

- in an extreme emergency, e.g. severe fetal distress or maternal haemorrhage
- where there is a contraindication to regional anaesthesia
- where the patient refuses to have a regional anaesthetic; this may be because of a previous bad experience with regional anaesthesia.

Currently, about 5–10% of caesarean sections in the UK are performed under GA. The main anaesthetic considerations are the risk of aspiration of acidic gastric contents (as little as 25 ml with pH < 2.5 may lead to a 50% mortality rate) and hypoxaemia resulting from airway difficulties. The previous sections on physiology of pregnancy, anatomy and antacid therapy have highlighted many of the problems that should be considered when a pregnant woman presents for a general anaesthetic. It is essential that a thorough pre-anaesthetic check is performed, with particular attention to the difficulties that may be encountered with tracheal intubation (see Table 52.5). It is mandatory that anaesthetists familiarize themselves with the operating theatre and the anaesthetic equipment (Table 52.6), in addition to the guidelines and equipment that are available for difficult and failed intubation. Drugs and equipment should be checked at the beginning of each period of duty on the delivery suite so that an emergency can be dealt with in a calm and ordered manner.

CAESAREAN SECTION

Preparation

1. Check the equipment again. Ensure that the suction equipment is working and that the table tilts head-down.
2. Perform a pre-anaesthetic check on the patient with particular attention to the airway and gastric contents.
3. Ensure that the assistant is ready.
4. Ensure that the patient is well positioned, paying particular attention to aortocaval compression and position for tracheal intubation.
5. Insert a 16 gauge i.v cannula and ensure that an infusion flows well.
6. Check that full routine monitoring is in use.
7. Preoxygenate the patient's lungs for 3 min using a well applied face mask.
8. Check that the assistant knows how to apply cricoid pressure.
9. Commence the anaesthetic using a rapid-sequence induction.

Table 52.5 Clinical methods to assess the airway

Mouth opening (5 cm interincisor gap, equivalent to two fingers breadth)
Mallampatti grade
Temporomandibular joint mobility (should be able to protrude lower incisors in front of upper incisors)
Neck mobility (90° flexion of head on neck)
Weight > 100 kg increases risk
Risk of airway oedema (increased by pre-eclampsia, stridor, URTI)

Technique

It is standard practice to use thiopental to induce anaesthesia in a dose of at least 4 mg kg^{-1}. This should be rapidly followed by succinylcholine 1–1.5 mg kg^{-1}. Cricoid pressure should be applied as consciousness begins to be lost and continued until the tracheal tube is confirmed to be in the trachea. Anaesthesia should be continued using nitrous oxide 50% and volatile agent in oxygen and positive pressure ventilation. Halothane or isoflurane are both commonly used and should be administered in a concentration of at least 0.5 MAC. Concentrations higher than 0.5 MAC cause excessive uterine relaxation, while lower concentrations predispose the patient to awareness. When using a circle breathing system, care is needed to prime the system with an adequate fresh gas flow and concentrations of the volatile agent, so that the desired 0.5 MAC level is reached quickly. If the fetus is compromised, there is evidence that the use of 100% oxygen with a volatile agent may be beneficial to the fetus by increasing oxygen transfer across the placenta. There is also increasing use of conventional gas ratios of nitrous oxide and oxygen (i.e. 66:33) from the beginning of the anaesthetic. This has become more common since the introduction of oximetry. After the delivery of the baby, an opioid, e.g. morphine, may be given with oxytocin, and an antibiotic to prevent wound infection. At this stage, the volatile agent may be increased towards 1 MAC, with 67% nitrous oxide. Additional non-depolarizing muscle relaxant (e.g. atracurium 25 mg) may be administered after the effect of the succinylcholine has worn off, as confirmed by a nerve stimulator. Residual neuromuscular block should be antagonized before tracheal extubation, with the patient in the lateral position and with a slight head-down tilt. Routine postoperative care in a fully equipped recovery area is essential. At this time, postoperative pain relief should be effective and the baby should be given to the mother whenever possible.

ASSESSMENT OF THE PREGNANT WOMAN PRESENTING FOR ANAESTHESIA AND ANALGESIA

Successive CEMD reports highlight the problems of women with intercurrent medical disease and the fact they are at increased risk in pregnancy and labour. There are many more women with a

Table 52.6 Equipment that should be available for general anaesthesia in a maternity unit

Two Macintosh laryngoscopes (one standard, one long blade)
Short-handled Macintosh laryngoscope (or 'Polio-blade' laryngoscope)
McCoy laryngoscope
Gum elastic bougie
Wide selection of tracheal tubes
Selection of oral and nasal airways
Laryngeal mask airway size 3
Percutaneous cricothyroidotomy kit

coincident significant medical problem becoming pregnant and it is important that these problems are recognized in the antenatal period. A good history should be taken. Recent developments in the national maternity record should facilitate significant medical problems being highlighted as the proposed record incorporates an extensive health questionnaire to be filled in by the woman and her midwife. The effect of the physiological changes of pregnancy on the disease must be recognized and appropriate investigations instigated.

Women with cardiac or respiratory disease need careful assessment, as the physiological changes of pregnancy and delivery may have a profound effect on the disease. Many of these women have good reserves for normal day-to-day activities but are unable to cope with the added stress of labour. Antenatal assessment often includes echocardiography, ECG and pulmonary function tests. Assessment of the medical record is particularly relevant where the woman has undergone surgery. Clear plans for labour and delivery need to be written in the record by all the medical team including the anaesthetist.

The other more common medical conditions occurring in women of child-bearing age are neurological disease, significant back problems including major surgery, drug allergies, previous anaesthetic problems and difficulties with tracheal intubation. Obesity, maternal age and smoking are also risk factors that should not be overlooked.

EMERGENCIES IN OBSTETRIC ANAESTHESIA

Emergencies in obstetric anaesthesia may be classified as follows:

- haemorrhage
- failed intubation
- pre-eclampsia and eclampsia
- total spinal or epidural block
- amniotic fluid embolus
- maternal and neonatal resuscitation.

HAEMORRHAGE

Significant bleeding occurs in 3% of all pregnancies and it may occur in either the antepartum or postpartum period.

Antepartum haemorrhage

Seventy per cent of all cases of antepartum haemorrhage result from placenta praevia and abruptio placentae.

Placenta praevia occurs when the placenta implants on the lower uterine segment and overlies the cervical os. It is assessed as being either anterior or posterior and the grade depends on the extent to which the placenta covers the os. In a grade 4 placenta praevia, the placenta covers the os, and in a grade 1 placenta praevia the placenta extends to the os. Significant bleeding may occur which may necessitate blood transfusion or urgent delivery. The potential estimate of the haemorrhage depends on the position of the placenta and this may be assessed by ultrasound scan. There are three factors that increase the potential for significant bleeding:

- In placenta praevia the veins on the anterior wall of the uterus are distended.
- If the placenta is anterior then the surgical incision extends through the placenta, causing significant haemorrhage.
- If the placenta covers the os then a raw area is left after its delivery. This area of the os does not have the ability to contract that the normal myometrium has, and may thus continue to bleed.

Women with diagnosed placenta praevia are usually delivered by elective caesarean section. As the condition may be associated with severe haemorrhage, which may be life-threatening, it is advisable that senior obstetric and anaesthetic staff are involved with the delivery of these patients. Blood should always be crossmatched. General anaesthesia is the technique of choice, but a consultant obstetric anaesthetist may consider regional anaesthesia in posterior grade 1 and 2 placenta praevia.

Abruptio placentae is defined as the premature separation of the placenta after the 20th week of gestation. It is associated with a perinatal mortality rate of up to 60%. Placental abruption may result in concealed or revealed haemorrhage. Typically the woman presents with abdominal pain, which may be severe, together with signs indicative of acute blood loss in proportion to the amount of blood lost. A trap for the unwary is that placental abruption may be associated with pre-eclampsia; therefore, if the pre-abruption arterial pressure was markedly elevated, the post-abruption BP may still appear normal, and so mask hypovolaemia. A large amount of blood loss is often associated with a consumptive coagulopathy and this occurs particularly with concealed haemorrhage.

Postpartum haemorrhage

Postpartum haemorrhage is the most frequent reason for surgery in the immediate postpartum period. Causes include:

- Retained placental tissue, including:
  - — placenta accreta: the placenta is abnormally adherent to the uterus but is normally placed (80% of cases)
  - — placenta increta: the adherence includes the myometrial muscle (15% of cases)
  - — placenta percreta: the adherence of the placental tissue extends right through to the peritoneal surface of the uterus (5% of cases). This is the commonest indication for caesarean hysterectomy.
- Uterine atony–the failure of the uterus to contract at the site of placental separation. The risk of uterine atony may be increased by:
  - — overdistension of the uterus (e.g. polyhydramnios, multiple gestation)
  - — prolonged (> 18 h) or precipitous (< 4 h) labour
  - — multiparity
  - — hypotension
  - — uterine infection
- Laceration of the birth canal – predisposing factors include instrumental delivery and a large infant.

Anaesthetic management of haemorrhage

Although regional anaesthesia has a role in the management of acute postpartum haemorrhage, the associated sympathetic block interferes with physiological compensatory mechanisms, potentially aggravating acute hypovolaemia. For this reason, GA is the preferred option in this situation.

Preoperative assessment

Estimation of the degree of blood loss is notoriously unreliable in the obstetric setting, and hence clinical estimation of the following signs of hypovolaemia should be undertaken:

- hypotension
- tachycardia > 120 beat min^{-1}
- urinary output < 0.5 min^{-1} kg^{-1}
- capillary refill time > 5 s
- anxiety, agitation or confusion
- transient or minimal response to 1–2 L crystalloid or 500 ml colloid fluid challenge.

The most recent triennial CEMD in the UK noted that deaths caused by haemorrhage had declined in this triennium, but that substandard management was identified in eight of 12 such deaths. Successive reports of the CEMD have highlighted the problems of haemorrhage and the need for each unit to have clear guidelines for major haemorrhage. Anaesthetists should be involved early in the management of such patients so that appropriate resuscitation, monitoring and planning for delivery may be developed.

The delivery suite team, including the anaesthetist, would:

- involve senior medical staff early
- request baseline haemoglobin and haematocrit
- place two large-gauge peripheral venous cannulae
- maintain circulating fluid volume
- administer group-compatible blood if possible or O-negative blood in a life-threatening situation
- consider insertion of invasive monitoring such as CVP or arterial monitoring
- involve the haematologist early for blood products and advice.

Intraoperative management

Rapid-sequence induction of GA is mandatory. Care with induction agents such as thiopental and propofol is required in hypovolaemic patients, as profound hypotension may ensue, leading to cardiovascular collapse. Ketamine 0.5–1 mg kg^{-1} stimulates the sympathetic nervous system and helps to preserve blood pressure during induction of anaesthesia.

Anaesthesia may be maintained with N_2O–O_2 mixtures and opioids such as fentanyl 1–2 μg kg^{-1} in boluses. Volatile agents should be administered cautiously because of the associated vasodilatation.

FAILED INTUBATION

Failed intubation reflects the relatively high incidence of airway difficulties in obstetric patients (approximately 1 in 300 compared with 1 in 2220 in non-pregnant patients). The increased incidence of difficult intubation in parturients is caused by changes in the soft tissues of the airway resulting in swollen upper airway mucosa, swollen and engorged breasts and full dentition. The decreasing use of general anaesthesia in obstetrics may lead to a relative lack of experience in this technique with increased anxiety for both junior and senior anaesthetists.

The modified failed laryngoscopy/intubation drill is an essential algorithm and should be displayed prominently in all obstetric theatres (Fig. 52.7). The essential points to take from the algorithm are to call for help when unexpected difficulty with laryngoscopy or intubation arises and to avoid repeated attempts at intubation without maintaining oxygenation. The placement of a laryngeal mask airway (LMA) may facilitate ventilation and, if used, cricoid pressure should be applied continuously.

PRE-ECLAMPSIA AND ECLAMPSIA

Hypertensive disorders (approximately 1 in 100 000 pregnancies) are among the leading causes of maternal mortality. Pre-eclampsia is defined as hypertension with proteinuria and pathological oedema after week 20. Eclampsia is defined as the occurrence of convulsions and/or coma during pregnancy not resulting from neurological disease.

Aetiology of eclampsia and pre-eclampsia

The aetiology is unknown, but current knowledge may be summarized as follows.

Immunological factors

In the normal placenta, the vascular bed is of low resistance. In pre-eclampsia there is abnormal migration of the trophoblast into the myometrial tissue and this leads to constriction of the spiral arteries which increases the resistance in the vascular bed. Prostacyclin and nitric oxide may be involved in this process.

Endothelial factors

Normotensive pregnant women demonstrate an increase in the activity of the renin–angiotensin–aldosterone system (RAAS) and a reduced response to exogenous angiotensin II. In pre-eclamptic women this does not occur and this has been linked to a lack of nitric oxide production by endothelial cells.

Platelet and coagulation factors

Endothelial dysfunction may lead to a lack of nitric oxide and prostacyclin, altering the balance of platelet function in favour of platelet aggregation.

Clinical presentation of pre-eclampsia

Clinically, pre-eclampsia is a multisystem disorder, and the predominant features in each system are as described below.

Cardiovascular system

Hypertension is defined as systolic arterial pressure >140 or diastolic >90 mmHg. Cardiac output and systemic vascular resistance are usually increased. Blood volume is decreased by up to 30% in severe cases, but with a normal CVP and pulmonary capillary wedge pressure (PCWP) unless there is pulmonary oedema. This may be attributable to vasoconstriction, and therefore the patient

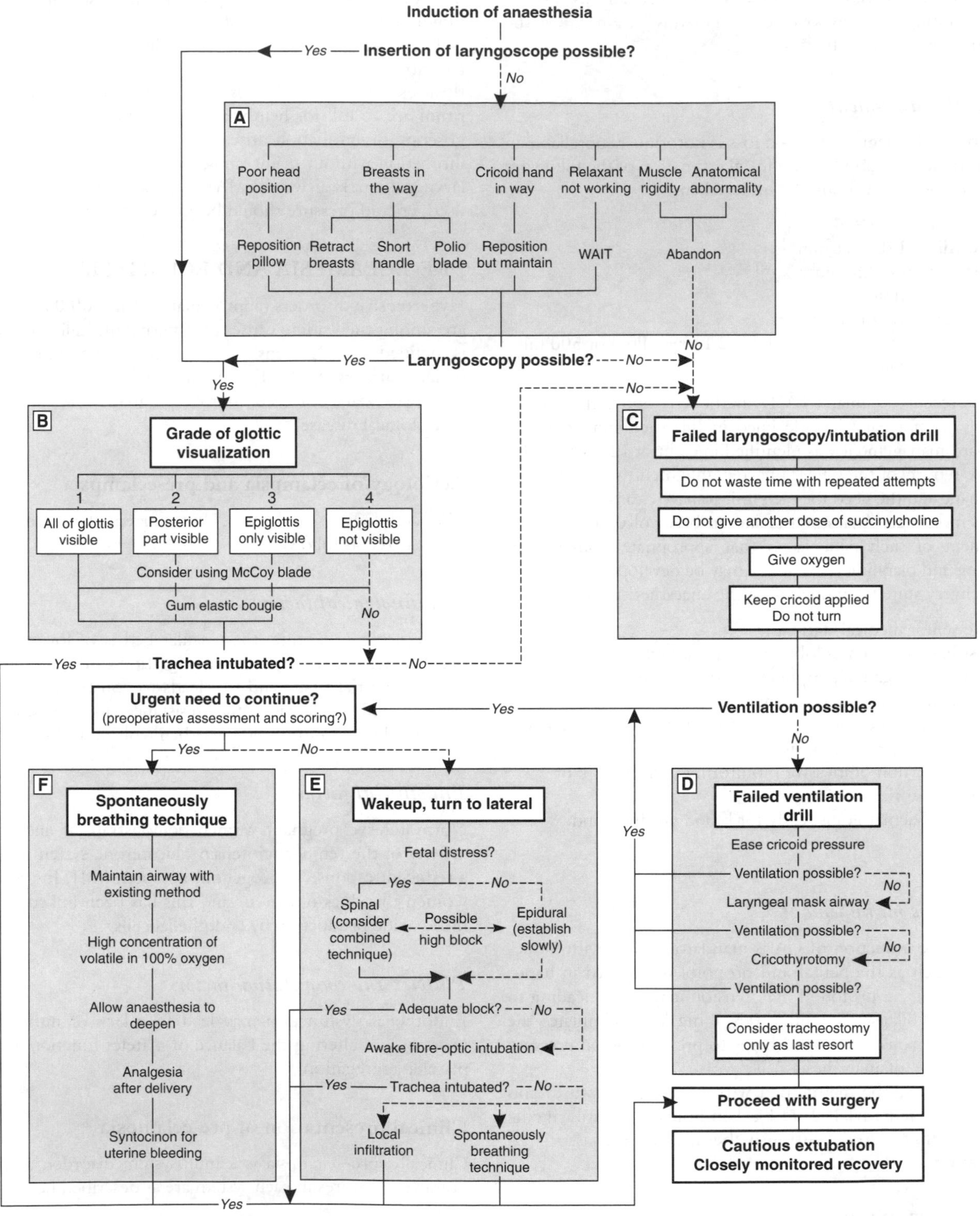

Fig. 52.7
Failed laryngoscopy/intubation drill.

is at risk of volume overload. Patients with pre-eclampsia may not have a raised arterial pressure, although it is significantly raised above baseline pressure at the beginning of pregnancy.

Central nervous system

Classically, this disease is accompanied by severe headache, visual disturbances and hyperreflexia. Seizures may occur without warning.

Renal system

Glomerular filtration rate is reduced by 25% compared with normal pregnant women, as a result of glomerular oedema, reducing the filtration efficiency such that proteinuria may occur. Although serum creatinine concentration rarely increases above normal, increased blood urea concentrations may be an early marker of deterioration.

Haematological system

Platelet and coagulation disorders may occur as discussed above. A rapidly decreasing platelet count is indicative of a worsening of pre-eclampsia, and low platelets may be associated with HELLP syndrome (haemolysis, elevated liver enzymes and low platelets). In general, a platelet count of 100×10^9 L^{-1} (taken within the last 12 h) and above is safe for insertion of an epidural catheter. At levels below this, a clotting screen is advised and the risks and benefits of regional block should be assessed.

Respiratory system

Pre-eclampsia increases the risk of airway oedema, which may make tracheal intubation hazardous. Pulmonary oedema may occur at any time, including up to 24 h after delivery, as a result of increased capillary permeability and decreased plasma oncotic pressure.

Management of pre-eclampsia

Obstetric management is designed to stabilize the mother and deliver the baby. It is essential that the mother is assessed and monitored carefully; this includes full biochemical and haematological screen, monitoring of arterial pressure, heart rate, fluid balance and oxygen saturation. High-dependency care is essential. Treatment of hypertension is essential and in the acute situation the drugs of choice are hydralazine, labetalol or nifedipine. Magnesium sulphate is used commonly in many parts of the world. Magnesium inhibits synaptic transmission at the neuromuscular junction, causing vasodilatation, and it also has a central anticonvulsant effect at the NMDA receptor. A loading dose of 4 g (in 100 ml saline) is given over 30 min, followed by a maintenance dose of 1–2 g h^{-1}. Serum concentrations must be monitored, with hourly assessment of peripheral limb reflexes. As serum concentrations increase above 10 mmol L^{-1}, there is progressive reduction in reflexes, respiratory arrest and asystole. The therapeutic range is 4–7 mmol L^{-1}.

Pre-eclamptic patients are vasoconstricted and hypovolaemic, so careful fluid administration is advisable during treatment of hypertension. There is continued debate concerning the suitability of crystalloid or colloid in these patients and a discussion of this is outside the remit of this chapter. It is important to remember that the woman may already be receiving antihypertensive therapy, e.g. methyldopa or nifedipine.

The role of epidural analgesia and anaesthesia in pre-eclampsia

Epidural analgesia is specifically indicated for labour analgesia in pre-eclampsia because:

- it provides excellent pain relief
- it attenuates the hypertensive response to pain
- it reduces circulating stress-related hormones and hence assists in controlling arterial pressure
- it improves uteroplacental blood flow
- these women have a higher incidence of caesarean section, and the presence of an epidural facilitates extension of the block.

If hypotension occurs, a crystalloid bolus (500 ml) may be administered, with the patient in a lateral tilt and receiving O_2. If this is not adequate, a bolus of ephedrine 3 mg may be given. Because of increased sensitivity of the circulation to exogenous vasopressors, caution is essential when administering ephedrine. Regional anaesthesia is the anaesthetic of choice if the woman is to be delivered by caesarean section, and although epidural anaesthesia has been the routine technique, there is increasing evidence to show that spinal anaesthesia or CSE may be the anaesthetic of choice for these women.

Eclampsia

If the woman has an eclamptic fit, the ABC of basic resuscitation should be commenced and it is essential that there is no compression of the aorta or vena cava during resuscitation. The treatment of eclampsia is 4 g magnesium sulphate by slow intravenous bolus as recommended in 1995 by the Eclampsia Trial Collaborative Group.

TOTAL SPINAL OR EPIDURAL BLOCK

Too large a volume of local anaesthetic or its inadvertent deposition in the subarachnoid space may lead to profound, extensive block. The time from injection of the anaesthetic solution to onset of symptoms depends upon the exact location of the injection:

- The effects of an epidural overdose are seen 20–30 min after the bolus.
- The effects of a subdural injection are seen 10–20 min after the bolus.
- The effects of a subarachnoid injection are seen within 2–5 min.

Local anaesthetic reaching the fourth ventricle results in cardiorespiratory arrest. Full resuscitation, including tracheal intubation and ventilation, external cardiac massage and vasopressors and inotropes are given as necessary. Spontaneous brain stem function returns as the excessively high block regresses over a period of 30 min to 4 h. However, when the mother has been stabilized, the baby is usually delivered by emergency caesarean section.

AMNIOTIC FLUID EMBOLISM

The incidence of amniotic fluid embolism is approximately 3 in 100 000 live births, but is associated with a high mortality. Amniotic fluid embolus has been described as a postmortem diagnosis depending on the pathological finding of fetal squames in the lung tissue. More recently, a clinical diagnosis has been used rather than a postmortem diagnosis. The woman presents with sudden collapse, usually after a rapid labour. Amniotic fluid in the maternal circulation causes hypotension and acute pulmonary oedema, followed rapidly by development of a consumptive coagulopathy and resultant haemorrhage. Management of this emergency involves resuscitation, with administration of oxygen and maintenance of the airway, including tracheal intubation and cardiopulmonary resuscitation, if necessary. Volume support with inotropes may be indicated. Treatment of the coagulopathy and intravenous fluids may be required. A protracted period of intensive care treatment may be necessary.

MATERNAL AND NEONATAL RESUSCITATION

Severe haemorrhage, amniotic fluid embolism, pulmonary embolus or other even more uncommon causes may result in an acutely collapsed mother. In these circumstances, immediate resuscitation is required, in the standard manner, but aortocaval compression should be avoided. Unsuccessful resuscitation is often caused by profound hypovolaemia. Caesarean section may be considered as part of the resuscitation in extreme situations; immediate delivery of the mother may dramatically improve her condition and the success of emergency resuscitation. The best chance of fetal survival in such circumstances is emergency delivery.

Neonatal resuscitation

The condition of the infant at birth may be assessed by:

- Apgar score – a clinical scale based on colour, heart rate, respiratory rate, capillary perfusion and tone of the limbs. It is obtained at 1 and 10 min after delivery, with maximum score being 10
- Umbilical cord vein pH, which is normally 7.25–7.35.

The process of resuscitation of the infant begins with gentle physical stimulation, suction of oral secretions and drying the baby. If there is little response and the heart rate is less than 80 beats min^{-1}, oxygen 100% is given by face mask. If respiration is inadequate and the heart rate is still less than 80 beats min^{-1}, ventilation is assisted at a rate of up to 60 breaths min^{-1} for 1 min by bag and mask. If the heart rate is still less than 80 beats min^{-1}, cardiopulmonary resuscitation is commenced, taking care not to cause damage to the delicate thoracic cage. This is continued with oxygenation and ventilation. Only if all of these measures fail to increase heart rate above 80 beats min^{-1} should the administration of epinephrine or atropine be considered. The newborn must be kept warm throughout.

More detailed neurobehavioral testing includes the NACS and Scanlon scoring systems.

ANAESTHESIA FOR INTERVENTIONS OTHER THAN DELIVERY

EXTRACTION OF RETAINED PRODUCTS OF CONCEPTION (ERPC)

Up to 20% of all confirmed pregnancies end in spontaneous abortion within the first trimester, and ERPC is indicated where there are retained placental products. These women are often very distressed and need sympathetic care. They should be assessed for blood loss, and although there is usually no problem, there is a significant risk of severe haemorrhage that may necessitate resuscitation, including blood transfusion. In the first trimester, anaesthesia is similar to that required for cervical dilatation and hysteroscopy. Anaesthesia may be induced with an i.v. induction agent, with or without a short-acting opioid such as fentanyl (1–2 μg kg^{-1}), and maintained via a face mask or LMA (as the procedure usually lasts 5–7 min) with the patient spontaneously breathing N_2O–O_2 and 1–2 MAC of volatile agent. Adequate depth of anaesthesia is required before cervical dilatation, as vagal stimulation in an inadequately anaesthetized patient may lead to bradycardia and laryngospasm. After cervical dilatation, the level of anaesthesia may be reduced to 0.5–1.0 MAC.

CERVICAL CIRCLAGE

This is a surgical procedure required occasionally for women with a history or active clinical features of an incompetent cervix, usually presenting as premature, precipitate labour. To reduce the risk of this occurring, a suture (Shirodkar suture) is placed around the cervix, in a procedure lasting 20–30 min. As this is usually performed in the second trimester or later, the anaesthetic considerations for any pregnant woman apply. Regional (spinal) anaesthesia is the technique of choice, with the required block height of T10–S5 being achieved using 1.5 ml hyperbaric bupivacaine with or without fentanyl 25 μg. If general anaesthesia must be undertaken, use of rapid-sequence induction is mandatory if the patient is at more than 12 weeks, gestation.

THE PREGNANT PATIENT WITH A SURGICAL (NON-OBSTETRIC) EMERGENCY

The incidence of general surgical emergencies is undiminished in pregnancy, and thus pregnant patients may require anaesthesia for laparotomy or any other procedure. If delivery is not anticipated, the anaesthetic technique should ensure good delivery of oxygen to the placenta. Use of depressant drugs such as opioids are not contraindicated. After the 13th week of gestation, the risk of regurgitation of gastric contents increases, so rapid-sequence induction should always be performed. It has been suggested that transvaginal ultrasound monitoring of the fetus may be useful.

EFFECT OF DRUGS ON THE FETUS

Drugs may have a harmful effect on the fetus at any time during pregnancy. In the early stages of pregnancy (at a stage when the woman may be unaware that she is pregnant), the conceptus is a rapidly dividing group of cells and the effect of drugs at that stage tends to be an all-or-none phenomenon, either slowing cell division where no harm is done or causing death of the embryo. Drugs may produce congenital malformations (teratogenesis), and the period of greatest risk is from weeks 3 to 11. In the second and third trimesters, drugs may affect the functional development of the fetus or have toxic effects on fetal tissues. Drugs given in labour or near delivery may adversely affect the neonate after delivery. Hence drugs should only be prescribed in pregnancy if the perceived benefit of the therapy to the mother outweighs the possible detrimental effects on the fetus. Drugs that have been extensively used should be prescribed in the lowest effective doses.

PHARMACOLOGY OF RELEVANT DRUGS

The detailed pharmacology of the drugs used during pregnancy is covered elsewhere in this textbook, but the following are of particular relevance.

Syntocinon (oxytocin)

Oxytocin is the posterior pituitary hormone responsible for effective uterine muscle contraction. It is indicated in a labour where the rate of progress is slow and immediately after delivery (either normal vaginal, instrumental or caesarean section) in order to cause placental delivery and closure of uterine vasculature. For augmentation or induction of labour, Syntocinon is usually administered via a syringe pump using an increasing dose as set out in the delivery suite guidelines. The usual dose to prevent postpartum haemorrhage is 10 international units (IU), but up to 40 IU may be infused over several hours to maintain myometrial contraction. It may also act on other types of vascular smooth muscle, resulting in hypertension. Syntocinon also has an antidiuretic hormone effect, so care should be taken if infused in dilute dextrose solution as hyponatraemia may occur.

Ergometrine

Ergometrine is also given to cause uterine contraction, usually in a dose of 500 μg. Ergometrine causes peripheral vasoconstriction, which may be severe, leading to hypertension and pulmonary oedema. It can cause nausea and vomiting as a result of its action on other types of smooth muscle and it is usually reserved for more severe cases of uterine atony. Ergometrine is contraindicated in pre-eclampsia.

Syntometrine

Syntometrine is a combination of ergometine 500 μg and Syntocinon 5 units. It is administered routinely by i.m. injection at the delivery of the anterior shoulder to assist in placental separation and reduction in postpartum haemorrhage.

Prostaglandins

Prostaglandins are a group of endogenous short polypeptides with a wide diversity of physiological functions. Their therapeutic use in obstetric practice is currently in medical termination of pregnancy. A prostaglandin-containing pessary may induce cervical dilatation and uterine contraction, expelling its contents. Prostaglandins may cause bronchospasm and also hypertension and are commonly used to 'ripen' the cervix in induction of labour.

Carboprost

Carboprost is a prostaglandin. It has an important role in the treatment of severe uterine atony unresponsive to Syntocinon or ergometrine. It is administered by i.m. injection and may be given into the myometrium at caesarean section.

Ritodrine

Ritodrine is occasionally given to arrest a premature labour. It is a β_2-adrenergic receptor agonist which relaxes uterine musculature and so prevents premature labour. The effect of ritodrine should be monitored carefully, as severe tachycardia and hypoglycaemia may occur.

FURTHER READING

Chestnut D H (ed) 1999 Obstetric anesthesia, 2nd edn. Mosby, St Louis

Datta S (ed) 1991 Anaesthetic and obstetric management of the high-risk pregnancy. Mosby-Year Book, St Louis

Eclampsia Trial Collaborative Group 1995 Which anticonvulsant for women with eclampsia? Evidence from the Collaborative Eclampsia Trial. Lancet 345: 1455–1463

Harmer M 1997 Difficult and failed intubation in obstetrics. International Journal of Obstetric Anesthesia 6: 25–31

Holdcroft A, Thomas T 2000 Principles and Practice of obstetric anaesthesia and analgesia. Blackwell Science, Oxford

MacEvilly E, Buggy D 1996 Back pain and pregnancy (review). Pain 64: 405–414

May A E (ed) 1994 Epidurals for childbirth. Oxford University Press, Oxford

Mushambi M C, Halligan A W, Williamson K 1996 Recent developments in the pathophysiology and management of pre-eclampsia. British Journal of Anaesthesia 76: 133–148

Reynolds F (ed) 2000 Regional anaesthesia in obstetrics. A millennium update. Springer, London

Why mothers die: a report of the triennial Confidential Enquiry into Maternal Death 1994–96

Yentis S M, Bridhouse A M, May A, Bogod D, Elton C 2000 Analgesia, anaesthesia and pregnancy. A practical guide. W B Saunders, London

53 Paediatric anaesthesia and intensive care

The differences in anatomy and physiology between children, especially infants, and adults have important consequences in many aspects of anaesthesia. The differences also account for the different patterns of disease seen in intensive care units (ICUs). Although major psychological differences persist throughout adolescence, a 10- to 12-year-old child may be thought of, anatomically and physiologically, as a small adult.

PHYSIOLOGY IN THE NEONATE

RESPIRATION

Control of respiration in newborn infants, especially premature neonates, is poorly developed. The incidence of central apnoea (defined as a cessation of respiration for 15 s or longer) is not uncommon in this group. The likelihood of this increases when the patient is given a drug with a sedative effect. Potentially life-threatening apnoea may occur. The incidence is reduced by postoperative administration of xanthine derivatives such as caffeine and theophylline which act as central respiratory stimulants Because of this problem, it is wise to admit for overnight oximetry and apnoea monitoring all children under 60 weeks post-conceptual age who have had surgical procedures, no matter how minor. Unlike the adult, hypoxia in the neonate and small child appears to inhibit rather than stimulate respiration.

The newborn has between 20 and 50 million terminal air spaces. At 18 months of age, the adult level of 300 million is reached by a process of alveolar multiplication. Subsequent lung growth occurs by an increase in alveolar size. The lung volume in infants is disproportionately small in relation to body size. Their metabolic rate is nearly twice that of the adult, and therefore ventilatory requirement per unit lung volume is increased. Thus they have far less reserve for gas exchange.

Before the age of 8 years, the calibre of the airways is relatively narrow. Airway resistance is therefore relatively high. Small decreases in the diameter of the airways as a result of oedema formation or respiratory secretions significantly increases the work of breathing. Elastic tissue in the lungs of small children is poorly developed. As a result of this, compliance is decreased. This has important consequences in that airway closure may occur during normal tidal ventilation, thereby bringing about an increase in alveolar–arterial oxygen tension difference ($P_{A\text{-}a}O_2$). This explains why P_aO_2 is lower in the infant than in the child. The decreased compliance results in ventilatory units with short time constants. Consequently, the infant is able to achieve adequate alveolar ventilation whilst maintaining a high respiratory rate. However, owing to the increased resistance and decreased compliance, the work of breathing may represent up to 15% of total oxygen consumption (Table 53.1). The high respiratory rate is necessary because the metabolic rate of the infant is nearly twice that of the adult. The high alveolar minute ventilation explains why induction and emergence from inhalation anaesthesia are relatively rapid in small children. The high metabolic rate explains why desaturation occurs very rapidly in children.

The ratio of physiological dead space to tidal volume V_d/V_t is similar to that of the adult at about 0.3. However, because the volumes are smaller, modest increases in V_d produced by equipment such as humidification filters may have a disproportionately greater effect (Table 53.2).

Ventilation in small children is almost entirely diaphragmatic. Because the ribs are horizontal, there is no bucket handle movement of the ribs as occurs in the adult. It is therefore important to appreciate that normal minute ventilation is respiratory rate-dependent.

It is important to appreciate that the infant's response to hypoxaemia can be bradypnoea and not tachypnoea as one would see in the adult.

CARDIOVASCULAR SYSTEM

The process of growth demands a high metabolic rate. It should therefore come as no surprise that infants and children have a

Table 53.1 Lung mechanics of the neonate compared with the adult

	Neonate	Adult
Compliance (ml cmH_2O^{-1})	5	100
Resistance (cmH_2O L^{-1} s^{-1})	30	2
Time constant (s)	0.5	1.3
Respiratory rate (breaths min^{-1})	32	15

Table 53.2 Respiratory variables in the neonate

Tidal volume (V_t)	7 ml kg^{-1}
Dead space (V_d)	(V_t) × 0.3 ml
Respiratory rate	32 breaths min^{-1}

higher cardiac index (compared with the adult) so that oxygen and nutrients can be delivered to actively growing tissues. The ventricles of neonates and infants are poorly compliant, so even though the ventricles of infants demonstrate the Frank–Starling mechanism, the main determinant of cardiac output is heart rate. Infants tolerate heart rates of 200 beats min^{-1} with ease (Table 53.3). Bradycardia may occur readily in response to hypoxaemia and vagal stimulation and it represents a decrease in cardiac output. Immediate cessation of the stimulus, and treatment with oxygen and atropine are absolutely crucial. A heart rate of 60 beats min^{-1} in an infant is considered a cardiac arrest and requires cardiac massage. Arrhythmias are rare in the absence of cardiac disease. The usual cardiac arrest scenarios are electromechanical dissociation and asystole, not ventricular fibrillation.

Even though infants and children have a higher cardiac index, arterial pressure tends to be lower than in adults because of a reduced systemic vascular resistance associated with an abundance of vessel-rich tissues in the infant. The pressure increases from approximately 80/50 mmHg at birth to the normal adult value of 120/70 mmHg by the age of 16 years. Children under the age of 8 years who are normovolaemic at the start of anaesthesia tend not to exhibit a decrease in arterial pressure when central neural blockade such as spinal anaesthesia is administered. They do not require fluid pre-loading as an adult would to avoid hypotension, because venous pooling tends not to occur as venous capacitance cannot increase much. The reasons for this are that the sympathetic nervous system is less well developed and so infants tend to be venodilated at rest. Second, they have a lower extremity to body surface ratio and as a consequence have a smaller venous capacitance.

As in all patients, the cardiovascular system must be carefully monitored. Pulse oximeter probes placed on the extremities provide a good index of peripheral perfusion. Auscultation of heart sounds, especially by an oesophageal stethoscope, is useful as the volume of heart sounds tends to be diminished as cardiac output decreases. Non-invasive measurement of arterial pressure is easily undertaken using an appropriately sized cuff. Complications preclude the use of invasive monitoring of arterial and central venous pressures for all but major cases.

Blood volume

The stage at which the umbilical cord is clamped determines the circulating blood volume of the neonate. Variations of up to +20% can occur. The average blood volume at birth is 90 ml kg^{-1}, and this decreases in the infant and young child to 80 ml kg^{-1}, attaining the adult level of 75 ml kg^{-1} at the age of 6–8 years. Blood losses of greater than 10% of the red cell mass should be replaced by blood, especially if further losses are expected. However, most children who have a normal haemoglobin concentration at the start of surgery can tolerate losses of up to 20% of their red cell mass. Children may tolerate a haematocrit of 25% and the decision to transfuse blood must be balanced against the risks, which include transmitted infection and antibody formation. The latter may cause problems in later life, especially to female children during child-bearing years.

Table 53.3 Variation in heart rates (beat min^{-1}) with age

Age	Mean value	Normal range
Neonate	140	100–180
1 year	120	80–150
2 years	110	80–130
6 years	100	70–120
12 years	80	60–100

Haemoglobin

At birth, 75–80% of the neonate's haemoglobin is fetal haemoglobin (HbF). By the age of 6 months, adult haemoglobin (HbA) haemopoiesis is fully established. HbF has a higher affinity for oxygen than HbA. This is demonstrated by the leftward shift of the oxygen haemoglobin dissociation curve (Fig. 53.1). Low tissue Po_2 and metabolic acidosis in the tissues result in the avidity of HbF for oxygen being reduced, thereby aiding delivery of oxygen. Alkalosis produced by hyperventilation results in less oxygen being available and it is therefore sensible to maintain normocapnia.

If blood transfusion is required, it is crucial that blood is filtered and warmed – the smaller the child, the more important this is. A syringe used via a tap in the intravenous giving set is probably the safest way of avoiding inadvertent overtransfusion. The circulating volume of a 1 kg neonate is of the order of 80 ml. Common sense dictates that blood loss should be carefully monitored, so swabs should be weighed and, if possible, all suction losses collected in a graduated container.

RENAL FUNCTION AND FLUID BALANCE

Body fluids constitute a greater proportion of body weight in the infant, particularly the premature infant, compared with the adult (Table 53.4). In an adult, most of the total body water is in the intracellular compartment. In a newborn infant, most of the total body water is in the extracellular compartment. With increasing age, the ratio reverses. Plasma volume remains constant throughout life at about 5% of body weight.

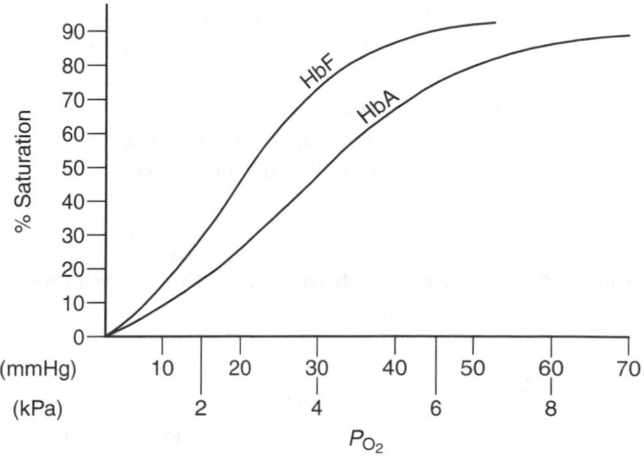

Fig. 53.1
Effects of fetal haemoglobin (HbF) on oxygen dissociation curve. HbA = Adult haemoglobin; Po_2 = Partial pressure of oxygen.

Table 53.4 Distribution of water as a percentage of body weight

Compartment	Premature	Neonate	Infant	Adult
ECF	50	35	30	20
ICF	30	40	40	40
Plasma	5	5	5	5
Total	85	80	75	65

ECF, extracellular fluid; ICF, intracellular fluid.

The kidneys are immature at birth. Both glomerular filtration rate (GFR) and subsequent reabsorption by the renal tubules are reduced. The GFR at birth is in the order of 45 ml min^{-1}/1.7 m^{-2}. This increases rapidly to about 65 ml min^{-1}/1.7 m^{-2} and then gradually approaches the adult value of 125 ml min^{-1}/1.7m^{-2} by the age of 8 years. Thus there is inability to handle excessive water and sodium loads. Overtransfusion may lead to pulmonary oedema and cardiac failure. The maturation in renal function is produced by hyperplasia in the first 6 months of life and then by a process of hypertrophy in the first year. Care must also be exercised when drugs eliminated by the renal route are used in infants; either reduced doses or an increased dosage interval should be used.

Poorly developed mechanisms exist for conserving water in the renal and gastrointestinal tract. Increased cutaneous water loss because of a large surface area to volume ratio through poorly keratinized skin may lead to a turnover of fluid in the infant of about 15% of total body water per day. Dehydration ensues very rapidly in an infant who is kept fasted.

FLUID THERAPY

An intravenous infusion delivering maintenance fluids should be in place for all neonates requiring surgery. Maintenance fluid requirements increase over the first few days of life (Tables 53.5 and 53.6). The normal infant requires of the order of 3–5 mmol kg^{-1} of sodium and an equivalent amount of potassium per day to maintain normal serum electrolyte concentrations. The ability of the infant's kidneys to eliminate excess sodium is limited. Exceeding this amount in the absence of loss results in hypernatraemia and its sequelae. Infants undergoing any procedure more than the briefest should also have their calorific needs addressed. This may be achieved by including dextrose-containing fluids in the regimen; failure to do so results in hypoglycaemia and ketosis.

Table 53.5 Fluid requirements in the first week of life

Day	Rate (ml kg^{-1} day^{-1})
1	0
2, 3	50
4, 5	75
6	100
7	120

Table 53.6 Maintenance fluid requirements

Weight (kg)	Rate (ml kg^{-1} day^{-1})
Up to 10 kg	100
10–20 kg	1000 + 50 × [weight (kg) − 10] ml
20–30 kg	1500 + 25 × [weight (kg) − 20] ml

This may occur rapidly because of the limited glycogen stores and high metabolic rate of the infant.

It is imperative that the anaesthetist recognizes and resuscitates the dehydrated infant appropriately before surgery. Clinical examination of skin turgor, tension of fontanelles, arterial pressure and venous filling may aid estimation of hydration, but electrolyte and haemoglobin concentrations and haematocrit, urine volumes and plasma and urine osmolalities should be monitored if problems of fluid balance exist (Table 53.7).

Intravenous fluids should be administered using a system that allows small volumes to be given accurately. This may vary from the anaesthetist injecting fluid using a syringe to microprocessor-controlled syringe driver pumps. The latter are preferable, as fluid is given at a steady rate and the anaesthetist's hands are free to tend to other tasks. During surgery, fluid administration should be increased to account for increased losses occurring through evaporation from exposed viscera and third space losses.

The intraosseous route may be used to carry out fluid resuscitation and drug therapy in shocked children. The needle should be inserted in an aseptic fashion to minimize the risk of osteomyelitis. Although various sites have been described for needle insertion, the proximal end of the tibia below the tuberosity is probably the easiest to perform. The intraosseous route is safer than attempting central venous cannulation in the shocked child in whom veins are difficult to discern. The usual fluid administered in this situation is

Table 53.7 Effects of dehydration in the young infant

	Mild	Moderate	Severe
Percentage loss of body weight	5%	10%	15%
Clinical signs	Dry skin and mucous membranes	Mottled cold periphery Depressed fontanelles Oliguria ++	Shocked Moribund Unresponsive to pain
Replacement	50 ml kg^{-1}	100 ml kg^{-1}	150 ml kg^{-1}

human albumin solution. This is given as a 10 ml kg^{-1} bolus and repeated until clinical improvement occurs.

TEMPERATURE REGULATION AND MAINTENANCE

Homeothermic animals possess the ability to produce and dissipate heat. Heat loss occurs by one of four processes: radiation, convection, evaporation and conduction. The environment in which the patient is situated governs the relative contribution of each. The neutral thermal environment is defined as the range of ambient temperatures at which temperature regulation is achieved by non-evaporative physical processes alone.

The metabolic rate at this temperature is minimal. The temperature of such an environment is 34°C for the premature neonate, 32°C for the neonate at term and 28°C for the adult.

Heat may be produced by one of three processes: voluntary muscle activity, involuntary muscle activity and non-shivering thermogenesis. Infants under the age of 3 months do not shiver. The only method available to increase their temperature in the perioperative period is non-shivering thermogenesis. The process is mediated by specialized tissue termed brown fat. It differentiates in the human fetus between 26 and 30 weeks of gestation. It comprises between 2 and 6% of total body weight in the human fetus and is located mainly between the scapulae and in the axillae. It is also found around blood vessels in the neck, in the mediastinum and in the loins. Brown fat is made of multinucleated cells with numerous mitochondria and has an abundant blood and nerve supply. Its metabolism is mediated by catecholamines. The substrate used for heat production is mainly fatty acids.

Radiation accounts for about 60% of the heat loss from a neonate in a 34°C incubator placed in a 21°C room. If the infant were in a thermoneutral environment of 34°C, the percentage loss by radiation would decrease to about 40% of the total heat loss, and, in addition, the total heat loss in this environment would be lower. The reason for this is that heat loss by radiation is a function of skin surface area and the difference in temperature between the skin and the room. The second major source of heat loss in the neonate is convection. This is a function of skin temperature and ambient temperature. The neonate possesses minimal subcutaneous fat that may act as thermal insulation and as a barrier to evaporative loss. A neonate has a body surface area to volume ratio about 2.5 times greater than the adult; thus a neonate may become hypothermic very rapidly.

If neonates are allowed to become hypothermic during anaesthesia, unlike adults they attempt to correct this by non-shivering thermogenesis. Metabolic rate increases and oxygen consumption may double. The increase in metabolic rate puts an additional burden on the cardiorespiratory system and this may be critical in neonates with limited reserve. The release of norepinephrine in response to hypothermia causes vasoconstriction, which in turn causes a lactic acidosis. The acidosis in turn favours an increase in right-to-left shunt, which causes hypoxaemia. As a result, a vicious positive feedback loop of hypoxaemia and acidosis is set up. The protective airway reflexes of a hypothermic neonate are obtunded, thereby increasing the risks of regurgitation and aspiration of gastric contents. The action of most anaesthetic drugs is potentiated by hypothermia. This effect is particularly important with regard to neuromuscular blocking drugs. The combination of hypothermia and prolonged action of these drugs increases the chances of the neonate hypoventilating after sugery.

Many precautions should be taken to ensure that the neonate's body temperature is maintained. First, the child must be transported to theatre wrapped up and in an incubator set at the thermoneutral temperature. The theatre should be warmed up to the thermoneutral temperature, ideally a few hours before the planned start of surgery. This interval allows the walls of the theatre to warm up and this reduces the net heat loss by radiation. One must appreciate that heat loss by radiation is a two-way process. The child loses heat by radiation to the walls and it also gains heat from the walls. All body parts that are not needed for insertion of cannulae and for monitoring should remain covered until the child has been draped with surgical towels. If the child has to be exposed, overhead radiant heaters may be used. During surgery, the child should lie on a thermostatically controlled heated blanket. Forced air warming systems are effective at maintaining the child's temperature during surgery; these work on the principle of blowing filtered warmed air into quilted blankets with perforations. This allows warmed air to come into direct contact with the patient. Simple measures such as using bonnets to reduce heat loss from the head are very effective. Intravenous fluids and fluids used to perform lavage of body cavities must be warmed. Anaesthetic gases should be humidified and warmed in order to preserve ciliary function and to reduce heat loss from the respiratory tract.

MONITORING

It is important in all procedures to measure temperature. For short procedures, an axillary temperature probe may be sufficient. In longer operations, core temperature should be measured at a variety of sites, such as rectal, bladder, nasopharyngeal and oesophageal. The oesophageal probe is often the preferred method as most modern oesophageal probes may be connected to a stethoscope. The anaesthetist is therefore able to listen to heart sounds in addition to recording the patient's temperature. When active heating methods such as cascade humidifiers and heated blankets are used, it is important that temperature gradients between the patient and the warming device are kept to less than 10°C. Failure to observe this may result in burns to the skin and the respiratory tract. In the ICU, simultaneous measurement of core and peripheral temperatures serves as a useful guide as to adequacy of the cardiac output. Decreases in cardiac output result in a reduction of blood flow to the peripheries and this is reflected in a core peripheral temperature gradient greater than 3–4°C.

PHARMACOLOGY IN THE NEONATE

DEVELOPMENTAL PHARMACOLOGY

Drugs given via the oral or rectal route are absorbed by a process of passive absorption. This process is dependent on the physicochemical properties of the drug and the surface area available for absorption. Most drugs are either weak bases or weak acids. The un-ionized portion of the drug therefore depends on the pH of the fluid in the gut. The gastric pH of the neonate is higher than that of the older child and adult. The consequence is that drugs inactivated by a low pH undergo greater absorption. Examples of these include antibiotics such as penicillin G.

Factors which determine the distribution of intravenously administered drugs include protein and red cell binding, tissue volumes, tissue solubility coefficients and blood flow to tissues. Neonates, in particular pre-term infants, have lower plasma concentrations of albumin. In addition, the albumin is qualitatively different in that its ability to bind drugs is lower than that of adult albumin. The concentration of α_1-acid glycoprotein is also lower in this group of patients; this protein is the major binding protein for alkaline drugs, which include opioid analgesics and local anaesthetics.

The blood–brain barrier is immature at birth; thus, it is more permeable to drugs. In addition, the neonate's brain receives a larger proportion of the cardiac output than does the adult brain. Consequently, brain concentrations of drugs are higher in neonates than in adults. For example, administration of morphine, which has low lipid solubility, results in high concentrations in the neonate's brain and therefore it should be used with caution and in reduced amounts in this age group.

In a neonate, total body water, extracellular fluid and blood volume are proportionally larger in comparison to an adult. This results in a larger apparent volume of distribution for a parenterally administered drug. This explains in part why neonates appear to require larger amounts of some drugs on a weight basis to produce a given effect. However, plasma concentrations tend to remain high for longer because they have smaller muscle mass and fat stores to which drugs redistribute.

The action of most drugs is terminated by metabolism or excretion through the liver and kidney. In the liver, phase I reactions convert the original drug to a more polar metabolite by the addition or unmasking of a functional group such as -OH, NH_2 or -SH. These reduction/oxidation reactions are a function of liver size and the metabolizing ability of the appropriate microsomal enzyme system. The volume of the liver relative to body weight is largest in the first year of life. The enzyme systems in the liver responsible for the metabolism of drugs are incompletely developed in the neonate. Their activity appears to be a function of postnatal rather than postconceptual age, because premature and full-term infants develop the ability to metabolize drugs to the same degree in the same period after birth. Adult levels of activity are achieved within a few days of birth. Phase II reactions that involve conjugation with moieties such as sulphate, acetate, glucuronic acid etc. are severely limited at birth. Most of these conjugation reactions are in place by the age of 3 months. The kidney ultimately eliminates most drugs. As mentioned above, GFR is lower in young children than in adults. However, by the age of 3 months the clearance of most drugs approaches adult values.

SPECIFIC DRUGS IN PAEDIATRIC ANAESTHESIA

Inhalation agents

Alveolar and brain concentrations of inhalation anaesthetic agents increase rapidly in children, because they have a greater alveolar ventilation rate in relation to functional residual capacity (FRC) and because of the preponderance of vessel-rich tissues. Induction and excretion of the agent at the termination of anaesthesia are more rapid.

The MAC value of anaesthetic agents changes with age. This is believed to be because of age-related differences in blood/gas solubility coefficients. From birth, MAC increases to a peak at the age of 6 months and then gradually declines until the adult value is reached. It is worth stating at this juncture that malignant hyperthermia has been reported or is possible with all the presently available volatile anaesthetic agents and that all potentiate the duration of neuromuscular blocking drugs.

Nitrous oxide

Nitrous oxide is used as a carrier gas for most inhalation anaesthetic agents. It is also used for its MAC-sparing effect. The effect is most marked with halothane with which a 60% reduction can be achieved. However, with the newer agents such as sevoflurane, only a 25% reduction may be produced. Thus, there would appear to be little to be gained by adding nitrous oxide to a sevoflurane anaesthetic. A major problem with nitrous oxide is its greater solubility compared with nitrogen. It diffuses into closed nitrogen-containing spaces at a greater rate than nitrogen leaves, thereby causing expansion. This effect is particularly important in lung lesions such as pneumothorax and congenital lobar emphysema. Expansion of the bowel in exomphalos or gastroschisis may make surgical reduction into the peritoneal cavity difficult.

Halothane

This agent has been the gold standard for induction of anaesthesia in children, because until recently its odour was one of the least pungent. It shares with all anesthetic agents the ability to depress the myocardium. However, it also slows heart rate, causing a decrease in cardiac output. It is therefore prudent to give an anticholinergic prior to its administration. Induction with halothane is smooth, and because most vaporizers allow 5 × MAC to be administered, it may be given in almost 100% oxygen. This is a useful feature when anaesthetizing a child with an airway problem. Another property which makes halothane useful in this situation is its prolonged action compared with the newer volatile agents, as it is undesirable that anaesthesia 'lightens' during instrumentation of the airway. In adult anaesthetic practice, repeat administrations of halothane within a period of less than 3 months may be associated with hepatic dysfunction and occasionally with fulminant hepatic failure. The exact mechanism of this toxic effect is not clear, but some have speculated that a reductive metabolite of halothane is responsible. Reductive hepatic metabolism of drugs is poorly developed in children and this may explain why this problem is extremely rare in children. However, if a child needs a second anaesthetic within 3 months of a first halothane anaesthetic, a risk–benefit assessment has to be undertaken. Economic considerations dictate that this is the most widely used inhalation agent for induction and maintenance of anaesthesia in children worldwide. As one might predict from its physical characteristics, emergence from halothane anaesthesia tends to take longer compared with the newer agents. It is acceptable to induce anaesthesia with halothane and then to use a less lipid-soluble agent for maintenance.

Enflurane

Induction with enflurane is not as smooth as that with halothane because of its pungent smell. It often induces breath-holding, coughing and laryngospasm. The high MAC value in children and the fact that it is not possible to give more that 2 × MAC with most vaporizers limit its value in paediatric anaesthetic practice. Because of epileptiform activity on the EEG when administered in high concentration to a hypocapnic patient, enflurane should be avoided in children with a history of seizures.

Isoflurane

Cardiac output tends to be well maintained when less than 1 MAC of this agent is used for maintenance of anaesthesia. However, because of its pungency, it is not a suitable agent for induction. All the adverse effects seen with induction with enflurane also occur with isoflurane, so in spite of the fact that it has a low blood/gas partition coefficient, induction tends to be slow. It may be used for maintenance of anaesthesia after halothane or intravenous induction.

Sevoflurane

The blood/gas partition coefficient of 0.68 results in rapid induction of anaesthesia with this agent and also a quick recovery. It is the least pungent of the currently available agents. It is possible to turn the vaporizer to its maximum output of 8% without experiencing significant problems of coughing, breath-holding or laryngeal spasm. There is little to be gained by including nitrous oxide during induction as the MAC-sparing effect on sevoflurane is not as great as with other agents. It is not unusual to observe slowing of the heart rate during induction, but it is not usually necessary to give an anticholinergic. Cardiac arrhythmias do not commonly occur during induction or maintenance with this agent. Economic considerations dictate that the agent is used mainly for induction, followed by a cheaper agent such as isoflurane for maintenance. Sevoflurane is an excellent choice for induction in children with upper airway obstruction, but it is probably wise to change over to halothane prior to instrumentation of the airway. The reason for doing this is so that the child does not 'lighten' during the procedure. The agent is partly degraded by soda lime to compound A which is nephrotoxic in rats because they possess the enzyme beta-lyase. This hazard would appear to be theoretical in humans.

Desflurane

The blood/gas partition coefficient of 0.42 suggests that induction should be rapid, but this is not so because desflurane is very irritant to the upper airway. It may be used for maintenance of anaesthesia with the benefit that emergence is very rapid. This may be particularly desirable in the ex-premature infant. Cost and the fact that the agent has to be delivered using a special vaporizer limit the use of this agent in paediatric practice.

Intravenous agents

The availability of topical local anaesthetic creams has resulted in venepuncture and cannulation being relatively atraumatic for children. As a consequence, intravenous induction has become more common.

Barbiturates

Thiopental is the most widely used in this class of agents. A dose of 5–6 mg kg^{-1} of a 2.5% solution is required in the healthy child. The main advantage of this agent is that injection into a small vein is pain-free. The agent can be given rectally using a 10% solution at a dose of 30 mg kg^{-1}, but induction and recovery tend to be slow with this technique.

Propofol

This agent may be used for both induction and maintenance of anaesthesia as part of a total intravenous technique. Although not common in paediatric anaesthetic practice, the technique of total intravenous anaesthesia using propofol is very useful in the child prone to malignant hyperthermia or the child with porphyria. Induction and maintenance doses tend to be larger in the younger healthy patient. The reasons for this are because of a larger central volume of distribution and because the clearance of the agent is higher compared with the adult. Pain on injection is a problem and this may be lessened by the addition of 0.2 mg kg^{-1} of lidocaine.

Ketamine

The current formulation of this drug is a racemic mixture of the S(+) and R(−) enantiomers. It is possible to separate the two enantiomers, although at present this does not appear to be a commercially viable proposition. The reason for doing this is that the S(+) enantiomer is twice as potent, recovery is quicker and the incidence of emergence psychic reactions is lower. One of the major advantages of ketamine is the intense analgesia it provides. The analgesia has both spinal and supraspinal components. Epidural administration of the drug in combination with local anaesthetic significantly prolongs the duration of analgesia compared with local anaesthetic alone. The lack of cardiovascular depression in vivo is a feature that allows the drug to be used for inducing anaesthesia in children with congenital heart disease. Occasionally, pulmonary vascular resistance may increase, and as a consequence pulmonary pressures also increase. Even though upper airway reflexes are relatively well preserved, aspiration of gastric contents may still occur. The drug has bronchodilator properties and may be used for sedating the child with status asthmaticus to allow artificial ventilation in the ICU. It is prudent to administer an anticholinergic when the drug is used for maintenance of anaesthesia, because increased salivation and bronchial secretions are potential problems. Emergence from ketamine anaesthesia is slower than with other agents. It may be accompanied by emergence phenomena such as hallucinations and unpleasant dreams. The incidence of these can be reduced by concurrent administration of a benzodiazepine.

Opioids

These may be used in large doses as the sole agent to provide stable haemodynamic conditions for children with cardiac disease. The major disadvantage of using this technique is that drug effects persist into the postoperative period, causing respiratory depression. As a result, postoperative mechanical ventilation is mandatory. Remifentanil is the newest of the synthetic opioids. It is unique in that its metabolism to a virtually inactive metabolite is by non-specific esterases in blood and tissue. The half-time of the drug is independent of the duration of infusion. There are few data on the use of this drug in infants and children, and at present it is unlicensed for use in children under the age of 2 years.

However, it is likely to be valuable in infants because of its lack of accumulation and short half-life.

Neuromuscular blocking drugs and their antagonists

The neuromuscular junction in infants is not mature. Electrophysiological studies demonstrate that the response of the junction is similar to what one might observe in a patient with myasthenia gravis. In other words, the junction is very sensitive to the effects of neuromuscular blockers. These drugs are polar and as a result distribute mainly to the extracellular space. Because this space is larger in the infant, the dose of drug required to depress twitch tension is similar or slightly larger than that required for adults on a dose/unit weight basis. The larger volume of distribution explains why drugs that depend on the kidneys or liver for elimination have a longer duration of action. Conversely, drugs such as atracurium which are degraded by a combination of ester hydrolysis and Hoffman elimination act for a shorter time because of the larger extracellular space.

Anticholinesterases are used to antagonize residual neuromuscular blockade. The appropriate anticholinergic to match the duration and onset should be combined with the anticholinesterase in order to minimize muscarinic side-effects. Atropine with edrophonium and glycopyrronium with neostigmine are the recommended combinations. The dose requirements are similar to those of adults and reversal should not be attempted in the presence of profound blockade. The edrophonium/atropine combination has a quicker onset of action and a shorter duration of action. This combination, although not readily available, might be more appropriate for reversing the currently widely used intermediate duration drugs.

Succinylcholine

This depolarizing neuromuscular blocking drug has the most rapid onset of action of any currently readily available agent. It is therefore the drug of choice for the patient with a full stomach and also for the treatment of laryngeal spasm. In the infant, it has the ability to cause bradycardia after only a single dose. It is wise to administer an anticholinergic before administration. A hyperkalaemic response is not seen after its administration to children with myelomeningocoele or cerebral palsy. It is one of the most potent triggers for malignant hyperthermia. The incidence of this increases if succinylcholine is preceded by a halothane induction. Fatal cardiac arrest has occurred in a small number of patients. It is presumed that these patients had unsuspected muscular dystrophies and that the drug caused massive muscle breakdown. As it is not possible to predict which patients might exhibit this response, it would appear to be wise to limit the use of the drug to patients with a full stomach and for the relief of laryngospasm.

Non-depolarizing agents

Onset and duration of action and the response in patients with renal and hepatic disease are probably the most important considerations when choosing one of these agents. Rocuronium has the most rapid onset of all the currently available agents. The onset of all these drugs may be increased by giving larger doses, but this is counterbalanced by a correspondingly longer duration of action. Currently a new amino-steroid, rapacuronium, is being evaluated in paediatric practice. Data suggest that its onset of action is similar to that of succinylcholine and that its duration of action is comparable with that of mivacurium. Mivacurium has the shortest duration of action of the currently available drugs. It is conceivable that, in the near future, succinylcholine may be replaced by a non-depolarizing drug. Mivacurium is best suited for the short surgical procedure, which usually matches its duration of action. Very occasionally, a patient may be cholinesterase-deficient in which case its duration is long. Atracurium, rocuronium and vecuronium have an intermediate duration of action, making them the most commonly used, as the duration of most paediatric operations falls into this category. Cis-atracurium and pancuronium are best reserved for the long procedure. Pancuronium is excreted renally and should be used with caution in the patient with renal failure. In spite of the fact that vecuronium and rocuronium are excreted by the liver, their duration of action is minimally affected by hepatic disease. Atracurium or cis-atracurium is the most obvious choice for patients with renal or hepatic disease, as elimination is altered minimally by organ failure.

ANAESTHETIC MANAGEMENT

PREOPERATIVE PREPARATION

For all elective surgery, it should be possible to prepare the child and family for what is to be expected in the perioperative period. This may be done in a wide variety of ways, including hospital tours, educational videotapes and pamphlets. The optimum choice depends on the age and intellectual ability of the child. Children possess great insight, and to attempt to keep forthcoming events secret is only likely to lead to mistrust and fear. All children should be visited preoperatively by the anaesthetist responsible for caring for them in the perioperative period. This is the opportunity not only to assess fitness for anaesthesia and surgery, but also, when appropriate, to allay anxiety, answer questions and to find out what the child's preferences are for mode of induction, pain relief etc.

Children who are systemically unwell should not have elective surgery. It is not unusual for a child to present with coryzal symptoms alone. There is an increased incidence of airway problems during anaesthesia; these children are more at risk of laryngeal spasm, breath-holding and bronchospasm, and in the postoperative period the chance of post-intubation croup is increased. The decision to proceed should be made only by a senior anaesthetist. Occasionally these symptoms precede a more serious upper or lower respiratory tract infection. In very rare cases, the viraemic phase of the illness may be associated with a myocarditis. Each case should be dealt with on its merits. Children who have active viral illnesses such as chickenpox should not have elective surgery, nor should children who have recently been immunized using live vaccines, for two reasons: first, there is an associated myocarditis or pneumonitis; and, second, to protect others on the ward who may be immunocompromised.

It is extremely important that the child is weighed before arrival in theatre, because body weight is the simplest and most reliable guide to drug dosage. Veins suitable for placement of cannulae should be identified and, if possible, local anaesthetic cream applied and covered with an occlusive dressing. If it has not been

Table 53.8 Estimates of children's weight

Age	Approximate body weight (kg)
Neonate	3
4 months	6
1–8 years	2 × age + 9
9–13 years	3 × age

possible to weigh the child, the weight may be estimated from the child's age (see Table 53.8).

PREOPERATIVE FASTING

Morbidity and mortality caused by aspiration of gastric contents are extremely rare in children undergoing elective surgery. What is becoming increasingly clear is that prolonged periods of starvation in children, especially the very young infant, are harmful. These children, who have a rapid turnover of fluids and a high metabolic rate are, at risk of developing hypoglycaemia and hypovolaemia. Research has shown that children allowed unrestricted clear fluids up to 2 h before elective surgery have a gastric residual volume equal to or less than that of children who have been fasted overnight. The essential message is that children should, rather than could, be given clear fluids up to 2 h before induction. Solids (including breast and formula milk) should not be given for at least 4 h before the anticipated start of induction. In the emergency setting, e.g. the child who has sustained trauma shortly after ingesting food, it is probably best (if possible) to wait 4 h before inducing anaesthesia. Clearly in this situation risk–benefit judgements have to be made. If it is surgically possible to wait 4 h, an i.v. infusion of a glucose-containing solution must be commenced and, if necessary, appropriate fluid resuscitation undertaken.

PREMEDICATION

The advent of local anaesthetic creams has reduced the necessity for sedative premedication. Currently two formulations are available:

- *EMLA* has been available for over a decade. Venepuncuture is usually painless if it has been applied and an occlusive dressing placed over the site at least 1 h before the planned procedure. It is wise to apply it over at least two locations marked by the anaesthetist in case the first attempt fails. It should not be used in the very small child or on mucous membranes because of the danger of systemic absorption of prilocaine that results in methaemoglobinaemia. It should not be left on the skin for more than 5 h. A major disadvantage of EMLA is that it causes some venoconstriction and this obscures the vein.
- *Tetracaine gel* is the other agent available for this purpose. It has the advantage of a quicker onset of action and also provides analgesia for a considerable period of time after the occlusive dressing has been removed. This is an advantage in the day-care unit, because it may be applied as part of the admission procedure for all the children, left on for about 45 min and then removed, as small children often object to the presence of the occlusive dressing.

Occasionally a sedative premedicant drug is required. This is particularly useful for the child who, in spite of good preoperative preparation, remains apprehensive. Currently the injectable form of midazolam given orally is gaining widespread popularity. The dose used is 0.5 mg kg $^{-1}$. An effect occurs within 10 min, with the peak at 20–30 min after administration. It may be used in the day case without a significant effect on discharge time. The bitter taste is a disadvantage. This should be eliminated when an oral formulation becomes available. One should err on reducing the dose if the patient is concurrently taking drugs that inhibit hepatic enzymes, because the duration of action of midazolam may be significantly prolonged.

An alternative to midazolam is oral ketamine in a dose 3–10 mg kg $^{-1}$. An antisialagogue (e.g. atropine 0.02 mg kg^{-1}) should be added to prevent excess salivation. The larger the dose, the more likely it is that the child may experience postoperative nausea and vomiting. If profound degrees of sedation are required, it is possible to combine midazolam and ketamine.

Intramuscular premedication is generally not tolerated well by children. Often it is the event in their hospital stay that they dislike the most. Rectal administration of induction agents such as thiopental has been used in doses of 25–30 mg kg^{-1}. This form of premedication may only be used under the direct supervision of the anaesthetist, as respiratory depression is a distinct possibility. A relatively new route for premedication administration is the intranasal route. This is particularly useful for the child who refuses to swallow an oral premedication. Drugs that have been used by this route include ketamine and midazolam in the doses mentioned above. It is not known at this stage how much of the drug goes through the cribriform plate directly into the central nervous system. Until this issue is clarified, it is best not to use this route routinely, because midazolam or its preservative and the preservative used with ketamine are neurotoxic when applied directly to neural tissue.

INDUCTION

It is important that the child is accompanied to the anaesthetic room by someone familiar. This person is usually a parent but it may be a ward play specialist with whom the child feels comfortable. It is equally important that whoever accompanies the child is not coerced into doing so. Children usually detect anxiety in their parents and this tends to have an adverse effect on their behaviour.

The person accompanying the child should be informed on the ward of what to expect in the anaesthetic room. For example, if an inhalation induction is planned, he or she should be made aware of some of the signs of the excitation phase that the child might exhibit. If an i.v induction is planned, the person should be made aware of how to assist the anaesthetist by distracting the child.

Unlike adult practice, it is not possible to have all the necessary monitoring devices placed on the child before induction. In most cases, it should be possible to place an appropriately sized pulse oximeter probe on a digit. Most children also allow the placement of a precordial stethoscope. The appropriate monitoring should be placed as soon as possible after the start of anaesthesia. The anaesthetist must always have an assistant present who is used to paediatric anaesthesia.

When inhalation induction is planned, clear, scented plastic masks are much more acceptable to little children than the traditional Rendell–Baker rubber masks. Clear masks allow respiration and the presence of vomitus to be observed. An alternative to using a mask is cupping one's hand over the face of the child while holding the T-piece. It is important to ensure that the flow of fresh gas is directed away from the child's eyes as anaesthetic gases may be irritant.

Airway management

The ratio of dead space to tidal volume tends to remain constant at about 0.3 throughout life in the healthy person. Anaesthetic apparatus such as connectors and humidification devices significantly increase dead space and should be kept to the minimum. This is especially important if the child breathes spontaneously during anaesthesia.

The Rendell–Baker masks were developed to fit around the facial anatomy of the child in an attempt to minimize equipment dead space. In fact, the flow of gas in a clear mask is such that the advantage of using Rendell–Baker masks is minimal. These masks are much more difficult to use than the clear ones with a pneumatic cushion. When using a face mask, it is important that the soft tissue behind the chin is not pushed backwards by the fingers, thereby obstructing the airway. The anaesthetist's fingers should rest only on the mandible.

The Jackson Rees modification of the Ayres T-piece is the breathing system traditionally used for children under 20 kg in weight. It has been designed to be lightweight with a minimal apparatus dead space. The apparatus may be used for both spontaneous and controlled ventilation. The open-ended reservoir bag is used for manual controlled ventilation. This mode of ventilation is especially useful in the neonate and infant, as one is able to detect changes in compliance produced by tube displacement. The reservoir bag also allows the application of continuous positive airway pressure for both the spontaneously breathing child and one undergoing ventilation. This may be helpful in improving oxygenation. The bag may be removed and an appropriate ventilator such as the Penlon 200 attached to the expiratory limb. A minimum gas flow rate of 3 L min^{-1} is required to operate this apparatus satisfactorily. Fresh gas flows of 300 ml kg^{-1} for spontaneous respiration and flows of 1000 ml plus 100 ml kg^{-1} for controlled ventilation usually result in normocapnia. It is difficult to scavenge the T-piece system. For the older child, it is satisfactory to use the Bain, Humphrey ADE or the circle absorber. It is easy to scavenge the waste gases from these systems with the resultant benefit of reducing pollution of the theatre environment. In addition, the circle system offers economic advantages because of the low fresh gas flows required.

The Guedel airway is a useful adjunct in maintaining the airway of a child undergoing anaesthesia. It is important that the appropriate size of airway is used. If an airway is too small or too large, it may obstruct the child's airway completely. A reliable way of selecting the correct size is to place the flange of the airway at the angle of the mouth. The correctly sized airway should reach the angle of the mandible. The tongue should be depressed using a depressor or even the blade of the laryngoscope and the airway inserted. The method used in adults of rotating the airway through 180° during insertion is not recommended for little children because of the possibility of damaging the pharynx and subsequently compromising the airway. It is important that all procedures involving the airway of a child, including suction of the pharynx, are performed under direct vision.

The laryngeal mask airway is a major advance in anaesthetic airway management. It does not protect the airway against aspiration of refluxed gastric contents. It should be used only when it is planned that the child is to breathe spontaneously during surgery. It follows that it is unwise to use the device when neuromuscular blocking drugs are used. The mask may be displaced easily, which may result in airway obstruction and gastric insufflation. With these provisos, it may be used for a variety of operations where in the past tracheal intubation would have been mandatory, such as squint correction tonsillectomy. Owing to the large cross-sectional area of the mask tube, airway resistance increases only a small amount, if at all. Masks are available to fit all children, including neonates. The neonatal (size 1) mask is not popular for several reasons. It is relatively difficult to insert; it may be displaced very easily and it increases apparatus dead space resulting in rebreathing and hypercapnia.

It is mandatory to intubate the trachea during artificial ventilation. Intubation of the trachea confers many advantages. The lungs are protected against aspiration of gastric contents, ventilation is controlled and bronchoalveolar toilet may be performed. Operations in the oral cavity of a small child are not possible without tracheal intubation. It is very difficult to maintain the airway of a neonate using an airway and a face mask for any but the shortest surgical procedure requiring general anaesthesia. It is usually wise to intubate the trachea electively in most situations. Insertion of a tracheal tube results in a reduction of the cross-sectional area of the airway. A 3.5 mm tube in a neonate causes an increase in resistance by a factor of 16. Neonates with a tracheal tube must undergo artificial ventilation in order to reduce the work of breathing.

The vocal cords should be visible in order to be certain of intubating the trachea. In order to be able to do this, the anaesthetist has to align three imaginary axes: one through the trachea, one through the pharynx and one through the mouth. In the older child and adult, this is usually achieved by placing a pillow under the head – the familiar 'sniffing the morning air' position. A layrngoscope blade is then put into the vallecula in front of the epiglottis and the laryngeal structures lifted. Because of anatomical differences, the technique needs to be modified for the infant. Infants have a head which is large and a neck which is short relative to the size of the body. Instead of placing a pillow under the head, it is usually necessary to place a small pad or pillow under the torso. An alternative is to ask the assistant to gently raise the torso off the surface on which the child is lying. The larynx of a child under the age of 2 years tends to sit higher in the neck opposite the vertebral bodies of C3–4, whereas in the older child it is opposite C5–6.This results in the larynx being more anterior during laryngoscopy. The epiglottis of the infant is relatively large and, because the cartilaginous support is not fully developed, tends to be floppy. The anaesthetist cannot usually elevate the epiglottis sufficiently in order to be able to see the vocal cords if a curved blade such as the Macintosh is used. Instead, the anaesthetist has to use a straight blade and place it on the posterior surface of the epiglottis whilst lifting. In addition to the above, gentle cricoid pressure helps to bring the three axes into alignment. This may be performed with the little finger of the left hand.

In the adult, the narrowest part of the airway is the glottic opening. In the child, the narrowest part is the cricoid ring which cannot be seen during laryngoscopy. It is very important that the correct size of tube is selected. If too big a tube is selected, the tracheal mucosa is damaged and the child may develop post-intubation croup; if it is too small, excessive leak makes positive pressure impossible. The ring forms a natural cuff around the tube, thereby eliminating the need for a pneumatic cuff. Generally, cuffed tubes are used only in children above the age of 10 years. The reason for this is that the pressure may render the underlying trachea ischaemic and subsequently lead to post-intubation croup. If possible, tracheal intubation should not be performed in children having day-case procedures. The laryngeal mask has eliminated the need for this.

The following formula is used to calculate the internal diameter of the appropriate size of tube:

$$(\text{age}/4) + 4 \text{ mm}$$

An alternative is to use a tube with an external diameter similar to that of the child's little finger. It is important that tubes with internal diameters 0.5 mm larger and smaller than the predicted size are readily available.

The tip of the tracheal tube should lie at the mid-trachea. For oral intubation, the measurement from the alveolar ridge to the mid-trachea is about (age/2) + 12 cm. An alternative is three times the internal diameter of the tube. For nasal intubation, the measurement is (age/2) + 15 cm.

For neonates, the best guide is related to weight (Table 53.9).

After intubation has been performed, the lung fields and epigastrium should be auscultated to confirm correct placement. Further confirmation of correct placement using a capnograph is essential. If intubation has been preceded by a period of difficult mask ventilation, it is not unusual for the stomach to become inflated. The inflated stomach decreases excursion of the lungs and results in arterial desaturation. If this has occurred, the stomach should be deflated by passing an orogastric tube, which is removed as soon as the task is complete.

Because children have a relatively short trachea, it is easy for the tube to become displaced and enter a main bronchus or for the trachea to become extubated. It is vital that the tube is well secured. It is best to use adhesive tape and secure the tube to the immobile maxilla rather than to the mandible. Preformed tubes such as the RAE are not recommended for the infant, because inadvertent bronchial intubation easily occurs.

MONITORING

There is no substitute for an experienced, vigilant anaesthetist directly observing the child. Changes in colour, inappropriate movement, respiratory obstruction and changes in respiratory pattern may be observed quickly and treated. A precordial stethoscope and pulse oximeter should always be attached before induction. The precordial stethoscope should be changed to an oesophageal one after the trachea has been intubated. The stethoscope is used as a qualitative measure of cardiac output. A volume-depleted infant has quiet heart sounds. The increase in intensity of the sounds after volume boluses may be discerned easily. Most oesophageal stethoscopes have a built-in temperature probe. If it is not possible to use this method to monitor temperature then an alternative site such as the rectum must be used. It is unwise to even consider extubating the trachea of a hypothermic infant. Ideally, ECG and arterial pressure monitoring should be in place before induction. In practice this is not always possible. Usually these devices are put in place as soon as the child is asleep. Capnography is mandatory for the child who has a tracheal tube or laryngeal mask.

Table 53.9 Estimates of tracheal tube size in neonates

Weight (kg)	Internal diameter (mm)	Length from alveolar ridge (cm)
1	2.5	7
2	3	8
3	3.5	9

DAY SURGERY

Day-case surgery confers many advantages in children. Children who are admitted to hospital often develop behavioural problems perhaps as a result of separation from parents and disruption of family life. These problems manifest as an alteration of sleep pattern, bedwetting and regression of developmental milestones.

Most children make excellent candidates for day-case surgery. They are usually healthy and the procedures performed are usually of short to intermediate duration. Only experienced surgeons and anaesthetists should undertake day-case surgery. Because this form of surgery is performed by experienced personnel, even ASA III patients may be considered. Children who are under 60 weeks post-conceptual age, those who have diseases that are not well controlled (e.g. poorly controlled epilepsy) and those with metabolic disease (e.g. insulin-dependent diabetes) that may result in hypoglycaemia should always be admitted electively for overnight stay.

Parents must be given clear written instructions well before the planned date of surgery. They should be told how long their child should be fasted before surgery. They should also be asked to make arrangements so that two responsible adults with their own transport accompany the child home.

Sedative premedication is rarely required for a child who has been well prepared. Children accompanied to the anaesthetic room by their parents usually remain calm. It makes sense to use agents with the shortest half-life. Regional anaesthesia performed at induction is useful in reducing the amount of anaesthetic needed intraoperatively and also provides excellent postoperative analgesia especially when long-acting agents such as bupivacaine or ropivacaine are used. Paracetamol and diclofenac given as suppositories at the end of surgery ensure that the child remains comfortable when the local anaesthetic has worn off. It is essential to seek the parent's informed consent for regional anaesthesia and rectal analgesics.

After surgery, the child should be allowed to recover in a fully equipped and staffed recovery ward. The child is returned to the day ward only when protective reflexes have returned. The child is discharged home when oral fluids are tolerated, but if the child has received intraoperative hydration, it is possible to ignore this criterion. Another yardstick used is whether the child has passed urine or not; this is particularly important if the child has been given a caudal block. Occasionally caudal blocks and inguinal blocks result in weakness of the leg. In this case, it is advisable to wait for the block to regress before discharging the child; clearly, this applies only to children who are walking. Ondansetron is useful in the treatment of postoperative nausea and vomiting, as the lack of any sedative effect is conducive to an early discharge. Children who have undergone tracheal intubation should remain on the day ward for at least 2 h to ensure that post-intubation croup does not occur.

Parents should be given an adequate supply of postoperative analgesics. It is crucial to emphasize the importance of giving analgesics pre-emptively 'by the clock' instead of waiting for the child to complain of pain.

SPECIFIC OPERATIONS IN THE NEONATE

INGUINAL HERNIA REPAIR

This is one of the commonest operations in the neonatal period. The incidence in this age group is highest amongst preterm infants. General anaesthesia is avoided preferably because of the risk of postoperative apnoea. The choice is between spinal and caudal epidural anaesthesia. Spinal anaesthesia offers the advantage of a quick onset with profound muscle relaxation in less than 2 min. Unfortunately the duration of action is very short – of the order of about 40 min. Addition of α_1-agonists such as phenylephrine and epinephrine may prolong the block to about 1 h. Caudal anaesthesia has a slower onset but lasts a long time so that bilateral hernia repair is easily possible. Large quantities of local anaesthetic have to be injected; total spinal anaesthesia and intravascular injection are potential problems. The child should have an intravenous cannula in situ, but unlike adult practice there is no need for volume preloading, nor is there a need to administer vasoactive drugs such as ephedrine.

PYLOROMYOTOMY

Pyloric stenosis usually presents in weeks 4–8 of life. A previously well male child develops projectile vomiting. Untreated, the child becomes severely dehydrated with a hypokalaemic, hypochloraemic metabolic alkalosis. As the obstruction is at the level of the pylorus, the body loses hydrogen and chloride ions but none of the alkaline small bowel secretions. The kidney is thus presented with a large bicarbonate load, which exceeds its absorptive threshold and this results initially in alkaline urine. As further fluid depletion occurs, the renin–angiotensin–aldosterone axis is activated in an attempt to preserve circulating volume. This results in an exchange of sodium ions for hydrogen and potassium ions, which leads to a paradoxical aciduria with a worsening hypokalaemia and metabolic alkalosis.

The initial management is placement of a nasogastric tube and an intravenous cannula. A solution of 5% dextrose in 0.45% saline to which 40 mmol L^{-1} of potassium chloride has been added is given at a rate of 6 ml kg^{-1} h^{-1}. The nasogastric tube is aspirated and the aspirate replace with 0.9% saline. The child is ready for surgery between 24 and 48 h after commencing this regimen. A normal potassium concentration and a bicarbonate concentration of 25 mmol L^{-1} are used to indicate that sufficient volume replacement has taken place.

In theatre, the child should have its stomach washed with warm saline until the aspirated fluid is clear. Induction should be smooth, by either the inhalation or intravenous route according to the experience of the anaesthetist. Postoperative analgesia is provided by wound infiltration followed by either rectal or oral paracetamol, depending on when the surgeon decides that the child may be fed.

TRACHEO-OESOPHAGEAL FISTULA AND OESOPHAGEAL ATRESIA

Six types of this condition (A–F) have been described. The commonest is C in which the proximal oesophagus ends as a diverticulum and the lower part exists as a fistula off the trachea just above the carina. Cardiovascular anomalies such as septal defects and coarctation of the aorta often coexist with this condition. An echocardiogram should always be performed before surgery. The corrective surgery should be performed as a matter of urgency as a one-stage repair. Delay results in soiling of the lungs and pneumonitis. Preoperatively the child should be nursed in an upright position to prevent soiling of the lungs by gastric fluid. It is important that a tube is placed in the diverticulum and continuous suction applied to aspirate the saliva that the child cannot swallow. If the lungs should become soiled then antibiotics and physiotherapy are required and the operation should be performed as soon as the child's condition has been optimized.

Inhalation induction is the preferred method. Positive pressure ventilation results in distension of the stomach and subsequent impairment of oxygenation. The tracheal tube should be inserted with the bevel facing up so that the posterior wall of the tube occludes the fistula. The tube should be inserted initially deeper than one predicts and then gently withdrawn until both lungs are being ventilated. Manual ventilation is recommended as surgical traction can easily occlude the neonate's soft trachea.

The lungs should be ventilated postoperatively in order that adequate amounts of analgesia may be given and also to prevent traction on the oesophageal anastomosis by movement of the head.

DIAPHRAGMATIC HERNIA

In this condition, the abdominal contents herniate through a defect in the diaphragm usually on the left side. The abdominal contents exert pressure on the developing lung and if the defect is large enough, the mediastinum is shifted to the right and the growth of the contralateral lung is also stunted. Repair of the hernia is not an emergency and the child should be managed medically. Problems that have to be managed include ventilation, acidosis and pulmonary hypertension. Surgery is considered when the child's condition has been optimized medically. Positive pressure ventilation by bag and mask may expand the abdominal viscera and should be avoided. Nitrous oxide should also be avoided for the same reason. The defect is usually repaired through an abdominal incision. It is not always possible to fit the viscera in the peritoneal cavity, in which case a silastic silo may be used and the contents gradually introduced. It is wise to avoid cannulation of veins in the lower extremity as the return of abdominal viscera increases the pressure in the inferior vena cava. Infants who present soon after birth with severe symptoms usually do not survive as they have inadequate amounts of lung tissue to sustain life.

EXOMPHALOS AND GASTROSCHISIS

Embryologically these are two separate conditions. However, both present similar challenges to the anaesthetist. The abdominal contents, which have herniated through the abdominal wall, offer a large surface area by which heat and fluid can be lost. It is imperative that the abdominal contents are placed into a clear sterile polythene bag as soon as possible after birth. The defects should be corrected as a matter of urgency. Nitrous oxide should be avoided to facilitate surgery and a nasogastric tube must be in place to decompress the stomach. If it is not possible to return all the viscera into the peritoneal cavity, a silastic silo may be used. It is usual to ventilate the child's lungs postoperatively because of the reduction in compliance caused by return of the viscera to the peritoneum. As with all congenital anomalies, associated abnormalities are described with these conditions, particularly with exomphalos.

POSTOPERATIVE CARE

Unless they are being admitted to an ICU, all children should be nursed in a properly equipped and staffed recovery unit. Oxygen should be administered until the child has good oxygen saturation breathing room air. The cardiovascular and respiratory systems should be monitored and interventions carried out appropriately. It is becoming increasingly popular to have a step-down area attached to the recovery unit. This is an area where the child may be accompanied by the parents but may still be monitored closely. The child is returned to the ward when warm, pain-free and haemodynamically stable. It is the anaesthetist's responsibility to ensure that appropriate analgesia and intravenous fluids have been prescribed.

INTENSIVE CARE

There are several reasons why children may have to be admitted to an ICU. Most children admitted are under the age of 2 years. The commonest reason for admission is because of established or incipient respiratory failure. Respiratory support usually takes the form of tracheal intubation and controlled ventilation.

Respiratory reserve is smaller in infants than in older children. Infants have a high requirement for oxygen. It is of the order of 7 ml kg^{-1} min^{-1}, whereas in the older child it is of the order of 3 ml kg^{-1} min^{-1}.

Respiration is predominantly by excursion of the diaphragm. The diaphragm in neonates has a lower percentage of type I muscle fibres and is therefore prone to fatigue easily if the work of breathing is increased. Although the infant airway is proportionally large compared with an adult airway, a given degree of airway oedema has a more profound effect on the infant's airway because of its smaller size. It is particularly important to recognize the signs of impending respiratory failure in the neonate and to intervene early before exhaustion occurs, without waiting for blood gas data. In this group, hypoxaemia results in a return to a fetal circulation and, as a consequence, worsening hypoxaemia, acidosis and death unless the cycle is broken. The signs include tachypnoea, grunting respiration and use of accessory muscles of respiration.

The diaphragm may be compromised in several ways. For example, corrective surgery for gastroschisis or diaphragmatic hernia results in diaphragmatic splinting because abdominal growth is insufficient to contain the entire bowel. Similarly, it may be splinted by distended loops of bowel such as in necrotizing enterocolitis.

The premature infant has a deficiency of surfactant. This results in alveolar instability and atelectasis. As a consequence, intrapulmonary shunting increases and lung compliance decreases. Mild cases may be treated conservatively with humidified oxygen. More severe cases require tracheal intubation and mechanical ventilation. The high pressures and high inspired oxygen concentrations required result in further damage to lung parenchyma. A significant number of children who have this treatment develop chronic lung disease of prematurity (previously termed bronchopulmonary dysplasia). A similar picture of reduced lung compliance is seen in infants who have aspirated meconium during delivery and also infants who are septicaemic.

The damage to lung parenchyma occurs as a result of shear injury associated with high peak inspiratory inflation pressures. Strategies that are used to limit this include the judicious use of PEEP in addition to high-frequency ventilation and oscillation. A major problem with high-frequency ventilation techniques is the difficulty of humidifying inspired gases adequately, which then leads to a severe tracheobronchitis.

Nitric oxide is a naturally occurring vasodilator with an extremely short half-life. When given by inhalation, it selectively dilates ventilated alveoli and thereby reduces pulmonary vascular resistance, without any systemic effects. It may therefore be used to match perfusion to ventilation. The selective pulmonary vasodilatation also leads to a reduction in the extent of right-to-left shunting. Nitric oxide is indicated for use in cases of persistent pulmonary hypertension associated with hyaline membrane disease, meconium aspiration syndrome, congenital diaphragmatic hernia and group B streptococcal sepsis.

Extracorporeal membrane oxygenation (ECMO) is a technique that has been developed from cardiopulmonary bypass technology. Blood is drained by gravity from a great vein. The vein most commonly used is the superior vena cava, entered via the internal jugular route. The blood then goes through a membrane oxygenator and is returned, using peristaltic pumps, back into the vena cava (in venovenous ECMO) or into the carotid artery (in veno-arterial ECMO). This technique may be used to 'rest' the lungs. It has been used successfully in hyaline membrane disease, meconium aspiration and in persistent pulmonary hypertension as in congenital diaphragmatic hernia. The technique has been most successful in children (rather than in adults) such as those who have severe viral or bacterial pneumonia, smoke inhalation and near drowning. Whilst the child is receiving ECMO, the lungs still require ventilation, albeit at much lower pressures and rates.

Severe upper airway obstruction is another reason for admission to the ICU. Acute epiglottitis is a disease caused by the organism *Haemophilus influenzae*. Intense glottic swelling occurs which may result in dysphagia. The child is usually aged between 2 and 7 years and is usually toxic, adopting a position of sitting forward and drooling saliva. The child must be taken straight to theatre for tracheal intubation to be performed before fatal total airway obstruction occurs. The child should not be upset, as crying worsens airway obstruction. Anaesthesia usually commences whilst the child is sitting on a parent's lap and the patient is then transferred to the operating table after becoming unconscious. An intravenous cannula is sited, atropine given and laryngoscopy performed when the child is adequately anaesthetized. Owing to the reduction in alveolar ventilation caused by the obstruction, induction takes longer than usual. Inhalation induction using halothane in oxygen alone is the method of choice, but only an experienced anaesthetist should carry out this procedure. An experienced ENT surgeon who can perform a tracheostomy should be present. The swollen epiglottis makes visualization of the vocal cords very difficult. Occasionally, the only clue as to the position of the laryngeal inlet is provided by bubbles emerging from the inlet with respiration – hence the importance of not giving neuromuscular blocking drugs. Initially oral intubation is performed, but this is often changed for a nasal tube when the airway has been secured. Antibiotic therapy is given and the child's trachea may usually be extubated after 2 days. The introduction of HIB immunization in infancy, to prevent *Haemophilus* meningitis, has resulted in the virtual disappearance of acute epiglottitis in the UK, as both conditions are caused by the same organism.

Laryngotracheobronchitis is another cause of upper airway obstruction in a child. The causative agent is usually one of the parainfluenza viruses. Occasionally it is caused by *Staphylococcus* bacteria. Croup (as this condition is commonly termed) is often managed conservatively with humidified oxygen. If the child is working very hard to breathe, tracheal intubation and controlled ventilation are indicated. It is preferable to intervene without waiting for biochemical evidence of respiratory failure. A tracheal tube 1 mm smaller than that predicted is required. Humidification of inspired gases is essential to keep the secretions thin so that they may be aspirated easily, as viscid secretions easily obstruct a small tube. The child's trachea may be extubated when an audible leak is heard around the tube when 20 cm of positive pressure is applied.

Paediatric intensive care is increasingly being centralized. A specialized retrieval team using ambulances designed for this purpose must be used for transfer from the receiving hospital to the paediatric ICU (PICU). It is incumbent on the receiving hospital to stabilize the child before transfer. This process includes tracheal intubation and intravenous cannulation. Nasotracheal tubes are generally preferred for several reasons. They are usually better tolerated than oral tubes and are also less likely to be displaced.

It is also of vital importance that the child is sedated adequately whilst in the ICU. The drugs that have been used most commonly are midazolam and an opioid such as morphine or fentanyl. Propofol is used widely for adults, but is not popular in PICUs in the UK, because of a few fatalities that occurred when it was used as the sole sedative agent in relatively high doses. The children developed a metabolic acidosis, lipaemic serum, hepatomegaly and ultimately multiorgan failure. Occasionally, neuromuscular agents have to be added to sedatives to help synchronization with the ventilator in children with severe respiratory disease. They may also be required to prevent an increase in intracranial pressure. It is crucial to establish that the child is well sedated before these drugs are used.

CARDIAC ARREST AND RESUSCITATION

The results of treating cardiac arrest in children are poor. If resuscitation results in survival, the incidence of significant neurological

Table 53.10 Paediatric resuscitation chart

	Age and weight						
	Neonate 3.5 kg	3 months 5 kg	1 year 10 kg	3 years 15 kg	6 years 20 kg	8 years 25 kg	12 years 40 kg
Tracheal tube							
Size (4 + age/4); cm	3.0	3.5	4.0	5.0	5.5	6.0	7.0
Length (oral); cm	9	10	11	13	14	15	17
Length (nasal); cm	11	13	14	16	19	20	22
Epinephrine 1: 10 000							
i.v./i.o./e.t.[a] 0.1 ml kg^{-1} repeated as necessary	0.5 ml	0.5 ml	1 ml	1.5 ml	2 ml	2.5 ml	4 ml
Sodium bicarbonate 8.4%							
1 ml kg^{-1} i.v.	3 ml	5 ml	10 ml	15 ml	20 ml	25 ml	40 ml
Atropine 500 μg in 5 ml							
0.2 ml kg^{-1} i.v./e.t.	1 ml	1 ml	2 ml	3 ml	4 ml	5 ml	8 ml
Calcium chloride 10%							
0.1 ml kg^{-1} i.v.	0.5 ml	0.5 ml	1 ml	1.5 ml	2 ml	2.5 ml	4 ml
Defibrillation (J)							
4 J kg^{-1}	10	20	40	60	80	100	160
Colloid volume (ml)							
10 ml kg^{-1} × 2–3 as necessary	35	50	100	150	200	250	400

i.v., intravenous; i.o., intraosseous; e.t., endotracheal.
[a] For endotracheal administration, give 10 times i.v. dose.
N.B. All drugs and fluids may be administered via the intraosseous route.

Drug infusions
Epinephrine: 0.03 mg kg^{-1} in 50 ml glucose 5%; start at 2 ml h^{-1}.
Dopamine: 3 mg kg^{-1} in 50 ml glucose 5%; 3–20 ml h^{-1}.
Dobutamine: 3 mg kg^{-1} in 50 ml glucose 5%; 5–20 ml h^{-1}.
Isoproterenol: 0.25 mg kg^{-1} in 50 ml glucose 5%; 1–4 ml h^{-1}.

impairment is high, probably because the arrest is usually preceded by a long period of hypoxaemia. In the adult, cardiac arrest is usually the result of an arrhythmia that requires immediate recognition and defibrillation. In the child, the commonest causes of cardiac arrest are hypoxaemia, hypovolaemia, electrolyte imbalance and drug overdose. It follows that if these conditions are prevented, cardiac arrest should not occur. Doses of appropriate drugs used in the management of cardiac arrest are shown in Table 53.10.

In infants it is recommended that the brachial pulse is palpated to confirm cardiac arrest. In older children, the carotid or femoral pulses are appropriate. One should not spend more than 10 s doing this. The chest should be compressed by one-third of its resting diameter. In infants, this is achieved using two fingers on the sternum. In the older child, the heel of one hand is used. After the age of 8 years, a two-handed technique as used in adults is appropriate.

Access to the circulation is vital in order for volume expansion and administration of drugs such as atropine and epinephrine. The intraosseous route should be used if a vein has not been cannulated within 90 s. The aspirate obtained should be sent for laboratory studies, including glucose, haemoglobin, urea and electrolyte concentrations and crossmatching of blood if necessary.

FURTHER READING

Baum V 1999 Anesthesia for genetic, metabolic and dysmorphic syndromes of childhood. Williams & Wilkins, Baltimore

British Journal of Anaesthesia 1999 Postgraduate educational issue: the paediatric patient. British Journal of Anaesthesia 83

Dalens B 1995 Regional anesthesia for infants, children and adolescents. Williams & Wilkins, Baltimore

McKenzie I et al 1997 Manual of acute pain management in children. Churchill Livingstone, Edinburgh

Motoyama E K, Davis P J 1996 Smith's anesthesia for infants and children. Mosby, St Louis

Peutrell J M, Mather S J 1997 Regional anaesthesia for babies and children. Oxford University Press, Oxford

Rowney D A, Doyle E 1998 Epidural and subarachnoid blockade in children. Anaesthesia 53: 980–1001

54 Dental anaesthesia

Anaesthesia and dentistry have a long historical association. Some of the first anaesthetics given were for dental extractions and the use of anaesthesia was quickly taken into dental practice in the late 19th century. Dental anaesthetic techniques have evolved in parallel with the changes in practice in other aspects of anaesthesia. The days of single operator anaesthetists and the 'black gas' induction (100% nitrous oxide) are now long gone. For many years, dental anaesthesia had been practised in a variety of sites varying from within dental schools to remote dental practices, with anaesthesia provided by anaesthetists, medical practitioners or indeed dentists.

Anaesthesia and dentistry cover three main types of surgery: first, outpatient anaesthesia for simple extractions of teeth, mainly in children ('dental chair anaesthesia'); second, day-case anaesthesia for straightforward extractions of molars or for minor oral surgery; and third, in-patient treatment for more complicated extractions or oral surgical procedures. These three areas of anaesthetic practice are covered in this chapter. In addition, sedation techniques are described, as they are likely to become of increasing importance as a result of the changes in dental anaesthetic practice in the UK.

The provision of dental anaesthetic and sedation services was the subject of a major report by the Department of Health (1991). The recommendations of this report have had far-reaching consequences on the provision of dental anaesthetic services and it has affected both anaesthetists and dentists. The recommendations within this report covered general anaesthesia, sedation and resuscitation. With regard to general anaesthesia, the report stated that its use should be avoided wherever possible and the same standards in respect of personnel, premises and equipment should apply wherever the anaesthetic is being administered. It further recommended that all anaesthetics should be administered by an accredited anaesthetist and that anaesthetic training should include specific experience in dental anaesthesia. It also made recommendations on the standard of equipment, techniques and facilities. In late 1998, the General Dental Council amended its guidance to dentists in respect of general anaesthesia. It strengthened its previous statement that 'general anaesthesia is a procedure which is never without risk' to a clear statement that general anaesthesia should only be considered if there is an overriding clinical need and alternative methods have been explained. The guidance also put greater emphasis on the responsibilities of the dentist in providing the equipment and staff to a level similar to that found in hospital. The effect of this ruling and the concurrent publication of *Standards and guidelines for general anaesthesia in dentistry* by the Royal College of Anaesthetists (1999) have effectively concentrated the provision of anaesthesia for dental surgery to centralized facilities. Both reports stated that sedation should be used in preference to general anaesthesia wherever possible and made further recommendations on training in sedation techniques and on the drugs and techniques to be used. The Department of Health report placed strong emphasis on the teaching, training and assessment of resuscitation skills and resuscitation facilities within dental practices.

OUTPATIENT DENTAL ANAESTHESIA

The use of general anaesthesia for outpatient dental extractions (exodontia) has decreased steadily in England and Wales from over 2 million per year in the mid-1950s to around 1.2 million per year in 1970 and down to less than 200 000 per year in 1990. This steady decrease reflects several factors including a general improvement in dental hygiene, a decreased number of practices providing general anaesthetic services and the increased use of local anaesthetic and sedation techniques. The use of general anaesthesia for dental extractions has been much more common in the UK than elsewhere in Europe or North America. Within the past few years in some centres, there has been an increase in the numbers attending for outpatient general anaesthesia. This may have reflected the change in practice, with more dental practitioners not providing an anaesthetic service and referring patients requiring general anaesthesia to a central resource. However, the expected increase in numbers referred to centres in the wake of the recent reports does not appear to have happened. In future the general anaesthetic outpatient dental service for an area will be provided in centres such as DGHs, dental schools or medical centres.

PATIENT SELECTION

The selection of patients presenting for dental chair anaesthesia should be the same as for patients undergoing any outpatient procedure, i.e. only healthy ASA grade I and II patients are appropriate. The preoperative screening of patients may be particularly difficult in a dental practice, but this is the situation in which careful selection of patients is of greatest importance. It is essential that the dental practitioners involved have some understanding of the anaesthetic implications of common medical conditions and are able to exclude patients with significant cardiac or respiratory disease, renal or hepatic impairment, bleeding disorders or a potentially difficult airway at the time of referral. Patients who do not meet these criteria should be referred to a specialist centre which has back-up facilities and should not be treated in a dental surgery.

The majority of patients are children between the ages of 4 and 10 years presenting for extraction of carious teeth. This group has a low incidence of systemic disease but a high incidence of respiratory tract infections. Dental problems requiring general anaesthesia are relatively uncommon under the age of 3 years, other than trauma to upper incisors ('A's and 'B's) resulting from a fall. In adults, the indications for general anaesthesia are fewer and include situations where local analgesia is ineffective, such as dental abscess. Another indication for general anaesthesia is for patients who are unable to cooperate with treatment under local analgesia because of mental impairment or physical disability. It is important that this group receives full preoperative assessment in view of coexisting disease and concurrent medication which may influence anaesthesia. The use of general anaesthesia as an option in adults who do not like dental treatment under local analgesia should be discouraged in favour of the use of sedation techniques (see below).

It is important that the nature of the dental surgical procedure undertaken is appropriate for a day case. This implies that the surgery should be of short duration and not so extensive that it is difficult to provide adequate postoperative analgesia.

The patient's social circumstances must be taken into account when offering outpatient treatment. The patient must be accompanied before and after the surgery and supervised by an adult for 24 h. Some patients may need time to make appropriate domestic arrangements.

EQUIPMENT

The site at which outpatient dental anaesthesia is administered should be equipped to the standards required in the day-case anaesthesia report and the Department of Health report; that is, the facilities for the anaesthetist and a surgeon should match those that would be provided in an in-patient theatre setting. For an anaesthetist, this is best dealt with under the areas of anaesthetic equipment, monitoring and resuscitation equipment.

The equipment necessary includes an anaesthetic machine which is capable of delivering a fast flow of 100% oxygen, should this be necessary (Fig. 54.1). Other facilities should include nitrous oxide and a vaporizer and an anaesthetic breathing system with which it is easy to provide assisted ventilation if required. If the patients regularly include children, a low-resistance circuit is required. Some older anaesthetic machines included on-demand breathing circuits. These were developed to minimize anaesthetic gas use when the anaesthetist carried gas cylinders from practice to practice and there is no indication for their current use. Modern machines such as those using a Quantiflex flowmeter provide a range of gas flows with mixtures ranging from 30 to 100% oxygen in nitrous oxide. Other equipment should include a variety of nasal and facial masks, oral and nasal airways, laryngoscopes with a variety of blades, including paediatric, and a range of oral and nasal tracheal tubes. A high-pressure suction unit should be available, preferably separate from the suction used by the dentist. The chair should be capable of head-down tilt and should be movable even in the event of power failure.

The minimum standards for monitoring during anaesthesia should be met (Table 38.17). Although most of the procedures in dental practice are short, it is very important that monitoring is used in each case. There is a high potential for airway obstruction resulting in hypoxaemia and also a relatively high incidence of cardiac arrhythmias especially when halothane is used. In practices where tracheal intubation is used, a capnograph is required.

A full range of resuscitation equipment must be available; this should include a defibrillator, an emergency drug pack (Table 54.1), facilities for intubation and full delivery of high-flow oxygen with positive pressure if necessary, e.g. an Ambu or Laerdal bag. The GDC guidelines specify that the anaesthetist, dentist and dental nurse are trained in resuscitation and attend regular refresher courses. It also recommends that they regularly practise resuscitation procedures as a team.

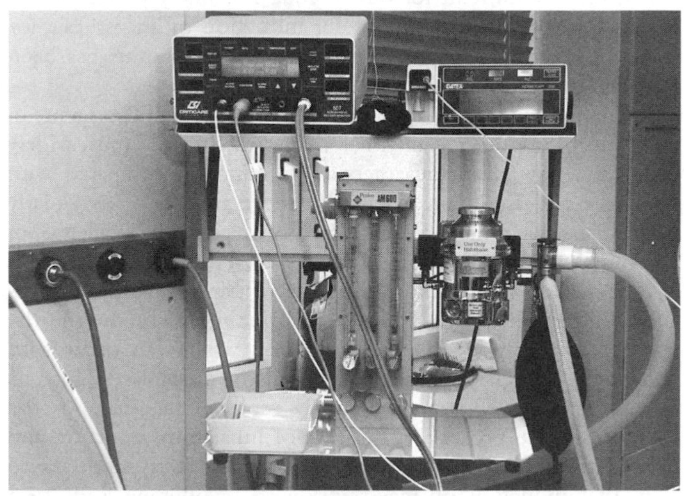

Fig. 54.1
Anaesthetic machine and monitoring suitable for dental anaesthesia.

Table 54.1 List of emergency drugs to be available in dental practices

Oxygen
Epinephrine
Lidocaine 1%
Atropine
Calcium chloride
Sodium bicarbonate
Glyceryl trinitrate (tabs or spray)
Aminophylline
Salbutamol inhaler
Chlorphenamine (chlorpheniramine)
Dextrose 50%
Hydrocortisone
Midazolam
Dextrose/saline infusion bag
Colloid infusion bag
Flumazenil*
Naloxone*

* Only if practice provides i.v. sedation.

POTENTIAL PREOPERATIVE PROBLEMS

- Presentation of poorly prepared or inappropriate patients requiring dental treatment.
- High proportion of patients are children who may have upper respiratory tract infection.
- Dental abscesses may lead to a difficult airway.
- Site may have inadequate facilities or equipment.

INDUCTION OF ANAESTHESIA

Anaesthesia may be induced by the inhalation or intravenous route. Traditionally, the inhalation route has been used for young children and the intravenous route for older children and adults. The introduction of EMLA cream has allowed the intravenous route to be used more frequently. However, EMLA cream should be applied 1 h before anticipated cannulation, which may be difficult for outpatients. For many years, methohexital was the drug of choice for induction of anaesthesia for dental outpatient practice. In the past few years, this has been replaced by propofol.

Inhalation induction has been described using all the agents in common use. Until recently, halothane was still the most widely used as it has advantages of ease of induction compared with enflurane and isoflurane which are more irritant – particularly isoflurane which may be associated with a high incidence of coughing and laryngospasm (Table 54.2). However, halothane is also associated with a high incidence of cardiovascular disturbances, in particular arrhythmias, which are more common in the presence of a raised P_aCO_2 , a situation which can occur with respiratory depression or if the airway is compromised. Since its introduction, sevoflurane has largely replaced halothane as the agent of choice because of the ease of inhalation induction and limited cardiovascular and respiratory effects. It is important to note that induction of anaesthesia with sevoflurane leads to a quicker and smoother loss of consciousness than with halothane, but the time to achieve surgical anaesthesia is the same or even slightly longer with sevoflurane (Table 54.3). The use of high concentrations of sevoflurane after loss of consciousness may be accompanied by marked sinus tachycardia, particularly in young children. The technique of inhalation induction with halothane followed by maintenance with enflurane has been described and this may have some advantages because of ease of induction with halothane and limitation of the cardiovascular effects by subsequent use of enflurane.

Induction of anaesthesia in younger children may be difficult if they become frightened or uncooperative. The risk of this can be minimized by a friendly explanation of what is going to happen and the use of some visual aid such as a well known cartoon character breathing into an anaesthetic mask. The induction can be made into a game such as blowing up a balloon (reservoir bag). It is often helpful to have one of the child's parents present during induction, having first explained to the parent the sequence of events and what is expected of him or her. The management of a screaming child who does not cooperate with either inhalation or i.v. induction is difficult. There is little to be gained and a lot of potential problems in holding the child down with a mask on the face. This is very distressing for the child, the parents and all the staff involved. The potential for problems during induction is high in a child who has a blocked nose and secretions from crying and who is distressed and tachycardic before the procedure starts. It is best in this situation to delay anaesthesia until the child is calm. This can usually be done by allowing the parents and the child to sit quietly for half an hour to discuss the problem. In the worst cases, it may be better to bring the child back on another day, perhaps using oral premedication.

Following either intravenous or inhalation induction, anaesthesia is maintained usually by spontaneous respiration of an inhalation agent, nitrous oxide and oxygen by nasal mask (Fig. 54.2). The use of incremental bolus doses of propofol to maintain anaesthesia during dental anaesthesia has been described and is the choice in some centres. Several studies have shown the benefits of using 50% inspired oxygen concentration in preference to 30%, as this has been shown to decrease the number and severity of hypoxaemic episodes.

Table 54.2 Induction of anaesthesia for dental extractions using halothane, enflurane or isoflurane; 50 children in each group (data based on Simmons et al 1989) SAP = systolic anterial pressure

	Halothane	Enflurane	Isoflurane
Induction time (min)	2.4	2.8	3.5
Respiratory problems (%) (cough, breath-holding, laryngospasm)	12	12	42
Ventricular arrhythmias (%)	14	0	0
Mean maximum increase in heart rate (%)	22	25	48
Mean maximum fall in SAP (%)	17	15	4

Table 54.3 Comparison of induction of anaesthesia, complications and recovery in children receiving sevoflurane or halothane (n = 50 in each group) for dental extractions (based on Paris et al 1997)

	Sevoflurane	Halothane
Time to loss of eyelash reflex (min)	1.5	1.9
Time to prop insertion (min)	3.9	3.5
Respiratory problem (n) (coughing, laryngospasm, etc.)	5	5
Arrhythmias		
Bigeminy (n)	0	15
Premature ventricular beats (n)	3	13
Time from end of operation to eye opening	7.3	7.8

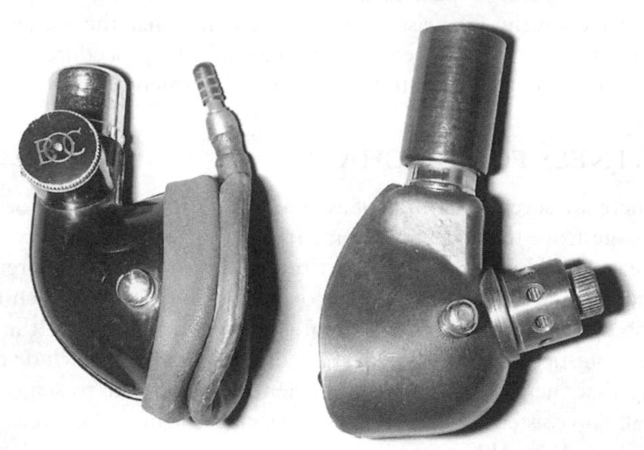

Fig. 54.2
Nasal masks used for dental anaesthesia.

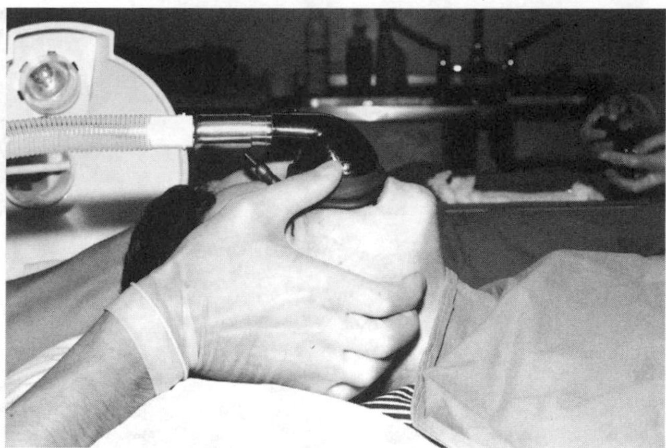

Fig. 54.3
Induction of anaesthesia using nasal mask over mouth and nose.

THE OPERATION

The sequence of events is as follows:

1. induction of anaesthesia
2. stabilization of the airway with a nasal mask (Fig. 54.3)
3. positioning of the gag or bite block by the dentist or anaesthetist
4. placement of a mouth pack to prevent debris from extracted teeth falling into the airway (Fig. 54.4)
5. extraction of teeth (Fig. 54.5), if necessary changing sides with repositioning of the bite block and pack
6. finishing the operation
7. turning the patient on to the side and recovery from consciousness.

As the airway is shared by the dentist and anaesthetist, it is important that both know the requirements of the other. The dentist requires, in turn, access to all four quadrants of the mouth and also some resistance to the pressure required for extraction of some teeth. In particular, in extraction of teeth from the lower jaw, the downward pressure required can potentially compromise the airway (Fig. 54.5). The anaesthetist needs to maintain the airway throughout the procedure using the nasal mask. This implies that the anaesthetist needs access to the upper half of the face to place the thumb on the nasal mask, and the airway is maintained by forward lift of the lower jaw with the fingers (Fig. 54.4). In placing the mouth gag, it is important not to use too large a size as this may make the airway more difficult to maintain. In placing the pack, it is also important that it is not sited too far posteriorly in the mouth such that it compromises the nasal airway (Fig. 54.4). The responsibility for placing the pack and gag varies from centre to centre between the anaesthetist and the dentist. Whoever places it, it is important that a patent airway is re-established after placement of the pack and gag, before any operative procedure starts. If at any point throughout the procedure there is a problem with the airway it is important that the anaesthetist can interrupt surgery until the airway is restored. At the end of the procedure, the packs are usually placed across the sockets to absorb any continuing bleeding, the gag is removed and the patient is placed in the left lateral position and given 100% oxygen to breathe.

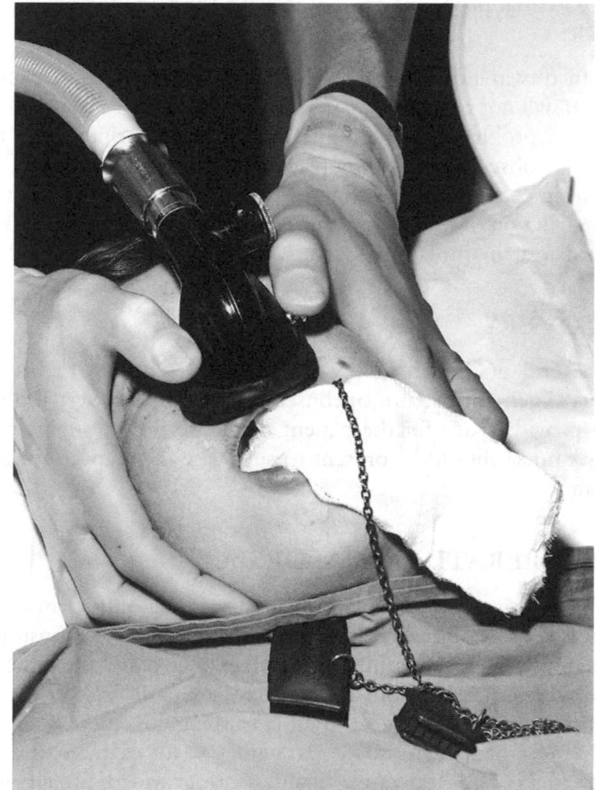

Fig. 54.4
The nasal mask has now been moved to cover the nose only and a gag and mouth pack inserted.

As in any general anaesthetic procedure, it is important that full resuscitative and support facilities are available immediately, in particular suction and facilities for oral tracheal intubation.

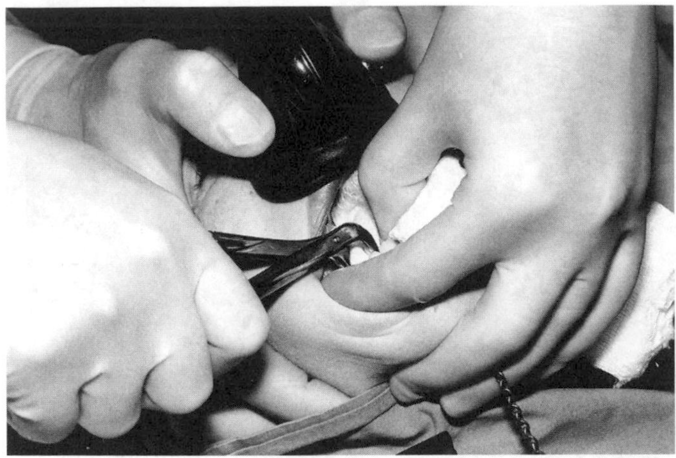

Fig. 54.5
Extraction of tooth from lower jaw. The dental pack is pushed to the left by the operator and the anaethetist maintains the airway by upward lift of the lower jaw to counteract the downward pressure exerted by the dentist.

PERIOPERATIVE PROBLEMS

The potential problems associated with the perioperative period include:

- difficulty in induction of anaesthesia in an uncooperative child who will not tolerate a mask or insertion of an i.v. cannula
- airway problems during induction because of irritant gases or airway obstruction, during placement of the gag and pack, during extractions or during early recovery
- obstruction of the airway by bleeding or bits of broken tooth
- cardiac arrhythmias.

RECOVERY

At the end of the procedure, the patient continues to breathe 100% oxygen until return of consciousness. The recovery facilities must provide space for the patient to recover in the supine position. A nurse should be present to supervise the recovery of each patient.

POSTOPERATIVE ANALGESIA

It is usual to give postoperative analgesics during outpatient dental extraction procedures. The amount of pain experienced postoperatively varies with the number of teeth extracted and the difficulty encountered in extraction. If there has been a difficult extraction of a tooth that has produced trauma to the gums, there is considerably more pain than simple extraction of, for example, a single upper incisor. Postoperative analgesia is provided usually with non-steroidal anti-inflammatory agents (NSAIDs) given orally in recovery or in the early postoperative period. The use of NSAIDs is ideal for postoperative dental pain, as some of the pain originates from the tissue swelling and these agents act in part by decreasing swelling. More recently, the use of a suppository which is inserted during anaesthesia has been described. Drugs given in this manner include paracetamol and diclofenac. It is appropriate to discuss the use of analgesic suppositories with the patient and/or the patient's parents preoperatively. Alternatively, paracetamol or ibuprofen may be given orally in a liquid form in recovery. Inability to control postoperative pain is one reason for admitting the patient postoperatively. Likewise, if it is anticipated that the surgery or extractions may produce considerable pain, the procedure may be deemed more appropriate for in-patient treatment.

FITNESS FOR DISCHARGE

There are several methods of assessing the patient's fitness for discharge from the recovery room. It is important that the patients are assessed by the medical practitioner and the dentist before discharge to identify any problems or potential problems which may arise. Assessment includes several clinical observations or the use of sophisticated tests of recovery. Clinical assessments include testing that the patient is alert and orientated, and able to stand and walk unassisted; simple scoring systems include the Steward's score and the Aldrete score.

POSTOPERATIVE PROBLEMS

The potential problems associated with the postoperative period may be classified under the headings of immediate or longer term.

Immediate

- hypoxaemia – secondary to diffusion hypoxaemia or airway problems
- airway problems – caused by laryngeal spasm, bleeding or debris in the airway
- vomiting.

Long-term

- continued bleeding
- postoperative pain and swelling
- nausea and vomiting.

DAY-CASE ANAESTHESIA

Developments in provision of day-case facilities have allowed an increasing number of dental procedures to be undertaken on a day-case basis. This differs from outpatient dental chair anaesthesia in that the patient goes through a formal admission to the hospital but is discharged home later in the day. The procedures for which this is appropriate are limited dental extractions, such as those of wisdom teeth, and minor oral surgical procedures including laser treatment.

PATIENT SELECTION

These patients are usually adults. They should be of ASA grade I or II and should comply with the standard criteria for selection of day-case patients. It is important to consider also the extent of the surgery involved and that a limitation may be the availability to provide adequate analgesia for the patient who is being discharged home. Therefore, caution should be exercised in undertaking extensive oral surgical procedures or difficult extractions of wisdom teeth. It is important that the patient is assessed formally by the anaesthetist before the anaesthetic so that appropriate investigations may be undertaken. This avoids unnecessary delays or cancellation on the day of surgery. Ideally, the patients should be assessed at a preoperative anaesthetic clinic.

ANAESTHETIC TECHNIQUE

The patient should arrive early on the morning of surgery, fasted and accompanied. If appropriate, the patient may be given an oral premedicant, such as temazepam, to take at home before coming into hospital and this could be arranged at a preoperative assessment visit. The majority of patients, however, do not receive premedication. A full admission clerking of the patient should be made and the patient assessed by the anaesthetist.

The nature of the surgery involved dictates that the majority of these patients require nasotracheal intubation. As the majority of the patients involved are young, healthy and are mobilized early, the potential for post-succinylcholine muscle pains is high and the use of succinylcholine is best avoided. The advantages of succinylcholine in speed of intubation and in controlling the airway have to be weighed against the potential disadvantages. There are several methods of reducing the incidence of postoperative succinylcholine pains using pretreatment with a non-depolarizing relaxant, dantrolene or benzodiazepines. Many of these techniques have been shown to reduce the incidence of muscle pain but none completely abolishes it. The alternatives for achieving nasal tracheal intubation would be to use a non-depolarizing relaxant or, following intravenous or inhalation induction, to take the patient to a deep plane of anaesthesia breathing a volatile agent spontaneously. If the anaesthetist is satisfied that there is no preoperative indication of a difficult intubation, the use of a non-depolarizing relaxant is probably the easiest.

Following intravenous induction, the nasotracheal tube is inserted. There is a relatively high risk of causing nasal bleeding while inserting or removing a nasotracheal tube. Several measures have been described to minimize this, including the use of a soft rubber catheter pulled over the end of the tube to act as protection through the nose. The catheter is removed through the mouth before the tube is placed in the trachea. The anaesthetist should then place the throat pack in the back of the mouth, around the tracheal tube to prevent any blood or debris falling into the back of the larynx. It is extremely important that the tail of the throat pack is brought out of the mouth and secured in some way to make sure that it is removed at the end of surgery. If nasotracheal intubation has been achieved using a non-depolarizing relaxant, it is obvious that maintenance is with intermittent positive pressure ventilation with nitrous oxide, oxygen and a volatile agent. If succinylcholine has been used, there is a choice between spontaneous respiration following recovery from blockade or continuation with a non-depolarizing relaxant. If an inhalation method has been used to achieve tracheal intubation, it is possible to maintain anaesthesia with the patient breathing spontaneously. As the patient has to be at a relatively deep plane of anaesthesia for nasotracheal intubation and the nasotracheal tube is narrow (6–6.5 mm) because of the airway dimensions, this technique should only be used for short procedures, as carbon dioxide retention will occur. In the presence of halothane, this technique has a high potential for producing arrhythmias and is not recommended. If for any reason the trachea cannot be intubated successfully using the nasal route, e.g. because of a deviated septum or previous nasal injury, orotracheal intubation may be used. While this is not ideal for allowing the dentist access to the operation site, it is an acceptable technique and the orotracheal tube can be moved carefully from one side of the mouth to the other to allow access to the appropriate quadrants. Similarly, the use of a laryngeal mask and spontaneous ventilation has been described, but this also limits dental access.

At the end of surgery the patient should be turned to the left lateral, head-down position before tracheal extubation.

EXTUBATION

The trachea may be extubated while the patient is still quite deeply anaesthetised or when the patient is very light. In view of the potential for blood and secretions to drain into the larynx, it is recommended that the trachea is extubated during light anaesthesia and that the airway is maintained until that time using the nasotracheal tube.

Perioperatively, a small dose of a short-acting opioid may be used to provide analgesia for particularly painful procedures. It is also common practice to administer an NSAID perioperatively to produce postoperative analgesia. There are a number of options available for administration, including oral premedication, intravenous, intramuscular and suppositories. Many dental surgeons recommend the use of a dose of dexametasone (8 mg) given perioperatively to help reduce the swelling and hence the pain. If the surgery is limited to one or two quadrants, it is appropriate to perform a local analgesic block during or at the end of surgery to help provide postoperative analgesia. However, it is not appropriate to produce local analgesic blocks in all four quadrants as this would create difficulties in swallowing secretions and in talking.

The patient should be recovered in a supine position and, when appropriate, allowed to sit up and then gradually to mobilize. It is appropriate that discharge does not occur until the patient is fully recovered and should take place a minimum of 2 h postoperatively. Additional postoperative analgesia may be provided, if required, with regular oral medication such as a paracetamol/codeine mixture. It is important that the patient is assessed by a medical practitioner and dentist before discharge and that the patient has good pain control, has no evidence of continuing bleeding and is fully orientated. On discharge, the patient should be accompanied and should be given a set of written instructions for the postoperative period with regard to operating machinery, drinking alcohol and being accompanied. It is important that, should there be any problems, the patient has a contact telephone number to seek advice. As with all day-case procedures, should a problem arise peri- or postoperatively, such as continued bleeding or persistent uncontrolled pain, there must be an easily implemented procedure which would allow overnight admission of the patient to hospital.

IN-PATIENT DENTAL ANAESTHESIA

Surgical procedures of a more invasive nature are managed more appropriately on an in-patient basis. These procedures may include impacted wisdom teeth where considerable surgery is anticipated and also oral surgical procedures on the gums and jaw. In this latter group, the anaesthetist must be particularly aware of the potential for difficulty in achieving tracheal intubation produced by limitation of jaw movement at the temporomandibular joint. It is very important in the preoperative assessment to make a full assessment of the airway. Limitation of jaw movement produced by pain or swelling cannot be relied upon to decrease after blockade with a muscle relaxant.

In general, in-patient dental cases are managed with nasotracheal intubation following intravenous induction. However, if difficulty is anticipated with the airway, an awake fibreoptic intubation or an inhalation induction should be considered. Following nasotracheal intubation, a throat pack is placed around the tracheal tube by the anaesthetist. Some oral surgical procedures use lasers and a laser-protected tracheal tube may be required.

These operations can be painful and the perioperative use of a short-acting opioid and NSAID is recommended. Postoperatively the patient may require i.m. or i.v. opioids with a PCA.

SEDATION

The move away from the use of general anaesthesia for dental procedures has been accompanied by increasing use of sedative techniques to permit dental procedures to be carried out under local analgesia in patients who are anxious or who are having more invasive procedures carried out. Although dentists receive training in the use of sedation, it is likely that with its increasing use, anaesthetists may be called on to provide sedation for patients undergoing dental procedures. The Department of Health (1991) report defined sedation as:

> A carefully controlled technique in which a single intravenous drug, or a combination of oxygen and nitrous oxide, is used to reinforce hypnotic suggestion and reassurance in a way which allows dental treatment to be performed with minimal physiological and psychological stress, but which allows verbal contact with the patient to be maintained at all times. The technique must carry a margin of safety wide enough to render unintended loss of consciousness unlikely. Any technique of sedation other than as defined above would be regarded as coming within the meaning of dental general anaesthesia.

The important aspects of this definition are that it states that a *single* i.v. drug is used, that it is only *part of an overall technique* of reassurance for the patient, that *verbal contact* is maintained throughout the procedure and that a *wide safety margin* from loss of consciousness is essential. These definitions imply that the use of a benzodiazepine in combination with an opioid for a surgical procedure is regarded as general anaesthesia and not as sedation.

There are two techniques which are used: intravenous use of small doses of benzodiazepines and, less commonly, inhalation of low concentrations of nitrous oxide in oxygen (termed *relative analgesia*).

INTRAVENOUS SEDATION

The aim of this technique is to have a patient who is feeling no anxiety, who is cooperative though drowsy, yet who is easily rousable. The procedure starts with intravenous cannulation and attachment of a pulse oximeter. Increments of benzodiazepine, usually midazolam, are given, and the amount titrated to the patient's response. Midazolam has largely replaced diazepam as the benzodiazepine used for these procedures as it has the advantage of a shorter half-life and no active metabolites. This implies that the patient has less postoperative sedation and is ready for discharge more promptly. The end-point for titration of midazolam and diazepam may be the onset of Verrill's sign, which is drooping of the eyelids (ptosis). This is thought by some authors to be too deep a level of sedation and they use an end-point at which the patient starts to have a delayed response to verbal command. It is important that verbal contact is not lost at any stage.

The use of intravenous sedation with midazolam is occasionally associated with the occurrence of dreams which may be of a sexual nature. These may be very distressing to the patient and can lead to misunderstandings with the operator. There are two recommendations which should be followed to minimize this risk: first, the maximum dose of midazolam should be limited to 0.1 mg kg^{-1}; and second, the operator should always be accompanied throughout the procedure by another person, usually the practice nurse.

Midazolam should be administered slowly and it must be remembered that there is a lag time before the onset of its sedative effect. When the appropriate level of sedation has been reached, local analgesia can be injected in the usual manner and the procedure can start. The initial dose of midazolam produces amnesia which may persist for 10–15 min and a longer period of anxiolysis. As the anxiolysis is the main reason for administering the drug, top-up doses should not be required too frequently. The patient should be monitored continuously using the pulse oximeter and it is important that the operator communicates regularly with the patient to assess the degree of awareness and comfort. At the end of the procedure, the patient should be given adequate time to recover before discharge. Flumazenil should be used only in the situation of accidental overdosage of benzodiazepines and not as a routine method of reversing sedation. The criteria for fitness discharge that would apply to a patient receiving a general anaesthetic should also apply to those who receive intravenous sedation, i.e. they should be accompanied home and should not operate machinery or drive for the first 24 h.

INHALATION SEDATION

Inhalation sedation involves the use of low inspired concentrations of nitrous oxide in oxygen and is also termed *relative analgesia*. The technique has been used in both adults and children but requires a degree of cooperation from the patient and significant input from the operator to make the technique work. The aim of the technique is to titrate a dose of inspired nitrous oxide which produces a light level of sedation and mild analgesia. This allows procedures to take place under subsequent local anaesthetic block. This technique may be useful in patients who have 'needle phobia' for local analgesic injections in the mouth. It is important for this procedure that the patient has been selected appropriately and understands what is involved. A nasal mask, which can be clipped round the head, is used and an initial concentration of 5–10% nitrous oxide in oxygen inhaled. This is stepped up in 5% increments to a maximum of 30% to provide an appropriate level of sedation and cooperation. The use of higher concentrations of nitrous oxide may lead to restlessness and occasionally aggression in the patient. A Quantiflex flowmeter is very useful for administration of nitrous oxide in this technique, because when the initial flow has been set, the relative concentrations of nitrous oxide and oxygen can be varied using a single dial. During onset of sedation, it is important that the operator maintains verbal communication and assists in establishing anxiolysis to allow placement of the local block and commencement of the procedure. Recovery from this technique is rapid and it has the advantage compared with intravenous sedation that, following a short recovery period, the patient is ready for discharge early and there is less restriction on mobility in the first 24 h.

Relative contraindications to the use of relative analgesia include a blocked nose, deafness, inability to cooperate through either physical or mental disability, active neurological disease or severe respiratory disease.

FURTHER READING

Church J A, Pollock J S S, Still D M, Parbrook G D 1991 Comparison of two techniques for sedation in dental surgery. Anaesthesia 46: 780–782

Department of Health 1991 Report on an expert working party on general anaesthesia, sedation and resuscitation in dentistry. Department of Health, Dental Division, London

General Dental Council. Maintaining standards: Guidance to dentists on professional and personal conduct. Revised Nov 1998

Paris S T, Cafferkey M, Tarling M, Hancock P, Yate P, Flynn P 1997 Comparison of sevoflurane and halothane for outpatient dental anaesthesia in children. British Journal of Anaesthesia 79: 280–284

Rood J P, Healy T E J 1990 The dental day case unit. Clinical Anaesthesiology 4: 799–806

Royal College of Anaesthetists 1999 Standards and guidelines for general anaesthesia in dentistry. Royal College of Anaesthetists, London

Seward G R 1990 The use of nitrous oxide–oxygen inhalation sedation with local analgesia as an alternative to general anaesthesia for dental extractions in children. British Dental Journal 168: 467–470

55 Anaesthesia for plastic, endocrine and vascular surgery

PLASTIC SURGERY

Plastic surgery includes the reconstitution of damaged or deformed tissues (congenital abnormalities or resulting from trauma, burns or infection), removal of cutaneous tumours or cosmetic alteration of body features. Division or removal of the abnormality often necessitates skin grafting. Major plastic surgery includes the formation and repositioning of free and pedicle grafts and the movement of skin flaps.

GENERAL CONSIDERATIONS

Many of these procedures have important common features. Patients may be physically deformed and attention should be directed to their psychological state, which is influenced by long periods of confinement and rehabilitation, concern over disfigurement or loss of limb function and occasionally chronic pain. The presence of local or generalized infection, and the patient's state of nutrition and haematocrit, should be considered, as they are important factors in postoperative outcome. Surgery is often prolonged, requiring special attention to patient positioning, anaesthetic technique, blood and fluid replacement therapy, and maintenance of body temperature. Postoperative pain may be severe, particularly from donor skin graft sites. Pain is usually peripheral rather than visceral in origin and local anaesthetic techniques are very useful.

Anaesthesia should be administered using humidified gases in a warmed theatre environment. To avoid protracted recovery from anaesthesia for prolonged procedures, an insoluble volatile agent which undergoes minimal biotransformation (e.g. isoflurane, desflurane or sevoflurane) is preferable. Nitrous oxide may produce marrow depression with exposure of more than 8 h duration and an oxygen/air mix should be substituted. A total intravenous technique may be used, although the vasodilatation produced by volatile agents may be beneficial to surgical outcome. Fluid balance should be maintained scrupulously. Haemorrhage is a common occurrence during plastic surgery, and blood transfusion is frequently required. However, blood rheology studies suggest that microvascular flow is optimal with a haematocrit of approximately 0.3. Overtransfusion should be avoided, and normothermia, normovolaemia and cardiac output maintained, to maximize peri- and postoperative perfusion of the surgical site.

The patient must be positioned to avoid ligament strain and pressure on skin over bony prominences. Pressure areas should be protected with soft padding and a ripple mattress; lumbar support is useful. An arterial cannula is often required for measurement of arterial pressure. Measures should be taken to prevent DVT formation. When surgery has been completed, wound dressing and bandaging may be lengthy procedures. Bandages may be applied around the trunk and the patient must be lifted carefully to avoid injury.

Cosmetic surgery of the face, tattoo removal, breast augmentation and removal of unwanted adipose tissue are usually performed on healthy patients.

HEAD AND NECK

Tracheal intubation is mandatory for surgery in this area and a reinforced tube should be used. Tumours or scarring of the neck, deformity of facial bones and cleft palate make tracheal intubation particularly difficult. The airway should be assessed carefully before anaesthesia, any difficulties anticipated and a complete range of equipment should be available. The administration of muscle relaxants in such patients may be unwise before the airway is secured by intubation; the use of local anaesthesia for awake intubation or an inhalational technique should be considered. The method of maintenance is determined by the condition of the patient, the type and duration of surgery (frequently prolonged) and the experience and preference of the anaesthetist. Venous drainage is improved and bleeding reduced in head or neck surgery if the patient is positioned in a 10–15° head-up tilt. Hypotensive techniques may also be indicated (see Ch. 56). It is important to protect the eyes from pressure, the ears from blood and other fluids and the endotracheal tube and anaesthetic tubing from dislodgement. It may be difficult to monitor chest movement and access to the arms may be impossible. An i.v. infusion with extension tubing is essential; there should be access to a three-way tap for injection of drugs. A foot should be exposed to allow the anaesthetist to monitor colour, capillary filling and arterial pulse.

TRUNK

Problems encountered in surgery on the trunk include the adoption of unusual postures and their attendant risks, haemorrhage, prolonged operation and restrictive dressings applied after surgery.

LIMBS

Local anaesthesia (e.g. by blockade of nerve plexuses in the neck, axilla and groin) may be an advantage in terms of analgesia and vasodilatation for surgery on upper or lower limbs. The duration of some plastic surgical operations and the use of a surgical tourniquet to provide a bloodless field may preclude some techniques, but prolonged neural blockade may be achieved using a catheter technique and by using an agent with a prolonged action (e.g. bupivacaine). Bier's block is of limited value because of tourniquet pain, and cuff deflation may be required by the surgeon to identify bleeding points. Intravenous sedative drugs or light general anaesthesia are useful adjuncts to help the patient tolerate a prolonged procedure. Specific nerve blocks may be useful; for example, blockade of the femoral and lateral cutaneous nerve of thigh provides good analgesia for skin graft donor sites during and after operation.

Surgical techniques of reimplantation and microsurgical repair of the limbs are well established and make specific demands upon the anaesthetist. These include maintenance of general anaesthesia for up to 24 h, control of vascular spasm and provision of optimum conditions for postoperative recovery. Vascular spasm in an isolated limb may be prevented by preoperative i.v. regional sympathetic blockade using guanethidine 15–20 mg, heparin 500 units and prilocaine 0.5% to a suitable volume.

BURNS

Death in victims of fire is usually caused by hypoxaemia, resulting either from a reduction in inspired oxygen concentration in a smoke-filled atmosphere or from poisoning by products of combustion. Carbon monoxide has an affinity for haemoglobin over 200 times greater than that of oxygen and high concentrations cause reduced oxygen carriage in the blood. The oxygen dissociation curve is distorted and shifted to the left, resulting in reduced oxygen delivery to the tissues. Inhalation of smoke particles and other toxic compounds, e.g. hydrogen cyanide, hydrogen sulphide and ammonia, contribute to pulmonary and systemic toxicity. In addition, there may be direct thermal injury to the airway with ciliary damage, mucosal oedema, loss of surfactant and epithelial destruction. These may result in mucosal sloughing, alveolar oedema and ventilation/perfusion mismatch.

The aim of immediate treatment is to secure the airway and administer high-flow oxygen; tracheal intubation and IPPV with 100% oxygen may be required to maintain an adequate P_aO_2. Such patients require humidification of inspired gas, physiotherapy and bronchial suction; bronchodilators and PEEP may be necessary. Newer techniques include bronchial lavage. Early signs suggestive of upper airway burns include facial or intraoral burns, singed facial or nasal hair, carbonaceous sputum, wheeze, hoarseness or stridor. The latter two are important as they may indicate impending airway obstruction; the airway must be urgently secured by tracheal intubation. Pulse oximeters are unreliable in determining tissue oxygenation as they cannot distinguish between oxyhaemoglobin and carboxyhaemoglobin. Most burns are extremely painful and carefully titrated intravenous opioids are usually required.

Tissue burns produce rapid fluid shifts and formation of oedema, particularly during the first 36 h. The resulting depletion of intravascular volume is greatest in the first few hours and it is essential that a fluid replacement regimen is started as early as possible in order to avoid hypovolaemic shock and acute renal failure. Fluid regimens based on that of Muir and Barclay are still widely used. Recent concerns regarding the safety of albumin solutions may lead to increased use of crystalloid-based regimens such as the Parkland formula, which is prevalent in the USA (Table 55.1). The type of resuscitation fluid used is less important than the early commencement of therapy. The pathophysiology of fluid shifts is complex, and volume replacement should be modified appropriately in response to alterations in urine output, plasma osmolality, vital signs and body temperature. Haematocrit, and serum urea and electrolyte concentrations should be monitored.

The hormonal response to burning results in a hypercatabolic state with tachycardia, hyperpnoea and hyperpyrexia.

After the eschar has formed, there is loss of pure water from the body surface with a resultant increase in plasma concentration of aldosterone. The patient is at risk of water depletion and relative sodium overload. In addition, there is a rapid increase in serum potassium and urea concentrations (caused by cellular disruption in damaged tissue) and haemolysis, and these are accentuated by acidosis caused by infection. In the natural course of recovery, kalliuresis and anaemia result from continuing haemolysis of red cells.

Sepsis frequently develops following severe burns, often leading to widespread metabolic derangement, multiorgan failure and death. The excessive inflammatory response to trauma and infection is associated with cytokine activity, notably tumour necrosing factor α, interleukin-1 (IL-1) and IL-6. Persistently elevated IL-6 concentrations are associated with a poor prognosis.

The anaesthetist may be involved with burn victims at an early stage when hypoxaemia or airway compromise is life-threatening and basic resuscitation is required. If sepsis and multiorgan failure develop, the patient must be admitted to an intensive therapy unit. General anaesthesia may be required for:

- early excision of damaged tissue
- excision of granulation tissue and subsequent grafting
- changes of dressing
- reparative plastic procedures to relieve contractures, permit limb function or correct deformities.

Table 55.1 Fluid regimens for burned patients

1. Estimate/measure weight
2. Estimate percentage area of burn using 'rule of nines' for adults and 'rule of tens' for children
3. Proceed with regimen if >15% burns in adults or >10% in children
4. Muir & Barclay formula:
   Requirements in each time period = body weight (kg) × % burns × 0.5 ml
   Fluids (human albumin solution 4.5%) according to formula in *each* of the following periods:
   0–4 h
   4–8 h
   8–12 h
   12–18 h
   18–24 h
   24–36 h
   In addition, water as 5% dextrose is required at 1–2 ml h^{-1}.
5. Parkland formula:
   Requirements in first 24 h = body weight × % burn × 4
   Fluids given as Ringer's lactate alone, 50% within first 8 h, 50% between 8 and 24 h

Recovery from burns trauma may be protracted. The anaesthetist must be aware of the probable requirement for multiple administrations of general anaesthesia, frequent use of opioid analgesics in the early stages and the importance of psychological support throughout the patient's stay in hospital.

Anaesthetic problems

Airway

Obtaining a secure airway in a patient with head and neck burns is vital but may be extremely challenging. In the initial stages, airway obstruction may occur. Most anaesthetists would use an inhalation induction in the conscious patient, although raw, painful tissues may render proper application of a face mask difficult. A rapid-sequence induction using a depolarizing muscle relaxant drug may be inadvisable (see below). Later, as soft tissues fibrose and distort, the range of movement in the neck and temporomandibular joints may become grossly restricted and render laryngoscopic intubation impossible. Tracheostomy is generally undesirable because of the risk that infection may spread to damaged skin. Awake intubation may be necessary.

It may be difficult to secure the tracheal tube in place. Several ingenious methods have been devised, such as suspension of the anaesthetic breathing system from the ceiling, the use of umbilical tape to tie the tube in place and wiring the tube to the upper teeth.

In the early stages of the patient's treatment, and after prolonged surgery, the pharynx should be examined closely before tracheal extubation. Oedema may form in the soft tissues around the base of the tongue and cause respiratory obstruction when the tracheal tube is removed.

Ventilation

Mechanical ventilation should be used in the severely burned patient and careful monitoring of ventilation is required. Metabolic rate may be doubled in a patient with 40% burns. This results in large increases in oxygen consumption and carbon dioxide production; i.v. nutrition increases the latter. Inhalation injury causes increased scatter of $\dot{V}/\dot{Q}$ ratios. A sophisticated ventilator, capable of providing PEEP and minute volumes up to 30 L min^{-1}, is required.

Fluid balance

The modern practice of early tissue excision is accompanied by extensive and rapid blood loss, in addition to the fluid balance problems mentioned above. Crossmatched blood must be available before surgery and it is wise to have two large-gauge venous cannulae in situ and facilities for warming infused fluids.

Monitoring

Cutaneous burns may make conventional monitoring (e.g. ECG electrode or blood pressure cuff placement) difficult. The potential for rapid blood loss during early phase surgery is an indication for invasive arterial pressure monitoring. Urine output and body temperature should be monitored. Central venous or pulmonary artery catheterization may be required in the presence of extensive burns, although catheter-related sepsis is a hazard.

Temperature loss

Heat loss is increased from a burned area by evaporation and inability of cutaneous vessels to constrict and prevent radiation. The anaesthetist should minimize heat loss during anaesthesia and surgery by use of a warming blanket, foil blanket, blood warmer, gas humidifier and an ambient theatre temperature and humidity of 27°C and 50%, respectively.

Anaesthetic drugs

Personal preference and the problems of repeated administration of anaesthesia govern the choice of anaesthetic agent. An inhaled nitrous oxide/oxygen mixture (Entonox) and i.v. ketamine are useful for analgesia during burns dressings. However, it is not safe to assume that the airway is preserved during ketamine anaesthesia and it is also wise to premedicate the patient with an antisialagogue. Diazepam may control the emergence hallucinations suffered by some patients who receive ketamine. Intravenous opioids (by infusion, boluses or patient-controlled analgesia) are effective alternatives. The disposition and action of many drugs are affected following burns, e.g. there is a resistance to the effects of non-depolarizing muscle relaxants.

Succinylcholine should be avoided in burned patients. In the presence of muscle damage, its administration may cause release of potassium into the circulation in concentrations sufficient to cause cardiac arrest. It is thought that the most dangerous period in this respect is between 4 days and 10 weeks after thermal injury.

SURGERY FOR TUMOURS OF THE ENDOCRINE SYSTEM

Amine precursor uptake and decarboxylation (APUD) cells originate from neuro-ectoderm and are distributed widely throughout the body. They synthesize and store neurotransmitter substances, including serotonin, ACTH, calcitonin, melanocyte-stimulating hormone (MSH), glucagon, gastrin and vasoactive intestinal polypeptide. Neoplastic change within these cells produces the group of tumours termed apudomas, e.g. carcinoid, pancreatic islet cell tumour, pituitary and thyroid adenoma, medullary carcinoma of thyroid and small cell carcinoma of the lung. These may be orthoendocrine or paraendocrine – the former produce amines and polypeptides associated normally with the constituent cells, while the latter secrete substances produced usually by other organs. There are two orthoendocrine apudomas which may produce significant difficulty for the anaesthetist.

CARCINOID TUMOUR

Carcinoid tumours arise in the enterochromaffin cells of the intestinal tract, are usually benign and occur most commonly in the small bowel or appendix. However, they may arise at any site in the gut and rarely in the gall bladder, pancreas or bronchus. Malignant change occurs in 4% and may produce hepatic secondaries, which are potentially resectable. Carcinoid tumours secrete a variety of vasoactive peptides and amines (e.g. kinins, serotonin, histamine and prostaglandins) which have a variety of effects on vascular, bronchial and gastrointestinal smooth muscle activity. They are normally metabolized in the liver and carcinoid disease may be asymptomatic unless the mediators reach the systemic circulation from hepatic metastases or a non-portal primary, e.g. bronchus, producing the clinical symptoms of carcinoid syndrome.

Kallikrein acts on circulating plasma kininogen to produce bradykinin and tachykinins. Bradykinin is a potent vasodilator which causes flushing, bronchospasm and increased intestinal motility and contributes to hypotension and oedema. Adrenergic stimulation and alcohol ingestion increase the production of bradykinin. The treatment of bronchospasm in a patient with carcinoid syndrome should therefore be with aminophylline and not epinephrine. Serotonin (5-hydroxytryptamine, 5-HT) causes abnormal gut motility and diarrhoea. It has positive inotropic and chronotropic effects on the myocardium and produces vasoconstriction and bronchospasm. It may cause endocardial fibrosis, leading to pulmonary and tricuspid stenosis or regurgitation (although bronchial carcinoid tumours may lead to left-sided cardiac valvular lesions). Histamine secretion may cause bronchoconstriction and flushing. Acute attacks of carcinoid syndrome may also be precipitated by fear or hypotension.

Diagnosis is confirmed by high urinary excretion of 5-hydroxyindoleacetic acid (5-HIAA), a metabolite of 5-HT. A liver scan may show filling defects caused by secondary tumours.

Management

Patients may receive drugs to alleviate the symptoms of diarrhoea, flushing and bronchospasm, but specific agents are available to inhibit synthesis, prevent release or block the actions of the mediators released by the tumour. However, the definitive treatment of carcinoid tumours is surgical removal. The most important drug is the somatostatin analogue, octreotide, which improves both symptoms and biochemical indices, and is useful in the prevention and management of perioperative hypotension and carcinoid crisis. Somatostatin (half-life 1–3 min) is secreted naturally by the pancreas and regulates gastrointestinal peptide production by inhibiting the secretion of growth hormone, thyroid-stimulating hormone (TSH), prolactin and other exocrine and endocrine hormones. Octreotide, the octapeptide analogue of somatostatin, has a longer half-life, high potency and low clearance, and may be given i.v. or s.c. The usual s.c. dose is 50–200 μg every 8–12 h. It is useful for symptom relief in other conditions, notably acromegaly, VIPoma and glucagonoma. It may produce gastrointestinal side-effects, gallstones and impaired glucose tolerance.

5-HT antagonists (ketanserin, methysergide) and antihistamines, e.g. ranitidine, chlorphenamine (chlorpheniramine), are also used. Cyproheptadine has both antihistamine and anti 5-HT actions.

Conduct of anaesthesia

The main perioperative problems are:

- fluid and electrolyte imbalance
- severe cardiovascular instability – marked hypotension or hypertension may occur, particularly during tumour manipulation
- bronchospasm
- possible cardiac valvular lesions.

Perioperative management should be in close cooperation with both physician and surgeon, and the patient's regular medication should be continued up to the time of surgery. Hypovolaemia and electrolyte disturbance should be corrected before operation, and anxiolytic premedication with minimal cardiovascular disturbance is desirable; oral benzodiazepines are often used alone or together with antihistamines, although oversedation should be avoided. Octreotide must be continued and may be introduced as premedication 50–100 μg s.c. 1 h before surgery in patients not already receiving it.

A smooth anaesthetic technique is essential, and techniques which may cause hypotension, including epidural and subarachnoid block, should be used with extreme caution. Sudden bronchospasm, arrhythmias and extreme fluctuations in arterial pressure may take place. Drugs which release histamine (e.g. thiopental, morphine, atracurium and curare) should be avoided and succinylcholine should not be used as it can cause peptide release. Careful intravenous induction of anaesthesia with etomidate or propofol should be accompanied by measures to obtund the potentially exaggerated pressor response to tracheal intubation. Non-depolarizing muscle relaxants with minimal histamine release and cardiovascular stability, such as vecuronium or rocuronium, are preferable, and anaesthesia should be maintained with opioids (e.g. fentanyl), inhaled nitrous oxide and a volatile agent. Bronchospasm may be resistant to treatment, and a flow-generator type ventilator capable of delivering the inspired gases at high pressure should be used.

Continuous monitoring of ECG and direct arterial pressure should be commenced before induction of anaesthesia. Major fluid shifts may occur during surgery, and the effects of circulating peptides may distort the physiological response to hypovolaemia. Central venous pressure (CVP) measurement is advisable when large blood loss is likely, and pulmonary artery catheterization may be required in patients with cardiac complications. Intraoperative hypotension may be severe and should be treated with intravenous fluids and octreotide 10–20 μg i.v. Sympathomimetic drugs may cause α-mediated peptide release and are best avoided. Hypertension is usually less severe and usually responds to increased depth of anaesthesia, β-blockade or ketanserin.

Close cardiovascular monitoring and good analgesia are required postoperatively and the patient should be observed in a high-dependency or intensive therapy unit. The use of epidural analgesia is controversial, but an epidural infusion of fentanyl alone or with bupivacaine 0.1% has been used successfully.

PHAEOCHROMOCYTOMA

Phaeochromocytomas are derived from chromaffin cells which secrete catecholamines (predominantly norepinephrine, but also epinephrine and occasionally dopamine), which occur in less than 0.1% of middle-aged hypertensive patients. The majority present as a single benign tumour of the adrenal medulla, but 10% may be found in ectopic sites, e.g. paravertebral sympathetic ganglia. Approximately 10% of phaeochromocytomas are malignant, and 10% are bilateral. They may be associated with multiple endocrine adenomata (MEA) and other syndromes (Table 55.2).

Table 55.2 Associations of phaeochromocytoma with other syndromes

MEA II (Sipple's syndrome)
Phaeochromocytoma
Hyperparathyroidism
Medullary cell thyroid carcinoma
MEA III (mucosal neuroma syndrome)
Mucosal neuromata
Phaeochromocytoma
Medullary cell thyroid carcinoma
Marfan's syndrome (occasionally)
Von Recklinghausen's disease (multiple neurofibromatosis)
Von Hippel–Landau disease (retinocerebral haemangioblastoma)
Tuberous sclerosis

The clinical features depend on the quantity of hormones secreted and on which is predominant. Norepinephrine-secreting tumours tend to present with severe refractory hypertension, headaches and glucose intolerance; circulating blood volume is reduced and vasoconstriction occurs. Epinephrine-secreting tumours tend to cause paroxysmal palpitations, anxiety and panic attacks, sweating, hypoglycaemia, tachycardia, tachyarrhythmias and occasionally high-output cardiac failure. Malaise, weight loss, pallor and psychological disturbances may occur, and end-organ damage (e.g. retinopathy, nephropathy) may arise as a consequence of hypertension. They present several problems to the anaesthetist (Table 55.3).

Diagnosis

Diagnosis is important as the mortality of patients undergoing surgery with an unsuspected phaeochromocytoma is up to 50%. It is confirmed by measurement of high plasma and urine concentrations of free catecholamines. Alternatively, 24-h urinary excretion rates of catecholamine metabolites may be used. These comprise metanephrines and 3-methoxy-4-hydroxymandelic acid (HMMA; also known as vanillylmandelic acid [VMA]), derived from the action of monoamine oxidase, and homovanillic acid (HVA) derived from the activity of catecholamine orthomethyltransferase. In addition, pentolinium or clonidine suppression tests may be used. Localization of tumours greater than 1 cm in diameter may be achieved by computed tomography (performed without intravenous contrast media which may precipitate release of hormone) or magnetic resonance imaging (MRI). Confirmation of the identity and position of an adrenal mass is by uptake of [^{131}I] *meta*-iodylbenzylguanidine (MIBG) monitored by gamma camera.

Preoperative preparation

Medical treatment of the effects of the tumour must be achieved before surgery. α-Adrenergic antagonists are used commonly to counteract the increased peripheral vascular resistance and reduced circulating volume, and phenoxybenzamine (non-competitive, non-selective), prazosin and doxazosin (α_1-selective, competitive antagonists) have been used successfully. Non-competitive α-antagonists are preferable, as surges of catecholamine concentrations, occurring particularly during tumour handling, do not overwhelm the effects of a non-competitive drug. Phenoxybenzamine is given in increasing titrated doses over 2–3 weeks before surgery, starting at a dose of 10 mg b.d. and going up to a usual dose 40–50 mg b.d. In this way, the circulating volume expands gradually with normal oral intake of fluid. Side-effects include initial postural hypotension, tachycardia, blurred vision and nasal congestion. A β-adrenergic antagonist may be required later to control tachycardia, but acute hypertension, cardiac failure and acute pulmonary oedema may occur if it is introduced without prior α-blockade because of unopposed α-mediated vasoconstriction. Propranolol, metoprolol and atenolol are useful agents if β-blockade is required. Labetalol is favoured by some physicians, but its β-effect predominates and α-antagonists should be administered first. Occasionally, phenoxybenzamine or phentolamine may be given by i.v. infusion (frequently on a daily basis for the 3 days preceding surgery). In this event, intravascular volume must be monitored by measurement of CVP, and i.v. colloids are often required to maintain a normal circulating volume. Alternatively, catecholamine synthesis may be suppressed actively by administration of alpha-methyl-*p*-tyrosine, a tyrosine hydroxylase inhibitor. This drug may be very successful in controlling catecholamine effects but may cause severe side-effects, including diarrhoea, fatigue and depression. The use of magnesium sulphate has been reported; it suppresses catecholamine release from the tumour and adrenergic nerve endings but has a narrow therapeutic window and plasma Mg^{2+} concentrations should be monitored.

Table 55.3 Anaesthetic considerations in patients with phaeochromocytoma

Preoperative
Hypertension
Vasoconstriction with reduced circulating volume
Pharmacological stabilization
α-blockade
β-blockade
Control of catecholamine synthesis
End-organ damage
Intraoperative
Severe cardiovascular instability, particularly:
— at induction of anaesthesia and tracheal intubation
— during tumour handling
— following ligation of venous drainage
Postoperative
Hypotension
Hypoglycaemia
Somnolence, opioid sensitivity
Hypoadrenalism
LV dysfunction

Preoperative investigations depend on the patient's physical condition, but the possibility of end-organ damage should be considered. Nephrectomy may be required to completely remove the tumour and renal function should be assessed preoperatively. Echocardiography may also be useful.

Conduct of anaesthesia

Sudden, severe hypertension (due to systemic release of catecholamines) may occur during tumour mobilization and handling, and severe hypotension may occur after ligation of the venous drainage of the tumour, particularly if preoperative preparation has been inadequate. Marked fluctuations in arterial pressure may also occur during induction of anaesthesia and tracheal intubation. Sedative and anxiolytic premedication is useful; agents used for induction and maintenance should be selected on the basis of cardiovascular stability, and drugs which have the ability to provoke histamine (and hence catecholamine) release are best avoided (Table 55.4). Monitoring of ECG, CVP and direct arterial pressure must be commenced *before* induction of anaesthesia. The exact choice of individual anaesthetic drugs is less important than careful conduct of anaesthesia, which may be induced by slow administration of thiopental or etomidate and maintained with nitrous oxide in oxygen, supplemented by either enflurane or isoflurane. The use of moderate doses of opioids (e.g. fentanyl 7–10 $\mu g\ kg^{-1}$) may aid cardiovascular stability. Drugs should be immediately available to treat acute hypertension (e.g. sodium nitroprusside [SNP], glyceryl trinitrate [GTN] or phentolamine), tachycardia or arrhythmias (e.g. esmolol) and hypotension (e.g. ephedrine, methoxamine, phenylephrine). Perioperative epidural analgesia may attenuate some of the cardiovascular responses, except during tumour handling, and is useful for postoperative analgesia. However, it should be used judiciously to avoid hypotension. Postoperative problems may include hypotension, hypoglycaemia, somnolence and opioid sensitivity, and hypoadrenalism. Invasive monitoring should be continued for 12–24 h after surgery and the patient must be nursed in a high-dependency or intensive care unit.

Table 55.4 Drugs to avoid in patients with phaeochromocytoma

Atropine
Succinylcholine
d-Tubocurarine
Atracurium
Pancuronium
Droperidol
Morphine
Halothane

MAJOR VASCULAR SURGERY

Anaesthesia for major vascular surgery is a complex subject, and only some of the features of the commoner vascular procedures are described: elective and emergency repair of abdominal aortic aneurysm, lower limb revascularization and carotid endarterectomy.

Patients presenting for major vascular surgery have a high incidence of coexisting medical disease, in particular:

- ischaemic heart disease
- hypertension
- congestive cardiac failure
- pulmonary disease
- renal disease
- diabetes mellitus.

Cardiac complications (myocardial infarction, arrhythmias and cardiac failure) are the commonest causes of morbidity and death after vascular surgery (see Chs 35 and 40) and it is vital that any coexisting medical conditions are optimized preoperatively. The patient may have recently undergone arteriography and the injection of large volumes of radio-opaque dye may cause renal dysfunction. Investigations should include ECG, chest X-ray, full blood count and serum urea and electrolyte concentrations in all patients, but more invasive or specialized tests may be required (see Ch. 34). Exercise tolerance is a useful indicator of functional cardiac status, but many vascular patients are limited by intermittent claudication or old age and may have a sedentary lifestyle. In this case, a patient with severe coronary artery disease may have no symptoms of angina and a normal resting ECG.

ABDOMINAL AORTIC ANEURYSM

The incidence of abdominal aortic aneurysms increases with age; they occur in 2–4% of the population over the age of 65 years. The risk of rupture increases with the size of the aneurysm. The mortality from a ruptured aortic aneurysm is 90% overall, and in those who survive until emergency surgical repair can take place, the mortality is still 50%. The mortality from elective repair is 10–20% and consequently there are screening programmes to identify those patients with small asymptomatic aneurysms. Elective surgery is indicated when the aneurysm exceeds 5.5 cm in diameter. Surgery involves replacing the aneurysmal segment with a tube or bifurcated prosthetic graft, depending on the extent of iliac artery involvement. In all cases, the aorta must be cross-clamped (see below) and a large abdominal incision is required. Surgery is prolonged and blood loss may be massive. These factors contribute to the high morbidity and mortality of this procedure.

Elective repair

Consideration should be given to the collection and storage of the patient's own blood in the weeks preceding surgery. This may then be used as autologous blood transfusion perioperatively. All vasoactive medication must be continued up to the time of surgery and an anxiolytic premedication is advantageous. A β-blocker in addition may decrease the incidence of perioperative myocardial ischaemia.

An arterial and two large intravenous cannulae should be placed before induction of anaesthesia, with monitoring of ECG and pulse oximetry. Cardiovascular changes at induction may be decreased by the administration of 500–1000 ml of crystalloid immediately before careful injection of the intravenous induction agent. After muscle relaxation, the trachea is intubated (see below) and anaesthesia continued using a balanced volatile/opioid technique. Perioperative epidural analgesia is favoured by many anaesthetists and may be commenced before or after induction of anaesthesia (see below).

Several important considerations apply to patients undergoing aortic surgery (Table 55.5).

The following are required:

- two large (14-gauge) cannulae for infusion of warmed fluids
- arterial catheter for intra-arterial pressure monitoring and blood sampling for acid–base and blood gas analysis
- central venous catheter for measurement of right atrial pressure
- continuous ECG monitoring for ischaemia (CM5 position) ±

Table 55.5 Major anaesthetic considerations for patients undergoing aortic surgery

Elderly patients with a high incidence of coexisting medical disease
Cardiovascular instability during induction of anaesthesia, aortic cross-clamping and aortic unclamping
Large blood loss and fluid shifts during and after surgery
The consequences of prolonged surgery in patients with coexisting disease
Marked heat and evaporative fluid losses from exposed bowel
Potential postoperative impairment of respiratory, cardiac, renal and gastrointestinal function

ST-segment analysis
- oesophageal or tympanic membrane temperature probe
- urinary catheter
- nasogastric tube.

All possible measures should be undertaken to maintain body temperature, including heated mattress and overblanket, warmed intravenous fluids, and warmed and humidified inspired gases. The ambient temperature should be warm and the bowel may be wrapped in clear plastic to minimize evaporative losses.

Three specific stimuli may give rise to cardiovascular instability during surgery:

Tracheal intubation. Laryngoscopy and tracheal intubation may be accompanied by marked increases in arterial pressure and heart rate which may precipitate myocardial ischaemia in susceptible individuals. This response may be attenuated by the i.v. administration of a β-blocker (e.g. esmolol 1.5 mg kg^{-1}) or a lipid-soluble opioid (e.g. alfentanil 500–600 μg) before intubation.

Cross-clamping of the aorta. Clamping of the aorta causes a sudden increase in systemic vascular resistance (afterload). This increases cardiac work and may result in myocardial ischaemia, arrhythmias and left ventricular failure. The degree of cardiovascular disturbance depends on the site of aortic cross-clamping and is greater at the supracoeliac compared with the infrarenal level. Vasodilators (e.g. SNP or GTN) are often infused just before clamping to obviate these problems.

While the aorta is clamped, distal blood flow is dependent on the collateral circulation. The lower limbs, large bowel and kidneys suffer variable degrees of hypoxia during which inflammatory mediators are released from white blood cells, platelets and capillary endothelium. These mediators include oxygen free radicals, neutrophil proteases, platelet-activating factor, cyclooxygenase products and cytokines, including interleukins.

Aortic declamping. Declamping of the aorta causes a sudden decrease in afterload with reperfusion of the bowel, pelvis and lower limbs. The inflammatory mediators are swept into the systemic circulation causing vasodilatation, metabolic acidosis, increased capillary permeability and sequestration of blood cells in the lungs. Mannitol may be beneficial in countering some of these effects. Hypotension after aortic declamping may be severe unless circulating volume has been well maintained. If relative hypervolaemia is produced during the period of clamping by infusion of fluids to produce a CVP of greater than 12–14 mmHg (and perhaps administration of GTN or SNP until shortly before clamp release), declamping hypotension is less of a problem and metabolic acidosis may be diminished. Renal blood flow decreases even when an infrarenal cross-clamp is used, and measures to maintain renal function are often required. The most important measure is the maintenance of extracellular fluid volume (CVP >12–14 mmHg). Mannitol, low-dose dopamine or furosemide may also be administered, although the evidence for their efficacy is conflicting.

Bleeding is a problem throughout the operation but may be particularly severe at aortic declamping as the adequacy of vascular anastomoses is tested. In addition to red cells, specific clotting factors are often required. Some surgeons prefer to reserve the use of clotting factors until the anastomoses are complete and most of the anticipated blood loss has occurred. Many patients are elderly and are unable to tolerate the large heat loss which occurs through the extensive surgical exposure, which necessitates displacement of the bowel outside the abdominal cavity. Hypothermia causes vasoconstriction, which may cause myocardial ischaemia, delayed recovery and difficulties with fluid management during rewarming, as large volumes of intravenous fluid may be required. Therefore all measures should be taken to prevent hypothermia.

In the more compromised patient, e.g. with ischaemic heart disease and poor left ventricular function, a pulmonary artery catheter should be used to measure cardiac output and monitor fluid management and left ventricular preload. Trans-oesophageal echocardiography is sometimes used. Preservation of an optimal preload reduces the incidence of precipitous decreases of arterial pressure after aortic declamping.

The postoperative period

Repair of abdominal aortic aneurysm should be conducted only in hospitals with adequate facilities. Postoperatively, the patient should be transferred rapidly to a high-dependency or intensive care unit, where full monitoring is resumed and ventilation continued with oxygen-enriched humidified air. IPPV is required until body temperature has increased to normal levels, the consequent vasodilatation has been treated with i.v. fluids and adequate analgesia achieved. Close attention is paid to cardiovascular, respiratory and renal function and to signs of continued blood loss from oozing.

Emergency repair

The principles of management are similar to those discussed above. However, the patient may be grossly hypovolaemic and often arterial pressure is maintained only by marked systemic vasoconstriction and the action of abdominal muscle tone acting on intra-abdominal capacitance vessels. Resuscitation with intravenous fluids before the patient reaches the operating theatre should be judicious, as hypertension may increase the extent of haemorrhage. The patient is prepared and anaesthetized on the operating table. While 100% oxygen is administered by mask, all monitoring catheters and two large-gauge i.v. cannulae are inserted under local anaesthesia. The surgeon then prepares and towels the patient ready for surgery and it is only at this point that anaesthesia is induced using a rapid-sequence technique. When muscle relaxation occurs, systemic arterial pressure may decrease precipitously and immediate laparotomy and aortic clamping may be required. Thereafter, the procedure is similar to that for elective repair.

The prognosis is poor for several reasons. There has been no preoperative preparation and most patients have concurrent disease. There may have been a period of severe hypotension, resulting in impairment of renal, cerebral or myocardial function. Massive blood transfusion, with its own attendant risks, is usually required. Postoperative jaundice is common because of haemolysis of damaged red cells in the circulation and in the large retroperitoneal haematoma which usually develops after aortic rupture. In addition, postoperative renal impairment and prolonged ileus often occur, frequently prolonging artificial ventilation for several days.

Endovascular aortic aneurysm repair

Endovascular repair of aortic aneurysms is a new technique which involves the transfemoral or transiliac placement of a balloon expandable stent-graft to exclude the aneurysm from the circulation from within the lumen of the aorta. It is performed via groin incisions and the aorta is temporarily occluded from within, rather than being cross-clamped. The cardiovascular, metabolic and respiratory consequences are reduced in comparison with conventional surgery. The anaesthetic considerations are the same, however, as the patients have the same incidence of coexisting disease, and blood loss may be large. If endovascular repair is not technically feasible, conversion to open surgery may be required, at which point the patient may be already anaemic, hypovolaemic and hypothermic. In this case, the mortality may be high. The technique is in its infancy and its long-term success is not known.

SURGERY FOR OCCLUSIVE PERIPHERAL VASCULAR DISEASE

Peripheral reconstructive surgery is performed in patients with severe atherosclerotic arterial disease, causing ischaemic rest pain, tissue loss (ulceration or gangrene), severe claudication with disease at specific anatomical sites (aortoiliac, femoropopliteal, popliteal or distal), or failure of non-surgical procedures. Most are heavy smokers and suffer from chronic pulmonary disease and polycythaemia. It should be assumed that all patients have widespread arterial disease. Exercise tolerance is limited by claudication, so patients may have severe coronary artery disease despite few symptoms and a normal resting ECG. Many have had angioplasties first and surgery may be reserved for those with the most severe disease.

Bypass of aortoiliac occlusion

Aortic bifurcation grafting is performed to overcome occlusion in the aorta and iliac arteries and to restore flow to the lower limbs. Anaesthetic management is similar to that required for surgery of aortic aneurysm. However, the occlusive nature of the disease results in the development of collateral vessels, and where possible, it is normal surgical practice to side-clamp the aorta, maintaining some peripheral flow, and to declamp the arteries supplying the legs in sequence. Thus the cardiovascular and metabolic changes are less severe than during aneurysm surgery.

Peripheral arterial reconstruction

The commonest peripheral arterial grafts inserted are those between axillary and femoral, or femoral and popliteal, arteries. Grafts are autologous vein or synthetic (e.g. Dacron or PTFE). Axillofemoral bypass surgery is performed in those not considered fit for aortic surgery, and these patients are often particularly frail. All these operations are prolonged and an IPPV/relaxant balanced anaesthetic technique is suitable. Particular care must be paid to the maintenance of normothermia, and administration of intravenous fluids. Hypothermia or hypovolaemia may cause peripheral vasoconstriction, compromising distal perfusion and postoperative graft function. Blood loss through the walls of open-weave grafts may continue for several hours after surgery and cardiovascular status should be monitored closely during this time. Epidural analgesia may be used alone or as an adjunct to general anaesthesia. Epidural anaesthesia has no effect on graft function (a meticulous anaesthetic technique is more important), but it provides effective postoperative analgesia. However, i.v. heparin is usually administered during surgery (see below) and this may increase the risk of an epidural haematoma if a catheter has been introduced. Oxygen therapy should be continued for at least 24 h after surgery, and monitoring in a high-dependency unit is often required.

CAROTID ARTERY SURGERY

Carotid endarterectomy is performed to prevent disabling stroke in patients with atheromatous plaques in the common carotid bifurcation or internal carotid artery. Most strokes from plaques in these sites are embolic. The underlying pathology is usually atherosclerosis, and most patients are elderly, with hypertension and generalized vascular disease. Cerebral autoregulation may be impaired and cerebral blood flow is therefore proportional to systemic arterial pressure. The main risk of surgery is the production of a new neurological deficit, which may be fatal or cause permanent disability. However, cardiovascular complications account for most of the other (non-stroke) morbidity and mortality. Carotid endarterectomy is unusual in that it is a preventative operation with well-defined indications based on the results of large-scale randomized studies performed in Europe and the USA. In patients with a previous stroke and a carotid stenosis >70%, the benefits of surgery outweigh the risks, whereas in those with mild stenosis (< 30%), the risks outweigh the benefits and medical treatment with antiplatelet drugs is preferred. Therefore the patients presenting for surgery are those with the most severe disease, and

Table 55.6 Factors which may be associated with increased perioperative risk in patients undergoing carotid endarterectomy

Increased risk	Decreased risk
Age	Asymptomatic
Female sex	Ocular symptoms only
Hypertension	Receiving antiplatelet therapy
Cardiovascular disease	
Diabetes	
Smoking	
Hyperlipidaemia	
Recent or progressive neurological symptoms	
Contralateral carotid stenosis	

the potential benefits are only realized if the overall perioperative mortality and morbidity are low (< 5%).

Of the potential perioperative risk factors (Table 55.6), only female sex, age >75 years, systolic hypertension and neurological status have repeatedly been implicated when specifically studied.

During surgery, the carotid artery is clamped, during which cerebral perfusion is dependent on collateral circulation via the Circle of Willis. A temporary shunt is usually inserted to bypass the site of obstruction, minimizing clamping time and the period of potential cerebral ischaemia. Several methods are available to assess cerebral blood flow during clamping, before proceeding with the endarterectomy. If flow is adequate, some surgeons prefer not to use a temporary shunt. The methods used include:

- transcranial Doppler ultrasonography of the middle cerebral artery
- measurement of arterial pressure in the occluded distal carotid segment (the 'stump' pressure)
- neurological assessment in the awake patient following clamping under local anaesthesia
- monitoring the EEG
- recording somatosensory evoked potentials
- measurement of jugular venous oxygen tension.

The primary aim of anaesthesia is to maintain cerebral perfusion during carotid clamping, using a technique which provides cardiovascular stability and allows rapid recovery at the end of surgery to facilitate early postoperative neurological assessment. Residual postoperative effects of anaesthesia may confuse the diagnosis of intraoperative embolism or ischaemic change. Rapid swings in arterial pressure are common because of the effects of surgical manipulation and clamping on carotid sinus baroreceptor and vagal reflexes. An intra-arterial cannula is mandatory for monitoring of arterial pressure, which should be maintained particularly during carotid clamping. The airway is not accessible during surgery, and tracheal intubation with a well-secured reinforced endotracheal tube is advisable. Anaesthesia should be induced cautiously using an intravenous agent and maintained with a balanced technique using an inspired oxygen concentration of 50% in air or nitrous oxide (100% inspired oxygen produces cerebral vasoconstriction) with isoflurane. All anaesthetic agents should be short-acting, and remifentanil, alfentanil or low dose fentanyl (100–200 μg) are useful adjuncts. Hypotension may potentially occur after induction and during the placement of cerebral monitoring, but it should be treated promptly and under no circumstances should it be allowed to persist. Vasopressors (e.g. ephedrine 3–6 mg, or methoxamine 0.25–0.5 mg increments) are frequently required and should be drawn up before induction of anaesthesia. A high P_aO_2, normocapnia and normothermia should be maintained. Blood loss and fluid requirements are usually modest. Postoperatively, pain is unusual and the combination of wound infiltration with local anaesthetic with a non-steroidal anti-inflammatory analgesic during surgery is effective.

The use of local or regional anaesthesia for carotid endarterectomy has its advocates. Its principal advantage is that the patient's neurological status can be directly assessed without the need for additional monitoring, and a vascular shunt may be obviated. Anaeshesia is provided by a combination of deep and superficial cervical plexus blocks with or without supplementary local anaesthetic infiltration by the surgeon. However, the patient must lie flat and remain still for the duration of the procedure, which may be prolonged, and deep cervical plexus blockade may be associated with significant complications (e.g. phrenic nerve palsy or accidental dural puncture). Overall, there is no evidence that neurological or cardiovascular outcome is improved by these techniques, compared with general anaesthesia.

Patients should be monitored in a high-dependency environment for several hours postoperatively. Approximately 30% of patients require control of postoperative hypertension, which may be severe and compromise the graft or cause intracranial haemorrhage. Intravenous β-blockers or an infusion of GTN, hydralazine or SNP may be required.

HEPARIN

Centres in the UK differ in their use of heparin during vascular surgery. In units where it is used systemically, a dose of 100 units kg^{-1} is given i.v. after preclotting the graft (where material such as Dacron is used) and at least one circulation time should elapse before arterial clamping begins. Some vascular surgeons rely solely on the local use of heparinized saline. If i.v. heparin is to be used, the anaesthetist should ensure that any epidural catheter has been sited at least 1 h before the heparin is given, and to wait for at least 3 h before catheter removal. In some centres, the anaesthetist may be asked to antagonize the heparin with protamine (0.5 mg per 100 units heparin) before termination of surgery.

CARDIOVERSION

DC cardioversion is an effective treatment for some re-entrant tachyarrhythmias, which may produce haemodynamic instability and myocardial ischaemia and which do not respond to other measures. Atrial fibrillation of less than 6 months' duration, atrial flutter, supraventricular tachycardia and ventricular tachycardia may be converted to sinus rhythm, although maintenance of sinus rhythm depends usually on the subsequent use of drugs. Cardioversion has little effect on contractility, conductivity or excitability of the myocardium, and has a low incidence of side-effects or complications.

Pre-anaesthetic assessment

Patients may present with a chronic arrhythmia for elective cardioversion or as an emergency *in extremis* with a life-threatening arrhythmia. They may have other serious cardiovascular pathology such as rheumatic disease, ischaemic heart disease, recent myocardial infarction or cardiac failure. Digitalis therapy predisposes to post-cardioversion arrhythmias; in some centres, it is withheld for 48 before cardioversion. If DC cardioversion is required in a patient receiving digoxin, the initial DC dose should be low (e.g. 10–25J) and increased if necessary. In some patients there is a significant risk of embolic phenomena, e.g. those with:

- mitral stenosis and atrial fibrillation of recent onset
- atrial fibrillation and a dilated cardiomyopathy
- a prosthetic mitral valve
- a history of embolic phenomena.

These patients should receive prophylactic anticoagulants for 2–3 weeks before cardioversion, and anticoagulation should be continued afterwards. Accurate knowledge of the medical and drug history and thorough clinical examination are essential before anaesthesia.

Cardioversion

DC electrical discharge passed through the heart depolarizes all excitable myocardial cells and interrupts abnormal pathways and foci. The attendant physician usually sites the electrodes anterolaterally with the patient supine, but the anteroposterior arrangement, with the patient in the lateral position, is sometimes used. The paddles should not be sited over the scapula, sternum or vertebrae and the skin must be protected with electrolyte jelly, saline-soaked gauze or any type of conducting pad.

The ECG monitoring lead chosen should demonstrate a clear R wave in order to synchronize the discharge away from the T wave and thus reduce the risk of development of ventricular fibrillation. If the arrhythmia does not convert after the first 50 J discharge, further shocks are given, using an increased energy discharge of up to 200 J.

Despite the use of synchronized discharge, ventricular fibrillation may be produced in the presence of hypokalaemia, ischaemia, digitalis intoxication and QT prolongation (caused by quinidine, tricyclic antidepressants or hyperalimentation).

Anaesthesia

Treatment should be carried out only in areas specifically designed for the purpose and with a full range of drugs, resuscitation and monitoring equipment available. These must be checked by the anaesthetist and patients prepared as for a surgical procedure.

ECG monitoring, oximetry and measurement of arterial pressure are instituted. A vein is cannulated and the patient's lungs are preoxygenated before induction of anaesthesia with an i.v. agent. The choice of agent is determined by the cardiovascular stability and recovery period required. If the patient is shocked, precautions to prevent aspiration of gastric contents should be taken and a rapid-sequence induction with cricoid pressure and tracheal intubation should be performed. However, many patients are admitted for elective cardioversion on a day-case basis, and a technique using i.v. propofol and spontaneous ventilation is suitable.

As soon as the patient is unconscious, the airway is secured and oxygenation maintained with a suitable breathing system. Before activation of the defibrillator, it is important to check that the patient is not in contact with any person or metal object. If repeated shocks are required, incremental doses of the anaesthetic may be given. The patient should be monitored carefully both during anaesthesia and after recovery of consciousness, in particular for evidence of recurrent arrhythmia, hypotension, pulmonary oedema, or systemic or pulmonary embolism.

FURTHER READING

Kinsella J (ed) Burns 1997 Clinical anaesthesiology, Vol 11 no 3. Baillière Tindall, London

Nimmo W S, Rowbotham D J, Smith G (eds) 1994 Anaesthesia, 2nd edn. Blackwell Scientific Publications, Oxford

Stoelting R K, Dierdorf S F 1993 Anesthesia and co-existing disease, 3rd edn. Churchill Livingstone, New York

Wildsmith A J, Bannister J (eds) 1999 Anaesthesia for major vascular surgery. Arnold, London

56 Hypotensive anaesthesia

The judicious use of deliberate hypotension is an important anaesthetic skill. Deliberate hypotension enables some complex operations to be undertaken in an almost bloodless environment. This may be important either if a small amount of blood loss interferes significantly with the surgeon's view of the operative field (e.g. during middle ear surgery), or in procedures which are so extensive that the magnitude of blood loss could be life-threatening in the absence of deliberate hypotension. Controlled hypotension also reduces complications resulting from major blood loss, including the risks of hypovolaemia and those associated with blood transfusion.

The factors which influence the safety of deliberate hypotension include the nature of the surgical procedure and the medical status of the patient. The prime concern is the safety of the patient and, despite a perceived surgical demand for hypotension, some patients have relative or absolute contraindications to deliberate hypotensive anaesthetic techniques. The duration of controlled hypotension should be limited to the shortest time necessary for safe surgery; arterial pressure should then be returned towards normal values to allow surgical haemostasis to be achieved.

Common indications for controlled hypotensive anaesthesia are shown in Table 56.1. The usual aim of hypotensive techniques is to reduce haemorrhage at the site of the operation. The most important means of minimizing haemorrhage is control of bleeding from arteries and veins by the surgeon. However, modification of the control systems which maintain arterial pressure homeostasis, together with careful positioning of the patient, can be used to assist the surgeon.

Table 56.1 Indications for controlled hypotensive anaesthesia

Expected major blood loss	Pelvic surgery for malignancy Head and neck surgery requiring reconstruction Large vessel vascular surgery Revision hip prosthetic surgery Reconstructive spinal surgery, e.g. scoliosis correction
Complex neurosurgery	Excision of intracranial or spinal meningiomas Arteriovenous malformations Pituitary surgery Craniofacial reconstruction
Microsurgery	Middle ear surgery Endoscopic sinus surgery Nerve and microvascular surgery Plastic free flap grafting
Intraocular surgery	Vitrectomy Choroidal surgery

BLEEDING

ARTERIAL BLEEDING

Incised arterial vessels do not vasoconstrict readily; therefore the normal haemostatic responses are incapable of controlling bleeding. The flow from damaged arterioles is related to the size of the vessels and the intraluminal pressure; reductions in vascular resistance or cardiac output (or both) reduce arterial pressure. Elevation of the cut end of the artery above the aortic root leads to a decrease in blood flow from the vessel. Arterial pressure decreases by approximately 1 mmHg for every 1 cm increase in vertical distance above the aorta.

Alterations in diastolic arterial pressure reflect the level of peripheral vascular tone. An increase in diastolic pressure resulting from tachycardia or release of catecholamines increases arterial bleeding. Hyperventilation, which reduces circulating concentrations of catecholamines, reduces arterial pressure, and therefore bleeding. However, hyperventilation results in vasoconstriction of cerebral arteries, and this limits the extent to which the arterial carbon dioxide tension may be reduced safely.

VENOUS BLEEDING

Venous congestion and pooling at the operative site may cause torrential haemorrhage, and it may be difficult to apply direct pressure to allow the haemostatic responses to occur (e.g. in haemorrhage from the epidural veins during spinal surgery). Manoeuvres which reduce venous pooling are important determinants of blood loss from veins. Elevation of the wound improves venous drainage, but this is not always possible during surgery, and may have disadvantages. For example, a head-up posture is often used during head and neck surgery. This leads to a reduction in venous pressure, and in haemorrhage at the operative site, but also causes a reduction in cardiac output because of the reduced venous return to the heart. In addition, the reduced venous pressure in the head and neck increases the risk of air embolism.

Obstruction to venous drainage by poor positioning, surgical retraction or large increases in intrathoracic pressure (e.g. because of coughing) must be avoided.

Hypoventilation during anaesthesia increases venous bleeding because hypercapnia causes dilatation of veins. It also increases circulating concentrations of catecholamines, making arterial hypertension more likely.

CONTROL OF ARTERIAL PRESSURE

The ability of anaesthetists to manipulate blood pressure safely depends on a clear understanding of the normal physiological control systems. The delivery of an adequate supply of oxygen and other nutrients to cells, and the removal of products of metabolism, are matched normally to the needs and metabolic activity of each organ. The potential volume of the total vascular compartment is far larger than the blood volume, and at any given time, some areas of the circulation are relatively inactive while others receive the majority of the blood flow. This regulation is achieved by the action of the sympathetic nervous system, by local vasoconstriction and by alterations in cardiac activity.

Drugs used to modify arterial pressure are reviewed extensively in Chapter 7.

CLINICAL CONSIDERATIONS

AUTOREGULATION

Blood flow to major organs such as the heart, brain and kidneys is maintained at a reasonably constant value by local autoregulation, which is effective throughout a range of arterial pressures. The lower limit of autoregulation in the cerebral and coronary circulations occurs in normal adults at a mean arterial pressure of 50–55 mmHg. Below this pressure, flow through the arteries decreases progressively with further decreases in the pressure gradient across the vessel. Renal glomerular filtration is affected in a similar fashion, leading to a decrease in urine production. Most of the studies of autoregulation have been undertaken in animals suffering from haemorrhagic shock, in which hypotension is associated with vasoconstriction. More recent studies in humans and in anaesthetized animals subjected to controlled hypotension suggest that autoregulation is maintained to lower limits of perfusion pressure, and that a larger safety margin exists before ischaemia occurs.

CONTRAINDICATIONS TO INDUCED HYPOTENSION (Table 56.2)

The development of arterial plaques and thickening of vessel walls which occur in patients with peripheral vascular disease limit the ability of arteries to either constrict or dilate. Blood flow through these vessels becomes dependent on the diameter of the lumen and the pressure gradient across the vessel. If the diameter of the lumen cannot be altered, then flow is related directly to arterial pressure. During controlled hypotension, the ability to autoregulate is lost, and perfusion of the organ served by the vessel may decrease to a level which results in ischaemia in some regions.

The delivery of oxygen is related to the haemoglobin concentration, and the presence of anaemia may result in ischaemia during controlled hypotension, even if autoregulation persists.

Table 56.2 Contraindications to hypotensive anaesthesia

Carotid artery stenosis
Previous ischaemic stroke
Recent subarachnoid haemorrhage with vascular spasm
Raised intracranial (or spinal) pressure compromising brain/cord perfusion
Untreated hypertension
Claudicating peripheral vascular disease
Fixed cardiac output – such as aortic stenosis or a cardiomyopathy
Ischaemic heart disease – angina or previous infarction
Renal impairment
Liver dysfunction
Hypovolaemia
Pregnancy
Glaucoma

The delivery of all nutrients, including oxygen, and the removal of the products of metabolism depend on an adequate cardiac output.

Patients with evidence of dysfunction of major organs, and those in whom the normal compensatory responses to hypotension are impaired, are also at increased risk of organ damage during controlled hypotension.

Consequently, patients with a history or clinical evidence of vascular disease should not be subjected to hypotension (deliberate or otherwise) during anaesthesia; this group includes patients who have suffered ischaemic strokes or recent myocardial infarction and those who have angina or peripheral vascular disease, especially associated with claudication. Caution is required in patients with untreated hypertension, hepatic or renal dysfunction, or autonomic neuropathy. Patients with poorly controlled glaucoma, anaemia or hypovolaemia are also at increased risk. Insulin-dependent diabetic patients may suffer from many of these conditions, even though they may be occult at the time of surgery, and controlled hypotension should be avoided if possible.

There are also groups of patients who have a relative contraindication to controlled hypotension. In these patients, it may be possible to use a controlled hypotensive technique, but very careful monitoring is required:

- The elderly are at increased risk because autoregulation, vascular damage and impaired autonomic control may lead to regional ischaemia in some organs during deliberate hypotension. One recommendation which has been made is that, in elderly patients, the mean arterial pressure should not be reduced below 80 mmHg (compared with the value of 50–55 mmHg which is acceptable in younger adults).
- There may be problems in maintaining oxygen delivery during hypotensive anaesthesia in patients with pulmonary disease, especially if there is evidence of reductions in preoperative oxygen tension or oxygen saturation. The reductions in pulmonary blood volume and perfusion pressure which occur during hypotensive anaesthesia may lead to marked increases in arteriovenous shunting and venous admixture. Patients with severe asthma, chronic obstructive airways disease, emphysema or neuromuscular or skeletal abnormalities are particularly at risk.
- Severe coronary artery disease leads to deranged autoregulation and areas of collateral circulation within the myocardium. The

areas of myocardium which are perfused normally may tolerate reduction in arterial pressure, but local damage can occur in the areas served by stenotic coronary arteries.
- In patients who have suffered a recent subarachnoid haemorrhage, spasm of the cerebral arteries often occurs, impairing autoregulation. Although controlled hypotension was used in the past during cerebral aneurysm surgery to reduce the risk of haemorrhage, it is now recognized that the reduction in cerebral perfusion pressure which accompanies deliberate hypotensive techniques leads to greater neurological damage and should be avoided.

MONITORING DURING CONTROLLED HYPOTENSION

The minimal monitoring standards required for patients in whom moderate hypotension is to be induced include ECG, arterial oxygen saturation, end-tidal carbon dioxide tension, temperature and non-invasive measurement of arterial pressure. Before hypotension is induced, there must be a period of cardiovascular stability. This, together with the time of, and response to, the administration of all hypotensive agents, must be recorded. The frequency of arterial pressure measurement is determined by the speed of onset of the hypotensive agent. If the anticipated effect is gradual (over 10–20 min), measurement of arterial pressure at intervals of 2–3 min is appropriate. If a hypotensive agent with a rapid onset of action is to be used, then invasive monitoring of arterial pressure is mandatory. Central venous pressure should be measured in situations in which hypotension is induced to avoid massive blood loss, because the combination of uncompensated haemorrhage and induced hypotension results in a high risk of damage to organs. Renal function becomes impaired as arterial pressure decreases, but there is little risk of ischaemic damage unless haemorrhage results in profound vasoconstriction because of catecholamine release. Urine output should be measured during long periods of deliberate hypotension, but it usually decreases significantly, or stops completely, when the perfusion pressure decreases below 80 mmHg.

It may be appropriate to monitor cerebral function during some operations conducted under hypotensive conditions. Techniques which can be used include visual or auditory evoked potentials, the bispectral index or modified Fourier analysis systems such as the cerebral function monitor or cerebral function analysing monitor.

Special care should be taken in positioning the patient before a procedure involving controlled hypotension because of the increased risks of skin ischaemia and pressure sores. These risks are increased still further if the patient becomes hypothermic, and steps should be taken to maintain a normal core temperature.

METHODS OF ACHIEVING CONTROLLED HYPOTENSION

A suggested method for producing controlled hypotension is shown in Figure 56.1.

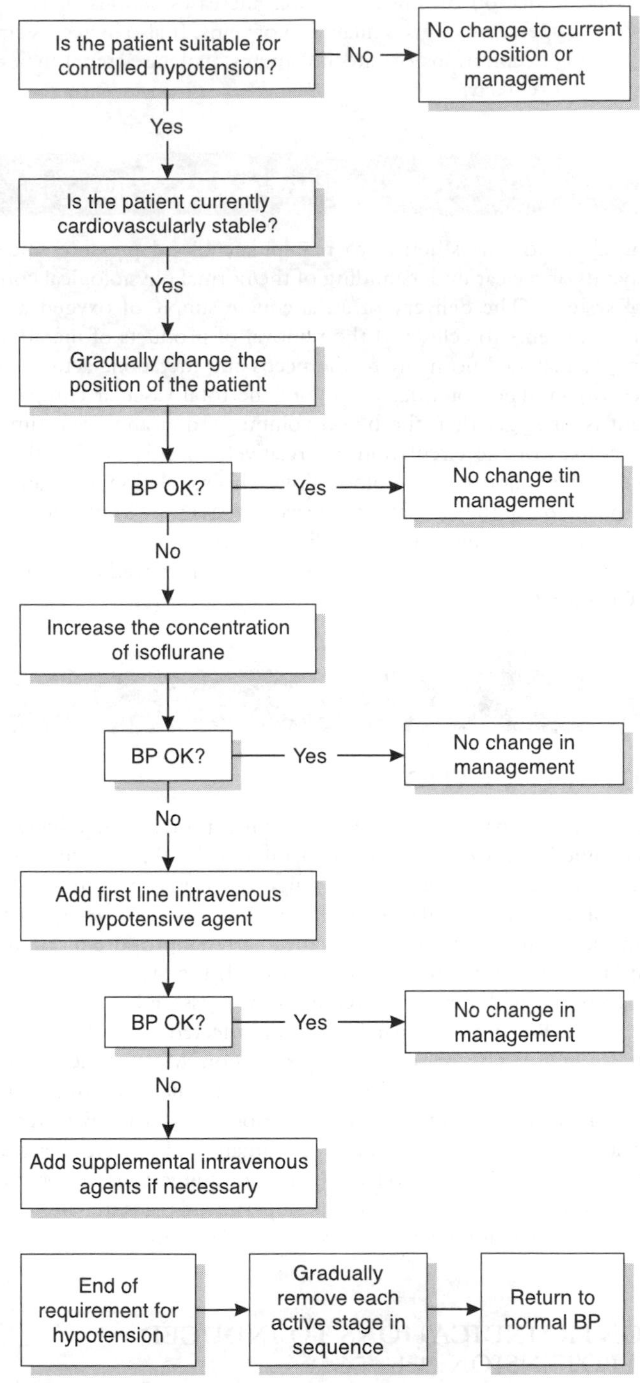

Fig. 56.1
A suggested scheme for controlled hypotension.

POSITIONING

The commonest method of enhancing a bloodless field by positioning is to elevate the operative site above the level of the heart. For example, during operations on the head or neck, a head-up tilt is often used. Sudden changes in posture may result in large alterations in arterial pressure, and these can elicit brisk reflex activity

Table 56.3 Hypotensive agents

Neurological depressants	General anaesthetic agents	Volatile anaesthetics Intravenous anaesthetics
Vasodilating agents	Direct acting	Sodium nitroprusside Glyceryl trinitrate Adenosine (ATP) Prostaglandin E_1 Hydralazine
	Indirect acting	Trimetaphan camsylate General anaesthetic agents
Cardiac depressants		β-Blockers General anaesthetic agents Calcium channel blockers

of the baroreceptor system. The best approach for operations on the head or neck is to elevate the head slowly, while also elevating the legs by 'breaking' the table. This prevents sudden pooling of blood in the legs.

Measurement of arterial pressure should be at the level of the brain, not the heart.

During spinal surgery, the patient is usually in the prone position. A variety of devices or frames is available to achieve a safe and stable position which allows free movement of the abdominal wall so that ventilation is not impaired and venous pressure is not increased. The frame is manipulated in such a way that the operative site is uppermost, to ensure good venous drainage. Poor positioning increases venous pressure because of compression or kinking of veins and may lead to torrential bleeding.

Any position in which the operative site is above the level of the heart carries with it a risk of venous air embolism. Retinal ischaemia can occur if the patient is in the prone position and pressure is applied to the eyes; this may result in blindness.

PHARMACOLOGICAL METHODS (Table 56.3)

The ideal drug for controlled hypotension during anaesthesia would have a very short duration of action. It would have a predictable dose–response curve to allow fine control of arterial pressure. It would not induce a steal phenomenon or uncouple oxidative metabolism. It would have an elimination pathway which was independent of hepatic or renal function, and would have little or no interaction with other drugs used during anaesthesia. There is no ideal agent available for the reduction of arterial pressure. Nevertheless, there are many drugs that may be used safely to reduce arterial pressure, and which result in a significant reduction in blood loss, particularly when combined with postural and other physiological measures (see Table 56.3). Spinal and epidural anaesthesia are often used to control arterial pressure. The local anaesthetic blockade of sympathetic efferent nerves results in arterial and venous vasodilatation in the area of the block and causes pooling of blood in dependent vessels. High sympathetic block also reduces cardiac output by affecting the sympathetic nerves to the heart; this may also reduce blood loss, but there is a risk with high spinal or epidural blocks that profound hypotension may occur. One of the disadvantages of spinal and epidural block is that there is a slow recovery time, and vasoconstrictor drugs may be required to return arterial pressure to normal.

Drugs used to induce controlled hypotension

Central nervous system depressants

Suppression of the baroreceptor reflex and depression of the vasomotor centre cause a progressive decrease in arterial pressure. Depression of local autonomic control also leads to a decrease in arterial pressure because of vasodilatation or cardiac depression. All anaesthetic drugs depress the cardiovascular system, although they vary in their precise actions; for example, halothane causes primarily depression of cardiac output, whereas isoflurane, desflurane and sevoflurane are predominantly vasodilators. These agents are preferable to halothane, because blood flow to essential organs is maintained better when hypotension is produced by vasodilators rather than a reduction in cardiac output.

The newer volatile anaesthetic agents sevoflurane and desflurane probably have no advantage over isoflurane. The administration of isoflurane in concentrations up to almost 2 MAC produces hypotension in healthy individuals by peripheral vasodilatation and a reduction in the baroreceptor reflex. These effects, combined with judicious positioning of the patient, provide safe and adequate hypotension for many procedures. At MAC values below 1, isoflurane maintains cerebral blood flow and reduces cerebral metabolism. It produces less cerebral vasodilatation than the other volatile anaesthetics, with the exception of sevoflurane, and therefore has a greater margin of safety in patients with raised intracranial pressure. However, higher concentrations lead to more vasodilatation and an increase in intracranial pressure. Coronary steal is a phenomenon in which areas of borderline perfusion may become ischaemic as a result of diversion of blood to normal areas of the heart if the blood vessels supplying these areas become dilated. Some studies have suggested that isoflurane can result in coronary steal, but the clinical significance appears to be minimal.

In elderly or hypertensive patients, the administration of high concentrations of isoflurane may result in a decrease in cardiac output and profound decreases in arterial pressure and tissue perfusion.

Enflurane is a potent myocardial depressant which also reduces vasoconstriction in the splanchnic circulation in response to activation of the baroreceptor reflex. These features make enflurane hazardous in patients with borderline organ perfusion, and its use is not recommended for hypotensive anaesthesia.

In many patients, an anaesthetic technique based on the use of a volatile anaesthetic agent and careful positioning of the patient ensures effective controlled hypotension. However, in some situations, it is necessary also to administer specific hypotensive drugs. These drugs are not anaesthetic agents but their effects may mask the signs of adequate anaesthesia. Consequently, it is essential to ensure that adequate anaesthesia is provided when these drugs are used.

Vasodilators

These drugs act primarily on vascular smooth muscle to cause a decrease in systemic vascular resistance; this in turn results in a decrease in arterial pressure for any given cardiac output. Many of the vasodilators act either by generating nitric oxide directly or by increasing its production. Nitric oxide interacts with and activates guanylyl cyclase. A cyclic GMP-dependent protein kinase is stimulated, causing an alteration to the phosphorylation of protein in smooth muscle cells. This leads to dephosphorylation of the light chain of myosin. It is the phosphorylation of the myosin light chain that regulates the contractile state of smooth muscles. The pharmacological and biochemical effects of the nitrovasodilators appear to be identical to those of 'endothelial-derived relaxing factor', which has been shown to be nitric oxide.

Peripheral vasodilators vary in their ability to maintain perfusion and oxidative coupling between metabolism and oxygen extraction. They are all administered intravenously, and most frequently by infusion. Invasive monitoring of arterial pressure is strongly recommended when these agents are used because of their potency and rapid action. The reduction in vascular resistance may increase cardiac output because of the reduced afterload, and this can limit the effectiveness of the drugs. Patients with autonomic dysfunction are unable to compensate for induced vasodilatation, and arterial pressure may fall precipitously. Caution should be exercised in patients who are known to suffer from autonomic abnormalities, such as patients with the Shy–Drager syndrome, or long-standing insulin-dependent diabetics.

Sodium nitroprusside. This has been used clinically to induce hypotension for over 50 years. It has five cyanide groups within its structure, and cyanide toxicity is a problem if it is used in high doses. It is a photosensitive compound which denatures directly to cyanide and nitric oxide. Both systemic and pulmonary circulations are dilated and this may result in progressive decreases in arterial oxygen saturation because of altered ventilation/perfusion ratios within the lung. The splanchnic vascular bed is also dilated, and pooling of blood in the splanchnic bed may cause extreme postural hypotension if the patient is repositioned. Younger adults tend to be tolerant to the effects of sodium nitroprusside because of catecholamine release mediated by the baroreceptor reflex. Elderly patients are often very sensitive to sodium nitroprusside and small doses may result in profound hypotension.

The onset of action of sodium nitroprusside is within 30 s, and the peak hypotensive effect occurs within 2 min. When the infusion is stopped, the clinical effect disappears within 3 min. The recommended maximum dose of sodium nitroprusside is 1.5 mg kg^{-1} and recommended infusion rates are 0.25–1.5 μg kg^{-1} min^{-1}. The risk of toxicity is high if the infusion rate exceeds 8 μg kg^{-1} min^{-1}, and if this rate is ineffective, alternative agents should be used or added.

Glyceryl trinitrate. This is an organic nitrate, and is one of a group of polyol esters of nitric acid. Its clinical action follows denitration to release nitric oxide, which in turn causes vasodilatation. Glyceryl trinitrate has been used to produce vasodilatation since 1879 (for the treatment and prophylaxis of angina). Low concentrations produce dilatation of veins to a greater extent than arterioles. Venodilatation results in decreased left and right ventricular chamber sizes and end-diastolic pressures, but there is little change in systemic vascular resistance. Systemic arterial pressure may decrease slightly; heart rate is usually unchanged. Pulmonary vascular resistance and cardiac output are both slightly reduced. Increasing concentrations of the drug leads to arterial vasodilatation and greater decreases in arterial pressure.

The avoidance of the potential toxicity of sodium nitroprusside and the chemical stability of glyceryl trinitrate make the latter drug a more common adjunct to volatile anaesthetics in inducing hypotension. Neither sodium nitroprusside nor glyceryl trinitrate has a significant effect on the baroreceptor reflexes, and reflex tachycardia is a common problem. This limits the use of both drugs, especially in young healthy adults.

Adenosine is believed to be a locally produced vasodilator and has been used clinically to induce controlled hypotension. The cardiovascular effects of adenosine include a dose-related increase in the conduction time along the bundle of His and an alteration in heart rate. Data from animal studies suggest that anaesthesia reduces the effect of adenosine on cardiac conduction, but infusions of adenosine triphosphate in humans have occasionally caused atrioventricular blockade which has resolved when infusion of the drug has ceased. Clinical experience with this agent is so limited that there is little to recommend its use at present.

Hydralazine. This drug relaxes predominantly resistance vessels. It has a gradual and prolonged action, taking up to 20 min to reach its maximal effect. It is usually administered as an intravenous bolus injection, and repeated if necessary every 20–30 min. It is used as an adjunct to hypotension induced by a volatile anaesthetic agent or glyceryl trinitrate and offers some protection from rebound hypertension.

Autonomic ganglion blocking drugs

Trimetaphan is the only member of this group of drugs still in clinical use; in the past, hexamethonium and pentolinium were also available. Trimetaphan acts within 2 min of the start of an infusion and is metabolized rapidly by plasma cholinesterases. It decreases the excitability of postganglionic neurones, largely at the nicotinic acetylcholine receptor sites. Its action at muscarinic receptors is minor. The major action of the drug is arterial vasodilatation, but blockade of sympathetic neurones induces the same postural changes which are seen in patients with autonomic dysfunction. Profound decreases in arterial pressure may follow changes in posture.

The predictable side-effects of increased concentrations of acetylcholine are undesirable and troublesome; they include tachycardia, bronchospasm, mydriasis, paralytic ileus, potentiation of muscle relaxants and retention of urine. The combination of a 10:1 mixture of nitroprusside and trimetaphan has been used successfully to achieve controlled hypotension during anaesthesia.

α-Adrenergic blocking drugs

There is little place for these drugs in current practice because the pure α-antagonists provoke marked reflex tachycardia which largely counteracts their effects in reducing blood loss. Phentolamine and urapidil are examples of this class of drug.

β-Adrenergic blocking drugs

These agents are useful in preventing or treating unwanted tachycardia during induced hypotension, although in high doses they can act as potent hypotensive agents in their own right. β-Blockers have little effect on pulmonary vessels and result in little change in intrapulmonary shunting, in contrast to drugs such as sodium nitroprusside. They are not recommended as sole hypotensive agents because of the marked depression of cardiac output which occurs when high doses are administered. Their principal use is as adjuncts to volatile anaesthetic agents or in combination with a vasodilator. The two most commonly used agents are labetalol and esmolol. Labetalol has both α and β affinity, with the β-effect being approximately seven times greater than the α-effect. Both labetalol and esmolol may be administered either by intravenous bolus injection or by continuous infusion. The time from injection to the peak effect for labetalol is 5 min, but it has a long half-life of 4 h and this causes difficulty in titrating its effect accurately. Esmolol has a much shorter half-life (9.2 min) because it is metabolized by an esterase in erythrocytes. It decreases plasma renin concentration but produces very marked cardiac depression at the concentrations necessary to be an effective sole hypotensive agent.

Other drugs

Calcium channel blocking drugs, e.g. nicardipine, have been used in clinical trials. They are reliable in inducing hypotension without a marked increase in heart rate, but the dosage must be titrated extremely carefully to avoid 'overshoot', because it is very difficult to reverse the effects of calcium channel blockers.

Prostaglandin E_1 has been used in Japan for controlled hypotension during neurosurgery and appears to be safe and reliable. It appears to be relatively free from side-effects, but is of only moderate potency. During neurosurgery, it maintains an appropriate balance between perfusion and oxygen demand.

REVERSAL OF CONTROLLED HYPOTENSION

The period of controlled hypotension should be the shortest necessary for safe, effective surgery. When controlled hypotension is no longer required, arterial pressure should be returned towards the preoperative value. This process should be controlled as carefully as the hypotensive technique itself.

Initially, the administration of 'second line' hypotensive agents such as intravenous vasodilators should be discontinued. This restores a more normal balance between circulating volume and capacity. The effects of the shorter-acting agents wane within 2–10 min. Next, the inspired concentration of volatile anaesthetic may be reduced to a normal anaesthetic value; this results in a further increase in arterial pressure towards normal. Finally, gentle repositioning restores normal perfusion.

Some patients still remain moderately hypotensive and it may be appropriate (e.g. to confirm haemostasis) to take active steps to restore arterial pressure to normal. It is important to emphasize that these steps should follow, and not substitute for, the three stages outlined above. Infusion of intravenous fluid or administration of ephedrine or methoxamine is usually effective.

Rebound hypertension may occur; this is treated most effectively with a short-acting intravenous drug such as the β-blocker esmolol. Persistent hypertension should be investigated carefully, because it is more likely to result from pain or hypothermia than clinically significant activation of the endocrine responses to hypotension.

CONCLUSIONS

The use of controlled hypotension remains an important anaesthetic skill, because the technique enables patients to benefit from surgery which could not be achieved satisfactorily without it. Safe use of the technique requires an understanding of basic physiology and pharmacology, in order to ensure that undue degrees of hypotension are not used when there is a medical contraindication. Surgical demand for a bloodless field cannot be allowed to override the clinical judgement of the anaesthetist, and some patients may suffer adverse consequences from any period of perioperative hypotension, controlled or otherwise.

FURTHER READING

Cole D J, Drummond J C, Shapiro H M, Zornow M H 1990 Influence of hypotension and hypotensive technique on the area of profound reduction in cerebral blood flow during focal cerebral ischaemia in the rat. British Journal of Anaesthesia 64: 498–502

Kick O, Van Aken H, Wouters P F, Verbesselt K, Van Hemelrijck J 1993 Vital organ blood flow during deliberate hypotension in dogs. Anesthesia and Analgesia 77: 737–742

Toivonen J, Kuikka P, Kaukinen S 1993 Effects of deliberate hypotension induced by labetalol with isoflurane on neuropsychological function. Acta Anaesthesiologica Scandinavica 37: 7–11

57 Neurosurgical anaesthesia

Neurosurgical procedures include elective and emergency surgery of the central nervous system, its vasculature and the cerebrospinal fluid (CSF), together with the surrounding bony structures, the skull and spine. Almost all require general anaesthesia. Apart from a conventional anaesthetic technique which pays meticulous attention to detail, the essential factors are the maintenance of cerebral perfusion pressure and the facilitation of surgical access by minimizing blood loss and preventing increases in central nervous tissue volume and oedema.

APPLIED ANATOMY AND PHYSIOLOGY

The skull is a rigid closed 'box', except in neonates and infants before the various component bones have fused together. The skull contains the brain, cerebral blood supply and CSF, and an increase in the space occupied by one of these components must be compensated for by a decrease in volume of one of the others. Failure of this mechanism leads to a rise in intracranial pressure. The normal brain weighs about 1400 g, and the total intracranial volumes of CSF and blood are 100 and 150 ml, respectively. The most important factors producing a rise in intracranial volume and therefore pressure are: for the brain, cerebral tumours, cysts and abscesses; for the vasculature, traumatic haematomas and vasodilatation caused by an elevated P_aCO_2; and for the CSF, obstruction to the normal circulation leading to hydrocephalus.

CEREBROSPINAL FLUID

The brain and spinal cord are surrounded by three meningeal layers: the pia, the arachnoid and the dura mater. The first of these layers is closely applied to the brain and between it and the arachnoid is the subarachnoid space containing the circulating CSF. This space is enlarged in parts of the brain to form ventricles, which contain both CSF and areas for secretion of this fluid, the choroid plexuses. CSF circulates in the subarachnoid space surrounding both the brain and the spinal cord and is reabsorbed by the arachnoid villi which lie mainly in the superior sagittal sinus over the surface of the brain. It is essential that circulation of CSF is unimpeded, because obstruction of the foraminae leading to and from the ventricles or to the aqueduct of Sylvius causes local accumulation of CSF and hydrocephalus.

In the normal adult, there are 120 ml of CSF, of which about 50 ml are in the spinal subarachnoid space. Its composition is similar to protein-free plasma and it is formed at the rate of 0.3–0.5 ml min^{-1}. The functions of CSF are both to buffer the brain against movements of the skull and to surround certain parts of the brain with a fluid capable of fluctuation in its concentration of ions, e.g. sodium, potassium and bicarbonate. Changes in CSF bicarbonate concentration are responsible for alterations in respiratory rate and volume mediated via the chemoreceptors. Some drugs can pass into CSF while others cannot, since its formation is one of selective secretion. The normal CSF pressure is about 120 mmH_2O in the recumbent position.

INTRACRANIAL PRESSURE

With normal cerebral compliance, the intracranial pressure (ICP) is 100–150 mmH_2O (8–12 mmHg) in the horizontal position. In the erect posture, ICP falls initially, but then, due to a decrease in reabsorption, the pressure returns to normal. ICP is related directly to intrathoracic pressure and has a normal respiratory swing. It is increased by coughing, straining and positive end-expiratory pressure. In cases of reduced cerebral compliance, small changes in cerebral volume produce large changes in ICP and such critical changes can be induced by drugs used during anaesthesia (e.g. halothane, isoflurane and sodium nitroprusside – see below), elevations in P_aCO_2 and posture, as well as by surgery and trauma (Fig. 57.1).

CEREBRAL BLOOD FLOW

The brain is dependent for its blood supply on four main arteries – the internal carotids and the vertebrals, the latter joining to form

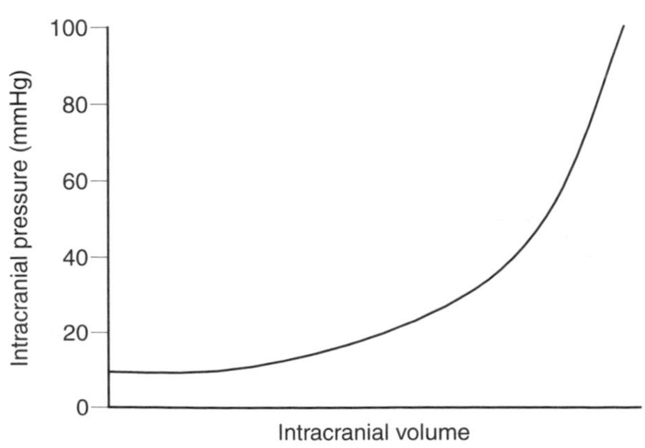

Fig. 57.1
The intracranial pressure/volume relationship.

the basilar artery. These vessels anastomose at the base of the brain, forming the circle of Willis which then gives off the anterior, middle and posterior cerebral arteries. Because of this anastomotic link, the brain can survive with occlusion of one or even two of its main arteries. Under normal conditions, the brain receives about 15% of the cardiac output, which corresponds to a cerebral blood flow (CBF) of 50 ml per 100 g tissue or 600–700 ml min^{-1}. The cerebral circulation is able to maintain a constant blood flow between mean arterial pressures of 60 and 140 mmHg by the process of autoregulation. This is mediated by a primary myogenic response involving local alteration in the diameter of blood vessels in response to changes in transmural pressure. Above and below these limits, or in the traumatized brain, autoregulation is impaired or absent, so that cerebral blood flow is related directly to cerebral perfusion pressure (CPP) (Fig. 57.2). This effect is also seen in association with cerebral hypoxia and hypercapnia, in addition to acute intracranial disease and trauma.

As CPP falls as a result of systemic hypotension or an increase in ICP, CBF is maintained until the ICP exceeds 30–40 mmHg. The Cushing reflex increases CPP in response to this rise in ICP by producing reflex systemic hypertension and bradycardia, despite these compensatory mechanisms also producing an increase in ICP. In the treatment of closed head injuries, where both ICP and mean arterial pressure are being monitored, it is essential to control the resultant CPP by vasopressor therapy where cerebral perfusion is borderline, since even transient absence of flow to the brain may produce focal or global ischaemia with infarction.

Figure 57.2 also demonstrates that haemorrhagic hypotension associated with excess sympathetic nervous activity results in a loss of autoregulation at a higher CPP than normal, while the use of vasodilators to induce hypotension shifts the curve to the left, maintaining flow at lower levels of perfusion pressure. Vasodilators also differ in their effect, so that autoregulation is preserved at a lower CPP with sodium nitroprusside than with autonomic ganglionic blockade (e.g. trimetaphan).

Cerebral metabolic rate also affects CBF; the increased electrical activity associated with convulsions produces an increase in lactic

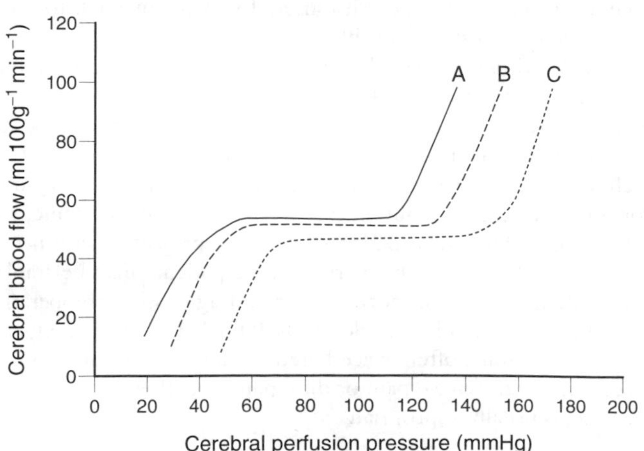

Fig. 57.2
Autoregulation of cerebral blood flow. A, drug-induced vasodilatation; B, normal; C, hypertension or haemorrhagic hypotension.

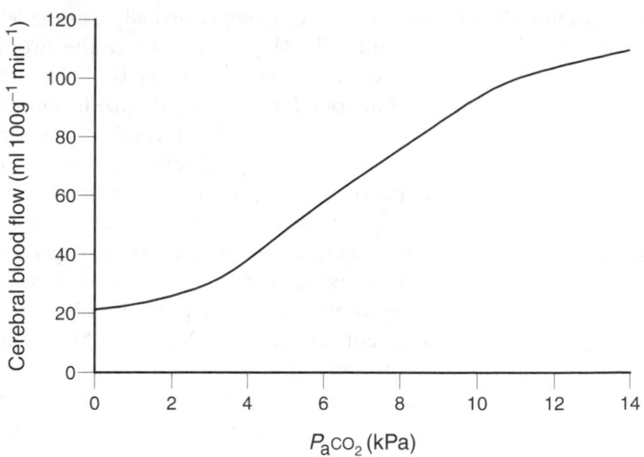

Fig. 57.3
The effect of increasing P_aCO_2 on cerebral blood flow.

acid and other vasodilator metabolites. This, together with an increase in CO_2 production mediated possibly via changes in CSF pH, produces an increase in CBF. Conversely, cerebral metabolic depression, in association with either deliberate or accidental hypothermia or induced by drugs, reduces CBF.

CEREBRAL METABOLISM

The overall energy consumption of the brain is relatively constant, whether during sleep or in the awake state, and represents approximately 20% of the oxygen consumption at rest, or 50 ml min^{-1}. Cerebral metabolism relies on glucose supply via the cerebral circulation as there are no stores of metabolic substrate. This is why the brain can tolerate only short periods of hypoperfusion or circulatory arrest before irreversible neuronal damage occurs. The brain also metabolizes amino acids, including glutamate, aspartate and γ-aminobutyric acid (GABA), together with release and subsequent inactivation of neurotransmitters.

The energy production of the brain is related directly to its rate of oxygen consumption, and the cerebral metabolic rate for oxygen ($CMRO_2$) is used to measure this index of cerebral activity. By the Fick principle, $CMRO_2$ is equal to the CBF multiplied by the arteriovenous oxygen difference. Although this is a quantitative measurement, where there is failure of oxygen or glucose supply and ATP production is less than its utilization, an alteration in $CMRO_2$ does not indicate the nature or extent of the problem.

Although barbiturates have been used to reduce cerebral metabolic rate, propofol and benzodiazepines have a similar, although less profound, effect. All are used in the sedation of patients with head injury and postoperative neurosurgical patients, and the choice is related more to the anticipated duration of sedation than to differences in the effects of the drugs, with the exception of prolonged barbiturate coma induced by infusion of thiopental.

EFFECTS OF OXYGEN AND CARBON DIOXIDE ON CBF

Carbon dioxide is physiologically the most important cerebral vasodilator. Even small increases in P_aCO_2 produce significant increases in CBF and therefore ICP. There is virtually a linear relationship between P_aCO_2 and CBF (Fig. 57.3). Over the normal range, an increase of P_aCO_2 by 1 kPa increases CBF by 30%. Conversely, hyperventilation to a P_aCO_2 of 4 kPa produces cerebral vasoconstriction and a decrease in ICP, although this is compensated for by an increase in CSF production over a more prolonged period of hyperventilation, such as that used in the treatment of head injuries. This is why there is no advantage in aggressive hyperventilation regimens in head injury management; indeed, the vasoconstriction induced may be detrimental to the recovery of a severely compromised brain. Hyperventilation below a P_aCO_2 of 4 kPa has little acute effect on ICP, and 2.5 kPa should be regarded as the absolute minimum, since below this level, the vasoconstriction induced leads to a fall in jugular bulb oxygen saturation. At a P_aCO_2 above 10 kPa, the increase in CBF becomes less marked.

Unlike the acute effects of carbon dioxide, alterations in P_aO_2 have little effect on CBF over the normal range. It is only when P_aO_2 falls below about 7 kPa that cerebral vasodilatation occurs and further reductions are associated with dramatic rises in CBF (Fig. 57.4).

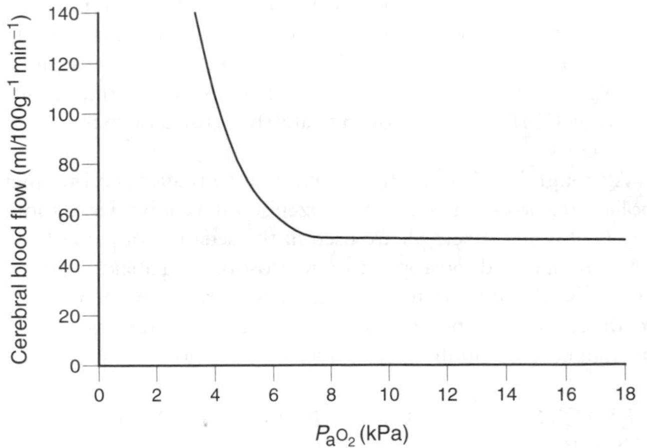

Fig. 57.4
The effect of decreasing P_aO_2 on cerebral blood flow.

ANAESTHESIA FOR ELECTIVE INTRACRANIAL SURGERY

GENERAL PRINCIPLES

Most intracranial operations involve a craniotomy, i.e. removal of a flap of bone to gain access to the brain substance beneath. Operative treatment may range from the removal of either an intracerebral or an extracerebral tumour to the clipping of an arterial aneurysm in the region of the circle of Willis, but anaesthesia for all these operations has many important factors in common. A smooth, uncomplicated technique is essential, avoiding increases in venous blood pressure, carbon dioxide concentration or arterial pressure while at the same time avoiding a decrease in cerebral oxygenation.

Most anaesthetists use a technique of intraoperative analgesia with fentanyl, alfentanil or remifentanil, neuromuscular blockade with vecuronium, rocuronium or atracurium, and IPPV. Low inspired concentrations of volatile anaesthetic agents, particularly isoflurane, are also used frequently, although particular care must be taken before the skull is open, since by inducing cerebral vasodilatation, they inevitably produce a rise in ICP. Many of these patients, particularly those with an intracerebral tumour, already have a markedly reduced cerebral compliance and a further increase in ICP may compress the brain severely (Fig. 57.1).

Patients with raised ICP are prone to nausea and vomiting and for this reason some anaesthetists intubate the trachea using a 'rapid sequence induction' technique to avoid possible regurgitation.

It is extremely important to ensure adequate fixation of the tracheal tube and intravascular cannulae and to protect the eyes, because access to the head and limbs is severely restricted during the operation. Continuous monitoring of the electrocardiograph and vascular pressures is essential; direct arterial pressure, central venous pressure and temperature monitoring are normally used, together with continuous measurement of oxygen saturation, and end-tidal carbon dioxide and inspired anaesthetic agent concentrations.

It is important to ensure that the patient is transferred to the recovery room with no residual neuromuscular blockade or opioid-induced respiratory depression, as either may produce critical increases in ICP related to hypercapnia and hypoxaemia (Figs 57.3 and 57.4).

PREOPERATIVE ASSESSMENT AND PREMEDICATION

Intracranial tumours

The preoperative condition of patients who present for craniotomy varies enormously. The level of consciousness ranges from completely awake and orientated to comatose; some patients are confused, disorientated, euphoric or aggressive. The anaesthetist must always assume that any abnormal behaviour is related to the patient's condition and not place too much reliance on what the patient says if it appears to conflict with previous history. In particular, apparently unrelated medical conditions may be forgotten, such as diabetes and hypertension, and patients may fail to mention previous anaesthetic problems.

Patients with intracranial tumours are usually taking steroids (normally dexamethasone 4 mg every 6–8 h), which may in turn precipitate a latent diabetic state, requiring insulin during the acute episode. Most patients have some symptoms of raised ICP, such as headache, nausea, vomiting or visual disturbances. Anticonvulsant therapy, usually with phenytoin or carbamazepine, will have been prescribed to patients who have presented with fitting or who are thought to be at risk. Some patients may be frankly dehydrated, but it is important to avoid aggressive preoperative fluid therapy since this may elevate ICP further. Many patients are extremely anxious, often exacerbated by mild confusion, and premedication with temazepam or diazepam, together with metoclopramide, is usually appropriate.

Vascular lesions

These include intracranial aneurysms, arteriovenous malformations and meningiomas. Congenital lesions are frequently seen in young and previously fit patients. Arteriosclerotic aneurysms occur in the older age group and may be associated with other, more widespread cardiovascular disease. Subarachnoid haemorrhage is now graded from 1 (in which the patient is symptom-free) to 5 (in which the patient is unconscious). Although clipping should prevent the risk of further bleeding, significant perioperative morbidity and mortality result from vasospasm, which may occur pre- or postoperatively. The current trend is to undertake emergency cerebral angiography and clipping of aneurysms in grade 1 and 2 patients, but to wait the conventional 10-day period in the remainder. Vasospasm is reduced or prevented by intravenous infusion of the calcium channel blocker nimodipine, which is started preoperatively in most patients.

An alternative method of treating cerebral aneurysms by interventional radiological 'coiling' is being evaluated at present in several neurosurgical centres. This appears to be very effective, particularly in the case of technically difficult or inaccessible aneurysms, such as those affecting the basilar artery. As many of the risks of open aneurysm surgery apply equally in this situation, a full, conventional neurosurgical anaesthetic technique should be used, including direct arterial pressure monitoring. If technical problems or aneurysm rupture occur, immediate transfer to theatre for emergency craniotomy may be necessary.

Patients with intracerebral haemorrhage range from complete lucidity to confusion and the preoperative assessment must take this into account. Those in the older age group may be receiving drugs with cardiovascular effects and are also frequently treated with aspirin, which may be a contraindication to urgent craniotomy. Those with a meningioma should be treated like patients with any intracranial space-occupying lesion. Benzodiazepine and antiemetic premedication is again appropriate in almost all patients, many of whom are quite aware of the severity of their condition.

EFFECTS OF DRUGS AND ANAESTHETIC TECHNIQUES

Induction of anaesthesia

With appropriate preoperative care, assessment and premedication, most patients arrive in the anaesthetic room sedated and without a grossly elevated ICP. Intravenous induction should always be used whenever possible, even in difficult children where a stormy inhalation induction might be detrimental to a pre-existing high ICP. An intravenous infusion of an isotonic electrolyte solution should be started through a large-bore intravenous cannula before induction.

Both thiopental and propofol reduce ICP and are suitable induction agents. The intravenous anaesthetic should be given with an appropriate dose of short-acting opioid and a neuromuscular blocking agent to facilitate a smooth induction and tracheal intubation, avoiding hypoxaemia and hypercapnia. It is equally important to remember that cerebral perfusion may be reduced in association with a raised ICP, and therefore an induction technique which produces significant hypotension may critically reduce cerebral perfusion in patients with a space-occupying lesion (SOL) or intracranial and subarachnoid haemorrhage associated with vasospasm.

Appropriate techniques for reducing the hypertensive response to laryngoscopy and intubation, such as supplementary thiopental, intravenous lidocaine (1–2 mg kg^{-1}), β-adrenoceptor blockade or supplementary opioids, are particularly appropriate when acute hypertension might precipitate secondary rupture of an aneurysm. Tracheal intubation should be preceded by topical anaesthesia of the trachea and larynx with lidocaine and should be with an armoured latex tracheal tube. Careful positioning of the tube is vital because any intraoperative flexion of the neck may result in intubation of the right main bronchus if the tube is initially too close to the carina. Nasogastric intubation is also used in patients in whom gastric aspiration may be needed and a pharyngeal pack is necessary if pharyngeal bleeding is likely to occur, e.g. during trans-sphenoidal hypophysectomy.

Positioning

Many neurosurgical operations are long, and positioning of the patient to facilitate optimum access, while preventing hypothermia and pressure sores or peripheral nerve injury, is very important. Supratentorial cranial surgery involving the frontal or frontotemporal areas is performed with the patient supine, while parietal and occipital craniotomies are carried out in the lateral or three-quarters prone (park bench) position. In all cases, care must be taken to avoid neck positions which impede venous drainage, because this may elevate intracranial venous pressure, while arterial compression, particularly in the elderly, may precipitate vertebrobasilar insufficiency.

In the fully prone position, which is used for surgery of the foramen magnum and cervical spine, the patient is supported on chest and iliac crest blocks or a purpose-built frame, both of which allow unimpeded respiratory movements and avoid abdominal compression. The use of 'jelly packs' on top of the support blocks greatly reduces the incidence of pressure damage, which can be serious in the frail and elderly. In the prone position, pressure areas can develop over the facial bones, particularly around the eyes; again, careful padding is vital. Eye protection is usually effected by taping, adhesive foam padding and the use of Polyfax eye ointment together with meticulous care to prevent skin cleaning solutions applied by the surgeon from entering the eyes. The head is shaved either partially or totally, usually under anaesthesia, and the skin is cleaned before transferring the patient to the operating theatre. Prevention of infection is essential because postoperative intracranial sepsis, although rare, is difficult to treat and can be fatal.

Active methods of protection against deep venous thrombosis (DVT), such as subcutaneous unfractionated or low-molecular-weight heparin, are not usually employed despite the significant risk of DVT in this group of patients. The risks of perioperative haemorrhage tend to outweigh the advantages in the majority of patients, but thromboembolism (TED) stockings and pneumatic compression (Flotron) leggings are a useful compromise.

Heat loss

Prevention of heat loss during prolonged surgery, and particularly in children, is accomplished by using either a 'space blanket' or wrapping the patient in 'bubble wrap' through which a small operative window is cut. Intravenous fluids are warmed and inspired gases are humidified. A warm air or water blanket is also effective unless the patient is prone and supported on blocks. It may be advantageous to allow the patient to cool a little in cases where a reduction in cerebral metabolism would be beneficial.

Maintenance of anaesthesia

The basis of anaesthesia for neurosurgery is mild hyperventilation with 66% nitrous oxide in oxygen to a P_aCO_2 of 3.5–4.0 kPa, supplemented with an opioid analgesic (e.g. fentanyl 2–3 μg kg^{-1}) and isoflurane 0.5–1.0%. The choice of neuromuscular blocking agent should take account of the length of operation and the relative need for normo- or elective hypotension; while pancuronium may be useful, particularly in elderly patients lying prone, it may be prudent to use an alternative agent to prevent excessive hypertension in, for example, aneurysm surgery. The advantage of longer-acting drugs is that neuromuscular blockade wears off gradually, minimizing the risk of intraoperative coughing and straining. A nerve stimulator is important if shorter-acting drugs are used intermittently or by infusion, to avoid difficulty in reversal or recurarization and consequent hypoventilation in the recovery period.

The initial part of a craniotomy is painful, but once the bone flap is reflected and intracranial surgery begins, pain is not an important feature again until closure of the wound. For this reason, supplementary intraoperative opioids in large doses are unnecessary and the use of a low concentration of isoflurane is sufficient to maintain anaesthesia. The use of isoflurane also prevents any possible awareness and consequent hypertensive response.

Reflex vagal stimulation can occur, particularly following stimulation of the cranial nerve roots or during vascular surgery around the circle of Willis and the internal carotid artery. This may necessitate immediate anticholinergic therapy with atropine to avoid severe bradycardia or even asystole.

Maintenance of normal arterial pressure is important in all patients, but can be a particular problem during induction in elderly patients who are turned lateral or three-quarters prone. Hypotension, with the consequent reduction in cerebral perfusion, should be treated by infusion of a moderate volume of fluid, but it is advisable to administer a vasopressor such as ephedrine at an early stage.

The use of air/oxygen mixtures in place of nitrous oxide is advocated by a number of neurosurgical anaesthetists. There are obvious contraindications to the use of nitrous oxide, e.g. pneumocephalus, intracranial cysts and following air encephalography (rarely performed since the advent of CT and MRI scanners). In addition, some anaesthetists believe that nitrous oxide should be avoided in situations where air embolism is a possibility, e.g. posterior fossa surgery.

Continuous total intravenous anaesthesia with propofol and alfentanil or remifentanil infusions is also gaining in popularity because it allows rapid postoperative recovery and assessment, avoids shivering and reduces the incidence of postoperative nausea and vomiting. It is particularly valuable in situations where the patient is required to wake up and move to command intraoperatively, e.g. during spinal surgery and trigeminal nerve radiofrequency lesion generation (see below). There are potential difficulties with hypotension and hypoventilation in such patients, but in expert hands, these are not major problems.

Fluid replacement therapy

Most patients who present for elective intracranial operations are satisfactorily hydrated preoperatively. The main exceptions are those with high ICP associated with nausea and vomiting, and patients with general debility and cachexia. The main intraoperative distinctions between patients are related to the underlying pathology. Cerebral tumours are associated with oedema and raised ICP, and therefore such patients require moderate fluid restriction, e.g. 1.5 L day^{-1} for a 60 kg female or 2 L day^{-1} for a 70 kg male.

Cerebrovascular surgery is associated with vasospasm and therefore blood flow is the prime prerequisite. A normal circulating blood volume is essential if the perfusion pressure is to be maintained, and although a slight fall in haematocrit to about 0.30 is optimal for perfusion, adequate colloid replacement must be given. Patients who have undergone aneurysm surgery do not require fluid restriction; indeed, some are given a volume expansion regimen using a mixture of low- and high-molecular-weight colloids (Haemaccel and Hespan) together with crystalloid to improve perfusion which may be limited by vasospasm.

Supplementary drug therapy

In addition to the normal anaesthetic drugs, care must be taken to continue or even supplement specific neurological drug therapy. Patients with a tumour or some vascular lesions may already be receiving anticonvulsants (usually phenytoin or carbamazepine), but others may require intravenous phenytoin perioperatively, depending upon the site of surgery. Patients receiving high-dose steroids need peri- and postoperative dexamethasone; the normal dose is 4 mg 6-hourly with 8–12 mg as an intraoperative bolus. Perioperative antibiotics are administered to all patients; a common choice is cefuroxime 1.5 g, which may need to be repeated during long operations.

Monitoring during neurosurgical anaesthesia

Monitoring should be instituted before induction; in patients in whom cardiovascular instability may be a problem, this should include invasive vascular monitoring.

Electrocardiographic (ECG) monitoring and measurement of oxygen saturation, together with non-invasive blood pressure monitoring, are essential in all patients.

It may be desirable to set up direct arterial pressure monitoring via a radial artery cannula under local anaesthesia prior to induction, although this may already have been established in acutely traumatized and head-injured patients. Arterial cannulation is now employed routinely in all intracranial operations, for surgery of the cervical spine, and in other situations in which rapid fluctuations in arterial pressure may occur. It also facilitates arterial sampling for blood gas and acid–base balance measurements.

Central venous pressure measurement should be used where major blood loss is expected, and during posterior fossa or cervical spine surgery, in which air embolism can occur (see below). Accurate placement of the tip of the catheter in the right atrium is important if aspiration of air is likely to be attempted.

Temperature monitoring (either oesophageal or rectal) is employed during many cases, particularly those which may be prolonged.

Oxygen saturation and end-tidal carbon dioxide concentration are monitored continuously in all patients. The latter has made a dramatic difference to the safety and quality of neurosurgical anaesthesia because alterations in carbon dioxide tension have such a profound effect on CBF and ICP.

Inspired anaesthetic agent and gas monitoring is now used routinely for all major neurosurgical cases.

A precordial or oesophageal stethoscope can be used to auscultate cardiac and respiratory sounds and also abnormal flow murmurs produced by air embolism. An oesophageal stethoscope is used more frequently in children.

Mechanisms for reducing ICP

The methods used commonly to limit increases in ICP or electively to reduce it include drugs, ventilation, posture and drainage. The use of diuretics such as 10–20% mannitol or furosemide is designed to deplete the intravascular fluid volume and subsequently reduce CSF production. Direct drainage of CSF may be accomplished either by lumbar puncture or by direct puncture of the cisterna magna or lateral ventricles. Hypercapnia must be prevented by the use of IPPV, while moderate hyperventilation produces cerebral vasoconstriction and a reduction in cerebral blood volume. Volatile anaesthetic agents such as isoflurane and other vasodilators (e.g. sodium nitroprusside) must be used cautiously, particularly before the skull is open.

Elective hypotension

Although elective hypotension was formerly one of the mainstays of cerebrovascular surgery, its use has diminished considerably in recent years, because of the increasing appreciation that cerebral perfusion is all-important. Most aneurysm surgery in now carried out at normotension; indeed, if the patient has an element of cerebral vasospasm, any reflex hypertension should be maintained. This concept has been made easier to implement by the simultaneous use of nimodipine.

If elective hypotension is required, the choice of technique is determined by the anticipated duration of induced hypotension. The main indications are to facilitate dissection and clipping of a difficult and inaccessible aneurysm or arteriovenous malformation, in which case a low pressure is needed for only a short period and sodium nitroprusside is the drug of choice. To reduce continuous and excessive blood loss in, for example, spinal surgery, moderate hypotension induced by isoflurane in increasing concentration or an autonomic ganglion blocker such as trimetaphan is more suitable; the emphasis must be on perfusion because spinal cord oxygenation is also critical and excessive hypotension may lead to anterior spinal artery thrombosis. The dose of sodium nitroprusside should be limited to 10 $\mu g\ kg^{-1}\ min^{-1}$ or 1.5 $mg\ kg^{-1}$ as a total intraoperative dose. Tachyphylaxis is occasionally a problem with sodium nitroprusside, but frequently occurs with trimetaphan.

SPECIAL PROBLEMS

Cerebrovascular surgery

Although aneurysm surgery is the largest component in this group, arteriovenous malformations and intracranial–extracranial anastomotic operations are also important. Meningiomas are formed from abnormal blood vessels and tend to produce symptoms related to a space-occupying lesion, rather than specific vascular problems. Nevertheless, their extreme vascularity, combined with difficult access, may make severe haemorrhage and blood volume replacement a significant factor.

The current trend in cerebrovascular surgery is for the maintenance of a normal cerebral perfusion pressure in all situations, which, combined with nimodipine, will produce adequate cerebral blood flow. Although fluid replacement therapy may be all that is required, mild peripheral vasoconstriction with ephedrine may be necessary in the often prolonged interval between induction and incision. Thereafter, induced hypotension is seldom employed and a colloid/crystalloid perfusion regimen to an optimal haematocrit of 0.30 is ideal (see above). Nimodipine therapy interacts with inhalation anaesthetic agents, particularly isoflurane, to enhance their hypotensive effects and may need to be discontinued temporarily during induction until surgery has started. Postoperative nimodipine therapy is continued for several days until the risks of vasospasm are past and this is often also the case with removal of arteriovenous malformations.

Blood entering the CSF either as a result of the initial haemorrhage or during operation is an extreme irritant. Its presence may cause large increases in plasma catecholamine concentrations with corresponding hypertension and vasospasm. Blood which clots in the aqueduct of Sylvius causes obstruction to CSF flow and non-communicating hydrocephalus, necessitating temporary ventricular drainage or ventriculoperitoneal shunt.

Pituitary surgery (hypophysectomy)

The pituitary fossa is approached either through a frontotemporal craniotomy in the case of large suprasellar tumours, or through the nose or ethmoid sinus for smaller lesions. The importance of pituitary surgery lies in the endocrine abnormalities such as acromegaly, which may be caused by an adenoma, or those which result from surgical hypophysectomy, such as diabetes insipidus. In addition, pituitary ablation may be used in the treatment of hormone-dependent tumours such as ovarian or breast neoplasms; in these conditions, the patients may be frail, cachectic and anaemic as a result of disseminated carcinoma.

Glucocorticoid replacement is all that is required in the immediate perioperative period; mineralocorticoid requirements increase only slowly over the subsequent days. Diabetes insipidus can present in the immediate postoperative period and requires stabilization with vasopressin until the degree of the imbalance is known.

Acromegalic patients who present for pituitary surgery may pose considerable difficulties in tracheal intubation and venous access. If the transoral, nasal or ethmoidal approaches are used for surgery, a pharyngeal pack must be inserted and the airway protected meticulously to prevent aspiration of blood and CSF.

CSF shunt insertion and revision

The majority of patients who present for insertion or revision of ventriculoperitoneal shunts are children with congenital hydrocephalus, usually resulting from spina bifida. Some patients require a permanent shunt after intracranial haemorrhage or head injury, particularly the elderly. The major anaesthetic considerations lie in the presentation of a patient with severely raised ICP who may be drowsy, nauseated and vomiting, with resultant dehydration. Compensatory systemic hypertension to maintain cerebral perfusion may also be present.

Rapid-sequence induction may be indicated to avoid aspiration; the increase in ICP due to succinylcholine is of secondary importance. Artificial ventilation to control P_aCO_2 is essential to prevent further increases in ICP, and volatile anaesthetic agents should be used sparingly for the same reason. When the ventricle is first drained, a rapid decrease in CSF pressure can result in an equally rapid reduction in arterial pressure, which no longer needs to be elevated to maintain cerebral perfusion. Adequate venous access is then important to allow rapid resuscitation in response to this severe but temporary hypotension.

The distal end of the shunt is usually introduced intraperitoneally, particularly if infection is a potential problem. Ventriculo-atrial shunts have largely been superseded because of arrhythmias during their insertion. When a ventriculo-atrial shunt is inserted, the anaesthetist may be asked to confirm correct positioning of the distal end by priming it with saline and attaching an ECG lead to observe changes in waveform during advancement of the catheter.

Relief of chronic pain

Although peripheral nerve blocks are normally performed in the pain clinic, severe intractable pain is sometimes relieved only by dorsal cordotomy or rhizotomy. Both techniques involve upper thoracic laminectomy to expose the spinal cord, with the patient prone as for decompressive surgery. Some patients are extremely frail, and positioning them to avoid pressure sores is particularly important. A number also have an element of autonomic neuropathy, with resultant cardiovascular instability. Neurological ablation produces intense temporary stimulation, and adequate anaesthesia and analgesia are particularly important during the process of nerve section.

Treatment of trigeminal neuralgia

This extremely debilitating condition is usually treated medically with large doses of carbamazepine. However, surgical lesions of the trigeminal ganglion are performed when the side-effects of medical treatment become unacceptable. Lesions of the ganglion are achieved by radiofrequency or injection of either phenol or alcohol. All of these techniques are very painful and require general anaesthesia. Current techniques involve anaesthetizing the patient while the ganglion is identified radiologically, waking the patient up to identify correct placement of the needle, and then re-anaesthetizing the patient during generation of the lesion or neurolytic injection. Propofol and alfentanil anaesthesia using a laryngeal mask provides optimal conditions. If the CSF is entered during localization of the ganglion, nausea frequently occurs and vomiting with the patient in the supine position should be anticipated.

A recent development in the treatment of trigeminal neuralgia has been the demonstration of an abnormal vascular loop compressing the trigeminal nerve in the posterior cranial fossa. A small craniotomy and decompression of the nerve is extremely successful in curing the symptoms; the problems of anaesthesia and surgery in this area are highlighted below.

Posterior fossa craniotomy

Surgery in the posterior cranial fossa involves lesions of the cerebellum and fourth ventricle. In addition, this position facilitates operations on the foramen magnum and upper cervical spine.

In the past, some surgeons favoured the sitting position because this produced superb venous drainage, relative hypotension and excellent operating conditions. The patients were frequently allowed to breathe a volatile anaesthetic agent (usually trichloroethylene) spontaneously so that changes in their respiratory pattern could be used to monitor the progress of fourth ventricular surgery in the region of the respiratory centre. This posed several major anaesthetic problems. Patients in the sitting position are prone to hypotension, which results inevitably in poor cerebral perfusion. Air embolism is also a severe potential problem because, when the skull is opened, many of the veins within the bone are held open and, if the venous pressure at this point is subatmospheric, air may enter the veins, leading to systemic air embolism.

For these reasons, the sitting position is no longer used other than in exceptional circumstances and posterior fossa surgery is carried out in the 'park bench' position; operations on the cervical spine are performed with the patient prone and supported on blocks (see above). Although this change has diminished the risks of cerebral hypoperfusion and consequent hypoxia, air embolism is still a potential problem. The operative site, particularly with a moderate head-up tilt, is still above the level of the heart and the veins are still held open by the surrounding structures.

Detection and treatment of air embolism

The mainstay of detection is vigilance and a high index of suspicion. The main period of risk is when the posterior cervical muscles are cut and the craniectomy is being performed. Bone is usually removed as a craniectomy in the posterior fossa rather than by raising a bone flap. Although the incidence of major air embolism is vastly lower than when the sitting position was used, small amounts of air still enter the circulation quite frequently. The severity of the problem depends upon the volume of air entrained and the fact that air bubbles expand in the presence of nitrous oxide.

The main practical method of detection is by end-tidal carbon dioxide monitoring, because the airlock produced in the pulmonary circulation results in a rapid reduction in CO_2 excretion (usually together with a fall in oxygen saturation). Arterial pressure decreases and cardiac arrhythmias are frequently seen. The use of an oesophageal stethoscope permits auscultation of the classic 'mill-wheel' murmur with large quantities of air, but requires continuous listening. Doppler ultrasonography is probably the most accurate method of early detection, before the embolus leaves the heart, but frequently suffers from interference.

In practice, provided that the sitting position is not used, large air emboli are uncommon. Treatment consists of preventing further entry of air by telling the surgeon, who immediately floods the operative field with saline, lowering the level of the head and increasing the venous pressure by jugular compression to raise intrathoracic pressure. Ideally, the air should be trapped in the right atrium by placing the patient in the left lateral position; it is then occasionally possible to aspirate air through a central venous catheter, which is commonly inserted in posterior fossa explorations. Vasopressors are sometimes required until the circulation is restored; occasionally full cardiopulmonary resuscitation is necessary.

RECOVERY FROM ANAESTHESIA AND POSTOPERATIVE ANALGESIA

The majority of patients are allowed to wake up as usual at the end of operation in a dedicated neurosurgical recovery room. It is essential to avoid hypercapnia or hypoxaemia, both of which may increase ICP; cerebral compliance following surgical intervention is often critical, particularly following removal of a space-occupying lesion or traumatic haematoma.

Complete reversal of non-depolarizing neuromuscular blockade must be achieved and judicious use of intraoperative opioids should remove the need for administration of naloxone. Doxapram may be used, although its cardiovascular side-effects also increase ICP. After major procedures or when severe oedema is likely, elective postoperative ventilation may be necessary.

ANAESTHESIA FOR EMERGENCY INTRACRANIAL NEUROSURGICAL PROCEDURES

The main indications for emergency intracranial surgery are bleeding as a result of trauma, which may be exacerbated in patients on anticoagulant drugs, including aspirin. Intracranial haematomata may arise either epidurally, subdurally or intracerebrally and may accumulate either rapidly or slowly. Many patients who present for anaesthesia are unconscious or semiconscious and irritable as a result of raised ICP and cerebral compression. The anaesthetic maintenance technique is similar to that used for elective intracranial surgery, consisting of a short-acting intravenous opioid, neuromuscular blockade with vecuronium or rocuronium and IPPV to a P_aCO_2 of 4 kPa. This is preceded by tracheal intubation facilitated with succinylcholine to avoid regurgitation and CO_2 retention in a patient with a potentially full stomach and raised ICP. Although succinylcholine has been shown to increase ICP in the normal brain, its effect in a non-compliant situation is less certain; more importantly, the risk of aspiration far outweighs that of a transient increase in ICP.

If the patient is unconscious, the initial anaesthetic requirements may be small. In the past, decompression of an intracranial haematoma through burr holes was often conducted under local anaesthesia. This method of treatment has been superseded by a full craniotomy and evacuation of the haematoma, because, if necessary, the bone flap can be left out or allowed to 'float' free, providing a method of decompression in the case of severe oedema. Burr holes are usually performed under local anaesthesia for the diagnosis and treatment of chronic subdural and epidural haematomata.

As the patient's brain is decompressed, the level of consciousness may lighten considerably and it may be necessary to deepen anaesthesia to prevent the patient becoming aware. It is important to avoid long-acting opioid analgesics because these may mask the eye signs and the level of consciousness, which are used to follow the progress of cerebral trauma postoperatively. Virtually all patients with head injury have had an emergency CT scan as part of their initial management. Many have undergone tracheal intubation and ventilation of the lung for this procedure and are subsequently kept anaesthetized and taken straight to the operating theatre for surgery to decompress the brain. It is important to remember that, with an expanding intracranial haematoma, speed is of the essence if cerebral damage is to be minimized or avoided. While adequate anaesthetic time must be taken to ensure safety, excessive delays may seriously affect the overall result of decompression and make the difference between a good and merely a moderate recovery.

The maintenance technique selected is influenced to an extent by the decision either to wake the patient immediately postoperatively (usually considered appropriate only in the case of an acute epidural haematoma in a young patient) or to use elective postoperative ventilation for 24 h. In the former case, the usual conditions mentioned earlier for elective neurosurgery apply; in the latter, generous short-acting opioid administration and neuromuscular blockade will prevent ICP increases in an intubated patient, particularly during transfer to the intensive care unit or by ambulance to another hospital.

MANAGEMENT OF THE HEAD-INJURED PATIENT

Head injuries and their subsequent treatment and rehabilitation represent a considerable proportion of neurosurgical practice. The immediate management must involve meticulous attention to the prevention of any secondary brain injury; little can be done about the primary insult to the brain or spinal cord. In recent years, the awareness of both the medical profession and the general public has had a profound effect on general resuscitation simply by improving airway management in the unconscious patient. The basic rules of head injury care are as follows:

1. *Initial airway maintenance*, remembering that oxygenation is initially more important than tracheal intubation.
2. *Assessment of any craniofacial injury,* together with the possibility of associated damage to the cervical spine. When in doubt, assume that the neck is unstable.
3. *Immediate assessment of other injuries,* particularly thoraco-abdominal, with appropriate emergency treatment.
4. *Further airway management,* including tracheal intubation. This must be accomplished without excessive neck manipulation and should be performed by an experienced person. It is important to make intubation as atraumatic as possible; consequently, sedation and neuromuscular blockade should be used irrespective of the level of consciousness, except in the most severe situation. The benefits of succinylcholine far outweigh the potential risks. Nasotracheal intubation is contraindicated in patients with a potentially fractured base of skull.
5. *Sedation and analgesia, and neuromuscular blockade.*
6. *Detailed assessment of thoracic, abdominal and limb injuries* and appropriate therapy to stabilize the patient's cardiovascular and respiratory systems before transfer to the CT scanner and X-ray room.
7. *Invasive arterial pressure monitoring,* together with ECG, end-tidal CO_2 and pulse oximetry. All of these are important in the early detection of deterioration in ICP, cardiovascular stability or respiratory function. A contused, oedematous and non-compliant brain tolerates only minimal changes in oxygen supply or carbon dioxide tension before ICP rises still further.

8. *After CT scan,* many patients are transferred directly to the neurosurgical operating theatre for evacuation of haematoma or insertion of an intraventricular catheter or epidural pressure monitor. Some patients who are scanned in peripheral hospitals have their scans relayed to the main neurosurgical centre. The patient is then transferred directly by ambulance to the neurosurgical operating theatre, but both cardiovascular and neurological stability must be achieved before the journey. Realistically, this involves the transfer of a sedated, intubated and ventilated patient, pretreated with mannitol to minimize acute increases in ICP.

INTENSIVE CARE OF HEAD-INJURED PATIENTS

The main benefits of intensive care are in the provision of optimal conditions to allow recovery from the primary cerebral injury while minimizing any secondary damage. In practice this means:

Sedation. This is best achieved with an infusion of either propofol or midazolam together with an opioid (usually morphine or alfentanil). Thiopental may be beneficial in cases of severely compromised cerebral blood flow and metabolism (see above).

Ventilation. It is particularly important in patients suffering from multiple trauma, especially with the combination of head and chest injuries, to ensure optimal oxygenation in the face of pulmonary contusion. This is normally achieved by the use of IPPV and may involve the use of positive end-expiratory pressure, the effects of which on the non-compliant brain are probably not as severe as in the normal situation, whereas the damage caused by hypoxaemia could be fatal. There is no evidence to suggest that severe hyperventilation improves outcome, and the main benefits of ventilation are therefore the prevention of hypercapnia and the provision of adequate cerebral oxygenation.

Detailed neurological assessment. This centres on the Glasgow Coma Scale, which is based upon eye opening, and verbal and motor responses (Table 57.1). Each response on the scale is assessed numerically; the lower the number, the more impaired is the response. The numbers are summated to produce a score. The lowest score is 3 and the highest 15.

ICP monitoring. It is very helpful to be able to monitor the effectiveness of therapy against ICP, and in particular to demonstrate an effective cerebral perfusion pressure. ICP increases in response to stimulation, physiotherapy, tracheal suction, etc., but should return to the pre-stimulation value within 5–10 min. Frequent and prolonged increases in ICP demonstrate a low cerebral compliance and the need for further sedation and ventilation. If weaning from mechanical ventilation is started and ICP rises and remains elevated, the patient should be re-sedated and the lungs ventilated for a further 24-h period.

It is beneficial to nurse head-injured patients in a 15° head-up tilt to assist in ICP reduction, provided that coexisting conditions permit.

Adequate fluid therapy and nutrition. Although otherwise fit patients with an isolated head injury have very low metabolic requirements, many fail to absorb from the gastrointestinal tract because of the effects of sedative and opioid drugs or simply secondary to head trauma; associated hypoxaemia exacerbates the problem. It is sometimes necessary to introduce parenteral nutrition, particularly in patients who are catabolic from coexisting injuries. As in elective patients at risk from elevated ICP due to cerebral oedema, head-injured patients are also at risk from excessive intravenous fluid therapy. Fluid restriction to a similar degree is appropriate, and if large amounts of fluid have been given during initial resuscitation, a gentle drug-induced diuresis with furosemide to create an overall negative fluid balance (or at least to prevent a positive balance) may be appropriate. Fluid overload also impairs oxygenation further in potentially hypoxic patients with combined head and chest injuries, or following aspiration at the time of head injury. The use of mannitol 20% tends to be reserved for the emergency treatment of raised ICP rather than the treatment of simple fluid overload.

High-dependency nursing care. Provision of appropriate care for the unconscious patient, even when breathing spontaneously, is difficult, and demands a high intensity of nursing care. Intensive or high-dependency care centralizes nursing, medical and monitoring resources to provide optimal care of the head-injured patient.

Table 57.1 The Glasgow coma scale

Clinical sign	Response	Score
Eyes open	Spontaneously	4
	To verbal command	3
	To pain	2
	No response	1
Best motor response to verbal command or to painful stimulus	Obeys	6
	Localizes pain	5
	Flexion withdrawal	4
	Abnormal flexion (decorticate rigidity)	3
	Extension (decerebrate rigidity)	2
	No response	1
Best verbal response	Orientated, converses	5
	Disorientated, converses	4
	Inappropriate words	3
	Incomprehensible sounds	2
	No response	1
Total	Minimum 3, maximum 15	

ANAESTHESIA FOR NEURORADIOLOGICAL PROCEDURES, CT AND MRI SCANNING

This is discussed in detail in Chapter 48.

SURGERY OF SPINE AND SPINAL CORD

Many neurosurgical procedures involve surgery in the region of the spinal cord, usually either for the decompression of nerves as a result of a prolapsed intervertebral disc or degenerative arthritis, or for the decompression of the cord when the spinal canal is occupied by tumour.

ANAESTHESIA FOR CERVICAL SPINE SURGERY

The cervical spine can be approached from either the anterior or the posterior route, depending largely upon the site of cord compression. Although the posterior approach is less likely to damage any vital structures, the patient must lie prone, and hypotension, blood loss and access, particularly in a large individual, may all cause problems.

Preoperative assessment is perhaps one of the most important in neurosurgical anaesthetic practice, because an unstable cervical spine is a major reason for the proposed surgery. In many patients, the neck is relatively unstable as soon as it is either flexed or extended, and the patient may be in a cervical collar or even neck traction. Bony degeneration from rheumatoid or osteoarthritis produces severe cord compression. However, with regard to tracheal intubation, the neck tends to be unstable in flexion and relatively stable in extension in most patients. It is essential to assess the range of neck movement fully with the collar removed, either in the ward or in the anaesthetic room, in addition to the assessment of the ease of tracheal intubation. It is doubly unlucky to have a difficult intubation in a patient with an unstable neck! If problems are anticipated, the normal 'difficult intubation' drill should be followed, using the methods with which the anaesthetist is most familiar. Severe ankylosing spondylitis involving the neck probably presents the most awkward problem, related to the rigid immobility of the cervical spine. Additional factors which apply particularly in rheumatoid patients include anaemia, steroid therapy, fragile skin, and renal and pulmonary problems.

ANTERIOR CERVICAL DECOMPRESSION WITH OR WITHOUT FUSION (CLOWARD'S OPERATION)

This technique involves exposing the anterior aspect of the cervical vertebral bodies and their interposing discs through a collar incision and drilling out a cylinder of bone and disc down to the posterior longitudinal ligament. The cord is decompressed microscopically through this hole, which is then filled with a bone dowel from the hip to produce a fusion. Single or multiple levels are involved, but the neck may be quite rigid for future intubation if several adjacent fusions are carried out.

Apart from the potential problems of tracheal intubation, anaesthesia is relatively straightforward, although pneumothorax is a potential problem with operations at the C7–T1 level. Retraction of the oesophagus and, more particularly, the carotid sheath and sinus may produce severe temporary cardiovascular disturbance (usually sinus bradycardia), which can be prevented by surgical instillation of local anaesthetic around the carotid artery. Postoperative haemorrhage may lead to acute airway obstruction.

POSTERIOR CERVICAL LAMINECTOMY

When these operations were performed in the sitting position, all the problems associated with posterior fossa surgery in this position also occurred. Patients are now placed prone, with the neck flexed, and in a slightly head-up posture to reduce haemorrhage. Nevertheless, bleeding from the nuchal muscles is often a problem and air embolism is still a potential risk. The main difficulties, as in all spinal surgery in the prone position, arise from epidural venous bleeding, and the waveform of IPPV can have a significant effect. It is important to have an intrathoracic pressure of zero for the majority of the expiration phase (a difficulty with some pressure generators such as the Manley). In addition, prolonged cord compression can result in an autonomic neuropathy which may produce significant hypotension both at induction and when the patient is turned into the prone position.

Cervical laminectomy is often accompanied by posterior fusion with either bone or metal. Many permanent designs such as the Ransford loop or Halifax clamp are used, and all produce immediate postoperative stability.

ANAESTHESIA FOR THORACOLUMBAR DECOMPRESSIVE SURGERY

In most instances, patients are placed in the prone position, either supported on chest and iliac crest blocks or in the 'jack-knife' position. A technique employing IPPV is essential because these procedures often take a long time. However, because raised ICP is not a problem, it is often sufficient to ventilate the lungs with a volatile anaesthetic agent unless this causes a decrease in systemic arterial pressure. A balanced anaesthetic technique is normally quite satisfactory, with the proviso that many patients, particularly the elderly, become hypotensive when placed prone. Considerable vagally mediated bradycardia can arise from nerve root stimulation during surgery, and pancuronium is particularly useful in both these situations. Vecuronium may be too short-acting for spinal surgery unless given by infusion.

As the spine is an extremely vascular area, hypotensive anaesthesia is used occasionally to decrease bleeding, and particularly the venous ooze in the operative field. This is also considerably reduced if the operative site can be placed above the level of the heart – another advantage of the patient lying prone. The magnitude of blood loss during bony surgery involving laminectomy is often sufficient to require blood transfusion and is very different from the peaceful conditions associated with lumbar microdiscectomy in the young, healthy adult!

Thoracic discs and tumours such as neurofibromata are occasionally approached by the transthoracic route, involving thoracotomy and a combined approach with the patient in the lateral position. Endobronchial intubation and one-lung anaesthesia may be needed to facilitate access in this situation.

LASERS

While lasers are used increasingly for tissue dissection and cautery, particularly in neurosurgery, their use demands specialized anaesthetic techniques because the laser beam burns through most substances, including tracheal tubes. The beam is reflected off impermeable structures such as retractors, producing damage in its path. Theatre staff must wear eye protection during laser surgery, even when they are remote from the beam, which usually passes through the operating microscope. Lasers must not be used in the presence of inflammable gases or vapours because the heat generated may ignite the gas, producing an explosion.

POSTOPERATIVE NEUROSURGICAL CARE

Although many patients who have undergone spinal or intracranial surgery are awake and conscious in the immediate postoperative period, some still require active, intensive treatment. This is important particularly in patients who have raised ICP (or when ICP is liable to rise) and in those who have undergone cerebral aneurysm surgery, when postoperative vasospasm may be a problem. Elective postoperative ventilation to control cerebral oxygenation and to produce a mild decrease in ICP is often employed, with continuous monitoring of both arterial and intracranial pressures. If vasospasm is present, specific vasodilator therapy with nimodipine is continued, together with a hyperperfusion regimen as described earlier, to prevent local areas of cerebral ischaemia which may result in hemiplegia. In general, postoperative opioids are avoided following craniotomy or upper cervical spine surgery, intramuscular codeine phosphate being used most commonly to provide analgesia, together with an antiemetic, e.g. metoclopramide, to treat the nausea which occurs frequently.

Surgery of the thoracic and lumbar spine, particularly involving fusion with an autologous bone graft, is associated with significant postoperative pain. Intramuscular opioids, non-steroidal anti-inflammatory drugs and patient-controlled analgesia have all been used to good effect. Systemic rather than regional analgesia is preferable because the graft donor site is often the most painful area. Urinary retention is a frequent neurological problem, which is exacerbated by anaesthesia, and temporary or intermittent catheterization may be required.

If the spine is stable postoperatively, early mobilization is encouraged unless there is a major neurological deficit which prevents it. Patients with unstable spinal conditions are nursed on a variety of special purpose-built beds and frames for significant periods. In this situation, the risks of hypostatic pneumonia, deep venous thrombosis and pulmonary embolism are considerable.

FURTHER READING

Mini-Symposium 1994 The brain. Current Anaesthesia and Intensive Care 5(1)

Van Aken H (ed) 1995 Neuroanaesthetic practice. BMJ Publishing Group, London

Walters F J M, Ingram S, Jenkinson J 1994 Anaesthesia and intensive care for the neurosurgical patient, 2nd edn. Blackwell Scientific Publications, Oxford

58 Anaesthesia for thoracic surgery

Thoracic anaesthesia offers particular anaesthetic challenges:

- control of the airway during bronchoscopy
- protection of the airway in patients with oesophageal disease, lung abscess, bronchopleural fistula or haemoptysis
- positioning a double-lumen tracheal tube to maintain anaesthesia in the lateral position with the chest opened and one lung collapsed
- postoperative care of a patient after lung tissue resection.

In common with major surgery at other sites, thoracic patients frequently have:

- parenchymal lung disease in addition to their presenting complaint
- a painful wound after surgery
- the potential for substantial haemorrhage
- the need for intravenous fluids after surgery.

Diagnosis, staging and resection of intrathoracic malignant disease occupy a large part of thoracic surgical practice. There is also a need for drainage and obliteration of an expanded pleural space to remove infection, prevent lung collapse and re-accumulation of air or liquid in the pleural space. Resection of bullous lung disease may improve the respiratory mechanics of the chest where there is parenchymal lung disease elsewhere.

PREOPERATIVE ASSESSMENT

HISTORY AND EXAMINATION

Thoracic patients often exhibit the respiratory symptoms of cough, sputum, haemoptysis, breathlessness, wheeze and chest pain, or oesophageal symptoms of dysphagia, pain and weight loss. Other common chest features are hoarseness, superior vena cava obstruction, pain in the chest wall or arm, Horner's syndrome, cyanosis and pleural effusion. Lung tumours may cause extrathoracic symptoms by metastatic spread, principally to brain, bone, liver, adrenals and kidneys, or by endocrine effects such as finger clubbing, hypertrophic pulmonary osteoarthropathy, Cushing's syndrome, hypercalcaemia, myopathies (e.g. Eaton–Lambert syndrome), scleroderma, acanthosis and thrombophlebitis.

Anaemia, cardiac disease and lung disease may all cause breathlessness. To distinguish between loss of lung tissue and reversible airways disease, the patient's own history of daily activity may reveal diurnal variation in breathlessness and associated symptoms of sputum, stridor and wheeze. Symptoms may conflict with the results of pulmonary function tests which require voluntary effort, if the tests have been performed ineffectively. Wheeze during expiration and stridor during inspiration are likely to result from airway obstruction below and above the thoracic inlet, respectively.

Production of sputum is the most common stimulus of cough, which is therefore almost universal in cigarette smokers. A dry cough may result from tumour or external compression of the upper airways.

Oesophageal tumours are associated with dysphagia. The restriction on ingestion of food exacerbates the cachexia of malignant disease. At induction of anaesthesia, patients are at risk of regurgitation of food and secretions from above the oesophageal obstruction.

Preoperative features of weight loss and protein-calorie malnutrition, and hypoalbuminaemia make postoperative pulmonary infection, multi-organ failure and delayed wound healing more likely. Patients with pre-existing chronic lung disease are more likely to suffer postoperative pulmonary complications.

Cyanosis may result centrally from intrapulmonary shunting caused directly by diseased tissue or because of lung collapse consequent to proximal airway obstruction. Peripheral cyanosis is possible in the face and arms if the superior vena cava becomes obstructed by mediastinal spread.

Many thoracic major surgical procedures are preceded by rigid bronchoscopy, which requires a clinical assessment of upper airway patency at the preoperative visit. Forced ventilatory effort by the patient may elicit stridor or wheeze, and palpation of the neck and inspection of the airway demonstrated on chest radiograph may reveal tracheal abnormality.

DIFFERENTIAL DIAGNOSIS

Preoperative investigations are required to confirm a diagnosis and stage the disease, in order to assess if the disease is resectable. Tumours are staged by assessing the spread of the primary tumour, presence of local lymph node spread and distant metastases (TNM staging). Further tests to assess physiological reserve are required to determine if the patient is operable.

INVESTIGATIONS

A variety of preoperative investigations are likely to have been performed to determine resectability. The chest radiograph may reveal changes months before symptoms are manifest. Of symptomatic patients, 98% have chest radiograph abnormalities. Lung tumours are central in 70% of patients and may show collapse or cavitation more peripherally in the lung. Tumours are commonly

3–4 cm in size by the time of presentation. Other features include tracheal deviation, superior vena cava obstruction, pleural effusions and air-filled cavities.

Tumour diagnosis and staging involves sputum cytology, bronchoscopy, needle biopsy, mediastinoscopy and mediastinotomy. Computed tomography (CT) and magnetic resonance imaging (MRI) of the chest may reveal the spread of disease. Biochemistry, bone scans and ultrasound scans of the abdomen may detect metastatic disease. Barium studies and oesophageal ultrasound are similarly able to diagnose and stage carcinoma of the oesophagus.

Preoperative pulmonary function testing by spirometry may help in assessment of risk before lung resection. Testing may involve the whole lung or attempt to distinguish between lung function in different lung regions.

Whole-lung testing

Spirometry using voluntary effort, pulse oximetry and arterial blood gas tensions breathing on air are influenced by the function of the whole lung.

Spirometry tests only the mechanical bellows function of the lung. Testing relies on voluntary effort and effective technique by the patient. From total lung capacity, the patient exhales to residual volume to measure the forced vital capacity (FVC). This is reduced in restrictive lung disease, such as cryptogenic alveolar fibrosis. The volume of gas exhaled forcibly in the first second gives the forced expiratory volume in 1 s (FEV_1). By definition, FEV_1 measures function when the lung is expanded well. In health, patients can exhale 70–80% of their vital capacity in 1 s, the FEV_1%. The remainder of the vital capacity may take another 2 s to exhale. With obstructive lung disease, the FEV_1% is reduced below 70% and the time taken to exhale the vital capacity is prolonged. The FEV_1% of patients with restrictive lung disease is preserved, although the absolute value of FVC, and therefore the volume exhaled in 1 s, is reduced. Values of 2 L for FVC and 1.5 L for FEV_1 offer a lower limit when screening for pneumonectomy. An FEV_1 of 1.0 L is cautionary for single lobectomy, because a whole-lung FEV_1 > 800 ml after surgery is about the amount a patient requires to avoid being dependent on mechanical ventilation.

Using whole-lung spirometry to predict postoperative lung function may be invalidated if the regional function of the lung is not known. For example, a patient with a FEV_1 of 1.5 L may have the same or better FEV_1 after lobectomy if the main bronchus of the affected lobe was occluded completely at the time of testing before surgery. The oxygenation of blood of such a patient may be improved by the removal of a non-functioning lung or lobe through which considerable right-to-left shunt existed.

Regional lung function

Ventilation/perfusion lung scans offer an indication of regional lung function. The relative contribution of the two separate lungs may be determined horizontally, but vertically within a lung, regions are indicated as upper, middle and lower zones rather than individual lobes or lung units.

Invasive assessment

For patients with borderline lung function for whom surgical resection offers great prognostic advantage, the risks and discomfort of invasive assessment of regional lung function may be worth the information obtained of likely residual function after surgery. Balloon occlusion of a main pulmonary artery before surgery or clamping a pulmonary artery during surgery allows some assessment of pulmonary artery pressures and oxygenation after resection. Inadequate blood oxygenation, arterial carbon dioxide tensions greater than 6.0 kPa and mean pulmonary artery pressures greater than 25 mmHg at rest, or greater than 35 mmHg with exercise, indicate inadequate function and increased operative risk.

Any intrathoracic operative procedure places an immediate burden on the right ventricle. Diagnosis of a failing right ventricle or coexisting pulmonary artery hypertension may render a patient's chest pathology inoperable.

TREATMENT

Before surgery, patients should be motivated to stop smoking and lose excess weight. Reversible airway narrowing should be treated with bronchodilators such as salbutamol, terbutaline, theophylline, inhaled steroids or sodium cromoglycate. By giving antibiotics to treat chest infection, and loosening and removing bronchial secretions with inhaled nebulized water aerosols, chest physiotherapy and postural drainage, the incidence of pulmonary complications is reduced. Overnight, stopping smoking improves bronchial reactivity and reduces carboxyhaemoglobin concentrations. Eight weeks after cessation of smoking, the excessive production of mucus is reduced; this makes tracheobronchial clearance easier and improves small airway function.

ANATOMY

The bronchial tree and the views obtained when facing the patient are illustrated in Figure 8.6 (p. 106). The trachea leads from the cricoid cartilage below the larynx at the level of the sixth cervical vertebra (C6) and passes 10–12 cm in the superior mediastinum to its bifurcation at the carina into left and right main bronchi at the sternal angle, T4/5. During inspiration, the lower border of the trachea moves inferiorly and anteriorly. The trachea lies principally in the midline, but is deviated to the right inferiorly by the arch of the aorta. The oesophagus is immediately posterior to the trachea and behind it is the vertebral column. The wall of the trachea is held patent by 15–20 cartilaginous rings deficient posteriorly where the trachealis membrane, a collection of fibroelastic fibres and smooth muscle, lies. It is wider in transverse diameter (20 mm) than anteroposteriorly (15 mm). The trachea passes from neck to thorax via the thoracic inlet at T2.

The right main bronchus is larger and less deviated from the midline than the left. The origin of the right upper lobe bronchus arises laterally 2.5 cm from the carina, whereas the origin of the left upper lobe arises laterally after 5 cm. These dimensions determine the relative ease of isolating each lung and ventilating them independently using double-lumen endobronchial tubes.

The oesophagus is a continuation of the pharynx at the level of the lower border of the cricoid cartilage (C6) 15 cm from the incisor teeth. It passes immediately anterior to the thoracic spine and aorta until descending through the oesophageal hiatus of the diaphragm at T10, to the left of the midline at the level of the seventh rib. There are four slight constrictions, at its origin, as it is crossed by the aorta and left main bronchus and at the diaphragm at 15, 25, 27 and 38 cm from the incisors.

RADIOGRAPHIC SURFACE MARKINGS

The apices of the lungs extend 2.5 cm above the clavicle where middle and inner thirds meet. Lung borders descend behind the medial end of the clavicle to the middle of the manubrium. The lung border is behind the body of the sternum and xiphisternum before sweeping inferiorly and laterally down to the level of the 11th thoracic vertebra. On the left at the level of the horizontal fissure at the fourth costal cartilage (T7), the medial border of the lung is displaced to the left of the sternal edge in the cardiac notch. The oblique fissure descends from 3 cm lateral to the midline at T4, inferiorly and anteriorly to the sixth costal cartilage 7 cm from the midline. The diaphragmatic reflection of the pleura extrudes below the lung to the lower border of T12.

The anatomy of structures important in local anaesthetic blocks to treat pain after surgery – the transverse superficial cervical nervous plexus, intercostal nerves, paravertebral sympathetic chain and epidural space – are detailed elsewhere (Ch. 11).

INDUCTION AND MAINTENANCE OF ANAESTHESIA

All currently available anaesthetic agents may be, and have been, used in anaesthetics for thoracic surgery. They are used in a way that is compatible with a strategy to maintain anaesthesia and haemodynamic stability during the procedure, while allowing the patient to breathe spontaneously in relative comfort immediately after surgery is complete. Large doses of opioid drugs i.v. are unlikely to achieve all these aims. Thoracic surgery patients may demonstrate sensitivity to drugs used in anaesthesia because of debility from the extent of their disease or from systemic effects, such as prolonged effects of neuromuscular blocking drugs in patients with Eaton–Lambert syndrome associated with carcinoma of the bronchus.

LATERAL THORACOTOMY

Many thoracic procedures are performed through a posterolateral thoracotomy incision between the fifth and eighth ribs. Patients have to be positioned on their side with the neck flexed, dependent shoulder brought forward and the arm raised under the pillow to protect shoulder and brachial plexus. The upper shoulder is flexed to 90° and the arm supported. Hips and knees are flexed together with a pillow between the legs. Padding, strapping, lower leg compression devices and diathermy pad complete the preparation for surgery (Fig. 58.1). Positioning with the chest flexed laterally away from the operative side on a bean bag which is then aspirated of air, or breaking the operating table can improve surgical access. The upper wrist has a tendency to flex, so radial artery cannulae give less trouble on the dependent side. Peripheral and jugular vein cannulae are more accessible on the operative side.

THE LATERAL POSITION

In health, with the chest erect, the right lung takes 55% of the pulmonary blood flow and the left lung 45%. In the right lateral position, the right lung takes 65% and the left lung 35% because of the influence of gravity. In the left lateral position, differences are reversed; the right lung takes 45% and left lung 55%. These changes persist under anaesthesia.

However, anaesthesia does affect the changes to ventilation of the two lungs in the lateral position. Awake, there is more ventilation to the dependent lung; similarly, the bases receive proportionately more ventilation than the apices when the chest is erect. The dependent lung has a less negative intrapleural pressure than the upper lung and is on a more favourable part of the pressure–volume curve. A change in pressure produces a greater change in volume in the dependent lung than the upper lung. Under anaesthesia, conditions for ventilation between the two lungs are reversed. Functional residual capacity is reduced. With paralysis of the diaphragm, the mechanical advantage of the greater curve of the lower diaphragm is lost and the lower lung is compressed by the mediastinum and abdominal contents. Awkward positioning on the operating table may further impede the lower lung. The lower lung is now on a less favourable position on the pressure–volume curve and any change in pressure produces greater change in the volume of the upper lung than the dependent lung. Anaesthesia therefore produces much worse ventilation/perfusion mismatch in the lateral position, with more blood going to the dependent lung and more ventilation going to the upper lung. Application of positive end-expiratory pressure up to 10 cmH_2O reverses the changes in ventilation and tends to restore ventilation to the dependent lung.

ONE-LUNG ANAESTHESIA

The principal indications for one-lung anaesthesia are:

- isolation of the lungs
- ventilation of one lung alone
- bronchopulmonary alveolar lavage
- collapse of one lung to allow surgical access to other structures.

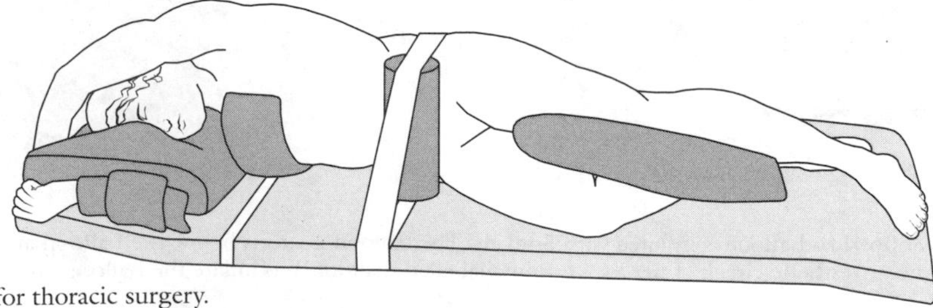

Fig. 58.1
Patient in right lateral position for thoracic surgery.

Isolation of a diseased lung with sepsis or haemorrhage may be necessary to protect the healthy lung. When there is inadequate ventilation of both lungs because of a large bronchopleural or bronchocutaneous fistula, a large unilateral bulla or because the compliance of two lungs is so different they require independent ventilation, satisfactory oxygenation may be obtained by ventilation of one lung alone. Pulmonary alveolar proteinosis may be treated by bronchoalveolar lavage. This requires that only one lung be lavaged with liquid at a time, whilst the other is protected. Video-assisted pulmonary and pleural surgery, and intrathoracic, non-pulmonary surgery such as oesophageal, aortic and spinal surgery may require the lung to be collapsed to allow access to the operative structures.

Ventilation of one lung alone may require either a double-lumen tracheal tube (Fig. 58.2), a bronchial blocker (Fig. 58.3) or an endobronchial tube. The double-lumen tube has greatest flexibility to allow changes from ventilation of two lungs to one lung then back to two lungs during or at the end of surgery. It allows aspiration of the main bronchi independently, and insufflation of oxygen to the non-ventilated lung. It has a larger external diameter than the bronchial blocker or endobronchial tube and may be difficult to position correctly where tracheal and bronchial anatomy is distorted. The two separate lumens are narrow and present a high resistance to spontaneous ventilation. This is overcome by positive pressure ventilation, but a single-lumen tube may have to be substituted at the end of surgery if resumption of spontaneous ventilation is not immediate. An endobronchial blocker with a hollow lumen allows insufflation of oxygen, some suctioning and may be used with a jet ventilator, which overcomes some of the disadvantages of the technique. The Rüsch bronchial blocker illustrated in Figure 58.3 (the 360601) has a 170 cm long, 2 mm stem (outside diameter) with a central lumen to a 2.75 mm diameter balloon, which accepts 5 ml air. It may be passed down a bronchoscope with a lumen greater than 2.8 mm diameter or the 15 mm tapered connector with a 1.8 mm seal shown.

POSITIONING DOUBLE-LUMEN ENDOBRONCHIAL TUBES

Double-lumen endobronchial tubes provide an effective means of isolating each lung to protect the other from blood and secretions.

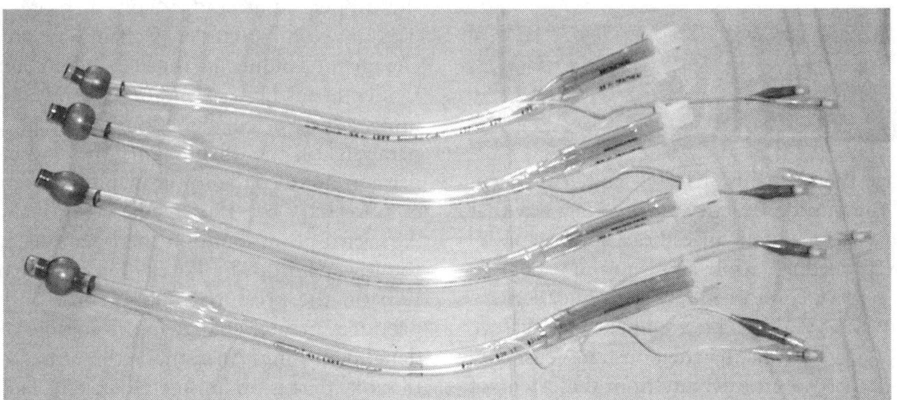

Fig. 58.2
Four left-sided Bronchocath double-lumen endobronchial tubes with balloons inflated from 35 FG (uppermost) to 41 FG (lowest).

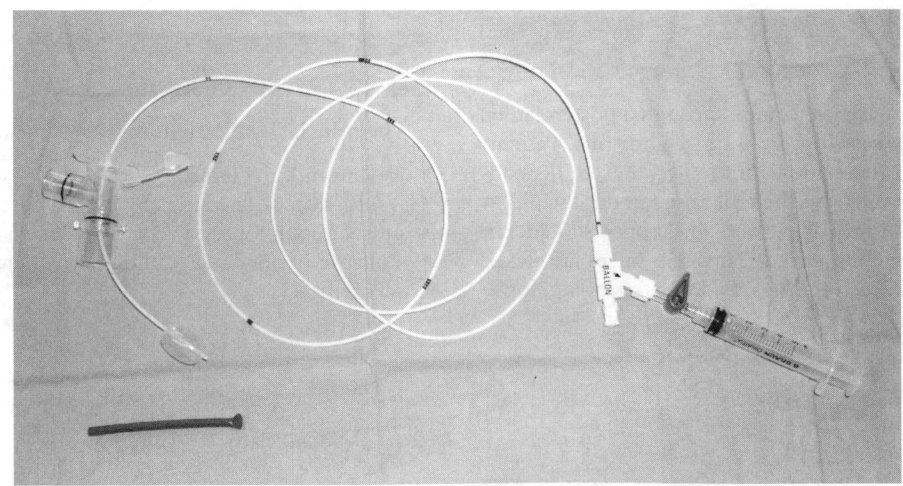

Fig. 58.3
A Rüsch 6 FG bronchial blocker (360601) – balloon is inflated with 5 ml air. The balloon guard is below the balloon and the stem passes through the 1.8 mm seal in the connector for the anaesthetic circuit. Luer-lock fittings (labelled 'balloon') to inflate the balloon and aspirate/inflate down the central lumen are on the right.

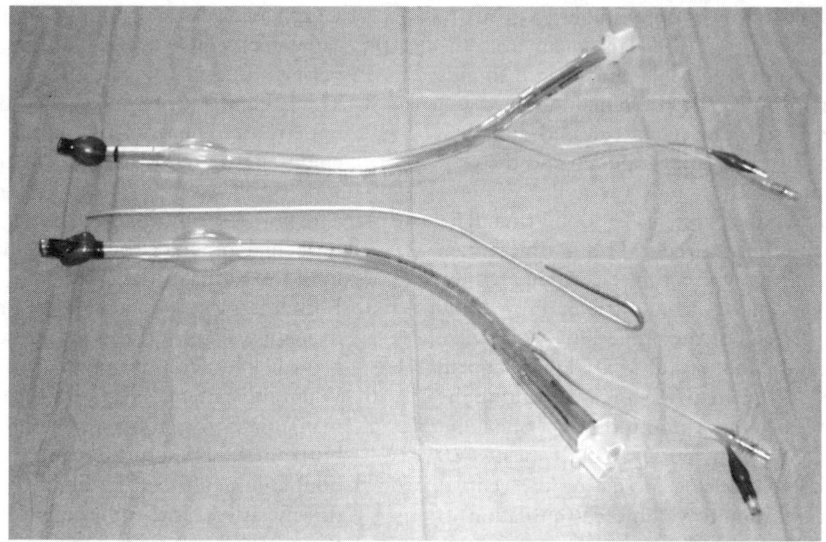

Fig. 58.4
Left (upper) and right (lower) 39 FG double-lumen endobronchial tubes are shown with a flexible introducer, which may be used to shape the tube to enable insertion.

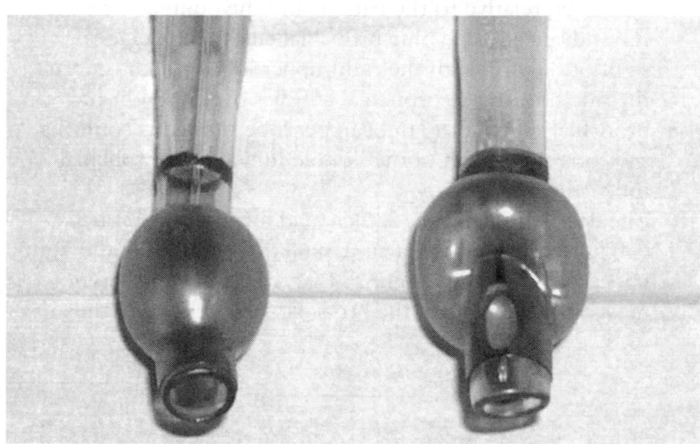

Fig. 58.5
Bronchial balloons inflated on left-sided (left) and right-sided (right) endobronchial double-lumen tubes. The right tube is eccentric and shows the side lumen to allow inflation of the right upper lobe.

They allow ventilation of one lung only, or both lungs independently. Being longer and with lumens more narrow than single-lumen tracheal tubes, they have a greater resistance to air flow. They are therefore not usually suitable for spontaneous ventilation. Disposable polyvinyl chloride tubes (Fig. 58.4) have substantially replaced the re-usable red rubber Robertshaw double-lumen tubes. Sizes of tube in common use in adult practice range from 35 to 41 French gauge (FG). Sizes 37–39 are usually suitable for men and 37 for women, but sizes 41 and 35 are available for individuals at extremes of the range of adult build. Left- and right-sided versions of double-lumen endobronchial tubes are necessary (Fig. 58.4) as they are curved anteroposteriorly and the balloon of the right bronchial tube is fenestrated to conduct gases down the right upper lobe bronchus, which would otherwise be occluded by the cuff of the tube (Fig. 58.5). The left upper lobe bronchus arises 2.5 cm further down the main bronchus than the right, so it is less likely to be occluded by the balloon of the bronchial tube.

Positioning double-lumen endobronchial tubes correctly is a skill learned quickly with practice. The task is usually straightforward, but however experienced the anaesthetist, great difficulties may be encountered with some patients. An incorrectly positioned double-lumen endobronchial tube may rapidly compromise the supply of oxygen to the lungs during thoracic surgery, with disastrous results. The correct position of double-lumen endobronchial tubes may be confirmed by clinical means or by using an intubating fibreoptic laryngoscope.

Clinical means

The patient lies supine on a level operating table with the head supported on a single pillow pulled clear of the shoulders to flex the neck and extend the head. After induction of anaesthesia and muscle relaxation, the larynx is identified by laryngoscopy. The double-lumen endobronchial tube is held at 90° to its eventual anatomical position, to align the curve of the bronchial lumen anteroposteriorly. The bronchial lumen is passed between the cords until it rests within the trachea. The double-lumen endobronchial tube is then rotated 90° back to point the bronchial lumen towards its intended bronchus. The head is turned away from the side of the bronchial lumen and the double-lumen endobronchial tube advanced gently until resistance is encountered and the bronchial tube is thought to be in the correct position. The tracheal cuff is then inflated and the lungs ventilated manually through both lumens of the tube. Visible movement of both sides of the chest, detection of a recognizable trace of exhaled carbon dioxide, breath sounds auscultated in both axillae and an unchanging pulse oximetry reading reassure the anaesthetist that the airway is controlled. Difficulties encountered whilst isolating individual lungs may be addressed whilst returning to this position of control.

The tracheal lumen of the breathing circuit is then clamped and the circuit distal to the clamp opened to air. Breath sounds are confirmed on the bronchial side. Two or more millilitres of air are then injected into the bronchial cuff until the leak of air from the tracheal tube is no longer audible or palpable, and breath sounds auscultated over the side opposite to the bronchial lumen cease. The tracheal lumen is then closed, the clamp released and then applied to the bronchial circuit; the circuit is opened and the procedure is repeated to confirm that chest movement and air entry occur to the tracheal side and not the bronchial side and that there are no air leaks from the anaesthetic circuit. The double-lumen endobronchial tube is then secured with a tube tie at the teeth by a clove hitch, and the tube tie is knotted round the neck by a bow to enable its quick release at the end of the procedure.

When each lumen of the double-lumen tube (DLT) is clamped, there should be a detectable increase in airway pressure during the breathing cycle when the tidal volume is directed down one lung. The peak airway pressure may then be controlled below 30 cmH_2O by reducing the tidal volume and increasing the ventilatory rate whilst maintaining the minute volume of ventilation. If there is no change on the ventilator or airway pressure gauges when one lumen of the tube is clamped, the bronchial lumen is likely to end in the trachea or else there is a substantial leak past the bronchial cuff. The position of the DLT should always be rechecked after the patient has been subjected to any changes in position, e.g. from supine to lateral etc.

Using the fibreoptic intubating laryngoscope

Confirming the correct position of a double-lumen endobronchial tube using a fibreoptic intubating laryngoscope should avoid many problems encountered with ventilation of the lungs during thoracic surgery. However, if parenchymal lung disease is so extensive that one lung is insufficient to keep tissues oxygenated, if pneumothorax develops on the side of the ventilated lung, or if the double-lumen tube is subsequently dislodged, problems with ventilation may still be encountered. A practical solution to the conflict between the costs and time for each use and cleaning of the fibreoptic intubating laryngoscope and the benefits of positioning the double-lumen endobronchial tube correctly may be reached by:

- using left-sided double-lumen endobronchial tubes for all operations except left lung resections
- confirming correct position of left-sided double-lumen endobronchial tubes clinically
- using the fibreoptic intubating laryngoscope to confirm the correct position of left-sided double-lumen endobronchial tubes where clinical testing does not demonstrate correct position conclusively, and correct position of all right-sided double-lumen endobronchial tubes.

Vascular cannulae and epidural catheters may be inserted before or after induction of anaesthesia depending on clinical need. If bronchoscopy precedes thoracotomy then one sequence of events might be as follows:

1. Anaesthesia is induced for bronchoscopy, followed by insertion of a double-lumen endobronchial tube into the trachea. The tracheal cuff is inflated and ventilation of both lungs confirmed as anaesthesia is maintained.
2. Peripheral venous, arterial, central venous and urinary catheters are inserted as required, if not already in place before induction of anaesthesia.
3. The patient is turned onto the side with the operative side uppermost. The neck and hips are flexed to insert the epidural catheter; otherwise the patient is positioned for surgery.
4. The fibreoptic intubating laryngoscope is passed down the bronchial lumen of the double-lumen endobronchial tube until the carina is identified.
5. Both lungs are ventilated if the bronchial lumen connector makes a seal around the laryngoscope; otherwise the bronchial lumen is clamped.
6. When the patient is lying on the side, the anaesthetist manipulates the laryngoscope tip in a vertical plane (i.e. horizontal section in the patient). For a right-sided double-lumen tube, the tip of the laryngoscope is directed downwards (to the right main bronchus) and advanced until the orifice of the right upper lobe bronchus is identified. Positioning the double-lumen tube often leaves the orifice of the right upper lobe bronchus covered by the tip of the bronchial tube (Fig. 58.6).
7. The tracheal cuff is then deflated, the laryngoscope is held fixed relative to the patient and the double-lumen tube advanced. The blue bronchial cuff then occludes sight of the orifice of the right upper lobe bronchus until the side hole in the bronchial cuff lies over it. Sight of bronchial rings of the right upper lobe bronchus confirms the correct position of the double-lumen endobronchial tube (Fig. 58.7).
8. The double-lumen tube is then held firm and the bronchial cuff inflated with 2 ml of air. Uninterrupted sight of the right upper lobe bronchus confirms that this manoeuvre has not moved the side hole of the bronchial tube relative to the

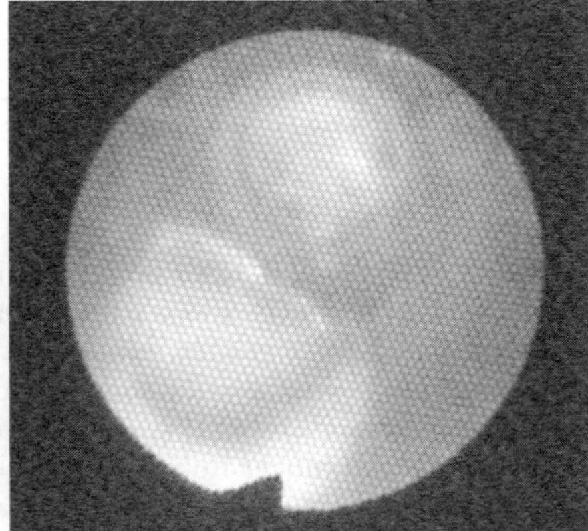

Fig. 58.6
Distal opening of bronchial lumen at 12 o'clock shows right middle and lower bronchi. The side opening of the bronchial lumen at 7 o'clock is against the wall of the right main bronchus and is not over the right upper lobe bronchus. The patient is lying on the right. Orientation: left, cephalad; upper, left; right, caudad; lower, right.

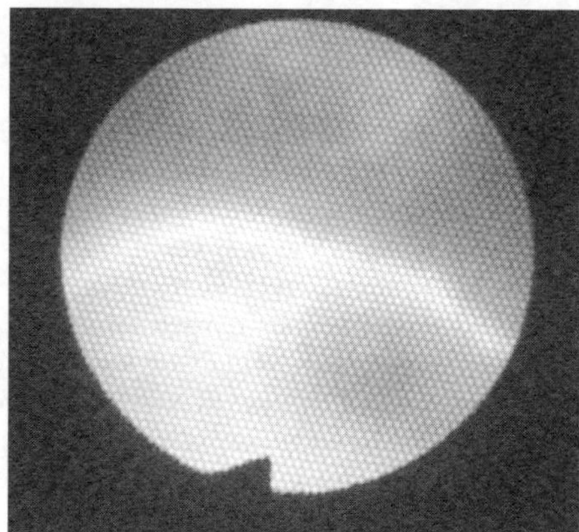

Fig. 58.7
The double-lumen tube has been repositioned so that the side opening of the bronchial lumen at 6 o'clock is now over the right upper lobe bronchus. The patient is lying on the right. Orientation: left, cephalad; upper, left; right, caudad; lower, right.

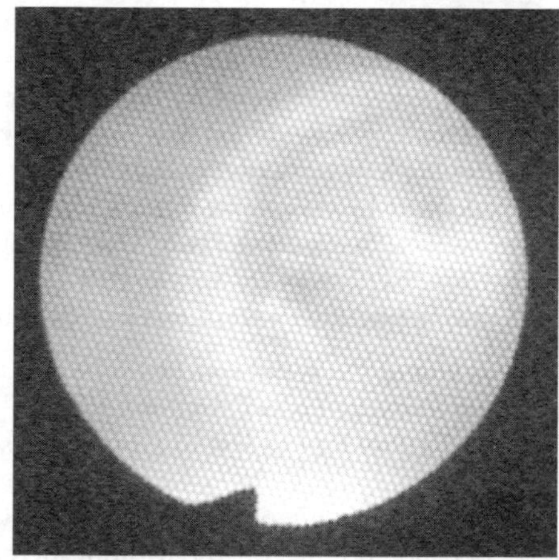

Fig. 58.8
Distal opening of bronchial lumen at 3 o'clock shows right lower and middle lobe bronchi. The dark colour at 9 o'clock is the bronchial lumen cuff. The patient is lying on the right. Orientation: left, cephalad; upper, left; right, caudad; lower, right.

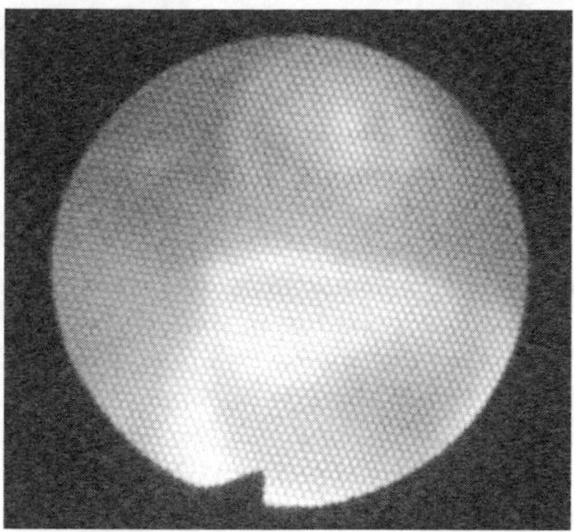

Fig. 58.9
The intubating laryngoscope is withdrawn to show the right middle and lower lobe bronchi through the distal opening at 12 o'clock and the right upper lobe bronchus through the side opening at 6 o'clock. The patient is lying on the right. Orientation: left, cephalad; upper, left; right, caudad; lower, right.

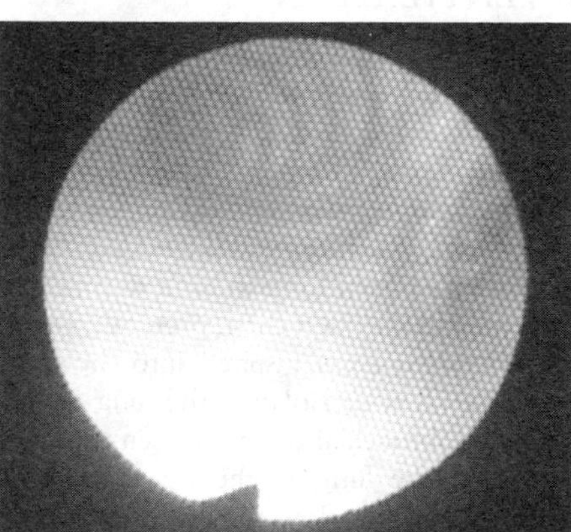

Fig. 58.10
The intubating laryngoscope has been passed down the tracheal lumen. The carina passes from 2 o'clock anteriorly to 6 o'clock posteriorly. The left main bronchus is to the left at 10–12 o'clock. On the other side of the carina, the dark crescent confirms that the inflated bronchial cuff is not herniating over the left main bronchus and the bronchial tube to the right of the cuff passes down the right main bronchus. The patient is lying on the right. Orientation: left, cephalad; upper, left; right, caudad; lower, right.

bronchus. The bronchi to the right middle and lower lobes may be seen through the distal lumen of the bronchial tube (Fig. 58.8). Withdrawing the intubating laryngoscope may give a view of the origins of all three lobar bronchi (Fig. 58.9).

9. The double-lumen tube is then held against the teeth or gums of the maxilla, the mark on the tube there is noted and the laryngoscope is removed from the bronchial lumen. Without moving it, the tube is tied with a clove hitch over this mark and the tube tie tied round the neck with a bow.
10. The tracheal cuff is then inflated with 5 ml of air and the fibreoptic laryngoscope is then passed down the tracheal lumen until the carina is identified again. The bronchial lumen is seen to pass down the correct main bronchus and the bronchial cuff in its main bronchus is seen to be inflated, but not herniating to impinge over the lumen of the other main bronchus (Fig. 58.10).
11. The laryngoscope is removed from the tracheal lumen and both lungs are ventilated.
12. Bronchial and tracheal lumens are clamped in turn, observing airway pressures, leaks and the extent of ventilation of each lung.

Passing a suction catheter down the bronchial lumen before starting removes secretions faster than is possible through the suction port of the fibreoptic intubating laryngoscope. Lubrication of the laryngoscope with water-soluble jelly aids its passage down both lumens and prevents the tube being dislodged when the laryngoscope is withdrawn. A receiver of warm water with detergent aspirated through the suction port reduces fogging of the tip of the laryngoscope. Warm soapy water provides a ready supply of fluid to unblock the suction port during the procedure and flush it through at the end, so that the suction port does not block with encrusted aspirate before there is an opportunity to clean the laryngoscope.

Clinical testing is specific – a problem detected with the position of the endobronchial double-lumen tube is very likely to predict a real problem if left uncorrected before surgery begins. However, it is not very sensitive. Inadequate isolation of one lung and excessive airway pressures may well be encountered after apparently successful positioning of the tube. Correct alignment of the fenestration in the bronchial cuff over the origin of the right upper lobe bronchus is particularly difficult to predict by clinical means alone.

MODE OF VENTILATION

Surgery through a thoracotomy wound with the patient breathing spontaneously causes the same problem as trauma patients experience with large open chest wounds. The pleural space with the chest open is at atmospheric pressure. During inspiration, gas flows from trachea and lung in the open chest into the dependent lung. During expiration, the flow is reversed, causing the lung in the open chest to inflate. Gas is transferred from lung to lung during the paradoxical ventilation of the lung in the open chest, preventing excretion of carbon dioxide and rendering gas inspired into the dependent lung hypoxic. Packing the chest or isolating the lung in the open chest with a blocker or endobronchial double-lumen tube may stop paradoxical ventilation of the lung in the open chest. Both devices increase the resistance to gas flow to the dependent lung, and so mechanical one-lung ventilation is usual during thoracic surgery.

PHYSIOLOGICAL CHANGES

With one lung perfused but not ventilated, a substantial right-to-left shunt should produce significant hypoxaemia. Because of the greater solubility of carbon dioxide and its more linear dissociation curve, the gradient from arterial to alveolar partial pressure of carbon dioxide is smaller than that for oxygen. Increasing alveolar ventilation of the ventilated lung reduces arterial carbon dioxide tension without substantially increasing arterial oxygen tension. Because of the flat portion of the oxygen dissociation curve, when haemoglobin is saturated fully, a further increase in alveolar oxygen tension improves only the trivial amount of oxygen in free solution and has no effect on the oxygenation of the blood in the non-ventilated lung. Hence this does not improve hypoxaemia caused by right-to-left shunt.

The severity of hypoxaemia observed is much less than that expected were regional perfusion to remain unaltered. As observed above, the lateral position directs more blood to the dependent lung because of gravity. In the non-ventilated lung, alveolar hypoxia results in increased vascular resistance, which directs more blood to the dependent ventilated lung, further reducing shunt and hypoxaemia. This protective change is termed hypoxic pulmonary vasoconstriction (HPV) and it is impaired by anaesthetic agents in experimental models. However, in clinical practice, other compensatory mechanisms in the intact human lung reduce shunt.

HPV has no effect if the alveolar oxygen tension is either 100 or 0%, or if the alveolar oxygen tension is the same throughout all lung units. It is more likely to have an effect with the 20–30% of cardiac output which shunts through the non-ventilated lung during one-lung anaesthesia. HPV effects are also maximal when pulmonary artery pressures and mixed venous oxygen saturation tensions are normal. The results of excessively high or low pulmonary artery pressures exceed the marginal changes in pulmonary artery pressures obtained by HPV. Similarly, an abnormally low mixed venous oxygen tension caused by low cardiac output or high oxygen consumption by, for example, hyperthermia or shivering has greater influence than any changes possible with HPV. High peak and end-expiratory ventilation pressures in the dependent lung increase its pulmonary vascular resistance and overcome any benefits of HPV in the non-ventilated lung. Excessive alveolar pressures may increase dead space by producing a region of lung which is ventilated but not perfused.

Volatile anaesthetic agents and pulmonary vasodilators such as glyceryl trinitrate, sodium nitroprusside, isoproterenol, dobutamine and nitric oxide have all been demonstrated to inhibit HPV. However, clinically there are far more variables than in the controlled conditions of the experimental laboratory bench. Poor positioning of the patient which compromises blood flow to the dependent lung, malposition of a double-lumen endobronchial tube, low cardiac output caused by inadequate blood volume replacement or impediment to blood flow by surgical manipulation may have a greater influence on hypoxaemia than the effects of changes in HPV.

Hypoxaemia during one-lung anaesthesia may be minimized by:

- correct positioning of the endobronchial tube
- increasing inspired oxygen concentration to 50%
- a tidal volume of 10 ml kg^{-1} or less to avoid increasing dead space
- positive end-expired pressure of no more than 5–10 cmH_2O to minimize dependent lung collapse without increasing vascular resistance
- maintaining cardiac output and pulmonary artery pressures near the normal range.

Insufflation of oxygen to the non-ventilated lung either at atmospheric pressure or with continuous positive alveolar pressure of 5 cmH2O should avoid the need for pharmacological intervention such as inhaled nitric oxide to the ventilated lung. During lung resection, when the pulmonary artery is clamped, the adequacy of gas exchange should be reassessed. The loss of shunt through diseased lung tissue may limit the loss of lung function expected after removal of lung tissue.

ANAESTHESIA FOR THORACIC SURGERY PROCEDURES

RIGID BRONCHOSCOPY

Rigid bronchoscopy in thoracic surgery is performed most often to obtain tissue diagnosis and determine if a lesion may be resected. Other indications include removal of foreign bodies and secretions, and control of haemorrhage. Therapeutic procedures such as laser therapy, bronchial stenting and alveolar lavage may be performed through a rigid bronchoscope.

Anaesthesia must permit the passage of a straight rigid bronchoscope of up to 9 mm external diameter, allow oxygenation and removal of carbon dioxide, avoid awareness, and control movement, coughing and reflex haemodynamic responses to mechanical stimulation of the tracheobronchial tree. This may be achieved by spontaneous ventilation, apnoeic oxygenation or, more usually, positive pressure jet ventilation. Spontaneous ventilation avoids inhaled foreign bodies being propelled more distally into the bronchial tree. However, it offers much less control than when neuromuscular blockade is used, and anaesthesia sufficient to cause respiratory depression is required to control reflex responses to bronchoscopy. Apnoeic oxygenation may be achieved by delivering oxygen into the conducting airways by a catheter and relying on diffusion down a concentration gradient from oxygenated airways to alveoli, where oxygen is absorbed continuously. Although effective in maintaining oxygenation measured by pulse oximetry, arterial carbon dioxide tension increases by 0.5 kPa min^{-1}. Using apnoeic oxygenation, enough time may be available to complete the surgical procedure, but eventually, assisted or spontaneous ventilation has to resume to ventilate the alveoli.

Positive pressure ventilation may be performed by intermittent occlusion of the bronchoscope or, more conveniently, by high-pressure jet ventilation using a Sanders Venturi technique. Oxygen at 400 kPa is released by a trigger held by the anaesthetist through a narrow orifice of 18–14G. The gas is directed through the jet at the operator end of the bronchoscope towards the patient end. The high-pressure jet entrains atmospheric air and inflates the chest. Care must be taken to avoid pulmonary barotrauma by limiting delivery of oxygen under pressure to short intermittent bursts according to the chest movement observed and ensuring that there is a large unobstructed opening at the observer end of the bronchoscope to allow gas under pressure to escape from the conducting airways. Oxygenation may be monitored by pulse oximetry. Intermittent ventilation may usually be restricted to times when the operator is not looking down the bronchoscope.

With the patient supine, removal of the pillow or extension of the neck by lowering the head of the operating table may be necessary to allow the bronchoscope to pass down the trachea. Antisialagogue premedication dries oropharyngeal secretions and aids visibility. Induction of anaesthesia by inhalation of volatile anaesthetic agents may be necessary occasionally to confirm that adequate ventilation may be achieved under anaesthesia where there is some obstruction to the upper airways. Depolarizing or competitive neuromuscular blocking agents may be used according to the needs of the patient or intended procedure. Topical local anaesthetics and systemic opioids with a rapid onset of action help to obtund the haemodynamic response to bronchoscopy. Intermittent positive pressure ventilation with a Venturi device requires a total intravenous anaesthetic technique.

Local trauma and bleeding are the most common complications. Ventilation after bronchoscopy may be impaired by persisting effects of anaesthetic drugs or compromise to the upper airway. A chest radiograph in the recovery room may provide early detection of pneumothorax or air in the mediastinum.

RIGID OESOPHAGOSCOPY

Fibreoptic oesophagogastroduodenoscopy is performed usually as an outpatient procedure under sedation, without demands for anaesthetic assistance. Rigid oesophagoscopy under general anaesthesia presents the anaesthetist with patients who are at risk of aspirating gastric contents. Patients with achalasia may have large volumes of fetid fluid accumulated in their oesophagus. All oesophagoscopy patients should undergo rapid-sequence induction with the suction catheter to hand and suction switched on. In patients with achalasia, there should be an attempt to drain the oesophagus before anaesthesia, which should be induced in a steep head-up tilt or in the left lateral position.

When anaesthesia has been induced and the cuff of the tracheal tube inflated to protect the airway, the tracheal tube should be passed to the left-hand side of the tongue to allow the oesophagoscope to be inserted behind where the tracheal tube usually lies. The tracheal tube is then taped or tied securely, and then held at all times by the anaesthetist. This prevents the tracheal tube being dislodged by the operator or the withdrawal of the oesophagoscope on most occasions, and makes the anaesthetist aware immediately of dislodgement of the tracheal tube, regurgitation of fluid into the oropharynx or requests for the tracheal cuff to be deflated as the oesophagoscope is passed through the cricopharyngeal sphincter.

Manipulations to the head or neck may be required to pass the oesophagoscope. Damage to the teeth or mucosal surfaces may occur. When the oesophagoscope has passed down the oesophagus, anaesthesia may be maintained with the patient breathing spontaneously. At the end of the procedure, patients should be awake and able to cough and protect their own airway before tracheal extubation, which takes place with the patient lying on the left side with suction apparatus and trained assistance ready to hand as at induction of anaesthesia.

Perforation of the oesophagus is an unusual but serious complication. Patients should have been awake for 1 h after oesophagoscopy without complaint of chest discomfort and have an unchanged chest radiograph before ingestion of oral fluids resumes.

CERVICAL MEDIASTINOSCOPY AND ANTERIOR MEDIASTINOTOMY

Both procedures are used to stage the extent of spread of intrathoracic malignancy or obtain a tissue diagnosis. Ventilation of both lungs through a single-lumen tracheal tube is usually adequate and surgical access may be improved by resting the shoulders on a sandbag and the head on a head ring.

Analgesia after surgery may be helped by infiltration of the wound by local anaesthetic, or transverse superficial cervical plexus and intercostal nerve blocks. Whilst the procedures are usually straightforward, there is always the potential for significant haemorrhage, damage to surrounding structures, and compromise to the airway from haematoma after surgery.

VIDEO-ASSISTED THORACOSCOPIC SURGERY (VATS)

Improvements in imaging and thoracoscopic instruments have allowed more elaborate procedures than biopsy such as lung resection, lung reduction surgery, pleurectomy and sympathectomy. The video image is magnified on monitors, but so too is movement and there is little space within the chest for instruments and camera lenses. A collapsed motionless lung may be essential, thereby requiring one-lung anaesthesia.

Pain after VATS procedures is less intense and prolonged than after posterolateral thoracotomy. Patients are much more comfortable after the chest drain is removed than thoracotomy patients at the same stage after surgery. A single paravertebral block at the level of the chest drain and intercostal incisions with bupivacaine 0.5% 20 ml followed by oral analgesia may be sufficient to allow patients to take deep breaths and cough after thoracoscopic surgery.

PULMONARY LOBECTOMY

One-lung anaesthesia allows dissection in a field disturbed only by the movement of the mediastinum. Inflation of the lung temporarily may help to identify the lung fissures. Passive insufflation of the collapsed lung either through a suction catheter or with 5 cm continuous positive airway pressure may augment oxygenation achieved by one-lung anaesthesia. Surgical traction on mediastinal structures and disturbance to the mediastinum by surgeons' hands, instruments or retractors may cause bradycardia, interruption of the venous return to the heart or compression of the chambers of the heart.

When the bronchial stump is closed and haemostasis secured, the chest may be filled with warm saline and the airway pressure held at 40 cmH_2O to test the integrity of the stump.

When chest drains are in position, the remaining lobe(s) are reinflated by applying gentle positive pressure to the anaesthetic breathing system. Observing the pleural surface confirms if all superficial lung tissue is reinflated. As the chest is closed, a subatmospheric pressure of 5 kPa is applied to the chest drains via an underwater seal. A significant air leak through damaged lung becomes apparent immediately if the ventilator reservoir collapses or if a reduction in the expired minute volume is detected by the ventilator alarm. The suction is then disconnected from the chest drains and reapplied when the patient resumes spontaneous breathing. Chest drains are then left without being clamped until the remaining lung has re-expanded fully, drainage has ceased and there is no air leak, when the chest drains are removed.

PNEUMONECTOMY

The operative lung should be collapsed as soon as skin disinfection and draping begin. Problems with oxygenation may then be apparent early in the procedure. Borderline oxygenation may improve when the pulmonary artery is clamped and shunt through the lung to be resected is interrupted. Intrapericardial dissections for tumours which have extensive local spread pose a risk of sudden, substantial haemorrhage. The integrity of the stump of the main bronchus may be tested when the lung has been removed (as after lobectomy).

When the chest is closed at the end of surgery, the remaining lung is fully inflated and the chest drain to the pneumonectomy space is clamped. Clamps are released for 5 min every hour to ensure that no air, blood or excess fluid accumulates in the pneumonectomy space. Leaving the chest drains open continuously may lead to a reduction in the pneumonectomy space and the mediastinum being shifted to the operative side as the remaining lung becomes hyperinflated with consequent respiratory embarrassment. The pleural space fills with serosanguinous fluid after pneumonectomy and fibroses subsequently, reducing the size of the space.

PLEURECTOMY AND PLEURODESIS

Recurrent pneumothorax or pneumothorax which fails to respond to conservative measures may require pleurectomy to re-expand the lung and prevent recurrence. Pleurectomy and talc pleurodesis are usually possible by thoracoscopy. Pain after pleurectomy is much greater than after diagnostic thoracoscopic procedures even with the same number of intercostal wounds. Patients may require the same analgesia as if the procedure had been performed via a thoracotomy wound.

EMPYEMA

Patients may remain remarkably well despite large collections of purulent material in the pleural space. Collections may arise after pulmonary infection, oesophageal rupture, and following thoracoscopy and thoracotomy. Chest drainage before surgery may reduce the volume of pleural fluid, but organized infection has to be removed by open surgery. There may be considerable blood loss during decortication of an empyema.

LUNG CYSTS AND BULLAE

Bullae are thin-walled, air-filled cavities within the lung which communicate slowly with the bronchial tree. In the presence of bullae, there is always the potential for tension pneumothorax under positive pressure ventilation, and the creation of a bronchopleurocutaneous fistula after insertion of a chest drain.

Similar changes in size may occur during anaesthesia with liquid-filled cysts. There is the added risk of soiling parenchymal lung tissue elsewhere with the liquid should the cyst rupture.

BRONCHOPLEURAL FISTULA

Although most common after lung resection surgery, bronchopleural fistulae may occur after acute respiratory distress syndrome (ARDS) and any intrathoracic sepsis. The chest should be drained before induction of anaesthesia to reduce the amount of purulent fluid in the chest cavity and avoid the prospect of tension pneumothorax. Anaesthesia should be induced with the affected side dependent, followed by prompt endobronchial intubation of the main bronchus on the unaffected side, in order to isolate the healthy lung from contamination by purulent secretions from the affected side. One-lung ventilation allows surgery on the affected side. Should there still be lung tissue on the affected side, high-frequency jet ventilation offers a means of keeping inflated and ventilating lung tissue in the presence of a large air leak, with mean intrathoracic pressures lower than with conventional intermittent positive pressure ventilation.

TRACHEAL SURGERY

Unless cardiopulmonary bypass is used, there must be a changing sequence of means of ventilating the lungs during surgery and measures to keep the neck flexed after surgery to avoid tension on the tracheal repair before it heals.

Until the tracheal lesion is resected, airway obstruction must be overcome during the early stages of anaesthesia. Maintaining spontaneous ventilation initially allows assessment of the adequacy of assisted ventilation under anaesthesia. With the lesion exposed, ventilation of one or both lungs through an incision in the trachea distal to the lesion allows resection of the lesion and repair of the posterior wall of the trachea. A narrow tracheal or endobronchial tube passes through the larynx beyond the anastomotic site, and then allows space for repair of the anterior wall of the trachea. Suturing the chin to the skin over the sternum keeps the neck in flexion until the tracheal anastomosis heals.

TRACHEOSTOMY

The neck is extended by placing a sandbag under the shoulders and securing the head on a head ring. The pharynx should be aspirated when surgical dissection of the trachea is complete, because incision of the second and third tracheal rings frequently bursts the cuff on the tracheal tube. The tracheal tube is then withdrawn sufficiently far to allow insertion of the tracheostomy tube, but is not withdrawn from the trachea. This retains a means of ventilating the lung and a conduit into the trachea to replace the tracheal tube over a gum elastic bougie should initial attempts to introduce the tracheostomy tube be unsuccessful. When the tracheostomy tube is positioned correctly, it is connected to a sterile catheter mount within the draped area and then to the anaesthetic system, which may be draped subsequently. The sandbag is removed before the neck wound is sutured.

Pneumomediastinum and pneumothorax may occur intraoperatively because of damage to the posterior tracheal wall. Haemorrhage and damage to other structures may occur immediately, or later as a result of the effects of pressure from a malpositioned tracheostomy tube.

OESOPHAGEAL SURGERY

Oesophagectomy is often preceded by oesophagoscopy with all the attendant risks of pulmonary aspiration. Thoracic approaches to the oesophagus may require one-lung ventilation to provide access for surgery. Oesophagectomy may take some hours and be associated with considerable fluid loss into the wound and surrounding tissues.

After surgery, effective analgesia is necessary to enable the patient to expand the chest and cough effectively. Patients should be nursed sitting or supported on pillows to avoid regurgitation of gastrointestinal fluid and subsequent aspiration. Total parenteral nutrition is not required as a routine, but may be necessary in the presence of postoperative complications such as mediastinitis from an anastomotic leak.

POSTOPERATIVE CARE

Pulmonary function is impaired after thoracic surgery beyond any changes expected after lung resection. There is a 35% reduction in functional residual capacity after lung resection, which takes 6–8 weeks to recover to preoperative values. However, thoracic surgery patients should be able to breathe spontaneously immediately after anaesthesia and surgery. A need for mechanical ventilation after surgery is likely to result from problems in patient selection, or during surgery and anaesthesia intraoperatively. The advantages of mechanical ventilation can be obtained during surgery. The lungs may be expanded under direct vision of the pleural surface and the bronchial tree aspirated. A mini-tracheostomy tube may be inserted through the cricothyroid membrane at the end of surgery, with the trachea extubated and the lungs ventilated through a laryngeal mask, to help aspiration of the trachea of patients unable to cough effectively. Prolonged mechanical ventilation exposes thoracic patients to regional lung collapse and nosocomial pulmonary infection.

A high inspired oxygen concentration to overcome hypoxaemia is usually required for the first 24 h after surgery and during sleep at night until chest drains are removed (assessed by pulse oximetry). Patients breathing air with a P_aCO_2 greater than 6.0 kPa before surgery are at increased risk of ventilatory failure after surgery and require oxygen therapy tailored to response. Most other patients benefit from oxygen 40–60% by clear plastic face mask or nasal prongs.

The posterolateral thoracotomy wound is exceedingly painful. Untreated, each breath provokes pain. To minimize pain, respiration is rapid and shallow. Analgesia sufficient to permit deep inspiration and productive coughing without respiratory depression is necessary to restore adequate spontaneous ventilation after thoracic surgery. Continuous epidural analgesia or (if that is contraindicated) paravertebral nerve blockade is more likely to achieve these aims than systemic opioid analgesia. Epidural local anaesthetic or opioids, or mixtures of the two, may be infused through a catheter introduced between the fifth and eighth thoracic vertebrae, depending on the sites of wound and chest drains, and the size and alignment of the intervertebral spaces. Bupivacaine 0–15 mg h^{-1}, or fentanyl 0–50 μg h^{-1}, alone or in combination, may be given as continuous infusions or background infusions and additional patient-controlled demands.

After oesophageal surgery, oral fluids are withheld for some days whilst a nasogastric tube drains the stomach. After lung resection in the morning, patients may be able to manage some food in the evening. Fluids i.v. are required for the first 24 h, although less is given than after other forms of major surgery. Maintenance fluids are restricted to avoid pulmonary oedema in remaining lung tissue that has been handled or through which there is a relatively increased pulmonary artery flow after lung resection. Ringer lactate solution 10 ml kg^{-1} h^{-1} in theatre and dextrose/saline 1 ml kg^{-1} h^{-1} thereafter, with the equivalent of saline 0.9% 500 ml in 24 h, provide maintenance fluids; blood and colloid may be added to replace further losses and support the circulation.

Patients are likely to be cold after thoracic surgery as a result of lying in theatre covered only by sterile drapes and with the chest open during surgery. Simple means to conserve heat during surgery by warming i.v. fluids and humidification of inspired gases, followed by convective warming blankets in the recovery room, may restore body temperature to normal soon after surgery is finished.

FURTHER READING

Bastin R, Moraine J-T, Bardocsky G et al 1997 Incentive spirometry performance. Chest 111: 559–563

Benumof J L 1995 Anaesthesia for thoracic surgery, 2nd edn. W B Saunders, Philadelphia

Benumof J L, Alfery D D 2000 Anesthesia for thoracic surgery. In: Miller R D (ed) Anesthesia, 5th edn. Churchill Livingstone, Philadelphia, PA, pp 1665–1752

Schroeder D 1999 The preoperative period summary. Chest 115: 44–46S

Sherry K 1996 Management of patients undergoing oesophagectomy. The report of the National Confidential Enquiry into Perioperative Deaths 1996/1997. Nuffield Provincial Hospitals Trust, London, p 57–61

Shimizu T, Kinouchi K, Yoshiya I 1997 Arterial oxygenation during one lung ventilation. Canadian Journal of Anaesthesia 44: 1162–1166

Youngberg J A, Lake C L, Roizen M F, Wilson R S 2000 Cardiac, vascular and thoracic anaesthesia. Churhill Livingstone, Philadelphia

Zibrak J D, O'Donnell C R, Marton K 1990 Indications for pulmonary function testing. Annals of Internal Medicine 112: 763–71

59 Anaesthesia for cardiac surgery

The cardiac surgical theatre, with its profusion of personnel, monitors and support equipment, is often intimidating to the trainee anaesthetist. However, the principles of anaesthetic care are similar to those elsewhere, the principal difference being that essential organ perfusion is achieved artificially when the heart itself is the object of surgery. Operations are termed 'open heart' when the functions of the heart and lungs are assumed by an extracorporeal pump and gas exchange unit (cardiopulmonary bypass, CPB). During 'closed' operations, cardiac and pulmonary functions remain intact and anaesthetic management is similar to that for thoracic surgery.

Excluding the insertion of pacemakers, more than 30 000 cardiac operations are undertaken each year in the UK in NHS hospitals. These include approximately 3500 for congenital abnormalities, 5000 for acquired valvular disease and 28 000 for ischaemic heart disease.

CONGENITAL CARDIAC ABNORMALITIES

These occur at a rate of 6–8 per 1000 live births. Correction of a third may be undertaken by closed operation, but the remainder, including septal defects, valve abnormalities and cyanotic lesions such as Fallot's tetralogy, require CPB.

ACQUIRED VALVULAR DISEASE

Stenosis or incompetence occurs and most commonly involves the mitral and aortic valves. Surgery usually comprises replacement with an artificial valve. This may be a mechanical prosthesis with a tilting disc or a tissue valve (usually a pig valve) specially mounted and prepared (heterograft). Prosthetic valves are reliable but necessitate the patient receiving anticoagulants for life. This is not usually necessary when porcine heterografts are used, but re-operation is common due to valve failure after about 10 years.

ISCHAEMIC HEART DISEASE

The concept of revascularizing ischaemic myocardium was introduced nearly 30 years ago with the insertion of a portion of saphenous vein from aorta to coronary artery distal to a stenosis (Fig. 59.1). Since then, coronary artery bypass grafting (CABG) has become the most commonly performed cardiac operation. The internal mammary artery is routinely used as a graft conduit. Complete arterial revascularization is increasingly common, using arteries such as the radial and epigastric arteries.

Angina is relieved in 80–90% of patients, but life expectancy is not increased in all groups when compared with medical treatment. Short-term prognosis is improved by surgery only in patients with disease of the left main coronary artery or its two principal branches, triple-vessel disease or impaired left ventricular function, but this improvement is not sustained.

Surgical options in the treatment of ischaemic heart disease have increased with the advent of new techniques such as coronary artery surgery without CPB, minimally invasive cardiac surgery and transmyocardial laser revascularization. Excluding the laser

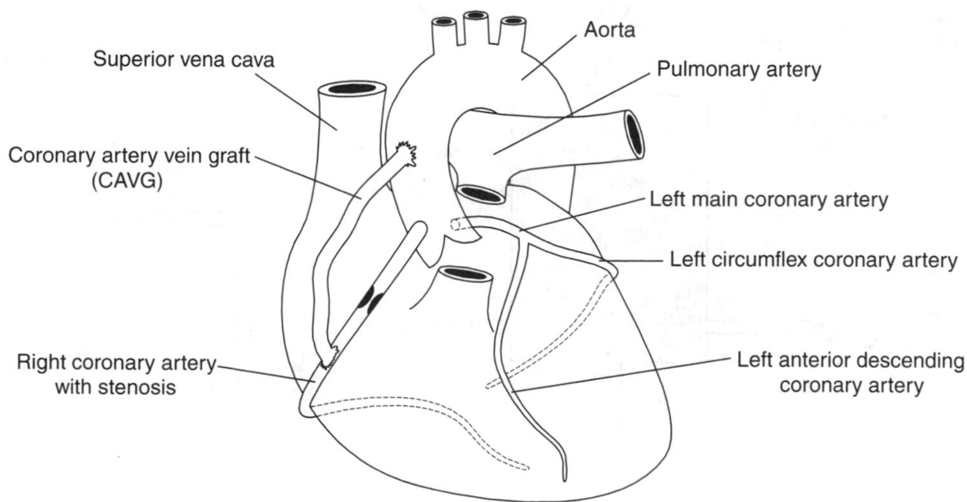

Fig. 59.1
Diagrammatic representation of coronary arteries and CAVG. 'Triple' vessel disease includes right, left circumflex and left anterior descending arteries.

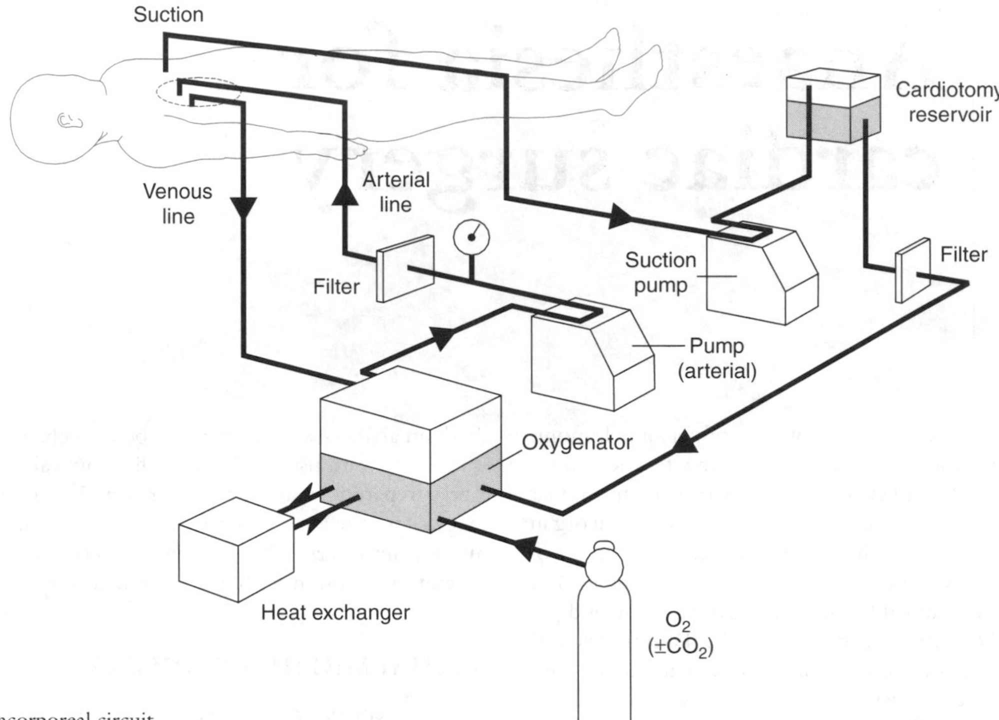

Fig. 59.2
Components of extracorporeal circuit.

procedure, these operations involve cardiac surgery on a beating heart and/or the use of parasternal incisions or multiple laparoscopic ports with video assistance. Anaesthetic management of all these newer procedures is broadly similar to that detailed later in this chapter, but haemodynamic instability caused by handling of the heart or severe ventricular dysfunction is more common.

EXTRACORPOREAL CIRCULATION (ECC)

The essential components of ECC comprise:

- pumps
- an oxygenator
- connecting tubes and filters
- fluid prime of these components.

These are normally arranged as shown in Figure 59.2. Blood from the venous side of the circulation, the venae cavae or right atrium, is drained by gravity to a venous reservoir and thence to a gas exchange unit (oxygenator) where oxygen is delivered to, and carbon dioxide removed from, the blood. The 'arterialized' blood is pumped into the arterial side of the circulation, usually into the ascending aorta. The heart and lungs are thus 'bypassed' or isolated and their function maintained temporarily by mechanical equipment remote from the body. A heat exchanger in the oxygenator varies the temperature of blood rapidly and redundant or spilled blood in or around the bypassed heart can be drained and returned to the venous reservoir for oxygenation and subsequent return to the circulation.

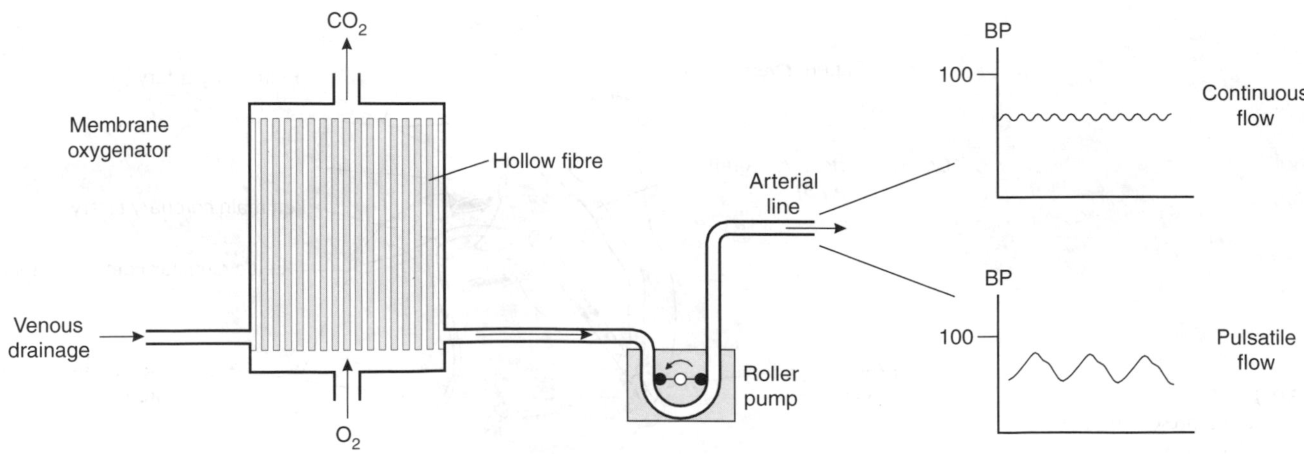

Fig. 59.3
Diagrammatic representation of a membrane oxygenator.

Pumps

Roller pumps displace blood around the circuit by intermittent compression of the circuit tubing during each sweep. By intermittent acceleration of the roller head, a 'pulsatile' waveform may be achieved, but there is no evidence that this more physiological flow improves overall outcome.

Oxygenator

Membrane oxygenators (Fig. 59.3) comprise a semipermeable membrane which separates gas and blood phases and through which gas exchange occurs. They cause less damage to blood components than bubble oxygenators, which are now used infrequently.

Connecting tubes, filters, manometer, suction

These must be sterile and non-toxic and should damage blood as little as possible. Increasingly, they are coated with heparin. A filter should also be incorporated in the arterial line to remove gas emboli which would pass directly to the aorta. Suction pumps are supplied to vent blood collecting in the pulmonary circulation or left ventricle during bypass and also to remove spilled blood from the pericardial sac. The blood is collected in the 'cardiotomy' reservoir, filtered and returned to the main circuit. This suction also causes damage to blood components.

Fluid prime

Originally it was anticipated that connection of the circulation to an external circuit would necessitate the extracorporeal circuit being filled with anticoagulated whole blood. This increases exposure to donor blood and may lead to incompatibility reactions. However, it became clear that this was unnecessary as the body tolerates a relatively low haematocrit. When CPB is commenced and the patient's blood is mixed with an ECC comprising clear fluid (fluid prime), the haematocrit decreases to approximately 20–25%. Although oxygen content is reduced, availability may be increased by improved organ blood flow resulting from reduced blood viscosity. In some patients (low body weight, children or those with a low preoperative haemoglobin in whom dilution would reduce the haematocrit to below 20%), blood may be added to the prime. In the normal adult, 'clear' primes are used almost exclusively (usually compound sodium lactate solution). Most units have individual recipes for addition to the prime (e.g. colloid solutions, mannitol, sodium bicarbonate and potassium) to achieve an isosmolar solution of physiological pH.

PREOPERATIVE ASSESSMENT

Most patients presenting for cardiac surgery have undergone comprehensive cardiological investigation and are taking medications. In addition to the routine investigations undertaken before any operation, specialized techniques are used to assess the cardiac lesion and degree of resultant dysfunction. The results of these investigations permit the anaesthetist to identify patients at particular risk where extra care and monitoring are required.

EXERCISE ELECTROCARDIOGRAPHY

Various stress protocols are used whereby a standard exercise test provokes ischaemic changes and symptoms. Changes in rhythm, rate, arterial pressure and conduction are recorded. The anaesthetist identifies the most useful ECG leads to monitor during surgery and may note the rate–pressure product (heart rate × systolic arterial pressure) at which ischaemia occurs, although this is unreliable under anaesthesia.

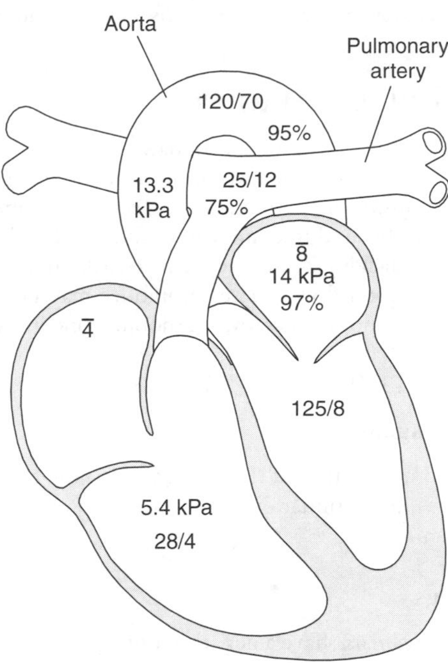

Fig. 59.4
Diagram of catherization values in a normal adult: pressures (mmHg), oxygen saturations (%) and tensions (kPa).

CARDIAC CATHETERIZATION

Considerable information may be obtained from catheterization:

- Evidence of failing function or of gradients across stenosed valves may be identified by pressure monitoring.
- Oximetry of blood at different sites indicates if shunts are present (Fig. 59.4).
- Cardiac output may be measured.
- The injection of radio-opaque dye into aorta or ventricles assesses incompetence of valves and the efficiency of ventricular contraction (ejection fraction) and wall motion:

$$\text{Ejection fraction (EF)} = \frac{\text{end-diastolic volume} - \text{end-systolic volume}}{\text{end-diastolic volume}}$$

- Injection of dye into coronary arteries defines the anatomy of the coronary circulation and the degree of patency or sites of stenosis.

ECHOCARDIOGRAPHY

Ultrasound is used to identify myocardial motion and valvular function. Preoperatively, this may be performed using a transthoracic or trans-oesophageal approach. The latter involves passing an ultrasound probe into the oesophagus under sedation. The proximity of the heart and oesophagus allows high-quality 'real time' images of the anatomy and function of the heart. Doppler techniques allow recognition of the direction and velocity of blood flow and are valuable in the diagnosis of acute valvular disease, e.g. failure of a prosthetic valve.

RADIONUCLIDE IMAGING

By imaging the activity of an appropriate radioisotope as it passes through the heart or into the myocardium, ventricular function and myocardial perfusion may be assessed. Technetium images blood volume and may be used to demonstrate abnormal wall motion and EF. Thallium, which is taken up by the myocardium, may be used to assess regional blood flow. These techniques may be used before and after exercise and/or therapy, e.g. dobutamine infusion.

PREOPERATIVE DRUG THERAPY

β-Blocking agents

Continued administration of these drugs up to the time of surgery is desirable, as discontinuation may increase the risk of preoperative infarction.

Other drugs

Calcium antagonists. have a negative inotropic effect but, as with the β-blockers, it is preferable to continue therapy throughout the perioperative period
Nitrates should be continued and may be included in the premedication if indicated.
Digitalis. In most centres, digoxin is discontinued 24–48 h before surgery to diminish digoxin-associated arrhythmias after surgery.
Diuretics should be continued until the day before surgery.
Anticoagulants, including aspirin, are usually stopped several days before surgery to permit coagulation to return towards normal. If there is a high risk of embolism, anticoagulants should be continued and coagulation defects treated postoperatively with transfusion of blood products.
Angiotensin-converting enzyme (ACE) inhibitors are prescribed for hypertension and cardiac failure. They can produce significant vasodilatation and hypotension intraoperatively. Perioperative use varies from unit to unit – they may be stopped up to 1 week before surgery or continued until the day of operation.
Potassium-channel activators are increasingly prescribed for the treatment of angina and these may be continued up to the day of operation.

OTHER INVESTIGATIONS BEFORE SURGERY

Haemoglobin

Haemoglobin should be adequate (> 11 g dl^{-1}) to prevent excessive haemodilution during bypass.

Coagulation

Clotting studies should be performed before surgery. Specific defects require correction before surgery, or alternatively the appropriate blood products should be made available.

Electrolytes

Serum potassium concentration should be within normal limits.

Urea and creatinine

Raised concentrations indicate an increased risk of renal failure postoperatively. Adequate urine output should be ensured after operation.

Liver function tests

Abnormal values may indicate congestive cardiac failure.

ASSESSMENT OF RISK

The mortality rate associated with cardiac surgery is diminishing but is still significant. Operative mortality for coronary artery surgery is relatively constant at 2–3%, but valve surgery is usually associated with a mortality of 3–10%. When more extensive surgery is undertaken, e.g. multiple valve replacement or coronary artery vein graft (CAVG) plus valve replacement, mortality rate increases.

Patients with an increased risk of perioperative complications may be identified during preoperative assessment. Increased risk is associated with the following factors:

- age > 65 years
- female sex
- recent unstable angina or myocardial infarction
- emergency surgery or re-operation
- poor left ventricular function as shown by:
  - — left ventricular end-diastolic pressure > 18 mmHg
  - — ejection fraction < 30%
  - — dyskinetic wall motion
- increasing number of vessels affected
- other system disease, e.g. diabetes mellitus, cerebrovascular and peripheral vascular disease, renal failure and obesity.

MONITORING

Extensive and accurate monitoring is essential throughout the perioperative period for the safe practice of cardiac surgery.

ECG

ECG should be monitored throughout the perioperative period. The ideal system is one which allows simultaneous multiple lead monitoring or at least switching between leads II and V5, for accurate identification of ischaemia. Rate and rhythm should also be observed.

Systemic arterial pressure

Arterial cannulation is mandatory, and not only permits direct measurement but also facilitates sampling of arterial blood for analysis. The preferred site is a radial artery.

Central venous and left atrial pressures

Right-sided filling pressure should be monitored by a catheter placed into the superior vena cava.

Controversy persists regarding the necessity to monitor left heart filling pressure in all patients via a flow-directed pulmonary artery catheter (PAC) inserted at or before induction. In some countries, there is enthusiasm for commencing full invasive monitoring before anaesthesia, but most anaesthetists in the UK undertake this only in poor-risk patients.

Cardiac output

Cardiac output (CO) may be measured by thermodilution using a PAC. Calculation of cardiac output and cardiac index, together with the derivatives of stroke work, pulmonary and systemic vascular resistances and tissue oxygen flux, permits the most accurate assessment of cardiological therapy. Modified PACs allow the real-time measurement of CO, mixed venous oxygen saturation and right ventricular function.

CO may also be measured by Doppler techniques using specialized oesophageal probes, but this is less accurate than thermodilution techniques.

Echocardiography

During anaesthesia, trans-oesophageal echocardiography is very useful. Abnormal motion of the ventricular wall detected in this way is a reliable index of myocardial ischaemia and can guide drug therapy or indicate the need for further surgical revascularization. Doppler techniques may be useful during valve surgery, e.g. to determine if an incompetent mitral valve has been adequately repaired.

EEG

A simple guide to cerebral activity and perfusion may be obtained from the various forms of processed EEG monitor. Interpretation is difficult in the hypothermic patient and the value of this technique is uncertain. Similar caveats apply to the monitoring of evoked potentials.

Temperature

Core temperature should be monitored from the nasopharynx, which approximates to brain temperature. Core–peripheral temperature gradients may give some guide to peripheral perfusion.

Biochemical and haematological analysis

Facilities should be available for immediate analysis of blood gas tensions, acid–base balance, serum potassium and blood glucose concentrations.

Measurement of packed cell volume and coagulation status should also be available. Activated clotting time (ACT) can be measured quickly in the operating theatre using the Haemochron apparatus (normal = 100–120 s), but access to the haematology laboratory should be rapid for assessment of a full clotting screen. Thromboelastography – the assessment of viscoelastic changes in blood during clotting – is increasingly used to assess haemostatic function in theatre.

Display

ECG, pressure waveforms and a digital output of heart rate and pressures should be displayed clearly on a screen visible to both surgeon and anaesthetist.

PATHOPHYSIOLOGICAL CONSIDERATIONS

The anaesthetist should have a clear understanding of the fundamental principles of cardiac physiology. Accurate monitoring reveals alterations in cardiac function and permits the anaesthetist to manipulate factors which ensure adequate pump output (Fig. 59.5) and myocardial blood supply.

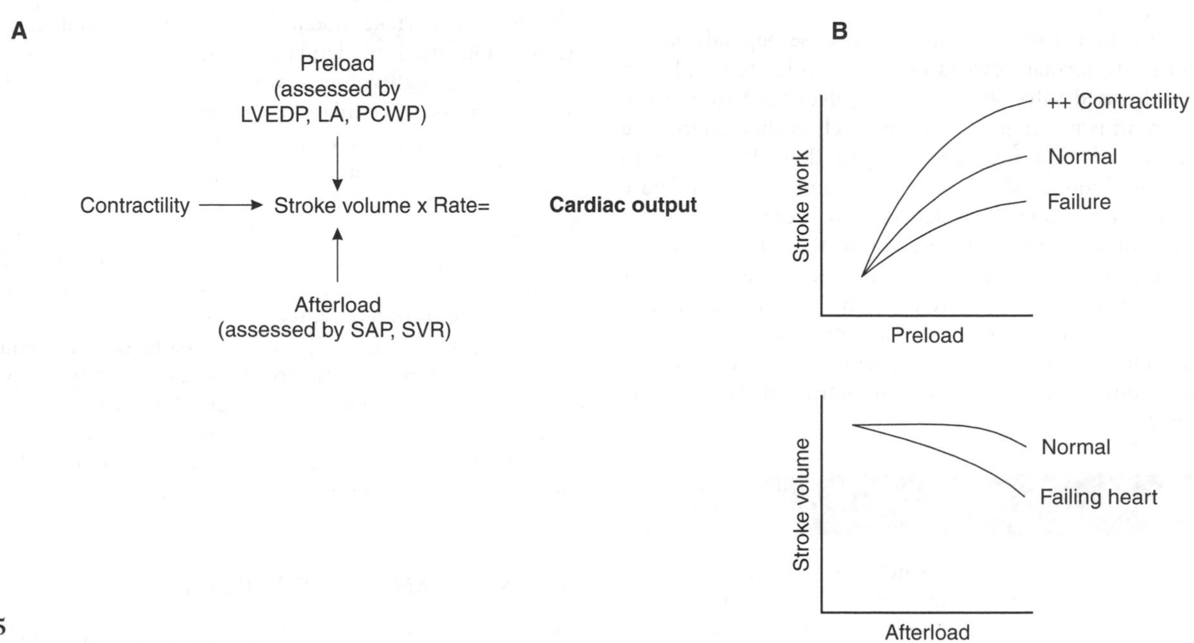

Fig. 59.5
Important aspetcs of mechanical function.

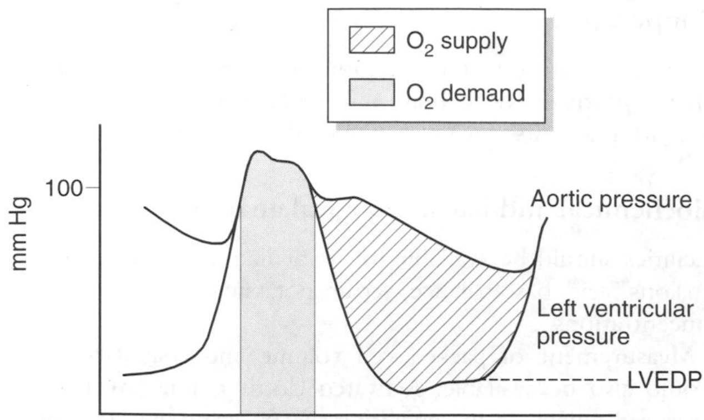

Fig. 59.6
The factors which determine myocardial oxygen supply and demand.

Preload and contractility determine the amount of work that the heart can perform. In the failing heart, the afterload determines how much work is expended in overcoming pressure compared with that used to provide forward flow. Thus cardiac output may be increased either by increasing preload or contractility, or by reducing afterload. However, oxygen consumption is raised by increasing heart rate, contractility, preload or afterload. Augmentation of cardiac output by increasing preload or contractility may thus have a detrimental effect on oxygen balance. However, reduction of afterload may increase cardiac output while simultaneously reducing oxygen demand.

Adequate coronary perfusion demands maintenance of diastolic aortic pressure at adequate levels. Oxygen supply to the myocardium occurs predominantly in diastole and is dependent on the gradient between diastolic aortic pressure and intraventricular pressure, and on the diastolic time. The portion of myocardium most at risk of developing ischaemia is the left ventricular endocardium. Figure 59.6 illustrates how these variables bear on oxygen supply and demand in the myocardium and how a satisfactory supply/demand ratio may be preserved.

Care of the patient with valvular heart disease depends on the valvular lesion. Abnormal heart rates are not tolerated well by a heart with a diseased valve. Incompetent valves tend to perform better if afterload is maintained at a low level, as this reduces the regurgitant fraction and increases forward flow. Patients with valvular stenosis require adequate preload and do not tolerate rapid reduction in peripheral resistance. This is especially true of patients with aortic stenosis where most of the afterload to left ventricular ejection is caused by the stenosed valve itself. This afterload is fixed and cannot be reduced by lowering peripheral resistance. Vasodilatation in these patients produces marked hypotension and results in failure of perfusion of the hypertrophied myocardium with no increase in forward flow through the stenosed valve.

ANAESTHETIC TECHNIQUE

There is no single preferred anaesthetic technique for cardiac surgery. The choice of a specific agent is less important than the care with which the drug is administered and its effects monitored.

PREMEDICATION

The most important preoperative preparation comprises a full explanation to patients of what is about to occur and their development of rapport with, and confidence in, the nursing and medical staff.

Most patients (particularly those with poor cardiovascular reserve) may be sedated preoperatively with an oral benzodiazepine (lorazepam 2–4 mg or temazepam 20–50 mg). In the particularly anxious patient, heavy sedation may be required to prevent increases in heart rate and arterial pressure before operation. A combination of an oral benzodiazepine and an intramuscular opioid is satisfactory. Patients receiving glyceryl trinitrate (GTN) may benefit from its administration as a transdermal patch at the time of premedication.

INDUCTION

All drugs and equipment should be ready and the theatre and bypass circuit available for immediate use before the patient arrives in the anaesthetic room.

Before induction, ECG electrodes should be applied and the ECG trace displayed. Arterial and large-gauge venous cannulae should be inserted under local anaesthesia. The lungs should be preoxygenated.

Induction may be achieved in a variety of ways. The standard agents may be given in small doses (e.g. thiopental 1–3 mg kg^{-1}, etomidate 0.05–0.2 mg kg^{-1}), or large doses of an opioids (e.g. morphine 1–4 mg kg^{-1}, fentanyl 10–100 μg kg^{-1}) may be administered with a benzodiazepine to obtain unconsciousness. A combination of these techniques may be used; consciousness is obtunded by an opioid in moderate dose and hypnosis is then produced by a small dose of an induction agent. An alternative is a target-controlled infusion of propofol with the target concentration increased in small steps, perhaps accompanied by an infusion of a short-acting opioid such as alfentanil or remifentanil.

As consciousness is lost, a muscle relaxant is administered and ventilation supported when necessary. Almost all currently available relaxants have been used during cardiac surgery. The objective is to undertake tracheal intubation without cardiovascular stimulation and thus adequate analgesia/anaesthesia is required. A low-pressure high-volume cuffed tracheal tube should be used. Positive pressure ventilation is continued, usually with an oxygen/air mixture or 50% nitrous oxide in oxygen.

Percutaneous cannulation of a subclavian or internal jugular vein is performed using a multilumen catheter to allow monitoring and infusion. Nasopharyngeal and peripheral temperature probes are applied and a urinary catheter inserted. Mechanical ventilation is continued with a breathing system containing a humidifier and bacterial filter.

Previously identified 'poor risk' patients may require more extensive monitoring of pressures and cardiac output before induction and catheters are inserted under local anaesthesia. Induction should be undertaken in theatre with the full team ready for immediate surgery. Adequate sedation must be provided during insertion of invasive monitoring catheters.

MAINTENANCE – PRE-BYPASS

During this period, surgical procedure involves preparation of the patient, skin incision, sternotomy and insertion of arterial and venous bypass cannulae. Anaesthetic management is designed to maintain stability of heart rate and arterial pressure, particularly at moments of profound stimulation, notably skin incision and sternotomy. If a technique based on i.v. opioids or volatile anaesthetics has been chosen, then additional i.v. analgesic drug or inhalation anaesthetic should be given before stimulation, remembering that the negative inotropic actions of volatile anaesthetics may be undesirable in those with poor ventricular function. The tendency of isoflurane to produce a 'coronary steal' (the diversion of blood *away from* ischaemic muscle) is not of clinical importance when it is part of a balanced anaesthetic technique and provided hypotension is avoided. Alternatively, the infusion rates of alfentanil or remifentanil may be increased temporarily as necessary, perhaps accompanied by increased target concentrations of propofol.

Arterial blood gas tensions, serum potassium concentration, haematocrit and the activated clotting time (ACT) should be measured when surgery is under way and conditions are stable. Before cannulation for bypass lines, heparin (300 units kg^{-1}; 3 mg kg^{-1}) should be injected into a secure central catheter of proven patency. In some units, the surgeon injects heparin directly into the left atrium before cannulation. ACT measurement should be repeated 3 min after injection of heparin; the value should exceed four times normal. Cardioplegia should be prepared and stored at 4°C.

When preparations are complete, the bypass pump commences and circulation is assumed by the extracorporeal circuit.

MAINTENANCE – ON BYPASS

Two factors complicate the provision of anaesthesia during cardiopulmonary bypass. Firstly, haemodilution, hypotension, non-pulsatile flow and hypothermia may alter the pharmacokinetics of drugs administered previously. Secondly, by short-circuiting the lungs, bypass prevents conventional inhalation anaesthesia. Techniques therefore include administration of bolus doses of an opioid or benzodiazepine, administration of a volatile agent into the gas flow of the oxygenator or continuous intravenous infusion of propofol. Additional doses of muscle relaxant may also be given. When full pump oxygenator flow is reached and ventricular ejection ceases, ventilation is suspended.

Surgery is preceded usually by cross-clamping the aorta to isolate the heart and prevent backflow. In the case of valvular surgery, the appropriate valve is exposed, excised and a new valve sutured in place. During coronary artery vein grafting, the distal anastomoses are usually completed first and, following release of the cross-clamp to permit restoration of myocardial perfusion, the proximal anastomoses are constructed using a portion of the aorta isolated by a side-clamp (Fig. 59.7).

Myocardial preservation

Most surgical techniques on the heart require an immobile heart. On bypass, the aorta is cross-clamped between the aortic cannula and the aortic valve, thus isolating the heart from the flow of oxygenated blood. During aortic cross-clamping, ischaemic damage to the myocardium can be minimized by attempts to reduce myocardial oxygen consumption. Currently, techniques of myocardial preservation include hypothermia to reduce basal metabolic rate and cardiac arrest to reduce oxygen requirements to a minimum, the latter usually achieved by injecting 500–1000 ml of crystalloid cardioplegic solution around the coronary arteries. Many cardioplegic solutions are available; the majority contain potassium and a membrane-stabilizing agent, e.g. procaine. Some centres infuse warm blood-based cardioplegic and reperfusate solutions continuously to minimize ischaemic and reperfusion injuries and improve delivery of oxygen and other substrates to the myocardium.

Cooling is achieved by the use of ice-cold cardioplegia and by pouring cold fluid (4°C) into the pericardial sac and into the heart chambers if they have been opened. If the heart is cooled to 15°C, it withstands total ischaemia for approximately 1 h. The technique used most commonly at present involves moderate hypothermia of

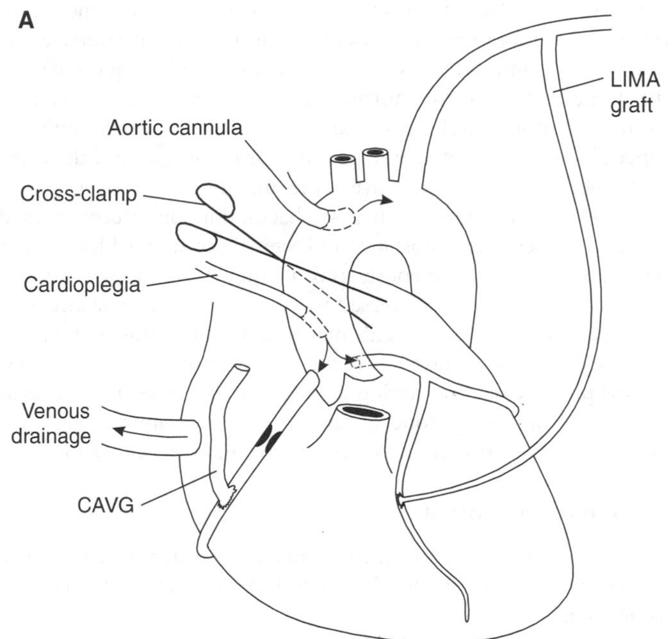

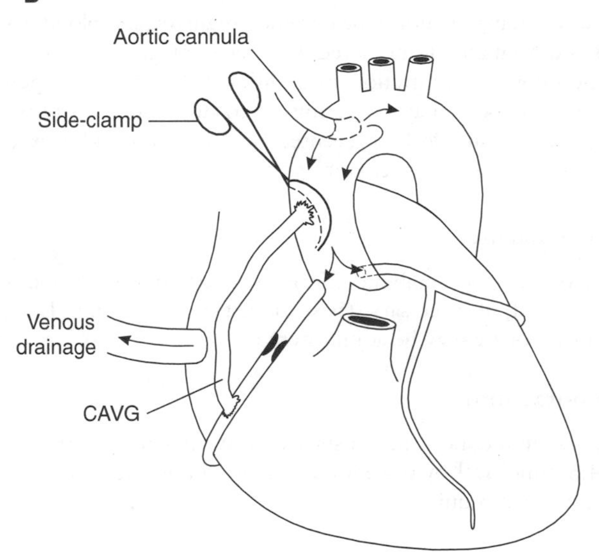

Fig. 59.7
Arrangement of cross-clamp, cardioplegia and anastomoses. **A** A left internal mammary artery (LIMA) graft **B** Vein graft with side clamp on aorta.

the body to 32°C and local cooling of the myocardium to a temperature of 15–18°C. If cross-clamping times are prolonged, cardioplegic cooling must be repeated if spontaneous cardiac contraction resumes.

A modification to this traditional technique has been the combination of local cooling of the heart with body temperatures of 33–37°C during CPB in an attempt to limit postoperative hypothermia.

Perfusion on bypass

At normothermia, a pump flow of 2.4 L min^{-1} m^{-2} of body surface area is required to prevent inadequate perfusion of the tissues. The pressure achieved within the vascular system is dependent on pump output and systemic vascular resistance. Controversy exists regarding optimum perfusion pressure, as essential organs, particularly the brain, may be damaged if mean arterial pressure is < 45 mmHg. Unfortunately, perfusion is difficult to assess clinically, especially in the hypothermic patient. Urine output and the cerebral function monitor may give some guidance.

Following the onset of bypass, haemodilution causes marked decreases in peripheral resistance and arterial pressure, which in most instances resolve spontaneously in 5–10 min. If this does not occur, arterial pressure may be increased by raising systemic resistance with a sympathomimetic agent, e.g. methoxamine 1–5 mg by bolus or phenylephrine by infusion. Frequently, peripheral resistance and arterial pressure increase during the hypothermic period of bypass as a result of increasing concentrations of catecholamines and then decrease as active rewarming results in profound vasodilatation.

Coagulation control

Adequate anticoagulation must be maintained during CPB; ACT should be measured every 30 min and extra heparin administered as necessary.

Oxygen delivery

Arterial blood samples should be obtained regularly and blood gas tensions and haematocrit measured. Oxygen carriage is dependent on haemoglobin concentration in addition to adequate oxygen tension. Haematocrit may be permitted to decrease to 20% but further reduction should be prevented by the addition of packed cells or blood to the bypass circuit.

Acid–base balance

The development of metabolic acidosis suggests that perfusion is inadequate and, if necessary (base deficit > 6–8 mmol L^{-1}), sodium bicarbonate may be administered.

Serum potassium

Serum potassium concentration should be maintained at approximately 4.5 mmol L^{-1} by the administration of potassium chloride (10–20 mmol) as required.

RESTORATION OF SPONTANEOUS HEARTBEAT

When the cross-clamp has been removed, oxygenated blood again flows into the coronary arteries, washing out cardioplegia and repaying the oxygen debt. Usually, the heart regains activity spontaneously. In a minority of patients, it starts to beat in sinus rhythm but reverts usually to ventricular fibrillation; internal defibrillation is required to convert fibrillation to sinus rhythm and is successful only if pH, serum potassium concentration, oxygenation and temperature are approaching normal values. The heat exchanger in the oxygenator is used to raise the temperature of blood, but peripheral temperature is often depressed for some time. If a spontaneous heartbeat cannot be maintained, pacing wires should be attached to the epicardium to initiate activity artificially.

At this stage, full bypass is maintained and although the heart is beating, there is little ejection from the ventricles. It is wise at this time to pause, ensure that all air has been vented from the heart chambers, wait until core temperature exceeds 36°C and rest the heart before it is required to pump again.

TERMINATION OF BYPASS

When body temperature exceeds 36°C, metabolic indices are normal and a regular heartbeat is present, the establishment of spontaneous cardiac output is attempted. An increasing volume of venous return is diverted into the right atrium past the extracorporeal cannulae by constricting the venous return catheter to the pump. Blood is now passing again through the pulmonary circulation and mechanical ventilation should be restarted; 100% oxygen is given, as the gas-exchanging efficiency of the lung is unknown at this stage and any air bubbles which have not been vented enlarge in volume if nitrous oxide is introduced.

Any output or ejection from the left ventricle gives a 'blip' on the arterial pressure trace after a QRS complex. If the myocardium is contracting satisfactorily, pump flow is reduced cautiously and the heart, now receiving all the venous return, achieves normal output. At this time, small doses of ephedrine, epinephrine or calcium chloride may provide a temporary inotropic stimulus.

Arterial pressure is the most easily measured index of successful termination of bypass but is a derivative of cardiac output and peripheral resistance. If there is doubt regarding pump efficiency, cardiac output should be measured and peripheral resistance derived.

If CPB is discontinued successfully, preload should be optimized (left atrial pressure 12–15 mmHg) by infusion of as much as possible of the residual fluid contained in the pump circuit. This is facilitated by the administration of vasodilators such as GTN. If cardiac output is inadequate, the circulation is reassumed by the extracorporeal pump and the heart allowed more time to recover.

Low output

If the heart is unable to generate sufficient output to maintain body perfusion after preload has been optimized, further action is required. An increase in contractility is produced by inotropic drugs. The simplest is a bolus of dilute epinephrine, but the most commonly used drugs are dobutamine, dopamine (both 2–20 μg kg^{-1} min^{-1}) or epinephrine (0.05–0.2 μg kg^{-1} min^{-1}) by infusion. If heart rate is slow, isoproterenol (0.02–0.2 μg kg^{-1} min^{-1}) may be indicated in some patients.

All these drugs tend to precipitate tachyarrhythmias; epinephrine and dopamine also cause vasoconstriction in high doses. They all increase myocardial oxygen demand and may precipitate infarction in patients with ischaemic heart disease.

Alternatively, a phosphodiesteras inhibitor may be given. These drugs act by inhibiting phosphodiesterase type III found in cardiac muscle, thus reducing the breakdown of cyclic AMP. Milrinone and enoximone are the most commonly used examples. They improve myocardial performance and are potent arterial and venous dilators. By reducing afterload, they not only reduce myocardial oxygen demand but also, in the failing ventricle, augment forward flow into the aorta. Administration is by bolus dose during CPB after aortic cross-clamp removal and subsequently by intravenous infusion. If ventricular dysfunction is severe, the phosphodiesterase inhibitors can be combined with a catecholamine as the two groups of drugs have complementary actions.

If these pharmacological methods fail to produce an adequate cardiac output, the intra-aortic balloon pump (IABP) may be used.

Intra-aortic balloon pump

The principle of the IABP is illustrated in Figure 59.8. If the balloon in the aorta is inflated immediately after systole, diastolic filling pressure is augmented and myocardial oxygen balance improved. Inflation also displaces blood from the aorta and increases peripheral flow. The balloon is deflated immediately before systole and this creates a low pressure in the aorta as ventricular output commences, reducing afterload (and thus oxygen consumption) and at the same time augmenting output.

COAGULATION CONTROL

When the bypass cannulae have been removed, residual effects of heparin are antagonized with protamine. Protamine 1 mg (or less) is given for each 100 units of heparin; the dosage may be titrated using the ACT. The drug should be given slowly, especially if there is residual hypovolaemia or raised pulmonary vascular resistance. Protamine may produce systemic hypotension rapidly, as a result of peripheral vasodilatation, but may also cause pulmonary vasoconstriction. In excessive dosage, it has anticoagulant effects.

Heparin is not the only factor which may cause bleeding during and after bypass. Contact of blood with foreign surfaces in the bypass circuit and suction tubing causes consumption of clotting factors and of platelets. Thus, if heparin appears to have been reversed satisfactorily and unexplained bleeding persists, a full clotting screen should be performed, including estimation of platelet numbers. Clotting factors may be replaced by the infusion of fresh frozen plasma and/or cryoprecipitate and platelet concentrate should be infused if the platelet count is less than $60 \times 10^9 L^{-1}$.

Surgically, the period following termination of bypass is concerned with prevention of haemorrhage and closure of the chest with drains in situ. In addition to the maintenance of unconsciousness, the anaesthetist must ensure the efficiency of myocardial performance, oxygen balance and peripheral perfusion together with correction of metabolic, biochemical, haematological or temperature abnormalities.

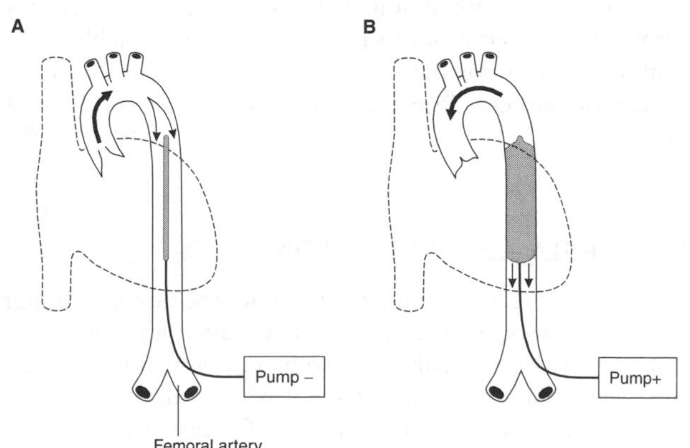

Fig. 59.8
Intra-aortic balloon pump. **A.** Systole. **B.** Diastole.

CONTROL OF THE CIRCULATION AFTER BYPASS

Despite measures to protect the myocardium during bypass, the heart suffers some deterioration in function and its contractility is reduced for 8–24 h. Thus, it operates on a lower Frank–Starling curve (see Fig. 59.5) and requires a higher preload to produce the same output. The contractility of the myocardium later improves and this increased efficiency permits a reduction in preload.

In addition, the peripheral circulation usually remains vasoconstricted for several hours postoperatively. In patients with reasonable ventricular function, hypertension may thus occur after bypass, especially in operations involving the aortic valve. The increased afterload results in additional myocardial oxygen consumption and tends to reduce cardiac output.

Reduction of peripheral resistance and systemic arterial pressure by a vasodilator (e.g. sodium nitroprusside or GTN) protects suture lines from damage, decreases oxygen demand, increases cardiac output if preload is not reduced excessively, improves peripheral perfusion and accelerates warming.

Conversely, some patients are very vasodilated after CPB, with cardiac output normal or even increased. This reflects a whole-body inflammatory response to CPB with the release of numerous vasoactive mediators. Treatment is with a norepinephrine infusion.

OTHER ASPECTS OF MAINTENANCE AFTER BYPASS

In addition to maintaining cardiac function and oxygen supply to the tissues during this period, the anaesthetist should ensure that normality is regained as soon as possible, and maintained, in respect of the following.

Temperature

Core temperature is raised easily on bypass via the oxygenator. However, the efficiency of rewarming the peripheral tissues depends on the patient's weight, total flow rate and peripheral perfusion. After bypass, there is often a decrease in core temperature (after-drop).

Biochemical monitoring

Essential monitoring includes blood gas tensions, acid–base balance, serum potassium concentration and haematocrit.

Cardiac rhythm

Heart block

Epicardial pacing lines should be inserted if AV dissociation occurs, traditionally to allow ventricular pacing. Atrial pacing (for bradycardia) or AV sequential pacing (for heart block) ensures that the atrial contribution to ventricular filling is not lost. Infusion of isoprenaline may improve ventricular rate as a temporary measure.

Supraventricular arrhythmias

Direct current cardioversion is the most convenient treatment when the chest is open. After chest closure, options include amiodarone, β-blockade, verapamil, adenosine or digoxin.

Ventricular arrhythmias

The threshold for arrhythmias is reduced by hypokalaemia and serum potassium concentration should be maintained above 4.5 mmol L^{-1}. If ventricular arrhythmias persist, lidocaine is the drug of first choice.

TRANSFER TO POSTOPERATIVE ITU

It is normal to prolong the same level of support and monitoring undertaken during surgery into the postoperative period. The duration of this care depends on the individual patient's response to surgery and speed of recovery.

Transfer of the patient from theatre to the intensive care unit may involve journeys along corridors and into lifts. It is essential that controlled ventilation is continued and ECG, arterial oxygen saturation and arterial pressure monitored during transfer. Battery-powered infusion pumps are essential to allow uninterrupted vasoactive drug infusions during transfer.

POSTOPERATIVE INTENSIVE THERAPY

The facilities and staff used to treat patients after cardiac surgery vary considerably. Some hospitals nurse these patients in a general ITU or specialist cardiac ITU, while others have cardiac surgery recovery areas where early tracheal extubation is normal.

Regardless of location, there should be a well-practised routine for the care of patients after surgery. Usually, ventilation of the lungs and full cardiovascular monitoring are recommenced immediately. The principles of care in this phase are similar to those described for the period of anaesthesia after termination of bypass.

HAEMODYNAMIC CARE

On return to ITU, attention is usually directed towards achieving vasodilatation, reduction of afterload and maintenance of preload. Blood transfusion is required if the haematocrit is less than 35%. Urine output may be maintained with diuretics, but usually a spontaneous diuresis occurs in response to the crystalloid load received in theatre. Serum potassium concentration must be monitored carefully and abnormalities corrected.

The majority of patients stabilize and regain adequate peripheral perfusion over the succeeding 3–4 h, permitting the level of cardiovascular support to be reduced.

In a minority of patients, low cardiac output requires the continued use of inotropic agents, vasodilators and, if necessary, IABP for some time.

BLOOD LOSS

This should be measured accurately. If excessive (300–400 ml h^{-1}), it may be necessary to re-operate on the patient. Attention to the coagulation system is required and additional protamine or coagulation factors prescribed as necessary. The most sinister complication of excessive bleeding is cardiac tamponade, which requires rapid thoracotomy and evacuation of blood from the chest. If deterioration occurs rapidly, thoracotomy must be undertaken in the ITU.

VENTILATION

In the 1960s, morphine anaesthesia for valve surgery in patients with poor ventricular function dictated that postoperative ventilation was required for 18–24 h. Later, the aims of postoperative ventilation were to avoid shivering following hypothermic bypass and to prevent hypoxaemia and hypercapnia during the period of haemodynamic instability which is common in the first few postoperative hours. These aims were generally achieved by assisting ventilation for 4–8 h and this remains current practice in most units. Thus, when the patient's arterial pressure, peripheral perfusion and core and peripheral temperatures are satisfactory, urine output is good, blood loss is less than 100 ml h^{-1}, and the patient is conscious and can maintain satisfactory blood gases with an inspired oxygen concentration of 50% or less, a trial of spontaneous ventilation is indicated. If respiratory volumes are adequate and the patient is not distressed, the trachea may be extubated.

However, some centres aim for earlier extubation. The trachea is extubated either in theatre or within 2 h of surgery, provided that the criteria for extubation detailed above are met. This demands changes in the practices of all those caring for cardiac surgery patients. Cross-clamp and bypass times must be brief. Active vasodilator therapy during rewarming minimizes temperature afterdrop following cardiopulmonary bypass. Anaesthetic techniques incorporating infusions of short-acting agents are suitable.

Unfortunately, some patients still require prolonged ventilation after cardiac surgery. Principles of their care are as detailed in Chapter 60.

ANALGESIA AND SEDATION

The anaesthetic technique used determines the timing of administration of postoperative analgesia. Even after high-dose opioid techniques, patients usually show some response in the first 2–3 h after surgery and it is useful to assess cerebral function at this stage in case damage has occurred. Pain relief is produced most commonly with i.v. opioids either by bolus dose or by continuous infusion supplemented with a propofol infusion for sedation. Recovery is rapid after the propofol infusion is stopped and this may facilitate early extubation.

An alternative is epidural infusion analgesia if a catheter has been sited preoperatively. Concerns over the risk of epidural haematoma in patients who are fully anticoagulated after catheter insertion have prevented the widespread use of this technique. The results of ongoing studies are awaited.

Just as important as pharmacological support is the human rapport which should be achieved between staff and patient.

FURTHER READING

Kaplan H A, Reich D L, Konstadt S N (eds) 1999 Cardiac anesthesia, 4th edn. W B Saunders, Philadelphia

Wasnick J D 1998 Handbook of cardiac anesthesia and perioperative care: a demythologized approach. Butterworth-Heineman,Boston

60 The intensive care unit

The intensive care unit (ICU) is the hospital facility within which the highest levels of continuous patient care and treatment are provided. The Department of Health NHS Executive defines intensive care as 'a service for patients with potentially recoverable conditions who can benefit from more detailed observation and treatment than can safely be provided in general ward or high dependency areas'.

The optimal size of an ICU in terms of bed numbers relates to the number of acute beds in the hospital. In the UK, this is generally 1–2% of the total number of acute beds. The design of ICUs varies from hospital to hospital but they are characterized by being designated areas in which there is a minimum nurse:patient ratio of 1:1 in addition to a nurse in charge at all times, 24 h cover by resident medical staff and the facilities to support organ system failures. High-dependency units (HDUs) are designated areas with a nurse:patient ratio of 1:2 in addition to a nurse in charge at all times, continuous *availability* of medical staff either from the admitting speciality or from the ICU, and an appropriate level of monitoring and other equipment. ICUs and HDUs may be either separate geographical entities or may be combined, with the beds occupied and staffed according to the prevailing need for ICU or HDU levels of care.

The physical space for each bed in an ICU is greater than on an ordinary ward because several nurses may need to treat a patient simultaneously and bulky items of equipment often need to be accommodated. Each bed area is supplied with piped oxygen, vacuum suction, medical compressed air and sometimes nitric oxide. The plethora of electronic monitors requires at least 12 electric power sockets (with emergency back-up electrical supply) at each bed. Sufficient bedside storage space is needed for drugs and disposable equipment. Each bed area should be equipped with a self-inflating resuscitation bag to enable staff to maintain artificial ventilation if the mechanical ventilator or gas supply fails.

WHO SHOULD BE ADMITTED?

The cost of providing ICU services is very high, and the resource is finite. ICU care must be directed towards patients who are most likely to benefit. It is equally important to identify patients who are not ill enough to benefit, and those who will die despite ICU treatment. ICU admission is indicated for:

- patients requiring, or likely to require, advanced respiratory support (see below) alone
- patients requiring support of two or more organ systems
- patients with co-morbidity who require support for an acute reversible failure of another organ system.

CATEGORIES OF ORGAN SYSTEM SUPPORT

Advanced respiratory support

- Mechanical ventilatory support (excluding mask continuous positive airways pressure, CPAP) or non-invasive ventilation.
- The possibility of sudden deterioration in respiratory function requiring immediate tracheal intubation and mechanical ventilation.

Basic respiratory monitoring and support

- The need for an inspired oxygen concentration of more than 40%.
- The possibility of progressive deterioration to the point of needing advanced respiratory support.
- The need for physiotherapy to clear secretions at least 2-hourly.
- Patients in whom the tracheal tube has been removed recently after a prolonged period of intubation and mechanical ventilation.
- The need for mask CPAP or non-invasive ventilation.
- Patients whose trachea is intubated to protect the airway but who do not need mechanical ventilation.

Circulatory support

- The need for vasoactive drugs.
- Support for circulatory instability caused by hypovolaemia from any cause unresponsive to modest volume replacement.
- Patients resuscitated after cardiac arrest where ICU or HDU care is considered clinically appropriate.

Neurological monitoring or support

- Central nervous system depression sufficient to compromise the airway and impair protective reflexes.
- Invasive neurological monitoring.

Renal support

- The need for acute renal replacement therapy.

ADMISSION TO ICU

The decision to admit a patient to ICU must take other factors into account. The referral should ideally be on a consultant-to-consultant basis and no patient should be admitted or refused admission without discussion with the ICU consultant.

The reversibility of the patient's illness must be considered; if it is not reversible, and incompatible with life, then the patient should not be admitted. Such decisions are not made easily and occasionally it is necessary to admit the patient and to provide active treatment for a period of time to assess the response.

The treatment must benefit the patient; subjecting a patient who is dying to mechanical ventilation and cardiovascular resuscitation merely to preserve organs for donation is not ethical, moral or legal.

Intensive care cannot reverse chronic ill health, and admission may be inappropriate for a patient who has significant co-morbidity which severely limits quality and length of life. However, some patients adapt to co-morbidity to the extent that they accept a quality of life which others would regard as unendurable; denying such patients admission based on the presence of co-morbidity alone is difficult to justify, and the patient's views must be respected.

If possible, the consultant should discuss with the patient and the relatives the range of treatment options and possible outcomes. However, acutely ill patients can rarely discuss details of their care, and relatives may find it difficult to make an objective judgement.

If a patient has made an Advance Directive ('Living Will') then its contents must be respected.

DISCHARGE FROM ICU

The patient should be discharged when the condition(s) that necessitated admission have been treated successfully and when organ failure has resolved. Discharge should be to an area which provides an appropriate level of care. It is unusual for an ICU patient to be discharged directly to the ward without receiving a period of 'step-down' high-dependency care within the ICU to determine that the clinical course is evolving satisfactorily. Thereafter, discharge may take place to either a HDU or the ward as determined by the patient's clinical condition. Many ICUs offer a 'critical care outreach team'; one of its functions is to follow up recently discharged ICU patients.

Approximately 25% of ICU patients die in the ICU, often as a result of treatment limitation in the face of continued deterioration despite maximal appropriate supportive therapy. In such patients, palliative and compassionate care should be continued in the ICU if death is imminent, although if death is inevitable but likely to be delayed, it may be appropriate to transfer the patient to a non-ICU/HDU area for terminal care.

STAFFING CONSIDERATIONS

THE ICU CONSULTANT

Difficult therapeutic and ethical policy decisions may be required at any time in the ICU. It is essential that they are taken by an individual whose previous experience allows a reasonable assessment of the likely outcome and whose therapeutic expertise is likely to give the patient the optimal chance of recovery. The ICU consultant, if not physically present in the unit, must always be available by telephone and should not be involved in any activity which precludes his or her attendance there within 30 min. Because of the critical nature of ICU patients' illnesses, the ICU consultant expects to be informed immediately of any significant change in their condition. The consultant's base speciality is relatively unimportant, but appropriate training and experience are crucial.

THE ROLES OF THE ICU RESIDENT

Communication

Although medical involvement with therapy in the ICU is greater than anywhere else in the hospital except the operating theatre, it should be appreciated that the major proportion of the care which patients receive in the ICU is provided by nursing staff, who have greatly extended roles, experience and responsibility. ICU nursing staff have undertaken specific training to enable them to perform titration of fluid replacement, analgesia, inotropic drug therapy and weaning from mechanical ventilation. The route by which complex instructions and information are transmitted between medical and nursing staff is of vital importance. A system in which a relatively junior clinician serves as a 'final common pathway' for all instructions works well in practice provided that the doctor involved is present within the unit at all times so that the nurses may obtain clarification of instructions, report changes in status and receive immediate help in emergencies. When the patient, relatives or friends are spoken to, it is vital that the nurse is present and takes part in the discussions. The content of such discussion must be recorded accurately in the patient's notes.

Confusion is minimized if the nursing staff take orders only from the unit staff and not directly from visiting clinicians, however eminent, even if they are nominally in charge of the patient. This is to ensure that the nurses who execute orders are able to confer with the person who gave them in case of difficulties. In addition, many patients may be under the care of several clinical teams (e.g. multiply injured patients may be treated by a selection from the orthopaedic, general, neuro-, dental, plastic or urological surgeons), so that it is essential that one individual is available to draw attention to, and when necessary harmonize, often conflicting therapeutic regimens. The ICU resident, because of his or her continuous presence in the unit, should be better informed about the patient's recent diagnostic results, physiological status and therapeutic responses than any visiting clinician and should attempt to use current knowledge to guide treatment along rational lines. The ICU consultant must be available to support the resident if conflict occurs, and also to deal with clinical problems.

The department which provides the unit staff differs from hospital to hospital; units serving primarily a single speciality (e.g. cardiac surgery or neurosurgery units) are usually staffed by the speciality involved, whereas most general ICUs are staffed by the anaesthetic department, which is well used to providing round-the-clock emergency services.

Therapeutic functions

The resident is the first doctor consulted by the nursing staff. It is necessary to decide rapidly whether the problem is within the resident's expertise or if more experienced help should be obtained. The number of occasions when immediate emergency action is required should be relatively small for patients already under the care of experienced ICU nurses (e.g. unforeseen circulatory collapse, accidental tracheal extubation), but resuscitative measures are often required for patients at the time of admission to the unit. The ICU consultant must be informed of any impending admission so that the therapeutic plan can be discussed. Decisions to exclude patients from the ICU should not be taken by the junior resident alone.

Most calls from the unit to the resident are the result of alterations in measurements or observations rather than a major catastrophe. Tracheal intubation and obtunded consciousness make direct communication with many patients extremely difficult, so that assessment of their problems is based primarily on clinical observation and interpretation of patterns of change in physiological status. The resident should remember that the majority of intensive care nurses (and especially the sisters and charge nurses) have an enormous amount of 'bedside' experience with critically ill patients and considerable reliance should be placed on their observations.

Assessment of patients

ICU patients often have multiple pathologies which interact with each other and with any co-morbidity. When dealing with a newly admitted emergency patient, assessment and resuscitation often take place simultaneously and follow the standard pattern of recognizing and dealing with problems in the order of airway, breathing and circulation. The resident should heed *all* the patient's problems and the responses to the treatments instigated. When called to a patient, the resident should begin to assess the patient's condition by thorough clinical examination in a systematic manner to ensure that nothing is missed. An example of such a system and some of the matters that the resident should consider under each heading is shown in Table 60.1.

Full assessment and examination of each patient, even if stable, should be carried out at least daily. The physiological status of critically ill patients can change very quickly and the majority of the parameters measured in ICU are displayed on large paper charts on an hourly basis. Modern electronic data capture systems collect information much more frequently, and allow staff to identify both acute changes and slower trends.

The ICU resident must be familiar with the equipment and documentation used within the unit. Accurate chart review is an essential part of assessment and treatment planning. Any changes to treatment must be recorded accurately and contemporaneously so that the effects of the changes can be observed.

CLINICAL GUIDELINES

It is impossible to provide a comprehensive review of all the conditions requiring ICU care and full treatment regimens for such conditions in one chapter. The following sections present a set of guidelines designed to help the resident in the fundamental processes of managing respiratory and cardiovascular failure, which are the two commonest reasons for admission to ICU.

RESPIRATORY PROBLEMS

Who should receive artificial ventilation?

Patients who are unable to maintain adequate levels of oxygenation or who develop hypercapnia may be candidates for mechanically assisted ventilation, provided that their pulmonary pathology is potentially reversible. Ventilatory failure may have developed already (in which case arterial blood gas values are abnormal) or may be judged as likely to occur (when blood gas values may be normal but the patient is 'exhausted').

Hypoxaemia

The commonest indication for artificial ventilation of a patient's lungs in the ICU is inability to maintain a satisfactory P_aO_2. There are many pathological conditions which produce hypoxaemia, but all have the same basic problem – an area (or areas) of lung with greater pulmonary blood flow than alveolar ventilation. Blood flow through areas of lung from which ventilation is completely absent is said to be 'shunted' and hypoxaemia caused by this mechanism shows little improvement when the inspired oxygen concentration is increased. Some clinical conditions which are associated frequently with hypoxaemia, and common responses to therapy, are listed in Table 60.2. Central cyanosis (seen best in the lips) shows that significant hypoxaemia is present, but if moderate anaemia (Hb < 10 g dl^{-1}) is present, as it is in many ICU patients, severe hypoxaemia (P_aO_2 < 6 kPa) may occur without obvious cyanosis.

The initial treatment of hypoxaemia is the administration of oxygen by face mask. At least 40% oxygen should be given, either by means of a fixed-performance mask (e.g. 40, 50 or 60% Ventimask) or by supplying at least 6 L min^{-1} of oxygen to a variable-performance mask (e.g. Hudson). Low-concentration fixed-performance masks and other devices which deliver 24–35% oxygen should be reserved for use in patients with chronic lung conditions in whom hypoxic drive may be maintaining ventilation. The effect of oxygen therapy should be assessed continuously by pulse oximetry and blood gas analysis should be carried out after 30 min. This gives a more reliable measure of oxygenation as well as providing information regarding the P_aCO_2 and acid–base status.

If P_aO_2 remains below 7 kPa in a patient with previously healthy lungs, the inspired oxygen concentration should be increased and blood gases measured again after 20 min. In addition, measures to combat infection, pulmonary oedema or bronchospasm should be introduced as appropriate, analgesia given if indicated and chest physiotherapy started. Mechanical ventilation is indicated if P_aO_2 does not remain above 7–8 kPa. A decreased level of consciousness and/or airway compromise may mandate early tracheal intubation and mechanical ventilation. If these are absent, administration of oxygen by mask CPAP should be tried if there are no contraindications.

Mask CPAP. A tightly applied face mask with a high-volume, low-pressure soft plastic rim held in place by a special harness is connected to a circuit delivering an air/oxygen mixture of the required F_iO_2. The flow rate of fresh gas into the circuit must be sufficient to keep the positive pressure set by the expiratory valve (2.5–10 cmH_2O) almost constant throughout the respiratory cycle with only a minimal pressure decrease during inspiration. Various commercial systems using Venturi or bellows systems are available but they consume large amounts of fresh gas. For CPAP to be successful, the patient must receive adequate analgesia, be alert and cooperative, and have no facial injuries (including a basal skull fracture). Patients often find the tight-fitting mask uncomfortable and require short periods of respite with an ordinary fixed F_iO_2 mask. At higher levels of CPAP (> 7.5 cmH_2O), the work of

Table 60.1 An example of a system for assessment of ICU patients

A.	Airway	Is the airway patent or at risk? What do I need to do to secure it? Is the cervical spine at risk? Type of tracheal tube? Position? How long has it been in place? Time for tracheostomy? Type of tracheostomy tube? Security of tube? What is coming up the tube? Cuff pressure?
B.	Breathing	Spontaneous ventilation – rate, depth, character, etc.? Mode of ventilation? Mechanical ventilation parameters? Inspired oxygen concentration? PEEP or CPAP level? Position of patient? Nitric oxide or other adjuncts? Clinical examination findings? Arterial blood gas analysis? Chest X-ray or other imaging?
C.	Circulation	ECG, pulse, blood pressure, CVP? Haemodynamic data, e.g. cardiac index, SVRI, PVRI, PCWP, etc.? Inotropic or other vasoactive drugs? Heart sounds? Fluid balance, plasma osmolality? Peripheral circulation/oedema?
D.	Disability/depth of sedation	Sedation score or Glasgow Coma Score? Focal neurology? Pupils? Fitting? Cerebral function monitors? Other specialized neurological monitors, e.g. ICP, jugular bulb saturation or transcranial Doppler?
E.	Equipment	Is it all working, calibrated and accurate? Is there any other monitoring that would safely give useful information?
F.	Fluids	How much and what fluid to give? Fluid balance 24 h/cumulative? Fluid output from where? Fistulae, drains, wounds? What is it – quality and quantity?
G.	Gut	Is it working? Can I use it to feed the patient? Prokinetic drugs? Dietary supplements/stress ulcer prophylaxis? Nasogastric tube aspirate/drainage? Wounds healing or not? Stomas – viable working or not? Bowel activity?
H.	Haematology	Check *all* blood results, haematology, clotting, biochemistry, serology. Is there any additional blood test that can help? Is transfusion required?
I.	Imaging	X-rays? Ultrasound, CT scanning? MRI? Echocardiography? Doppler? Nuclear medicine?
J.	Joints and limbs	Fractures, dislocations, other trauma? DVT and appropriate prophylaxis?
K.	Kelvin	Temperature and temperature chart?
L.	Lines	Examine all catheters/cannulae (intravenous, intra-arterial and others) and ask yourself: When placed? Where placed? Are they necessary? Replacement or removal? Signs of sepsis?
M.	Microbiology	Aggressive microbiological surveillance: swabs, blood cultures, sputum, bronchoalveolar lavage, drain fluid, urine, removed line tips. Strict asepsis and cross-infection avoidance – touch a patient, wash your hands. Check results daily. Directed antimicrobial therapy only. Antibiotic levels, doses and course duration. Make friends with your microbiologist: joint daily ward rounds
N.	Nutrition	All patients need feeding. Enteral nutrition is best. Nasogastric feeding, oral, percutaneous gastrostomy, jejunal feeding, intravenous feeding?
O.	Other consultants	Nobody knows everything – arrange appropriate specialist opinions. Let the patient's general practitioner and hospital consultant know one of their patients is in the ICU
P.	Pain relief and psychological support	Prescribe analgesia by appropriate routes, intervals and doses. Talk to your patient always, even if there is a depressed level of consciousness. Explain procedures simply and carefully. Give sedation and psychotropic drugs if indicated
Q.	Question	If you are unsure of what to do, ask your consultant. You should never undertake a task for which you have been inadequately trained
R.	Relatives	Keep relatives fully informed, be honest when discussing prognosis, ask for information on past medical history and daily activity if appropriate. Always hold discussions away from the bedside unless the patient is fully aware/autonomous and can participate. Always hold discussions with the patient's nurse present and document your comments
S.	Skin	Examine skin for perfusion, wounds, signs of systemic disease or infection. Pressure area care, mouth care etc.
T.	Trauma and transport	Multiple trauma patients require multidisciplinary management. Trauma patients may not have had a complete secondary survey; late diagnosis of unrecognized problems may cause significant morbidity and mortality. Transport of ICU patients within or between hospital requires the same level of care and monitoring that they receive in the ICU itself
U.	Universal precautions	Owing to the plethora of infectious diseases transmitted by blood and other bodily fluids, all staff should be aware of the necessity of wearing gloves, aprons and occasionally face guards when performing invasive procedures
V.	Visitors	These may be the patient's relatives or other medical personnel involved in the patient's care. Visiting colleagues should be treated with respect and courtesy, but ultimately all changes to therapy *must* be discussed with the ICU consultant
W.	What to do	When the patient has been fully assessed, you must formulate a plan to deal with his or her problems. This plan must be documented clearly in the notes and discussed with the bedside nurse. Parameters must be agreed within which the nurse is able to vary the components of the therapeutic regimen according to the patient's response and outside which you need to reassess the patient. Time is an important part of your plan and regular reassessment is essential
Y.	Why?	Every time you review the patient, ask yourself why the patient was admitted and what the active problems are now. Keep on track and forget nothing!

breathing against the expiratory valve may result in an elevation of P_aCO_2, and CPAP alone is generally not effective in most cases of respiratory failure associated with hypercapnia.

If the patient does not have a functioning nasogastric tube, then air swallowing and gastric dilatation may be a problem and hinder diaphragmatic excursion or provoke regurgitation.

Table 60.2 Some causes of hypoxaemia and usual responses to therapy

Clinical condition	Response to therapy		
	O_2 by mask	IPPV	Need for PEEP
1. Pulmonary oedema			
(a) cardiac	Fair	Good	Uncommon
(b) permeability	Poor	Fair	Often needed
2. Asthma (bronchodilators may make worse)	Good	Good but technically very difficult	Uncommon
3. Chronic bronchitis	Fair (Ventimask)	Good	Uncommon
4. Emphysema	Good (Ventimask)	Good	Rare, beware pneumothorax
5. Pneumonia			
(a) lobar	Poor	Poor	Try, often disappointing
(b) bronchial	Fair	Good	Useful
6. Pulmonary contusion	Fair	Fair	Often needed, beware pneumothorax
7. Right-to-left intracardiac shunts	Poor	Disastrous	Never
8. Retained secretions	Poor	Good, access for suction important	Helpful
9. 'Exhaustion'	Not accepted	Good	Uncommon

Patients who are unable to maintain adequate oxygenation often have a pulmonary problem which is associated with other pathology. Persisting inability to cough effectively because of pain and/or weakness leads to retention of secretions and progressive alveolar collapse. The prophylactic use of tracheal intubation and intermittent positive pressure ventilation (IPPV) has become common in patients who normally produce significant quantities of bronchial secretions and whose ability to cough has been impaired by injury or operation to the chest and/or upper abdomen. Patients in whom pain rather than weakness is the major defect may often be managed more conservatively if first-class pain relief is provided (e.g. by epidural or i.v. infusion of opioid), together with physiotherapy, and the use of nasal airways or selective use of minitracheotomy to facilitate suction.

Hypercapnia

Carbon dioxide clearance is related directly to alveolar ventilation. Causes of inadequate ventilation, together with the likely duration of the disability, are listed in Table 60.3. It may be inappropriate to start IPPV in clinical situations where ventilatory insufficiency cannot be reversed by therapy. For some patients, non-invasive (i.e. non-intubational) forms of respiratory support (NIRS) are applicable. The types of NIRS used most widely are non-invasive positive pressure ventilation (NIPPV) by mask and negative pressure ventilation (NPV). NIPPV and NPV have been used successfully in the management of patients with non-traumatic causes of ventilatory failure, particularly for home ventilation of patients who chronically retain carbon dioxide or who have high spinal injury, and who do not have a permanent tracheostomy but require nocturnal ventilation. NIPPV uses a portable electrically powered volume- or pressure-cycled ventilator to deliver synchronized positive pressure breaths via a tight-fitting nasal or full face mask held in place by a harness. NPV requires a made-to-measure 'cuirass' which is worn over the chest and sealed at the neck and waist. This is connected to a pump which cyclically produces negative pressure within the cuirass; the intrathoracic pressure is exceeded by atmospheric pressure and air flows into the chest. The pump then cycles to atmospheric pressure and expiration occurs as a result of the normal elastic recoil of the lungs and chest wall. The device is essentially a miniature version of the old cylindrical 'iron lung'.

Patients whose dysfunction is described in the lower part of Table 60.3 are likely to make vigorous efforts to maintain normocapnia, while those in whom the dysfunction may be described broadly as 'neurological' are usually unable to make any significant improvement to minute volume despite a progressive increase in P_aCO_2. Mechanical ventilation is required usually if P_aCO_2 exceeds 7 kPa in patients who habitually maintain a P_aCO_2 in the normal range (4.7–5.3 kPa), or if P_aCO_2 increases by more than 2 kPa above the patient's usual level.

Exhaustion is indicated by a pattern of laboured, rapid, shallow breathing which is often accompanied by deterioration in the level of consciousness. This situation may occur in a wide range of clinical conditions, including cardiac failure and severe septicaemia, when the institution of artificial ventilation may be followed by an improvement in oxygenation, a reduction in pulse rate and reversal of a trend towards metabolic acidosis. When it occurs in conjunction with myocardial failure, a disproportionate amount of the limited cardiac output is used to maintain ventilation, and artificial ventilation may allow adequate perfusion of vital organs to be resumed. Mechanical ventilation is probably required if the respiratory rate remains at or above 45 breaths min^{-1} for more than 1 h.

Mechanical ventilation

Tracheal intubation

To enable IPPV to be carried out effectively, a cuffed tube must be placed in the trachea either via the mouth or nose, or directly through a tracheostomy. In the emergency situation, an orotracheal tube is usually inserted. If the patient is conscious, anaesthesia should be induced carefully with an appropriate dose of i.v. induction agent and muscular relaxation produced, usually with succinylcholine. The full range of adjuncts for difficult intubation should be available.

The critically ill patient is often exquisitely sensitive to i.v. anaesthesia, and cardiovascular collapse may occur; consequently, full resuscitation equipment must be immediately available.

If the patient is unconscious, a muscle relaxant alone may be necessary (but not obligatory) to facilitate the passage of the tube; however, an i.v. induction agent and muscle relaxant should always be used in patients with severe head injury to prevent an increase

Table 60.3 Some causes of inadequate spontaneous ventilation

Site of dysfunction	Common causes	Probable duration of inadequacy
A. Patients usually unable to increase ventilation (appear passive)		
1. Respiratory centre	Brain injury (coning)	Permanent
	Pharmacological depression (e.g. opioids, barbiturates)	Hours (depends on drug)
2. Upper motor neurones	High spinal damage (above C4)	Permanent
3. Lower motor neurones	Poliomyelitis	Weeks but may be permanent
	Polyneuritis	Months
	Tetanus	Weeks
4. Neuromuscular junction	Myasthenia gravis	Weeks or months
	Neuromuscular blockers	Minutes or hours
5. Respiratory muscles	Myopathies, dystrophies	Permanent
B. Patients who attempt to increase ventilation (appear dyspnoeic)		
6. Chest wall		
(a) Deformity	Kyphoscoliosis	Permanent
	Burn eschars	Until incised
(b) Damage	Rib fractures	Days or weeks
7. Lungs – reduced compliance	Pulmonary fibrosis	Permanent
	ARDS	Days or weeks
8. Airways – increased resistance	Upper airway obstruction: croup, epiglottis	Until relieved
	Lower airway obstruction:	
	asthma	Days
	bronchitis and emphysema	Permanent

in intracranial pressure (ICP) during laryngoscopy and tracheal intubation.

Many patients are hypoxaemic, and it is essential that 100% oxygen is administered before tracheal intubation.

After muscle relaxation has been induced, the tube should be inserted by the route which is associated with the least delay.

If the patient is unconscious and the victim of blunt trauma, when cervical spine injury is a possibility, the cervical spine should be immobilized during intubation using manual in-line immobilization (MILI). Using this technique, oral intubation is safe even in the presence of biomechanical instability of the cervical spine. If the patient has a rigid neck collar in place before intubation, MILI should be applied and the collar removed to facilitate laryngoscopy, and then replaced before discontinuing MILI.

Cricoid pressure should be applied to minimize the risk of aspirating gastric contents. A sterile, disposable plastic tube with a low-pressure cuff should be used. The tube should be inserted such that the top of the cuff lies not more than 3 cm below the vocal cords. The proximal end of the tube should then be cut so that the incompressible plastic connector lies between the incisor teeth if an oral tube is used, or in the external nares if nasal intubation is selected.

Nasotracheal intubation is less popular than formerly in the ICU because of increased recognition of the risk of sepsis from sinusitis.

The head should be placed in a neutral or slightly flexed position (on one pillow) after tracheal intubation and a chest X-ray taken to ensure that the tip of the tube lies at least 5 cm above the carina.

Bronchial intubation is the commonest dangerous complication during mechanical ventilation as the tracheal tube may migrate down the trachea when the patient is moved during normal nursing procedures. Intubation of the right main bronchus cannot be detected reliably by observation of chest movements or by auscultation of the chest because of the exaggerated transmission of breath sounds during IPPV, although absent or asynchronous chest movement may occur when pulmonary collapse has taken place. Bronchial intubation is one of the causes of a sudden decrease in compliance, and restlessness and coughing often occur if the end of the tube irritates the carina. If this is suspected, the tube should be withdrawn gradually by up to 5 cm while lung compliance and chest expansion are observed carefully. The position of the tube should always be confirmed by a chest radiograph.

When the upper airway or larynx is obstructed and conventional tracheal intubation is not possible (e.g. occasional cases of epiglottitis or laryngeal trauma), the emergency airway of choice is cricothyroidotomy. Tracheostomy is employed more commonly as a planned procedure to make management easier and more comfortable in patients who require ventilation for prolonged periods (e.g. tetanus, poliomyelitis, Guillain–Barré syndrome) or to aid weaning. In such cases, it is performed as a formal operation under general anaesthesia after the airway has been secured using a tracheal tube. In most ICUs, percutaneous dilatational tracheostomy is employed. This technique can be performed at the bedside, often using bronchoscopic control. It should be undertaken only by fully trained staff.

Management of patients undergoing ventilation

The aims of IPPV are to maintain adequate oxygenation of the tissues with an inspired oxygen concentration of less than 50% and to maintain the $P_{a}CO_2$ at a satisfactory level without causing iatrogenic lung injury or cardiovascular compromise.

Arterial oxygenation

This is controlled by manipulating the inspired oxygen concentration and by varying the end-expiratory pressure. Figure 60.1 describes measures that may be used to maintain arterial oxygenation within the desired limits (P_aO_2 = 10–15 kPa and S_aO_2 > 95%). Pulse oximetry is a useful continuous monitor, but does not reliably reflect small but significant changes in P_aO_2. Inspired concentrations of oxygen exceeding 50–60% should be avoided for more than a few hours if possible because of the risk of oxygen-induced pulmonary damage. However, in severe hypoxaemia, it may be necessary to ignore this risk.

Carbon dioxide tension

This is controlled during conventional ventilation by changing the respiratory rate and/or tidal volume. It is desirable to minimize the changes in P_aCO_2 (especially if initially elevated), because too rapid a reduction may lead to decreases in cerebral blood flow, cardiac output and arterial pressure. In patients with normal or low P_aCO_2 before IPPV, minute volume should be adjusted to produce a P_aCO_2 of 4.5–5 kPa, a value at which spontaneous ventilatory efforts should be minimal. If the initial P_aCO_2 is high, its value should not be reduced by more than 1 kPa h^{-1} and, if raised chronically (e.g. in chronic bronchitis), it should not be reduced below the patient's own 'normal' level when well. If the P_aCO_2 is below 4 kPa, minute volume should be reduced by decreasing the respiratory rate. Because P_aCO_2 increases relatively slowly, at least 1 h should elapse before contemplating further changes in minute volume.

Mode of ventilation

Intermittent positive pressure ventilation (IPPV), or controlled mandatory ventilation (CMV), is the basic mode of mechanical ventilation used during balanced anaesthesia, but it is rarely used in its simplest form in the ICU. When CMV is used, the ventilator is set to deliver a fixed tidal volume at a fixed rate to produce a fixed minute ventilation sufficient to ensure adequate CO_2 elimination. Any attempt by the patient to take a spontaneous breath during any

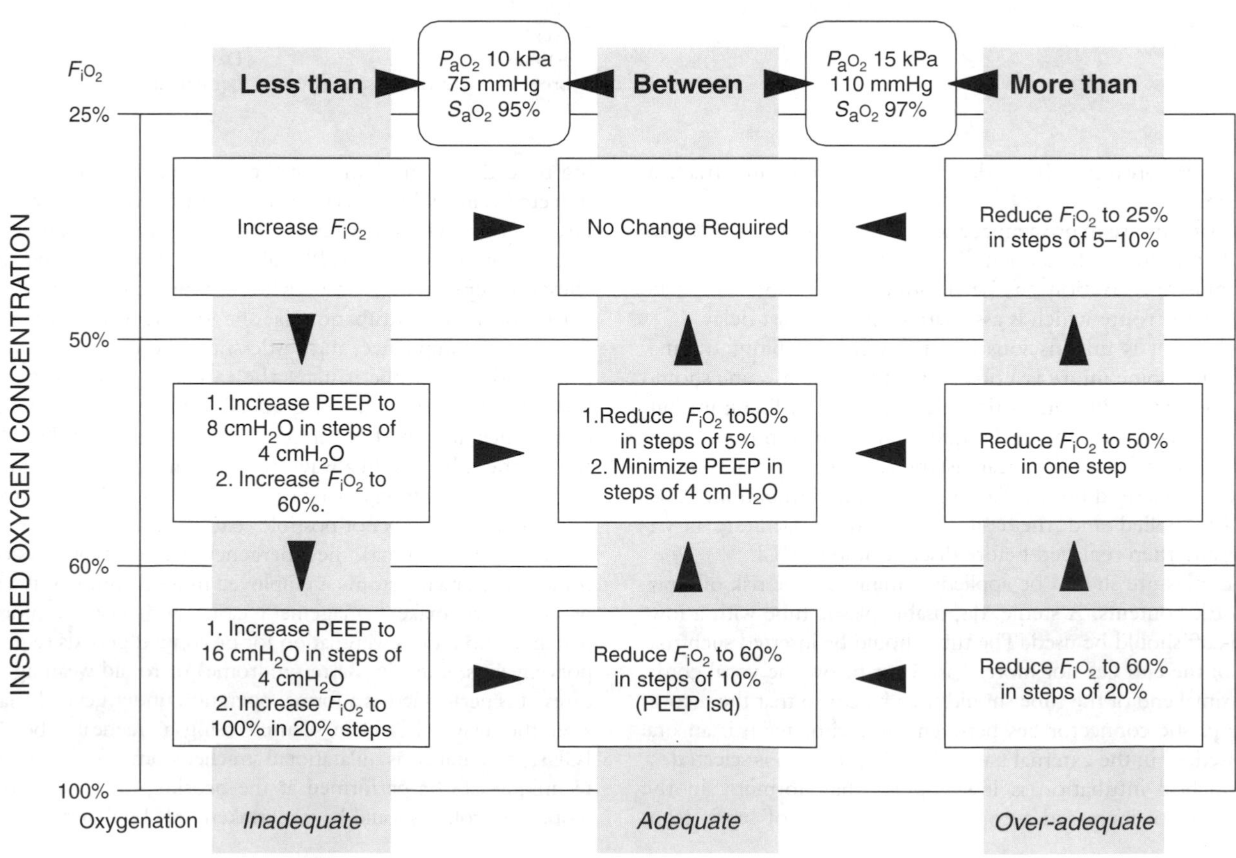

Fig. 60.1
Control of arterial oxygenation. To use this diagram: 1. Measure the inspired oxygen concentration (F_iO_2) and arterial blood gases and find appropriate box on diagram. 2. Adjust F_iO_2 and/or positive end-expiratory pressure (PEEP) as suggested. Where more than one action is proposed, proceed in the order described. In general, the greater the deviation from adequacy, the larger the steps required. 3. Repeat measurements after 20–30 min and read just if necessary. NB: If PO_2 is measured on samples of mixed (or central venous) blood before and after adding or increasing PEEP, effect of PEEP on cardiac output and oxygen flux may be assessed (see text).

part of the respiratory cycle is unsuccessful. In addition, the ventilator continues to deliver mandatory breaths, even if the patient is attempting to breathe; consequently, very high inflation pressures may be generated if the ventilator cycles to inspiration while the patient is coughing or attempting to breathe out, resulting in impaired gas exchange, a risk of barotrauma to the lung and depression of cardiac output. To enable patients to tolerate CMV, it is often necessary to provide deep sedation and, in some cases, to administer a neuromuscular blocking drug. Oversedation of critically ill patients tends to decrease cardiac output by depressing myocardial function or by vasodilatation; this is a risk particularly in patients who have received inadequate fluid resuscitation, in the elderly, and in other patients with myocardial dysfunction. Drug-induced paralysis in ICU patients can result in very unpleasant memories and, if used for a long period, may result in prolonged impairment of neuromuscular function, with muscle wasting, weakness and increased difficulty in weaning from mechanical ventilation.

Modes of ventilation have been developed which allow preservation of the patient's own respiratory efforts by detecting an attempt by the patient to breathe in and synchronizing the mechanical breath with spontaneous inspiration; this technique is called synchronized intermittent mandatory ventilation (SIMV). If no attempt at inspiration is detected over a period of some seconds then a mandatory breath is delivered to ensure that a safe total minute volume is provided. Another technique is called pressure support ventilation (PSV). When PSV is employed, each spontaneous breath is detected and then assisted by delivering gas until a pre-set level of positive pressure is achieved. The technique is, in essence, patient-triggered, pressure-limited ventilation and may be used only if the patient has a normal intrinsic respiratory rate.

These more advanced techniques allow satisfactory levels of ventilation without the need to provide deep sedation, and with a lower mean intrathoracic pressure than occurs using CMV. Consequently, less sedation is required, respiratory muscle tone is preserved, there is greater cardiovascular stability and the risk of barotrauma is reduced.

The choice of the best mode of ventilation for an individual patient often changes at different periods in the disease process, and the technique which provides the best gas exchange is often found only by trial and error.

Ventilator-induced lung injury (VILI)

When pulmonary pathology has resulted in the development of acute lung injury (ALI) or adult respiratory distress syndrome (ARDS), either directly or indirectly as a result of a cytokine-mediated systemic inflammatory response, then the lung is particularly at risk of secondary injury as a result of injudiciously aggressive ventilatory strategies using conventional modes of ventilation. Attempts to achieve 'normal' arterial blood gas tensions often require the use of very high tidal volumes, high respiratory rates and high peak inflation pressures. Many ventilators are capable of delivering these pre-set variables regardless of the compliance or resistance of the lungs. If all the alveolar subunits of the lungs had normal and equal compliance, the tidal volume would be distributed equally. However, diseased lung is non-homogeneous; some units have normal compliance and others have poor compliance with long time constants. Some alveolar subunits are available to be ventilated and others are not. As a result of the inhomogeneity, the more normal alveolar subunits are ventilated preferentially and subjected to pressures which cause overdistension; both high tidal volumes and high pressure can cause overdistension. Overdistension injury resulting from excessively high tidal volumes is termed 'volutrauma' and overdistension injury resulting from excessive pressures is termed 'barotrauma'.

In extreme cases of barotrauma, gas from overdistended, ruptured alveoli forms interstitial pulmonary emphysema and tracks along the adventitia of intrapulmonary blood vessels. Eventually, the gas bubbles coalesce as they migrate centrally and mediastinal emphysema occurs.

If the process persists, gas bursts through the mediastinal pleura to cause a pneumothorax. Unrecognized pneumothorax is a serious complication during positive pressure ventilation because the volume of the pneumothorax enlarges with each breath and tension pneumothorax may occur rapidly.

Even if pneumothorax does not develop, repeated overdistension of alveoli by high tidal volumes may contribute to a deterioration of the underlying lung problem. The cyclical opening and closing of the alveoli result in a shearing injury. Exudative pulmonary oedema may form as a result of increased alveolar permeability; compliance decreases further, and the tidal volume is displaced to more normal alveoli so that the injury is propagated. The insult is probably increased by concurrent oxygen toxicity as a result of the use of high $F_{I}O_2$ in an attempt to preserve an adequate arterial oxygen tension.

Lung protective ventilatory strategies

The end-points of the pathophysiology of VILI and the pathophysiology of diseased lung injury are identical and it seems reasonable to prevent exacerbation of lung injury by the adoption of a lung protective ventilatory strategy. The mechanism of VILI suggests that the avoidance of overdistension, shear stress injury and oxygen toxicity should be the main strategies of such a technique.

Pressure and volume limitation strategy

A reduction in volutrauma may be achieved theoretically by the use of low tidal volumes during ventilation. Classically, relatively large tidal volumes (10–12 ml kg^{-1}) have been used to ensure normocapnia in the range of 4.5–5.5 kPa, but in the presence of the lung inhomogeneity, this leads to overdistension, high peak inspiratory pressures and the production of VILI. Reducing the tidal volume to 6–8 ml kg^{-1} and limiting peak inspiratory pressure in the presence of poorly compliant lung result in a decreased incidence of overdistension and a reduction in transalveolar pressure. Overdistension does not seem to occur if the transalveolar pressure is kept below 35 cmH_2O, which equates to a plateau airway pressure of 35–45 cmH_2O. The main disadvantage of pressure limitation (also called pressure-controlled ventilation, PCV) is that minute ventilation is decreased and hypercapnia occurs; however, this may be acceptable if the probability of survival is improved ('permissive hypercapnia'). The low lung volumes generated during PCV increase the tendency of alveoli to collapse and this must be countered by a concurrent lung recruitment strategy.

Lung recruitment strategy

Shear forces induce alveolar damage because of the cyclical opening and subsequent closure of alveoli. Collapse of alveoli at end-expiration at low or zero PEEP produces the maximum degree of alveolar injury. The use of higher levels of PEEP tends to hold alveoli open, stops them collapsing totally at end-expiration and limits the shear forces applied. The level of PEEP required to prevent collapse and to recruit unopened alveoli is difficult to calculate on an individual basis, although an estimate can be made from the patient's pressure/volume static compliance curve (see p. 112) by choosing the lower inflection point on the ascending limb or the upper inflection point on the descending limb. However, constructing such curves by the application of successively increasing tidal volumes and measuring the pressure that each volume generates is not very physiological and the PEEP level produced is probably not appropriate to all of the various alveolar time constants present in an inhomogeneous diseased lung. Arbitrary incremental levels of PEEP may be applied at, say, 4, 8, 12 and 16 cmH_2O to determine the level which produces the best oxygenation for a given F_IO_2 with the least cardiovascular compromise. Alternative strategies for recruiting closed or semi-closed alveolar subunits involve giving an occasional single large tidal breath and holding end-inspiration for 20 s.

The effects of PEEP on the circulation should be monitored by observing trends in arterial pressure and by measuring changes in the oxygen concentration in mixed (or central) venous blood. The supply of oxygen available to the body (the oxygen flux) is the product of the cardiac output and the arterial oxygen content. PEEP often increases the arterial oxygen content but may depress cardiac output so that oxygen flux is reduced. If this happens and total body oxygen consumption remains unchanged, less oxygen is returned to the heart and the oxygen content in the mixed (or central) venous blood decreases. If venous oxygen saturation does decrease after the application of (or an increase in the level of) PEEP, then:

1. PEEP should be reduced by 5 cmH_2O
2. inspired oxygen concentration should be increased by 10%
3. measurements of arterial and venous PO_2 should be repeated after 20 min.

Alternative modes of ventilation

For simple elective postoperative ventilation in patients with non-diseased lung, the modes described above are usually adequate, but occasionally, as the lung becomes more diseased, alternative modes of ventilation must be used. Taking into account the mechanism of VILI and the theoretical advantages of avoiding overdistension and shear injury while promoting lung recruitment, it is possible to formulate alternative strategies for ventilating injured lungs. The aim should be to use a ventilatory mode that opens underventilated alveolar units, keeps them open for as long as possible to allow optimal gas exchange at volumes and transalveolar pressures which do not induce secondary lung injury or produce haemodynamic instability, and then allows exhalation to a lung volume and positive end-expiratory pressure which prevent alveolar collapse and allow adequate carbon dioxide excretion.

Pressure-controlled inverse ratio ventilation

For an alveolar subunit of a given compliance, a high pressure applied for a short time produces volume expansion which may be equal to that produced by a lower pressure applied for a longer period. PCV may be used with a range of I:E ratios, from the 'normal' 1:2 to the equal ratio 1:1 or inverse ratios of 2:1 or even 3:1. Pressure-controlled inverse ratio ventilation (PCIRV) offers theoretical advantages in terms of lung protection and recruitment, particularly when combined with PEEP in some patients with poor lung compliance and alveoli with long time constants. The improvement in oxygenation which often occurs may be the result of reduced arteriovenous shunt, decreased ventilation–perfusion mismatch or increased functional residual capacity as a result of intrinsic PEEP developing due to the short expiratory phase. While the development of intrinsic PEEP has some advantages in terms of alveolar recruitment, too much, particularly in the presence of bronchospasm or other obstruction to expiration, may promote volutrauma. Where evidence of increasing intrinsic PEEP is found, the expiratory time should be increased.

The use of PCIRV is not tolerated by unsedated patients because the inverse I:E ratio is a very uncomfortable pattern of ventilation. High doses of sedative drugs and occasionally neuromuscular blocking drugs are required to facilitate the optimal pattern of ventilation.

In chest trauma with coexisting blunt myocardial injury, sedation to the required depth often requires inotropic support to maintain cardiac output. Hypovolaemic patients may suffer a decrease in cardiac output particularly at inverse ratios of 3:1 as a result of the prolonged positive intrathoracic pressure. Trauma patients with a head injury and raised ICP in combination with lung contusion form a not infrequent group of patients where a lung protective ventilatory strategy with permissive hypercapnia is at odds with the need to control P_aCO_2 to low normocapnia for ICP control.

Tracheal gas insufflation and PCIRV

In some patients with very poor lung compliance, the short inspiratory time associated with the use of PCIRV may result in a tidal volume so small that the anatomical and equipment dead spaces come to represent a large proportion of the tidal volume, resulting in a progressive increase in P_aCO_2. The dead space may be washed out by placing a catheter coaxially in the tracheal tube to lie with its tip just above the level of the carina. Tracheal gas insufflation (TGI) flushes out the dead space, so that gas rebreathed from the dead space contains no CO_2. Correct positioning of the catheter is vital, because movement of the catheter may cause damage to the tracheal mucosa. The catheter gas must be humidified and the inspired oxygen concentration should be the same as that of the gas delivered by the ventilator.

High-frequency ventilation

High-frequency oscillation (HFO) uses a tidal volume lower than dead space volume. Small tidal volumes are generated by pistons or electromagnetic diaphragms to produce oscillatory gas flows at rates of between 150 and 3000 breaths min^{-1}. HFO combined with recruitment manoeuvres is currently under investigation in both adults and children. The concept has potential advantages in patients with established barotrauma or bronchopleural fistulae where very low mean airway pressures may be advantageous.

Prone positioning

Despite the use of high $F_{I}O_2$, PEEP and optimal PCIRV, some patients become progressively more difficult to oxygenate. Another strategy to improve ventilation is to place the patient in the prone position. The improved gas exchange was thought to occur as gravity redistributed blood from the dorsal regions of the lungs, where atelectasis had developed, to the anterior segments where alveoli were more recruitable. Recent work has suggested that the improvement is related to changes in regional pleural pressure. In the prone position, pleural pressure becomes more uniform and reduces ventilation–perfusion mismatch. The technique is not popular with nursing staff because it is very labour-intensive; four people are needed to turn the patient and great care is required to ensure that the airway and vascular catheters/cannulae are not dislodged.

Inhaled nitric oxide

Nitric oxide (NO) is an ultra-short-acting pulmonary vasodilator which improves oxygenation by dilating pulmonary vessels adjacent to the best ventilated alveolar units. When given by inhalation, it is delivered preferentially to the more recruited alveoli of the inhomogeneous lung and diffuses rapidly out of the alveoli to the pulmonary capillaries, causing relaxation of vascular smooth muscle and dilatation of the blood vessel. It is rapidly bound and inactivated by haemoglobin (in 110–130 ms) and its vasodilator effects are therefore limited to the pulmonary circulation.

The blood flow past underventilated alveoli is normally reduced as a result of the hypoxic vasoconstrictor response, but the improved blood flow induced by NO in the vessels adjacent to open alveoli reduces the resistance of vessels in areas of the lung which are well ventilated, increasing the proportion of blood which perfuses these areas. This results in a net reduction in intrapulmonary shunt and an increased $P_{a}O_2$. Patients with very severe hypoxaemia may be saved from a hypoxic death, while in moderate hypoxaemia, it may be possible to reduce $F_{I}O_2$, thereby reducing the risk of oxygen toxicity.

NO is administered in concentrations of 5–20 parts per million (ppm) in patients whose oxygenation has failed to improve despite optimization of PCIRV, PEEP and prone positioning; the dose used should be the lowest which is effective in achieving a 20% improvement in $P_{a}O_2$:$F_{I}O_2$ ratio. In high concentrations (> 100 ppm), NO is highly reactive and toxic, and the delivery system used must conform to rigid safety standards. During the use of NO, the concentration of methaemoglobin in the blood and the inspired nitrogen dioxide concentration must be measured. NO therapy is expensive and potentially dangerous. It improves oxygenation in the short term in about 50% of patients but the effect is often transient.

Extracorporeal gas exchange (ECGE)

This technique, also termed extracorporeal membrane oxygenation (ECMO), represents the final option if all other avenues of providing ventilatory support have failed. Partial cardiopulmonary venovenous bypass is initiated using heparin-bonded vascular catheters, and extracorporeal oxygenation and carbon dioxide removal are achieved using a membrane oxygenator. A low-volume, low-pressure, low-frequency regimen of ventilation is continued to contribute to respiration. The concept is that by providing adequate oxygenation and carbon dioxide removal with minimal ventilation, the lungs are 'rested' and lung healing is more likely to occur. Its use in trauma patients is particularly difficult as any active bleeding is worsened because the extracorporeal circulation system requires anticoagulation. Currently, in the UK, the availability of ECGE in adults is limited to a few centres carrying out evaluative research.

Assessment of ventilated patients

A checklist for 'troubleshooting' the patient undergoing artificial ventilation is shown in Figure 60.2.

Attempts to breathe out of phase with the ventilator may cause significant problems with oxygenation and carbon dioxide clearance, and may generate very high peak airway pressures. The first priorities are to exclude and, if necessary, correct hypoxaemia or hypercapnia (Figs 60.1 and 60.2) and to detect any adverse effects or complications of ventilation. When these problems have been excluded, a change in sedation, analgesia or mode of ventilation, or rarely the use of neuromuscular blockade, may be indicated.

Reassurance, analgesia and sedation

All but a few patients require some sedation or analgesia while receiving IPPV through a tracheal tube. Ideally, patients should require only light sedation, except when unpleasant or painful procedures are performed, so that they can understand and cooperate with therapy. The experienced ICU nurse explains exactly what is happening, reassures and develops methods of communication that do not distress the patient. Such explanations should be brief, as attention span is short in the sick, and should be repeated frequently because memory is impaired. Regular assessment and formal sedation scoring (Table 60.4) should be carried out to avoid oversedation and the associated risks of cardiovascular depression and delayed recovery of consciousness.

The use of sedative drugs to treat pain, or the use of analgesic drugs to produce sedation, almost invariably results in an overdose and in prolongation of recovery. Sedative and analgesic drugs should be given in a ratio appropriate to the needs of the individual patient for anxiolysis and the treatment of pain. Midazolam and propofol are the drugs used most commonly to produce sedation; midazolam is cheaper, but propofol results in more rapid recovery, particularly after prolonged periods of infusion.

Table 60.4 An example of a sedation scoring system for use with intensive care patients

Inadequate	Anxious and agitated or restless, or both
Desired	Cooperative, orientated and tranquil Responds to command only Brisk response to light glabellar tap or loud auditory stimulus
Too deep	Sluggish response to light glabellar tap or loud auditory stimulus No response to light glabellar tap or loud auditory stimulus

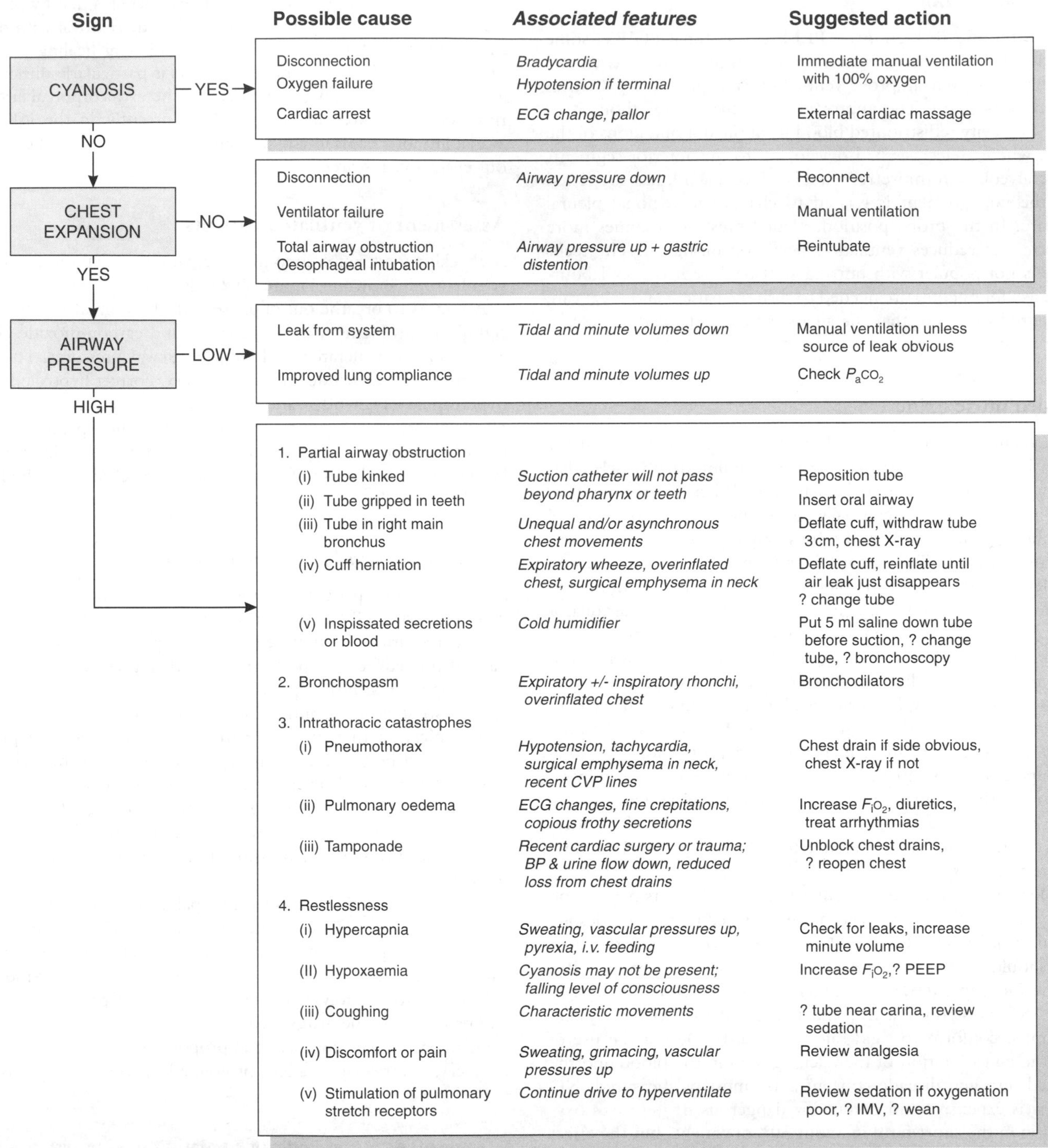

Fig. 60.2
Checklist for the patient undergoing ventilation.

Morphine and alfentanil are used widely to provide analgesia; alfentanil has a shorter elimination half-life and is useful if weaning from mechanical ventilation is anticipated within the next few hours. Continuous infusions of remifentanil (an ultra-short-acting opioid analgesic) or dexmedetomidine (an α_2-agonist) are under investigation. Metabolism of sedative drugs and accumulation of metabolites normally excreted in the urine result in wide variability in the effects of these drugs not only among individuals but also at different stages of illness in each patient.

Weaning from mechanical ventilation

Weaning is the process by which the patient's dependence on mechanical ventilation is gradually reduced to the point where spontaneous breathing sufficient to meet metabolic needs may be sustained. Because of the adverse effects of mechanical ventilation, weaning should be undertaken at the earliest opportunity.

Pressure support modes

The newer modes of ventilation such as pressure support ventilation or assisted spontaneous breathing on modern microprocessor-controlled ventilators allow the patient to participate actively in ventilation much earlier in the resolution of lung failure than was possible previously. These modes detect a patient's attempt to breathe spontaneously, synchronize with it and support it to a preset level of positive pressure. At low levels, this compensates for the resistance of the tracheal tube and breathing system; at higher levels, it allows the patient to generate an adequate tidal volume with minimal effort. These modes of ventilation are appropriate only for patients with a relatively normal respiratory rate and normal I:E ratio. The level of pressure support can be reduced gradually as the patient's ventilatory capabilities improve, and when the level of pressure support has been reduced to the value of PEEP, the patient has been weaned to CPAP. The use of such systems allows lower levels of sedation and avoidance of neuromuscular blocking drugs, and reduces disuse atrophy of the respiratory muscles. Weaning is thus a dynamic process in which the mode of ventilation changes from one which necessitates no participation by the patient to one in which mechanical assistance is reduced by titration against the patient's capability to sustain adequate gas exchange.

T-piece methods

Not all ICUs use these 'step-down' modes of ventilation routinely. An alternative is to use trials of spontaneous breathing with CPAP using a simple T-piece system. Periods of spontaneous breathing are allowed without any mechanical support and mechanical ventilation is restarted if the patient shows objective signs of diminished respiratory function. The periods of spontaneous breathing are increased progressively until tracheal extubation is possible.

There is conflicting evidence regarding the superiority of one method over the other and it seems likely that the mode of weaning needs to be individualized in the same manner as the mode of ventilation by taking into account the needs of the patient and the stage of the underlying disease.

If the need for mechanical support is likely to be prolonged, tracheostomy is often performed to prevent the adverse effects of prolonged orotracheal intubation and to facilitate weaning by reducing dead space, work of breathing and the need for sedation, while improving clearance of secretions and rendering re-ventilation easy if necessary..

Optimizing weaning

Although weaning is undertaken as early as possible in all patients, the chances of success are greatly increased if certain preconditions are met:

- The original requirement for mechanical ventilation has resolved.
- Sedative and analgesic drugs have been reduced to doses which do not depress ventilation.
- Inspired oxygen concentration is less than 50%.
- CO_2 elimination is not a problem and there is no respiratory acidosis.
- There is no metabolic acidosis.
- Nutritional status, trace elements, minerals, etc. are normal.
- Sputum production is minimal or sputum clearance good.
- Neuromuscular function is adequate.
- The patient is calm, cooperative and pain-free.
- There is no high-grade fever.

Monitoring during weaning

Respiratory rate, tidal volume, oxygen saturation, P_aCO_2 and P_aO_2 should be monitored and variables should be set beyond which weaning should be discontinued. When setting such variables, it is important to remember that the levels of P_aO_2 and P_aCO_2 should reflect the pre-morbid 'normal' values, which are often higher than the physiological norm. Although these vital signs offer objective criteria, the appearance of restlessness, tiredness, confusion, sweatiness, use of accessory muscles and generally abnormal respiratory patterns often occur before changes in vital signs and should be heeded as a warning sign that weaning has been unsuccessful.

CARDIOVASCULAR FAILURE

Although actual or expected ventilatory failure is the commonest reason for admission to the general ICU, cardiovascular failure is a frequent finding in the critically ill patient. When associated with pulmonary problems, the effects of cardiovascular insufficiency may be exacerbated because of reduced oxygenation of blood. Cardiovascular failure may be acute or chronic. When it develops rapidly (e.g. heart failure after myocardial infarction or peripheral circulatory failure after haemorrhage), it is termed 'shock' and, unless the condition is corrected rapidly, admission to ICU is necessary. Shock is a state in which the circulation is unable to provide adequate perfusion to meet the metabolic needs of the tissues. Unchecked, shock leads to generalized tissue hypoxia and multiple organ dysfunction. When reperfusion occurs, a secondary insult can worsen the initial injury. Cardiovascular monitoring and support in the ICU aim to pre-empt the development, or provide early recognition, of circulatory shock followed by rapid and effective support of the circulation to prevent the downward spiral into multiple organ failure.

Cardiovascular monitoring

It is possible to monitor the cardiovascular system clinically by the volume of the pulse, skin temperature, capillary refill, detection of tachycardia and sweating, or by identifying surrogate markers of cardiac output such as urine output. Biochemical evidence of established tissue hypoxia, such as metabolic acidosis with a raised blood lactate concentration, is another indicator of shock but may also occur in other forms of metabolic derangement. These are all late insensitive signs of shock, and significant delays in treatment, with an adverse effect on prognosis, occur if reliance is placed on them.

In critically ill patients, alterations in preload, cardiac function and afterload may occur very quickly and unpredictably, so that real-time measurement of these changes is vital to ensure early intervention and assessment of the effect of therapeutic interventions.

ECG

The ECG is monitored routinely in ICU patients although the presence of a bedside nurse has reduced the requirement for automatic arrhythmia detection systems of the type found in coronary care units.

Systemic arterial pressure

This may be measured intermittently by a conventional or automated sphygmomanometer or continuously by direct intra-arterial recording from the radial, brachial, dorsalis pedis or femoral arteries. Percutaneous arterial cannulation is used widely to monitor arterial pressure (Fig. 60.3) and to give ready access to arterial blood samples. Enormous technical efforts are being made to design non-invasive systems which may make invasive procedures less necessary, but at present their accuracy and dependability are inadequate in critical situations. Direct intra-arterial measurement is vital if inotropic or other vasoactive drugs are being used.

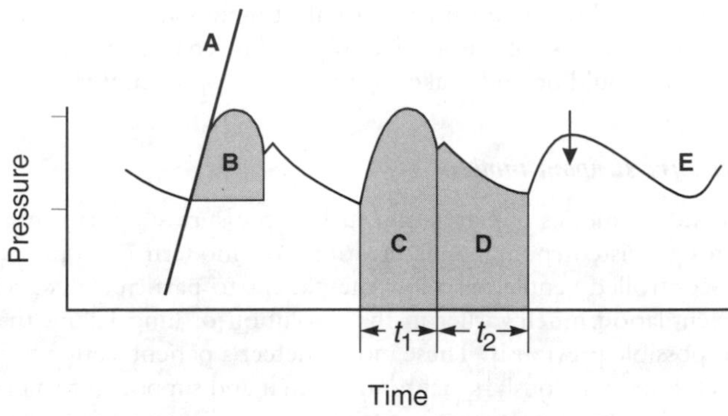

Visible sign	*Physiological effect*
A - rate of pressure increase	Myocardial contractility
B - area under pressure	Stroke volume
C - systolic pressure x time(t_1)	Myocardial oxygen consumption
D - diastolic pressure x time(t_2)	Myocardial oxygen supply
E - loss of waveform detail	Catheter occlusion (flush it!)

Fig. 60.3
Information to be gained from the arterial pressure signal.

Central venous pressure (CVP)

This may be measured from a catheter introduced into the superior vena cava and connected to an electronic manometer. Multi-lumen catheters allow secure access for infusions of various drugs which may be incompatible with each other and for administration of intermittent sedatives without fear of inadvertent flushing in of inotropic or other drugs; they also provide a dedicated route for temporary intravenous nutrition. The pressure transduced from the catheter is not usually useful as an absolute value; trends over a period of time are much more important, although rapid changes in response to administration of vasoactive or inotropic drugs, or fluid challenges, may also be significant. CVP readings must be interpreted in the knowledge that a high reading may be caused by high pulmonary artery pressure, high intrathoracic pressure or some other pulmonary abnormality, and not necessarily by cardiac abnormality or volume overload.

Pulmonary artery pressure (PAP)

This is measured by insertion of a flow-directed pulmonary artery catheter (PAC). The information gained from measurement of pulmonary capillary wedge pressure (PCWP) permits a distinction to be drawn between pulmonary oedema from high left atrial pressure (when PCWP is high) and that caused by increased permeability of pulmonary capillaries (when PCWP is not elevated). This may be helpful particularly in patients with multiple injuries and pulmonary problems, severe septicaemia or actual or incipient left ventricular failure.

PACs are used also to provide information relating to other haemodynamic variables such as cardiac output measured by thermodilution or continuous methods. Some types of PAC also give a continuous reading of mixed venous oxygen saturation. Computerized monitoring systems use these measurements to provide a wide range of derived parameters which may assist in resuscitation and treatment.

The indications for insertion of a PAC include:

- patients who require inotropic/vasoactive drug therapy
- assessment of fluid loading in SIRS/sepsis, after massive blood loss or other situations in which balancing preload and afterload is difficult, e.g. severe eclampsia with hypertension, pulmonary oedema and oliguria
- diagnosis of non-cardiogenic pulmonary oedema in ARDS
- pre-optimization of high-risk patients before surgery.

Complications of PAC insertion include those of central venous cannulation, but in addition they include arrhythmias during insertion, valve erosion causing a sterile or infective vegetation, pulmonary infarction, rupture of pulmonary artery and massive haemorrhage.

Before acting on the values measured using a PAC, its position must be checked on a chest X-ray. The tip of the catheter should lie in a zone in the pulmonary vasculature where pulmonary capillary pressure should exceed alveolar pressure. In addition, PCWP should be less than the mean pulmonary artery pressure, and the PO_2 of a sample of blood in the wedged position should be greater than mixed venous PO_2. Other pitfalls in practice are that high intrathoracic pressures falsely elevate PCWP – 5 cm of PEEP increases PCWP by 1 mmHg. This change is exaggerated further if the tip of the PAC is in a zone of low pulmonary blood flow or if the patient is hypovolaemic. Mitral regurgitation gives a falsely high value of PCWP as a result of the large v-wave; measuring the pressure at the top of the a-wave is more accurate. As the catheter warms and becomes thermolabile, it tends to migrate distally even when the balloon is deflated; if this occurs, it must be withdrawn until a pulmonary artery trace is identified, because prolonged wedging may cause pulmonary infarction. The balloon should always be deflated passively after measuring PCWP and the catheter must never be withdrawn with the balloon inflated as this may cause vascular rupture.

A recent retrospective analysis of a large US database has suggested that there may be increased mortality in patients with PACs as compared with controls. This may reflect the now abandoned practice of 'goal-directed therapy' and further prospective randomized trials are underway. A PAC should not be inserted unless the potential benefits to the patient exceed the risks.

Trans-oesophageal echocardiography (TOE)

Because of the potential risks of PACs, the assessment of cardiac function by non-invasive means has been expanding in recent years. A Doppler ultrasound probe passed into the oesophagus to lie alongside the descending arch of the aorta allows continuous measurement of velocity waveforms. The area under the recorded waveform may be converted to an estimate of stroke volume using a nomogram, while the acceleration and peak velocity of the rising curve are related to cardiac output. The data may be improved if the ejection fraction is measured simultaneously. The 'flow time' (the duration of the systolic flow) is related to circulating volume and peripheral resistance. Information may also be obtained relating to global left ventricular function and the presence of any structural abnormality. The response to fluid challenges is readily seen in real time without exposing the patient to the risks of a PAC; this may be useful in high-risk surgical patients who require optimization of cardiovascular function before surgery.

Gastric tonometry

The gut functions at relatively low levels of perfusion and oxygenation compared with other tissues and is at risk of ischaemia when the body attempts to compensate for a low cardiac output from any cause by vasoconstriction of the splanchnic circulation. Mucosal acidosis may be used as an early marker of shock. A gastric tonometer consists of a catheter with a silastic balloon at its tip which is inserted into the stomach or colon to lie against the wall. The balloon is filled with saline, and over a period of time CO_2 from the gut wall dissolves in the saline. The $P\text{CO}_2$ in the saline is assumed to be the same as the $P\text{CO}_2$ in the gut mucosa. The $P\text{CO}_2$ in the saline and the arterial bicarbonate concentration are entered into the Henderson–Hasselbalch equation to calculate intramucosal pH (pHi). The lower the pHi, the greater is the degree of ischaemia.

Cardiovascular support

Whatever the cause of cardiovascular failure, the aim of treatment is to restore organ perfusion and oxygenation to their pre-morbid levels. This may be achieved only by manipulating preload, myocardial contractility, heart rate and afterload. Therapy must be rapid, if irreversible organ damage is to be avoided.

The first step is to ensure that there are no airway or breathing problems before adjusting preload with optimization of fluid therapy monitored using the methods described above. When preload has been optimized, persisting evidence of shock is treated with appropriate inotropic or other vasoactive drugs; careful monitoring is essential because each patient's response varies.

The choice of drug is determined by the patient's underlying pathophysiology; where low cardiac output persists, dobutamine or epinephrine may be used, while cardiac failure with pulmonary oedema may require vasodilators or intra-aortic balloon counterpulsation. Blood flow may need to be redirected (e.g. by use of dopexamine to promote splanchnic blood flow). If a high-output, vasodilated state exists after fluid loading (e.g. in SIRS/sepsis), a vasoconstrictor such as norepinephrine should be used. The drugs and doses must be titrated against the patient's response with the aim of achieving a normal haemodynamic state.

In the general ICU population, the pursuit of supranormal values of oxygen delivery and cardiac output confers no survival benefit and increases mortality in some groups of patients. Stimulating a diseased myocardium with increasing doses of inotropes merely leads to tachycardia, arrhythmias, myocardial ischaemia and decreased survival. The use of inotropic and other vasoactive substances must be coupled with simultaneous optimization of preload and afterload.

If metabolic acidosis is severe (base deficit >15 mmol L^{-1}), the response to inotropes is often reduced; metabolic acidosis which persists after fluid resuscitation and correction of tissue hypoxia may require treatment with sodium bicarbonate and renal support.

SUPPORT OF OTHER SYSTEMS

Renal support

Primary renal disease is a rare cause of admission to the ICU, whereas secondary renal disease causing oliguria is very common in ICU patients. This stems from the extreme sensitivity to oxygen deprivation of those portions of the renal tubules that lie in the medulla. These normally work at the lowest level of the oxygen cascade and suffer early if tissue perfusion is reduced. Prevention of dysfunction progressing to established renal failure depends upon preservation of perfusion and avoidance of hypoxia. Cardiac output, perfusion pressure and intravascular volume should be optimized before considering any other renal support, such as a diuretic. The use of low-dose dopamine has been abandoned; it merely acts as a diuretic and is subject to the same restrictions.

Sudden cessation of urinary output should be regarded as being caused by obstruction until proved otherwise. All drugs should be reviewed for possible nephrotoxic effects and their doses adjusted if cumulation is a problem. Any life-threatening complication such as hyperkalaemia should be treated appropriately until definitive renal support can be arranged. In patients with rhabdomyolysis from any cause, aggressive fluid loading combined with alkalinization of urine and administration of mannitol may protect the kidney from further damage. Other renal protection regimens are unproven. Infusion of a loop diuretic is used in some ICUs to reduce distal tubular oxygen consumption in patients with non-oliguric renal failure.

Renal replacement therapy (RRT)

The absolute indications for RRT are uncontrollable hyperkalaemia, acidaemia, severe salt and water overload unresponsive to diuretics in the presence of good urine volume, and severe uraemia or anuria unrelated to obstruction. In most ICUs, continuous venovenous haemofiltration (CVVH) is used with a pump and filter in an extracorporeal circuit connected via a double-lumen vascular catheter placed in a central vein. These systems rely on the production of large volumes of what is essentially 'glomerular filtrate' by ultrafiltration of water and small solutes through the filter's semipermeable tubules. Accurate i.v. replacement with an equal volume of specific replacement fluid is required to maintain fluid balance; replacing slightly less allows the equivalent amount of water to be removed from the patient. In very catabolic septic patients, the ultrafiltration effect may be enhanced by passing dialysis fluid through the filter via a separate channel in a counter-current manner (continuous venovenous haemodiafiltration, CVVHD). The use of continuous slow techniques is tolerated better than intermittent haemodialysis in unstable ICU patients.

Neurological support

Despite the wide range of pathologies that require patients to be admitted to the ICU for specialized neurological support, some specific treatment regimens are common to them all.

Irrespective of the primary cause of neurological damage, secondary injury may be caused by hypoxaemia, hypotension, hypercapnia and metabolic disturbances. Consequently, the airway should be secured, the lungs ventilated to achieve a $P_{a}CO_2$ of 4–5 kPa, the inspired oxygen concentration adjusted to sustain a $P_{a}O_2$ in excess of 12 kPa and appropriate steps taken to maintain blood pressure within the normal range. Intravenous administration of glucose should be avoided and insulin should be administered intravenously if the blood glucose concentration exceeds 11 mmol L^{-1} because hyperglycaemia increases the risk of secondary brain injury. The plasma osmolality and serum sodium concentration should be monitored carefully because hypo-osmolality of the plasma creates an osmotic gradient across the blood–brain barrier and may provoke cerebral oedema.

In patients with raised ICP, it may be appropriate to monitor cerebral perfusion pressure (CPP) by direct measurement of ICP and mean arterial pressure. ICP should be maintained within the normal range if possible; sudden increases may occur in patients who are restless or hypertensive, and adequate sedation and analgesia are usually important components of therapy. CPP may be increased by judicious fluid loading and the use of pressor agents. However, high arterial pressure should be avoided, because many patients with brain injury have impaired cerebral autoregulation and a high CPP may result in increased cerebral oedema.

Administration of neuromuscular blockers is rarely required except to prevent shivering if surface cooling has been used in an attempt to decrease cerebral metabolic rate.

Cerebral blood flow may be monitored using radioisotope methods, or estimated using transcranial Doppler techniques, jugular venous bulb oxygen saturation or tissue oxygen electrodes placed within the skull.

Electrical activity of the brain may be monitored using techniques such as compressed spectral array or the analysing cerebral function monitor.

In modern neurosurgical ICUs, a combination of these techniques is often used to produce multimodal analysis of brain function, and therapy is adjusted to maximize oxygen delivery, minimize oxygen consumption, preserve cerebral blood flow and normalize ICP.

GENERAL INTENSIVE CARE

Visitors to ICUs often focus on the technology and fail to appreciate the intensity of the nursing and paramedical support needed for each patient. Skin care, tracheal suction, stress ulcer prophylaxis, DVT prophylaxis, turning, washing, eye, mouth and bowel care, mobilization and passive movement, and psychological support to the patient (and relatives) take considerable patience and skill and are important contributors to good outcome.

All ICU patients need nutrition as soon as possible, regardless of the reason for admission. Very few ICU patients are able to take a normal diet. There is increasing evidence that early enteral nutrition improves outcome and some evidence that specific diet supplements such as glutamine may improve immune function and survival. With the exception of patients with gastrointestinal obstruction, prolonged paralytic ileus, short bowel syndrome or enterocutaneous fistula, the majority of ICU patients can be fed via the enteral route within 48 h. A fine-bore nasogastric tube may be inadequate in some patients and a nasojejunal tube, feeding jejunostomy or percutaneous gastrostomy may be used. Parenteral feeding is the route of last resort but is better than nothing.

Of all ICU patients who die after spending more than 5 days in the ICU, 80% die in a manner which involves sepsis. Cross-infection is a particular risk and strict asepsis and personal hygiene are vital. The emergence of multiresistant microorganisms is an increasing problem and is conquered best by control of cross-infection, good aseptic techniques and regular microbiological surveillance, with swabs, blood cultures and other samples being taken at every opportunity. The widespread use of prophylactic or broad spectrum antibiotics is to be avoided.

OUTCOME AFTER INTENSIVE CARE

Intensive care has developed without much research into its efficacy in terms of improved survival and quality of life after discharge. Very few of the procedures performed commonly in the ICU have been subjected to scientific scrutiny, but it would be impossible ethically to allocate critically ill patients randomly to receive either ward or ICU care in an attempt to conduct a prospective controlled trial of the ICU process as a whole. Consequently, observational audit methods have been developed to compare actual outcome with predicted outcome in terms of survival. In the near future, all ICUs in the UK will be required to gather data to assess their performance. These methods require an objective scoring system which can assess severity of illness reproducibly and which takes into account the case mix of the ICU. Survival or death after ICU is influenced not only by the quality, timing and type of care, but also by the age of the patient, the severity of illness, the presence of co-morbidity, the illness which precipitates admission and the presence of any emergency or elective treatment given before admission.

The Intensive Care National Audit Research Centre (ICNARC) used the acute physiology and chronic health evaluation (APACHE) score developed by Knauss to compare ICU mortality and total hospital mortality among 22 057 ICU patients between 1995 and 1998 in 62 ICUs in England and Wales. The data showed an average mortality of 20.6% in ICUs and a total hospital mortality of 30.9%, but the mortality in different hospitals varied threefold. Because of the problems of case mix variability, these scoring systems are best used for comparative audit so that deviations from the norm may be identified and investigated, or for evaluative research; for example, severity of illness could be used to stratify patient groups into those with similar predicted outcomes of death so that the success or failure of a specific intervention may be evaluated within a homogenous group of patients.

Scoring systems should not be used to individualize treatment decisions within the ICU. The higher the APACHE score, the less likely a patient is to survive. For example, a 71-year-old man admitted to ICU after emergency abdominal aortic aneurysm repair may have physiological abnormality and co-morbidity which gives him an

Table 60.5 Recognition of brain stem death. Brain stem death may be assumed if: (a) the answer to each of the ten questions is 'no'; and (b) the assessment is repeated with the same results after at least 4 h. If the answer to any of the questions is 'yes' or 'don't know', active treatment must be continued

1. Is there any doubt as to the cause of the coma and brain damage (e.g. trauma, cerebrovascular accident, drowning)?
2. Has the patient received (or taken) any drugs which could have either depressed the central nervous system (e.g. alcohol, sedatives, hypnotics, analgesics) or impaired his or her muscular capabilities (e.g. muscle relaxants)?
3. Are there any metabolic or endocrine disturbances which could affect neural function (e.g. blood glucose changes, uraemia, hepatic dysfunction)?
4. Is the patient's temperature less than 35°C? (Midbrain failure is often followed by a rapid decrease in temperature, but hypothermia itself may induce coma. If the temperature is below 35°C, active warming must be started and further cooling minimized with 'space blankets'.)
5. Do the pupils react to light?
6. Are there corneal reflexes?
7. Do the eyes move during or after caloric testing?
8. Are there motor responses in the cranial nerve distribution in response to painful stimulation of the face, trunk or limbs?
9. Does the patient gag, cough or otherwise move following the passage of a suction catheter into the nose, mouth or bronchial tree?
10. Does the patient show any respiratory activity at all when the arterial carbon dioxide tension exceeds 7 kPa (checked on an arterial sample)?

APACHE score of 22. For this *condition*, with this score, the probability of death is 60.5%, but the probability of death for this *patient* cannot be predicted; he or she may be one of the 39.5% who survive! Thus, at their present level of accuracy, scoring systems cannot be used alone to identify patients in whom continued treatment is futile.

ICU care is supportive rather than curative and has the ability to prolong the process of dying. This is not in the best interests of a patient who continues to deteriorate despite maximal supportive therapy. In such patients, the continuation of treatment is both futile and unethical. About 70% of deaths in ICUs occur after limitation of treatment. This is not euthanasia; the patient dies of the underlying disease process when the supporting therapies are withdrawn. The identification of patients in whom there should be a change from aggressive supportive therapy to compassionate, palliative care is difficult. Opinions may vary as to what constitutes futility, the timing of the change to palliative care and the nature of the treatments to be withdrawn. There is variability among countries, and among ICUs within the same country.

In terms of predicting which patients are unlikely to survive, those who are comatose and unresponsive after severe brain damage are amongst the easier to distinguish. The signs of 'brain stem death' are well recognized and a scheme of assessment is shown in Table 60.5. If brain stem death is a likely diagnosis, the possibility of organ donation should always be considered and discussed with the patient's family. It is best if these discussions are initiated by ICU staff who are experienced in dealing with bereaved relatives.

Assessments of functional disability, quality of life and return to work among patients who have survived an admission to the ICU are more difficult to quantify than death, but the small numbers of studies which have been undertaken suggest that mortality is significantly higher than would be expected in matched individuals for several years, that a significant proportion of patients report impaired quality of life and that many remain unable to work for prolonged periods after discharge. However, the majority of patients survive and return to a reasonable quality of life.

Improving outcome

Many patients who undergo elective or, more commonly, emergency surgery receive inadequate preoperative preparation in respect of volume resuscitation or cardiovascular support. These patients are particularly at risk from hypovolaemia and myocardial ischaemia in the perioperative period, and suffer an exaggerated stress response. These factors amplify postoperative SIRS because of decreased organ perfusion. There is increasing evidence that outcome may be improved in high-risk surgical patients if blood volume and cardiovascular function are optimized preoperatively.

The fact that the most seriously ill patients are now nursed in specialized areas has resulted in 'de-skilling' of ward-based nursing and medical staff. The increased throughput of surgical patients, together with the reduction in the working hours of trainee medical staff, has resulted in a risk that patients may deteriorate in the ward unnoticed, or that their deterioration may be treated inadequately, so that there may be great difficulty in resuscitation when the true severity of the patient's condition is recognized. The total hospital mortality of patients admitted to the ICU from other hospital wards (45%) is significantly greater than the mortality among patients admitted from the accident and emergency department (30%) or from the operating theatre (20%).

There is therefore a need for an area within the hospital which can provide an intermediate level of care. These areas are usually called high-dependency units (HDU). The development of HDUs should proceed in tandem with education of ward-based medical and nursing staff and with the development of 'critical care outreach' teams. Increasingly, the barriers between ICU, HDU and the post-anaesthesia care unit (PACU) will become blurred so that critically ill patients can receive the level of care most appropriate for the severity of their illness and the progress of their disease at all times during their stay in hospital.

FURTHER READING

Craft T, Nolan J, Parr M 1999 Key topics in critical care. BIOS Scientific Publishers, Oxford

Hillman K, Bishop G 1996 Clinical intensive care. Cambridge University Press, Cambridge

Singer M, Grant I S 1999 ABC of intensive care. BMJ Publications, London

Webb A R, Shapiro M, Singer M, Suter P 1999 Oxford textbook of critical care. Oxford University Press, Oxford

61 Management of chronic pain

Recent advances in the understanding of the fundamental mechanisms involved in the transmission and modulation of noxious impulses have significantly extended the range of assessment tools and treatments clinicians offer to patients with pain. The majority of medical pain specialists in the UK are anaesthetists. Historically, anaesthetists have been responsible for the relief of pain in the perioperative period and have developed skills in percutaneous neural blockade. This expertise, developed originally for local anaesthetics, was then extended to neurolytic agents. Initially, pain clinics started as nerve-blocking clinics and most pain management clinics continue to be directed by anaesthetists. However, with increasing awareness of the complexity of the pain experience, there has been recognition that other health care professionals have a significant role in the management of patients with chronic pain. A multidisciplinary approach involving anaesthetists and other health care professionals is being offered increasingly to patients with pain.

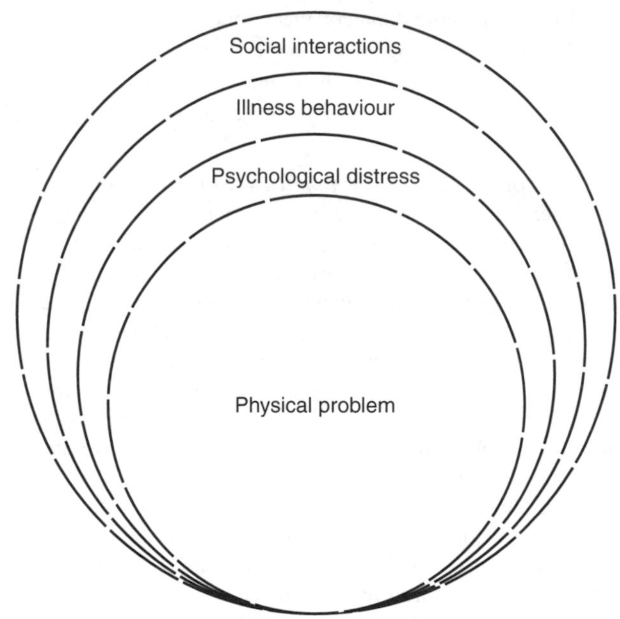

Fig. 61.1
An illustration of pain as a biopsychosocial phenomenon.

DEFINITION OF PAIN

Everyone has experienced pain, but it has been difficult to define this sensation satisfactorily. One description is 'what the patient says hurts'.

The International Association for the Study of Pain (IASP) defines pain as 'an unpleasant sensory and emotional experience associated with actual or potential tissue damage, or described in terms of such damage'.

This definition emphasizes that pain is not only a physical sensation but also, ultimately, a subjective psychological event. It accepts that pain can occur in spite of negative physical findings and investigations.

Pain has sensory, cognitive and motivational-affective dimensions and has been described as a biopsychosocial experience as illustrated in Figure 61.1. This must be taken into account when assessing and planning a treatment strategy for the patient with pain.

THE PARADIGM OF PAIN

Pain management concerns postoperative, acute and chronic pain and cancer-related symptom control in children and adults. A joint report of the (then) College of Anaesthetists and the Royal College of Surgeons highlighted the need to improve standards of postoperative pain management and many hospitals have established acute pain teams. However, many hospitalized patients suffer from acute non-postoperative pain. This may be caused by trauma, burns or acutely painful medical conditions (e.g. cardiac pain, osteoporotic spinal collapse). Some medical conditions may cause recurrent acute painful episodes such as sickle-cell crisis or acute exacerbations of chronic pancreatitis. Unrelieved acute pain may lead to chronic pain. Chronic pain is described as pain following an episode of tissue damage which persists after the time when healing is expected to be complete. This is usually taken arbitrarily as 3 months. However, chronic pain is a complex biopsychosocial phenomenon and a single pathophysiological explanation is not available for many chronic non-malignant pain states. Cancer-related pain problems may present to the anaesthetist for management as a hospital in-patient or outpatient, in a hospice or in the home. There are many common areas within the management of acute and chronic pain, and increasingly pain is viewed as a continuum rather than two separate entities, with subsequent merging of management techniques and staff.

Postoperative, recurrent, chronic persistent and cancer-related pain also occurs in children. Difficulties in pain assessment and unsubstantiated fears and myths regarding pain in children and its treatment have led to less than optimal management. Recommendations for the management of pain in children have been published recently and are detailed in the further reading section.

EPIDEMIOLOGY OF CHRONIC PAIN

The true incidence of chronic pain in the UK is unknown. Attempts have been made to study this, but obtaining a true picture is difficult because many patients with chronic pain seek help from a range of medical practitioners and complementary therapists. It has been estimated that 7% of the population suffer chronic pain at any one time. Back pain represents the largest group in most surveys. Back pain is the main reason for 20% of all visits to a GP and is cited as the cause for 45 million certified days off work annually. The annual cost of NHS treatments for back pain is nearly £500 million, plus half as much again for non-NHS treatments.

Pain is experienced by 20–50% of patients with cancer at the time of diagnosis and by up to 75% of patients with advanced disease.

CLASSIFICATION OF PAIN

Pain may be classified according to aetiology.

NOCICEPTIVE PAIN

Nociceptive pain results from tissue damage causing continual nociceptor stimulation. It may be either somatic or visceral in origin.

Somatic pain

Somatic pain results from activation of nociceptors in cutaneous and deep tissues, such as bone. Typically, it is well localized and described as aching, throbbing or gnawing. Somatic pain is usually sensitive to opioids.

Visceral pain

Visceral pain arises from internal organs. It is characteristically vague in distribution and quality and is often described as deep, dull or dragging. It may be associated with nausea, vomiting and alterations in arterial pressure and heart rate. Stimuli, such as crushing or burning, which are painful in somatic structures often evoke no pain in visceral organs. Mechanisms of visceral pain include abnormal distension or contraction of smooth muscle, stretching of the capsule of solid organs, hypoxia or necrosis and irritation by algesic substances. Visceral pain is often referred to cutaneous sites distant from the visceral lesion. One example of this is shoulder pain resulting from diaphragmatic irritation.

NEUROPATHIC PAIN

Neuropathic pain is caused by functional abnormality of the peripheral and/or central nervous system. It is characteristically dysaesthetic in nature and patients complain of unpleasant abnormal sensations. There may be marked allodynia, i.e. a normally non-painful stimulus, such as light touch, provokes pain. Pain may be described as shooting or burning and may occur in areas of numbness. Neuropathic pain may develop immediately after nerve injury or after a variable interval. It is often persistent and relatively resistant to opioids. There is a tendency for a favourable response to centrally modulating medication, such as anticonvulsants and tricyclic antidepressants.

There are many causes of neuropathic pain. Central pain is associated with lesions of the central nervous system, such as infarction and trauma. Lesions in the peripheral nervous system include peripheral nerve injuries, peripheral neuropathies and tumour infiltration.

Sympathetically maintained pain

Pain that is maintained by sympathetic efferent innervation or by circulating catecholamines is termed sympathetically maintained pain (SMP). It may be a feature of several pain complaints. Sympathetic nerve block provides at least temporary reduction of pain, but current thinking is that this does not imply a mechanism for the pain. Thus, the condition previously termed 'reflex sympathetic dystrophy' has now been renamed 'complex regional pain syndrome type I', as not all patients with this clinical diagnosis have relief of pain following sympathetic nerve block.

Complex regional pain syndrome (CRPS) type I is a syndrome that can develop in a limb after mild soft tissue trauma or a fracture (Fig. 61.2). The pain is characteristically burning in nature and associated with allodynia (abnormal sensitivity of the skin). It is associated at some point with swelling, abnormal sweating and changes in skin blood flow. Atrophy of the skin, nails and muscles can occur and localized osteoporosis may be demonstrated on X-ray or bone scan. Movement of the limb is usually restricted as a result of the pain and contractures may result. Treatment is directed at providing adequate analgesia to encourage active physiotherapy and improvement of function. In cases with sympathetically maintained pain, sympathetic nerve block may be part of this treatment strategy.

Complex regional pain syndrome type II is a condition that has the features described above, but which occurs after partial injury of a nerve or one of its branches.

SOMATOFORM PAIN DISORDER

This is a currently accepted psychiatric diagnosis, which can be used when there is substantial evidence that psychological factors are judged to have an important role in the onset, severity, exacer-

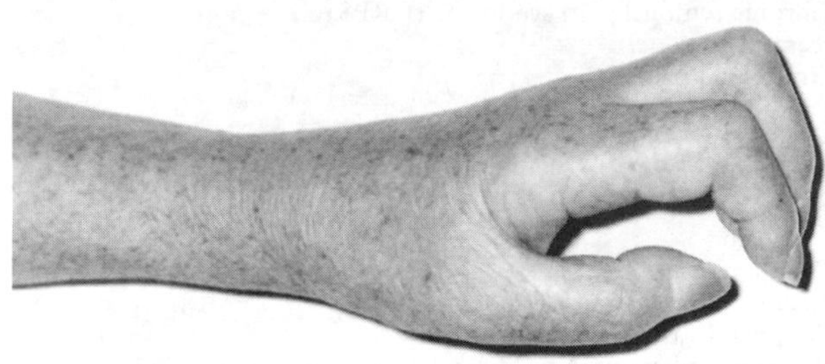

Fig. 61.2
Complex regional pain syndrome type 1 following Colles' fracture.

bation or maintenance of the pain. Strict diagnostic criteria must be fulfilled before such a diagnosis can be made and this should be made by or in conjunction with a psychiatrist. Chronic pain is usually the cause and not the result of psychiatric symptoms.

PAIN MANAGEMENT CLINIC

In the pain management clinic, patients present with pain resulting from many different pathological processes. Some examples of common painful conditions are listed in Table 61.1.

ASSESSMENT

Comprehensive assessment of patients with pain is a vital first step. Pain is a generally a symptom rather than a disease. Efforts should be made to investigate, diagnose and, if possible, treat the underlying cause of the pain before using empirical pain-relieving techniques. Patients attending a pain management clinic may be referred by either their hospital consultant or their GP but this maxim should be followed.

The key elements of a pain history should be ascertained using a structured interview. Assessment should include:

- location, verbally or using a pain diagram
- mode of onset and frequency
- aggravating factors
- relieving factors
- quality, e.g. burning, shooting – use McGill Pain Questionnaire
- intensity, e.g. verbal rating scale, visual analogue scale, faces pain scale (children)
- previous treatments
- concurrent medical illnesses
- current medication (analgesics and others)
- basic psychological/psychiatric assessment
- patient's own ideas as to causation
- impairment and disability.

Many patients, especially those with malignancy, have more than one site of pain and separate histories should be taken for each complaint as their aetiology may differ. Particular care and skill are needed when taking a pain history from children and the elderly.

An appropriate physical examination relevant to the pain complaint should be performed. Special reference might be made to tender points and trigger points in muscles and scars, neurological deficit and signs implicating involvement of the sympathetic nervous system including vasomotor, sudomotor and trophic changes.

Occasionally further laboratory, radiological and electrophysiological tests might be needed for full evaluation.

Basic psychological assessment can be made by the clinician, sometimes aided by questionnaires. Levels of anxiety, depression and coping ability are some of the elements that can be measured using appropriate tools. If full psychological evaluation is indicated, it should be performed either by a psychiatrist or by a clinical psychologist, preferably one who is an integral member of the pain management team.

Chronic pain affects not only the patient, but also the family. Patients with chronic pain become depressed, anxious and medication-dependent. They lose their jobs, financial security and social status. Their relationships deteriorate. Interviewing of the patient's relatives or close friends may be important in assessing the impact of the pain on family dynamics and lifestyle.

From the history, examination, investigations and previous diagnosis, the pain complaint should be classified. Full explanation of the pain complaint and the results of investigations should be discussed with the patient. A patient-led problem list should be formulated and patient expectations for treatment should be explored and, if necessary, rationalized. The limitations of the medical model of disease for some chronic pain complaints should be explained. A treatment plan should be jointly formulated with the patient after discussion of the available treatments and the potential benefits and side-effects of those options.

Table 61.1 Some common painful conditions

Malignant aetiology
Primary tumours
Metastases
Treatment-related, e.g. post-surgery pain
Non-malignant aetiology
Musculoskeletal
Back pain
Neuropathic
Trigeminal neuralgia
Postherpetic neuralgia
Brachial plexus avulsion
Radicular pain of spinal origin
Peripheral neuropathy
Chronic regional pain syndrome (CRPS)
Visceral
Urogenital pain
Pancreatitis
Post-surgery
Phantom pain
Stump pain
Scar pain
Post-laminectomy
Ischaemic
Peripheral vascular disease
Raynaud's phenomenon/disease
Intractable angina
Headaches

METHODS OF MANAGEMENT OF CHRONIC PAIN

Chronic pain is a complex phenomenon and often multifactorial in aetiology. Several methods of treatment may therefore be used in the same patient, either concomitantly or sequentially.

MEDICATION

Many patients in pain are prescribed analgesic drugs. The pharmacology of these agents is fully discussed elsewhere (Ch. 18) and only aspects of particular relevance to their use in chronic pain are mentioned below.

Non-steroidal anti-inflammatory drugs

Non-steroidal anti-inflammatory drugs (NSAIDs) interfere with the production of prostaglandins and prostacyclins by inhibiting the enzyme cyclooxygenase. They possess analgesic and anti-inflammatory action and are used widely in the management of mild to moderate pain, particularly of somatic origin. They may be very effective for painful bone metastases and useful in dysmenorrhoea, arthritis and musculoskeletal pain. They may be used orally or as a suppository. Side-effects may be a problem, especially in the elderly.

McQuay & Moore (1998) have assessed the efficacy of topical NSAIDs for chronic painful conditions using the concept of number-needed-to treat (NNT). An NNT value of 1 describes an event that occurs in every patient given the treatment but in no patient in the comparator group. NNTs of 2–4 indicate effective treatments. Published randomized control trials on chronic painful conditions (mainly knee osteoarthritis) have studied over 1000 subjects using either topical NSAIDs or placebo and found that, for analgesic effects from topical NSAIDs, the NNT was 3.1.

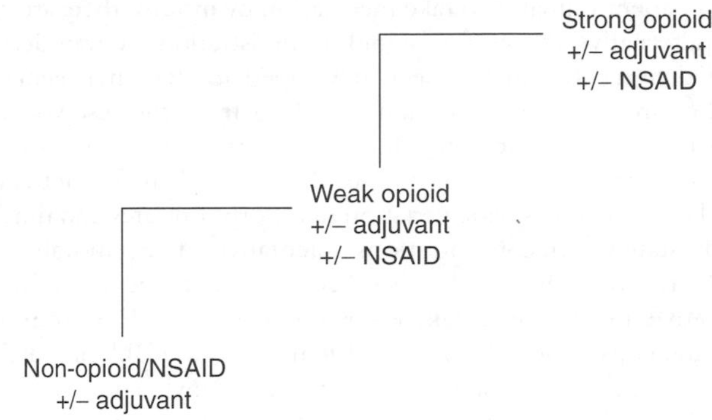

Fig. 61.3
The WHO analgesic ladder.

Opioid analgesics

Cancer pain

Approximately 70% of patients with advanced cancer develop significant pain before death. Most cancer pain responds to pharmacological measures and successful treatment is based on simple principles that have been promoted by the World Health Organization and are extensively validated. Analgesic drugs should be taken 'by mouth', 'by the clock' (i.e. regularly) and 'by the analgesic ladder' (Fig. 61.3). Cancer pain is continuous and medication must be taken regularly. It is given orally unless intractable nausea and vomiting occur or unless there is a physical impediment to swallowing. The first step on the 'analgesic ladder' is a non-opioid, such as paracetamol, aspirin or an NSAID. If this is inadequate, a weak opioid such as codeine is added. The third step is substitution of the weak opioid by a strong opioid. Inadequate pain control at one level requires progression to an drug on the next level, rather than to an alternative of similar efficacy. Adjuvant analgesics, such as tricyclic antidepressants or anticonvulsants, may be used at any stage.

Using these strategies, pain can be controlled successfully in about 90% of patients with cancer pain without resorting to other interventions.

Morphine is the strong oral opioid of choice. Immediate-release oral morphine, either as a liquid or in tablet form, is given every 4 h, if necessary in increasing dosage, until pain is controlled. When the required daily dose has been established, it is usual to convert to sustained-release morphine tablets, which need to be taken only once or twice daily. In addition, immediate-release morphine elixir or tablets should be prescribed for breakthrough pain. The dose of morphine necessary to treat breakthrough pain is one-sixth of the total daily morphine requirement.

Education of the medical and nursing professions, and also the patient and family, is still necessary to ensure that adequate doses of opioids are prescribed and taken. Health care professionals often overestimate the side-effects of morphine. Respiratory depression is uncommon when morphine is prescribed for cancer pain. Surveys have shown that patients are concerned about side-effects of morphine, especially tolerance, addiction, constipation and drowsiness. Tolerance does not appear to be a problem clinically. Many patients with static disease take the same dose of morphine for long periods of time. Disease progression may necessitate an increase in dose, but there is no upper limit to the dose of morphine and pain control is usually regained without difficulty. Addiction (psychological dependence) does not occur in patients with cancer pain, and if the pain is relieved by other means, such as radiotherapy or a nerve block, many patients will stop their opioids. Nausea and vomiting may occur when morphine is first commenced and an antiemetic can be prescribed for the first week after commencing this medication, but often it may then be stopped. Sedation and cognitive impairment may occur as the dose is increased but usually resolve. However, there is no tolerance to the constipating effect of morphine and laxatives need to be taken regularly.

Efforts should be made to reassure both patients and relatives of the efficacy and safety of morphine analgesia in both the short and the long term to ensure that medication is taken.

Alternative opioids and alternative routes of administration. Hydromorphone is an alternative opioid which has been recently licensed for use in the UK, although it has been available for several years in North America. It is used orally and is more potent than morphine, with 1.3 mg of hydromorphone being equivalent to 10 mg of morphine. When administered orally, hydromorphone reaches its peak effect more rapidly than morphine and has a slightly shorter duration of action. Immediate-release and sustained-release preparations are available. Hydromorphone is normally used if morphine is not tolerated.

Methadone is a potent opioid analgesic and also an *N*-methyl-D-aspartate (NMDA) receptor antagonist. Methadone is absorbed rapidly by the oral route and has a long half-life that may range from 13 to 51 h. Initial dosing must be monitored carefully as relatively small doses of methadone may be needed in comparison with the previous opioid dose. When repeated doses are given, the drug accumulates and after the first few days the frequency of administration may need to be reduced to twice or thrice daily. Methadone should be considered a third-line drug indicated for cancer pain that appears poorly responsive to morphine, diamorphine, fentanyl or hydromorphone in spite of dose escalation and the use of adjuvant drugs. Methadone is available as tablets, linctus and injection.

If a patient is unable to take medication by mouth, there are various alternative routes for opioid administration. A transdermal drug delivery system has been developed for fentanyl. Fentanyl patches are stuck onto the skin and drug from the reservoir diffuses through the rate-controlling membrane and forms a subcutaneous depot from which the drug is taken up into the circulation. There is wide variation in absorption rates and time to steady-state serum concentrations of fentanyl. After removal of the patch, the terminal half-life has been shown to be 17 ± 2.3 h, indicative of the time taken for the drug to clear from the subcutaneous depot. Transdermal fentanyl is available in patches that deliver 25, 50, 75 and 100 μg h^{-1} of fentanyl. They should be placed on unbroken skin usually on the upper body and need to be changed every 72 h. They are suitable for patients who cannot or prefer not to take oral medication or who are intolerant of morphine. However, the delay in onset of analgesia makes them unsuitable for treatment of acute pain. Immediate-release morphine should be prescribed in appropriate dosage for breakthrough pain.

Continuous subcutaneous administration is another alternative method of administration if oral medication cannot be taken. A small portable battery-operated syringe driver fitted with a 20 ml syringe containing the total daily opioid dose is usually used. Because of its greater solubility, diamorphine is the drug of choice for this route of administration in the UK. A conversion ratio of 3 mg oral morphine to 1 mg subcutaneous diamorphine is used.

Morphine suppositories are available for rectal administration.

Opioids can be administered spinally, either epidurally or intrathecally, for:

- patients whose pain is controlled effectively by oral opioids but who suffer intolerable unacceptable side-effects, such as drowsiness or vomiting
- patients whose pain cannot be controlled by the use of oral or systemic opioids.

Only a small proportion (less than 2%) of patients with cancer pain are candidates for spinal opioids. Much smaller doses of drug are required when given spinally and thus side-effects are minimized. The daily dose of morphine via the epidural route is 1/10 of the oral 24-h dose and the intrathecal dose is 1/10 of the epidural dose. Contraindications to the insertion of a spinal catheter are similar to those in the acute situation. Side-effects, such as respiratory depression, itching and urinary retention, that cause such concern in the opioid-naive patient are rare in cancer patients who have been chronically exposed to systemic opioids.

The field of spinal opioid therapy is sufficiently new that guidelines for selection of route (intrathecal or epidural), choice of drug (opioid or opioid/local anaesthetic combination), administration protocol (intermittent bolus or continuous infusion) and equipment (tunnelled or totally implanted catheter and reservoir) are still being formulated.

Before introducing this technique, it is essential to devise formal protocols and an education programme for hospital, hospice and primary care nurses and doctors to facilitate management of the patient in any of these settings.

Non-cancer pain

Weak opioid drugs, e.g. dihydrocodeine, are useful for moderate pain. However, they may be taken in excess, and often with only little benefit, by the patient with chronic non-malignant pain. Treatment in the pain management clinic may involve weaning the patient off such medication.

The use of strong opioids in non-malignant pain is controversial. There is conflict about whether opioids are effective and whether or not they are safe. There is some evidence that opioids relieve pain and improve function in patients with non-cancer pain. However, there are other studies that conclude that chronic opioid therapy exacerbates psychological distress, impairs cognition and worsens outcome. The controversy is also compounded by the perceived risk of psychological dependence (addiction). Guidelines for the use of opioids in non-malignant pain have been formulated in several countries and work is being undertaken in the UK to produce clinical guidelines.

Adjuvant analgesics

These are drugs that have primary indications other than pain but are analgesic in some painful conditions.

Oral corticosteroids

The mechanism by which corticosteroids produce analgesia is unknown. They reduce inflammatory mediators, specifically prostaglandins. They reduce peritumour oedema in neoplastic tissue, thus relieving pain by reducing pressure on adjacent pain-sensitive structures. They are administered for cerebral metastases, spinal cord compression, superior vena caval compression and neural infiltration or compression. In addition, they are prescribed for their euphoric effect and to stimulate appetite for patients with cancer.

Anticonvulsants

Anticonvulsants are used in the treatment of neuropathic pain. The precise mechanism of action is unclear. They have a stabilizing effect on neuronal cell membranes, possibly by inactivation of sodium channels. They may also facilitate GABA (γ-aminobutyric acid)-mediated inhibition and decrease activation of NMDA receptors. Gabapentin, carbamazepine and phenytoin have a product licence for use in neuropathic pain and trigeminal neuralgia.

For anticonvulsants in a variety of neuropathic pains, the NNT for more than 50% relief is approximately 2.5, indicating that they are effective. Sedation and ataxia are common side-effects of some of these drugs and may limit dose escalation, especially in the elderly. Serious complications (mainly haematological) may occur.

Tricyclic antidepressants

Tricyclic antidepressants have an important role in the management of pain, independent of their effect on mood. Tricyclic drugs reduce the reuptake of the amine neurotransmitters norepinephrine and 5-hydroxytryptamine into the presynaptic terminal, increasing the concentration and duration of action of these substances at the synapse and thereby enhancing activity in the descending inhibitory pain pathway.

Animal models of acute pain have consistently demonstrated the antinociceptive effect of tricyclic drugs. Controlled clinical trials have shown beneficial results in postherpetic neuralgia, diabetic neuropathy, atypical facial pain and central pain. The NNT for effectiveness for antidepressants in neuropathic pain is about 2.5.

The effective dose of a tricyclic drug for analgesia is usually lower than that required for depression (although a dose–response for analgesia has been demonstrated) and analgesia is apparent in 3–4 days compared with 3–4 weeks for antidepressant effects. Amitriptyline is the commonest tricyclic drug prescribed as an analgesic and the normal starting dose is 10–25 mg *nocte*. Side-effects include sedation (which can be beneficial), constipation and a dry mouth. Other tricyclic drugs used as analgesics include imipramine and prothiaden. Selective serotonin reuptake inhibitors, such as fluoxetine, appear to be less effective analgesics.

Antiarrhythmic drugs

Systemic local anaesthetic infusions have been used diagnostically and therapeutically for chronic neuropathic pain. Lidocaine 5 mg kg^{-1} given intravenously to patients with painful diabetic peripheral neuropathy in a double-blind cross-over study has been demonstrated to produce analgesia. Unfortunately, the effect is short-lived. Oral mexiletine has been used successfully in diabetic peripheral neuropathy.

Ketamine

Ketamine is an NMDA receptor antagonist; it has been used successfully as an analgesic via intravenous, subcutaneous and oral routes. Psychometric side-effects may be a problem.

Capsaicin cream

Capsaicin is an alkaloid derived from chillies. It depletes substance P in local sensory nerve terminals. Local application may alleviate pain in painful diabetic peripheral neuropathy, osteoarthritis and psoriasis. It has also been suggested for postherpetic and intercostobrachial neuralgia.

NEURAL BLOCKADE IN PAIN MANAGEMENT

Nerve blocks have been performed for many years in the management of pain. A nerve block comprises an injection of a local anaesthetic (sometimes combined with steroid) or a neurolytic agent around a peripheral or central sensory nerve, a sympathetic plexus or a trigger point. Correct use of nerve blocks in the treatment of chronic pain requires an experienced practitioner with a thorough knowledge of anatomy and an understanding of pain syndromes. Neural blockade should be undertaken in appropriate locations by clinicians who are fully acquainted with the techniques involved and who are competent to manage the complications that may arise. The use of radiological control and contrast media is strongly advocated to confirm accurate needle placement.

Potential sites for neural blockade are demonstrated in Figure 61.4, and indications for neural blockade are listed in Table 61.2. Some comments about commonly performed nerve blocks are made in the section below. For a full description of the techniques of neural blockade, the reader should consult suggested texts in the further reading section.

Table 61.2 Indications for neural blockade

Nerve block	Indications
Trigger point injections	Myofascial pain, scar pain
Somatic nerve block	Nerve root pain, scar pain
Trigeminal nerve block and branches	Trigeminal neuralgia
Stellate ganglion block	SMP, CRPS
Coeliac plexus block	Intra-abdominal malignancy, especially pancreas
Superior hypogastric plexus block	Malignant pelvic pain
Lumbar sympathetic block	Ischaemic rest pain SMP, CRPS Phantom and stump pain
Epidural steroids	Nerve root pain, benign or malignant
Intrathecal neurolytics	Malignant pain
Percutaneous cervical cordotomy	Unilateral somatic malignant pain, short life expectancy

SMP, sympathetically maintained pain; CRPS, complex regional pain syndrome.

Local anaesthetics

Local anaesthetics have been injected into muscle trigger points for the relief of myofascial pain and it has been shown that prolonged relief of pain can result from a series of local anaesthetic blocks to peripheral nerves. It is unclear why pain relief may persist after the duration of pharmacological action.

Corticosteroids

Corticosteroids have been shown to block transmission in normal unmyelinated C fibres and to suppress ectopic neural discharges in experimental neuromas. They are sometimes added to local anaesthetics when injected into trigger points, typically those in painful scars.

Epidural steroids

Epidural steroids have been used since 1962 for nerve root pain. A recent meta-analysis of all randomized controlled trials has concluded that epidural administration of corticosteroids is more effective in reducing lumbosacral radicular pain (in both the short and long term) than placebo. In addition, McQuay & Moore (1998) have addressed the question 'How well do they work?' by investigating the short-term (1–60 days) and long-term (12 weeks–1 year) efficacy of epidural steroids for sciatica. They used the NNT as a measure of clinical benefit. The NNT for short-term, greater than 75% pain relief was just under 7.3. This means that for seven patients treated with epidural steroids, one will obtain more than 75% pain relief in the short term who would not have done so had he or she received the control treatment (placebo or local anaesthetic). The NNT for long-term (12 weeks–1 year) improvement was about 13 for 50% pain relief.

However, the use of epidural steroids is not without potential hazards and controversy. The most common side-effects relate not to the steroid but to technical aspects of the technique. There have been reports of dural tap (2.5%), transient headache (2.3%) and transient increase in pain (1.9%). As with any spinal technique, an aseptic technique must be used and the usual contraindications observed. Methylprednisolone acetate and triamcinolone are the

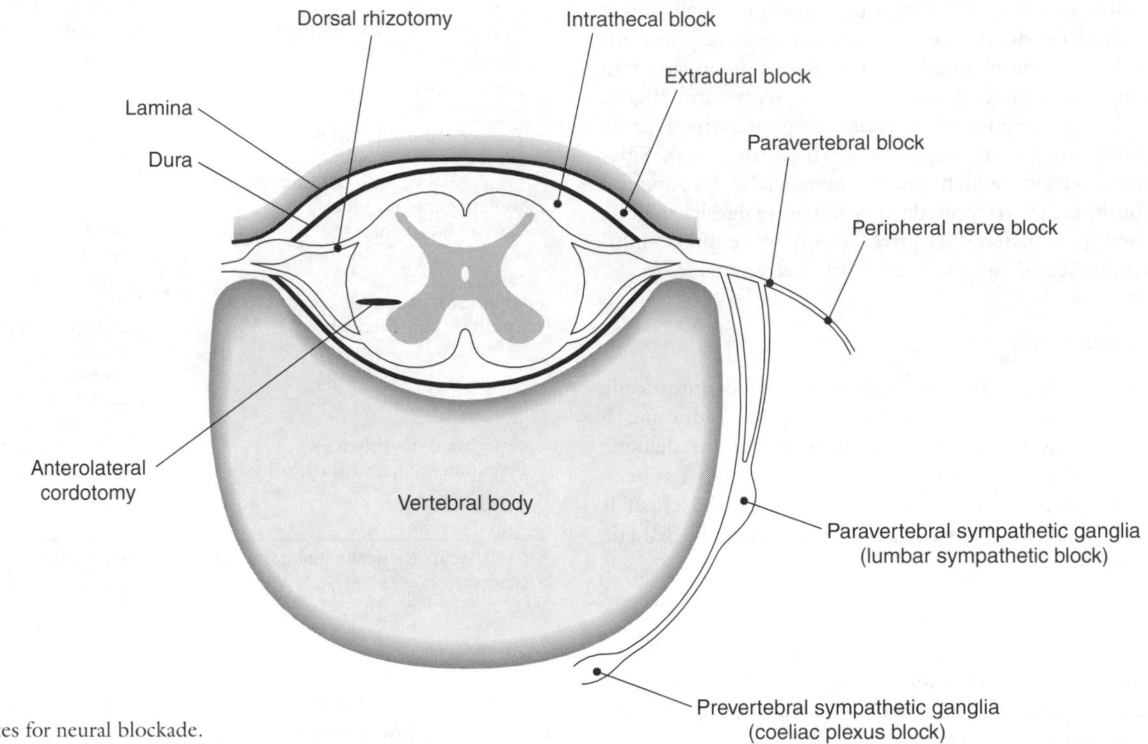

Fig. 61.4
Potential sites for neural blockade.

steroids most commonly used. It has been shown that neither of these preparations is deleterious when injected into the epidural space. However, they may have harmful effects if injected inadvertently into the subarachnoid or subdural space.

Before an epidural steroid injection is undertaken, the patient should receive a consultation during which the perceived merits, expectations, risks and possible complications are fully explained. This should include an explanation that the steroid preparation is being used outside of its product licence. The doctor should be satisfied that the procedure is indicated, that appropriate neurological examination and investigations have been performed and that there is no contraindication to the procedure. Written consent should be obtained. Arrangements should be made for the outcome to be formally monitored by the doctor who prescribed the procedure or the one who performed it. Provision should be made for an earlier consultation if necessary.

Lumbar and cervical facet blocks

Chronic back and neck pain are common complaints in pain management clinics. Lumbar and cervical facet joints have been considered to be potential sources. Injections of steroid into both lumbar and cervical facet joints are commonly performed procedures, although there is controversy about long-term benefit. Radiofrequency lesions of the facet nerves have been suggested for longer-term relief.

Sympathetic nerve blocks

Visceral nociceptive afferents travel in the sympathetic nervous system to the spinal cord. Visceral pain tends to be less opioid-sensitive than somatic pain. Percutaneous sympathetic blocks may therefore be useful in the management of severe cancer-related visceral pain that is poorly controlled with opioids or controlled only with intolerable side-effects.

Percutaneous coeliac plexus block using 50% alcohol is one of the most commonly used and effective blocks performed for cancer pain. It is used for pain resulting from upper gastrointestinal neoplasms, in particular carcinoma of the pancreas. Radiological screening, either X-ray or CT, is mandatory, although this in itself does not ensure absence of complications. Hypotension, especially postural hypotension, should be anticipated and managed appropriately. Serious complications are rare, although paraplegia has been reported.

The superior hypogastric plexus innervates the pelvic viscera. Superior hypogastric plexus block with phenol has been used for pelvic pain from cervical, prostatic, colonic, rectal, bladder, uterine and ovarian malignancy and rectal tenesmus.

Chemical lumbar sympathectomy using phenol is performed for inoperable ischaemic leg pain. Radiological screening using contrast medium is necessary to ensure correct needle placement. The complication rate is low, the most common complication being genitofemoral neuralgia, with the reported incidence varying from 4 to 15%.

Stellate ganglion and lumbar sympathetic block with local anaesthetic is sometimes helpful in the treatment of sympathetically mediated pain, CRPS types I and II, amputation stump and phantom pain.

Intravenous regional sympathetic block with guanethidine

Hannington-Kiff described the intravenous regional guanethidine technique in 1974 and it has become a popular method of treating CRPS. The technique is the same as intravenous regional analgesia (IVRA), but with the addition of guanethidine 10–20 mg. It has been postulated that guanethidine initially releases norepinephrine from the peripheral sympathetic adrenergic terminal and then blocks reuptake, thus depleting norepinephrine stores. However, a recent systematic review of the randomized controlled studies of intravenous regional guanethidine block in the treatment of CRPS failed to show evidence of effectiveness.

Neurolytic techniques

Neural destruction can be produced with alcohol, phenol, heat or cold. In general, the use of neurolytic techniques has diminished in the last two decades. There are many reasons for this, including the improved use of analgesic drugs, the recognition that the effect of neuroablative procedures is often transient, the development of neurostimulatory techniques and appreciation of the cognitive and behavioural elements of pain. The clinical indications for neurolytic techniques are limited to patients with cancer pain and a few selected non-cancer conditions. Careful thought with regard to the potential benefits and risks of the procedure, appropriate patient selection and fully informed consent is essential before performing a neurolytic procedure.

Chemical neurolysis

The commonest neurolytic agents employed are phenol and ethyl alcohol. Phenol acts by coagulating proteins and destroys all types of nerves, both motor and sensory. It is available in water or in glycerol. Its most frequent indication is for lumbar sympathetic block for peripheral vascular disease. Large systemic doses cause convulsions followed by central nervous system depression and cardiovascular collapse. Alcohol is the neurolytic agent of choice for coeliac plexus block when the large volume required prohibits the use of phenol. It has a higher incidence of neuritis than phenol and is not used for other blocks.

Radiofrequency lesions

A destructive heat lesion can be produced using a radiofrequency current. The radiofrequency electrode comprises an insulated needle with a small exposed tip. A high-frequency alternating current flows from the electrode tip to the tissues, producing ionic agitation and a heating effect in tissue adjacent to the tip of the probe. The magnitude of this heating effect is monitored by a thermistor in the electrode tip. Damage to nerve fibres sufficient to block conduction occurs at temperatures above 45°C, although in practice most lesions are made with a probe tip temperature of 60–80°C. An integral nerve stimulator is used to ensure accurate placement of the probe. Whereas the spread of neurolytic solutions is unpredictable, radiofrequency lesions are more precise. The size of the lesion depends on the tip temperature, the duration of the current and the length of the exposed needle tip.

Radiofrequency lesions of the trigeminal nerve may be used to treat trigeminal neuralgia in the elderly patient whose pain is uncontrolled by anticonvulsant drugs and who is unsuitable for microvascular decompression.

Cryotherapy

Lesions may be produced in the nervous system by cold, using a cryoprobe. The Joule–Thompson effect (using nitrous oxide as the refrigerant gas) produces cooling. The probe tip may reach a temperature of –75°C. There is complete functional loss after a cryolesion; however, recovery can be expected after several weeks and this may have advantages in certain situations.

STIMULATION-INDUCED ANALGESIA

Transcutaneous electrical nerve stimulation, spinal cord stimulation, deep brain stimulation and acupuncture may produce stimulation-induced analgesia.

Transcutaneous electrical nerve stimulation

Transcutaneous electrical nerve stimulation (TENS) has been used widely since Melzack and Wall proposed the gate control theory in 1965. They postulated that large-diameter primary afferents exert a specific inhibitory effect on dorsal horn nociceptive neurones and that stimulation of these fibres would alleviate pain. Conventional TENS produces high-frequency, low-intensity stimulation which relieves pain in the area in which it produces paraesthesia. Stimulation variables of TENS can be altered to produce low-frequency acupuncture-like TENS, which, unlike conventional TENS, produces analgesia, which is antagonized by naloxone.

A small battery-powered unit is used to apply the electrical stimulus to the skin via electrodes (Fig. 61.5). These are placed over the painful area, on either side of it or over nerves supplying the region, and stimulation is applied at an intensity that the patient finds comfortable. Adverse effects are minimal, with allergy to the electrodes or gel being the commonest problem encountered. TENS is used for a variety of musculoskeletal and neuropathic pains and has recently been advocated in refractory angina. Tolerance to TENS does sometimes occur. It may be possible to overcome this by changing stimulation variables.

TENS has also been used for acute postoperative pain and for analgesia for the first stage of labour. However, there is evidence of lack of analgesic effect in both these areas, although women using it as a method of pain relief tend to favour it for future births. Whilst studies have shown clear benefit from the use of TENS in chronic pain, there is a general lack of evidence for effectiveness of TENS rather than evidence of lack of effect.

Spinal cord stimulation

Spinal cord stimulation (SCS) has been advocated as a reversible non-ablative method for the management of intractable pain, especially that of neuropathic origin, when pharmacotherapy has failed. Electrical stimulation may be applied to the spinal cord via electrodes implanted surgically or positioned percutaneously in the epidural space under X-ray control. To be effective, the stimulating electrode must be positioned to produce artificial paraesthesiae in the distribution of the pain. It is usual practice for the patient to undergo a period of trial stimulation. Patients showing substantial improvement in pain relief and other outcome measures can be considered for permanent implantation of a battery-

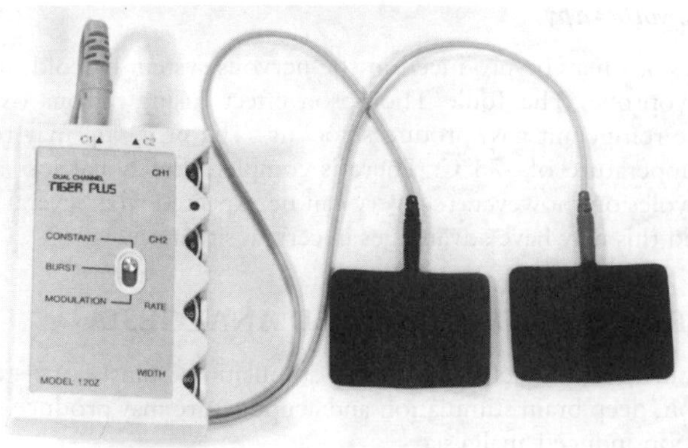

Fig. 61.5
A transcutaneous electrical nerve stimulator.

driven stimulus generator. The patient uses a magnet to activate the stimulator. The equipment is expensive and a proportion of patients obtain good relief initially only to have their pain return after some months.

SCS has also been demonstrated to promote local blood flow and ischaemic ulcer healing in patients with peripheral vascular disease. More recently, spinal cord stimulators have been implanted for angina. Studies have confirmed fewer ischaemic episodes, reduced frequency of hospital admissions and improved quality of life. Concern has been raised that SCS may mask the pain of myocardial infarction, but this is not the case and mortality rates in patients with stimulators are similar to those of the general population with coronary artery disease

Acupuncture

The Chinese have known for 4000 years that inserting needles at specific points in the body produces analgesia. According to Chinese philosophy, *ch'i*, the life force, circulates around the body in pathways termed meridians. Injury and illness can block the flow of *ch'i*, causing pain and disease. Acupuncture is believed to release these blocks and balance the energy of the patient. Traditionally, acupuncture points are stimulated by the insertion of fine needles which are then rotated manually or stimulated by heat (moxibustion) or electrically. For acupuncture analgesia to be effective, the patient should experience a numbing heavy sensation, called *te-ch'i*, spreading from the acupuncture site. However, it is clear that it is not necessary to use traditional acupuncture sites to obtain analgesia. Several studies have shown that needling can produce pain relief whether applied to specified acupuncture points or to sham points.

Acupuncture may be considered to produce high-intensity, low-frequency stimulation. It is postulated that there exists both a segmental and a non-segmental mechanism for acupuncture analgesia, but these have yet to be clarified. Naloxone has been shown to reverse acupuncture analgesia

Acupuncture has become an accepted treatment in many pain management clinics, especially for musculoskeletal pain. However, the results of clinical trials have been conflicting. This is caused, in part, by difficulty in designing randomized, controlled, double-blind trials. Three systematic reviews have examined the effectiveness of acupuncture in chronic non-malignant pain. These show an effect, but it is often short-lived (3 days).

Single-needle acupuncture to the P6 point on the wrist is antiemetic in postoperative nausea and vomiting, morning sickness and in patients receiving cytotoxic drugs.

PSYCHOLOGICAL TECHNIQUES

Pain is not merely a sensation of tissue damage, but a complex interaction of biochemical, behavioural, cognitive and emotional factors. Chronic pain patients become anxious, depressed, distressed, functionally impaired and lose self-esteem. These important aspects should be addressed in the pain management clinic. A clinical psychologist is an essential member of the pain management team. A cognitive and behavioural approach investigates how thoughts (often negative) and behaviours (often maladaptive) reinforce the chronic pain state. Cognitive and behavioural techniques can be used to reduce the helplessness and hopelessness of the pain patient and to increase the level of functioning and emotional well-being in spite of the pain.

Pain management programme

A pain management programme is a psychologically based rehabilitative treatment for patients with chronic pain which remains unresolved by currently available medical or other physically based treatments.

The aim of a pain management programme is to reduce the disability and distress caused by chronic pain by teaching sufferers physical, psychological and practical techniques to improve their quality of life. It aims to enable patients to be self-reliant in managing their pain. It differs from other treatment provided in the pain clinic in that pain relief is not the primary goal.

A pain management programme is facilitated by a multidisciplinary health care team. Key clinical staff include an anaesthetist, a clinical psychologist, a physiotherapist and an occupational therapist, all trained in pain management. Information and education about the nature of pain and its management, medication review and advice, psychological assessment and intervention, physical reconditioning, advice on posture, and graded return to the activities of daily living are components of pain management programmes.

EVIDENCE-BASED PRACTICE

There is an increasing drive for evidence-based medicine and for offering to patients only those interventions that are known to be effective. For many of the procedures that are commonly used in the pain management clinic, the evidence is not available and further work is required to gather this evidence. However, the effectiveness of some of the interventions used for chronic pain has been studied and the results are summarized in Table 61.3.

COSTS OF PAIN MANAGEMENT SERVICES

There is little information on the costs of pain management services. A detailed study of the costs incurred by users of speciality pain clinic services in Canada has shown that users incur less direct health care costs than non-users with similar conditions. Similar results were shown by a small study of NHS pain clinic attendees. This showed that the pain clinic covered its costs by reducing consumption elsewhere within the trust and by reducing GP consultations and private treatments. The available data indicate that pain clinics result in direct health care savings of over £1000 per patient per year and that total savings may be twice the cost of running the chronic pain service.

Advances in knowledge of pain pathophysiology by scientists and increasingly close cooperation between them and clinicians have led to a better understanding of mechanisms sustaining chronic pain and an increase in therapeutic options. In addition, the increasing acceptance by the medical profession and the general public of the importance of psychological factors in chronic pain has opened up new treatment opportunities. There is evidence of the effectiveness of many of the treatments used in the management of chronic pain, but further work is needed on those interventions where information is lacking and in identifying which patients may benefit most from specific treatments.

Table 61.3 Effectiveness of some of the interventions used for chronic pain

Effective interventions (of those studied)
Minor analgesics
Anticonvulsant drugs
Antidepressant drugs
Systemic local anaesthetic-type drugs for neuropathic pain
Topical NSAIDs in rheumatological conditions
Topical capsaicin in diabetic neuropathy
Epidural corticosteroids for back pain and sciatica
Psychological interventions
Interventions studied where evidence is lacking
TENS in chronic pain
Relaxation
Spinal cord stimulation
Ineffective interventions (of those studied)
Intravenous regional sympathetic block with guanethidine
Injections of steroids in or around shoulder joint

FURTHER READING

Cousins M J, Bridenbaugh P O (eds) 1998 Neural blockade in clinical anesthesia and management of pain. Lippincott, Philadelphia

Dolin S J, Padfield N L, Pateman J A (eds) 1996 Pain clinic manual. Butterworth-Heinemann, Oxford

Grady K M, Severn A M 1998 Key topics in chronic pain. BIOS Scientific Publishers, Oxford

Kaye P 1995 A–Z pocketbook of symptom control. EPL Publications, Northampton

McQuay H J , Moore R A 1998 An evidence-based resource for pain relief. Oxford University Press, Oxford

Southall D (ed) 1997 Prevention and control of pain in children. A manual for health care professionals. BMJ Publishing Group, London

Stannard C F, Booth S 1998 Churchill's Pocketbook of Pain. Churchill Livingstone, Edinburgh

Twycross R 1997 Symptom management in advanced cancer. Radcliffe Medical Press, Oxon

Waldman S D, Winnie A P 1996 Interventional pain management. W B Saunders, Philadelphia

Wall P D Melzack R (eds) 1999 A textbook of pain. Churchill Livingstone, Edinburgh

62 Cardiopulmonary resuscitation

Cardiopulmonary resuscitation (CPR) is required when the supply of oxygen to the brain is insufficient to maintain function. Oxygen delivery is dependent upon cardiac output, haemoglobin concentration and saturation of haemoglobin with oxygen; this depends predominantly on respiratory function. CPR is required most commonly after cardiac arrest, respiratory arrest or a combination of the two.

CEREBRAL HYPOXIA

The brain is more sensitive to hypoxaemia than any other organ, including the heart. It has a limited facility for anaerobic metabolism and cannot store oxygen. Hypoxaemia is tolerated remarkably well in the normal individual, as cerebral blood flow increases substantially to compensate for reduced oxygen carriage in blood. In contrast, ischaemia (e.g. circulatory arrest) or hypoxaemia in a patient unable to increase cerebral blood flow (e.g. cerebrovascular atherosclerosis or a low cardiac output state) results in the rapid onset of anaerobic metabolism. The cerebral cortex is damaged permanently by ischaemia of more than 3–4 min duration. Thus, although a patient may survive an episode of circulatory arrest, permanent impairment of cerebral function may result if cerebral oxygen delivery is not restored within 3–4 min of the initial cessation of blood flow. The commonest cause of brain damage after cardiac arrest is delay in starting resuscitation. Therefore, when circulatory arrest has occurred, it is essential to start CPR as rapidly as possible.

CARDIOPULMONARY RESUSCITATION

Guidelines for the performance of cardiopulmonary resuscitation have been published by the European Resuscitation Council (1998a) and the Resuscitation Council (UK). These guidelines were developed from the 1997 International Liaison Committee for Resuscitation advisory statements that were based on specific scientific evidence, where available, or supported on the basis of common sense or ease of teaching and skill retention.

BASIC LIFE SUPPORT

Assessment (Fig. 62.1)

Approach the patient ensuring that there is no danger from the surrounding environment. Assess the level of responsiveness by gently shaking the patient and shouting 'Are you all right?' If the patient is unresponsive then shout for help and commence basic life support immediately (see Fig. 62.1).

Airway

In the unresponsive patient, open the airway by tilting the head back and lifting the jaw forwards (Fig. 62.2). This displaces the tongue, the most common cause of airway obstruction, from the back of the pharynx. In cases of suspected cervical spine injury, the airway should be opened by using the jaw thrust manoeuvre only, whilst maintaining in-line cervical spine immobilization. Head tilt and neck extension must never be used in this situation.

Breathing

With the airway held open, check for breathing by:

- *Looking* – to see if the chest wall is moving or if the abdominal wall is indicating an obstructed airway by a seesaw movement.
- *Listening* – over the mouth for sounds of air movement or for added sounds indicating an obstructed airway.
- *Feeling* – over the mouth with the side of the face for signs of air movement indicating effective breathing.

Allow 10 s to check for breathing.

If the patient is not breathing then you must call for help at this stage. The only exception to this rule is where the patient is a child or the cause of the collapse is trauma or drowning. In these exceptional circumstances, basic life support continues with rescue breathing before calling for help.

Call for help

It is essential to get help at an early stage. Therefore, if you are alone and the patient is not breathing, it is important to leave the patient at this stage and to go and telephone for help. After help has been summoned, return immediately to the patient and continue basic life support. Alternatively, if there is someone with you, ask him or her to go for help whilst you continue resuscitation. It is important to insist that this person returns to inform you of the response of the emergency team.

Rescue breathing

If the patient is unresponsive and is not breathing, ventilate the patient's lungs with two expired air breaths. With the airway held open, pinch the nostrils closed. Take a full breath and seal your lips

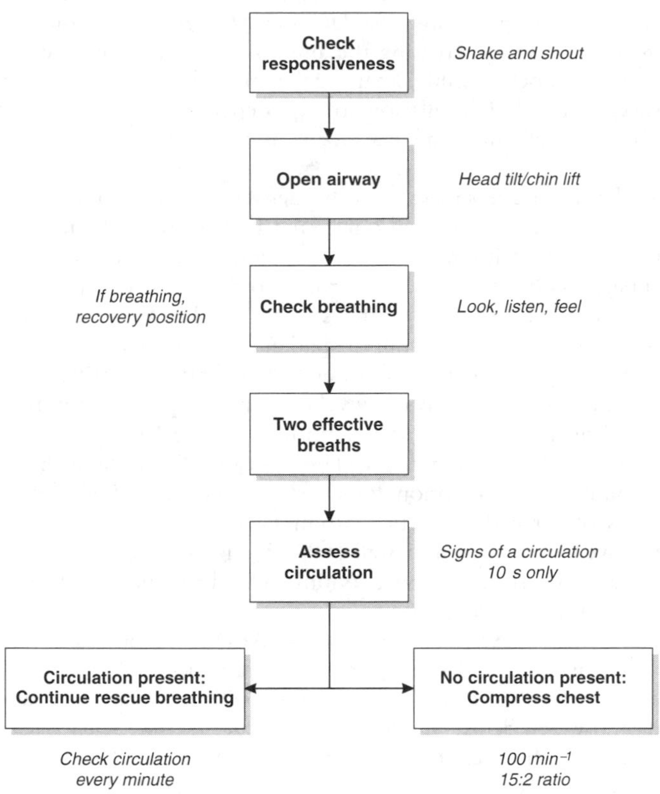

Fig. 62.1
Basic life support.

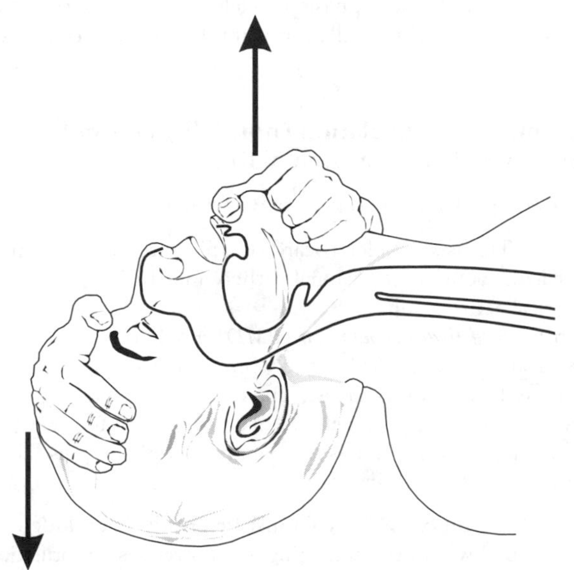

Fig. 62.2
Backward tilt of the head stretches the anterior neck structures and thereby lifts the base of the tongue off the posterior pharyngeal wall.

over the patient's mouth. Blow steadily into the patient's mouth, sufficiently to see the chest expand. Each breath should take approximately 2 s for a full inflation. Maintaining the airway, take your mouth away from the patient and allow the chest to deflate in expiration. Repeat this manoeuvre to give two ventilations. If two effective rescue breaths have not been achieved after five attempts at ventilation then the rescuer should proceed to the next stage of basic life support.

Circulation

Basic life support continues with a pulse check. This is carried out by feeling for the carotid pulse in the neck for 10s. Despite the apparent simplicity of the pulse check, studies have shown that both lay rescuers and health care professionals have difficulty in making an accurate pulse check. Therefore the guidelines now include the statement that starting chest compressions should be considered without delay in the patient showing no obvious signs of life following expired air ventilation.

If there is no pulse or there are no signs of life, start chest compressions immediately.

Chest compressions

Chest compressions are performed on the lower third of the sternum, two fingers breadth above the xiphisternum. The overlapping heels of both hands are used to compress the chest by depressing the sternum approximately 4–5 cm at a rate of 100 compressions min^{-1}. After 15 compressions, give two expired air breaths.

Continue basic life support, 15 chest compressions with two expired air ventilations, until advanced life support arrives. Do not interrupt basic life support to perform further assessments of the patient unless the patient shows signs of recovery.

Respiratory arrest

If the patient is not breathing but has a pulse, perform 10 expired air breaths before leaving the patient to telephone for help. This sequence should also be used if the cause of the collapse is trauma or drowning. On returning to the patient, recheck the breathing and the pulse. If a pulse is present, continue expired air breathing at a rate of 10 breaths min^{-1}, but recheck the pulse at regular intervals. Commence full basic life support if the pulse stops.

Mechanisms of action of chest compressions

The original theory of the action of chest compressions was that the heart was squeezed with each depression of the sternum between the sternum anteriorly and the vertebral column posteriorly. Each compression of the heart pumped blood around the circulation (the heart pump theory).

A later theory, the chest pump theory, uses the concept that each chest compression raises the intrathoracic pressure. This raised pressure is transmitted to the intrathoracic vessels; the arteries, being thick-walled, retain and transmit this pressure, whereas the veins, being thin-walled, collapse. The result is a pressure gradient between the arterial and the venous systems and thus a forward flow of blood around the circulation.

Basic life support only provides 15–20% of normal cardiac output and should be regarded as 'buying time' until the commencement of advanced life support.

ADVANCED LIFE SUPPORT

By following the basic life support procedure described above, the early telephone call for help should result in the prompt arrival of the equipment and personnel needed to perform advanced life support. In adult resuscitation where the most common cause is ventricular fibrillation, the early use of a defibrillator has been demonstrated as having a definite effect on eventual survival.

In specialized in-hospital areas, e.g. the operating theatre, the intensive care unit or the coronary care unit, the time to defibrillation is negligible. In these situations, it is recommended that if a defibrillator is immediately to hand, defibrillation should not be delayed for the initiation of basic life support.

ADVANCED LIFE SUPPORT ALGORITHM

(Fig. 62.3)

The algorithm illustrates the recommended pathway for adult advanced life support (ALS). It begins by emphasizing the importance of establishing basic life support and then continues by recommending a precordial thump. The precordial thump has been shown to be effective in some witnessed cardiac arrests.

The next stage of treatment depends on the rapid assessment of the patient's cardiac rhythm. The patient must be connected to a cardiac monitor (or defibrillator) and the cardiac rhythm assessed. If the electrocardiographic rhythm is compatible with a cardiac output then the pulse must be assessed carefully.
The treatment pathway splits into two specific limbs:

- ventricular fibrillation (VF)/pulseless ventricular tachycardia (VT)
- Non-ventricular fibrillation (Non-VF)/non-pulseless ventricular tachycardia (non-VT).

Ventricular fibrillation (VF)/pulseless ventricular tachycardia (VT)

This is the most common arrhythmia associated with sudden cardiac arrest in adults. The treatment is defibrillation and the survival rate from cardiac arrest has been shown to be related directly to the interval between collapse and the first defibrillation. It is essential, therefore, that rapid and accurate assessment of the presenting cardiac rhythm be made early in the treatment process.

Defibrillation is delivered as a series of three direct current (DC) shocks at 200, 200 and 360 J. Subsequent defibrillation attempts are made at 360 J. The shocks are delivered via self-adhesive contact pads or manually applied paddles. The electrodes/paddles are applied to allow the maximum current flow through the myocardium. One electrode is applied to the right of the upper sternum below the clavicle and the other is centred over the fifth left intercostal space in the midclavicular line (corresponding to the cardiac apex near the position of ECG leads V4/V5).

An initial DC shock at 200 J causes minimal myocardial damage and is adequate to achieve success in most recoverable situations, especially when delivered within the first few minutes after the collapse. This first DC shock decreases the thoracic impedance, thus increasing the amount of energy from the second DC shock at 200 J that reaches the heart. The chance of success of each defibrillation attempt depends on many dynamic variables including the waveform and vectors of myocardial activity.

The first three shocks must be delivered in a rapid sequence and should be interrupted only if the ECG shows a rhythm that is consistent with myocardial perfusion. Therefore, following application of the contact electrodes to the chest, the defibrillator is charged and the operator shouts 'stand clear'. Any oxygen source is disconnected from the patient. Following a visual check that no-one is touching the patient, the operator defibrillates the patient and immediately checks the resultant rhythm. If ventricular fibrillation persists, the defibrillator is recharged and the patient is defibrillated again. This is repeated for three shocks without any interruption for chest compressions. Following a series of three defibrillation attempts, the manual paddles are removed from the chest wall (self-adhesive pads can be left in place) and basic life support continued for 1 min before a further series of shocks are given.

Automated external defibrillators (AEDs) are now available. These machines voice prompt the operator through a series of actions leading to defibrillation. These sophisticated machines also diagnose ventricular fibrillation or fast ventricular tachycardia, indicate to the operator the need to defibrillate and charge to the appropriate number of joules. The operator then defibrillates the patient by pushing the relevant button and the machine recycles through its programme, following the universal ALS algorithm illustrated (Fig. 62.3), prompting the operator to the appropriate action. The simplicity of the AED belies its sophistication; not only can it diagnose and treat VF/VT faster than manual defibrillation methods, but it can also be used by non-medical operators trained in its use. Some AED models are using a biphasic defibrillation waveform. These biphasic models have been shown to be extremely effective at defibrillation using lower levels of delivered energy.

Non-ventricular fibrillation (non-VF)/non-pulseless ventricular tachycardia (non-VT)

Non-VF/non-VT may be one of two rhythms:

- *Asystole.* This is a flat electrocardiograph trace indicating no ventricular activity. Occasionally, there may be P wave electrical activity only.
- *Electromechanical dissociation (EMD).* EMD or pulseless electrical activity (PEA) has the worst prognosis of all rhythms associated with cardiac arrest. The diagnosis is made when the electrocardiogram shows electrical activity consistent with cardiac activity but there is no palpable peripheral pulse (i.e. pulseless electrical activity).

To make this diagnosis, VF/VT must be positively excluded. The right-hand pathway of the algorithm is followed, as defibrillation is not indicated as a primary intervention. Survival from these non-VF/VT rhythms is poor, with an overall survival rate of 10–15% of that of VF/VT rhythms.

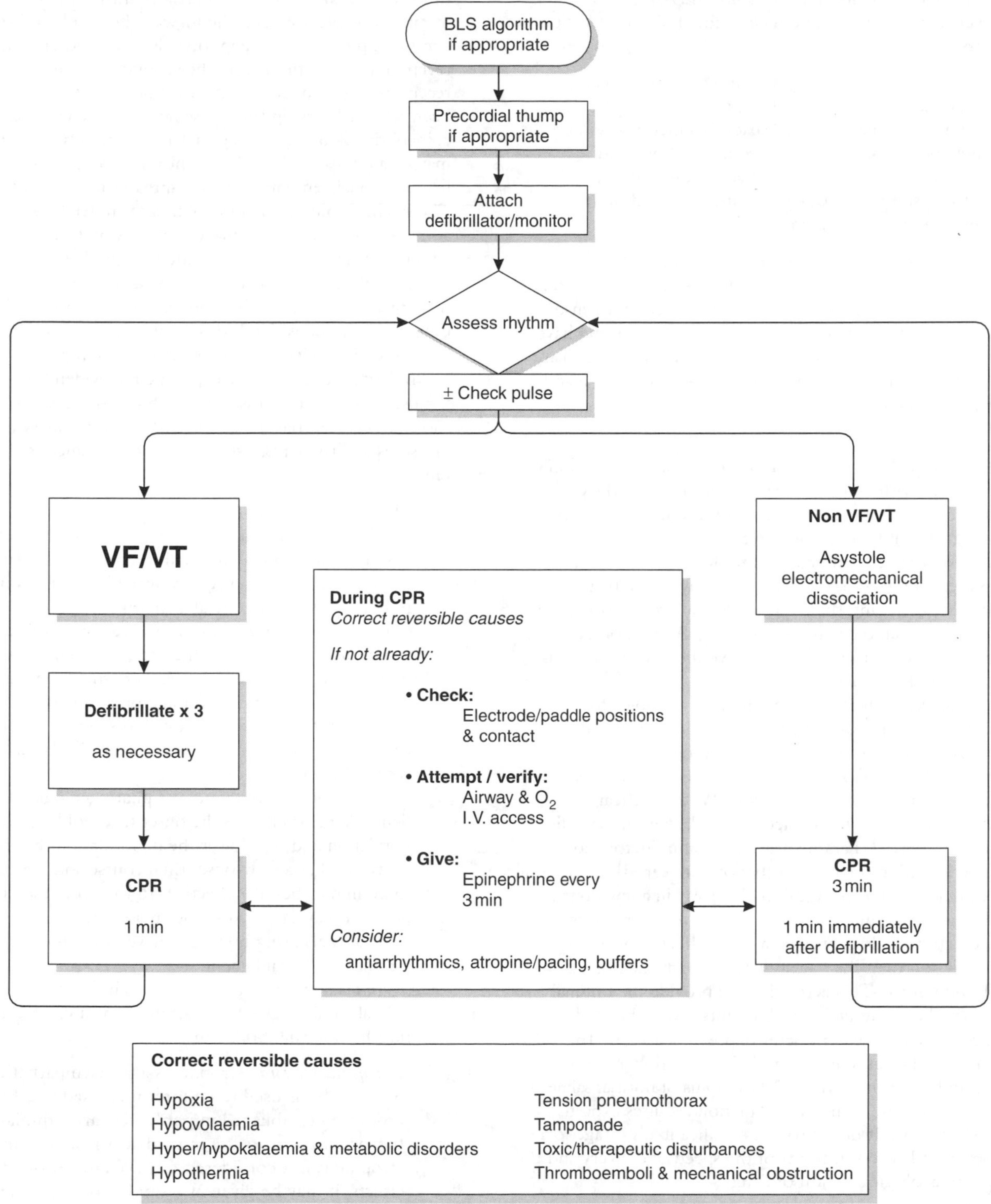

Fig. 62.3
Advanced life support.

The treatment of cardiac arrest when either asystole or EMD is diagnosed is continued basic life support in cycles of 3 min whilst other resuscitative methods are applied. After 3 min, the patient is rapidly reassessed and the appropriate pathway followed.

ACTIONS TO BE TAKEN DURING CPR

There are a series of actions to be taken during resuscitation that are common to both pathways of the algorithm. These are summarized in the box between the two pathways on the diagram (Fig. 62.3).

1. *Correct the reversible causes of the cardiac arrest.*
The reversible causes are described as the 'four Hs' and 'four Ts' of resuscitation:

Hypoxia	Tension pneumothorax
Hypovolaemia	Tamponade
Hypo/hyperkalaemia and metabolic disorders	Toxic/therapeutic disorders
Hypothermia	Thromboembolic and mechanical obstruction

Each of these should be looked for and excluded or, if diagnosed, specifically treated.

2. *Check the electrode/paddle position and contact.*
Electrocardiographic rhythm assessment is fundamental to the use of the ALS algorithm. Therefore, it is essential to ensure that the electrode/paddles are positioned correctly and have effective contact. Rhythms associated with cardiac arrest can be mimicked by movement artefact, lead disconnection and electrical interference.

3. *Attempt/verify:*
   (i) ***Airway and O_2.*** Securing the airway and ventilation of the lungs with a high concentration of inspired oxygen are of major importance. Ventilation can be carried out using a self-inflating bag, valve and mask. The level of inspired oxygen can be raised to 50% by attaching an oxygen supply at 5–6 L min^{-1} directly to the bag, or to 90% by increasing the oxygen flow rate to 8–10 L min^{-1} and adding an oxygen reservoir bag. An oral or nasal airway may be inserted to improve the efficiency of bag, valve, mask ventilation.

   Tracheal intubation is the method of choice for securing the airway. Tracheal intubation ensures that oxygen is delivered directly to the lungs, eliminates leaks and gastric insufflation and protects the airway from the regurgitation of gastric contents. When tracheal intubation has not been achieved, a laryngeal mask airway can be inserted. Paramedics, nurses and doctors not experienced in tracheal intubation can learn the technique of insertion of a laryngeal mask airway in a few hours. Whilst the laryngeal mask does not provide full airway protection, it does provide a more effective airway and ventilation than the bag, valve and mask system.

   (ii) ***Venous access.*** This is required to provide the optimal method of drug delivery. Attempts should be made to cannulate a large peripheral vein with a 14G or 16G cannula. Drugs administered via the peripheral route should be flushed with a 20 ml bolus of normal saline (0.9%). Central venous cannulation requires expertise and training. It does provide significant advantages over peripheral access in terms of the speed of delivery and the pharmacological action of drugs.

4. *Give epinephrine every 3 min.*
Epinephrine 1 mg (10 ml of 1 in 10 000 solution or 1 ml of 1 in 1000 solution) is given intravenously every 3 min. Epinephrine is used in resuscitation mainly for its α-adrenergic receptor stimulant effects. This α-adrenergic action causes peripheral vasoconstriction, raises the systemic vascular resistance, raises the end-diastolic filling pressure and thus improves coronary perfusion. In addition, epinephrine is believed to 'stiffen' the major vessels leading away from the heart, thus aiding in the transmission of the raised intrathoracic pressure and the forward flow of blood (the chest pump theory). Epinephrine also has β-adrenergic receptor activity, stimulating the chronotropic and inotropic receptors of the myocardium. If venous cannulation has not been achieved early in the resuscitation sequence, then epinephrine 2–3 mg, diluted in 10 ml normal saline (0.9%) may be administered via the tracheal route and followed by five additional ventilations to aid spread throughout the lungs. The tracheal route is inferior to direct venous drug administration as the pharmacodynamics of drugs administered via the tracheal route is unpredictable.

   Although epinephrine remains the drug of choice, there is no clinical evidence that it improves survival or neurological outcome in humans. High-dose epinephrine, 3 or 5 mg, is not recommended as its use has not resulted in improved overall survival rates. There is little experimental evidence to support the use of other vasopressor drugs, but vasopressin has been shown in clinical trials to significantly raise coronary perfusion pressures and to increase the return of spontaneous circulation rates.

5. *Consider:*
   (i) ***Antiarrhythmic drugs.*** The use of antiarrhythmic drugs has been recommended to aid electrical defibrillation, to prevent the reoccurrence of ventricular fibrillation and to terminate serious electrical arrhythmias.

   Lidocaine has been used in the treatment of resistant ventricular fibrillation. Clinical trials and animal studies have shown that lidocaine offers no improvement in survival from ventricular fibrillation and may actually raise the threshold for defibrillation. Lidocaine is advocated to prevent the reccurrence of ventricular fibrillation after successful defibrillation.

   Bretylium has been used as a pharmacological defibrillator. It elevates the onset threshold for ventricular fibrillation and may lower the defibrillation threshold. Bretylium has a slow-onset time course and may take up to 20 min to be fully effective. In the post-resuscitation phase, it may cause profound hypotension and EMD. Clinical trials using bretylium have not demonstrated any significant clinical benefit.

   Amiodarone does prevent ventricular arrhythmias and animal studies have demonstrated that it can reduce the threshold for defibrillation.

   (ii) ***Atropine/pacing.*** Atropine is a parasympathetic nerve blocker and is used to counter increased vagal tone. Its use is well established in peri-arrest arrhythmias, but the evidence for its use in cardiac arrest is equivocal. As atropine is not considered to have any serious adverse effects, it may be given as a single dose of 3 mg intravenously. This dose is sufficient to effectively block vagal activity.

   Electrical pacing of the heart can be attempted where there is P-wave activity evident. Percutaneous or pervenous pacing can be attempted depending on the local skills and available equipment. Although pacing has been of benefit in the emergency management of severe bradycardias, it has not been shown to be successful in asystole. This may be a failure in technique or, alternatively, it may be that pacing is only considered at too late a stage in the resuscitation sequence, probably when the myocardium is beyond electrical stimulation. Repeated chest thumps (external cardiac percussion) may generate ventricular complexes where myocardial contractility has not been compromised. If a detectable cardiac output is not detected using repeated chest thumps then conventional basic life support must be performed.

(iii) ***Buffers.*** In prolonged resuscitation the patient may become increasingly acidotic. This is especially so when initial basic life support has been delayed, ventilation has not been performed effectively (respiratory acidosis) or chest compressions have not been successful in achieving a satisfactory flow of blood (metabolic acidosis). In most cases, establishing effective basic life support maintains the acid–base status quo without further intervention.

Where basic life support procedures have been established and the patient's lungs have been effectively ventilated, any associated acidosis may be reversed pharmacologically by administration of buffer solution such as sodium bicarbonate solution. There is little evidence to support the routine administration of buffers. A volume of 22.4 ml of gaseous carbon dioxide is produced for every 1 mmol of carbon dioxide produced by buffering activity. Therefore, if the lungs are not perfused and ventilated effectively, a severe respiratory acidosis occurs. Furthermore, rapid diffusion of carbon dioxide into cells results in a paradoxical intracellular acidosis. Finally, the hyperosmolarity and high sodium ion concentrations in sodium bicarbonate solution may exacerbate cerebral oedema. The recommendation for the use of buffers is therefore limited to severe acidosis, where the pH is less than 7.1 and the base excess is greater than –10 mmol L^{-1}. Sodium bicarbonate is usually administered as an intravenous 50 ml bolus of an 8.4% solution (50 mmol of HCO_3^- ion). Following administration of sodium bicarbonate, the intravenous cannula must be flushed carefully, as residual sodium bicarbonate inactivates epinephrine administered subsequently. Sodium bicarbonate is only recommended routinely in patients with pre-existing metabolic acidosis, hyperkalaemia, or tricyclic antidepressant or phenobarbital overdose.

PERI-ARREST ARRHYTHMIAS

Although this chapter deals with the management of cardiac arrest, an essential part of the strategy must include the prevention and treatment of the potentially fatal arrhythmias that occur in the peri-arrest period. The guidelines for management of these arrhythmias are presented in three algorithms. These algorithms do not provide a treatment strategy for every known peri-arrest rhythm but merely provide a guide to the initial recognition and management of these arrhythmias. It must be emphasized that where the clinician does not have the required experience or skill, further expert help must be summoned.

Bradycardia (Fig. 62.4)

A bradycardia is defined as a ventricular rate of below 60 beats min^{-1}. The algorithm for bradycardia may be summarized as (European Resuscitation Council 1998):

If there is a risk of asystole, pace immediately; if there is no perceived risk of asystole but the haemodynamic state of the patient is poor, give atropine and pace only if this is ineffective; if there is no perceived risk of asystole and the patient is not compromised haemodynamically to an important degree then only observation is required.

Broad complex tachycardia (Fig. 62.5)

A broad complex tachycardia is nearly always ventricular in origin. However, it may be difficult to distinguish a rapid broad complex tachycardia from a supraventricular tachycardia. Little harm results if a supraventricular tachycardia is treated as a ventricular one, whereas the converse may result in very serious consequences. The algorithm for broad complex tachycardia may be summarized as (European Resuscitation Council 1998):

If there is no pulse as a result of the arrhythmia the condition should be treated as cardiac arrest using the ventricular fibrillation/ventricular tachycardia protocol for cardiac arrest. If there is a pulse but inadequate perfusion then cardioversion is required as soon as possible. If there is a broad complex tachycardia without adverse haemodynamic disturbance then routine antiarrhythmic therapy should be used with cardioversion only if this fails.

Narrow complex tachycardia (Fig. 62.6)

A narrow complex tachycardia is nearly always a supraventricular arrhythmia. Although a narrow complex tachycardia is generally regarded as less hazardous than a broad complex tachycardia, it is a recognized trigger for ventricular fibrillation in susceptible patients. The algorithm for narrow complex tachycardia may be summarized as (European Resuscitation Council 1998):

For regular arrhythmic supraventricular tachycardias (that almost always have heart rates faster that 140 min^{-1}), vagal manoeuvres or adenosine may be tried first, but if these are not successful, in the presence of adverse signs the recommended strategy is cardioversion. Without adverse signs there is a choice of routine antiarrhythmics that include a short acting β blocker, digoxin, verapamil and amiodarone. Atrial fibrillation is a special case: rigid guidelines cannot be readily applied, and expert help may be prudent when the rate is persistently over 130 beats min^{-1}.

AFTERCARE

For every 10 in-hospital resuscitation events, three patients survive the initial resuscitation procedures, two survive the next 24 h, 1.5 survive to be discharged from hospital and one patient lives for 1 year after the initial event. These simple statistics illustrate the initial success rate of resuscitation and emphasize the need for careful post-resuscitation care.

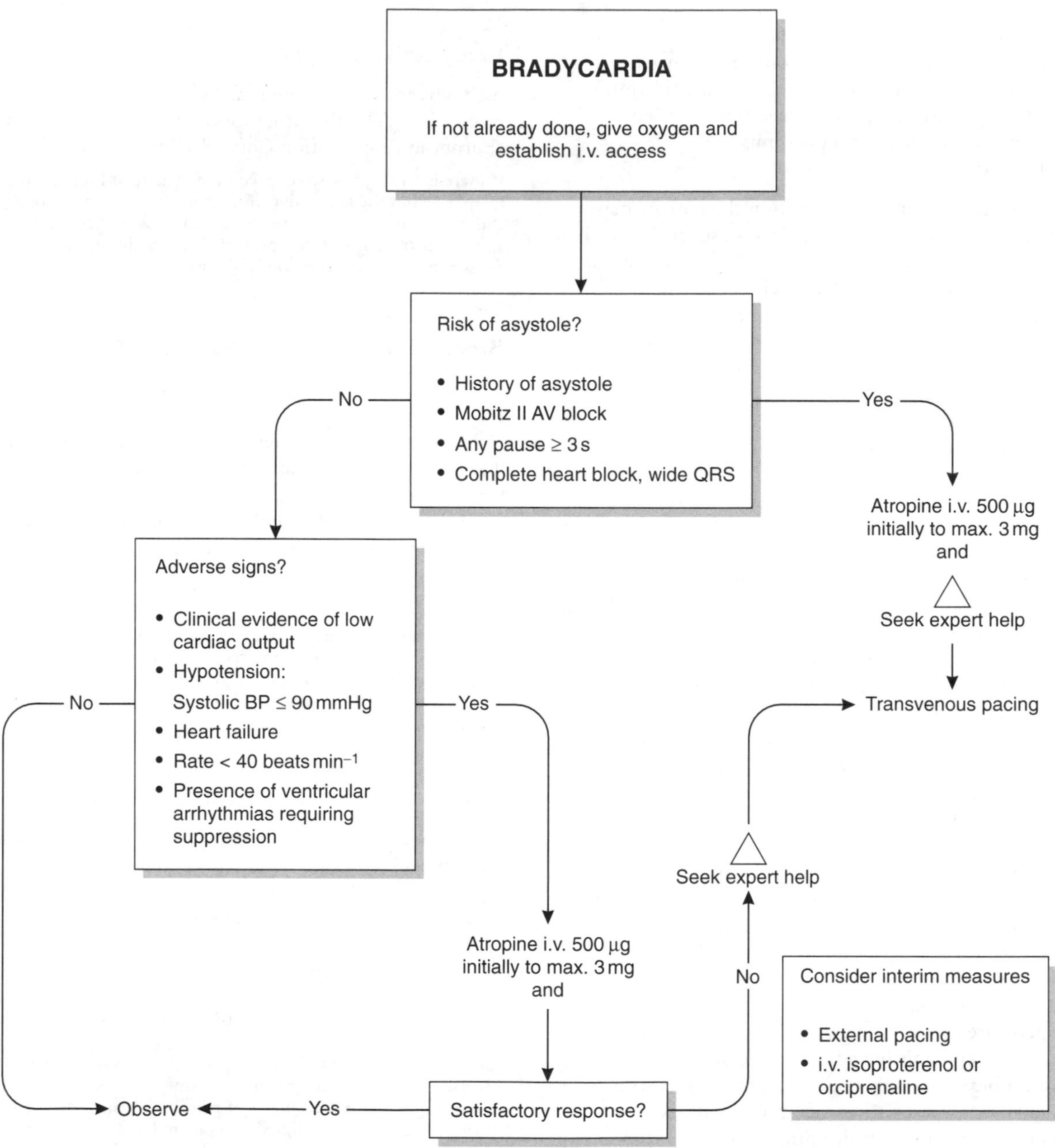

Fig. 62.4
Treatment of bradycardia.

Following resuscitation, all patients should be cared for in a specialized unit, e.g. an intensive care or a coronary care unit. Careful monitoring of vital functions must be established and abnormalities in serum electrolyte concentrations corrected to prevent reccurrence of the event. In a few patients, the event may have been extremely rapid and little additional care is required. The majority will require further circulatory and respiratory support.

CARDIOVASCULAR SYSTEM

Optimizing and stabilizing myocardial function is essential in the post-arrest phase. It is also essential to minimize cerebral ischaemia resulting from cerebral vasospasm, and overcoming this by maintaining a mean arterial pressure of greater than 90 mmHg may place undue strain on the heart and compromise cardiac function. Therefore, balancing the requirements of cerebral perfusion

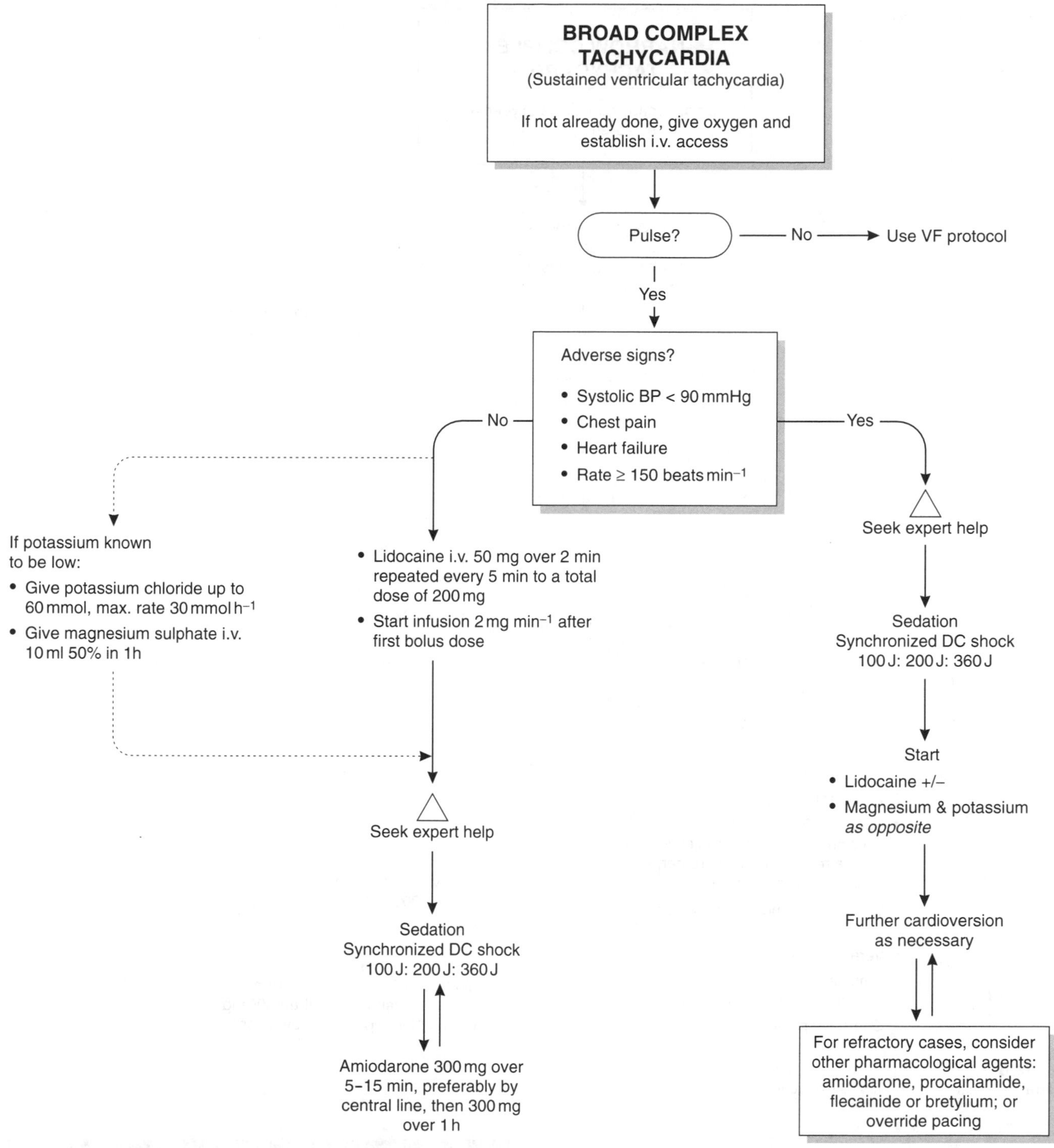
BROAD COMPLEX TACHYCARDIA
(Sustained ventricular tachycardia)
If not already done, give oxygen and establish i.v. access
Pulse?
No
Use VF protocol
Yes
Adverse signs?
• Systolic BP < 90 mmHg
• Chest pain
• Heart failure
• Rate ≥ 150 beats min−1
No
Yes
If potassium known to be low:
• Give potassium chloride up to 60 mmol, max. rate 30 mmol h−1
• Give magnesium sulphate i.v. 10 ml 50% in 1h
• Lidocaine i.v. 50 mg over 2 min repeated every 5 min to a total dose of 200 mg
• Start infusion 2 mg min−1 after first bolus dose
Seek expert help
Sedation
Synchronized DC shock
100 J: 200 J: 360 J
Amiodarone 300 mg over 5–15 min, preferably by central line, then 300 mg over 1 h
Seek expert help
Sedation
Synchronized DC shock
100 J: 200 J: 360 J
Start
• Lidocaine +/–
• Magnesium & potassium as opposite
Further cardioversion as necessary
For refractory cases, consider other pharmacological agents: amiodarone, procainamide, flecainide or bretylium; or override pacing

Fig. 62.5
Treatment of broad complex tachycardia.

against myocardial function using afterload reduction therapy and direct pharmacological myocardial stimulation requires meticulous monitoring The insertion of an indwelling arterial cannula is mandatory to monitor beat-by-beat blood pressure. Arterial blood samples can also be obtained for blood gas analysis, electrolyte estimation and acid–base balance. A pulmonary artery catheter or trans-oesophageal Doppler monitor may aid in reestablishing the haemodynamic status of the patient, and transoesophageal echocardiography may provide more detailed information on overall cardiac performance.

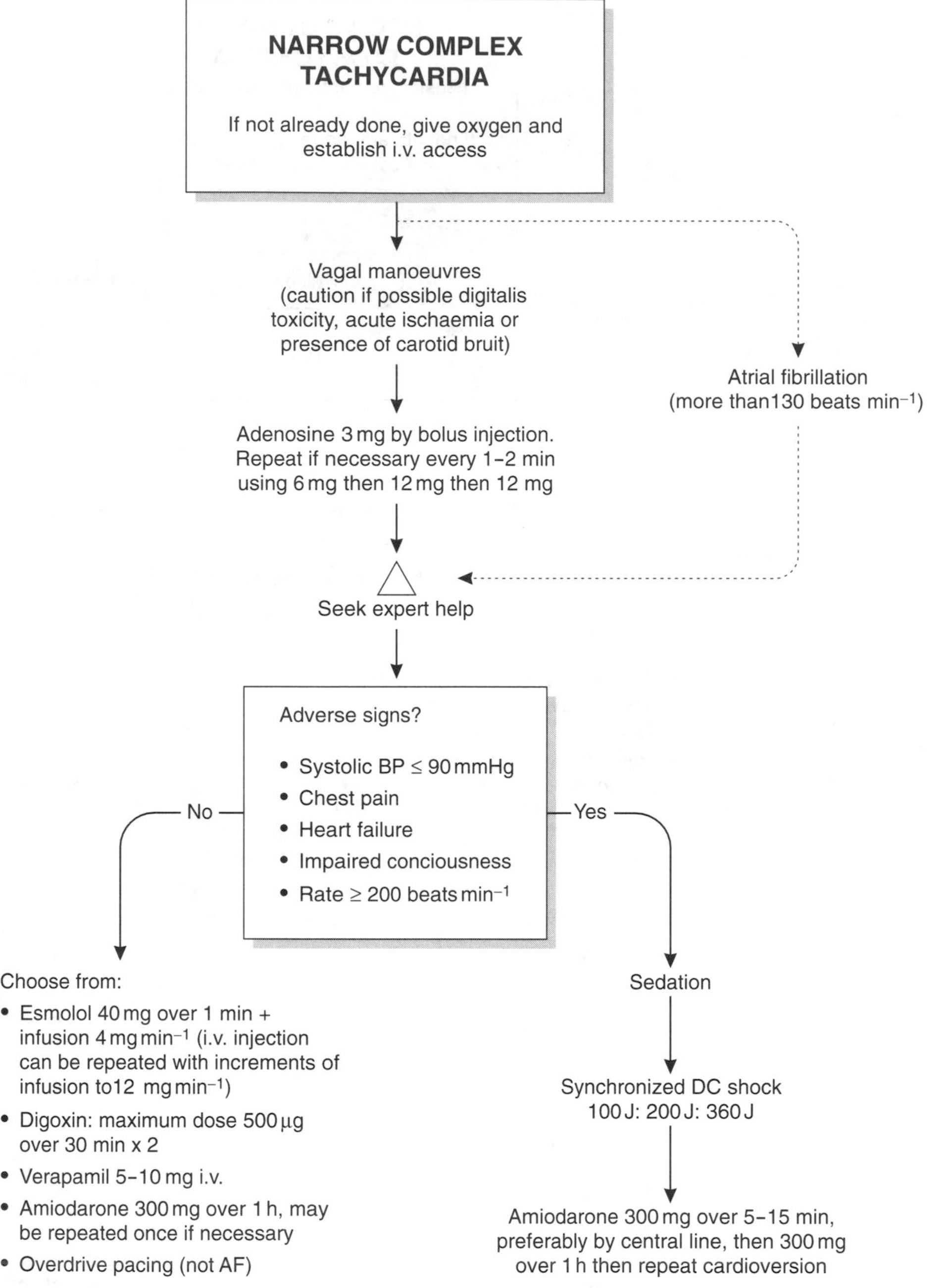

Fig. 62.6
Treatment of narrow complex tachycardia.

RESPIRATORY SYSTEM

All patients must have a chest X-ray and blood gas analysis after CPR. Lung dysfunction is produced during resuscitation for reasons that may include inhalation of vomit, lung contusion, fractured ribs and pneumothorax. Pulmonary oedema may occur in the presence of heart failure and after head injury, drowning or smoke inhalation. Oxygen therapy for at least 24 h should follow any episode of circulatory arrest. If overt respiratory failure supervenes, more intensive treatment is required, including tracheal intubation and a planned period of artificial ventilation.

PREVENTION OF CARDIAC ARREST

The commonest causes of cardiac arrest during surgery are hypoxaemia and haemorrhage. Hypoxaemia may occur with alarming rapidity during periods of apnoea or respiratory obstruction, particularly in obstetric patients and young children; in the latter, bradycardia is an important premonitory sign. Steady and persistent haemorrhage may pass unnoticed until the patient deteriorates suddenly from hypovolaemia. Other causes include overdose with hypotensive or local anaesthetic agents, exogenously administered epinephrine and the injudicious use of intravenous induction agents in the presence of pre-existing hypovolaemia. Dental anaesthesia has been associated with the sudden development of malignant arrhythmias and cardiac arrest. Vagal reflexes affecting the heart may be involved in surgery on the eye, rectum, carotid sheath or upper respiratory tract.

Generally, the outcome after abrupt cardiac arrest is good if the event is recognized rapidly and treatment is prompt and effective.

INITIATING AND TERMINATING CPR

Resuscitation should be attempted in all patients. The decision 'not to attempt resuscitation' is a complex one and must be based on local guidelines. These guidelines should include the following:

- The decision not to resuscitate should be made by a senior doctor who should consult others as appropriate.
- The decision should be communicated to medical and nursing staff, recorded in the patient's notes, and reviewed at appropriate intervals.
- The decision should also be shared with the patient's relatives.
- Other appropriate treatment and care should be continued.

The decision to terminate resuscitation depends on several variables. The results from resuscitation where the initiation of basic life support has been delayed, e.g. remote sites or no bystander response, are extremely poor. Similarly, survival is rare if the time to advanced life support procedures is longer than 30 min. Evidence of cardiac death or cerebral damage is important, as these events affect the resulting quality of life. However, each case must be assessed individually and the decision not to proceed agreed by all the resuscitation team. The decision to terminate resuscitation can be made in patients with an ultimate poor prognosis or those who are suffering from end-stage disease. Age itself is not a prognostic indicator, although survival of patients over the age of 80 years is not as good as in younger patients, probably because of underlying disease.

Hypothermia does confer some protection against the effects of hypoxia. Resuscitation should continue for longer than for normothermic patients and certainly until active rewarming has established a viable central body temperature. Resuscitation should also be prolonged in patients who have taken sedative, hypnotic or narcotic drugs before cardiac arrest, as these drugs are also believed to provide protection against the effects of hypoxia. Finally, resuscitation must continue until the reversible causes of cardiac arrest (the four Hs and four Ts) have been treated.

FURTHER READING

Colquhoun M, Handley A, Evans T (eds) 1999 ABC of resuscitation, 4th edn. BMJ Books, London

European Resuscitation Council (Bossaert L, ed.) 1998a Guidelines for Resuscitation. Elsevier, Amsterdam

European Resuscitation Council 1998b Working group on basic life support. Resuscitation 37: 67–80

European Resuscitation Council 1998c Working group on advanced life support. Resuscitation 37: 81–90

European Resuscitation Council 1998d Paediatric basic life support. Resuscitation 37: 97–100

European Resuscitation Council 1998e Paediatric advanced life support. Resuscitation 37: 101–102

Appendices

Appendix Ia: Abbreviations used in text and appendices

α	adrenoceptor type (after Ahlquist)
ABO	nomenclature for blood groups (after Landsteiner)
ACD	acid citrate dextrose
ACE	angiotensin-converting enzyme
ACh	acetylcholine
ACT	activated clotting time
ACTH	adrenocorticotrophic hormone
ADH	antidiuretic hormone
ADP	adenosine diphosphate
AER	auditory evoked response
AHF	antihaemophilic factor (factor VIII)
AIDS	acquired immunodeficiency syndrome
AIP	acute intermittent porphyria
ALS	advanced life support
ALT	alanine aminotransferase
AMP	adenosine monophosphate
AMPA	γ-amino-3-hydroxy-5-methyl-4-isoxazole proprionate
ANP	atrial natriuretic peptide
ANS	autonomic nervous system
APACHE	acute physiological and chronic health evaluation
APTT	activated partial thromboplastin time
ARDS	acute respiratory distress syndrome
ASA	American Society of Anesthesiologists
Asp	L-aspartate
AST	aspartate aminotransferase
AT	antithrombin
ATP	adenosine triphosphate
AUC	area under curve
AV	atrioventricular
β	adrenoceptor type (after Ahlquist)
B	bone marrow-dependent (as in B cells)
BM	Boehringer Mannheim (makers of BM Stix blood glucose testing strips)
BP	boiling point
BP	*British Pharmacopoeia*
BSA	body surface area
BW	body weight
BZ	benzodiazepine
C	cervical or coccygeal vertebra
C	content
°C	degrees Celsius
C_x	clearance of x
C	compliance
C_3F_8	perfluoropropane
Ca	calcium
$CaCO_3$	calcium carbonate
cAMP	cyclic adenosine monophosphate
CaO	calcium oxide
CAVG	coronary artery vein graft
CBF	cerebral blood flow
CC	closing capacity
CCT	central conduction time
CCU	coronary care unit
CDH	Christiansen Douglas Haldane (effect)
CEPOD	Confidential Enquiry into Perioperative Deaths (UK)
CFAM	cerebral function analysing monitor
CFM	cerebral function monitor
CGRP	calcitonin gene-related peptide
CHO	carbohydrate
CI	cardiac index (cardiac output/body surface area)
CK	creatine kinase
Cl	clearance (of drug)
cm	centimetre (10^{-2} m; not a unit in the SI system)
cmH_2O	centimetres of water
$CMRO_2$	cerebral metabolic rate for oxygen
CMV	cytomegalovirus
CNS	central nervous system
C_0	concentration at time = 0
CO	cardiac output
CO_2	carbon dioxide
cp	centipoise
CPAP	continuous positive airways pressure
CPB	cardiopulmonary bypass
CPD	citrate phosphate dextrose
CPD–A	citrate phosphate dextrose with adenine
CPK	creatine phosphokinase
CPP	cerebral perfusion pressure
CPPV	continuous positive pressure ventilation
CPR	cardiopulmonary resuscitation
^{51}Cr	chromium atom – isotope weight 51 Da (radiolabelled)
CRB	chain recombinant technology using bacteria (insulin)
CSF	cerebrospinal fluid
C_{ss}	concentration at steady state
C_t	concentration at time *t*
CT	computed tomography
CTM	cricothyroid membrane
CV	closing volume
CVP	central venous pressure
Δ	delta – minimal increment (of)
δ	delta opioid receptor
D	dose (of drug)
d	density
d	deci (one-tenth part)
Da	dalton (measure of atomic weight)
D&C	dilatation and curettage (of uterus)
DAP	diastolic arterial pressure
DBS	double burst stimulation
DC	direct current
DCR	dacrocystorhinostomy
DDAVP	desmopressin

DFP di-isopropyl fluorophosphonate
DoH Department of Health
DIC disseminated intravascular coagulation
DNA deoxyribonucleic acid
Dopa Deoxyphenylalanine
2,3-DPG 2,3-diphosphoglycerate
dTC dextrotubocurarine
DVT deep vein thrombosis
ECC extracorporeal circulation (heart bypass)
ECF(V) extracellular fluid (volume)
ECG electrocardiogram
ECM external cardiac massage
ECT electroconvulsive therapy
EDTA ethylenediaminetetra-acetic acid
ED_x effective dose for x% of population
EC European Community
EEG electroencephalogram
EF ejection fraction
EMD electromechanical dissociation (PEA)
EMG electromyogram
EMLA® eutectic mixture of local anaesthetic
EMMV extended mandatory minute ventilation (or volume)
EMP enzyme modified porcine (insulin)
EMO Epstein and Macintosh (of Oxford)
ENNS early neonatal neurobehavioural score
ENT ear, nose and throat
EP evoked potential
EPI Eysenck personality inventory
EPP end-plate potential
ERPOC evacuation of retained products of conception
ESWL extracorporreal shock wave lithotripsy
EUA examination under anaesthesia
EVR endocardial viability ratio
F Faraday's constant
FDP fibrin degradation products
$Fe^{2+(3+)}$ iron ionized – ferrous (ferric) ion
FEV_1 forced expiratory volume (in 1 s)
FF filtration fraction
FFA free fatty acid
FFP fresh frozen plasma
FGF fresh gas flow
$F_{I}O_2$ fractional inspired oxygen concentration
FRC functional residual capacity
FSH follicle-stimulating hormone
FVC forced vital capacity
g gram
G6PD glucose-6-phosphate dehydrogenase
GABA γ-aminobutyric acid
GFR glomerular filtration rate
GH growth hormone
GI gastrointestinal
Glu L-glutamate
Gly glycine
GMP glutamate monophosphate
GTN glyceryl trinitrate
h hour
H^+ hydrogen ion
H_1 histamine – type 1 receptor
H_2 histamine – type 2 receptor
HAFOE high air flow oxygen enrichment
Hb haemoglobin
HbA adult haemoglobin
HbF fetal haemoglobin
HbNH carbamino haemoglobin
HBsAg hepatitis B surface antigen
hCG human chorionic gonadotrophin
HCO_3^- bicarbonate ion
H_2CO_3 carbonic acid
Hct haematocrit
HDU high-dependency unit
He helium
HFFDV high-frequency forced diffusion ventilation
HFJV high-frequency jet ventilation
HFOV high-frequency oscillatory ventilation
HFPPV high-frequency positive pressure ventilation
HFV high-frequency ventilation
Hg mercury
5-HIAA 5-hydroxyindoleacetic acid
HIV human immunodeficiency virus
HLA human leucocyte antigen
HOCM hypertrophic obstructive cardiomyopathy
HPA hypothalamopituitary axis
hPL human placental lactogen
HPV hypoxic pulmonary vasoconstriction
HR heart rate
5-HT 5-hydroxytryptamine (serotonin)
HTLV human T cell leukaemia virus
Hz hertz (cycles per second)
I infusion rate
IABP intra-aortic balloon pump
ICF(V) intracellular fluid (volume)
ICP isometric contraction period; intracranial pressure
ID internal diameter
I/E inspiratory/expiratory
IgA immunoglobulin type A (γ-globulin A)
IgE immunoglobulin type E (γ- globulin E, reagin)
IgG immunoglobulin type G (γ-globulin G)
ILM intubating laryngeal mask (airway)
i.m. intramuscular
IMV intermittent mandatory ventilation
INR international normalized ratio
IOP intraocular pressure
IPPV intermittent positive pressure ventilation
IRP isometric relaxation period
ISA intrinsic sympathomimetic activity
ITU intensive therapy unit
i.v. intravenous
IVC inferior vena cava
IVF in vitro fertilization
IVRA intravenous regional anaesthesia
J joule
κ kappa – opioid receptor type
K kelvin
K^+ potassium ion
KCCT kaolin cephalin clotting time
kg kilogram
K^+_i potassium ion (inside cell)
K^+_o potassium ion (outside cell)
kPa kilopascal
l length
L (*n*) lumbar vertebra (number *n*)
LAP left atrial pressure
LATS long-acting thyroid stimulator
lb in^{-2} pounds per square inch
LDH lactate dehydrogenase
LH luteinizing hormone
LISS low ionic strength saline
lm lumen
LMA laryngeal mask airway
LMN lower motor neurone
ln natural logarithm (to base e)
log logarithm(to base 10)

LOS	lower oesophageal sphincter
LSCS	lower-segment Caesarean section
LVEDP	left ventricular end-diastolic pressure
μ	micro (10^{-6}); Mu opioid receptor type
μV	microvolts
m	metre
mA	milliampere
MAC	minimum alveolar concentration (for anaesthesia)
MAO	monoamine oxidase
MAOI	monoamine oxidase inhibitor
MAP	mean arterial pressure
MC	Mary Caterill (name of proprietary mask)
MC	monocomponent – 'free of impurities' (as in insulin)
MCV	mean corpuscular volume
MEAC	minimum effective analgesic concentration
MEPP	miniature end-plate potential
mg	milligram
Mg^{2+}	magnesium ion
MH	malignant hyperthermia
MI	myocardial infarction
min	minute
ml	millilitre
mm	millimetre
mmHg	millimetres of mercury
MMPI	Minnesota multiphasic personality inventory
MMV	mandatory minute ventilation
mN	millinewton
mol	mole
mosmol	milliosmole
MRI	magnetic resonance imaging
ms	millisecond
MSH	melanocyte-stimulating hormone
mV	millivolt
MVP	mean venous pressure
MW	molecular weight
η	viscosity
N	newton (unit of force)
N/A	not available; not applicable
NO	nitric oxide
N_2O	nitrous oxide
Na	sodium
Na^+	sodium ion
NACS	neurological & adaptive capacity score
Na/K-ATPase	sodium- and potassium-dependent adenosine triphosphatase
NEEP	negative end-expiratory pressure
NH_3	ammonia
NH_4^+	ammonium ion
NHS	National Health Service (UK)
NMDA	*N*-methyl-D-aspartate
NMR	nuclear magnetic resonance
NSAID	non-steroidal anti-inflammatory drug
NTD	neural tube defects
O_2	oxygen
ODC	oxyhaemoglobin dissociation curve
ODP	operating department practitioner
osmol	osmole
π	pi (= 3.14159)
π_{BC}	oncotic pressure in Bowman's capsule
π_{CAP}	oncotic pressure in capillary
P	electrocardiographic nomenclature
P_{50}	oxygen tension which results in a haemoglobin saturation of 50%
Pa	pascal (unit of pressure)
P_A	alveolar partial pressure (of gas)
P_a	arterial partial pressure (of gas)
P_B	barometric pressure
PAFC	pulmonary artery flotation catheter
PAH	*para*-aminohippuric acid
PAP	pulmonary artery pressure
PAOP	pulmonary artery occlusion pressure (= PCWP)
P_{BC}	hydrostatic pressure in Bowman's capsule
PCA	patient-controlled analgesia
P_{CAP}	hydrostatic pressure in capillary
PCWP	pulmonary capillary wedge pressure
PDPH	post-dural puncture headache
PE	pulmonary embolus
$P_{\bar{E}}$	mean expired partial pressure
$P_{E'}$	end-expired partial pressure
PEA	pulseless electrical activity (EMD)
PEEP	positive end-expiratory pressure
PEFR	peak expiratory flow rate
PF	pathological fibrinolysis
PG(X)	prostaglandin type (X)
pH	hydrogen ion activity (negative logarithm to base 10 of the measured hydrogen ion concentration)
P_I	inspired partial pressure
PIFR	peak inspiratory flow rate
pK_a	expression of dissociation constant in an equilibrium (negative logarithm to base 10 of the dissociation constant)
PMGV	piped medical gases and vacuum systems
PONV	postoperative nausea and vomiting
ppm	parts per million
PRN	*pro re nata* (as needed)
PRP	platelet-rich plasma
PTA	plasma thromboplastin antecedent (factor IX)
PTF	post-tetanic facilitation
PTP	post-tetanic potentiation
P_tCO_2	transcutaneous oxygen partial pressure
PTT(K)	partial thromboplastin time (kaolin)
PVC	polyvinyl chloride; premature ventricular contraction
PVR	pulmonary vascular resistance
$\dot{Q}_t$	total liquid flow in unit time
QRS	elctrocardiographic nomenclature
ρ	rho (= density)
r	radius (of circle or sphere)
R	universal gas constant
RA_x	renal artery concentration of *x*
RAP	right atrial pressure
RAST	radioallergosorbent test
RBF	renal blood flow
RDS	respiratory distress syndrome
Re	Reynolds number (dimensionless)
REM	rapid eye movement
RH	relative humidity
Rh(x)	Rhesus blood group (major phenotype x)
RLF	retrolental fibroplasia
RNA	ribonucleic acid
RPF	renal plasma flow
RPP	rate–pressure product
RQ	respiratory quotient
RSD	reflex sympathetic dystrophy
RV	residual volume
RV_x	renal vein concentration of *x*
s	second
S	saturation (of haemoglobin)
SA	sinoatrial
SAB	subarachnoid block
SAGM	saline adenine glucose mannitol
SAP	systolic arterial pressure
s.c.	subcutaneous

SDP	subdural pressure
SF_6	sulphur hexafluoride
SG	specific gravity
SH	sulphydryl group
SI	*Système International d'Unités*
SIMV	synchronized intermittent mandatory ventilation
SIADHS	syndrome of inappropriate antidiuretic hormone secretion
SIIFT	syndrome of inappropriate intravenous fluid therapy
SNP	sodium nitroprusside
SOL	space-occupying lesion
SR	slow release
SRS–A	slow-reacting substance of anaphylaxis
SSRI	selective serotonin reuptake inhibitor
STOP	surgical termination of pregnancy
STP	standard temperature and pressure
SV	stroke volume
SVC	superior vena cava
SVP	saturated vapour pressure
SVT	supraventricular tachycardia
T	thymus-dependent (T cells)
T	temperature
$t_{1/2\alpha}$	α half-life (distribution half-time)
$t_{1/2\beta}$	β half-life (elimination half-time)
T_3	tri-iodothyronine
T_4	thyroxine
TA	titratable acid
TBG	thyroxine-binding globulin
TBW	total body water
TEC®	temperature controlled (vaporizer)
TENS	transcutaneous electrical nerve stimulation
TEPP	tetraethyl pyrophosphate
TFA	trifluoroacetyl
TISS	therapeutic intervention severity score
TIVA	total intravenous anaesthesia
TLA	translumbar aortography
TLC	total lung capacity
Tm	tubular maximal reabsorption
TMJ	temporomandibular joint
TMP	trimetaphan camsylate
TNS	transcutaneous nerve stimulation
TOF	train of four
TPR	total (systemic) peripheral resistance
TSH	thyroid-stimulating hormone
TURP	transurethral resection of prostate
TWC	total water content
TXA_2	thromboxane A_2
U	urine concentration
UK	United Kingdom
URT(I)	upper respiratory tract (infection)
USA	United States of America
V	volt
V	volume
$\dot{V}_t$	volume per unit time (gas flow)
v	velocity
V4R	mobile chest lead in electrocardiography (position 4 reversed)
VC	vital capacity
V_d	dead space (ventilation);volume of distribution
$V_{d(ANAT)}$	anatomical dead space
$V_{d(PHYS)}$	physiological dead space
VF	ventricular fibrillation
VFP	ventricular fluid pressure
VIC	vaporizer in circuit
VIE	vacuum insulated evaporator
VIP	vasoactive intestinal peptide
VOC	vaporizer out of circuit
VT	ventricular tachycardia
V_t	tidal volume
vWF	von Willebrand factor
W	watt

Appendix Ib: SI system

The *Système International d'Unités* (SI system) has been developed to reduce the large number of units in everyday physical use to a much smaller number, with standard symbols.

The seven base units are derivatives of the MKS system of physical measurement:

Length	metre	m
Mass	kilogram	kg
Time	second	s
Electric current	amp	A
Thermodynamic temperature	kelvin	K
Amount of substance	mole	mol
Luminous intensity	candela	cd

Any other units are derived units and may be expressed by multiplication or division of base units:

Volume	cubic metre	m^3			
Force	newton	N	$kg\ m\ s^{-2}$	=	$J\ m^{-1}$ (J/m)
Work	joule	J	$kg\ m^2\ s^{-2}$	=	N m
Power (rate of work)	watt	W	$kg\ m^2\ s^{-3}$	=	$J\ s^{-1}$ (J/s)
Pressure (force/area)	pascal	Pa	$kg\ m^{-1}\ s^{-2}$	=	$N\ m^{-2}$ (N/m^2)

X^{-1} has been used in preference to the solidus (/), either of which is specified in the standard.
Non-standard units such as the litre (L), day, hour and minute may be used with SI but are not part of the standard.

VOLUME

The SI unit of volume is the cubic metre, but for medical purposes the litre (L or dm^3) is retained.

TEMPERATURE

A temperature difference of 1 kelvin (1 K) is numerically equivalent to 1 degree Celsius (1°C). In everyday use the degree Celsius is retained. The Fahrenheit scale is no longer used medically. It is being phased out of use with the general public.

The magnitude of a unit is expressed by the addition of standard prefixes and symbolic prefixes. The magnitude of SI units usually changes by 10^3 per step:

Fraction	SI prefix	Symbol	*Multiple*	SI prefix	Symbol
10^{-1}	deci	d	10	deca	da
10^{-2}	centi	c	10^2	hecto	h
10^{-3}	milli	m	10^3	kilo	k
10^{-6}	micro	μ	10^6	mega	M
10^{-9}	nano	n	10^9	giga	G
10^{-12}	pico	p	10^{12}	tera	T
10^{-15}	femto	f			
10^{-18}	atto	a			

It can be seen that the SI handling of 'kilogram' is non-standard; the name of the base unit already contains a preficacial multiple. Names of decimal multiples and submultiples of the unit of mass are formed by attaching prefixes to the word 'gram'.

MOLES

$$\text{Moles} = \frac{\text{weight in g}}{\text{molecular weight}}$$

$$\text{Thus 1 mol } H_2O = \frac{18 \text{ g}}{18}$$

18g H_2O = 1 mol

For univalent ions, moles and equivalents are numerically equal, but for multivalent ions the number of equivalents must be divided by the valency to obtain the molar value. Thus 10 mEq Ca^{2+} = 5 mmol Ca^{2+}.

MOLES/OSMOLES

Strictly the SI unit of osmolality should be the mole, this representing the calculated number of particles/molecules in solution. However, the osmole is also used; this is the measured osmolality (the number of osmotically active particles per kilogram of solution). Thus, the molar value for osmolality is theoretical, while the osmolar value is empirical.

Appendix II: Inhaled anaesthetic agents – physical properties

Name	Formula	MW (Da)	BP (°C)	SVP (kPa, 20°C)	MAC (%)	Flammable in O_2	Ostwald solubility coefficients at 37°C			
							Blood/gas	Fat/blood	Oil/gas	Oil/H_2O
Nitrous oxide	N_2O	44	–88	(5300)	105	0	0.47	2.3	1.4	3.2
Halothane	$CF_3CHClBr$	197	50	32	0.75		2.5	51	224	220
Enflurane	$CHFClCF_2$ O CF_2H	184.5	56	23	1.7	6	1.9	36	98	120
Isoflurane	CF_3CHCl O CF_2H	184.5	49	32	1.15	6	1.4	45	91	174
Desflurane	CF_2H O $CFHCF_3$	168	23.5	89	7.3	18–21	0.42	27	18.7	
Sevoflurane	$CH(CF_3)_2$ O CH_2F	200	58.5	21	2.0		0.59	48	54	
Chloroform	$CHCl_3$	119	61	21.3	0.5		10		260	100
Cyclopropane	$CH_2CH_2CH_2$	42	–33	638	9.2	2–60	0.45		11.5	34.4
Diethyl ether	C_2H_5 O C_2H_5	74	35	56.5	1.9	2–82	12	5	65	3.2
Ethyl chloride	C_2H_5Cl	64.5	13	131	2.0	4–67	3.0			
Fluroxene	CF_3CH_2 O $CHCH_2$	126	43	38	3.5	4	1.4		48	90
Methoxyflurane	$CHCl_2CF_2$ O CH_3	165	105	3	0.2	5–28	13	38	950	400
Trichloroethylene	$CHClCCl_2$	131	87	8	0.17	9–65	9		960	400

MW, molecular weight; BP, boiling point; SVP, saturated vapour pressure; MAC, minimum alveolar concentration.
Drugs listed below the line have no product licence in the UK and are of historical interest only. MAC values are for young adults; MAC is higher in children, and decreases in older adults.

Appendix III: Cardiovascular system

NORMAL VALUES

Blood flows	% of cardiac output	Flow (ml min^{-1}) (70 kg man)
Heart	4	200
Brain	14	700
Liver	25	1250
Kidneys	24	1200
Lung	3	150
Muscle	19	950
Skin	5	250
Fat	5	250
Remainder	1	50
Total	100	5000

ECG times

P wave	< 0.10 s
PR interval	0.12–0.20 s
QRS time	0.05–0.08 s
QT time	0.35–0.40 s
T wave	< 0.22 s

Pressures (mmHg)

	Range	Mean
Central venous pressure (CVP)	0–8	4
Right atrial (RA)	0–8	4
Right ventricular (RV)		
Systolic	14–30	25
End-diastolic (RVEDP)	0–8	4
Pulmonary arterial (PA)		
Systolic	15–30	23
Diastolic	5–15	8
Mean ($\overline{PAP}$)	10–20	15
Pulmonary artery wedge (PAWP)		
Mean	5–15	10
Left atrial (LA)	4–12	7
Left ventricular (LV)		
Systolic	90–140	120
End-diastolic (LVEDP)	4–12	7

Derived haemodynamic variables

Variable		Typical value (70 kg)
Cardiac output (CO)	SV × HR	5 L min^{-1}
Cardiac index (CI)	$\frac{CO}{BSA}$	3.2 L min^{-1} m^{-2}
Stroke volume (SV)	$\frac{CO}{HR} \times 1000$	80 ml
Stroke index (SI)	$\frac{SV}{BSA}$	50 ml m^{-2}
Systemic vascular resistance (SVR)	$\frac{MAP - CVP}{CO} \times 80$	1000–1200 dyn s cm^{-5} (not SI unit)
Pulmonary vascular resistance (PVR)	$\frac{\overline{PAP} - LAP}{CO} \times 80$	60–120 dyn s cm^{-5} (not SI unit)
Left ventricular stroke work index (LVSWI)	$\frac{1.36\,(MAP - LAP) \times SI}{100}$	50–60 g m m^{-2}
Rate–pressure product (RPP)	SAP × HR	9600
Ejection fraction (EF)	$\frac{ESV - EDV}{EDV}$	> 0.6

BSA, body surface area; HR, heart rate; MAP, mean arterial pressure, CVP, central venous pressure; $\overline{PAP}$, mean pulmonary arterial pressure; LAP, left atrial pressure; SAP, systolic arterial pressure; ESV, end-systolic volume; EDV, end-diastolic volume.

VASOACTIVE INFUSIONS

Drug	Dilution	Typical dosage range
Sympathomimetic drugs		
Dobutamine (β_1)	Into glucose 5% 500 ml 250 mg = 500 μg ml^{-1}	1μg – 40 μg kg^{-1} min^{-1}
Dopamine (low – δ) (moderate – δ, β_{1+2}) (high – α, β_1)	Into glucose 5% 500 ml 200 mg = 400 μg ml^{-1} *or* 800 mg = 1600 μg ml^{-1}	1μg – 5 μg kg^{-1} min^{-1} (low) 5–10 μg kg^{-1} min^{-1} (moderate) > 15 μg kg^{-1} min^{-1} (high)
Dopexamine (β_2, δ)	Into glucose 5% or saline 0.9% 50 ml 40 mg = 800 μg ml^{-1}	500 ng – 6 μg kg^{-1} min^{-1}
Epinephrine (low – α, β_{1+2}) (higher – α)	Into glucose 5% 500 ml 5 mg = 10 μg ml^{-1}	Start at 20–50 ng kg^{-1} min^{-1} Most respond to < 200 ng kg^{-1} min^{-1} > 500 ng kg^{-1} min^{-1} leads to excess vasoconstriction
Isoproterenol (β_{1+2})	Into glucose 5% 500 ml 4 mg = 8 μg ml^{-1}	10–400 ng kg^{-1} min^{-1}
Metaraminol (α)	Into glucose 5% 500 ml 50 mg = 100 μg ml^{-1}	100 ng–1 μg kg^{-1} min^{-1} (infrequent use as infusion)
Norepinephrine (α, β_1)	Into glucose 5% 500 ml 4 mg = 8 μg ml^{-1}	50–200 ng kg^{-1} min^{-1}
Phenylephrine (α)	Into glucose 5% 500 ml 25 mg = 50 μg ml^{-1}	100–500 ng kg^{-1} min^{-1}

VASOACTIVE INFUSIONS (Cont.)

Miscellaneous

Amiodarone (Wolff–Parkinson–White syndrome or refractory tachycardias)	Into glucose 5% 250 ml – *not* 0.9% saline 150 mg = 600 μg ml^{-1}	40 μg kg^{-1} min^{-1} for 2 h Max. 1.2 g in 24 h
Disopyramide (membrane stabilization)	Into glucose 5% or saline 0.9% 450 ml 500 mg = 1000 μg ml^{-1}	5–7 μg kg^{-1} min^{-1}after loading dose – see data sheet or *British National Formulary*
Flecainide (membrane stabilization)	Into glucose 5% or saline 0.9% 500 ml 150 mg = 300 μg ml^{-1}	4 μg kg^{-1} min^{-1} after loading dose – see data sheet or *British National Formulary*
Glyceryl trinitrate (venous and arteriolar dilator)	Into glucose 5% or saline 0.9% to 50 ml (depends upon source) 5–10 mg = 100–200 μg ml^{-1} – do not give into Viaflex or other polyvinyl chloride containers – ideally use syringe pump	10–200 μg min^{-1} (0.2–3 μg kg^{-1} min^{-1})
Isosorbide dinitrate (venous and arteriolar dilator)	Into glucose 5% or saline 0.9% 45 ml 5 mg = 100 μg ml^{-1} – do not give into Viaflex or other polyvinyl chloride – ideally use syringe pump	30–120 μg min^{-1} (0.6–2 μg kg^{-1} min^{-1})
Lidocaine (membrane stabilization)	Into glucose 5% or saline 0.9% 500 ml 1 g = 2 mg ml^{-1} = 2000 μg ml^{-1}	25–50 μg kg^{-1} min^{-1} after loading dose – see data sheet or *British National Formulary*
Mexiletine (membrane stabilization)	Into glucose 5% or saline 0.9% 500 ml 250 mg = 500 μg ml^{-1}	500 μg min^{-1} after loading dose – see data sheet or *British National Formulary*
Sodium nitroprusside (arteriolar and venous dilator)	Into glucose 5% or saline 0.9% 500 ml 50 mg = 100 μg ml^{-1}	0.5–8 μg kg^{-1} min^{-1} (for hypertensive crisis) 0.1–1.5 μg kg^{-1} min^{-1} (for hypotensive anaesthesia)

Appendix IVa : Chemical pathology – biochemical values

These values are given for example only – each reporting laboratory provides reference values for its own population and method. This is especially true of enzyme assays. Values given are those obtained from Chemical Pathology in Warwick, where these are available. No inference should be made about the molecular weight of a substance by reference to US and SI values

Name	US units	SI units
Amino acid nitrogen	4–8 mg%	3–6 mmol L^{-1}
Ammonia	80–110 μg%	<50 μmol L^{-1}
Amylase	80–180 Somogyi units%	70–300 IU L^{-1}
Base excess	± 2 mEq L^{-1}	± 2 mmol L^{-1}
Bicarbonate		
Actual	22–30 mEq L^{-1}	22–30 mmol L^{-1}
Standard	21–25 mEq L^{-1}	21–25 mmol L^{-1}
Bilirubin – total	0.3–1.1 mg%	3–18 μmol L^{-1}
Buffer base (pH 7.4, P_aCO_2 5.3, Hb 15 g dl^{-1})	48 mEq L^{-1}	48 mmol L^{-1}
Calcium		
Total	8.5–10.5 mg% (4.5–5.7 mEq L^{-1})	2.25–2.6 mmol L^{-1}
Ionized	4–5 mg%	1.0–1.25 mmol L^{-1}
Chloride	95–105 mEq L^{-1}	95–105 mmol L^{-1}
Cholesterol	140–300 mg%	3.6–7.8 mmol L^{-1}
Cholinesterase, plasma (pseudocholinesterase)	Dibucaine number > 80% usually normal Dibucaine number <20% usually homozygote for atypical cholinesterase	
Copper	80–150 μg%	13–24 nmol L^{-1}
Urinary copper	15–50 μg per 24 h	0.2–0.8 μmol per 24 h
Cortisol		
0900 h } radioimmunoassay	9–23 μg $litre^{-1}$	250–635 nmol L^{-1}
2400 h } technique	<7.2 μg%	<200 nmol L^{-1}
Neonatal (competitive protein-binding technique)	30 μg $litre^{-1}$	200–650 nmol L^{-1} <200 nmol L^{-1} 330–1700 nmol L^{-1}
Creatine (phospho)kinase (CK)	100 IU L^{-1} – male 60 IU L^{-1} – female	25–200 IU L^{-1} 25–150 IU L^{-1}
Creatinine	0.5–1.4 mg%	45–120 μmol L^{-1}
Epinephrine	100 pg ml^{-1}	0.55 nmol L^{-1}
Fibrinogen	150–400 mg%	1.5–4.0 g L^{-1}
Folate	3–20 ng ml^{-1}	3–20 μg L^{-1} 2.1–27 nmol L^{-1}
Glucose		
Fasting	55–85 mg%	4–6 mmol L^{-1}
Postprandial	<180 mg%	<10 mmol L^{-1}
γ-Glutamyl transpeptidase	7–25 IU L^{-1}	male: <50 IU L^{-1} female: <30 IU L^{-1}
Hydroxybutyrate dehydrogenase (HBD)		100–240 IU L^{-1}
Iodine – total	3.5–8.0 μg L^{-1}	273–624 nmol L^{-1}
^{131}I uptake	20–50% of administered dose in 24 h	
Iron	80–160 μg%	14–30 μmol L^{-1}
Iron-binding capacity	250–400 μg%	45–69 μmol L^{-1}

Name	US units	SI units
Lactate	0.6–1.8 mEq L^{-1}	0.6–1.8 mmol L^{-1}
Lactate dehydrogenase	30–90 IU L^{-1}	100–300 IU L^{-1}
Lead		<1.8 μmol L^{-1}
Magnesium	1–2 mg%	
	1.5–2.0 mEq L^{-1}	0.7–1.0 mmol L^{-1}
Methaemoglobin	<3% of total haemoglobin	
Nitrogen (non-protein) (urea + urate + creatinine + creatine	18–30 mg%	12.8–21.4 mmol L^{-1}
Norepinephrine	200 pg ml^{-1}	1.25 nmol L^{-1}
Osmolality	280–300 mosmol kg^{-1}	280–300 mmol kg^{-1}
Phosphate	2.0–4.5 mg%	0.8–1.4 mmol L^{-1}
	3.0–6.0 mg% (children)	1.0–1.8 mmol L^{-1} (children)
	<8.1 mg% (neonatal)	<2.6 mmol L^{-1} (neonatal)
Phosphatase		
Acid (total)	1–5 KA units%	1–9 IU L^{-1}
Acid (prostatic)		0–3 IU L^{-1}
Alkaline	3–13 KA units%	17–100 IU L^{-1}
Potassium	3.4–5.3 mEq L^{-1}	3.4–5.3 mmol L^{-1}
Protein		
Total	6.0–8.0 g%	60–80 g L^{-1}
Albumin	3.5–5.0 g%	35–50 g L^{-1}
Globulin	1.5–3.0 g%	15–30 g L^{-1}
Pyruvate	0.4–0.7 mg%	34–80 μmol L^{-1}
Sodium	133–148 mEq L^{-1}	133–148 mmol L^{-1}
Thyroxine (T_4)	4.7–11 μg%	52–140 nmol L^{-1}
Transaminase		
aspartate transaminase (AST)	5–40 unit.ml^{-1}	5–40 IU L^{-1}
alanine transaminase (ALT)		2–53 IU L^{-1}
Transferrin	220–400 mg%	2.2–4.0 g L^{-1}
Triglycerides (fasting)	71–160 mg%	0.8–1.8 mmol L^{-1}
Tri-iodothyronine (T_3)	90–170 ng%	0.8–2.5 nmol L^{-1}
T_3 uptake	95–117%	95–117%
Urea	15–48 mg%	2.5–8.0 mmol L^{-1}
Urea nitrogen (BUN)	10–20 mg%	7.1–14.3 mmol L^{-1}
Urate		
Men	4–9.5 mg%	225–470 μmol L^{-1}
Women	3–7.5 mg%	180–390 μmol L^{-1}

Appendix IVb:

Conversion chart – hydrogen ion concentration to pH

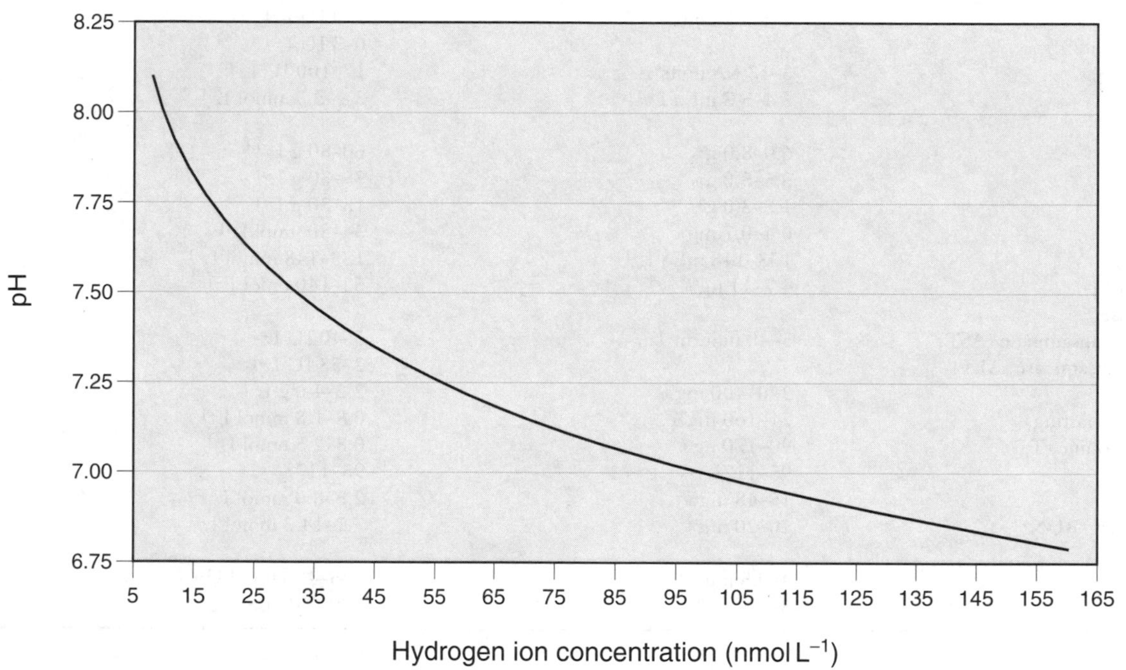

Appendix V: Haematology

NORMAL VALUES

Haemoglobin	
Men	13.5–18.0 g dl^{-1}
Women	11.5–16.5 g dl^{-1}
10–12 years	11.5–14.8 g dl^{-1}
1 year	11.0–13.0 g dl^{-1}
3 months	9.5–12.5 g dl^{-1}
Full-term	13.6–19.6 g dl^{-1}
Red blood cell count (RBC)	
Men	4.5–6.0 × 10^{12} L^{-1}
Women	3.5–5.0 × 10^{12} L^{-1}
White blood cell count (WBC)	4.0–11.0 × 10^{9} L^{-1}
Neutrophils	40–70%
Lymphocytes	20–45%
Monocytes	2–10%
Eosinophils	1–6%
Basophils	0–1%
Platelet count	150–400 × 10^{9} L^{-1}
Reticulocyte count	0–2% of RBC
Sedimentation rate	
Men	0–15 mm in 1 h
Women	0–20 mm in 1 h
Plasma viscosity	1.50–1.72 mPa s
Packed cell volume (PCV) and haematocrit (Hct)	
Men	0.4–0.55
Women	0.36–0.47
Mean corpuscular volume (MCV)	76–96 fl
Mean corpuscular haemoglobin concentration (MCHC)	31–35 g dl^{-1}
Mean corpuscular haemoglobin (MCH)	27–32 pg

COAGULATION TESTS

Activated clotting time (ACT; Haemochron type)	80–135 s
Antithrombin III	> 80% normal
Bleeding time (platelet function)	2–9 min
Clotting time (largely replaced by ACT)	2–9 min
D dimers	< 0.3 mg L^{-1}
Fibrinogen – plasma	1.5–4 g L^{-1}
INR (international normalized ratio warfarin therapy value)	
Therapeutic range for:	
Atrial fibrillation, deep venous thrombosis, pulmonary embolism, tissue heart valves	2–3
Mechanical heart valve	3–4.5
KCCT (also known as PTTK, APTT)	33–41 s
Heparin therapy value	1.5–2.5 × normal
If pregnant	1.5–2.0 × normal
Platelet count	150–400 × 10^9 L^{-1}
Prothrombin time	12–14 s
Thrombin time	circa 15 s

KCCT, kaolin cephalin clotting time; PTTK, partial thromboplastin time, kaolin; APTT, activated partial thromboplastin time.

COAGULATION SCREEN

WHAT TO CHECK?

Prothrombin time (PT)
Kaolin cephalin clotting time (KCCT)
Thrombin time (TT)
Fibrinogen
Platelet count

If all are normal, consider checking bleeding time and, in neonates, factor XIII concentration.

WHEN TO CHECK?

Elective patient

- With suspicious history (bleeding after cuts, previous surgery or dental extractions, easy bruising)
- With family history of bleeding problems
- Receiving anticoagulants – warfarin, heparin or aspirin, for example
- With intercurrent illness such as obstructive jaundice, liver disease, uraemia or leukaemia.

Emergency or intraoperative patient

With excessive bleeding despite apparent vascular integrity.

WHAT TO DO?

Possible cause	Treatment
PT and KCCT prolonged	
Drug effect (warfarin/coumarin)	Vitamin K FFP Coagulation concentrates
Obstructive jaundice	Vitamin K FFP
Liver disease	Vitamin K FFP
Haemorrhagic disease of the newborn	Vitamin K
Factor II, V, X deficiency	FFP Coagulation concentrates

WHAT TO DO? (*Cont.*)

Possible cause	Treatment
If TT is also prolonged	
Fibrinogen deficiency	Cryoprecipitate FFP
Are D-dimers increased?	
Disseminated intravascular coagulation (DIC)	Treat cause FFP Platelets ? Antithrombin III concentrate
Is KCCT prolonged?	
Heparin therapy	Stop therapy ? Reverse effect with protamine
Factor VIII deficiency – haemophilia	Factor VIII concentrate: high purity
Von Willebrand's disease	Vasopressin Factor VIII concentrate: intermediate purity
Factor IX deficiency	Factor IX concentrate
Factor XI or XII deficiency	FFP
Is PT prolonged (with normal KCCT)?	
Factor VII deficiency	FFP, factor VII concentrate
Is platelet count decreased ($< 100 \times 10^9$ L^{-1})?	
Peripheral destruction	
? Immune-mediated	Steroids
? DIC	Treat cause
? TTP or HUS	Platelets FFP ? Antithrombin III concentrate Plasma exchange
Inadequate production	
Marrow failure	Platelets
Is bleeding time prolonged?	
Von Willebrand's disease	Factor VIII concentrate: intermediate purity Vasopressin
Functional platelet disorder	
Inherited	Platelets
Acquired	Platelets
Uraemia	Dialysis/haemofiltration Cryoprecipitate
Drugs	

Always consult haematology colleague when uncertain.
FFP, fresh frozen plasma; TTP, thrombotic thrombocytopenic purpura; HUS, haemolytic uraemic syndrome.

Appendix VI
Fluid balance

FLUID COMPOSITION OF BODY COMPARTMENTS

Typical blood volume		*Total water content (TWC)*
Infant	90 $ml.kg^{-1}$	60% male (55% female) of body weight (18–40 years)
Child	80 $ml.kg^{-1}$	55% male (46% female) of body weight (> 60 years)
Adult male	70 $ml.kg^{-1}$	Volume of extracellular fluid 35% TWC
Adult female	60 $ml.kg^{-1}$	Volume of intracellular fluid 65% TWC

INTRAOPERATIVE FLUID REQUIREMENT — ADULT

(1) Initial volume	1.5 $ml.kg^{-1}.h^{-1}$ for duration of preoperative starvation
+ (2) Maintenance	1.5 $ml.kg^{-1}.h^{-1}$
+ (3) Operative insensible loss	e.g. 1–2 litre for abdominal surgery
+ (4) Blood loss	Replace with blood when loss exceeds 20% of estimated blood volume

FLUID, ELECTROLYTE AND NUTRITIONAL REQUIREMENTS

Minimum daily requirements per kilogram for adults, and children and infants. Neonates see Appendix IXc.

	Adults (per kg)	**Children and infants (per kg)**		**Adults (per kg)**	**Children and infants (per kg)**
Water	30–45 ml	100–150 ml	Mn^{2+}	0.1 µmol	0.3 µmol
Energy	30–50 kcal (0.15–0.21 MJ)	90–125 kcal (0.38–0.5 MJ)	Zn^{2+}	0.7 µmol	1.0 µmol
			Cu^{+}	0.07 µmol	0.3 µmol
Protein	0.7–1.0 g	2.2–2.5 g	Cl^{-}	1.3–1.9 mmol	1.8–4.3 mmol
Na^{+}	1–1.4 mmol	1–2.5 mmol			
K^{+}	0.7–0.9 mmol	2 mmol			
Ca^{2+}	0.11 mmol	0.5–1 mmol			
Mg^{2+}	0.04 mmol	0.15 mmol			
Fe^{2+}	1 µmol	2 µmol			

COMPOSITION OF COMMON INTRAVENOUS FLUIDS

Name	pH	Calculated[a] osmolality	Ions (mmol L^{-1}) Na$^+$	K$^+$	Cl	HCO_3^-	Misc.	CHO (g L^{-1})	Protein (g L^{-1})	MJ L^{-1}
Crystalloids										
Sodium chloride 0.9%	5.0	308	154	0	154	0	0	0	0	0
Glucose 5%	4.0	280	0	0	0	0	0	50	0	0.84
Glucose 4% + saline 0.18%	4.5	286	31	0	31	0	0	40	0	0.67
Glucose 5% + saline 0.45%	4.5	430	77	0	77	0	0	50	0	0.84
Lactated Ringer's (Hartmann's solution)	6.5	280	131	5	112	29 (as lact.)	Mg^{2+} 1 Ca^{2+} 1	0	0	0.038
Sodium bicarbonate 8.4%	8.0	2000	1000	0	0	1000	0	0	0	0

[a]Calculated value, assuming total dissociation of ions.

Name	pH	Oncotic pressure (mmH_2O)	Ionic content (mmol L^{-1}) Na$^+$	K$^+$	Cl$^-$	Misc.	CHO (g L^{-1})	Protein (g L^{-1})	MJ L^{-1}	Typical half-life in plasma
Colloids										
Gelatin (succinylated, Haemaccel)	7.4	370	145	5.1	145	Ca^{2+} 6.25, PO_4^{2-} Trace, SO_4^{2-} Trace	0	35	0	5h
Gelatin (polygeline, Gelofusine)	7.4	465	154	0.4	125	Ca^{2+} 0.4, Mg^{2+} 0.4	0	40	0	4 h
Dextran 70 in sodium chloride 0.9%	4–7	268	154	0	154	0	0	0	0	12 h
Dextran 70 in glucose 5%	3.5–7	268	0	0	0	0	50	0	0.84	12 h
Hetastarch (Hespan)	5.5	310	154	0	154	0	0	0	0	17 days
Pentastarch (Pentaspan)	5.0	320	154	0	154	0	0	0	0	18 h
Blood products										
Human albumin solution (PPF 4%)	7.4	275	150	2	120					
(20% salt-poor solution also available – ionic content varies with manufacturer)										
Whole blood	> 6.5	Na$^+$ depends on donor values. K$^+$ increases with storage time								
Plasma-reduced blood	> 6.5	Na$^+$ depends on donor value. K$^+$ higher than in whole blood, but total quantity *per unit* is similar								
SAGM blood	> 6.5		150		150	Adenine 0.6%, glucose 2.6%, mannitol 1.6%				

Accepted safe storage times at 4°C	
Heparinized blood	Only available for special applications
Acid citrate dextrose	21 days
Citrate phosphate dextrose	28 days
Citrate phosphate dextrose adenine	35 days
SAGM	35 days

SAGM, saline adenine glucose mannitol.

Appendix VII: Renal function tests

Clearance tests

Inulin clearance ≃ glomerular filtration	100–150 ml min^{-1}
Para-aminohippuric acid clearance ≃ renal plasma flow	560–830 ml min^{-1}
Creatinine clearance ≃ glomerular filtration rate (overestimates low glomerular filtration rate)	104–125 ml min^{-1}

Blood tests

Serum/plasma

Osmolality	280–300 mosmol kg^{-1}
Creatinine	45–120 μmol L^{-1}
Urea	2.7–7.0 mmol L^{-1}
Urea nitrogen	1.6–3.3 mmol L^{-1}

Urine tests

Osmolality	300–1200 mosmol kg^{-1}
Creatinine	8.85–17.7 mmol per 24 h
Sodium	50–200 mmol per 24 h

Comparative urinary values

	SG	Osmolality	U/P urea ratio	U/P osmolality
Normal	1000–1040	300–1200	>20:1	>2.0:1
Prerenal failure	>1022	>400	>20:1	>2.0:1
Renal failure				
Early	1010	<350	<14:1	<1.7:1
Late			<5:1	<1.1:1

SG, specific gravity; U, urine; P, plasma.

Appendix VIII: Pulmonary function tests

SPIROGRAM

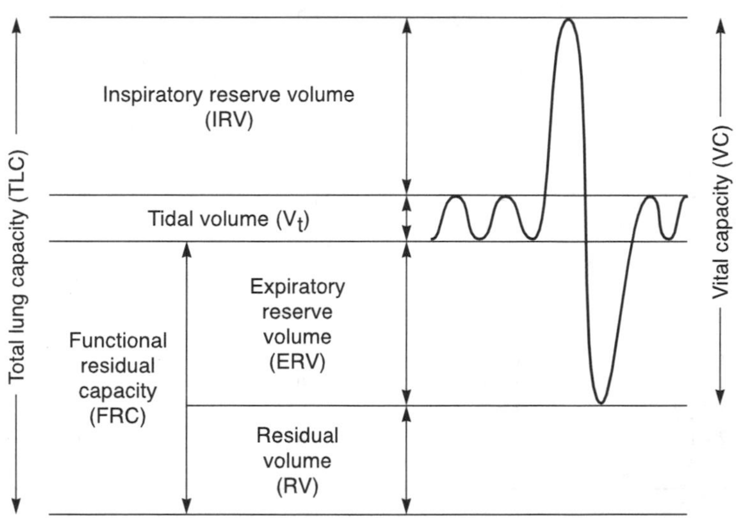

Volumes (ml) in 60 kg male

V_t	400 - 600
IRV	3300 - 3750
ERV	950 - 1200
FRC	2300 - 2600
RV	1200 - 1700
VC	3800 - 5000
TLC	5000 - 6500

Fig. VIII
Lung volumes in an average healthy male adult.

Commonly used abbreviations

Primary symbols

C = concentration of gas — blood phase
D = diffusing capacity
F = fractional concentration in the dry gas phase
P = partial pressure — gas
Q = volume of blood
R = respiratory exchange ratio
S = saturation of haemoglobin with oxygen or carbon dioxide
V = volume of gas
$\dot{X}$ = dot above symbol indicates 'per unit time'
$\bar{X}$ = bar above symbol indicates 'mean value'

Example: P_aO_2 = partial pressure of arterial oxygen

Secondary symbols

Usually typed as subscripts, capital letters indicate gaseous phase; lower-case letters indicate liquid phase.

A = alveolar
B = barometer
D = deadspace
E = expired
I = inspired
T = tidal
a = arterial
c = capillary (pulmonary capillary)
v = venous
p = peripleural

PULMONARY FUNCTION TESTS – FEMALES

Age (years)	Height (cm)	$FEV_{1.0}$ (L)	FVC (L)	$FEV_{1.0}$ /FVC (%)	PEFR (L min^{-1})
20	145	2.60	3.13	81.0	377
	152	2.83	3.45	81.0	403
	160	3.09	3.83	81.0	433
	168	3.36	4.20	81.0	459
	175	3.59	4.53	81.0	489
30	145	2.45	2.98	79.9	366
	152	2.68	3.30	79.9	392
	160	2.94	3.68	79.9	422
	168	3.21	4.05	79.9	448
	175	3.44	4.38	79.9	478
40	145	2.15	2.68	77.7	345
	152	2.38	3.00	77.7	371
	160	2.64	3.38	77.7	401
	168	2.91	3.75	77.7	427
	175	3.14	4.08	77.7	457
50	145	1.85	2.38	75.5	324
	152	2.08	2.70	75.5	350
	160	2.34	3.08	75.5	380
	168	2.61	3.45	75.5	406
	175	2.84	3.78	75.5	436
60	145	1.55	2.08	73.2	303
	152	1.78	2.40	73.2	329
	160	2.04	2.78	73.2	359
	168	2.31	3.15	73.2	385
	175	2.54	3.48	73.2	415
70	145	1.25	1.78	71.0	282
	152	1.48	2.10	71.0	308
	160	1.74	2.48	71.0	338
	168	2.01	2.85	71.0	364
	175	2.24	3.18	71.0	394

PULMONARY FUNCTION TESTS – MALES

Age (years)	Height (cm)	$FEV_{1.0}$ (L)	FVC (L)	$FEV_{1.0}$ /FVC (%)	PEFR (L min^{-1})
20	160	3.61	4.17	82.5	572
	168	3.86	4.53	82.5	597
	175	4.15	4.95	82.5	625
	183	4.44	5.37	82.5	654
	191	4.69	5.73	82.5	679
30	160	3.45	4.06	80.6	560
	168	3.71	4.42	80.6	584
	175	4.00	4.84	80.6	612
	183	4.28	5.26	80.6	640
	191	4.54	5.62	80.6	665
40	160	3.14	3.84	76.9	536
	168	3.40	4.20	76.9	559
	175	3.69	4.62	76.9	586
	183	3.97	5.04	76.9	613
	191	4.23	5.40	76.9	636

Pulmonary function tests – males (*Cont.*)

Age (years)	Height (cm)	$FEV_{1.0}$(L)	FVC (L)	$FEV_{1.0}$/FVC (%)	PEFR (L min^{-1})
50	160	2.83	3.62	73.1	512
	168	3.09	3.98	73.1	534
	175	3.38	4.40	73.1	560
	183	3.66	4.82	73.1	585
	191	3.92	5.18	73.1	608
60	160	2.52	3.40	69.4	488
	168	2.78	3.76	69.4	509
	175	3.06	4.18	69.4	533
	183	3.35	4.60	69.4	558
	191	3.61	4.96	69.4	579
70	160	2.21	3.18	65.7	464
	168	2.47	3.54	65.7	484
	175	2.75	3.96	65.7	507
	183	3.04	4.38	65.7	530
	191	3.30	4.74	65.7	551

FEV_1, forced expiratory volume in 1 s; FVC, forced vital capacity; PEFR, peak expiratory flow rate.

LUNG FUNCTION: ADULT AND NEONATAL VALUES

Examples

	Adult (65 kg)	Neonate (3 kg)
V_d	2.2 ml kg^{-1}	2–3 ml kg^{-1}
V_t	7–10 ml kg^{-1}	5–7 ml kg^{-1}
$\dot{V}_E$	85–100 ml kg^{-1} min^{-1}	100–200 ml kg^{-1} min^{-1}
Vital capacity	50–55 ml kg^{-1}	33 ml kg^{-1}
Respiratory rate	12–18 breath min^{-1}	25–40 breaths min^{-1}
P_aO_2	12.6 kPa (95 mmHg)	9 kPa (68 mmHg)
P_aCO_2	5.3 kPa (40 mmHg)	4.5 kPa (33 mmHg)

Appendix IX: Paediatrics

TRACHEAL AND TRACHEOSTOMY TUBE SIZE

Age (years)	TT and tracheostomy tube size ID (mm)	TT length (cm)	
		Oral	Nasal
Premature (by weight)			
1 kg	2.5	7	
2 kg	3.0	8	
3 kg	3.5	9	
0–3 months	3.0/3.5	10	
3–6 months	3.5	12	15
6–12 months	3.5	12	15
2	4.0	13	16
3	4.0	13	16
4	4.5	14	17
5	5.0	14	17
6	5.5	15	18
7	5.5	15	18
8	6.0	16	19
9	6.0	16	19
10	6.5	17	20
11	6.5	17	20
12	7.0	18	21
13	7.0	18	21
14	7.5	21	24
15	7.5	21	24
16	8.0	21	24
17	9.0	22	25
18	9.5	22	25
20	9.5	23	26

TT, tracheal tube; ID, internal diameter.

Below 8–10 years, non-cuffed tubes should be used.

It is always advisable to have available a tube one size smaller than calculated.

DOSAGE OF DRUGS IN COMMON ANAESTHETIC USAGE

Premedication

Atropine	20 μg kg^{-1}
Hyoscine	20 μg kg^{-1}
Glycopyrrolate	5 μg kg^{-1}
Diazepam	200–400 μg kg^{-1}
Droperidol	100 μg kg^{-1}
Trimeprazine	2 mg kg^{-1}

Intravenous induction

Propofol	3 mg kg^{-1}
Thiopental	5 mg kg^{-1}
Methohexital	1.5 mg kg^{-1}
Ketamine	2 mg kg^{-1}

Other induction routes

Ketamine intramuscular	10 mg kg^{-1}
Thiopental rectal	30 mg kg^{-1})
Methohexital rectal	25 mg kg^{-1})

Neuromuscular blocking drugs

Succinylcholine	2 mg kg^{-1}
Atracurium	300–500 μg kg^{-1}
Cis-atracurium	80–200 μg kg^{-1}
Mivacurium	250–400 μg kg^{-1}
Rocuronium	500–1200 μg kg^{-1}
Vecuronium	100 μg kg^{-1}
Tubocurarine	500 μg kg^{-1}
Pancuronium	80–100 μg kg^{-1}

Reversal of neuromuscular blocking drugs

Neostigmine	
Child	50 μg kg^{-1}
Neonatal	80 μg kg^{-1}
Atropine	20 μg kg^{-1}

Analgesics – intravenous/intramuscular

Morphine	200 μg kg^{-1}
Fentanyl	0.5–1.5 μg kg^{-1}
Alfentanil	2.5–5 μg kg^{-1}

Rectal

Diclofenac	2 mg kg^{-1} (for acute dosage only)

FLUID AND ELECTROLYTE BALANCE

Postoperative fluid and electrolyte requirements in infancy and childhood

Weight	Rate
Up to 10 kg	100 ml kg^{-1} day^{-1}
10–20 kg	1000 ml + (50 × [wt (kg) – 10]) ml kg^{-1} day^{-1}
20–30 kg	1500 ml + (25 × [wt (kg) – 20]) ml kg^{-1} day^{-1}

Fluid requirements in the first week of life

Day	Rate
1	0
2, 3	50 ml kg^{-1} day^{-1}
4, 5	75 ml kg^{-1} day^{-1}
6	100 ml kg^{-1} day^{-1}
7	120 ml kg^{-1} day^{-1}

Fluid and electrolyte requirements in infancy and childhood

	Age (years)										
	1 week	1	2	3	4	5	6	7	8	9	10
Weight (kg)	3.5	10	13	15	17	19	21	23	25	28	32
Insensible water loss (ml kg^{-1} day^{-1})	30	27.5	27	26.5	26	25	24	23	22	21	20
Water requirement (ml kg^{-1} day^{-1})	150	100	100	90	90	90	70	70	70	70	70
Na^+ requirement (mmol kg^{-1} day^{-1})	4	3	2.5	2	2	1.9	1.9	1.9	1.8	1.75	1.7
K^+ requirement (mmol kg^{-1} day^{-1})	2.5	2	2	2	2	1.75	1.75	1.5	1.5	1.5	1.5

These are basal requirements. Additional fluid (10–20%) is required during major surgery, in addition to replacement of overt losses. During the postoperative period, fluid requirements are increased in the presence of pyrexia. Fluid and electrolyte balance should be adjusted after measurement of serum electrolyte concentrations and serum osmolality.

Appendix X: Gas flows in anaesthetic breathing systems

System	Spontaneous ventilation	Intermittent positive pressure ventilation
Mapleson A (Lack or Magill)	Minute ventilation (MV; theoretically V_A) 80 ml kg^{-1} min^{-1}	2.5 × MV 200 ml kg^{-1} min^{-1}
Mapleson D (Bain or coaxial Mapleson D)	2–3 × MV 150–250 ml kg^{-1} min^{-1}	70 ml kg^{-1} min^{-1} for P_aCO_2 of 5.3 kPa 100 ml kg^{-1} min^{-1} for P_aCO_2 of 4.3 kPa
Mapleson E (Ayre's T-piece)	2 × MV	As Mapleson D Minimum of 3 L min^{-1} fresh gas flow
Mapleson F (Jackson Rees modification of Ayre's T-piece)	As Mapleson E	As Mapleson E

V_A alveolar minute volume; P_aCO_2, arterial carbon dioxide tension.

NORMAL VENTILATION VALUES FOR RESTING AWAKE SUBJECTS

Weight (Kg)	Minute volume (ml)	Tidal volume (ml)	Frequency (breath min^{-1})
Neonate 2	480	14–16	30–45
3	600	17–24	25–40
10	1680	80	21
20	3040	160	19
30	4080	240	17
40	4800	320	15
50	5200	400	13
60	5280	480	11
70	5600	560	10

Index